Textbook of Anaesthesia

Textbook of Anaesthesia

Edited by

A. R. Aitkenhead BSc, MD, FFARCS
Professor of Anaesthesia,
University of Nottingham Medical School,
Nottingham, UK

G. Smith BSc(Hons), MD, FFARCS
Professor of Anaesthesia,
University of Leicester School of Medicine, Leicester, UK

SECOND EDITION

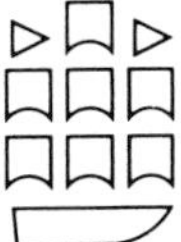

CHURCHILL LIVINGSTONE
EDINBURGH LONDON MELBOURNE AND NEW YORK 1990

CHURCHILL LIVINGSTONE
Medical Division of Longman Group UK Limited

Distributed in the United States of America by
Churchill Livingstone Inc., 1560 Broadway, New York,
N.Y. 10036, and by associated companies, branches
and representatives throughout the world.

First edition 1985
Reprinted 1985
Reprinted 1988
Second edition 1990
Reprinted 1990

ISBN 0 443 039577

British Library Cataloguing in Publication Data
Textbook of anaesthesia. — 2nd ed
1. Medicine. Anaesthesia
I. Aitkenhead, A. R. (Alan R.) II. Smith, G.
(Graham), *1941–* IV. Smith, G. (Graham), *1941–*
Textbook of anaesthesia
617'.96

Library of Congress Cataloging in Publication Data
Textbook of anaesthesia/edited by A. R. Aitkenhead,
G. Smith. — 2nd ed.
p. cm.
Includes bibliographies and index.
ISBN 0-443-03957-7
1. Anesthesiology. I. Aitkenhead, A. R. (Alan R.)
II. Smith, G. (Graham)
[DNLM: 1. Anesthesia. WO 200 T355]
RD81.T44 1990
617.9'6 — dc20
DNLM/DLC
for Library of Congress 89-7217
CIP

Printed in Great Britain at The Bath Press, Avon

Preface

The first edition of this book was intended to satisfy the needs of the new recruit into anaesthesia during the first 1–2 years in the specialty. In addition, it was hoped that it might provide suitable reading for anaesthetists studying for the (then) new Part 1 FFARCS examination (now Part 1 FCAnaes) and the European Diploma of Anaesthesiology. The response to the first edition was very encouraging and it clearly proved useful not only to the intended audience but also to a wider readership including medical practitioners giving occasional anaesthetics in rural areas or underdeveloped countries and non-medical staff involved full-time in anaesthesia. The success of the first edition has therefore stimulated us to produce a second.

The aims of this new edition are broadly similar to those of the first. However, as a result of our own awareness of some deficiencies in the first edition, and after receiving many helpful comments from reviewers and readers of the book, we have introduced several new chapters, undertaken major revision of chapters on pharmacology and practical aspects of anaesthesia, and updated the content of the remainder.

We have rewritten those chapters describing the pharmacology of intravenous and inhalation anaesthetics, and of drugs used to supplement anaesthesia. A new chapter outlining basic knowledge of physics, an important area for the trainee anaesthetist, has been incorporated to supplement the physics contained in the contributions on anaesthetic apparatus and monitoring; these chapters also have been revised very substantially, and this reflects the vital importance of a full understanding of all types of equipment employed in anaesthetic practice. The chapter describing the operating theatre environment has been expanded considerably to incorporate essential details of theatre design and to discuss briefly the medicolegal aspects of anaesthetic practice, which is assuming increasing importance worldwide.

Chapters on postoperative care, postoperative pain, local anaesthetic techniques and obstetric anaesthesia and analgesia have also been rewritten. In order to discuss in more detail the management of patients encountered frequently by the trainee anaesthetist, we have introduced new chapters describing anaesthesia for gynaecology, genito-urinary and orthopaedic surgery, radiological investigation and radiotherapy. There is also a new chapter on the management of fluid, electrolyte and acid-base balance. We have retained chapters that discuss more complex forms of surgery because trainees may be required to undertake some of these procedures from time to time, albeit under supervision. The appendices have been expanded and revised to provide ready access to detailed information which may be useful during pre-operative assessment and management of patients undergoing anaesthesia and surgery.

We are again grateful to our contributors, who have allowed us to undertake widespread revision of manuscripts in an attempt to obtain uniformity of style. We are indebted again to the publishers, Churchill Livingstone, who have arranged for redrawing of the substantial number of new figures. Our gratitude must be recorded to Mrs Rosaleen O'Brien, Principal Secretary in the University Department of Anaesthesia at Leicester, for substantial secretarial work.

We hope that this text will prove as popular as

the first edition, and will be used by trainees as a practical guide in the operating theatre and as the foundation of their theoretical learning. It may be valuable also as an 'aide memoire' for teachers in anaesthesia, and may be appropriate reading for undergraduates who undertake an elective period of training in anaesthesia, and for recovery room nurses.

Nottingham and Leicester, 1990

AA
GS

Acknowledgements

Many of the figures and diagrams incorporated in the text have been redrawn or modified from original diagrams appearing elsewhere. We therefore gratefully acknowledge permission from authors, publishers and editors in respect of the following:

Chapter 1
Fig. 1.15 *from* Lord Brock 1982 Lung abscess, 2nd edn. Blackwell Scientific Publications, Oxford. Fig. 1.21 *from* Lee, J A, Atkinson R C 1978 Lumbar puncture and spinal anaesthesia. Churchill Livingstone, Edinburgh. Figs 1.3, 1.4, 1.5, 1.10, 1.11, 1.12, 1.13, 1.14, 1.16, 1.17, 1.18, 1.19 and 1.20 *from* Ellis H, Feldman S 1977 Anatomy for anaesthetists, 3rd edn. Blackwell Scientific Publications, Oxford.

Chapter 3
Fig. 3.14 *from* Smith J J, Kampine J P 1980 Circulatory physiology — the essentials. Williams and Wilkins, Baltimore. Fig. 3.15 *from* Guyton A C 1967 New England Journal of Medicine 277: 805. Fig. 3.19 *from* Ledingham I McA, Hanning C D In (eds) Gray, T C, Nunn J E, Utting J F 1980 General anaesthesia, 4th edn. Butterworths, London. Fig. 3.20 *from* Prys-Roberts C 1980 The circulation in anaesthesia. Blackwell Scientific Publications, Oxford.

Chapter 5
Fig. 5.1 *from* Chapnick P 1973 Skin of ourselves. Science, April: 20. Figs 5.14, 5.16, 5.17, 5.28, 5.29 and 5.41 *from* Bell G H, Emslie-Smith D M, Paterson C R 1980 Textbook of physiology, 10th edn. Churchill Livingstone, Edinburgh. Figs 5.2, 5.3, 5.4, 5.5, 5.6 and 5.13 *from* Hendry B 1981 Membrane physiology and cell excitation. Helm Croom. Figs 5.7, 5.8 and 5.9 *from* Maze M 1981 Clinical implications of membrane receptor function in anaesthesia. Anesthesiology 55: 160. Fig. 5.10 *from* Braesrup C 1982 Neurotransmitters and CNS disease anxiety. Lancet 2: 1030. Fig. 5.12 *from* Spero L 1982 Neurotransmitters and CNS disease: epilepsy. Lancet 2: 1319. Figs 5.18, 5.19, 5.21, 5.22, 5.24, 5.25, 5.26 and 5.27 *from* Mitchell G A Essentials of neuroanatomy, 3rd edn. Churchill Livingstone, London. Fig. 5.20 *from* Green J H 1976 An introduction to human physiology, 4th edn. Oxford University Press, Oxford. Fig. 5.36 *from* Ganong W F 1979 Review of medical physiology, 9th edn. Lange Medical Publications, California. Fig. 5.23 *from* Patten J P 1977 Neurological differential diagnosis. Starke, London. Fig. 5.30 *from* Jessel T M 1982 Neurotransmitters and CNS disease: pain. Lancet 2: 1084. Fig. 5.31 *from* Lipton S 1979 The control of chronic pain. Fig. 5.32 *from* Gray T C, Nunn J F, Utting, J E (eds) 1980 General anaesthesia, 4th edn. Butterworth, London. Fig. 5.35 *from* Maynard D B, Jenkinson J L 1984 The cerebral function analysing monitor: initial experience, application and further development. Anaesthesia 39: 678–690. Fig. 5.37 *from* Branthwaite M 1980 Anaesthesia for cardiac surgery and allied procedures. Blackwell Scientific Publications, Oxford.

Chapter 9
Figs 9.1–9.9 *from* Eger E I 1982 Isoflurane (AErrane). Airco Inc.

Chapter 12
Fig. 12.3 *from* Churchill-Davidson H C 1965 Anesthesiology 26: 224.

Chapter 16
Figs 16.3 and 16.18 *from* Parbrook G D, Davies P D, Parbrook E O 1982 Basic physics and measurement in anaesthesia. Heinemann, London. Figs 16.5, 16.13 and 16.21 *from* Mushin W, Jones P L 1987 Macintosh, Mushin and Epstein's Physics for the anaesthetist, 4th edn. Blackwell Scientific Publications, Oxford. Fig. 16.6 *from* Ward C S 1985 Anaesthetic equipment: physical principles and maintenance, 2nd Edn. Baillière Tindall, Eastbourne.

Chapter 17
Figs. 17.5, 17.6, 17.9 and 17.27 *from* Ward C S 1985 Anaesthetic equipment: physical principles and maintenance, 2nd Edn. Baillière Tindall, Eastbourne. Fig. 17.17. Courtesy of Penlon Limited. Figs 17.20 *from* Mapleson W W 1960 The concentration of anaesthetics in closed circuits with special reference to halothane. 1: Theoretical study. British Journal of Anaesthesia, 32: 298. Fig. 17.36 by courtesy of Colgate Medical Ltd.

Chapter 20
Fig. 20.2 *from* Atkinson R S, Rushman G B, Lee J A 1982 A synopsis of anaesthesia, 9th edn. John Wright, Bristol. Fig. 20.3 *from* Lichtiger M, Moya F (eds) 1978 Introduction to the practice of anaesthesia, 2nd edn. Harper and Row, Hagerstown, Maryland.

Chapter 21
Figs 21.6 and 21.7 *from* Kidd J F 1988 Pulse oximeters: basic theory and operation. Care of the Critically Ill 4: 10. Fig. 21.9 *from* Ward C S 1975 Anaesthetic equipment: Physical principles and maintenance. Baillière Tindall, Eastbourne. Fig. 21.20B *from* Hinds C J 1987 Intensive care: a concise textbook. Baillière Tindall, Eastbourne. Fig. 21.22 *from* Huch R, Huch A 1976 Transcutaneous non-invasive monitoring of PO_2. Hospital Practice 2: 43. Fig. 21.26 *from* Simpson J C 1981 Monitoring during Anesthesia for Cardiac Surgery. In: Gerson G R (ed) Monitoring during Anesthesia. International Anesthesiology Clinics 19 (1): 137. Tables 21.6 and 21.7 *from* Sykes M K 1987 Essential monitoring. British Journal of Anaesthesia 59: 901.

Chapter 24
Figs 24.2 and 24.5 *from* West J B 1977 Pulmonary Pathophysiology — The Essentials. Blackwell Scientific Publications, Oxford.

Chapter 25
Fig. 25.1 *from* Hannington-Kiff J G 1981 Pain, 2nd edn. Update Publications Limited, London. Fig. 25.2 *from* Austin K L, Stapleton J V, Mather L E 1980 Multiple intramuscular injections: A major source of variability in analgesic response to meperidine. Pain 8: 47.

Chapter 26
Fig. 26.4 *from* Lichtiger M, Moya F (eds) 1978 Introduction to the practice of anesthesia, 2nd edn. Harper and Row, Hagerstown, Maryland. Figs 26.11 and 26.13 *from* Wildsmith J A W, Armitage E N (eds) 1987. Principles and practice of regional anaesthesia. Churchill Livingstone, Edinburgh. Fig. 26.12 *from* Ellis H, Feldman S 1977 Anatomy for anaesthetists, 3rd edn. Blackwell Scientific Publications, Oxford. Fig. 26.15 *from* Moore D C 1979 Regional block, 4th edn. Charles C. Thomas, Springfield, Illinois.

Chapter 30
Fig. 30.1 Courtesy of Siemens Limited.

Chapter 33
Fig. 33.1 *from* Moir D D 1976 Obstetric anaesthesia and analgesia. Ballière Tindall, London.

Chapter 37
Fig. 37.2 *from* Cole P In: Langton Hewer C, Atkinson R S 1979. Recent advances in anaesthesia and analgesia, Vol. 13. Churchill Livingstone, London.

Chapter 38
Fig. 38.3 *from* Kitahata L M, Galicich J H, Sato I 1971 Journal of Neurosurgery 34: 185.

Chapter 44
Fig. 44.1 *from* Feldman S, Ellis H 1975 Principles of resuscitation, 2nd edn. Blackwell Scientific Publications, Oxford. Figs 44.2 and 44.3 *from* Gilston A, Resnekov L 1971 Cardiorespiratory resuscitation. William Heinemann, London.

Appendix XI(b) *from* Cotes J E 1979 Lung function, 4th edn. Blackwell Scientific Publications, Oxford.

Contributors

Alan R. Aitkenhead BSc MB ChB MD FFARCS
Professor of Anaesthesia, University of Nottingham Medical School, Nottingham

Douglas S. Arthur MB ChB FFARCS
Consultant, Department of Anaesthesia, Royal Infirmary, Glasgow

David B. Barnett MB ChB MD FRCP
Professor of Applied Pharmacology and Therapeutics, University of Leicester School of Medicine, Leicester Royal Infirmary, Leicester

Allan G. H. Cole MB BS FFARCS
Consultant, Department of Anaesthesia, Leicester Royal Infirmary, Leicester

David R Derbyshire MB ChB FFARCS
Consultant, Department of Anaesthesia, Warwick General Hospital, Warwick

David Fell MB ChB FFARCS
Senior Lecturer, Department of Anaesthesia, Leicester Royal Infirmary, Leicester

Valerie A. Goat MB ChB MD FFARCS
Consultant, Nuffield Department of Anaesthetics, John Radcliffe Hospital, Oxford

Ian S. Grant MB ChB MRCP FRCP (Edin. & Glas.) FFARCS
Consultant, Department of Anaesthesia, Western General Hospital, Edinburgh

Ronald Greenbaum MB ChB FFARCS DObst RCOG
Consultant, Department of Anaesthesia, University College Hospital, London

Christopher D. Hanning BSc MB BS FFARCS
Senior Lecturer, University Department of Anaesthesia, Leicester Royal Infirmary, Leicester

Stephen A. Hudson MPharm MPS
Principal Pharmacist and Clinical Tutor, Western General Hospital and Strathclyde University, Glasgow

R. Hugh James MB BS FFARCS DTM&H DObst RCOG DA
Consultant, Department of Anaesthesia, Leicester Royal Infirmary, Leicester

Michael J. Jones MB ChB MRCP FFARCS
Lecturer, University Department of Anaesthesia, Leicester Royal Infirmary, Leicester

John H. Kerr BM BCh DM FFARCS
Consultant, Nuffield Department of Anaesthetics, John Radcliffe Hospital, Oxford

Alistair Lee MB ChB FFARCS
Senior Registrar, Department of Anaesthesia, Edinburgh Royal Infirmary, Edinburgh

D. Geoffrey Lewis BA MA MB BChir MD FFARCS
Consultant, Department of Anaesthesia, Leicester Royal Infirmary, Leicester

Una M. MacFadyen BSc MB ChB MRCP DCH
Lecturer, University Department of Child Health, Leicester Royal Infirmary, Leicester

Peter J. McKenzie MB ChB FFARCS
Consultant, Nuffield Department of Anaesthetics, John Radcliffe Hospital, Oxford

Christopher J. D. Maile MA MB BChir FFARCS
Consultant, Department of Anaesthesia, Worcester Royal Infirmary, Worcester

Walter S. Nimmo BSc MB ChB MD FFARCS FFARACS FRCP
Medical Director, Inveresk Clinical Research Unit, Edinburgh

John Norman PhD MB ChB FFARCS
Professor of Anaesthesia, University Department of Anaesthesia, Southampton General Hospital, Southampton

Timothy M. O'Carroll MB BS FFARCS DObst RCOG
Consultant, Department of Anaesthesia, Leicester Royal Infirmary, Leicester

David G. Raitt MB ChB FFARCS DA
Consultant, Department of Anaesthesia, Leicester Royal Infirmary, Leicester

Guy S. Routh MB BS FFARCS
Consultant, Department of Anaesthesia, Cheltenham General Hospital and Gloucestershire Royal Hospital, Gloucester

Graham Smith BSc MB BS MD FFARCS
Professor of Anaesthesia, University of Leicester School of Medicine, Leicester

John Thorburn MB ChB FFARCS DA DObst RCOG
Consultant, Department of Anaesthesia, Western Infirmary, Glasgow

Gerald C. Tresidder MB BS FRCS
Lecturer, Department of Anatomy, University of Leicester Medical School, Leicester

Douglas A. B. Turner MB ChB FFARCS
Consultant, Department of Anaesthesia, Leicester Royal Infirmary, Leicester

Mairlys Vater MB BCh FFARCS DA
Consultant, Department of Anaesthesia, Russells Hall Hospital, Dudley

Peter G. M. Wallace MB ChB FFARCS DObst RCOG
Consultant, Department of Anaesthesia, Western Infirmary, Glasgow

John Walls MB ChB FRCP
Consultant, Renal Unit, Leicester General Hospital, Leicester

Malcolm J. H. Wellstood-Eason MB ChB FFARCS
Consultant, Department of Anaesthesia, Leicester Royal Infirmary, Leicester

John A. W. Wildsmith MB ChB MD FFARCS
Consultant, Department of Anaesthesia, Edinburgh Royal Infirmary, Edinburgh

Sheila M. Willatts MB BS FRCP FFARCS DObst RCOG DA
Consultant, Department of Anaesthesia, Bristol Royal Infirmary, Bristol

J. Keith Wood MB ChB FRCP FRCPE FRCPath
Consultant, Department of Haematology, Leicester Royal Infirmary, Leicester

Contents

1. Anatomy 1
Gerald C. Tresidder

2. Respiratory physiology 23
D. Geoffrey Lewis

3. Cardiovascular physiology 43
Christopher D. Hanning

4. Outlines of renal physiology 63
John Walls

5. Physiology of the nervous system 77
Sheila M. Willatts

6. Maternal and neonatal physiology 111
Una M. MacFadyen

7. Haematology 125
J. Keith Wood

8. Principles of general pharmacology and pharmacokinetics 139
Walter S. Nimmo

9. Inhalational anaesthetic agents 153
Graham Smith

10. Intravenous anaesthetic agents 175
Alan R. Aitkenhead

11. Drugs used to supplement anaesthesia 193
Alan R. Aitkenhead

12. Neuromuscular blockade 211
John Norman

13. Drugs affecting the autonomic nervous system 225
David B. Barnett and Stephen A. Hudson

14. Miscellaneous drugs of importance in anaesthesia 241
Stephen A. Hudson and David B. Barnett

15. Local anaesthetic agents 257
John A. W. Wildsmith

16. Basic physics for the anaesthetist 269
Graham Smith

17. Anaesthetic apparatus 291
Graham Smith and Alan R. Aitkenhead

18. The operating theatre environment 323
Alan R. Aitkenhead

19. Preoperative assessment and premedication 333
Graham Smith

20. The practical conduct of anaesthesia 349
David Fell

21. Monitoring during anaesthesia 363
Mairlys Vater

22. Fluid, electrolyte and acid–base balance 389
Douglas A. B. Turner

23. Complications during anaesthesia 405
Timothy M. O'Carroll

24. Postoperative care 421
Alan R. Aitkenhead

25. Postoperative pain 449
Graham Smith

26. Local anaesthetic techniques 459
Alistair Lee and John A. W. Wildsmith

27. Anaesthesia for gynaecological, genitourinary and orthopaedic surgery 485
Allan G. H. Cole

28. Anaesthesia for ENT surgery 495
Timothy M. O'Carroll

29. Anaesthesia for ophthalmic surgery 501
Peter J. McKenzie

30. Anaesthesia for radiology, radiotherapy and psychiatry 507
Michael J. Jones

31. Day-case anaesthesia 519
R. Hugh James

32. Emergency anaesthesia 527
Douglas A. B. Turner

33. Obstetric anaesthesia and analgesia 541
John Thorburn

34. Paediatric anaesthesia and intensive care 555
Douglas S. Arthur

35. Dental anaesthesia 573
John Thorburn

36. Anaesthesia for plastic, endocrine and vascular surgery 583
David G. Raitt

37. Hypotensive anaesthesia 595
Valerie A. Goat

38. Neurosurgical anaesthesia 603
Ronald Greenbaum

39. Anaesthesia for thoracic surgery 615
Alan R. Aitkenhead

40. Anaesthesia for cardiac surgery 629
Peter G. M. Wallace

41. Intercurrent disease and anaesthesia 645
Ian S. Grant

42. The intensive therapy unit 677
John H. Kerr and Guy S. Routh

43. Relief of chronic pain 695
Malcolm J. H. Wellstood-Eason

44. Cardiopulmonary resuscitation 705
Christopher J. D. Maile

Appendices 715
David R. Derbyshire

Index 755

1. Anatomy

A knowledge of anatomy is important to the anaesthetist. In the conduct of anaesthesia it is required to enable him to cannulate veins and arteries, to undertake laryngoscopy for tracheal intubation or to undertake bronchoscopy for removal of aspirated material. It is also essential to know the anatomy relating to local anaesthetic nerve blocks. In addition, a sound knowledge of anatomy is necessary in cardiopulmonary medicine and to understand the surgeon's techniques and requirements.

Clearly, this short chapter cannot cover all the anatomical knowledge required of the anaesthetist. Its purpose is to describe in detail only those aspects relevant to the conduct of general anaesthesia and spinal anaesthesia and to indicate areas for further study in the standard textbooks of anatomy.

VENEPUNCTURE

Upper limb

The valved superficial veins form varying patterns, but the common arrangements are shown in Figures 1.1 and 1.2.

The arrangement of the arteries is less varied than that of the veins. However, developmental anomalies do occur and it is wise to inspect and palpate for arterial pulsation before undertaking venepuncture. An 'ulnar' artery may leave the brachial artery in the arm and, passing superficial to the common attachment of the superficial flexor muscles of the forearm, lie immediately deep to the median basilic vein — without the intervention of the bicipital aponeurosis. Similarly a 'radial' artery may arise proximally and be situated superficially in the forearm.

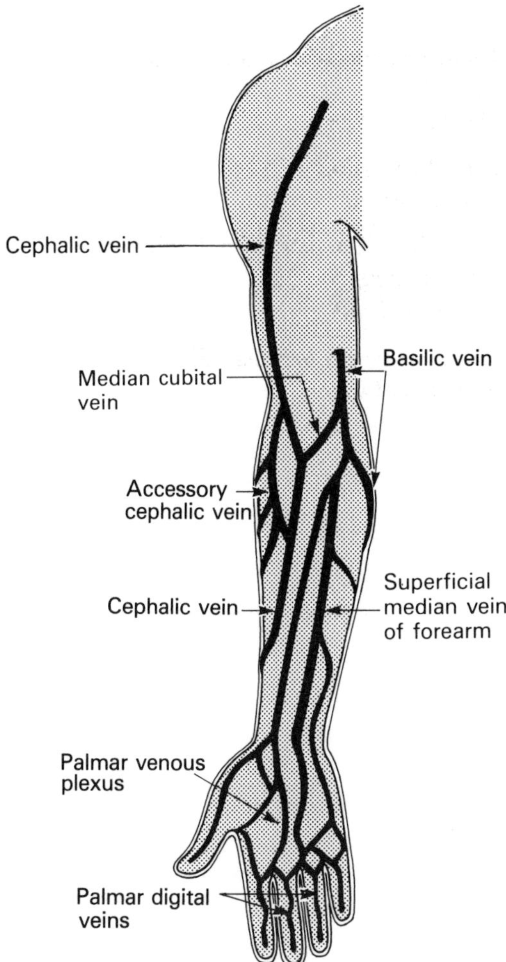

Fig. 1.1 Superficial veins of the right upper limb.

Metacarpal veins, lying superficially on the back of the hand, drain blood from the digits and hand (Fig. 1.2). These veins join together to form the

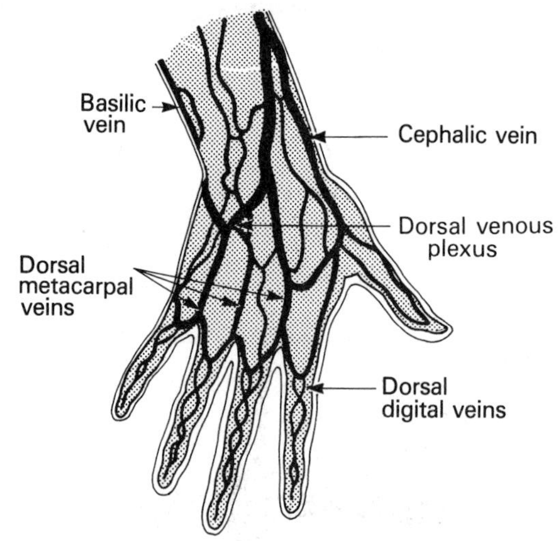

Fig. 1.2 Dorsal metacarpal veins of the right hand.

dorsal venous arch. From the lateral and medial ends of the dorsal venous arch, the blood is carried centripetally by the cephalic and basilic veins respectively. These veins also receive tributaries from the skin and superficial tissues of the forearm thus draining, respectively, the pre- and postaxial borders of the upper limb. The basilic vein, having received the brachial veins, continues as the axillary vein. The cephalic vein, after passing through the deltopectoral groove, drains into the axillary vein

Venepuncture may be performed at the following sites:

1. On the back of the hand and lateral aspect of the wrist in one of the dorsal metacarpal veins (Fig. 1.2).
2. On the anterior aspect of the forearm in the cephalic or median veins (Fig. 1.1), or one of their tributaries. Usually there are useful veins also on the posterior aspect.

It is preferable to cannulate veins on the back of the hand and on the forearm rather than those at the elbow because the cannula may be secured more easily in situ.

When a venepuncture is to be made at or below the elbow greater venous distension can be obtained in an obstructed vein if the front of the forearm is massaged by firm pressure from the wrist upwards. This delivers blood from the superficial veins and from the deep (communicating) vein (Fig. 1.3) which drains the deeper structures of the forearm. A conscious patient should be asked to flex and extend the digits forcibly several times and then to clench the fist firmly. Subsequently the forearm should be massaged from the wrist upwards.

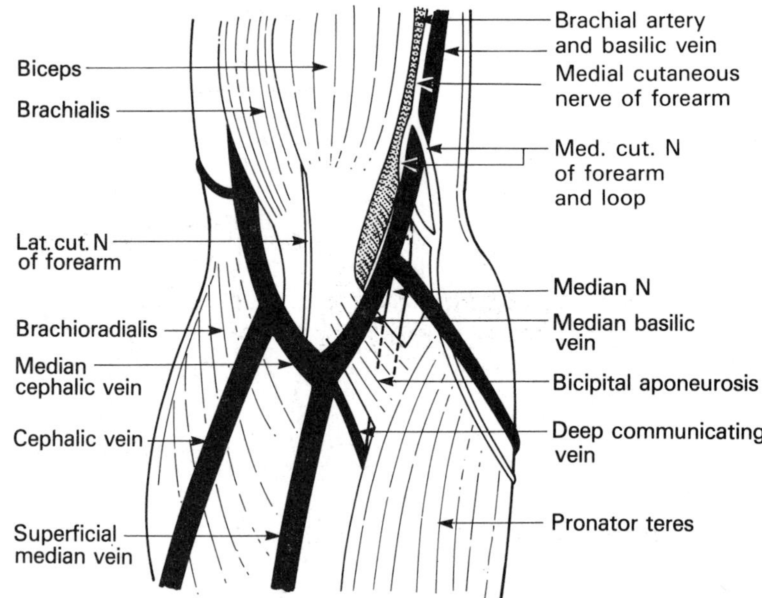

Fig. 1.3 Veins at the right elbow.

3. At the elbow in either the median cephalic or median basilic vein (Fig. 1.3). Usually the median basilic vein is the larger and more mobile of the two, but, if used inexpertly, there may be complications. If the needle is inserted too deeply, it may pass through the bicipital aponeurosis and penetrate the brachial artery. The pulsation of this artery can be felt immediately medial to the tendon of the biceps. Medial to the brachial artery lies the median nerve. An anomalous ulnar artery may lie just deep to the median cubital vein and be at risk if the vein is penetrated too deeply. Withdrawal of arterial blood in a pulsatile stream indicates that this has happened.

The medial cutaneous nerve of the forearm divides into its anterior and posterior branches at the elbow (Fig. 1.3) and sometimes these loop around the median basilic vein. Thus perivenous piercing with the needle, extravasation of fluid, or the occurrence of a haematoma at this site may damage nerve fibres and in the conscious patient cause acute pain along the inner border of the forearm.

4. Below the clavicle in the subclavian vein (Fig. 1.4). Use of the right subclavian rather than the left provides easier access to the superior vena cava and right atrium. The subclavian vein — the continuation of the axillary — runs from a point just below and medial to the midclavicular point. From here it arches upwards, then, passing downwards and forwards (Fig. 1.5) it joins the internal

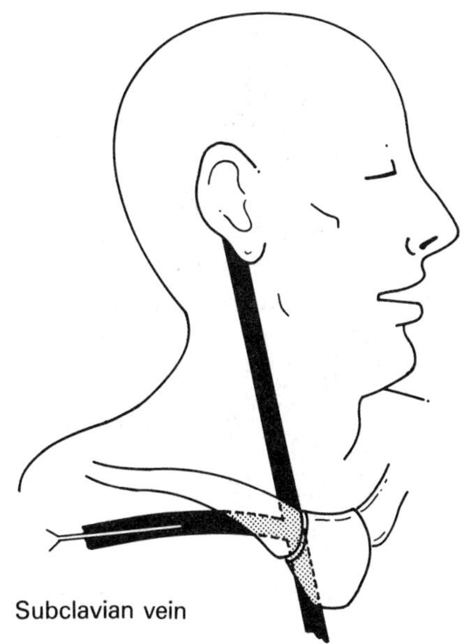

Fig. 1.4 Right subclavian and jugular veins.

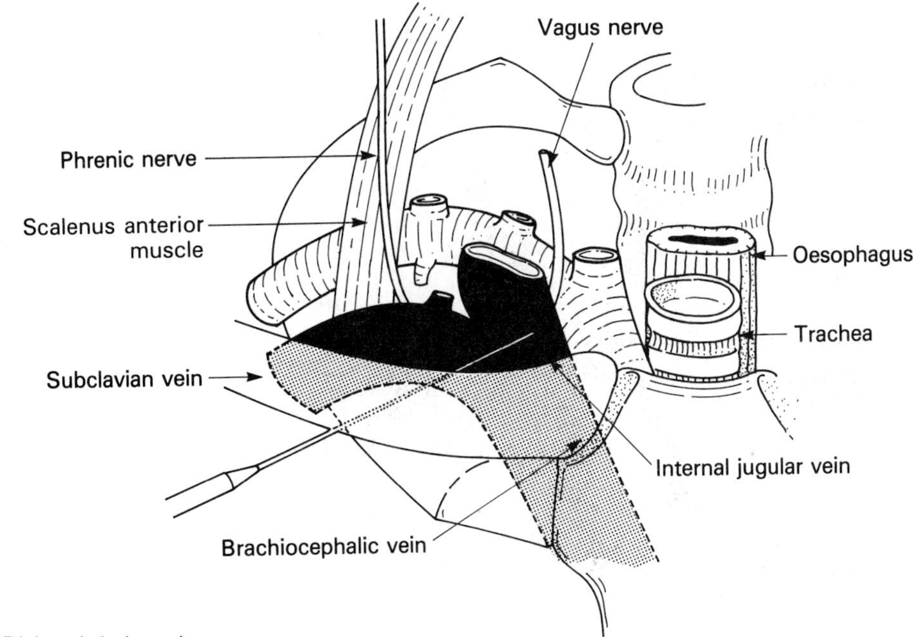

Fig. 1.5 Right subclavian vein.

jugular to form the brachiocephalic vein posterior to the sternoclavicular joint. The subclavian vein lies in a groove on the superior surface of the first rib. The subclavian artery lies above and behind the vein with the scalenus anterior tendon intervening. The phrenic nerve lies deep to the prevertebral layer of the cervical fascia covering the scalenus anterior. By puncturing the skin below the clavicle — at the junction of its middle and medial thirds — the needle is passed upwards and medially in the direction of the sternoclavicular joint. The vein should be entered at its confluence with the internal jugular vein.

Neck and head

Venepuncture may be performed above the clavicle in the external and internal jugular veins. For puncture of the external and internal jugular veins the patient should be lying in a slight Trendelenburg position with the head turned away from the side of puncture. This position provides easy access to and distension of the veins and minimises the risk of air embolism. Finger pressure just above the middle of the clavicle also produces distension of the external jugular vein.

The external jugular vein, receiving blood from the scalp and face, is formed by the union of the posterior auricular vein and the posterior division of the retromandibular vein (Fig. 1.6). It runs vertically downwards from just behind the angle of the mandible to pass posterior to the clavicle lateral to the sternocleidomastoid muscle, where it terminates in the subclavian vein. In its course it lies deep to the skin and the platysma muscle, and superficial to the investing layer of the deep cervical fascia and sternocleidomastoid muscle. Puncture of the vein should be made one finger's breadth above the clavicle.

The internal jugular vein (Figs 1.6 and 1.7) is the continuation of the sigmoid sinus. It runs from its superior bulb (dilation) just below the base of the skull to terminate posterior to the sternoclavicular joint, where its inferior bulb is joined by the subclavian vein to form the brachiocephalic vein. The internal jugular lies deep to the sternocleidomastoid muscle on the lateral side of the internal and common carotid arteries (Fig. 1.8).

It is safest to puncture the internal jugular vein using a 'high approach'. A common technique is to approach the vein at the apex of the triangle formed by the sternal and clavicular heads of sternocleidomastoid muscle (Fig. 1.8). This is found usually at the level of the cricoid cartilage. At this point a needle is directed downwards at an angle of 30° to the skin in the direction of the ipsilateral nipple. If the internal jugular vein is not encountered, the needle is redirected medially.

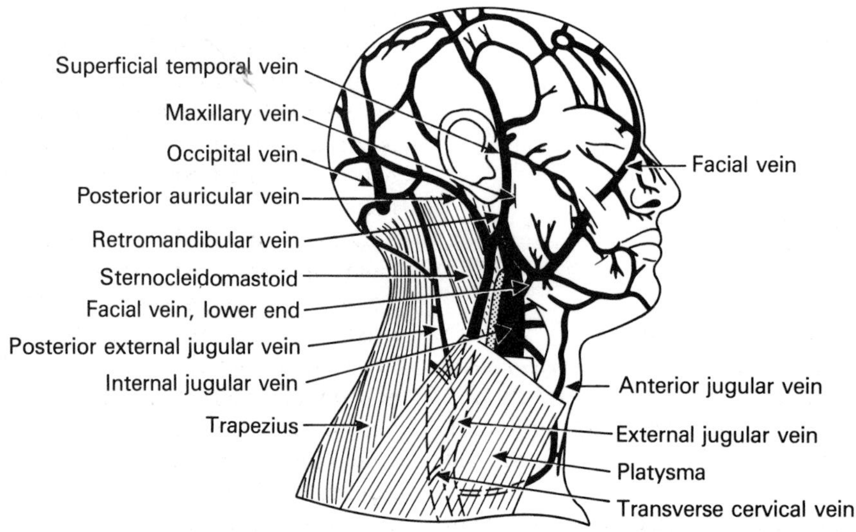

Fig. 1.6 Veins of right side of the head and neck.

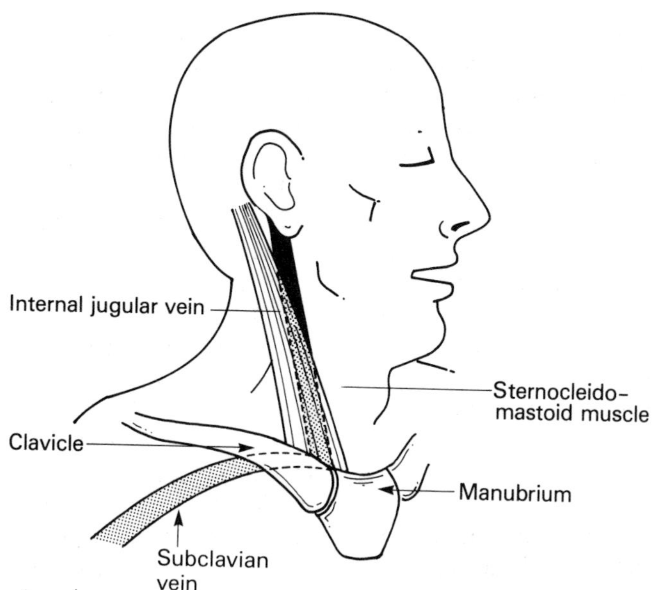

Fig. 1.7 Right internal jugular vein.

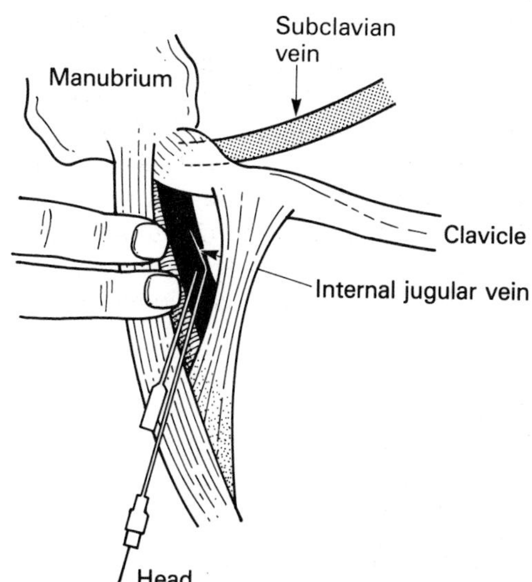

Fig. 1.8 Approach to the right internal jugular vein. Catheter inserted through cannula.

Complications include puncture of the common carotid artery, branches of the costocervical trunk, or the thoracic duct (on the left side) and damage to the sympathetic trunk. The 'high approach' reduces the chance of injury to the pleura and lung.

On the right side, cannulation of the right atrium is easy because the right internal jugular vein, brachiocephalic vein, superior vena cava and right atrium lie almost in a straight line.

Lower limb

There are several different patterns of the superficial saphenous system. Various direct and indirect communications exist between the long (great) and short (small) saphenous veins (Fig. 1.9). Throughout their courses these veins both receive tributaries from the skin and subcutaneous tissues and also give off perforating branches which join the deep veins. The perforating veins normally convey blood from the superficial to the deep system. All the veins of the lower limb have bicuspid valves which are arranged so that blood is directed towards the heart. The flow of blood may be reversed when varicosity of the veins is present.

Dorsal metatarsal veins, which receive blood from the toes, run together to form a dorsal venous arch which lies across the foot over the heads of the metatarsal bones. This dorsal network of veins also receives blood from the sole and sides of the foot. The medial end of the dorsal venous arch is continued as the long saphenous vein; the lateral end continues as the short saphenous. These veins respectively mark the pre- and postaxial borders of the lower limb.

The long saphenous vein lies with the

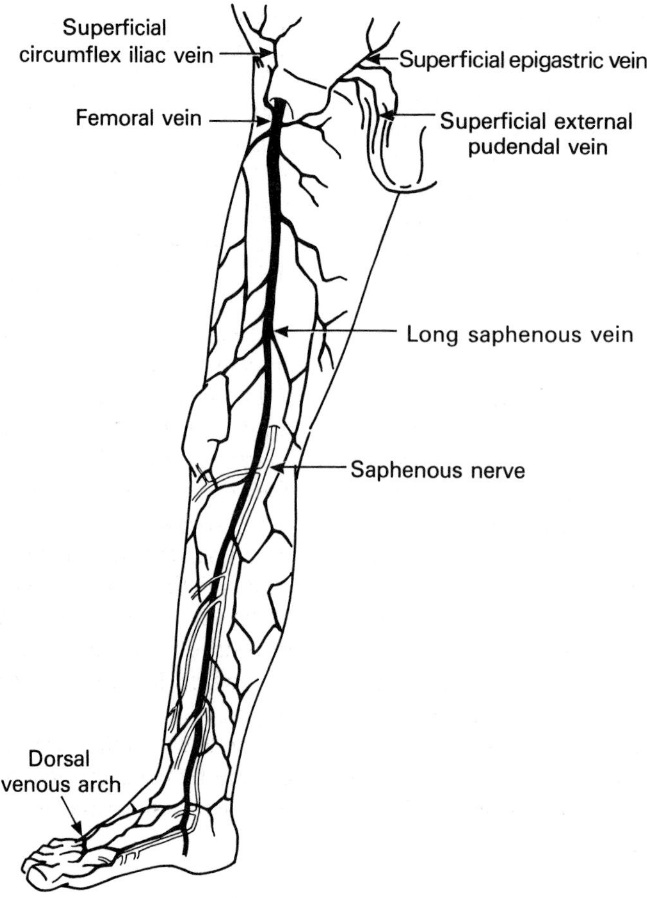

Fig. 1.9 Superficial veins of the right lower limb.

saphenous nerve immediately anterior to the medial malleolus at the ankle (Fig. 1.9). As the vein ascends (still accompanied by the saphenous nerve) along the medial side of the leg, it passes obliquely across the lower part of the tibia to become posteromedial at the medial condyles of the tibia and femur. From here, often accompanied by branches of the medial femoral cutaneous nerve, the vein passes upwards and obliquely forwards to pass through the saphenous opening of the deep fascia (which lies two finger breadths below and lateral to the pubic tubercle) to enter the femoral vein, which lies medial to the femoral artery. When puncturing the long saphenous vein, any perivenous probing with the needle or spread of injection fluid, or the occurrence of a haematoma, may damage the accompanying nerve and cause acute pain in the conscious patient.

Venepuncture may be performed:

1. On the dorsum of the foot in the dorsal venous arch or one of its tributaries (Fig. 1.9). This provides the best site in the lower limb for i.v. infusions in the operating theatre.
2. On the anteromedial aspect of the leg using either the long saphenous vein or one of its tributaries (Fig. 1.9). The saphenous vein has a thick wall and therefore a sharp needle is required. The lowest part of the vein, in its own fascial sheath, lies in direct contact with the periosteum over the tibia and care should be taken to avoid injuring these structures.

UPPER RESPIRATORY AIRWAY

The upper airway consists of passages extending from the anterior nares down to and including the larynx. The nasal cavity extends from the nostrils (anterior nares) to the posterior nares or choanae where it opens into the nasopharynx or postnasal space. The cavity is divided by the nasal septum into right and left halves. Each half consists of three regions.

The nose

The *nasal vestibule* lies just inside the nostril. It is the widest part (up to 1 cm) of the cavity. The vestibule is lined by skin which bears coarse hairs (the vibrissae) and sebaceous and sweat glands. At approximately 2 cm distance from the nostrils, the skin becomes continuous with the mucous membrane of the *respiratory region of the nasal cavity*. This membrane consists of columnar or pseudostratified ciliated epithelium with occasional goblet cells. Beneath the basal lamina lie mucous and serous glands with a vascular cavernous tissue containing arteriovenous communications.

The *olfactory region* is situated in the roof of the nasal cavity. This region is covered with olfactory epithelium extending over the superior part of the septum medially and the superior concha laterally.

The floor of the cavity is formed, from before backwards, by the hard palate comprising the palatal processes of the maxillae and in its posterior quarter the horizontal plates of the palatine bones. The soft palate is attached to the posterior margin of the hard palate. The floor is almost horizontal as it passes posteriorly; it is gently concave from side to side. These bones are covered by periosteum to which the thin overlying mucous membrane is intimately adherent.

The medial wall of the cavity is formed by the nasal septum. After the age of seven years, the septum is often deviated from the median plane. This diminishes the size of one half of the cavity and increases that of the other. The septum comprises the vomer bone and the perpendicular plate of the ethmoid bone. Anteriorly lies the septal cartilage. These structures are covered respectively by periosteum and perichondrium over which lies a thick layer of mucous membrane (Fig. 1.10).

The lateral wall of the nose is constituted on the outside by cartilage and bone. In front and below lie three nasal cartilages. The lower cartilages meet

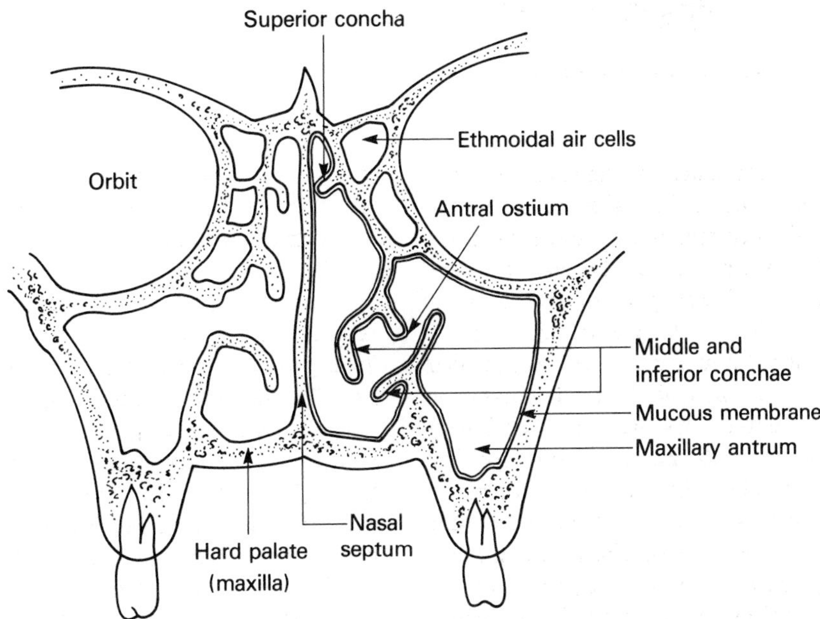

Fig. 1.10 Coronal section of the nasal cavities and sinuses.

in the midline forming the point of the nose. Above and posteriorly, the nasal bone and the frontal process of the maxilla form the remainder of the side wall. On the inside of the nose, the lateral wall of the nasal cavity (Fig. 1.11) is formed by the nasal surfaces of the maxilla anteriorly and inferiorly, posteriorly by the perpendicular plate of the palatine bone and superiorly by the ethmoid. From the latter the superior and middle conchae form projections into the cavity. The inferior concha is a separate bone articulating with the maxilla and palate. The lateral wall, formed mainly by the three projecting conchae, is covered by a thick and very vascular mucous membrane. Below each concha is a passage or meatus. The paranasal sinuses open into the meatuses — the posterior ethmoidal sinus opens into the superior meatus; the remainder open into the middle meatus. The nasolacrimal duct opens into the anterior part of the inferior meatus. Just beyond the posterior end of the inferior meatus above the level of the soft palate, in the nasopharynx, lies the opening of the pharyngotympanic (Eustachian) tube with the tubal tonsil attached to its posterior lip.

The *nasopharynx* or post-nasal space, in its upper part, is the direct posterior continuation of the nasal cavity. The nasopharynx lies just above and behind the soft palate which forms the anterior boundary in its lower part.

The rigid roof and posterior wall of the nasopharynx are formed by bones covered with periosteum and mucous membrane. Passing from above downwards are the body of the sphenoid, the basilar part of the occipital bone and the anterior arch of the atlas (Fig. 1.12). The lateral walls are composed of muscle (mainly the superior constrictor) and the thick pharyngobasilar membrane which is inelastic. Thus the airway through the nasopharynx is always kept patent for breathing. The cavity is lined by respiratory epithelium.

The nerve supply of the mucous membrane lining the nose and nasopharynx is derived mainly from cranial nerve V (trigeminal) and both sympathetic and parasympathetic parts of the autonomic nervous system.

Cranial nerve I (olfactory) carries the special sensation of smell from the roof and adjoining walls of the nose to the brain. The anterior ethmoidal branch of the ophthalmic division of the trigeminal nerve conveys afferent somaesthetic impulses from the anterosuperior quadrant of the lateral wall of the nasal cavity and the corresponding part of the septum. The remainder of the lateral wall and most of the medial (septal)

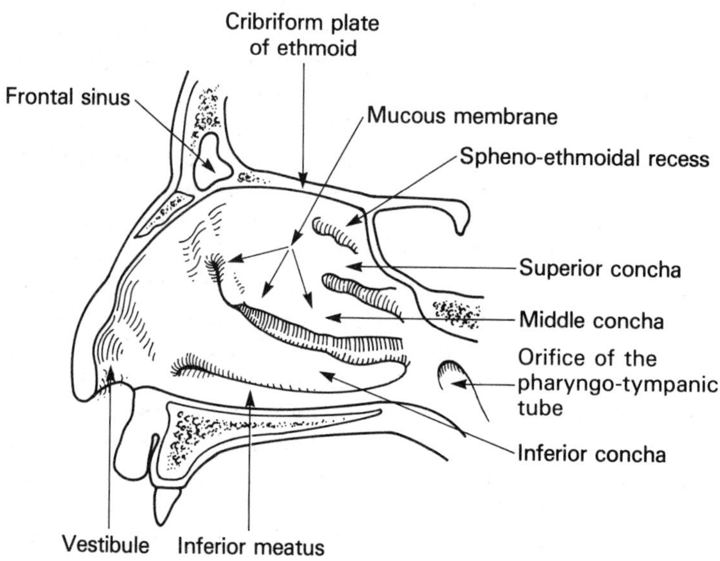

Fig. 1.11 Right nasal cavity: lateral wall.

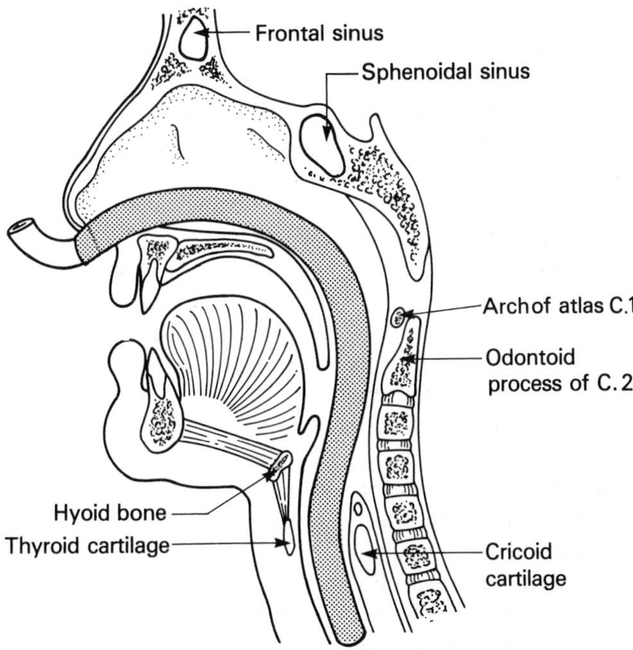

Fig. 1.12 Right side of the pharynx: intubated.

wall receives its sensory supply from branches of the pterygopalatine ganglion. This ganglion, lying in the pterygopalatine fossa, is suspended by two branches from the maxillary nerve, which is the second division of the trigeminal nerve. Additional nerves, branches of the maxillary and its anterior superior alveolar branch, supply the lateral wall and floor respectively.

The parasympathetic nerves conduct secretor impulses from the superior salivatory nucleus (in the pons) to the mucous and serous secreting cells in the mucous membrane of the nose and nasopharynx. These impulses pass via the nervus intermedius, along its continuing fibres forming the greater petrosal nerve, which is joined by sympathetic fibres. This nerve synapses in the pterygopalatine ganglion whence the postganglionic fibres pass, with the sensory branches of the ganglion, to the mucous membrane. Stimulation produces mucous and serous secretions.

Some afferent nerve fibres conveying the special sense of taste from the oral surface of the soft palate travel through the pterygopalatine ganglion into the greater petrosal nerve. These fibres are the peripheral processes of unipolar cells in the geniculate ganglion of cranial nerve VII (facial). The central processes travel in the nervus intermedius to join the fasciculus solitarius and synapse in its nucleus in the medulla oblongata.

The sympathetic nervous supply for the head has its cells of origin at the level of the first and second thoracic segments of the spinal cord. From here fibres pass upwards to synapse in the superior cervical sympathetic ganglion. The second neurone fibres pass along the wall of the internal carotid artery. Some of the sympathetic fibres, named the deep petrosal nerve, branch off to join with fibres of the greater petrosal nerve in the formation of the nerve of the pterygoid canal. The sympathetic fibres pass through the pterygopalatine ganglion without synapsing. They are distributed with the other branches of the ganglion to supply constrictor impulses to the smooth muscle in the walls of blood vessels.

The main arterial supply of the inside of the nose comes from the maxillary artery. The maxillary artery, a terminal branch of the external carotid artery, continues through the infratemporal fossa and eventually through the pterygopalatine fossa to give branches to the lateral and medial walls of the nasal and nasopharyngeal cavities. These arterial branches accompany branches of the pterygopalatine ganglion. Anterior and posterior ethmoidal arteries, branches of the ophthalmic artery, supply the upper part of the nasal cavity. The ascending pharyngeal artery (a vertically ascending branch arising from the origin of the external carotid artery) and the ascending palatine branch of the facial artery supply the nasopharynx and soft palate.

The veins draining the nose and nasopharynx correspond to the arteries. These veins pass through the pterygopalatine fossa to drain into the pterygoid plexus. This plexus of veins, which has valves, lies within and around the lateral pterygoid muscle. Two large vessels, the maxillary veins, pass backwards from the plexus and join the superficial temporal veins to form the retromandibular vein. Other venous communications are made with the facial and ethmoidal veins and the cavernous sinus.

Most of the lymphatic vessels draining the nasal and nasopharyngeal cavities pass either directly to the upper deep cervical lymph nodes or indirectly via the retropharyngeal and parotid nodes. Beneath the mucous membrane there is a collection of lymphoid tissue, the (naso) pharyngeal tonsil or 'adenoids'. This lies on the upper part of the posterior wall of the nasopharynx. The pharyngeal tonsil is prolonged laterally to join the tubal tonsil. In children, hypertrophy of the pharyngeal tonsil may obstruct the airway and, if the tubal tonsil enlarges, the pharyngotympanic tube may be obstructed.

Deviation of the nasal septum is a common occurrence. It results usually from direct trauma to the nose. Rarely it may occur before the age of seven years. There may be overgrowth of the cartilage alone, or excessive growth of the vomer and perpendicular plate of the ethmoid may lead to 'buckling' of the cartilage. Deviation of the septum can lead to occlusion of the nasal cavity into which it projects.

Deflections of the septum or hypertrophic rhinitis and vascular engorgement affecting the middle and inferior conchae may reduce the size of one or both nasal cavities. Nasal polyps growing from the mucosa overlying the conchae may also protrude into the upper and middle meatuses. Usually it is easy to pass a lubricated tube through a nostril and along the inferior meatus to enter the nasopharynx although any of these defects may make this difficult.

The mouth

The mouth is bounded externally in front and at the sides by the lips and cheeks; the vestibule of the mouth is the space between its external boundaries and the internal boundary provided by the teeth and gums. The remainder of the mouth constitutes the oral cavity which is separated from the nasal cavities above by the palate. The floor of the mouth is occupied mainly by the muscular tongue. Posteriorly, at the sides, the palatoglossal folds arch upwards and with the upper surface of the tongue form the oropharyngeal isthmus between the mouth and oropharynx.

The mouth is lined by mucous membrane covered with stratified squamous epithelium which continues on to the anteroinferior surface of the soft palate and over the whole tongue. Beneath the mucous membrane lie mucous glands.

The prehensile anterior part of the tongue is covered by filiform papillae. These provide a certain roughness (under the moist surface) and so facilitate the tongue being firmly gripped between finger and thumb. At the sides and tip of the tongue there are fungiform papillae which bear taste buds. Taste buds are found also in all vallate papillae. These lie dorsally at the V-shaped site of fusion of the derivatives of the embryological first and third branchial arches from which the definitive tongue is derived.

The muscles of the tongue are striated. Except for the palatoglossus muscles, supplied from the pharyngeal plexus, all the muscles of the tongue are supplied by cranial nerve XII (hypoglossal).

The mucous membrane over the anterior two-thirds of the tongue and the adjoining gums of the lower jaw is supplied by the lingual nerve — a branch of the mandibular division of the trigeminal nerve. Afferent impulses from the taste buds in the anterior two thirds of the tongue and floor of mouth pass along the chorda tympani nerve. The central processes of its cells, lying in the geniculate ganglion of cranial nerve VII, pass in the nervus intermedius to synapse in the nucleus solitarius.

The efferent parasympathetic supply to the salivary glands in the tongue and floor of the mouth takes origin from the superior salivatory nucleus in the pons. The nerves travel in the nervus intermedius, initially in company with the facial nerve, to continue in the chorda tympani nerve. These nerve fibres synapse in the submandibular ganglion whence the postganglionic fibres pass with the branches of the lingual nerve to convey secretor impulses to the salivary glands.

The *oropharynx* communicates anteriorly through the oropharyngeal isthmus with the upper part of the oral cavity. Superiorly, through the pharyngeal isthmus, it communicates with the nasopharynx. The former is closed by contraction of the palatoglossal muscles and by drawing the tongue backwards and upwards to press against the tensed soft palate. The pharyngeal isthmus is closed by contraction of the levator palati muscles; these raise the soft palate upwards and backwards against the highest fibres of the simultaneously contracting superior constrictor and palatopharyngeus muscles. In this action, the highest fibres of the palatopharyngeus form a ridge (of Passavant) as they encircle the pharynx between the superior constrictor and the lining layer of mucous membrane.

Anteroinferiorly the oropharynx is bounded by the back of the tongue. This has a smooth moist surface which facilitates the onward movement of a bolus. Beneath the mucous membrane are scattered nodules of lymphoid tissue, the lingual tonsils, which are prolonged laterally to join the palatine tonsil. The posterior third of the tongue extends from the vallate papillae to the two valleculae.

The (palatine) tonsil, lying between the palatoglossal arch (anteriorly) and palatopharyngeal arch (posteriorly), and the pharyngeal constrictor muscles form the lateral wall of the oropharynx. The constrictor muscles meet in a midline raphe posteriorly. At the level of the oropharynx the constrictors lie in front of the 2nd and 3rd cervical vertebrae. At the level of the upper free border of the epiglottis the oropharynx becomes continuous with the laryngopharynx.

The pharyngeal plexus of nerves and the pharyngeal plexus of veins lie on the outer surface of the middle constrictor muscle about the level of the hyoid bone. The former supplies sensory and motor nerves to the oropharynx. Cranial nerves IX (glossopharyngeal) and X (vagus), and sympathetic fibres, mingle to form the pharyngeal plexus. The sympathetic supply comprises postganglionic fibres with cell bodies in the superior cervical ganglion. The somaesthetic impulses leave the plexus to travel via the glossopharyngeal and vagal nerves. The unipolar cells of these nerves are in their superior ganglions. In the medulla the central processes from the superior ganglions pass to synapse in the caudal part of the nucleus of the spinal fasciculus of the trigeminal nerve. The 'gag' reflex in the unanaesthetised state is induced by touching the mucous membrane covering the posterior third of the tongue, soft palate or lateral and posterior walls of the oropharynx. Pathways from the nuclei in the medulla convey impulses to the nearby nucleus ambiguus and hypoglossal nucleus, leading to efferent motor impulses. These travel via cranial nerves IX, X and XII causing contraction of palatal, pharyngeal and lingual muscles, the effect of which is to close the pharynx completely.

Impulses of the special sense of taste also travel in cranial nerves IX and X; their unipolar cells are in their inferior ganglions and their central processes pass to synapse in the nucleus solitarius. Efferent parasympathetic fibres travel from the inferior salivatory nucleus (in the upper medulla) via the glossopharyngeal nerve. After synapsing in small ganglia in the mucous membrane of the oropharynx they convey secretor impulses to its mucous and serous glands.

The vascular supply of both the oro- and laryngopharynx is as follows. The arterial supply comes from the ascending pharyngeal, ascending palatine and tonsillar branches of the facial artery and branches of the lingual, superior and inferior laryngeal arteries. The venous drainage is into the pharyngeal plexus of veins which drains upwards to the pterygoid plexus and downwards into the internal jugular vein. Lymphatic drainage is to the deep cervical lymph nodes.

The *laryngopharynx* is the continuation of the oropharynx. In the upper part of the laryngopharynx, the paths for food and air cross. A bolus of food or fluid is projected downwards and backwards from the oral cavity through the oro- and laryngopharynx and into the oesophagus. In so doing it inevitably crosses the airway which is passing from the nasopharynx, downwards through the oropharynx and across the upper part of the laryngopharynx to pass forwards to the larynx.

As a result of this chiasma it is possible for fluid, food or foreign bodies taken into the mouth to pass down forwards into the larynx to reach the trachea and bronchi. In the conscious state this is prevented by the mechanism of deglutition. In this act respiration is momentarily suspended. The bolus is pushed onwards by successive contractions of the pharyngeal constrictor muscles (assisted by gravity). At the same time the larynx is elevated by contraction of the stylo-, salpingo- and palatopharyngeus muscles. This elevation assists in closing the laryngeal inlet. Further elevation of the larynx is achieved by raising the hyoid bone from which the larynx is suspended. Entrance through the inlet into the vestibule of the larynx is also restricted by being covered by the tilting of the epiglottis backwards and downwards.

In vomiting, particularly in the unconscious state when the reflex pathways are out of action, it is possible for the regurgitated gastric contents to be expelled up the oesophagus, through the cricopharyngeal 'ring' of muscle, into the laryngopharynx and then forwards across to the vestibule and so downwards through the larynx and trachea to the lungs.

It is also possible for air and material expectorated from the lungs and lower respiratory airways to enter the oesophagus and stomach. This is prevented normally by the sphincter-like contraction of the cricopharyngeal part of the inferior constrictor muscles.

Anteriorly, the upper limit of the laryngopharynx is marked by the upper free edge of the epiglottis. Bounding the sides of the inlet to the larynx are the aryepiglottic folds passing posteriorly to the arytenoid cartilages, which articulate inferiorly with the cricoid cartilage. At the sides the salpingo-, stylo- and palatopharyngeus muscles are passing downwards (within the inferior constrictor) to gain attachment to the posterior (vertical) border of the thyroid cartilage and to the fibrous layer of the wall of the pharynx. The overlapping inferior constrictor and the middle and superior constrictor muscles form the rest of the lateral and entire posterior wall of the laryngopharynx. Posteriorly the constrictors are in relation to the anterior longitudinal ligament which is adherent to the periosteum over the lower part of the 3rd cervical vertebra and the succeeding 4th, 5th and 6th vertebrae.

The lining mucous membrane extends laterally as folds from the sides of the epiglottis. Above, it covers the deep aspect of the thyrohyoid membrane, and below, the thyroid cartilage. Spreading backwards it lines the muscles forming the lateral and posterior walls of this part of the pharynx. A longitudinal furrow is formed on each side between the bulge of the larynx, covered by its posterolateral muscles and the overlying mucous membrane, and the concavity of the thyroid cartilage which contains it. These are the right and left piriform fossae (Fig. 1.13).

The larynx

The larynx is the continuation of the airway from the laryngopharynx to the trachea. The cavity of the larynx extends from its inlet to the lower border of the cricoid cartilage. In men its length is approximately 45 mm and its anteroposterior diameter 35 mm; in women, these measurements are approximately 35 mm and 25 mm respectively.

The framework of the larynx comprises cartilages, ligaments and membranes. The outer wall is made up in part by the following cartilages: thyroid; cricoid; paired arytenoids lying on the vertical lamina of the cricoid; the small paired corniculate and cuneiform cartilages; and the cartilage of the epiglottis (Fig. 1.14).

Extrinsic ligaments — thyrohyoid and cricotracheal — join the larynx to the hyoid bone above and to the trachea below. Intrinsic membranes form the inner tube of the 'skeleton' of the larynx.

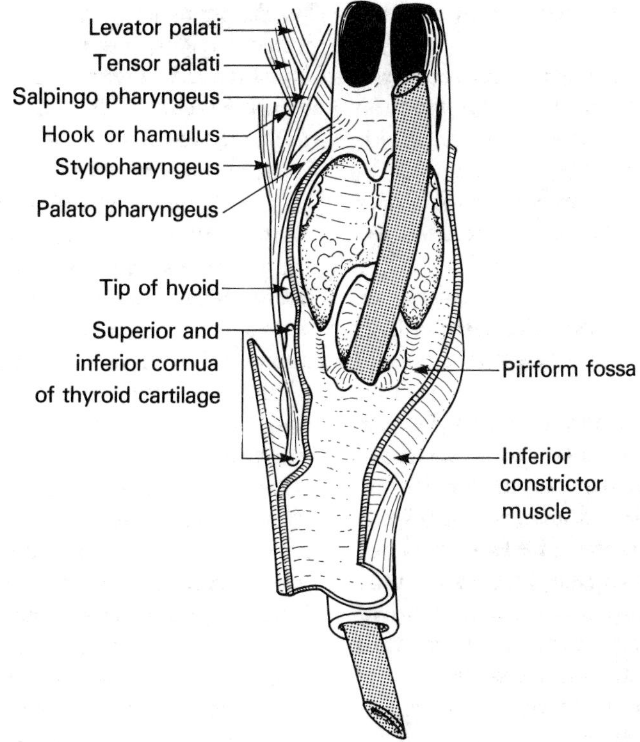

Fig. 1.13 The pharynx seen from behind: intubated.

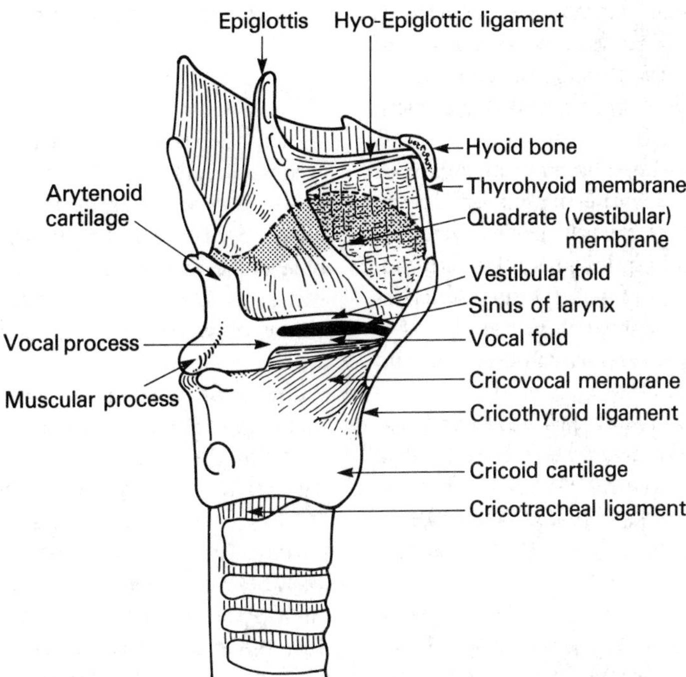

Fig. 1.14 Cartilages and ligaments of the larynx — from the right side.

There are two of these bilateral fibroelastic membranes: the upper one — the vestibular or quadrate membrane — extends between the arytenoid and thyroid cartilages and the epiglottis; its free lower border forms the vestibular fold. The fissure between the right and left folds is termed the rima vestibuli. The free upper border forms the aryepiglottic fold which encircles the almost vertical laryngeal inlet or aditus.

The lower membrane — the cricovocal or cricothyroid membrane — connects the cricoid and arytenoid cartilages to the thyroid cartilage. It is attached anteriorly in the notch of the thyroid cartilage and posteriorly to the tip of the anterior angle (the vocal process) of the arytenoid cartilage. Its free upper border forms the vocal fold. The slit, which becomes a space when the vocal folds are separated, is known as the rima glottidis. This is the narrowest part of the airway in the adult; in the infant, the trachea just below the level of the cricoid is the narrowest part. The lower thin part of the cricovocal membrane is attached to the superior border of the cricoid cartilage.

The vestibule of the larynx lies between the inlet and the rima vestibuli. The intrinsic muscles of the larynx run between attachments to the laryngeal cartilages and membranes. The two aryepiglottic muscles encircling the laryngeal inlet act as a sphincter. The two posterior crico-arytenoid muscles rotate the arytenoid cartilages around a vertical axis and draw them downwards and outwards. The effect of these movements is to separate the vocal folds and thereby widen the rima glottidis. The two actions of the posterior crico-arytenoids are antagonised by the lateral crico-arytenoid and transverse arytenoid muscles respectively: their contractions close the glottis.

There is a mucous membrane lining the larynx. Above, it is continuous with that of the laryngopharynx; it is attached loosely and has a stratified squamous surface. Over the vocal folds the mucous membrane is thin and intimately adherent. Below the folds, the mucous membrane has a ciliated columnar epithelium. Except over the vocal folds the mucous membrane contains many mucous glands.

Laryngeal branches of the superior and inferior thyroid arteries supply the larynx. The veins draining the larynx pass to the internal jugular and brachiocephalic veins. The vocal folds form a watershed for lymphatic drainage. Vessels pass upwards and downwards to join the deep cervical lymph nodes.

The fibres of the vagus nerve are distributed through its superior and recurrent laryngeal branches. These supply all the intrinsic muscles of the larynx with efferent motor impulses from the nucleus ambiguus. If one recurrent laryngeal nerve is partially damaged the vocal fold on the same side moves towards the midline because the paralysis affects mainly the posterior cricothyroid muscle. If the recurrent nerve paralysis is complete the affected vocal fold lies in the neutral (cadaveric) position and there is hoarseness of the voice. With increased adduction of the unaffected vocal fold the rima glottidis again approaches its normal shape and size and so the voice is restored. In bilateral partial paralysis the vocal folds are apposed (due to unopposed action by the adductors) thereby obstructing the airway and causing respiratory stridor or total airway obstruction. Bilateral complete paralysis leads to a valve-like obstruction as a result of the slack vocal folds flapping together. This is accompanied by respiratory stridor and there is also loss of voice because the vocal folds cannot be approximated.

All the somaesthetic impulses from the mucosa of the larynx are also conveyed, as afferents, in the two laryngeal nerves. With their unipolar cells in the superior ganglion of the vagus, the fibres pass to synapse in the caudal part of the spinal nucleus of the trigeminal nerve.

The parasympathetic efferent fibres of the vagus arise from the dorsal nucleus of the vagus. Travelling in the superior and recurrent laryngeal nerves they convey secretor impulses to the glands in the mucous membrane of the larynx. The sympathetic nerves travel along the arteries supplying the larynx. These postganglionic fibres pass to the arteries from the middle cervical ganglion.

The larynx and the succeeding trachea form midline structures in the neck. The vocal folds lie just below the notch of the thyroid cartilage behind the laryngeal prominence (Adam's apple). The upper poles of the thyroid gland are at the sides of the larynx. Posterolateral to the thyroid gland lie the great vessels of the neck. The gland

and the vessels are covered by the infrahyoid muscles and the sternocleidomastoid muscle, the deep cervical fascia, the platysma muscle and skin.

LOWER RESPIRATORY AIRWAY

The lower airway consists of the trachea and bronchi. The trachea is suspended from the cricoid by the cricotracheal ligament. This passes from the lower border of the cricoid to the first ring of the trachea and is continuous below with the fibrous membrane investing the tracheal rings. When the larynx is elevated in deglutition the upper part of the trachea also rises, its fibroelastic wall being stretched. Below, the trachea bifurcates about the level of the sternal angle — the joint between the manubrium and body of the sternum (level with the disc between the 4th and 5th thoracic vertebrae).

The trachea is freely moveable. It is a midline structure except above its bifurcation where it deviates slightly to the right side. It is 10–12 cm long. In deep inspiration, the trachea is lengthened (by 3–5 cm) by the drawing downwards of its bifurcation and the two principal bronchi. In the adult the diameter of the lumen is about 2.5 cm; in the infant the diameter is less than 3 mm.

A number (16–20) of C-shaped rings of hyaline cartilage maintain the patency of the fibroelastic membrane. Posteriorly, the circumference is flattened slightly by the presence of the unstriped trachealis muscle stretching between the ends of each cartilaginous ring. Contraction of this unstriped muscle narrows the lumen of the trachea and prevents its overdistension when the intraluminal pressure is raised, e.g. during abdominal straining. The trachea is lined by respiratory-type mucous membrane. There is a plentiful supply of mucous and serous glands.

Vagal (recurrent) laryngeal and sympathetic nerve fibres supply the trachea. The general somatic afferent fibres of the vagus have their cell bodies in its superior ganglion, and the central processes pass to synapse in the caudal part of the spinal nucleus of the trigeminal nerve. The general visceral afferent impulses are conducted to the nucleus solitarius; the cell bodies of these neurones are in the inferior ganglion of the vagus. Efferent parasympathetic fibres arise from the dorsal nucleus of the vagus to pass in its recurrent laryngeal branch to supply motor impulses to the unstriped trachealis muscle. Other efferent fibres convey secretor impulses to the glands in the lining of the trachea. Vasoconstrictor sympathetic fibres, with their cell bodies in the middle cervical ganglion, pass with the inferior thyroid artery and its branches to reach the trachea.

The inferior thyroid artery is the main arterial supply, although the bronchial arteries also contribute. The trachea is drained by veins emptying either directly into the brachiocephalic veins or indirectly via the inferior thyroid venous plexus. The lymph is drained to the lower deep cervical lymph nodes and to the pre- and paratracheal nodes.

In the neck the trachea lies immediately in front of the oesophagus. The recurrent laryngeal nerve lies in the groove between the two. Posterolateral to the trachea lies the carotid sheath with the thyroid gland intervening. The isthmus of the thyroid gland is anterior and adherent to the 2nd, 3rd and 4th tracheal rings.

In the superior mediastinum, the trachea continues to lie anterior to the oesophagus. In front, the brachiocephalic artery passes obliquely to the right and the left brachiocephalic vein crosses at or above the upper border of the manubrium. The pleural sacs overlap these vessels. On the left of the trachea, lower down, lies the arch of the aorta with the common carotid and subclavian arteries arising from it; on bronchoscopy the pulsation of the aorta is visible. The superior vena cava lies to the right of the trachea. On each side the nearby lung, covered by pleura, envelops the trachea and the structures surrounding it.

The bronchi (Fig. 1.15)

The trachea bifurcates behind the beginning of the arch of the aorta. The deep part of the cardiac plexus of autonomic nerves lies anterior to the bifurcation; below and on each side of the trachea lie tracheobronchial lymph nodes.

At the bifurcation arise the right and left primary (principal, main) bronchi. The right main

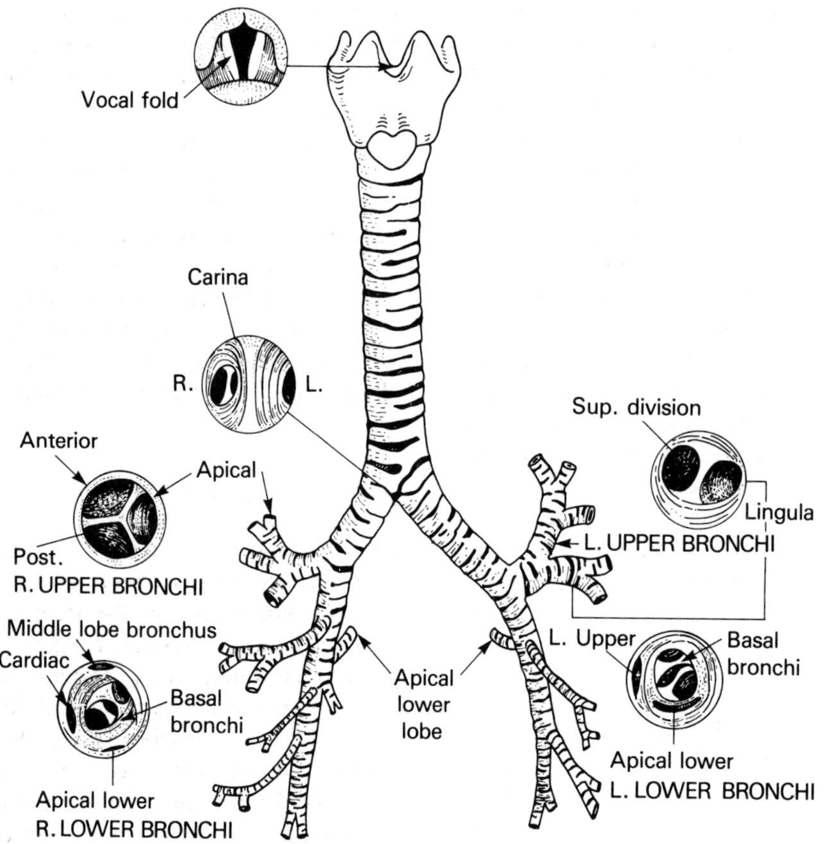

Fig. 1.15 Bronchial tree and views obtained at bronchoscopy.

bronchus continues more nearly in the vertical line of the trachea than does the left; its calibre is larger and its length (4.5 cm) shorter than that of the left (5 cm). The azygos vein arches over the upper aspect of the right bronchus; below initially and then crossing anterior to it is the right pulmonary artery. After the superior lobe (secondary) bronchus branches off, the main bronchus continues downwards for 2 cm, crossing posterior to the pulmonary vessels, to enter the hilum of the lung. There it gives off the middle lobe (secondary) bronchus and continues as the lower lobe (secondary) bronchus. Opposite, or just below, the opening of the middle lobe bronchus, the lower lobe bronchus gives off the apical (superior) bronchus to the upper segment of the lower lobe. The lower lobe bronchus continues for a further 2 cm to give off the other tertiary bronchi to the anterior, posterior, lateral and medial (cardiac) basal segments. The left main bronchus crosses obliquely beneath the arch of the aorta to lie anterior to the oesophagus and descending aorta. The bronchus at first passes behind and then below the left pulmonary artery to enter the hilum of the left lung where it divides into superior and inferior lobe (secondary) bronchi. On the left side, the superior lobe bronchus gives off the lingular bronchus; this is the equivalent of the right middle lobe bronchus. The segmental (tertiary) bronchi to the lower lobe are similar to those on the right except that the left medial (cardiac) basal bronchus, when present, is small and comes off with the anterior basal bronchus (Fig. 1.15).

The tertiary segmental bronchi from each lobar bronchus are given off to supply segments of the lobes. These structural units are known as bronchopulmonary segments; they are numbered, and are named in accordance with the part of the lung in which each lies. Each bronchopulmonary segment has its own bronchovascular supply. Surgically it is possible to develop planes of separation between segments. Thus segmental resections in addition to lobectomy or pneumonectomy may be carried out at operation.

On bronchoscopy the lining of the trachea and bronchi may be seen and the openings of the secondary lobar bronchi can be identified. The trachea appears as a glistening pinkish-red tube with spaced white rings (the underlying cartilages). Above its bifurcation, aortic arch pulsation can be seen anteriorly and on the left. At its bifurcation the carina appears as a sharp sagittal ridge. The right main bronchus separates off from the vertical at about 25° and the left at 45°. By inspection through a bronchoscope and using the figures on the face of a clock the following orifices can be identified at measured distances (average) from the carina.

Right side:
- Upper lobe bronchus: 3 o'clock at 2.5 cm
- Middle lobe bronchus: 12 o'clock at 4.5 cm
- Apical bronchus of lower lobe: 6 o'clock at 4.5 cm

Left side:
- Upper lobe bronchus: 9 o'clock at 5.0 cm
- Lingular bronchus: central at 5.5 cm
- Apical bronchus of lower lobe: 6 o'clock at 6.0 cm

The basic structure of the bronchi is similar to that of the trachea. The bronchi are supplied by bronchial arteries, usually branches from the descending aorta. The veins from the right bronchi drain into the azygos and those on the left enter the left superior hemiazygos vein. The lymphatic vessels of the bronchi drain to nodes at the hilum of the lung and then to the tracheobronchial group.

The pulmonary plexus of nerves supplies the bronchi. This plexus is formed from parasympathetic (vagal) and sympathetic contributions. The pulmonary plexus lies in front of and behind the root of the lung. Networks of nerves pass from the plexus to surround and supply the bronchi. The general visceral afferent fibres of the vagus have their cell bodies in its inferior ganglion; the central processes pass to synapse in the nucleus solitarius. The efferent vagal fibres conveying motor impulses to the unstriped bronchial muscle arise from the dorsal motor nucleus of the vagus. This nucleus also supplies secretor efferent impulses to the glands in the bronchi. The parasympathetic preganglionic branches of the vagus synapse in ganglia on the walls of the bronchi. The sympathetic supply originates from the 2nd to the 5th thoracic segments of the spinal cord. The postganglionic fibres take origin from synapses in the upper four thoracic ganglia.

SPINAL PUNCTURE

The vertebral canal in the vertebral column is triangular in cross-section. There are openings placed symmetrically at the sides through which the spinal nerves emerge. Anteriorly the wall of the canal is formed by the posterior surfaces of the bodies of the vertebrae (covered by periosteum) and of the intervertebral discs. Both these are covered (posteriorly) by the tough posterior longitudinal ligament. This ligament has serrated margins and narrows gradually as it descends. The serrations are widest where they are attached very firmly to the intervertebral discs. In the intervening narrow sections the ligament is attached to the periosteum over the upper and lower parts of the backs of the vertebral bodies. The posterior wall of the vertebral canal is formed by the anterior surfaces of the laminae (lined by periosteum) of the vertebrae and by the intervening ligamenta flava (Fig. 1.16). The latter, consisting mainly of yellow elastic tissue, extend medially from the capsules of the joints between the superior and inferior articular processes. The right and left ligaments meet each other medially, leaving small intervals in the midline for the passage of veins joining the internal and external vertebral venous plexuses. Each ligamentum flavum passes in an almost vertical plane from a ridge on the lower part of the anterior surface of a lamina above to the upper margin and adjoining posterior surface of the lamina below.

The deepest part of the thin interspinous ligament merges with the posterior aspect of the

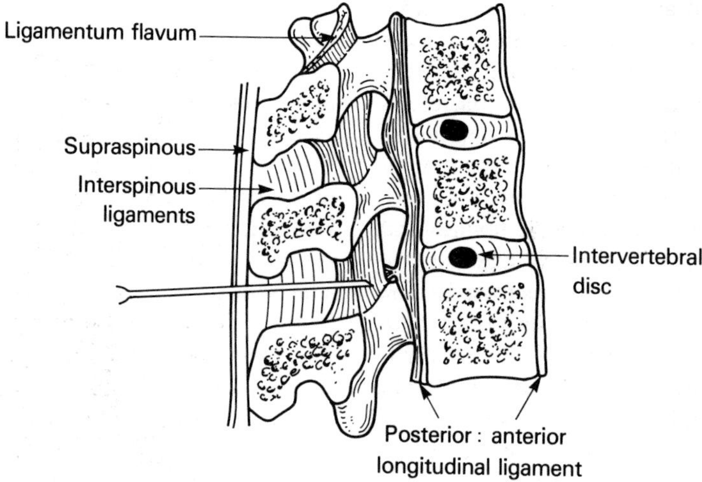

Fig. 1.16 Sagittal section of lumbar spine.

midline meeting of the ligamenta flava. Superficially the interspinous ligaments are continuous with the deep anterior borders of the supraspinous ligaments, which join the tips of the spinous processes. The ligamenta flava and the interspinous ligaments are thickest between the lumbar vertebrae. When opened up by flexion of the spine the space between successive spinous processes and laminae is greatest in the lumbar region.

The wall of the vertebral canal is incomplete at the sides. From the lateral borders of each vertebral body a pedicle projects posteriorly. The pedicles are shorter (in the vertical plane) than the height of the corresponding vertebra; thus an intervertebral foramen is produced between successive pedicles. In the intervertebral foramen lie the spinal nerve and dorsal root ganglion, covered by sleeves of all three meninges, which merge with the epineurium of the spinal nerve immediately lateral to the foramen. Spinal arteries, veins, lymphatics and fat also pass through the intervertebral foramen. Lining the vertebral canal is a layer of extradural fat in which lies the internal vertebral venous plexus.

Within the vertebral canal lies the dura mater, which is formed of dense fibrous tissue. The ensheathing sac of dura contains the spinal cord and nerve roots covered by the leptomeninges. As already indicated the dura mater and leptomeninges extend laterally as sheaths for the dorsal and ventral roots of each spinal nerve. Superiorly the spinal dura mater is a prolongation of the inner, investing layer of the cranial dura. It is attached around the circumference of the foramen magnum. The spinal dura is also attached to the posterior longitudinal ligament and periosteum overlying the backs of the bodies of the second and third cervical vertebrae. This attachment to the posterior longitudinal ligament continues down the length of the dura. By this means, the dural sac is held forwards against the backs of the vertebral bodies and intervertebral discs. Inferiorly the spinal dura mater extends down to the level of the lower border of the second piece of the sacrum where it is closely apposed to and merges with the arachnoid mater. From here it continues, with the arachnoid, as a cover of the filum terminale, which is the connective tissue projection of the pia mater from the apex of the conus medullaris. The filum terminale (after lying centrally in the cauda equina) emerges below the sacral hiatus and passes posterior to the sacrococcygeal joint to be attached to the dorsal aspect of the coccyx.

The arachnoid mater is a thin tubular membrane lining the dural sac. It envelops the spinal cord and nerve roots, which are covered by pia mater. Where it is in close relation to the spinal cord, the arachnoid is joined to the pia mater by delicate strands of connective tissue, the web-like appearance of which gives its name to the membrane. The cerebrospinal fluid is found between the arachnoid and pia mater. The spinal arachnoid and pia maters are continuations at their upper ends of the cranial leptomeninges.

The pia mater forms a very thin, intimate membranous cover to the spinal cord and nerve roots. Blood vessels run on the surface of the pia and pierce it to supply the cord. From right and left sides of the entire length of the spinal cord — from the foramen magnum to the second lumbar vertebra — the covering pia mater forms a fibrous flange midway between the ventral and dorsal nerve roots. This is termed the ligamentum denticulatum. Laterally the border projects with tooth-like processes which pierce the arachnoid to merge with the dura mater. This attachment of the ligamentum denticulatum fixes the spinal cord securely to the dura mater.

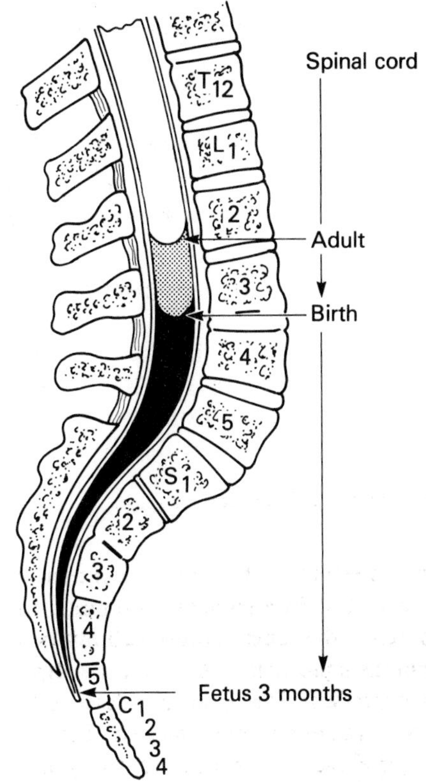

Fig. 1.17 Termination of spinal cord.

The spinal cord and nerves

The spinal cord continues from the medulla oblongata at the level of the foramen magnum. Inferiorly it terminates in a conically shaped apex called the conus medullaris (Fig. 1.17). In adults the termination of the cord varies, lying higher in women than men, commensurate with the shorter length of the trunk. Thus the cord ends, usually, at a level between the upper and lower borders of the second lumbar vertebra. In the neonate the apex of the conus medullaris lies between the 3rd and 4th vertebrae. In the elderly, the cord may descend to terminate at the third lumbar vertebra because of shrinkage of the intervertebral discs.

In the early embryo, the spinal nerves pass transversely through the intervertebral foramina at the same level as their segmental origin from the spinal cord. Because of disproportionate growth, most dorsal and ventral nerve roots pass obliquely downwards from their spinal segment to emerge as spinal nerves through their original, but now lower situated, intervertebral foramina. The obliquity is most marked for the lumbar and sacral nerve roots which are known collectively as the cauda equina. These, with the filum terminale, lie within the subarachnoid space.

The spinal cord is made up of centrally placed grey matter, which consists of nerve cells arranged usually in groups, and of white matter consisting of nerve fibres which, except for those ascending fibres conveying impulses of pain, are myelinated. The fibres are arranged in tracts and convey afferent nervous impulses upwards to the brain (ascending) and efferent impulses downwards from the brain (descending). The cauda equina consists of the centrally placed connective tissue filament called the filum terminale, most of the lumbar and all the sacral, dorsal and ventral nerve roots. These roots convey respectively afferent and efferent nervous impulses. The dorsal and ventral roots are myelinated. The nerve cells of the spinal cord do not regenerate if traumatised. The axons of the ascending and descending nerve fibres are covered by a myelin sheath. This, however, is produced by oligodendrocytes and not by Schwann cells so no regeneration occurs if the fibres are traumatised.

Thus, the spinal cord is held at its sides by its spinal nerves and is also attached laterally throughout its length to the dura matter by the ligamenta denticulata. The dura is attached anteriorly to the posterior longitudinal ligament and to the periosteum covering the backs of the vertebral bodies and the intervertebral discs, particularly the upper cervical ones.

Forward bending of the head and trunk with flexion at the occipito-atlantal joint and at the joints between all the vertebrae draws the spinal cord slightly upwards and forwards in the vertebral canal. This movement ensures that the conus medullaris lies as high as possible in the lumbar part of the dural sac. If lumbar puncture is carried out below the level of the 3rd lumbar spinous process in the adult, or the 4th in the infant, young child or elderly patient, the spinal cord cannot be injured by the needle. Besides ensuring the safety of the cord, full forward flexion stretches the supra- and interspinous ligaments and ligamenta flava and so opens up the spaces between successive spinous processes and laminae of the lumbar and 1st sacral vertebra; this effect is greatest between the 3rd and 4th lumbar spines. This allows the anaesthetist more room for manipulation of the needle at lumbar puncture.

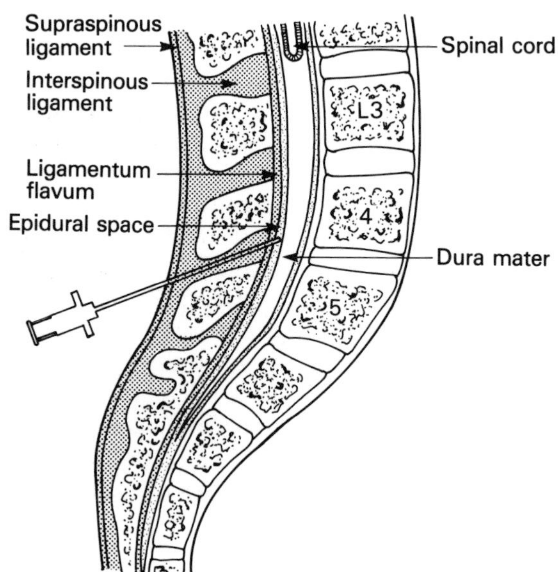

Fig. 1.18 Lower part of spinal cord and meninges.

The meningeal spaces

A number of spaces, actual or potential, exist within the vertebral canal. From without inwards they are:

1. The *extradural, epidural or peridural space*, which extends for the whole length of the spinal dura mater. It is closed superiorly at the foramen magnum. Inferiorly it opens into the cavity of the sacral part of the vertebral canal (Fig. 1.18). This cavity has a fluid capacity of approximately 25 ml. The extradural space lies between the inner surface of the vertebral canal and the outer surface of the dural sac. It is deepest posteriorly where the laminae and ligamenta flava meet in the midline; this feature is most marked in the lumbosacral part of the spine.

The extradural space contains loose fat and a plexus of veins. The fatty areolar tissue extends laterally for a short distance through the intervertebral foramen, surrounding the spinal nerve in its covering. The veins, which are valveless, form the internal vertebral venous plexus. Basivertebral veins, emerging from foramina in the middle of the backs of the vertebral bodies, join this plexus which is formed of two anterior and two posterior longitudinally running veins. These are joined, opposite each vertebra, by a series of venous rings encircling the dural sac; these transversely-running veins can be entered by a needle during lumbar puncture as they pass posterior to the dura. The plexus receives tributaries from the spinal cord and surrounding bones. It communicates, through the intervertebral foramina, with veins running the length of the vertebral column. Fluid injected into the sacral (Figs. 1.19 and 1.20) or lumbar parts of the extradural space may spread superiorly to the foramen magnum and laterally through the intervertebral foramina.

In the thoracic part of the spine the extension of the extradural space through the intervertebral foramina subjects it to pressures present in the thorax (Fig. 1.21). Any sustained or sudden increase of intrathoracic pressure produces a positive pressure within the extradural space. Deep inspiration lowers still further the negative, subatmospheric intrathoracic pressure transmitted to the extradural space. Pressure changes are most marked in the thoracic part of the extradural space, but extend down to the lumbar region.

2. The *subdural space* is a potential space lying

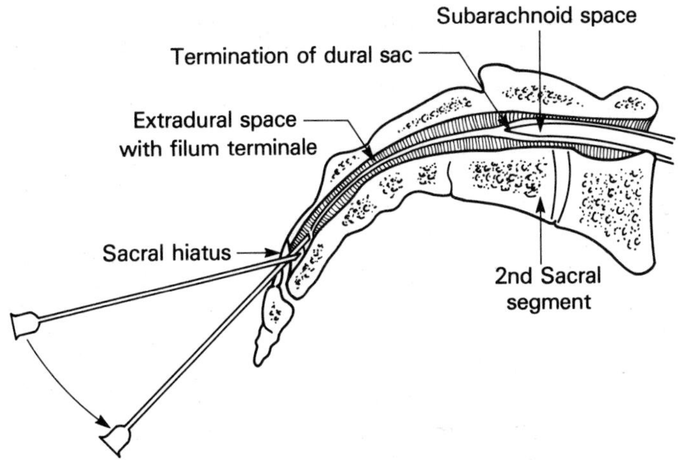

Fig. 1.19 Sacral part of extradural space.

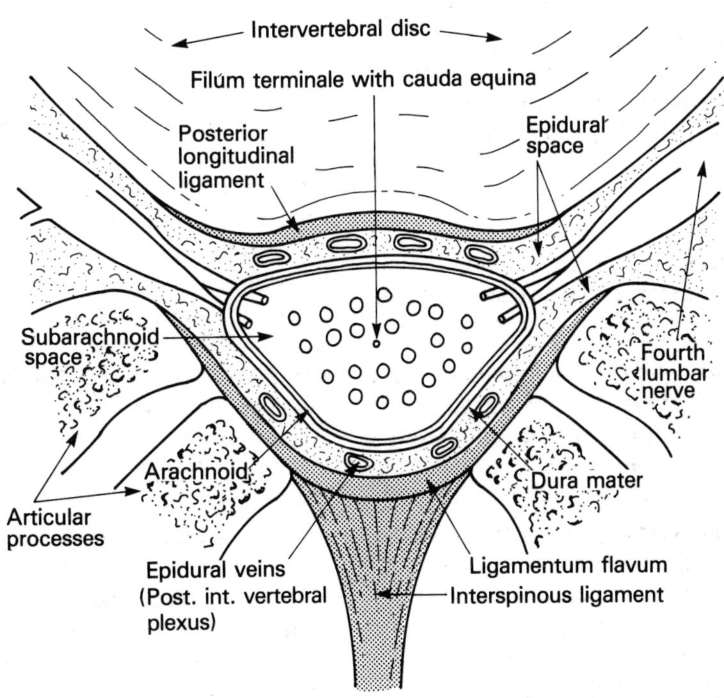

Fig. 1.20 Cross-section of vertebral canal.

between the dura and arachnoid maters. Between the surfaces of these membranes there are capillary and lymphatic vessels for the supply and drainage of the dura mater and extradural fat. Above, the space is in continuity with that between the cranial dura and arachnoid. At the sides, between these meninges, it extends to the intervertebral foramina. Below, it terminates

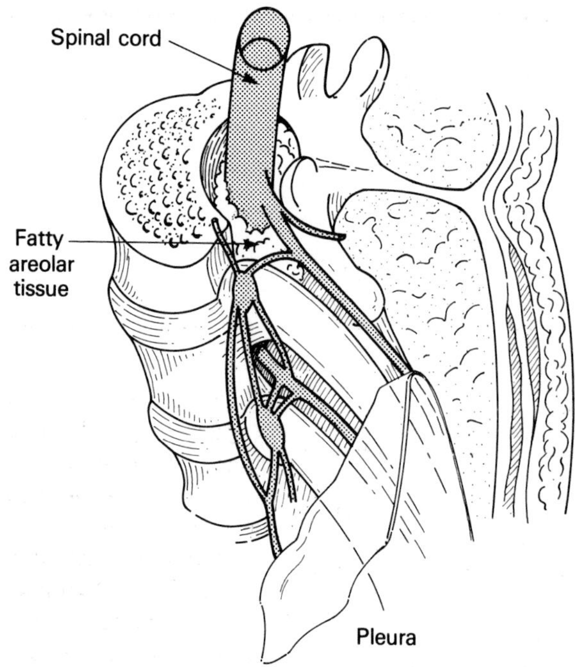

Fig. 1.21 Extrapleural extension of extradural space. The parietal pleura has been reflected to show the underlying structures.

where the dura and arachnoid fuse at the level of the 2nd sacral vertebra.

3. The *subarachnoid space* lies between the arachnoid mater, lining the dural sac, and the pia mater covering the spinal cord. It contains the cerebrospinal fluid. Superiorly the space is directly continuous with that around the brain. Laterally the fluid in the space extends to the intervertebral foramina surrounding the dorsal and ventral nerve roots of each spinal nerve (Fig. 1.20). Inferiorly the spinal subarachnoid space is larger than elsewhere. Here it contains the spinal cord, as the latter narrows towards its terminal conus medullaris, and the cauda equina. The space terminates below at the level of the second sacral vertebra, where the tube of arachnoid mater fuses with the inner surface of the lower limit of the dural sac (Fig. 1.19).

FURTHER READING

Brock R C 1952 Lung abscess, 2nd end. Blackwell Scientific Publications, Oxford

Ellis H, Feldman S 1988 Anatomy for anaesthetists, 5th edn. Blackwell Scientific Publications, Oxford

Last R J 1984 Anatomy — regional and applied, 7th edn. Churchill Livingstone, Edinburgh

Macintosh R, Lee J A 1985 Lumbar puncture and spinal analgesia, 5th edn. Churchill Livingstone, Edinburgh

Warwick R, Williams P L 1980 Gray's anatomy, 36th edn. Longman, Edinburgh

2. Respiratory physiology

CONTROL OF VENTILATION

The function of respiration is to convey oxygen to the cells and to remove the metabolic product, carbon dioxide. The principal control of ventilation resides in centres in the brain stem, and the activity of the respiratory centre is modified by central and peripheral receptors to permit adequate pulmonary gas exchange. Other reflexes arising from receptors in the lung and respiratory tract modify the pattern of ventilation.

Central control of ventilation

It is known that the essential areas involved in the control of respiration lie in the brain stem, since transection above this level leaves the respiratory rhythm intact. Microelectrode recordings suggest that the main respiratory nuclei lie bilaterally in the medulla. Three main groups have been identified:

1. Located in close proximity to the nucleus retroambigualis in the ventrolateral medulla are neurones which discharge during inspiration, expiration, and early in the inspiratory phase. These are upper motor neurones supplying the contralateral intercostal muscles. The inspiratory neurones inhibit those of expiration but reverse inhibition has not been shown.
2. A second group lies bilaterally in the dorsal medulla close to the nucleus solitarius. Two types of inspiratory activity have been noted, one of which parallels phrenic nerve discharge, and the other, lung inflation.
3. The third group is the nucleus ambiguus which contains the upper motor neurone cells of the glossopharyngeal and vagus nerves.

Experimental transection of the midpons produces deep breathing with a short expiratory phase; if, in addition, the vagi are cut, breathing is held in inspiration. This sustained gasp is termed apneusis. It is clear therefore that rhythmic ventilation is dependent on the upper pons. This rhythmicity is located in nucleus parabrachialis medialis (NPBM) which was previously known as the pneumotactic centre. Stimulation of dorsal NPBM shortens the phase (inspiration or expiration) during which it is applied; stimulation of the ventral portion shortens inspiration.

Although the evidence suggests that NPBM is essential for rhythmic ventilation, it appears that respiratory rhythm is not generated here. Indeed it has not been possible to locate a 'pacemaker cell', i.e. a rhythmically discharging neurone in phase with respiration but with no synaptic input. Recent hypotheses have suggested that the interconnections of the respiratory neurones may produce an unstable circuit which causes respiratory oscillations.

The effect of ventilation is to modify the O_2 and CO_2 tensions of arterial blood. Alterations in the levels of these variables stimulate chemoreceptors which, in turn, relay the information centrally and thereby modify ventilation. The preservation of normal Pa_{O_2} depends on peripheral chemoreceptors which respond to hypoxaemia whereas hypercapnia stimulates primarily brain stem receptors.

Peripheral chemoreceptors

The carotid bodies lie close to the carotid sinus, and the aortic bodies are grouped around the aortic arch. They consist of two types of specialised cell in extremely vascular tissue. The glomus cells (type 1 cells) are innervated by afferent fibres which convey centrally information on variations in blood gas tensions. A linear relationship has been noted between peripheral chemoreceptor discharge and CO_2 tension in arterial blood, but it is uncertain if the response is caused by a direct action of CO_2 or hydrogen ion (H^+) concentration. Receptor response has a hyperbolic relationship with Pa_{O_2}. The chemoreceptor response to both hypoxaemia and hypercapnia is not additive but multiplicative.

Type 2 cells and their processes surround the type 1 cells but have no known function.

Central chemoreceptors

Areas sensitive to changes in P_{CO_2} are located on the ventrolateral surface of the medulla, close to the site of emergence of cranial nerves VII–X. These areas are bathed in cerebrospinal fluid (CSF). A further area lateral to cranial nerve XII has a pH-dependent frequency of discharge. The final stimulus may be the extracellular H^+ concentration close to the receptor but, as its level varies with P_{CO_2} in both blood and CSF, P_{CO_2} is usually considered to be the stimulus.

Chemoreceptor effects

As the arterial oxygen tension decreases, ventilation shows little change until a level below 8 kPa is reached. The relationship between Pa_{O_2} and ventilation is exponential. Above a Pa_{O_2} of 8 kPa there is little response to steady state changes but increased ventilation has been noted with transient changes in oxygen tension.

Ventilation increases linearly as Pa_{CO_2} increases above 5 kPa; the slope is increased by hypoxaemia.

In summary, P_{CO_2} (or H^+ concentration) stimulates peripheral and central chemoreceptors; hypoxaemia stimulates the peripheral chemoreceptors but depresses the central chemoreceptors as a result of central hypoxia. The resultant effect of chemoreceptor activity is an increase in both the rate and depth of ventilation.

Modified chemoreceptive response

In some conditions, including chronic lung disease and exposure to high altitudes, abnormal responses are obtained from the chemoreceptors.

1. *High altitude*. At high altitude, the reduced atmospheric pressure results in a reduction in inspired, and thus arterial, oxygen tension. Unacclimatised subjects respond to hypoxaemia by hyperventilation, thus reducing Pa_{CO_2}. Acclimatisation results in a decrease in CSF [HCO_3^-] which lowers CSF pH at a given carbon dioxide tension, thereby increasing sensitivity to P_{CO_2}. However, this explanation is probably too simplistic, as the increase in ventilation is retained despite a progressive diminution in the response to hypoxaemia in subjects who have lived at high altitudes for many years.

2. *Chronic lung disease*. In chronic obstructive lung disease there is a reduced response to hypercapnia in 'blue bloater' patients in addition to that caused by mechanical factors. In contrast, 'pink puffers' retain their ability to respond to hypercapnia and hypoxaemia in the face of distressing effort.

Other lung receptors

1. *Airway stretch receptors* at the dorsal ends of the tracheal and bronchial rings are responsible for the Hering-Breuer reflex which, when elicited, terminates inspiration and prolongs expiration. The reflex is excited by inflation of the lungs. It is present in man but appears to vary in intensity from subject to subject. It is difficult to detect in anaesthetised man.

2. *Epithelial receptors* in the larynx and trachea cause coughing, laryngospasm and bronchospasm when stimulated. Stimulation of those in the bronchi causes hyperventilation in addition, and may be partially responsible for asthma.

3. *J receptors* in the alveolar wall close to the pulmonary capillary appear to respond to the presence of alveolar interstitial fluid. In pulmonary congestion and oedema, rapid shallow breathing and laryngeal constriction occur.

MECHANICS OF VENTILATION

The respiratory muscles perform the work of respiration. The most important muscle is the diaphragm which is assisted by the intercostal and abdominal muscles. The work of ventilation overcomes:

1. The elastic resistance of the tissues; work is proportional to the tidal volume;
2. The frictional resistance of the airways and viscous resistance of the tissues; work varies with gas flow;
3. The inertial resistance of the airways and tissues; work is related to the acceleration of the inflowing gas.

An indication of the amount of work required to overcome the elastic forces is given by the compliance. This is defined as the change in the volume of air in the chest for each kPa change of transthoracic pressure:

$$\text{Compliance } (C) = \Delta V/\Delta P$$

where ΔV is the change in volume of the thorax and ΔP is the change in transthoracic pressure.

The dynamic resistance to ventilation is produced by (2) and (3) above; however, the increased work required to overcome inertial resistance is generally ignored as being too small. The contribution of viscous resistance of the tissues is relatively small (20–30%) and relatively constant. The frictional resistance of the airways is more important and more variable, and is regarded generally as representing non-elastic resistance (P/rate of volume change [litre/s] where P is the transthoracic pressure).

Compliance

The compliance of the respiratory system comprises that of the conducting airways and that of the thorax and lungs.

The compliance of the respiratory airway

Any increase in tidal volume contributes to an increase in the inefficiency of respiratory exchange (respiratory deadspace). A figure of 0.02–0.04 litre/kPa has been suggested for airway compliance, most of which resides in the intrathoracic portion of the airways.

Compliance of the thorax

Both chest wall and lungs have elastic properties which interact to provide an overall value for total thoracic compliance. When a subject is relaxed at the end of a normal expiration, the retractive forces of the lung and the chest wall are in equilibrium. If both were allowed to find their own equilibrium in isolation the lung would contract and the chest expand, as occurs when the chest is opened. At the end of normal expiration in a relaxed subject, the volume of air in the lung is called the functional residual capacity (FRC). The values for FRC in the average man are 2900 ml when seated and 2100 ml when supine. Variables which alter lung compliance also alter FRC.

Lung compliance (C_L). This can be estimated by measuring the change in lung volume which occurs with a unit change of pressure across the lung wall (transmural pressure), i.e. the pressure difference between the alveolar space and the intrapleural space. This is performed when a steady state exists and is called the '*static lung compliance*'. In Figure 2.1 the relationship can be seen to be curvilinear, the radii of curvature being greater at lung volumes below FRC and close to total lung capacity; however, in the midrange, a constant value can be used as an approximation for lung compliance.

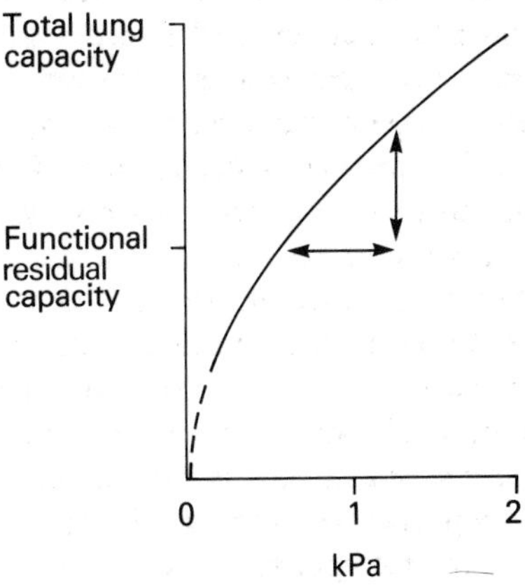

Fig. 2.1 Change in lung volume with change in transmural pressure.

Technically it is difficult to measure intrapleural pressure as the pleural space is only a potential space. It is customary to measure this pressure in the oesophagus using a balloon. In the erect subject, a 10 cm balloon is passed into the middle third of the oesophagus. In the supine position the weight of the mediastinal contents may cause the pressure recorded to be erroneously high and adjustment of the site of the balloon may be necessary.

The elastic retractive forces of the lung are caused by the elastic fibres of the lung parenchyma and the surface tension of the liquid/air interface in the alveoli. Indeed, approximately 50% of the elastic recoil is attributable to the elasticity of the parenchyma and approximately 50% to the surface tension forces.

This knowledge, however, is difficult to reconcile with the increase in surface tension which might be expected in alveoli which are diminishing in size during expiration if, as is generally assumed, alveoli mimic bubbles in their physical properties.

By Laplace's equation, the pressure P within a bubble (pascals) varies directly with surface tension T (mN/m) and indirectly with the radius of curvature r (mm) in the following manner:

$$P = \frac{2T}{r} \qquad (1)$$

As the radius of curvature of the alveolus falls, the pressure inside the alveolus rises; the small alveoli, having higher pressures, would empty into the larger alveoli, rendering the forces within the lung unstable. This does not occur in the lung because in the fluid lining of the alveoli there are surface-active substances called surfactant. These substances consist of phospholipids which are secreted by cuboidal cells with large nuclei at the junctions of septa (type II alveolar cells). As the alveolus decreases in size, the surface film becomes concentrated and the surface tension decreases to approximately 10 mN/m; as the alveolus increases in size, the surface tension rises to approximately 30–40 mN/m.

Lung compliance in the conscious erect average man is approximately 2 litre/kPa, and 1.5 litre/kPa in the supine position.

The compliance of the chest wall (C_{CW}). This is difficult to assess because of the activity of the respiratory muscles. It may be calculated theoretically by noting the change in lung volume which occurs during a unit change in the atmospheric–intrapleural pressure difference. This is complicated by the inevitable participation of the respiratory muscles in the conscious subject; if the measurement is conducted under anaesthesia, that in itself may bias the calculation. A value of 2 litre/kPa is usually suggested in the supine position but this may increase by 30% in the seated subject.

Total thoracic compliance (C_T). This is calculated from the change in lung volume which occurs with a unit change in the alveolar/ambient pressure gradient. An approximate value for an average man is 0.85 litre/kPa. Total thoracic compliance can be measured in conscious subjects only if they are trained to relax; therefore it is usually measured in paralysed anaesthetised subjects. (This is true also of chest wall compliance.)

The total compliance of the thorax is related to the other compliances as below:

$$\frac{1}{C_T} = \frac{1}{C_L} + \frac{1}{C_{CW}} \qquad (2)$$

Hysteresis. Elastic bodies exhibit a phenomenon termed hysteresis. This can be demonstrated in the lung. If lung volume above FRC is plotted during inflation against transmural pressure under static conditions, a curve is obtained. The relationship approximates to that of a straight line. However, if the process is repeated during deflation, the inflated lung shows a reluctance to deflate, i.e. the elastic retraction is smaller than expected, and the compliance is greater than expected (Fig. 2.2). This is caused mainly by changes in the surface tension forces and is more marked at the extremes of lung volume.

Static and dynamic compliance

The above discussion has been confined to static compliance which is an entity of importance in a basic scientific discipline such as physiology because it is an estimate of the elastic retractive

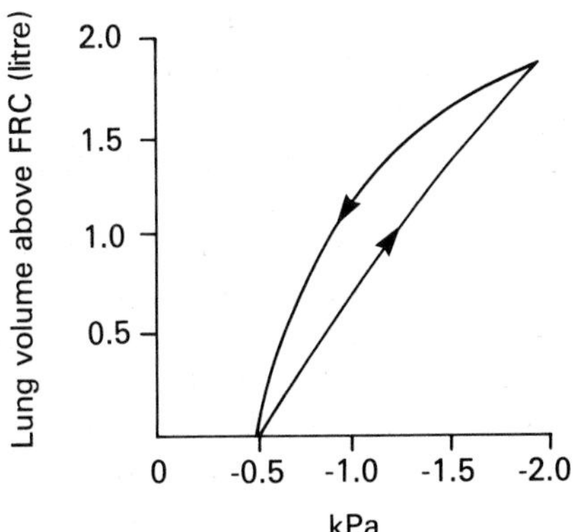

Fig. 2.2 Hysteresis in the lung demonstrated by a comparison of static compliances during inflation and deflation.

forces of the lung. The inflow of air is sufficiently slow to allow the redistribution of gas to be complete.

In a practical discipline such as anaesthesia, a different concept is more relevant. This is dynamic compliance which measures compliance when redistribution of gases *within* the lung is still taking place although the exchange of flow with the environment is zero. This is the situation which occurs at the end of inspiration and expiration in spontaneously breathing man.

The distribution of air within the lung is dependent only on the compliance of the alveoli when static compliance is measured, whereas the resistance to gas flow within regional airways influences dynamic compliance.

In Figure 2.3 the part of the lung with a low resistance to air flow and a low compliance fills rapidly and is termed a 'fast' alveolus; the part of the lung with a high resistance and a high compliance fills much more slowly and is termed a 'slow' alveolus. In this situation dynamic compliance is smaller than static compliance because the high airway resistance prevents complete filling of the high-compliance alveolus in the time available for the measurement of dynamic compliance. If a patient with chronic obstructive lung disease is anaesthetised, it might be observed that the lungs are 'uncompliant' on controlling ventilation. The dynamic compliance is reduced because of severe airways resistance but static compliance may be raised because of destruction of the lung septa.

Factors which influence compliance

1. *Body size.* Lung compliance varies with body surface area, height, weight, vital capacity, functional residual capacity and residual volume — all of which are related to body size. In order to make experimental data more widely applicable, specific compliance (lung compliance/FRC) is often calculated.

2. *Posture.* When the erect patient lies down, compliance decreases but specific compliance is unaltered.

3. *The volume history of the lungs.* A progressive decrease in lung compliance (of between 23% and 33%) has been recorded during quiet breathing. Deep breaths restore compliance to normal levels. This effect has been attributed to changes in alveolar configuration.

4. *Pulmonary blood volume.* A reduction in pulmonary blood volume, as may occur during IPPV, increases compliance.

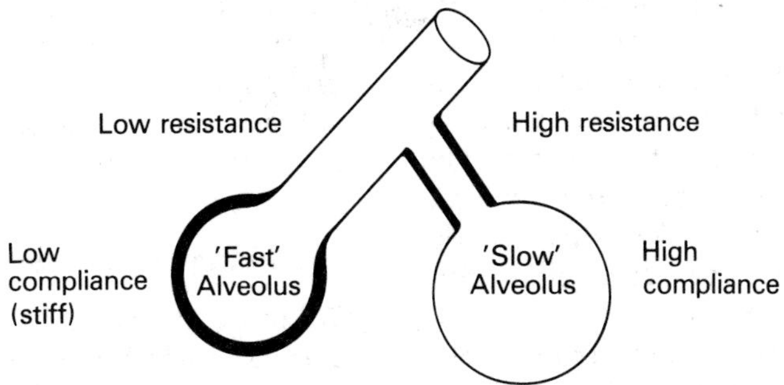

Fig. 2.3 Illustration of differential filling of alveoli in respiratory disease.

5. *100% oxygen at low tidal volume.* Lung compliance diminishes after breathing 100% oxygen for 2 min. This is not observed when air is breathed.

6. *Severe pulmonary disease.* Decreases in dynamic lung compliance have been recorded in chronic obstructive lung disease.

7. *Age.* There is little evidence that compliance or FRC varies with age.

The effect of anaesthesia on compliance

1. *Premedicant drugs.* Morphine has little effect on compliance. Anticholinergic drugs increase the compliance of the airways but little is known of their effect on lung parenchyma.

2. *General anaesthesia.* Dynamic lung compliance is reduced markedly after induction of anaesthesia and the institution of artificial ventilation. It is uncertain if this change is caused by anaesthesia alone or by anaesthesia and artificial ventilation because it is difficult to determine compliance in the spontaneously ventilating subject. A marked reduction in FRC has been recorded during anaesthesia (approximately 20%); a decrease in lung compliance seems the most likely explanation. There is little evidence that compliance falls progressively with time so the greater part of the decrease must occur in the first few minutes of anaesthesia. Hyperinflation or a 'sigh' during ventilation raises compliance briefly, probably by temporarily reducing pulmonary blood volume.

Closing capacity

The lung volume present after a maximum expiration is called residual volume (RV). At this minimum lung volume, there is a reduction in size of the airways and some airways in the lower lung regions close off. The closing capacity (CC) is the lung volume at which this closure is first recorded using a marker gas expirogram. A bolus of marker gas such as helium or xenon-133 is inspired at residual volume and the subject continues to inspire until the maximum lung volume (total lung capacity, TLC) is reached. The marker bolus is distributed preferentially to the upper lung regions because many of the airways in lower lung regions are closed at lung volumes approximating to residual volume. The trace shown in Figure 2.4

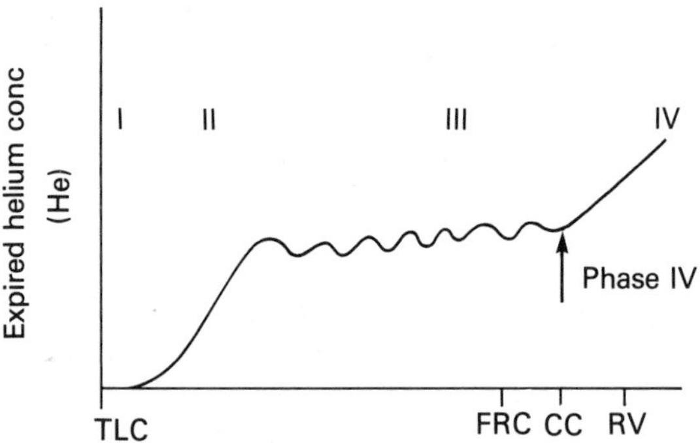

Fig. 2.4 Estimation of closing volume. A slow expiration has taken place after inhalation of a bolus of helium at residual volume. The arrow marks the start of phase IV.

may be divided into four phases: phase I has no marker gas as it consists of expired deadspace; phase II exhibits an increase in marker gas to a plateau; phase III is a plateau; phase IV shows a discrete increase close to residual volume. Phase III represents a mixture of gas from the upper lung areas (containing marker gas) and of gas from the lower lung areas (free of marker gas). When the airways of the lower lung areas close as residual volume is approached, expired gas empties predominantly from the upper lung areas and the concentration of marker gas rises. Closing capacity is the lung volume at which phase IV starts.

Closing capacity increases with age but is independent of body position. Its relationship to FRC is of great importance; if it exceeds FRC, there is some lower airway closure during tidal respiration. Under these circumstances, impaired oxygenation of blood takes place in the part of the lung where airway closure has occurred. Closing capacity in the supine position reaches FRC soon after 40 years of age; in the erect position it reaches FRC at approximately 60 years of age. As a considerable reduction in FRC has been recorded during anaesthesia, it is likely that the closing capacity exceeds FRC and impairs oxygenation during anaesthesia even in younger subjects.

Airway resistance

During inspiration in the spontaneously breathing subject, the chest wall and the lung expand. This causes a reduction in transthoracic pressure (P)

which enables the inspired air to overcome the elastic and resistive forces. It can be stated in the following simplified equation that:

$$\Delta P = \left(\underset{\text{(elastic)}}{\frac{V_T}{C}} + \underset{\text{(resistive)}}{R\dot{V}}\right) \times K \qquad (3)$$

where P is the applied pressure; C is compliance; V_T is tidal volume; $\dot{V}$ is flow rate; R is resistance; and K is a constant.

The resistance to airflow in the spontaneously breathing normal adult man is 0.05–0.2 kPa $\text{litre}^{-1}\,\text{s}^{-1}$, the value varying with the tracheobronchial anatomy and the type of gas flow.

The precise relationship between pressure and flow, i.e. the resistance to flow, is dependent on the type of flow — laminar, transitional or turbulent. Calculations of resistance assume that the flow is occurring in straight, smooth, cylindrical tubes which is patently not true when considering the tracheobronchial tree.

Flow characteristics

Laminar flow describes the movement of gas down straight tubes with a parabolic profile and is the most efficient system of moving gas. The relationship of the pressure decrease (ΔP) across the tube is expressed by the Hagen–Poiseuille law.

$$\Delta P = \frac{8\eta l\dot{V}}{\pi r^4} \qquad (4)$$

where r is the radius of the tube; l the length of the tube; $\dot{V}$ the flow rate; and η the viscosity of the gas.

As resistance is equal to $\Delta P/\dot{V}$, it also equals $8\eta l/\pi r^4$. If flow is turbulent, a much greater applied pressure is required, i.e. the resistance is greater. The possibility of turbulent flow occurring may be estimated by calculating Reynolds' number (Re).

$$\text{Re} = \frac{v\rho r}{\eta} \qquad (5)$$

where v is the linear velocity; r is the tube diameter and ρ is the gas density. If the tube diameter is large and the linear velocity high — as might be expected in the trachea — turbulent flow is more likely to occur. In turbulent flow the resistance to flow is greater than that with laminar flow and is increased more rapidly with increase of flow.

Cooper has suggested that if Reynolds' number is less than 1000, laminar flow is present in the tracheobronchial tree; if Reynolds' number exceeds 1500, flow is turbulent.

In the lung, Reynolds' number is likely to exceed its critical value in the trachea and larynx only during rapid ventilation; nonetheless the assumption that laminar flow is present is invalid because of the vortices which occur in the inspired air at each division of the bronchial tree.

As resistance to flow varies with both the flow rate and the flow characteristics, citing a value for airway resistance at one flow rate is of little value. A German physiologist Röhrer suggested an equation for use during transitional flow:

$$\Delta P = \underset{\substack{\text{laminar}\\\text{component}}}{k_1\dot{V}} + \underset{\substack{\text{turbulent}\\\text{component}}}{k_2(\dot{V})^2} \qquad (6)$$

where ΔP is the pressure decrease, $\dot{V}$ is the flow rate, k_1 is the constant for laminar flow and k_2 the constant for turbulent flow.

A more recent modification by Cooper enables a good approximation to be made in an expression of one term:

$$\Delta P = 2.4(\dot{V})^{1.3} \qquad (7)$$

which differs by less than 10% from equation (6) for flow rates between 0.2 and 3.0 litre/s.

Theoretical calculations suggest that the major part of the resistance resides in the larger airways and that resistance diminishes dramatically in the small airways (less than 2 mm internal diameter, i.e. generations 12–23 in the Weibel classification) to virtually zero in generations 18–23 in the Weibel nomenclature. Thus, even severe damage in very small airways may not be reflected in tests of airway resistance.

Factors which influence airway resistance

The upper airways make the greatest contribution to airway resistance. Therefore obstruction of the upper air passages by inhalation of foreign bodies, swelling or oedema of the mucosa caused by inflammation or neoplasm, or external pressure on the trachea increase airway resistance.

The lower airways (those less than 2 mm internal diameter) are the cause of increased resistance in chronic obstructive lung disease, e.g. chronic bronchitis and emphysema, and in acute disease, e.g. bronchial asthma. During spontaneous breathing in the normal subject, the pressure within the airways is greater than the intrapleural pressure throughout expiration. During active expiration, the intrapleural pressure may increase sufficiently to overcome the elastic recoil of the airway. This results in small airway collapse and air trapping distal to the closure. In chronic bronchitis and emphysema the loss of lung tissue reduces the elastic recoil and increases the likelihood of air trapping.

Airway closure may occur also in acute asthma because increased muscular activity and mucosal oedema may narrow the lumina of the bronchioles and predispose to airway closure during active expiration.

Moving from the erect to the supine position causes the functional residual capacity to diminish by almost 1 litre. This decrease in lung volume reduces airway diameter, thereby increasing airway resistance.

THE EFFECT OF ANAESTHESIA ON AIRWAY RESISTANCE

Premedicant drugs. Morphine may cause bronchial constriction by release of histamine. Anticholinergic drugs, e.g. atropine, increase anatomical deadspace by bronchodilation, and decrease airway resistance.

General anaesthesia. Airway resistance is markedly increased during anaesthesia. Much of this increase is produced by the tracheal tube and its connections, which have a resistance of 0.4–0.6 kPa $\text{litre}^{-1}\ \text{s}^{-1}$.

A more recently recognised factor is the decrease in functional residual capacity of approximately 20% after induction of anaesthesia. This may reduce the diameter of airways in the lung and thereby increases airway resistance. Healthy anaesthetised patients have an airway resistance of 0.3–0.6 kPa $\text{litre}^{-1}\ \text{s}^{-1}$. When the trachea is intubated, the resistance increases to 1 kPa $\text{litre}^{-1}\ \text{s}^{-1}$.

Some anaesthetic induction agents, including thiopentone, may cause bronchoconstriction. The belief that *d*-tubocurarine causes bronchoconstriction has not been substantiated.

THE INEFFICIENCY OF RESPIRATORY GAS EXCHANGE

Under normal circumstances the respiratory muscles ensure that an adequate volume of air reaches the lungs so that sufficient oxygen is supplied to, and carbon dioxide removed from, the pulmonary capillary circulation. An increase in metabolic rate is met by increased work of the respiratory muscles and heart.

The airways of the respiratory system branch repeatedly before ultimately reaching the alveoli. The Swiss anatomist Weibel counted 23 generations of airways. The airways situated immediately before those which take part in respiratory exchange are termed the terminal bronchioles. Generations 17 to 23 take part in respiratory exchange. The inspiratory gases pass by bulk flow to the end of the terminal bronchioles and then by rapid gaseous diffusion over the remaining small distance.

Factors which increase inefficiency include:

1. *Respiratory deadspace.* The respiratory system is inherently inefficient because the respiratory gases enter and leave the lungs via a common pathway as far as the terminal bronchioles. This is termed the anatomical deadspace. A proportion (usually 70%) of the tidal volume enters the alveoli and takes part in respiratory exchange. If some of these alveoli are no longer perfused — after, for example, a pulmonary embolus — an increased portion of the tidal volume is wasted. This results in hypercapnia unless the central drive increases ventilation. The magnitude of the compensatory increase reflects the extent of the inefficiency.

2. *Shunt.* A portion of the cardiac output passing from the right ventricle to the systemic circulation does not come into contact with alveolar gas, and is said to be shunted (anatomical shunt). Anatomical shunt results from Thebesian and bronchial venous blood flow in the normal subject but shunt may be increased in pathological conditions including lung collapse and cardiac conditions with right-to-left shunting. It amounts

to approximately 5% of cardiac output in normal awake man.

3. *Ventilation/perfusion ratio* ($\dot{V}_A/\dot{Q}_c$) *inequality.* The greater part of the lungs is both ventilated and perfused. However, some factors, e.g. gravity, affect the distribution of both ventilation and perfusion, causing some areas to be underventilated (low $\dot{V}_A/\dot{Q}_c$) and other areas to be overventilated (high $\dot{V}_A/\dot{Q}_c$). The overall effect is to increase hypoxaemia and hypercapnia.

4. *Diffusion.* If molecules of respiratory gases are impeded whilst diffusing from the alveoli across the alveolar capillary membrane to the capillary blood, the efficiency of respiratory gas exchange decreases.

5. *Hypoventilation.* Hypoventilation results from an inadequate response of the respiratory system to metabolic demands, and causes hypercapnia and hypoxaemia. It may result from muscular weakness or inadequate respiratory drive.

Some of these factors are considered in greater detail below.

Respiratory deadspace

A major concern in the care of anaesthetised patients, and of patients in the intensive therapy unit, is to ensure that both ventilatory exchange in the lungs and the transport of respiratory gases by the circulation are sufficient for the needs of the patient. As some overall index of the efficiency of respiratory gas exchange is necessary, Enghoff modified Bohr's deadspace equation so that the portion of ventilation not taking part in cardiorespiratory gas exchange, i.e. wasted ventilation, can be calculated. This is termed physiological deadspace ($V_{D,PHYS}$).

Bohr–Enghoff equation

$$V_{D,PHYS} = V_T \frac{(Pa_{CO_2} - P\bar{E}_{CO_2})}{(Pa_{CO_2} - PI_{CO_2})} \qquad (8)$$

where V_T is tidal volume; Pa_{CO_2} is arterial CO_2 tension; $P\bar{E}_{CO_2}$ is mean expired CO_2 tension and PI_{CO_2} is inspired CO_2 tension.

If the inspired CO_2 concentration is negligible and $V_{D,PHYS}$ is expressed as a proportion of tidal volume,

$$\frac{V_{D,PHYS}}{V_T} = 1 - \frac{P\bar{E}_{CO_2}}{Pa_{CO_2}} \qquad (9)$$

Physiological deadspace is increased in respiratory disease and during anaesthesia. It is the sum of anatomical and alveolar deadspaces.

Anatomical deadspace ($V_{D,ANAT}$) is a term used to describe the conducting airways of the respiratory tract which do not take part in respiratory gas exchange. In normal subjects, in whom alveolar deadspace is very small, anatomical deadspace and physiological deadspace approach the same value. It can be measured planimetrically using Fowler's method of plotting nitrogen concentration against expired volume after inhaling a breath of pure oxygen.

Alveolar deadspace ($V_{D,ALV}$), which cannot be measured directly, results from ventilated but unperfused areas of lung and from an inhomogeneity of ventilation/perfusion ratios within the lung; it varies approximately with the arterial to end-tidal CO_2 tension difference; however, during exercise the end-tidal CO_2 partial pressure (PE'_{CO_2}) may exceed the arterial tension because of increased CO_2 output.

Factors which influence deadspace in conscious man

1. *Anatomical deadspace;*

a. is increased with increase in size of the subject;
b. is greatest on standing, less when seated and least when supine;
c. is larger when the neck is extended and the jaw protruded: conversely it is less when the neck is flexed and the chin depressed;
d. varies directly with tidal volume (approximately 20–40 ml/100 ml tidal volume);
e. is increased by catecholamines, e.g. adrenaline and isoprenaline, and decreased by histamine and 5-hydroxytryptamine.

2. *Alveolar deadspace* usually has a volume which is close to zero in normal awake, spontaneously breathing man; it is increased if there are areas of lung in which ventilation exceeds perfusion.

Alveolar deadspace:

a. is increased in subjects who stand motionless for some minutes because perfusion of the lung apices diminishes;
b. is increased after haemorrhage or fat embolism;
c. is increased in pulmonary disease, e.g. emphysema.

Effect of anaesthesia on deadspace

1. *Anatomical deadspace.* Antisialagogue drugs increase anatomical deadspace. Hyoscine 0.4 mg i.m. results in a 33% increase in deadspace which may last in excess of 2 h.

There is little evidence that anatomical deadspace is increased as a result of induction of anaesthesia (unless an induction agent possessing anticholinergic properties is used).

The effect of muscular paralysis and IPPV on the conducting airways is poorly documented. Indirect evidence suggests that increases in deadspace occur.

2. *Alveolar deadspace.* Anticholinergic premedication reduces pulmonary artery pressure and increases alveolar deadspace by reducing perfusion of the apices of the lung.

There is little evidence that general anaesthesia results in an increase in alveolar deadspace. In addition there is no evidence for any progressive increase in deadspace with duration of anaesthesia. However, it is generally agreed that alveolar deadspace is greater in anaesthetised, artificially ventilated patients compared with unpremedicated, unanaesthetised controls.

Physiological deadspace also increases with decreasing inspiratory/expiratory (I/E) ratio although the greater part of this change is probably attributable to an increase in anatomical deadspace.

Ventilation/perfusion ratio inequality

Distribution of inspired gas in the lung.

Inspired gas is distributed unevenly in the lung. A progressive increase in ventilation occurs from the apex to the base of the lung in the erect subject. Ventilation per unit volume of lung is 50% greater at the base than at the apex. This discrepancy is caused by gravity, which distorts the shape of the lung causing relative compression at the base and increased transpulmonary pressure at the apex. On inspiration from FRC to TLC, the lower resting volume of the basal areas permits greater expansion.

It should be realised that an analogous situation exists in the supine subject. That part of the lung which lies superiorly is less well ventilated; however, since the anteroposterior diameter is much less than the distance from the root of the neck to the diaphragm, the differences in ventilation are less marked. In the lateral position, the dependent lung is better ventilated although this is not the case in the artificially ventilated subject (see p. 620).

Distribution of perfusion

Blood flow also increases from apex to base under the influence of gravity. If the lung is partitioned into three zones, the flow of pulmonary blood is dependent upon the relationship between alveolar pressure (P_A), arterial pressure (Pa) and venous pressure (Pv). This is explained most easily if we consider a special type of flow resistor named after Starling (Fig. 2.5). It comprises a length of flexible collapsible rubber tubing which passes through a rigid box.

The upstream pressure (Pa) may be overcome by the pressure in the box (P_A) which collapses the tubing and prevents flow, whatever the level of the downstream pressure (Pv). This situation occurs in the upper parts of the lungs, where alveolar pressure exceeds arterial pressure.

In the middle section, alveolar pressure exceeds venous pressure, but is less than arterial pressure ($Pa > P_A > Pv$); perfusion is dependent on the pressure difference $Pa–P_A$, and is independent of the venous pressure. This is known as the 'vascular waterfall' because, like a waterfall, the flow is independent of the downstream pressure.

In the lower zone, Pv exceeds P_A and perfusion depends entirely on the pressure difference on either side of the box ($Pa–Pv$).

A fourth zone at the base of the lung has been postulated, where perfusion is reduced because of increased pulmonary interstitial pressure affecting the larger vessels.

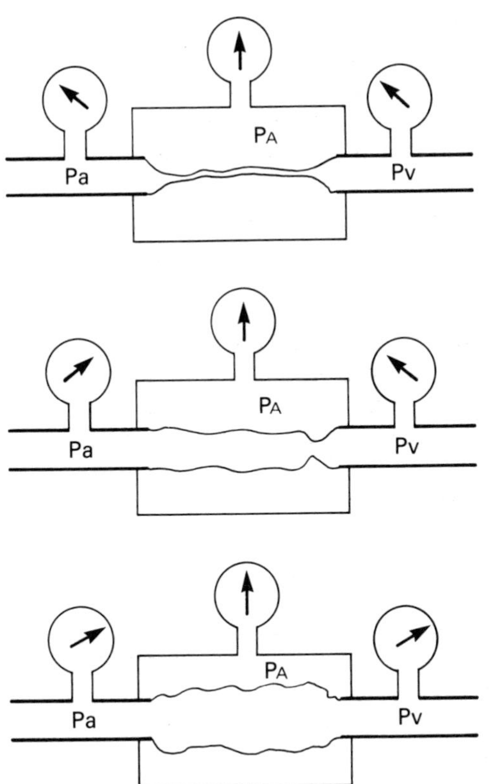

Fig. 2.5 Hydrostatic effects in the upper, middle and lower zones of the lung illustrated by the Starling resistor.

The gradient in pulmonary perfusion from the apex to the base is similar in direction to the distribution of ventilation but is greater in magnitude.

Similar changes in ventilation and perfusion exist in the supine subject but are less marked because the anteroposterior axis of the thorax is small compared with the distance from the apex to the base of the lung.

Ventilation/perfusion ratios ($\dot{V}_A/\dot{Q}_C$)

Radio-isotope techniques allow the inequality of ventilation and perfusion to be measured; results attained in an erect subject could be represented by those shown in Figure 2.6. A wide range of $\dot{V}_A/\dot{Q}_C$ values is obtained which would be greater if the lung were further subdivided. It should be appreciated that the average values of the $\dot{V}_A/\dot{Q}_C$ ratios belie the true effects of $\dot{V}_A/\dot{Q}_C$ ratios on respiratory efficiency.

Assessment of $\dot{V}_A/\dot{Q}_C$ ratios is difficult and requires elaborate equipment. In order to assess the effects of ventilation/perfusion inequalities, Riley and his colleagues proposed a mathematical simplification which assumes that inequalities of $\dot{V}_A/\dot{Q}_C$ ratios do not exist. A three-compartment

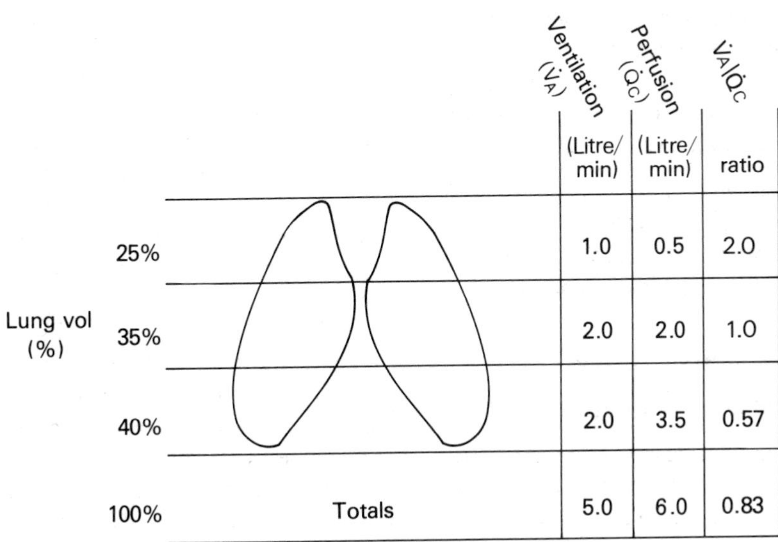

Fig. 2.6 Ventilation/perfusion ratios in an erect subject.

model of the lung was constructed which assumes that the arterial-alveolar CO_2 difference is negligible and unaffected by inhomogeneity of ventilation and perfusion. The alveoli can then be categorised into three groups:

1. Those ventilated but not perfused (alveolar deadspace).
2. Those ideally ventilated and perfused ('normality').
3. Those perfused but unventilated (venous admixture).

Using the Enghoff modification of Bohr's equation (equation 9) it is possible to calculate physiological deadspace. Since physiological deadspace = anatomical deadspace + alveolar deadspace, alveolar deadspace can be estimated. This will include not only true alveolar deadspace (unperfused alveoli) but an additional deadspace equivalent to the inefficiency caused by alveoli with high $\dot{V}_A/\dot{Q}_C$ ratios.

Shunt

An analogous assessment of alveoli with predominantly low $\dot{V}_A/\dot{Q}_C$ ratios can be calculated as shunt and added to true anatomical shunt. The sum is usually called *venous admixture*.

Venous admixture	= anatomical (or frank) shunt	+ 'shuntlike' effect (from areas of low $\dot{V}_A/\dot{Q}_C$)

Venous admixture is calculated from the 'shunt equation'

$$\frac{\dot{Q}_s}{\dot{Q}_t} = \frac{Cc'_{O_2} - Ca_{O_2}}{Cc'_{O_2} - C\bar{v}_{O_2}} \qquad (10)$$

where $\dot{Q}_s$ is venous admixture (litres/min), $\dot{Q}_t$ is cardiac output (litre/min), Cc'_{O_2} is the end-capillary oxygen content (ml/dl), Ca_{O_2} is the arterial oxygen content and $C\bar{v}_{O_2}$ is the mixed venous oxygen content.

The end-capillary oxygen content is calculated from the alveolar air equation (Table 2.1). A value for the alveolar oxygen tension is obtained; this is in equilibrium with the end-capillary oxygen tension from which the corresponding content can be derived.

Clinically, the alveolar – arterial oxygen partial pressure difference (A – a) P_{O_2} is often used as an approximation for venous admixture; however, a reduction in cardiac output causes a reduction in the mixed venous oxygen tension (if oxygen consumption remains constant) and by lowering arterial oxygen tension leads to an increase in this estimate of venous admixture.

If the Riley method of analysis is used, it would be convenient to differentiate shunt from low $\dot{V}_A/\dot{Q}_c$ ratio inequality. Theoretically, if the inspired oxygen tension is raised, venous admixture should be reduced if it is caused chiefly by a scatter of $\dot{V}_A/\dot{Q}_c$ ratios, but there should be no effect on true shunt. However, if a high concentration of oxygen is inspired it may cause

Table 2.1 Alveolar air equations

Ideal alveolar air	$P_AO_2 = P_{I_{O_2}} - \dfrac{Pa_{CO_2}}{R}$	where R = respiratory exchange ratio
Riley's equation	$P_AO_2 = P_{I_{O_2}} - \dfrac{Pa_{CO_2}}{R}[1 - F_{I_{O_2}}(1 - R)]$	
Filley's equation	$P_AO_2 = P_{I_{O_2}} - Pa_{CO_2}\left(\dfrac{P_{I_{O_2}} - P\bar{E}_{O_2}}{P\bar{E}_{CO_2}}\right)$	

Note: 1. Riley's equation assumes that inert gases are in equilibrium and the inspired oxygen concentration constant. Filley's equation permits lack of equilibrium for inert gases.

2. $P_{I_{O_2}} = F_{I_{O_2}} \times (P_B - P_{H_2O})$,
where $F_{I_{O_2}}$ = fractional inspired oxygen concentration
P_B = barometric pressure
P_{H_2O} = saturated vapour pressure of water at body temperature.

absorption collapse of the lung, increasing true shunt.

Effect of anaesthesia on venous admixture

Venous admixture, as measured by (A − a) P_{O_2}, increases after induction of anaesthesia whether ventilation is controlled or not. As yet it is uncertain if this increase in venous admixture is caused by an increase in true shunt or in $\dot{V}_A/\dot{Q}_c$ scatter. Isotope studies in the supine position fail to demonstrate sufficient $\dot{V}_A/\dot{Q}_c$ ratio inequality to account for the increase in venous admixture; thus by default it is assumed to be shunt. 'Micro-atelectasis', i.e. collapse in the absence of evidence by conventional radiography, may occur with anaesthesia.

A recent investigation assessed lung collapse in 13 supine patients by transverse computerised tomography. Concurrently, the distribution of $\dot{V}_A/\dot{Q}_c$ ratios was estimated by a multiple inert gas elimination technique to determine the degree of venous admixture. In spontaneously breathing anaesthetised patients, a close correlation occurred between the degree of collapse and the magnitude of venous admixture. Both collapse and venous admixture increased after ventilation was controlled.

The spatial inhomogeneity of ventilation and perfusion has been considered in detail because it has proved the most popular explanation for impairment of gas exchange. It is doubtful if this abnormality is of significance in anaesthetised supine subjects unless closing volume approaches functional residual capacity.

It is also possible that failure of the respiratory gases to mix completely during a respiratory cycle might increase the inefficiency of respiratory gas exchange. This is termed 'stratified inhomogeneity of ventilation and perfusion'. Its significance in the anaesthetised subject is uncertain but, theoretically, concentration gradients would be decreased by a low respiratory frequency and the introduction of a post-inspiratory pause.

A third possibility is that respiratory efficiency might diminish because of cyclical changes in alveolar CO_2 and O_2 partial pressures during the respiratory cycle, i.e. temporal inhomogeneity of ventilation and perfusion. This is negligible in conscious man but is increased during anaesthesia with spontaneous respiration because expiratory flow is exponential. When ventilation is controlled, greater inefficiency might be anticipated because lung volume is greater during the inspiratory phase and perfusion is reduced; perfusion is greatest in the expiratory phase when lung volume is small.

Alveolar-capillary diffusion

The limitation imposed on respiratory efficiency by the diffusion of CO_2 and O_2 across the alveolar–capillary membrane is believed to be small. Since CO_2 has a much higher water solubility than oxygen and can penetrate an aqueous medium 20 times more rapidly under normal circumstances (i.e. in the absence of a carbonic anhydrase inhibitor), impaired diffusion tends to cause hypoxaemia rather than hypercapnia.

The oxygen molecules follow a diffusion path from the alveoli across the membrane to the pulmonary capillaries because they diffuse from a high to a low partial pressure. Theoretically, hypoxaemia cannot occur in a normal subject at rest provided that the alveolar oxygen tension is normal. It was believed that respiratory exchange was limited by impaired diffusion in the alveolar–capillary block syndrome, e.g. fibrosing alveolitis and interstitial pulmonary oedema; however it seems likely that this inefficiency in gas exchange results from spatial inhomogeneity of ventilation and perfusion because of distortion of tissues. A diffusion defect can be expected (theoretically) if the cardiac output is raised, e.g. during exercise, because equilibrium may not be attained between gas in the alveoli and gas in the capillaries.

The measurement of transfer factor for carbon monoxide was believed to estimate diffusion defects. It now seems more likely that a reduction in transfer factor is caused by a decrease in pulmonary surface area (e.g. lung resection or emphysema), pulmonary arteriovenous shunting or spatial inhomogeneity of ventilation and perfusion.

Anaesthesia and controlled ventilation have little effect on transfer factor.

Summary

The chief factors responsible for inefficiency in respiratory gas exchange are hypoventilation, shunt and spatial inhomogeneity of ventilation and perfusion. The latter two factors are believed to be increased after induction of anaesthesia and control of ventilation; the contribution of stratified and temporal inhomogeneities is uncertain.

CONTROLLED MECHANICAL VENTILATION

The development of intensive therapy has resulted in increasing sophistication of methods of ventilatory support often directed to re-establishing spontaneous respiration in patients with poor lung function.

Conventional artificial ventilation of the lungs, also termed IPPV (intermittent positive pressure ventilation) is achieved usually with a tidal volume of 10–15 ml/kg at a rate, in adults, of 10–12 breaths/min. Early experiments suggested that IPPV resulted in pulmonary collapse, and 'artificial sighs' were incorporated into most ventilators allowing the tidal volume to double or triple in size once in 30–100 breaths. Later experimental evidence showed that such a manoeuvre is unnecessary.

In 1948 Cournand suggested that if the intrathoracic pressure increased, this would reduce pulmonary capillary flow and therefore cardiac output. Experimental evidence in dogs has shown that cardiac output does not decrease until the transpulmonary pressure exceeds 1 kPa, but that vena cava flow ceases at peak inspiration (3 kPa).

Efforts were directed to reducing the mean transpulmonary pressure by limiting the duration of inspiration and introducing a postexpiratory pause. There was little improvement because cardiac output diminished significantly with IPPV only in patients with autonomic blockade or decreased circulating volume. If the inspiratory period is reduced to less than 1 s, the efficiency of respiratory gas exchange decreases.

A subatmospheric pressure (NEEP — negative end-expiratory pressure) was used also to reduce the effects of IPPV on mean intrathoracic pressure. It reduces mean intrathoracic pressure but increases the risk of 'air trapping' in the lungs especially in patients with diseased terminal airways, e.g. emphysema. In addition, both dead-space and venous admixture increase.

The introduction of an expiratory airway resistance proved of great benefit. The main advantage of PEEP (positive end-expiratory pressure), is that it increases FRC, allowing tidal volume to be raised above closing capacity. This improves gas distribution within the lungs. It also decreases lung water in patients with incipient or frank pulmonary oedema, reduces left ventricular filling pressure and improves cardiac output. Theoretically, the increased intrathoracic pressure would be expected to reduce cardiac output but in practice this does not always occur.

In the absence of vasomotor instability and decreased circulatory volume, PEEP often increases arterial oxygenation with reduction of venous admixture. It is recommended when the lungs are 'poorly compliant', e.g. adult respiratory distress syndrome (ARDS) or mitral regurgitation. Nonetheless, the response to PEEP is unpredictable and each patient should be assessed individually to determine the net effect of increased FRC and potential decrease in cardiac output.

The application of an expiratory resistance during spontaneous respiration is termed CPAP (continuous positive airway pressure). This also appears most beneficial in patients with pulmonary disease and is used frequently in children with respiratory distress syndrome (RDS). If PEEP has proved successful in improving oxygenation during artificial ventilation, it is often advisable to use CPAP for a period following the resumption of spontaneous ventilation.

Weaning from controlled mechanical ventilation

Triggering

Triggering enables a patient to initiate a mechanical inflation by lowering the airway pressure, i.e. an attempted spontaneous ventilation. As weaning progresses, the subatmospheric pressure required to initiate a passive inflation is increased. By triggering ventilation in this way, there is less risk that the patient will 'fight' the ventilator whilst being weaned from controlled ventilation.

Synchronised intermittent mandatory ventilation (SIMV)

When the patient has started to breathe spontaneously, the frequency of the mandatory breaths delivered by the ventilator is gradually reduced. A double circuit is designed so that a patient can breathe spontaneously from one circuit whilst a second circuit conveys mandatory breaths from the ventilator. This is called intermittent mandatory ventilation (IMV). This method has the disadvantage that a mandatory breath might be superimposed upon a spontaneous breath. A recent improvement has allowed IMV to be synchronised with spontaneous respiration (SIMV). If a spontaneous breath occurs within a triggering period, i.e. just before the next mandatory breath is due, it triggers the preset mandatory breath; at other times the patient breathes spontaneously. Sophisticated ventilators enable the spontaneous minute volume to be compared with the total expired volume.

Extended mandatory minute volume (EMMV)

This recent development, also termed mandatory minute ventilation (MMV), allows the ventilator to adjust mandatory ventilation with reference to the patient's spontaneous respiration, whilst the patient is being weaned from the ventilator. Acceptable values for tidal volume and respiratory rate are preset on the ventilator. In the absence of spontaneous respiration they are delivered in the usual way (IPPV); if, however, the patient takes a spontaneous breath, the ventilator delays delivering the preset tidal volume. If sufficient spontaneous breaths are taken the ventilator does not ventilate the patient but, if the patient's respiratory efforts decline, mandatory breaths are again delivered by the ventilator.

Inspiratory assist

Some ventilators can supplement spontaneous breaths mechanically, preventing shallow ventilation. This triggering device is used with SIMV and EMMV.

High-frequency ventilation (HFV)

In recent years HFV has excited interest because it can produce good gas exchange by methods not previously explored. Sjöstrand classified HFV into three distinct groups (see also Table 2.2):

1. High-frequency jet ventilation (HFJV)
2. High-frequency positive pressure ventilation (HFPPV)
3. High-frequency forced diffusion ventilation (HFDV), or high-frequency oscillatory ventilation (HFOV)

1. *High-frequency jet ventilation (HFJV).* High-velocity gas is delivered through a small cannula inserted through the cricothyroid membrane or place within a tracheal tube. Air is entrained around the orifice by the Bernoulli principle. The respiratory frequency is 150–500 breaths/min and the tidal volume is generally less than the anatomical deadspace. It usually generates a pressure above atmospheric which is equivalent to a PEEP value of 0.5 kPa. It has been used during endos-

Table 2.2 High-frequency ventilation

	Frequency (cycles or breath/min)	Air entrainment	V_T (ml)	P_A
High frequency positive pressure ventilation (HFPPV)	60–150	NO	100–300	Higher
High frequency jet ventilation (HFJV)	150–300	YES	<150	Medium
High frequency forced diffusion (oscillatory) ventilation HFDV/HFOV	500–3000	NO	***	Lower

V_T = tidal volume set at ventilator.
P_A = alveolar pressure.
*** = immeasurable by conventional means.

copy in patients with bronchopleural fistula, during laryngeal surgery and for weaning patients from ventilators.

2. *High-frequency positive pressure ventilation (HFPPV)*. This technique uses conventional ventilators and the customary technique of tracheal intubation. It uses lower respiratory frequencies than HFJV (60–150 breaths/min) and tidal volumes of 100–300 ml. It differs from HFJV by not entraining air.

3. *High-frequency forced diffusion ventilation (HFDV)*, or *high-frequency oscillatory ventilation (HFOV)*. Sine wave oscillations of frequencies of 500 to 3000/min are used in conjunction with tidal volumes of a few millilitres. There is no bulk flow, so intrapulmonary pressure is low. Although oxygen need only be supplied to satisfy metabolic needs, CO_2 is usually removed by absorption.

The chief advantages of HFV are improved respiratory gas exchange and better patient acceptance of controlled ventilation. Circulatory depression in patients with cardiovascular instability might be expected to be reduced. The reduction of pulmonary barotrauma reported for this technique might prove useful if recent reports of bronchiolectasis, as a result of artificial ventilation with PEEP, are confirmed.

Both HFJV and HFDV need careful adjustment to ensure adequate CO_2 elimination.

BLOOD GASES

Oxygen transport

During spontaneous respiration in an atmosphere of P_{O_2} = 21 kPa, a normal individual exhibits an arterial P_{O_2} of approximately 13.3 kPa (Fig. 2.7). With a normal cardiac output, this results in an *oxygen flux* (arterial oxygen content × cardiac output) of 1 litre/min at rest, which can be raised to 15 litre/min on exercise. Most of this oxygen is carried in blood in chemical combination with haemoglobin. At normal arterial oxygen tension, haemoglobin is almost fully saturated (97.5%); thus increasing the oxygen tension has little effect on haemoglobin saturation.

A small proportion of oxygen is carried in solution (Table 2.3). In arterial blood at 37°C it is 0.0225 ml dl^{-1} kPa^{-1} which is approximately 0.3 ml/dl blood at normal arterial tension. In mixed venous blood, the oxygen tension is normally 5 kPa, and the dissolved oxygen approximately 0.1 ml/dl. Thus only 0.2 ml/dl blood is available to the tissues from oxygen dissolved in blood when breathing air. The importance of dissolved oxygen is that if the inhaled oxygen concentration is raised to 100% it increases the dissolved arterial oxygen to 2 ml/dl blood, although there is little effect on oxygen carriage by haemoglobin.

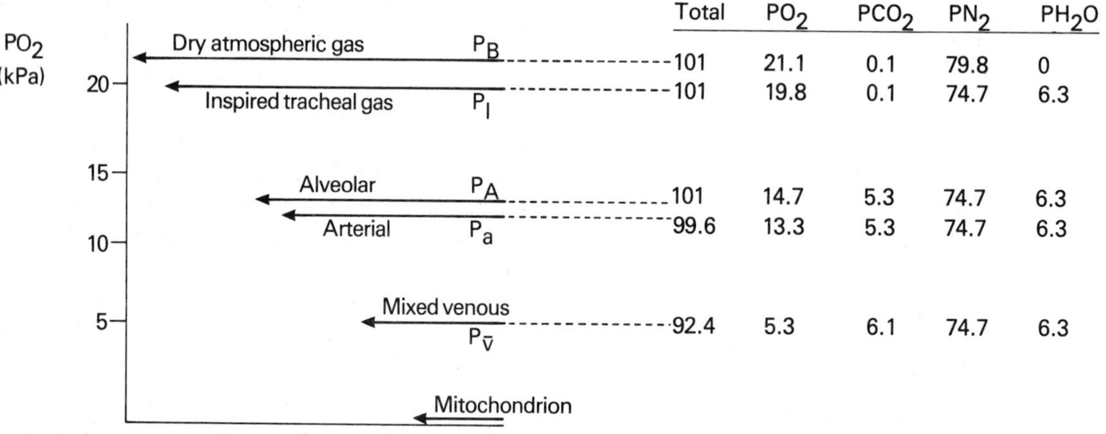

Fig. 2.7 The oxygen cascade.

Table 2.3 Arterial and mixed venous gas composition

	Arterial	Mixed venous
Oxygen tension (P_{O_2}) (kPa)	13.3	5.3
Oxygen content (ml/dl)		
Total	20	15
Attached to Hb	19.7	14.9
Dissolved	0.3	0.1
Carbon dioxide tension (P_{CO_2}) (kPa)	5.3	6.0
Carbon dioxide content (ml/dl)		
Total	50	54
Dissolved	2.5	2.9
Carbamino	2.5	3.7
HCO_3^-	45	47.4

Haemoglobin is a complex compound with a molecular weight of 64 500. It contains ferrous iron which forms reversible compounds with oxygen. The theoretical oxygen-carrying capacity of haemoglobin (Hüfner's constant) is 1.39 ml/g. However, because of impurities associated with haemoglobin, e.g. methaemoglobin, a value of 1.34 or 1.36 ml/g is used in practice.

The oxyhaemoglobin dissociation curve (ODC) in Figure 2.8 shows oxygen saturation of haemoglobin on the ordinate and oxygen tension on the abscissa. The position of the curve is defined by the oxygen tension when the haemoglobin saturation is 50% (P_{50}) under standard conditions. P_{50} varies between 3.5 and 3.9 kPa in normal subjects.

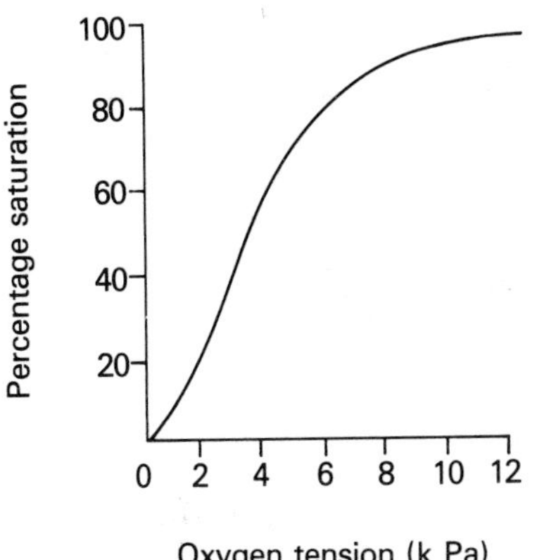

Fig. 2.8 The oxyhaemoglobin dissociation curve.

In venous blood the oxygen tension is normally 5 kPa and the haemoglobin saturation is 75%. In the tissues the P_{50} increases, i.e. ODC moves to the right, and more oxygen is released from the haemoglobin at a given tension. If the P_{50} decreases i.e. the ODC moves to the left, less oxygen is available. The affinity of haemoglobin for oxygen is influenced by the following factors:

1. *Bohr effect.* The Bohr effect is a shift to the right of the ODC, i.e. an increase in P_{50}, with increasing hydrogen ion concentration. The classical Bohr effect refers to changes in H^+ concentration resulting from alterations in P_{CO_2}. However, a similar shift of the curve takes place with an increase in H^+ concentration from other causes, e.g. metabolic acidosis. A decrease in H^+ concentration moves the curve to the left.
2. *2,3-DPG and CO_2 tension.* 2,3-Diphosphoglycerate (2,3-DPG) is produced by glycolysis and influences ion changes in the red cell. At constant H^+ concentration the interaction of 2,3-DPG and CO_2 tension reduces the affinity of haemoglobin for oxygen.
3. *Temperature.* Hypothermia shifts the ODC to the left whereas pyrexia shifts it to the right.

CO_2 carriage

Carbon dioxide is produced by tissue metabolism and conveyed by the venous circulation to the lungs. CO_2 is transported as:

1. *Dissolved CO_2.* The solubility of CO_2 in plasma is 0.5 ml dl^{-1} kPa^{-1}, and the dissolved CO_2 in arterial blood amounts to 2.5 ml/dl if the arterial tension is 5.3 kPa. The mixed venous tension is 6.0 kPa and this represents an increase in dissolved CO_2 of approximately 0.4 ml/dl blood.
2. *Bicarbonate.* Much of the gaseous CO_2 diffusing from the cells into the venous blood is rapidly hydrolysed to H_2CO_3 (carbonic acid) in the red cells. It then dissociates into H^+ and HCO_3^- ions. The bicarbonate diffuses into the plasma, and chloride diffuses into the red cells to maintain

electrical neutrality according to the Gibbs–Donnan equilibrium, as potassium ions cannot leave the red cell. The hydrogen ion is buffered by the reduction of haemoglobin, which normally takes place simultaneously, thereby producing basic forms of histidine on the haemoglobin molecule.

The hydrolysis of CO_2 to carbonic acid can be achieved in the required time only if it is catalysed. Carbonic anhydrase acts as catalyst for this reaction; 1 mol of carbonic anhydrase allows the hydration of 1 000 000 mol CO_2/min.

The movement of chloride into the red cells is known as the Hamburger, or 'chloride', shift; the latter term obscures the important fact that bicarbonate efflux from the red cells is the prime effect and the 'chloride shift' merely a compensatory phenomenon.

3. *Carbamino compounds.* CO_2 also combines with the amino residues of haemoglobin.

$$\begin{aligned} HbNH_3 &\rightleftharpoons HbNH_2 + H^+ \\ CO_2 + HbNH_2 &\rightleftharpoons HbNHCOOH \\ HbNHCOOH &\rightleftharpoons HbNHCOO^- + H^+ \end{aligned}$$

CO_2 carriage is increased in venous blood because partially reduced haemoglobin carries more carbamino compounds than oxyhaemoglobin; this portion is evolved in the lungs. It contributes approximately 10% to the increased CO_2 carriage in venous blood.

Haldane effect

The Christiansen–Douglas–Haldane effect relates to the diminished carriage of CO_2 when partially reduced haemoglobin, a weak acid and buffer, is converted to the stronger acid, oxyhaemoglobin. The CO_2 tension increases with oxygenation although the CO_2 content remains constant.

The decrease in CO_2 content in arterial blood is caused by the loss of the oxylabile carbamino carriage and the reduction in bicarbonate ion because of the diminished buffering of H^+ by haemoglobin.

LUNG FUNCTION TESTS (see Appendix XI page 750)

Defects of the mechanical properties of the lung can be assessed easily from simple tests. The readily available portable dry spirometers (e.g. Vitalograph) enable expiratory spirograms to be used in assessing disease. After a maximum inspiration, the expired air is exhaled as rapidly as possible. The total volume expired is the forced vital capacity (FVC) and that portion which is expired in the first second is the forced expired volume at one second ($FEV_{1.0}$). Both values have to be compared with standard values adjusted for age, height and sex. The ratio $FEV_{1.0}/FVC$ compensates for these variations. If a ratio of less than 70% is present, some obstruction of the larger intrathoracic airways is present.

The Wright peak flowmeter measures the peak expiratory flow rate (PEFR) which is sustained for 10 ms. The measurement of lung volumes in conjunction with the above measurement allows the differentiation of the major patterns of defects of lung mechanics. It is desirable to measure total lung capacity (TLC), functional residual capacity (FRC) and residual volume (RV); if one of these variables is measured the others can be computed easily. FRC, for example, may be assessed by the inhalation of a tracer gas (e.g. helium) and the result calculated from its subsequent dilution.

An obstructive pattern, present in chronic obstructive lung disease, shows a low $FEV_{1.0}/FVC$ ratio, low PEFR, low VC and high RV.

A restrictive pattern is seen after resection of the lung or some skeletal defects, e.g. kyphoscoliosis, and is revealed by a normal $FEV_{1.0}/FVC$ ratio, low PEFR, low RV and low VC.

More elaborate tests of mechanical function can be made using a body plethysmograph with an oesophageal balloon to measure intrapleural pressure. Measurements of pressure and volume may be plotted on an X/Y recorder or an oscilloscope. 'Dynamic compliance' can be calculated from the slope of the line joining 'no flow' points. The width of the loop indicates airway resistance; the area of the loop is affected by both compliance and resistance, and is related to the work performed by the respiratory muscles (Fig. 2.9).

Gas exchange can be assessed non-invasively by measurement of the transfer factor for carbon monoxide by the single breath or the steady state method. If the transfer factor is reduced, it suggests the presence of venous admixture or destruction of lung tissue. Decreased transfer

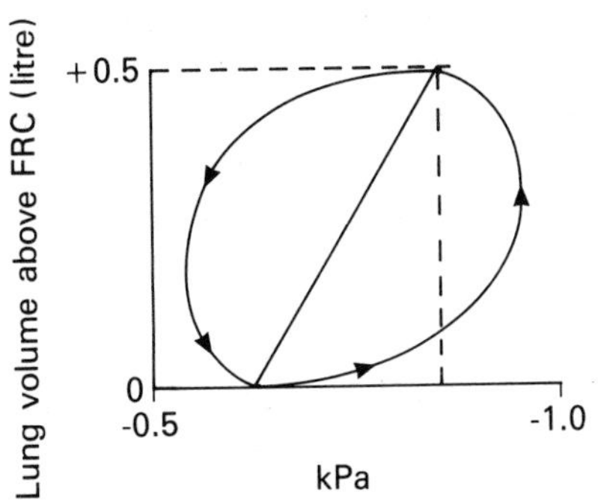

Fig. 2.9 Dynamic pressure/volume loops. Area indicates work performed against resistance. The slope of the line joining the no-flow points indicates compliance.

factor is found in diffuse pulmonary fibrosis, emphysema and pulmonary oedema. It seems unlikely that a defect of diffusion exists in these conditions and hypoxaemia results probably from spatial maldistribution of ventilation and perfusion. If severe respiratory disease is present (e.g. causing dyspnoea at rest) arterial blood gas analysis is required.

The assessment of acid–base balance — pH and base deficit — in conjunction with the blood gases, allows an estimation of the compensatory changes of acidosis and alkalosis which may serve as an index of the severity of respiratory inefficiency (see Ch. 22).

FURTHER READING

Cotes J E 1979 Lung function — assessment and application in medicine, 4th edn. Blackwell Scientific Publications, London

Nunn J F 1987 Applied respiratory physiology, 3rd edn. Butterworths, London

West J B 1982 Pulmonary pathophysiology — the essentials, 2nd edn. Williams & Wilkins, Baltimore

West J B 1985 Best and Taylor's physiological basis of medical practice, 11th edn. Williams & Wilkins, Baltimore

3. Cardiovascular physiology

The cardiovascular system may be considered under two major headings: the peripheral circulation, which adjusts blood flow to individual tissues, and the heart which generates the sum of the individual flows.

PERIPHERAL CIRCULATION

Under normal physiological conditions, blood flow through an organ is determined by its metabolic requirements. Blood flow per unit mass of tissue varies widely from organ to organ both in the basal resting state and at maximum flow (Fig. 3.1). Disease states, such as hypovolaemia and sepsis, and drug therapy, including anaesthesia, may interfere with autoregulatory mechanisms resulting in excessive or inadequate perfusion.

Blood flow rate is determined by the driving pressure (the difference between mean arterial pressure, MAP, and mean venous pressure, MVP), and the resistance to that flow.

$$\text{Flow} = \frac{\text{MAP} - \text{MVP}}{\text{Resistance}}$$

Resistance to blood flow is determined by three factors: calibre and length of the vessels, viscosity of blood and nature of the flow (turbulent or laminar).

Flow profile

In the absence of irregularities of the vessel wall (e.g. resulting from atheroma), flow in blood

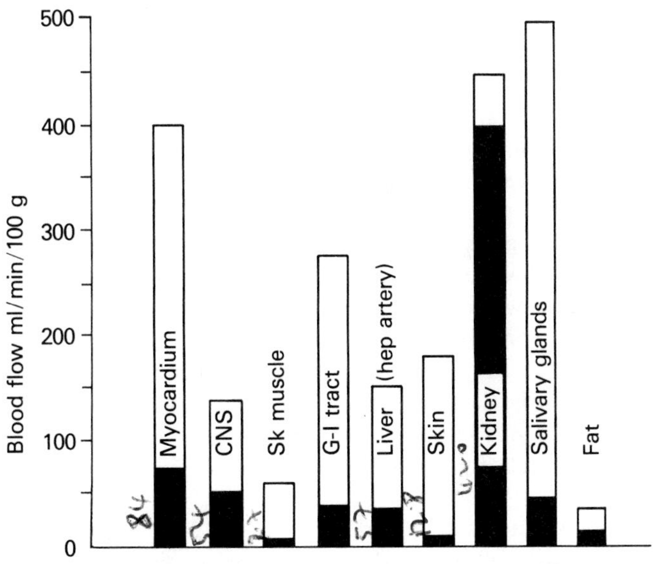

Fig. 3.1 Blood flow at rest (solid portion) and at maximum flow rate (total height) in various organs.

vessels is laminar. The relationship between driving pressure and flow under such conditions is expressed by the Hagen–Poiseuille formula:

$$\dot{Q} = \frac{\pi r^4 \Delta P}{8 l \eta}$$

where $\dot{Q}$ is the flow rate, r the radius of the vessel and l its length. ΔP is the driving pressure and η the blood viscosity. This relationship holds true only for steady flow of Newtonian fluids, i.e. those whose viscosity is independent of flow rate. These conditions do not apply to the cardiovascular system, where flow is pulsatile and blood viscosity is determined by flow rate. It is thus an oversimplification, but illustrates the critical role of the vessel radius in determining flow rate, since the relationship is to the *fourth* power of the radius.

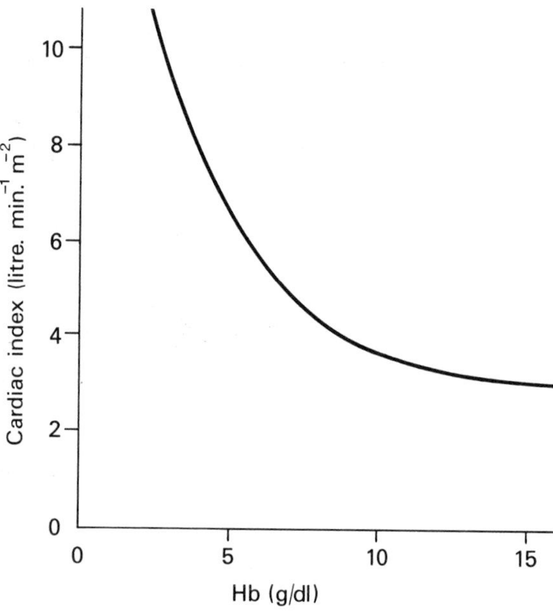

Fig. 3.2 Relationship between haemoglobin concentration and cardiac index in chronic anaemia.

Viscosity

Blood is a mixture of solutes (e.g. electrolytes and proteins) and particles (e.g. cells and chylomicrons). At low flow rates, the cells tend to aggregate, thus increasing viscosity. The subject is further complicated by the tendency of cells to concentrate in the centre of the blood vessel where the velocity is greatest. The haematocrit is therefore lowest at the periphery of the lumen where the velocity is lowest. Thus blood tends to act much more as a Newtonian fluid in vivo than in vitro. The tendency of erythrocytes to concentrate in the centre of a vessel results in a lower haematocrit in blood which enters side branches. This process is known as plasma skimming, and has obvious implications on flow rate and oxygen delivery.

Anaemia reduces oxygen carrying capacity and results in an increase in blood flow to maintain oxygen delivery. The increased flow rate is facilitated by reduced viscosity secondary to the reduced erythrocyte count. Clinically, there is little effect on cardiac index until the haemoglobin concentration decreases below 10 g/dl (Fig. 3.2), the usually accepted lower limit for routine anaesthesia.

Volatile anaesthetic agents increase blood viscosity by increasing the rigidity of the erythrocyte membrane. However, the effect is slight in comparison with the effect of anaemia and has no significant effect on tissue blood flow rates.

Blood viscosity is a complex subject and the reader is referred to Stuart and Kenny (1980) for a more extensive review.

Control of the peripheral circulation

Blood flow through the capillary beds is controlled by local mechanisms and, under normal circumstances, cardiac output adjusts to meet the total flow required. Regulatory mechanisms ensure that the perfusion pressure (arterial pressure) is maintained irrespective of changes in total flow and posture. During periods of stress, e.g. hypovolaemia, the regulatory mechanisms override local control to maintain the blood supply of essential organs including the brain, heart and kidney. These organs also possess autoregulation, i.e. a constant blood flow despite changes in perfusion pressure.

The capillary bed (Fig. 3.3)

Capillaries are composed of a single layer of endothelial cells which permit free exchange of

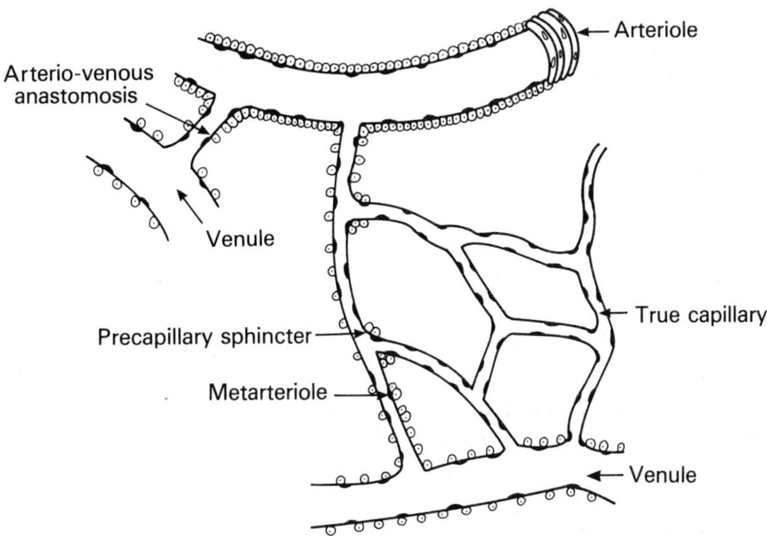

Fig. 3.3 Diagrammatic representation of the microcirculation.

nutrients and metabolites between tissues and blood. Not all capillaries are open at any one time and there are generally preferred routes through which blood flows predominantly.

In many tissues, there are also direct arterio-venous anastomoses. In the skin, these facilitate heat loss by increasing tissue flow rate without affecting capillary perfusion.

Control of flow through capillaries is effected by contraction and relaxation of the smooth muscle of the metarterioles and the precapillary sphincters. A number of metabolic factors including oxygen, ATP and hydrogen ions have been shown to affect capillary flow but the exact mechanism has not been elucidated.

Local regulation of flow by metabolites controls the distribution of blood flow within an organ, in addition to total flow.

Control of the systemic circulation

The systemic circulation is controlled by mechanisms which determine the distribution of blood flow according to priority rather than local needs, the maintenance of an adequate perfusion pressure and the adjustment of cardiac output by variations in the capacity of the circulation.

Arteriolar diameter

The calibre of the arterioles and precapillary sphincters determines blood flow to the peripheral circulation. The calibre depends upon the inherent tone of the smooth muscle, the activity of the autonomic nervous system, circulating hormones, and the local concentration of metabolites (Fig. 3.4).

Inherent tone

Smooth muscle generally exhibits spontaneous contraction in the absence of other stimuli and this is the likely source of inherent tone. Mechanical stretching of the muscle by pulsatile internal pressure may also initiate contractions. In general, those tissues with the poorest sympathetic innervation have the greatest inherent tone. For example vessels in skeletal muscle, brain and myocardium have a high tone whereas those in skin have a low inherent tone.

Autonomic nervous system (Chs 5 and 13)

Sympathetic adrenergic (Fig. 3.5). The adrenergic sympathetic fibres are the predominant pathway whereby the systemic circulation is

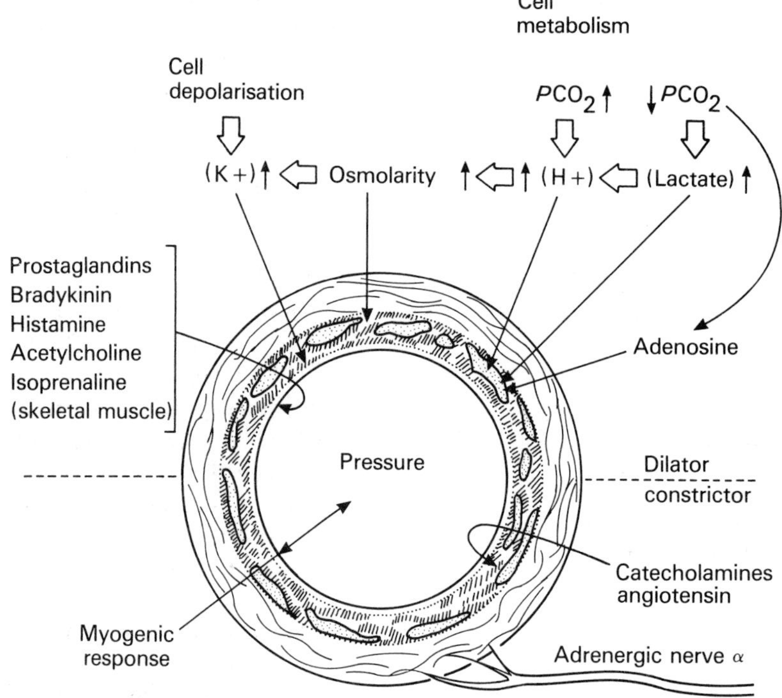

Fig. 3.4 Factors affecting vascular tone.

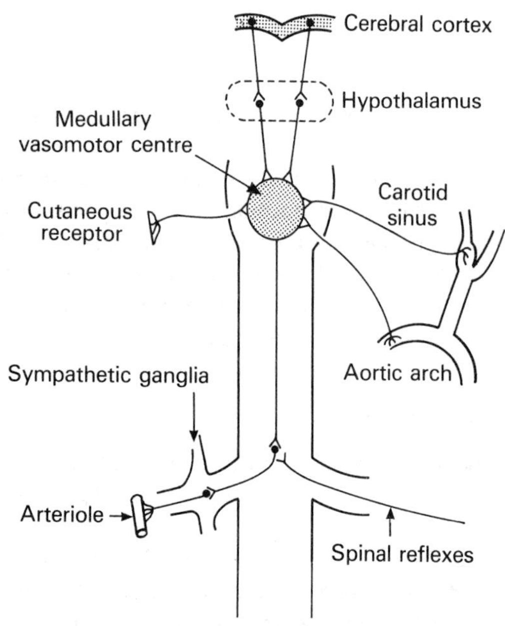

Fig. 3.5 The vasomotor centre.

controlled. The vasomotor areas in the medulla send descending fibres to the preganglionic cells in the thoracolumbar segment of the spinal cord. The preganglionic fibres synapse with postganglionic fibres in the ganglia of the sympathetic chain from which postganglionic fibres travel to vascular smooth muscle. The activity of the vasomotor centres is influenced by afferent impulses from many sensory areas including baroreceptors, chemoreceptors and skin, and from higher centres in the cortex and hypothalamus. The preganglionic cells in the spinal cord may also be influenced directly by higher centres and by reflex activity at spinal level.

The vasomotor centre is active continuously, resulting in a resting tone in vascular smooth muscle. Increased sympathetic activity does not affect all tissues equally. Tissues with the highest intrinsic vascular tone respond less well than those with a lower tone (Fig. 3.6). Thus with increased adrenergic sympathetic activity there is redistri-

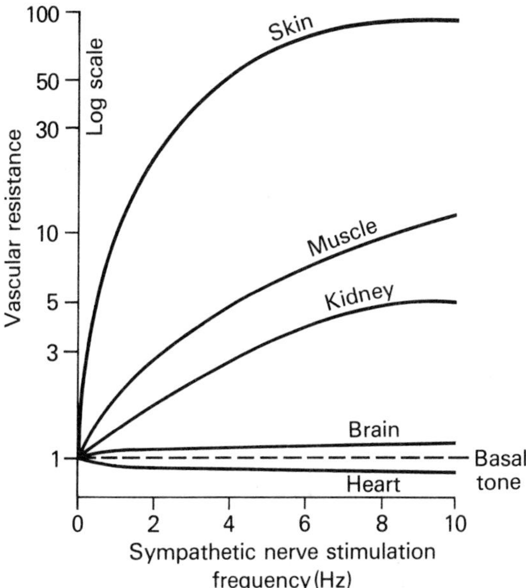

Fig. 3.6 The effect of sympathetic nervous stimulation on vascular resistance in various organs.

bution of blood from skin, muscle and gut to brain, heart and kidney.

Sympathetic cholinergic. Activation of sympathetic cholinergic fibres results in vasodilatation in skeletal muscle. These fibres are represented centrally in the cerebral cortex and are involved in the anticipatory response to exercise, the 'fight or flight' reaction. Stimulation of the appropriate area of the brain results in redistribution of blood flow from skin and viscera to skeletal muscle.

Dopaminergic receptors. Dopamine is a precursor of noradrenaline and has been shown to have a vasodilator effect on splanchnic and renal vessels mediated through specific receptors. This response is useful pharmacologically but the physiological role of such receptors is unclear.

Humoral control. Adrenaline and noradrenaline are released by the adrenal medulla and from adrenergic nerve endings. Their concentrations may increase dramatically during stress but they probably contribute little to cardiovascular control. Their prime role may be in the metabolic response to stress.

Angiotensin II is a potent vasopressor produced by the conversion of angiotensinogen by renin. Renin is released from the juxtaglomerular apparatus of the kidney in response to a reduction in systemic arterial pressure. Angiotensin II probably plays little part in acute regulation of the circulation but, by increasing the secretion of aldosterone, leads to retention of sodium and hence an increase in circulating volume.

Metabolic control

A number of metabolites influence the calibre of blood vessels, including CO_2, K^+ and H^+. Adenosine, bradykinin and prostaglandins are among the chemicals known to cause vasodilatation. It is likely that different tissues respond more readily to some compounds than others.

Induced hypocapnia resulting from hyperventilation results in generalised vasoconstriction and reduction in tissue blood flow which may be deleterious.

Hypoxia results in vasodilatation in all parts of the circulation except the pulmonary vessels, where vasoconstriction occurs. The vasodilatation is countered by reflex vasoconstriction mediated by the sympathetic nervous system resulting from stimulation of the chemoreceptors. This acts as a protective mechanism to increase blood flow to the brain.

Autoregulation

Blood flow through many organs remains almost constant over a wide range of perfusion pressure. In man, this phenomenon is most marked in the renal and cerebral circulations. The mechanism is unclear, although accumulation or washout of vasodilator metabolites seems a likely explanation. Alterations in the intrinsic tone of vascular smooth muscle have also been proposed.

Measurement of blood flow

The measurement of blood flow in absolute terms through tissues is technically difficult. However, the relationship between flow and oxygen consumption is of more importance. If the imbalance is severe, organ failure occurs and this may be manifest by oliguria, clouding of consciousness, etc. Clinically, it is useful to assess flow in the organ which is most accessible, viz. the skin. Clinical assessment of skin flow by capillary refill may be supplemented by the measurement of the gradient between core temperature and skin temperature, which is normally less than 5°C. Mixed venous oxygen tension may provide a global assessment of the adequacy of tissue perfusion. Normal mixed venous oxygen tension is 6 kPa, and values below 3.7 kPa are associated with a poor prognosis. The value must be interpreted with care particularly in the presence of arteriovenous shunting of blood, when the value may be elevated despite tissue hypoxia.

Capacitance vessels

The veins contain approximately 80% of the blood volume (Fig. 3.7). Venoconstriction and dilatation adjust the capacity of the circulation to maintain a balance with the blood volume, for example during hypovolaemia (vide infra) and with changes in posture. Impairment of venoconstriction by disease or drugs, e.g. antihypertensive agents, leads to a reduction in cardiac output and hypotension on standing (postural hypotension).

The calibre of the veins is adjusted by changes in sympathetic activity, mediated both by nervous and humoral stimulation. The postcapillary venules are also sensitive to local concentrations of metabolites in the same manner as the precapillary sphincters.

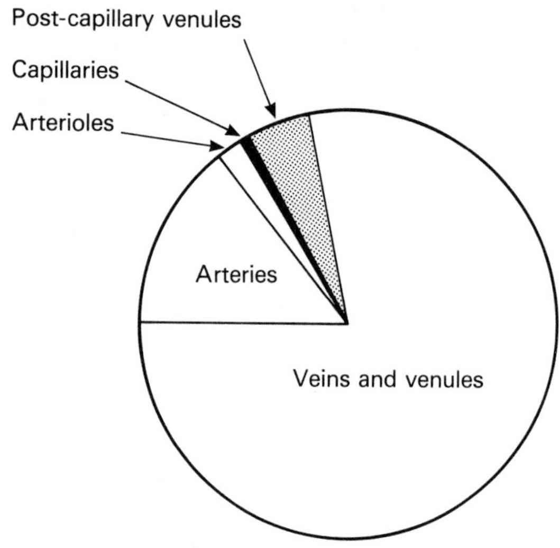

Fig. 3.7 Distribution of blood volume between different parts of the circulation.

Control of arterial pressure

Systemic arterial pressure is controlled closely in order to maintain the driving pressure necessary for tissue perfusion. The normal values vary with age and sex (Table 3.1) in addition to physiological changes including sleep. It must be stressed that although systemic arterial pressure may be measured readily the readings obtained should be interpreted with care. A normal or even elevated arterial pressure is no guarantee of

Table 3.1 Changes in arterial pressure, cardiac output and peripheral vascular resistance with age.

	Arterial pressure (mmHg)		Blood flow		Peripheral vascular resistance**	
Age (years)	Systolic/diastolic	Mean	Cardiac index* (litre min^{-1} m^{-2})	Cardiac output (litre/min)	(mmHg $litre^{-1}$ min^{-1})	(dyne s cm^{-5})
10	100/65	75	4.0	4.8	15	1150
20	110/70	85	3.7	6.7	12	950
30	115/75	90	3.4	6.1	14	1100
40	120/80	92	3.2	5.8	15	1200
50	125/82	95	3.0	5.4	17	1300
60	130/85	98	2.8	5.0	19	1500
70	135/88	102	2.6	4.7	21	1650
80	140/90	105	2.5	4.5	22	1800

* Assuming a body surface area of 1.2 m^2 at age 10 and 1.8 m^2 thereafter
** Assuming a CVP of 5 mmHg

adequate tissue perfusion. Mean arterial pressure (MAP) may be calculated from the formula:

$$\text{MAP} = \text{diastolic arterial pressure} + \frac{\text{pulse pressure}}{3}$$

Its value is determined by the product of cardiac output (CO) and total systemic peripheral resistance (TPR).

$$\text{MAP} = \text{CO} \times \text{TPR}$$

The units for expressing TPR are confusing. Traditionally, it has been expressed as dyne s cm^{-5} and more recently as N s m^{-5} (1 dyne s cm^{-5} = 100 N s m^{-5}).

$$\text{TPR (dyne s cm}^{-5}) = \frac{\text{MAP (mmHg)}}{\text{CO (litres/min)}} \times 80$$

Thus, if MAP = 100 mmHg and CO = 5 litre/min, TPR = 1600 dyne s cm^{-5}.

Mean arterial pressure is thus a balance between cardiac output and resistance to flow posed by the vascular beds.

Neurones in the medulla receive and integrate afferent impulses from the baroreceptors, chemoreceptors, skin, muscle and viscera, and from higher centres, the hypothalamus and cortex. Classically these neurones have been described as a discrete vasomotor centre but it is now thought that they are distributed in several regions of the medulla. Activity in these neurones leads to increased vasoconstrictor tone and thus an increased arterial pressure, provided that cardiac output does not decrease.

Baroreceptors

Arterial baroreceptors are located in the carotid sinus and the wall of the aortic arch. The nerve endings are not sensitive to pressure but to deformation of the arterial wall (stretch receptors). Stimulation of the baroreceptors leads to reflex reduction in vasoconstrictor and venoconstrictor tone, and to bradycardia. Arterial pressure is thus reduced by diminution of both total peripheral resistance and cardiac output. Conversely a reduction in baroreceptor activity leads to vaso- and venoconstriction and increased heart rate.

Other cardiovascular reflexes

The chemoreceptors located in the carotid and aortic bodies respond to hypoxaemia and to a lesser extent hypoperfusion. Chemoreceptor stimulation results in a general increase in cardiovascular sympathetic activity, increasing systemic arterial pressure.

A large number of stretch receptors have been described in the heart and great vessels but their role is unclear. Stimulation of receptors in the atria increases sympathetic activity thus aiding the increase in cardiac output which results from increased atrial pressure. Other atrial receptors appear to be responsible for regulation of blood volume by influencing ADH release and thus water balance.

Assessment of baroreceptor responses

The response to change in posture is a useful guide to the ability of a patient to respond to cardiovascular stress. This is of importance in patients with autonomic neuropathy (e.g. diabetics) and those receiving vasodilator drugs.

The Valsalva manoeuvre, a forced expiration against a closed glottis resulting in increased intrathoracic pressure and decreased venous return, is a convenient bedside assessment. In the normal individual, arterial pressure is maintained by a combination of tachycardia and vasoconstriction during the period of increased intrathoracic pressure (Fig. 3.8). On release of the raised intrathoracic pressure there is transient hypertension and bradycardia until the vasoconstriction is reversed. The heart rate response is easiest to detect and may be measured at the bedside.

The baroreceptors may be tested also by external stimulaton or by inducing a transient increase in arterial pressure by administration of a short acting vasopressor, e.g. noradrenaline. These tests are more suitable for research than for clinical evaluation.

THE HEART

Anatomy

The heart comprises four chambers; the right and left ventricles, which generate the energy to propel

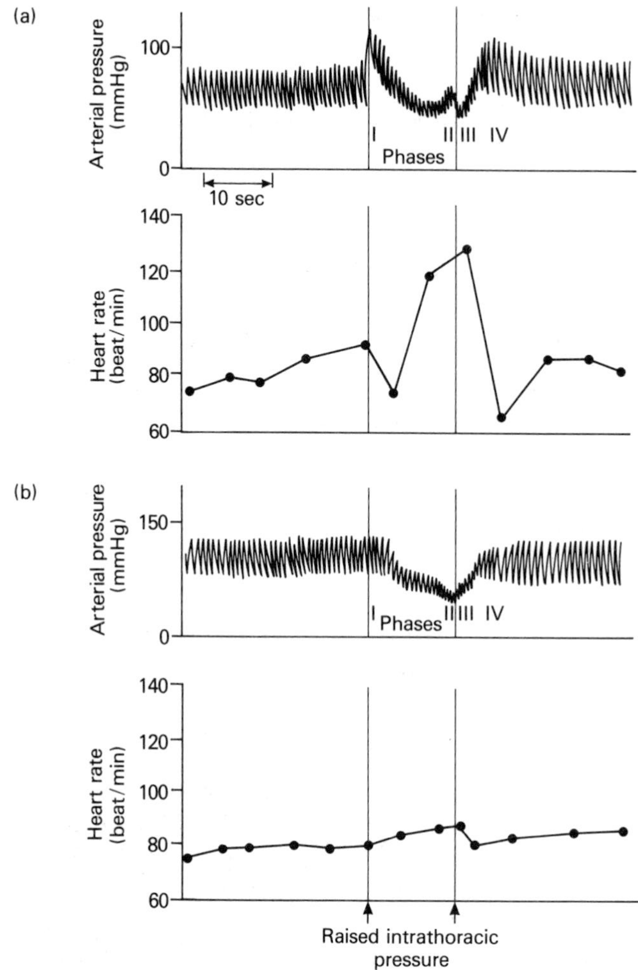

Fig. 3.8 Valsalva manoeuvre: (a) normal response; (b) patient with impaired cardiovascular control. See text for details.

the blood around the pulmonary and systemic circulations respectively, and the atria which serve as reservoirs for blood and as accessory pumps to augment ventricular filling. Uncompensated loss of atrial activity, e.g. atrial fibrillation, reduces cardiac output by approximately 35%.

Cardiac muscle has properties intermediate between those of skeletal and smooth muscle. It has cross-striations similar to those of skeletal muscle and in common with smooth muscle, exhibits spontaneous rhythmic contractions acting as a single unit or syncitium. The muscle fibres are arranged in an interdigitating spiral fashion to form the two ventricles. The left ventricle, which performs approximately six times as much work as the right, has a much thicker wall and is conical in shape. The right ventricular wall is thinner, and applied to the left ventricular wall (Fig. 3.9). The ventricular and atrial muscle fibres are inserted into a fibrous framework at the atrioventricular junction which provides an attachment also for the cardiac valves.

The cardiac valves ensure that blood flows only from atria to ventricles to arterial systems. The aortic and pulmonary valves act passively, opening in response to a pressure gradient between ventricle and artery and closing when the gradient reverses. The tricuspid and mitral valves are

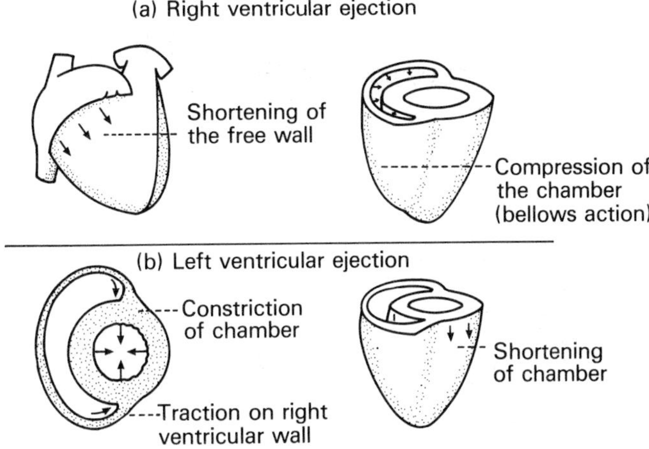

Fig. 3.9 Ventricular contraction. Note influence of left ventricular contraction on the right ventricle.

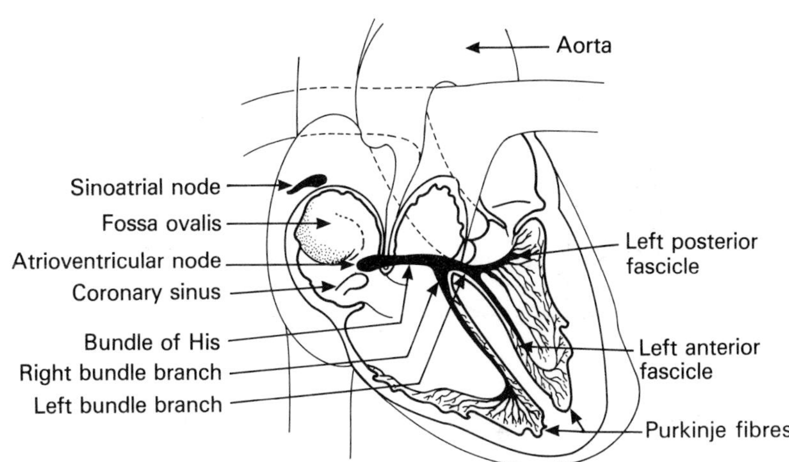

Fig. 3.10 The cardiac conducting system.

prevented from bulging back into the atria during ventricular systole by the papillary muscles and their chordae tendineae.

The conducting system (Fig. 3.10) comprises fibres of specialised muscle cells and is responsible for the initiation and spread of cardiac contraction. The sinoatrial (SA) node lies in the wall of the right atrium close to the superior vena cava. An impulse originating here sweeps through the atria, leading to atrial systole, and activates the atrioventricular (AV) node. The AV node is continuous with the AV bundle (bundle of His) which pierces the fibrous septum separating atria and ventricles. The AV bundle runs through the ventricular septum and divides into right and left bundles which supply their respective ventricles.

Electrophysiology of the heart

A normal heart beat is initiated by cells of the SA node. The wave of contraction passes around the atria through the AV node and bundle to the ventricles. Cells of the conducting system (pacemaker cells) exhibit spontaneous depolarisation resulting from a relative permeability to sodium ions (Fig. 3.11). At a threshold of −50 mV a sudden sharp depolarisation occurs which is propagated to other cells, initiating a heart beat. The rate of spontaneous depolarisation is fastest in the SA node which thus has the fastest intrinsic rate and normally determines heart rate. Inhibition of higher parts of the system may result in other cells, for example in the AV node or ventricles, acting as pacemaker at their own slower intrinsic rates. The heart rate is determined by the rate of spontaneous depolarisation which is increased by sympathetic activity and decreased by vagal activity. Extreme vagal activity may halt spontaneous depolarisation, resulting in asystole until an impulse is generated by a pacemaker cell further down the system (vagal escape).

The action potential of cardiac muscle differs markedly from skeletal muscle. The duration of depolarisation is approximately 200 ms (in contrast to 1–2 ms in skeletal muscle). Cardiac muscle is inexcitable during this period.

The electrocardiogram (ECG)

Electrical currents generated by cardiac muscle during depolarisation and repolarisation are reflected in changes of electrical potential at the skin. The magnitude and polarity of the potential at a particular point depends upon the mass of muscle contracting, and upon its orientation. The P wave reflects atrial depolarisation, the QRS complex ventricular depolarisation and the T wave ventricular repolarisation.

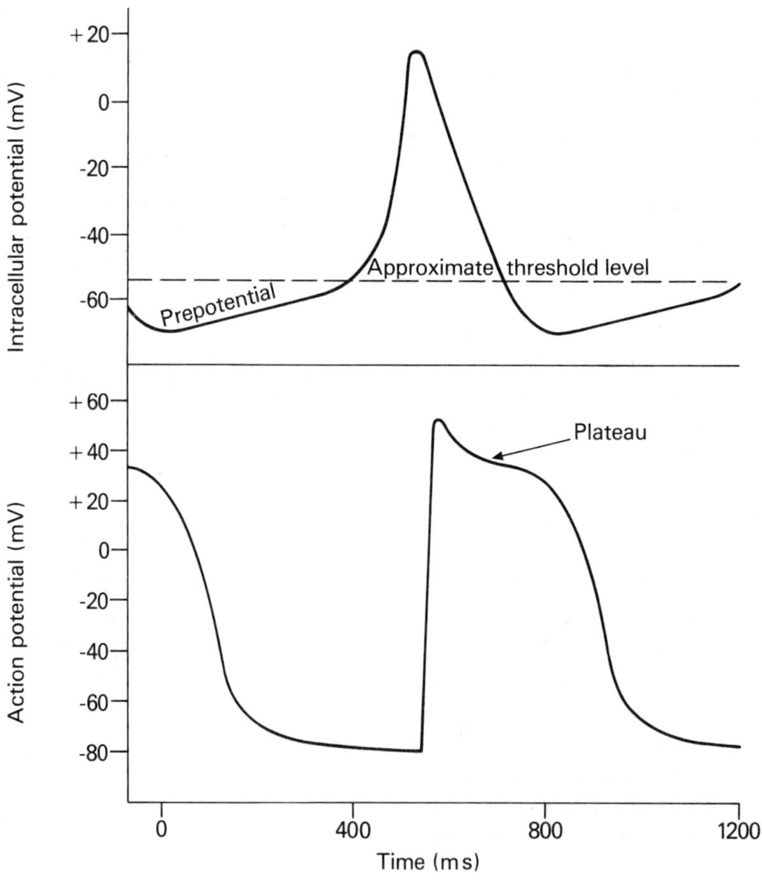

Fig. 3.11 Upper panel: transmembrane potential of a pacemaker cell; heart rate 75 beats/min. Lower panel: cardiac muscle action potential.

The ECG reflects the *electrical* activity of the heart and it may indicate rate and rhythm in addition to some indication of myocardial damage. It does *not* reflect the adequacy of mechanical contraction. Normal complexes may be observed in the absence of mechanical activity. For further information on the measurement and interpretation of the ECG, the reader is referred to one of the standard texts, e.g. Rollason (1975).

The cardiac cycle (Fig. 3.12)

A heartbeat is initiated by spontaneous depolarisation of an SA node pacemaker cell. A wave of depolarisation spreads over the atria, which contract. At this point, the atrioventricular valves are open and the ventricles are filling under the pressure of the venous return; the pulmonary and aortic valves are held closed by the pressure gradient between pulmonary artery or aorta and their respective ventricles. Atrial contraction augments ventricular filling as diastole nears its end. The wave of depolarisation passes through the AV node, along the AV bundle and spreads over the ventricles. Ventricular contraction (systole) follows. As ventricular pressure increases, the AV valves close and a phase of isometric contraction (i.e. increasing tension without shortening) begins. The aortic and pulmonary valves open as ventricular pressures exceed aortic and pulmonary arterial pressures and the ejection phase commences. Atrial repolarisation occurs during early systole and the atria refill with blood as they relax. Spontaneous depolarisation begins in the SA node.

Towards the end of systole, ventricular repolarisation occurs and the ventricles relax. The pulmonary and aortic valves close as pulmonary arterial and aortic pressures exceed the respective ventricular pressures, marking the end of systole. The closure of the AV valves and aortic and pulmonary valves is audible as the first and second heart sound respectively. The aortic valve normally closes before the pulmonary, splitting the second sound. Aortic valve closure is seen as the dicrotic notch on the aortic pressure waveform.

Relaxation is isometric until ventricular pressure is less than atrial pressure when the AV valves

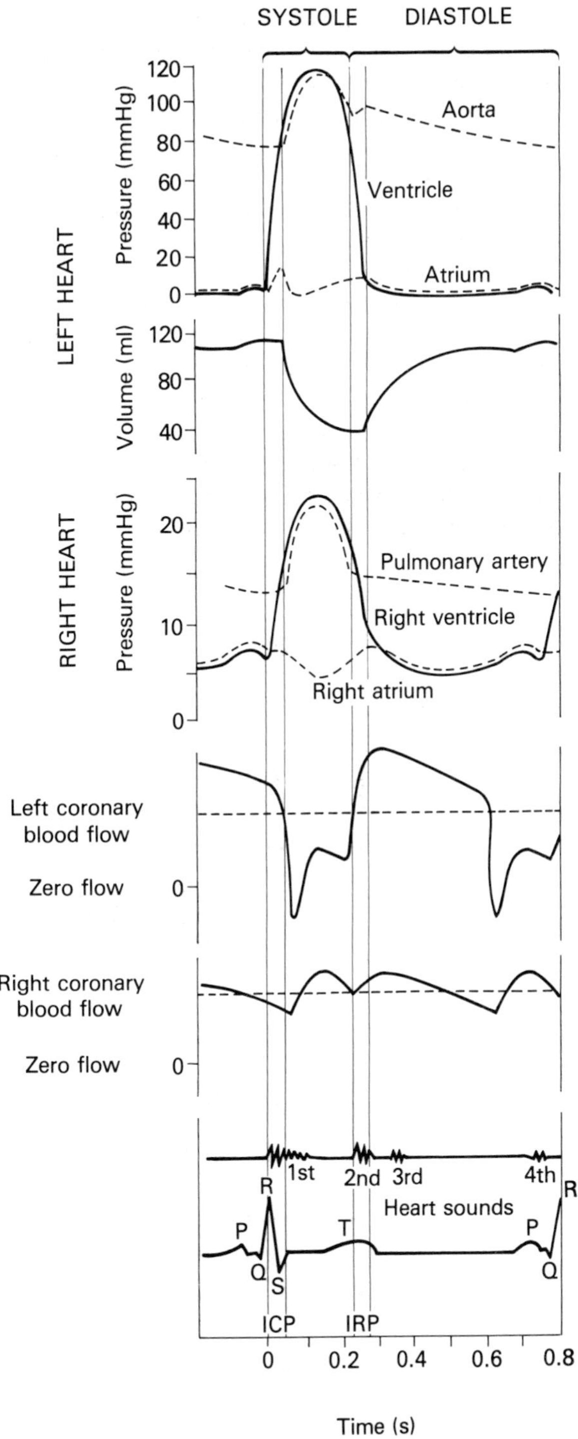

Fig. 3.12 The cardiac cycle. ICP = isometric contraction period. IRP = isometric relaxation period.

open and ventricular filling begins. Filling continues passively until the SA node initiates a further cardiac cycle. At a normal heart rate of 70 beats/min, a cardiac cycle occupies about 850 ms, of which approximately 220 ms is systole. Increased heart rates are accomplished almost entirely by a reduction in the duration of diastole (and ventricular filling). Thus, the atrial contribution to ventricular filling becomes proportionately more important as heart rate increases.

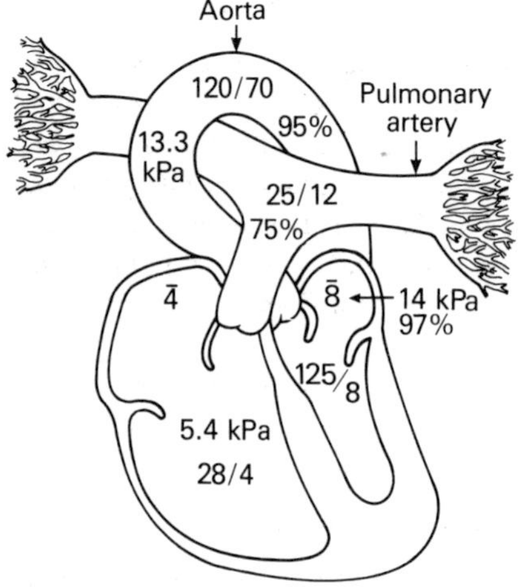

Fig. 3.13 Cardiovascular pressures, oxygen tensions and saturations.

The passage of cardiac catheters and the interpretation of the waveforms is possible only if the cycle of events and their temporal relationship is understood clearly. Figure 3.12 summarises these events. Normal intracardiac pressures and oxygen tensions are shown in Figure 3.13.

Coronary circulation (Fig. 3.14)

The myocardium is supplied by two coronary arteries, the right and left, which supply their respective ventricles. There is often a degree of overlap in the areas supplied but there is little communication between the two vessels. The arteries run over the surface of the heart giving off branches which penetrate the myocardium to supply the capillary beds. Venous drainage from the left ventricle passes via the coronary sinus into the right atrium; that from the right passes via the anterior cardiac vein also into the right atrium. In addition, a small proportion of the coronary flow (3–5%) drains directly into the ventricles through the Thebesian veins.

The normal coronary blood flow at rest is approximately 250 ml/min (80 ml/min per 100 g of tissue) and this may increase five-fold during maximal exercise (Fig. 3.1). Myocardial oxygen consumption is approximately 11 ml min^{-1} 100 g^{-1} compared with skeletal muscle at 8 ml min^{-1} 100 g^{-1}. Coronary venous Po_2 is very low (ap-

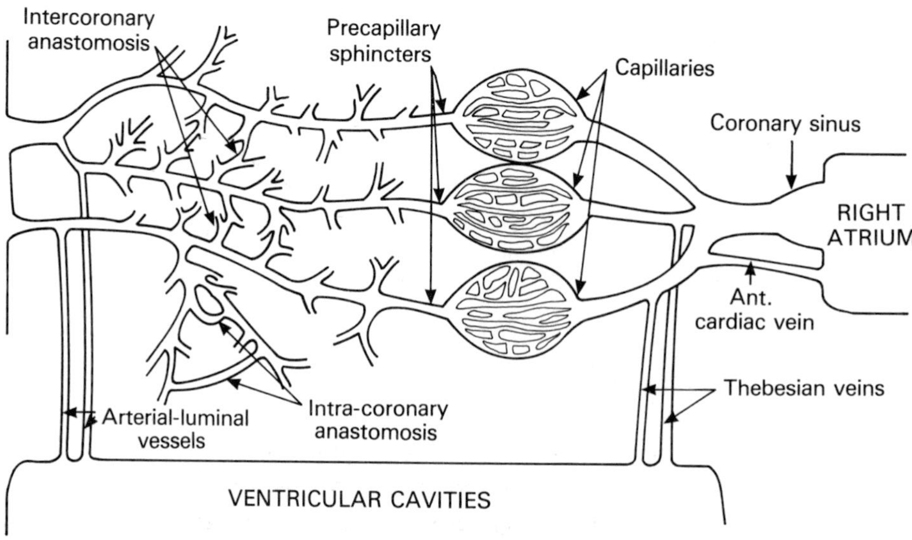

Fig. 3.14 Diagrammatic representation of the coronary circulation.

proximately 4 kPa (30 mmHg)). Thus increased oxygen consumption by the heart cannot be met by an increased extraction but must be accommodated by increased flow or an increase in myocardial efficiency. If increased flow cannot be achieved, increased extraction may result in tissue hypoxia. This feature of the coronary circulation is illustrated by the response to anaemia; if the oxygen carrying capacity of blood is halved (Hb 7 g/dl) and cardiac output is doubled then myocardial blood flow should *quadruple* if myocardial hypoxia is to be avoided.

The coronary circulation is unique in that blood flows principally during diastole because the intramyocardial vessels are compressed during systole (Fig. 3.12). Increased heart rate shortens diastole and may thus impair myocardial blood supply if flow rate cannot increase during diastole. The intramyocardial pressure is highest in the subendocardial region and lowest at the epicardium. An increased intraventricular pressure during diastole, as may occur during sudden hypertension, has a greater effect on flow through the subendocardial vessels and may result in subendocardial ischaemia.

Coronary blood flow is determined predominantly by myocardial metabolic activity. Although there are sympathetic fibres to the heart, changes in myocardial oxygen demand induced by sympathetic stimulation have a predominant effect on coronary vascular resistance in comparison with local vascular effects of the catecholamine transmitters. Although autoregulation occurs in the coronary circulation, this phenomenon may be difficult to demonstrate in vivo because of the changes in myocardial oxygen demand that accompany changes in perfusion pressure.

Cardiac output

Cardiac output ($\dot{Q}$) is the product of stroke volume (SV) and heart rate (HR).

$$\dot{Q} = SV \times HR$$

In a normal 70 kg man at rest, SV = 70 ml, HR = 70 beats/min and $\dot{Q}$ = 5 litres/min. In order to compare the cardiac output of patients of different size, the cardiac output per square metre of body surface area is often calculated. This is termed cardiac index (CI). For example, surface area = 1.7 m^2 in a 70-kg man, and:

$$CI = \frac{5}{1.7} = 3 \text{ litre min}^{-1}\text{ m}^{-2}$$

Control of cardiac output

The cardiac output is determined by the metabolic requirements of the body, and over a period of time it equals the venous return (Fig. 3.15). The

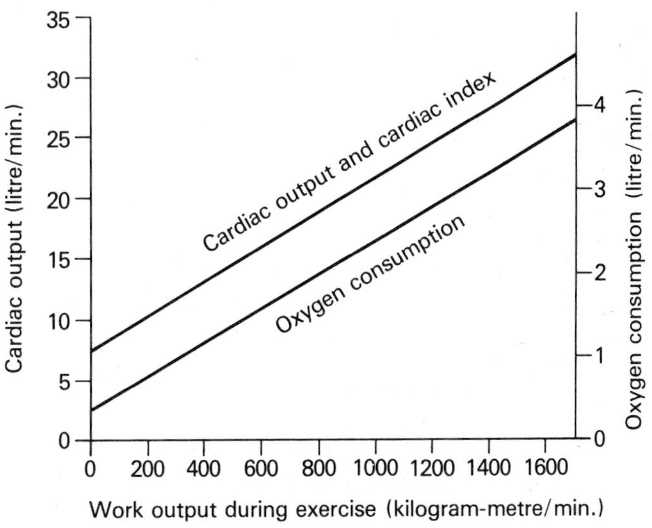

Fig. 3.15 Relationship between exercise, cardiac output and oxygen consumption.

outputs of the two ventricles must also be identical. A consistent difference of 1 ml between the right and left ventricular stroke volumes at a heart rate of 70 beats/min would lead to an imbalance of 1 litre in 14 min. The balancing of venous return and cardiac output, and of right and left ventricular outputs, is an intrinsic property of the myocardium, and occurs even in a denervated heart with a fixed rate. If this were not so, cardiac transplantation would be impossible and patients with cardiac pacemakers could not exercise.

In 1915 Starling stated the relationship between the force of cardiac contraction and muscle fibre length thus: 'The law of the heart is thus the same as the law of muscular tissue generally, that the energy of contraction, however measured, is a function of the length of the muscle fibre'. This intrinsic property of cardiac muscle enables the heart to balance venous return and cardiac output and the outputs of right and left ventricles. This mechanism alone compensates for increases in venous return of 200–300% above resting values. Further increases in venous return are met by increases in contractility of the muscle fibres and heart rate. These changes are mediated by the autonomic nervous system.

The mechanism is best understood if the effect of an increase in activity in a muscle group is considered. Increased metabolism in muscle leads to locally induced vasodilatation and increased blood flow. The increased flow rate increases venous return, which distends the right atrium and ventricle. The resulting increased force of contraction increases right ventricular stroke volume which leads to left ventricular distension. This in turn causes increased left ventricular stroke volume and an increase in cardiac output if heart rate remains constant. The increased cardiac output is maintained until reduced muscle metabolism leads to vasoconstriction, reversing the process. If the vasodilatation is sufficient to reduce peripheral vascular resistance, arterial pressure decreases transiently. Baroreceptor activity diminishes, and vasoconstriction and increases in heart rate and contractility occur, as a result of increased sympathetic activity. The increased heart rate and contractility lead to a further increase in cardiac output. In the case of muscular exercise, increased sympathetic activity may occur before the increase in venous return as the cerebral cortex 'anticipates' the activity.

Cardiac contractility

The force of contraction is determined by the initial fibre length (Frank–Starling mechanism) and by the ability of the cardiac muscle to contract at a given initial fibre length (*contractility*). These relationships are illustrated usually as a curve relating force of contraction to fibre length (Fig. 3.16), changes in contractility being shown as displaced but parallel curves.

Starling's law, as stated above, is almost impossible to validate in man because the two parameters (force of contraction and fibre length) cannot be measured directly. Consequently, parameters such as stroke volume, speed of contraction, maximum rate of rise of ventricular pressure, peak ventricular pressure, ejection fraction (stroke volume/end-diastolic volume) and

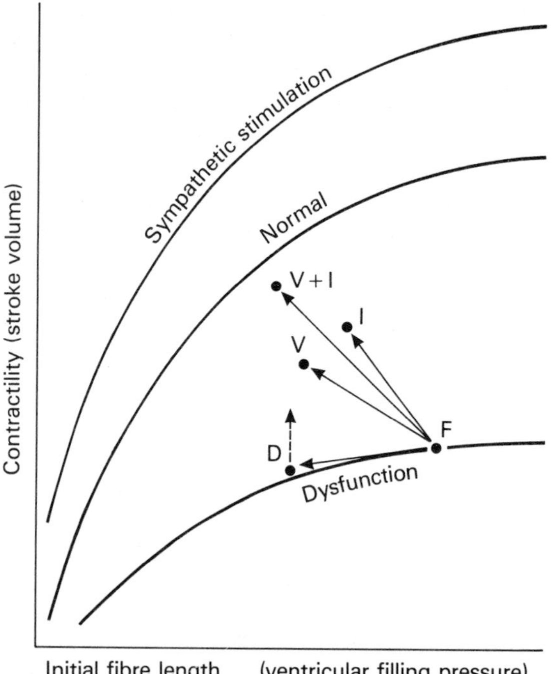

Fig. 3.16 Starling's law of the heart and changes in myocardial contractility. Letters and arrows signify effects of different treatments in cardiac failure. I = inotropic drugs; V = vasodilator drugs; V + I = combined use; D = diuretics. Broken arrow indicates that ventricular function may improve later.

stroke work (SV × [MAP − MVP]) have been used. All these parameters are indirect measures of the force of contraction and must be interpreted with care. For example, a leaking mitral valve results in a reduction in forward stroke volume despite an increase in left ventricular work.

Similarly, alternative parameters have been used to reflect initial fibre length. End-diastolic volume and pressure have been used widely. End-diastolic pressures, particularly right and left atrial pressures, require careful interpretation as the change in pressure with a given volume change depends upon the compliance of the chamber. Thus the pressure change in a stiff ventricle is greater than in a flabby ventricle for the same volume change.

Ventricular function curves based on the indirect parameters mentioned above are useful clinically in plotting the response to treatment but may be of limited value in determining deviations from normality.

Sympathetic stimulation is the most significant extrinsic factor which increases myocardial contractility. The effect may be induced by neuronal activity or by circulating endogenous or exogenous catecholamines. Both heart rate and contractility increase, with a parallel effect on cardiac output and myocardial oxygen consumption.

Calcium ions increase contractility, as do digoxin and insulin as well as all the sympathomimetic amines. Conversely, contractility is reduced by β-adrenergic blocking drugs, antiarrhythmic agents, the majority of general anaesthetics (vide infra) and an elevated extracellular potassium ion concentration.

Control of heart rate

Heart rate is determined by the rate of spontaneous depolarisation of the sinoatrial node. The resting heart rate is approximately 75 beats/min, and increases to 110 beats/min after total denervation, indicating the importance of inhibitory vagal parasympathetic activity. Thus cardiac acceleration may be achieved either by a decrease in vagal activity or an increase in sympathetic activity.

Increases in heart rate occur largely as a result of shortening of diastole. Excessive increases in heart rate impair ventricular diastolic filling such that stroke volume and cardiac output decrease. Similarly, cardiac output decreases if an increasing stroke volume is unable to compensate for a decreasing heart rate. In a normal heart, cardiac output is unimpaired between 40 and 150 beats/min although this range may be reduced considerably by disease.

Assessment of cardiac function

The best clinical indication of cardiac function is the state of the peripheral circulation. Simple methods of assessment, as discussed previously, are often adequate, and should be employed before more invasive techniques are contemplated.

Ventricular filling pressures

The pressure in the central veins (CVP) is equated with the right ventricular end-diastolic pressure. The pressure measured depends on venous return, the ability of the heart to respond, the state of filling of the circulation, and venous tone. Because CVP measurement is influenced by many factors and because the value noted depends critically on the zero point chosen, isolated readings are of little value. With any control system, the maximum information can be obtained by observing the effect of small perturbations. Thus the response of the CVP to small fluid challenges is more valuable than single readings. This is illustrated in Figure 3.17, where the upper panel illustrates the course of a young traumatised hypovolaemic patient who, with vigorous sympathetic activity, has induced such venoconstriction that CVP is elevated. Fluid challenges *decrease* the CVP as cardiac output increases and vasodilatation occurs. In contrast, the lower panel illustrates a patient with cardiac impairment. Fluid challenges produce a sustained elevation of CVP which on the second occasion exceeds the ability of the heart to respond, and active intervention is required.

In the examples given above, it is assumed that right and left ventricular function is comparable and that changes in CVP reflect changes in left atrial pressure (LAP) both in direction and magnitude. Clinically, there is often a marked disparity between the function of the two ventricles, and left ventricular filling pressures must be

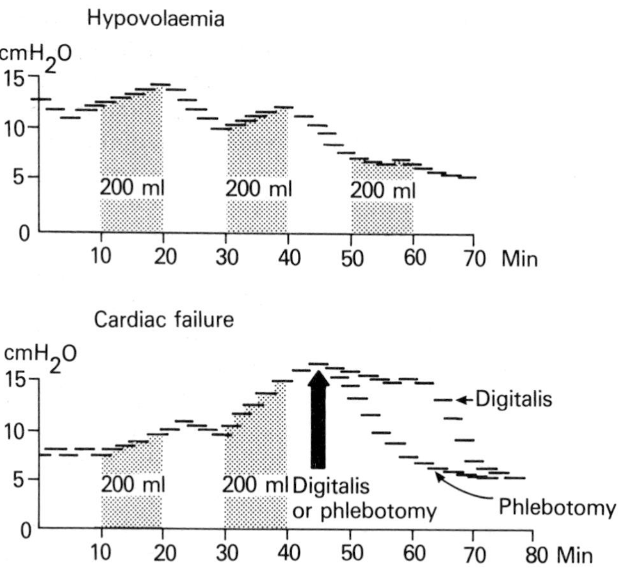

Fig. 3.17 Changes in central venous pressure with fluid replacement. Upper panel: hypovolaemia in a young patient. Lower panel: cardiac failure. See text for details.

measured more directly. This is achieved usually by floating into the pulmonary artery a balloon-tipped catheter which is then wedged in a branch (see Ch. 21). Since there is no flow through that segment of the pulmonary circulation, the pressure at the tip of the catheter (PCWP) equilibrates to a value close to LAP.

Cardiac output

The measurement of cardiac output is useful as part of an overall assessment of the circulation. Isolated measurements are of little value. For example, a cardiac output of 5 litres/min indicates excellent function after myocardial infarction but indicates failure in severe sepsis or major burns. Again, this measurement is most useful in assessing the response to therapy. The standard method of measurement is the Fick principle, namely that oxygen consumption ($\dot{V}_{O_2}$) equals the arteriovenous oxygen content difference $(A - V)C_{O2}$ multiplied by cardiac output ($\dot{Q}$).

$$\dot{Q} = \frac{\dot{V}_{O_2}}{(A - V)\ C_{O_2}} = \frac{250\ \text{ml/min}}{5\ \text{ml/dl}} = 5\ \text{litres/min}$$

This method is time-consuming and has been replaced in clinical use by thermal- or dye-dilution methods. The principal of these techniques is that a bolus of indicator is injected into blood entering the heart, where it mixes in the venous return. The concentration of indicator is measured downstream and plotted against time. As the mass of indicator is known, integration of the concentration curve may be used to derive the volume in which the indicator was distributed, the cardiac output. Cold glucose solution, the indicator in the thermal technique, is injected into the right atrium, and the decrease in blood temperature is sensed in the pulmonary artery by a thermistor, which is incorporated into a balloon-tipped catheter. Estimations may be repeated at frequent intervals.

Indocyanine green is the indicator used in the dye method. Sampling is usually from the radial artery through a detector cuvette. The initial dye has usually recirculated before the last dye has cleared the heart, thus obscuring the latter part of the decay curve. Modern cardiac output computers extrapolate from the first part of the curve, thus avoiding the problem of recirculation.

CARDIOVASCULAR RESPONSE TO DISEASE AND ANAESTHESIA

Hypovolaemia (Fig. 3.18)

Hypovolaemia is a common clinical problem. It is a result of imbalance between the blood volume and the capacity of the circulation and causes impaired tissue perfusion. It may be caused by loss of fluid, e.g. haemorrhage, or excessive vasodilatation, e.g. high spinal anaesthesia.

Loss of fluid reduces venous return, decreasing right atrial filling pressure and thus cardiac output. The resulting hypotension is countered by the baroreceptors, which increase heart rate and induce vaso- and venoconstriction. These measures maintain arterial pressure and minimise the decrease in cardiac output. Cardiac output is redistributed away from skin, muscles and viscera, and blood flow is maintained to heart and brain. Arterial pressure is maintained usually until approximately 20% of the blood volume is lost and cardiac output has diminished by 30%; thereafter it decreases progressively. Any drug which attenuates vasoconstriction or tachycardia, for example anaesthetic agents or β-blockers, results in earlier hypotension.

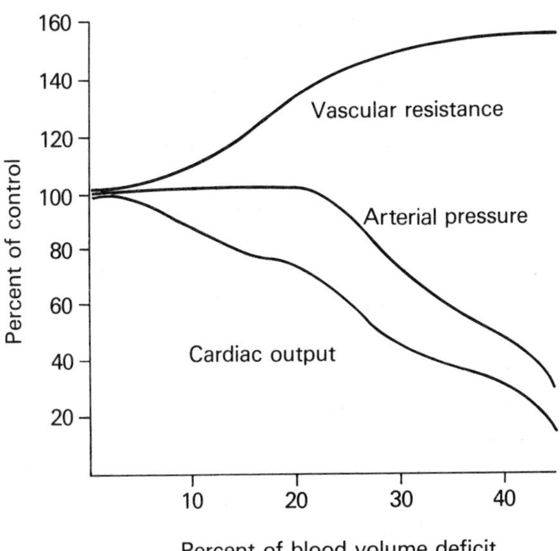

Fig. 3.18 Cardiovascular changes with progressive hypovolaemia.

Increased ADH and aldosterone secretion retain water and sodium, compensating for the fluid loss in the longer term. Reduction in capillary pressure results in translocation of fluid from the extracellular space into the circulation as a result of the oncotic pressure of plasma, further compensating for the hypovolaemia.

Severe or prolonged reduction in perfusion may lead to organ failure, for example renal failure. In addition, accumulation of tissue metabolites may result in local vasodilatation, overcoming the vasoconstriction and exacerbating the hypotension. This phase has been termed *'irreversible shock'* and represents clinically the phase when simple fluid replacement is inadequate to restore a normal circulation.

The initial management of hypovolaemia consists of replacement with the appropriate fluid. It is important that fluid is not given blindly but that a cycle of assessment, therapy, reassessment, further therapy and so on is initiated to ensure optimum replacement. This cycle is emphasised in Figure 3.19, which shows a suggested plan of management of circulatory failure.

Cardiac failure

The heart may fail as a pump for many reasons, e.g. ischaemia, trauma, drugs and sepsis. As the ventricles fail, stroke volume is reduced and baroreceptor activity increased. The resulting venoconstriction increases ventricular filling pressures and initial myocardial fibre length, and restores stroke volume towards normal. The reduced cardiac output results also in fluid retention. Eventually the myocardial fibres are unable to generate any further increase in contractility, and cardiac output diminishes rapidly. Venous pressures become so high that pulmonary and/or peripheral oedema occur.

Management of cardiac failure may be approached in three ways: optimisation of ventricular filling pressures, enhancement of contractility, and reduction of cardiac work. A reduction of filling pressure is necessary in most patients in right or left ventricular failure. This may be achieved by diuretics, venesection or venodilator drugs. Contractility may be enhanced by a variety

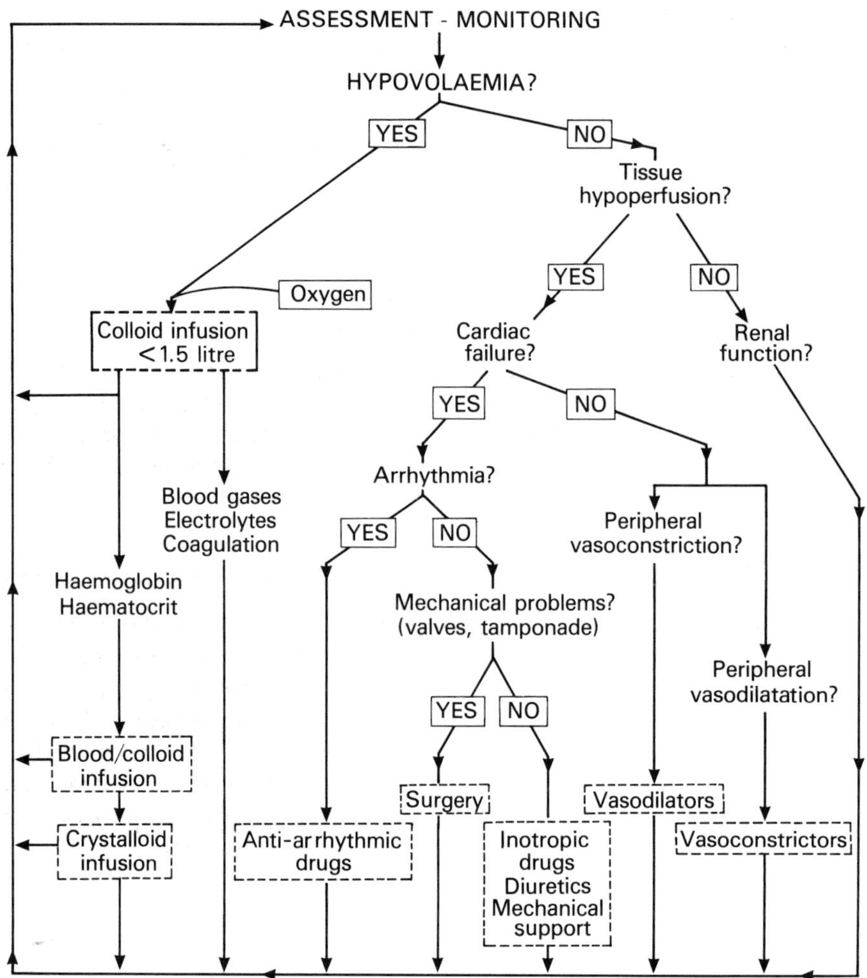

Fig. 3.19 Management of cardiovascular failure. The cycle of assessment, therapy and reassessment is emphasised.

of drugs (vide supra) but usually at the expense of increased myocardial oxygen consumption. Cardiac work is determined by the volume of blood pumped (cardiac output) and the resistance against which it is pumped (vascular resistance). The former is reduced already but reduction of the latter with vasodilators may enhance cardiac performance considerably. Such treatment must be given with care as excessive vasodilatation may result in severe hypotension and impairment of perfusion of vital organs. Filling pressures are often reduced by vasodilatation and may require adjustment.

Once again the need for a cycle of assessment therapy and reassessment is emphasised. Figure 3.16 shows the effect of various therapies on ventricular function.

Anaesthesia

All anaesthetic agents depress myocardial function in the isolated heart, but clinically the depressant effect may be countered or exacerbated so that the resultant effects on cardiac output may vary greatly (see Ch. 9).

Sympathetic activity

Ether, cyclopropane and ketamine increase sympathetic activity, with maintenance of cardiac output during light anaesthesia. In contrast, halothane and enflurane depress sympathetic activity leading to reduced contractility and peripheral vasodilatation. Halothane also enhances parasympathetic activity, resulting in bradycardia.

Ventilation

Artificial ventilation of the lungs may reduce venous return by increasing mean intrathoracic pressure. However, lighter planes of anaesthesia are usually used when IPPV is employed, and this may offset the reduction in cardiac output.

Changes in Pa_{CO_2} may have profound effects. Hypercapnia increases cardiac output by sympathetic stimulation and by peripheral vasodilatation. However, hypercapnia may induce ventricular arrhythmias in the presence of volatile anaesthetics, e.g. halothane. Hypocapnia induces peripheral vasoconstriction, increased vascular resistance and thus a reduction in cardiac output. Arterial pressure is usually maintained.

Surgical stimulation

Surgical stimulation results generally in increased sympathetic activity, counteracting the depressant effects of anaesthesia. Variations in arterial pressure with anaesthesia and surgical stimulation are often more pronounced in elderly or hypertensive patients. Some surgical stimuli, e.g. distension of viscera or traction on peritoneum, may induce vasodilatation and bradycardia, reducing arterial pressure and cardiac output.

Other drugs

Several drugs, e.g. opioids and muscle relaxants, cause peripheral vasodilatation by direct action on the vessels, histamine release or ganglion blockade. These actions may be unwelcome in some circumstances, while in others they may be used deliberately to induce arterial hypotension.

Subarachnoid and extradural anaesthesia

Subarachnoid and extradural anaesthesia block the sympathetic outflow and cause arteriolar and venous dilatation. Bradycardia results also if the cardiac fibres are involved ($T_1 - T_4$). In general, the circulation is well maintained provided that arterial pressure is prevented from decreasing excessively by the judicious use of volume replacement and vasopressors.

FURTHER READING

Braunwald E 1974 Regulation of the circulation (two parts). New England Journal of Medicine 290: 1124, 1420
Cohn J N, Franciosa J A 1977 Vasodilator therapy of cardiac failure. New England Journal of Medicine 297: 27
Gordon R J, Ravin M B, Daicoff G R 1979 Cardiovascular physiology for anaesthetists. Charles C Thomas, Springfield, Illinois
Guyton A C 1967 Regulation of cardiac output. New England Journal of Medicine 277: 805
Guyton A C 1981 The relationship of cardiac output and arterial pressure control. Circulation 64: 1079
Prys-Roberts C (ed) 1980 The circulation in anaesthesia. Blackwell Scientific Publications, Oxford
Rollason W N 1975 Electrocardiography for the Anaesthetist, 3rd edn. Blackwell Scientific Publications, Oxford
Scurr C, Feldman S (eds) 1982 Scientific foundations of anaesthesia, 3rd edn. Heinemann, London
Shimosato S 1981 Anesthesia and cardiac performance in health and disease. Charles C Thomas, Springfield, Illinois
Smith J J, Kampine J P 1980 Circulatory physiology — the essentials. Williams & Wilkins, Baltimore
Stuart J, Kenny M 1980 Blood rheology. Journal of Clinical Pathology 33: 417

4. Outlines of renal physiology

The kidney plays a vital role in maintaining homeostasis. It safeguards the stable internal environment necessary for each of the cellular components to function efficiently, despite a variable fluid and solute intake by the organism as a whole. Homeostasis is achieved by a combination of complex processes:

1. Excretion of the waste products of metabolism.
2. Production of hormones which influence other organs in the body.
3. Control of the extracellular fluid (ECF). This influences indirectly the intracellular composition in terms of volume, osmolality and acid–base status.

Before discussing the various components and functions of the kidney, it is necessary to consider briefly the body fluids and their compartments.

BODY FLUIDS AND COMPARTMENTS

Total body water in man is approximately 60% of total body weight, i.e. 42 litres of water for a 70 kg man. In females, total body water is approximately 10% less, because of the greater proportion of fat than in males; fat cells have a lower water content than other cells of the body. The water is distributed in various spaces or compartments.

Intracellular fluid

This is the largest water compartment in the body, representing two-thirds of total body water (approximately 28 litres).

Extracellular fluid

This constitutes the remaining one-third of total body water (14 litres) and may be subdivided further into two compartments:

1. Intravascular, i.e. within the plasma (4 litres).
2. Interstitial. This fluid (approximately 11 litres in volume) is outside the intravascular compartment and serves to 'bathe' individual cells.

The composition of the various fluids differs with the requirements of each compartment (Table 4.1). Sodium is the main cation in the extracellular compartment, whereas potassium is the principal cation of the intracellular compartment. This is achieved by the different permeability of cell membranes for some cations; the cell membrane is approximately 50 times more permeable to potassium than to sodium. Intracellular protein carries a negative charge which attracts the positively

Table 4.1 Composition and volume of body fluids according to compartment

	Intravascular (Plasma) 4 litres	Interstitial 10 litres	Intracellular 28 litres
Sodium (mmol/litre)	142	142	10
Potassium (mmol/litre)	5	5	150
Chloride (mmol/litre)	103	113	10
Bicarbonate (mmol/litre)	25	26	10
Protein (g/litre)	60–80	0	25
Osmolality (mosmol/kg H_2O	285	285	285

charged potassium ions. Most importantly, however, the sodium pump extrudes sodium actively from the cell in exchange for potassium with the use of the enzyme Na-K-ATPase.

The water content of plasma is 93%; the remainder comprises proteins, lipids and other large molecular weight substances. Therefore, the actual value for sodium concentration in intravascular water should be approximately 153 mmol/litre. In clinical practice, if the proportion of water is reduced, e.g. by large increases in protein, lipid or glucose concentration, the plasma sodium value is spuriously lowered; this is termed pseudohyponatraemia.

Cell membranes are permeable to water and there is a continual flux of fluid among the different body compartments at different rates of exchange. Two main mechanisms are responsible for these fluid shifts:

1. *Osmotic pressure*. Osmotic pressure is the pressure exerted by the number of particles in a solution. Osmolality, the usual term used in clinical practice, is defined as the number of milliosmoles per kg of water (mosmol/kg). Ions, being in greater abundance, exert a greater osmotic pressure. For example, 1 mmol of sodium chloride exerts an osmotic pressure of 2 mosmol, as each molecule is composed of 1 sodium and 1 chloride ion. Although of a larger molecular mass, proteins exert less osmotic pressure. Water moves freely across a semipermeable membrane and does so from an area of low osmolality to one of higher osmolality, i.e. the increase in osmotic pressure attracts water. This movement continues until the osmotic pressure is equal on both sides of the membrane. This mechanism is in effect between the intracellular and interstitial compartments. As shown in Table 4.1, the osmolality in the three compartments is identical. Any increase in intracellular osmolality increases water transport into the cell, thereby increasing its volume, and vice versa.

2. *Hydrostatic pressure*. This is the main mechanism for fluid movement across a capillary bed from the intravascular to the interstitial compartment. Figure 4.1 shows the various pressures exerted as the hydrostatic pressure decreases from 32 mmHg at the arterial end to 12 mmHg at the venous end of the capillary. The oncotic pressure exerted by plasma proteins represents a constant 'negative' pressure that draws fluid into the capillary. Thus, fluid moves out of the capillary at the arterial end and is withdrawn at the venous end. These hydrostatic pressures are known as Starling's forces. There is a small interstitial pressure, estimated to be approximately 2–5 mmHg, although it appears to have little or no effect on this mechanism unless the capillary, which may be damaged by some pathological process, leaks protein into the interstitium. If this occurs, then the interstitial pressure is increased and the existing balance of forces altered.

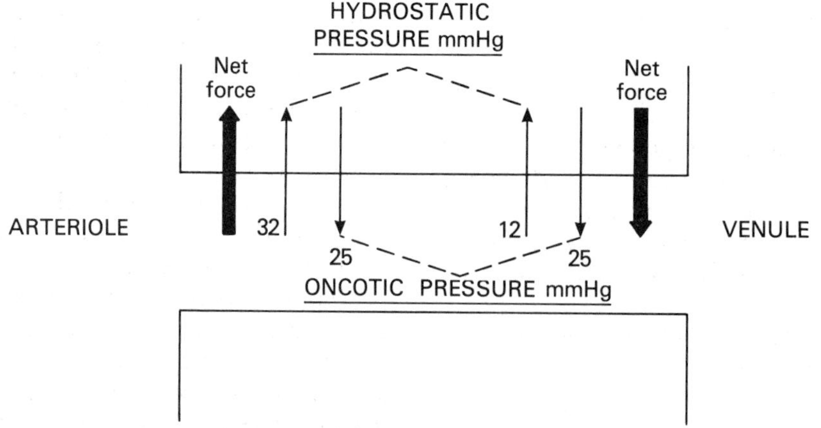

Fig. 4.1 Hydrostatic forces across a capillary wall (Starling's forces).

Renal blood flow

Before considering renal blood flow, it is necessary to understand the gross anatomy of the kidney. There are two populations of nephrons in the mammalian kidney:

1. *Cortical*. These nephrons (approximately 85% in man) lie within the cortex of the kidney and have short loops of Henle which dip only into the outer medulla.
2. *Juxtamedullary*. These nephrons, which constitute the remaining 15% in man, lie in the juxtamedullary area of the cortex, and are distinguished from their outer cortical neighbours by having long loops of Henle entering the inner medulla to participate in the diluting and concentrating mechanisms of the kidney.

The blood supply to the kidney is from the renal artery, which, having entered the renal pelvis, divides into a number of interlobar arteries. These further divide into the arcuate arteries and supply the small interlobular arteries from which the glomerular vessels arise. Each glomerulus is supplied by a single afferent arteriole which branches into a network throughout the glomerulus. It then reforms into a single vessel, the efferent arteriole. The efferent arteriole in turn forms branches around the proximal tubule (pars recta) and around the loop of Henle to form the vasa recta. It is possible for the efferent arteriole from one glomerulus to form the vasa recta of an adjacent tubule. The mesh of vessels then reforms into a single vessel which drains into the interlobular vein and thence to the renal vein.

Considering its size in relation to other organs of the body, the kidney is unique in receiving an extremely high blood flow (approximately 20–25% of cardiac output). This amounts to 500–600 ml/min to each kidney. Such a flow rate is necessary to carry sufficient oxygen for the high energy requirements of tubular processes, especially sodium reabsorption.

Renal plasma flow (RPF) may be measured using the Fick principle:

$$\text{RPF} = \frac{U_X V}{RA_X - RV_X}$$

where U_X = urine concentration of a substance x
V = urine volume
RA_X = renal artery concentration of the substance
RV_X = renal vein concentration of the substance

The commonest substance used is *para*-aminohippuric acid (PAH) which is cleared almost completely in one passage through the kidney. It is both filtered by the glomerulus and secreted by the renal tubule. In this instance, RV_X should be negligible and, as there is no extrarenal clearance of PAH, the expression may be modified as follows:

$$\text{RPF} = \frac{U_{PAH} V}{P_{PAH}} \text{ ml/min,}$$

where V = urine volume in ml/min
U_{PAH} = urine PAH concentration in mg/ml
P_{PAH} = plasma PAH concentration in mg/ml

Renal blood flow (RBF) may be calculated by adjusting the RPF for the haematocrit.

$$\text{RBF} = \frac{\text{RPF}}{1-\text{Hct}} \text{ ml/min,}$$

where Hct = haematocrit

As only 90% of PAH is extracted by the human kidney, the clearance of PAH (C_{PAH}) underestimates RPF by approximately 10%. In order to improve the accuracy of measurement it is possible to estimate RPF from the disappearance curve of intravenously injected ^{131}I-labelled PAH, eliminating the potential error introduced by timed urine collections.

The extrinsic control of RBF is influenced by the sympathetic nerve outflow from T4 to L2. Increases in sympathetic tone such as those produced by haemorrhage, shock, pain, cold or severe exercise produce vasoconstriction.

Some hormones (adrenaline, noradrenaline, antidiuretic hormone (vasopressin) in large non-pharmacological doses, serotonin and angiotensin) also reduce renal blood flow.

Within the kidney, RBF is redistributed to various anatomical areas. This has been demonstrated in animals using radioactive labelled tracers or microspheres and in man by the injection of radiolabelled inert agents (such as xenon or krypton) and measurement of their rate of disappearance over the kidney. From such studies in man, it has been shown that the cortex receives approximately 500 ml min^{-1} 100 g^{-1}, the outer medulla receives approximately 100 ml min^{-1} 100 g^{-1} and the inner medulla only 20 ml min^{-1} 100 g^{-1}. The lower medullary flow rate is necessary for the working of the counter-current mechanism.

There are two other properties that confer distinguishing features on the renal circulation. The first is that the mean glomerular capillary pressure is maintained at 45 mmHg, which is approximately 20 mmHg more than other capillary networks in the body. This is necessary for glomerular filtration (vide infra). The mean peritubular capillary pressure is only 15 mmHg and lower than intratubular pressure, thereby enhancing tubular reabsorption.

The second feature is autoregulation, which occurs in the cortex but not in the medulla and allows constant blood flow when renal perfusion pressure is altered. It is an intrinsic property of the renal vasculature, i.e. it is independent of nerves or hormones, and occurs over a range of systolic arterial pressure from 90–180 mmHg. Over this range glomerular filtration rate (GFR) parallels RPF, but glomerular filtration ceases when systolic arterial pressure decreases below 60 mmHg. The effects of autoregulation are achieved by changes in resistance in the afferent and efferent arterioles. When arterial pressure decreases, there is relative vasodilatation of the afferent arteriole and vasoconstriction of the efferent arteriole. This results in an increase in the fraction of plasma filtered (filtration fraction) and glomerular filtration is maintained. If arterial pressure increases, the vasoconstriction occurs in the afferent arteriole, with the opposite effects on filtration fraction.

The autoregulatory mechanism may be dampened by vasodilator drugs which act on smooth muscle vasculature, e.g. acetylcholine, dopamine, prostaglandins and the calcium channel blockers.

The exact mechanism of autoregulation is still a matter of debate. Originally it was believed to result either from mechanical factors, i.e. skimming of red blood cells and an increase in blood viscosity within the renal vasculature, or a response to overall increase in intrarenal pressure generated by changes in systemic arterial pressure. Current evidence now favours the 'myogenic theory' which states that the increase in smooth muscle contraction is produced by an increase in the intraluminal pressure, or in the tangential tension of the vascular wall. The role of locally generated vasoactive substances, e.g. angiotensin II, remains controversial.

Glomerular filtration

The process of glomerular filtration allows 180 litres/24 h or 120 ml/min of fluid and solutes to pass through the glomerular capillaries via the endothelial fenestrations, the glomerular capillary basement membrane and the pedicles of the podocyte into Bowman's space. The fluid which enters the proximal tubule from Bowman's space is an ultrafiltrate of plasma, i.e. it is virtually protein-free. Small amounts of albumin pass through the glomerular basement membrane but are reabsorbed almost entirely in the proximal tubule so that the final urinary concentration of albumin is less than 120 mg/24 h. The ease with which solutes pass through the glomerular basement membrane depends on their size, charge and possibly shape.

The filtering process is extremely efficient for substances of low molecular weight, i.e. the ratio of solute concentration between the plasma within the glomerular capillary and the fluid in Bowman's capsule is 1. As molecular weight increases, the amount of filtered solute decreases until a cut-off point at a molecular weight of 70 000 is reached, above which no further molecules pass. It should be noted that this range allows for a small quantity of albumin (molecular weight 69 000) to be filtered. The constituents of the glomerular basement membrane are mainly negatively charged sialoproteins which repel the negatively charged protein particles in plasma. It has been demonstrated that dextrans, with a molecular weight similar to some small proteins but with no charge, pass through the glomerular basement membrane 10–20% more efficiently. There is also some evidence that changes in molecular shape may facilitate the passage of some molecules through the membrane.

The forces required to drive glomerular filtration are similar to the Starling forces across capillary networks elsewhere in the body, although of a greater magnitude. The mean arterial pressure in the glomerular capillary is 45 mmHg compared with 20 mmHg elsewhere. As discussed previously, this is a result of the presence of a second resistance vessel, the efferent arteriole. Also, this pressure remains relatively constant over a wide range of systolic arterial pressure as a result of the process of autoregulation. Glomerular filtration rate (GFR) is a product of the forces driving filtration minus the forces opposing filtration and may be expressed thus:

$$\text{GFR} \propto (P_{\text{CAP}} + \pi_{\text{BC}}) - (P_{\text{BC}} + \pi_{\text{CAP}}),$$

where P_{CAP} = hydrostatic pressure in the glomerular capillary
P_{BC} = hydrostatic pressure in Bowman's capsule
π_{BC} = oncotic pressure in Bowman's capsule
π_{CAP} = oncotic pressure in glomerular capillary.

However, as π_{BC} is negligible, i.e. ultrafiltrate is virtually protein-free, the relationship may be rewritten:

$$\text{GFR} \propto P_{\text{CAP}} - P_{\text{BC}} - \pi_{\text{CAP}}$$

To convert this relationship into an equation, the sieving coefficient (K_f), i.e. the resistance to flow across the glomerular basement membrane, is introduced:

$$\text{GFR} = K_f\,(P_{\text{CAP}} - P_{\text{BC}} - \pi_{\text{CAP}})$$

Measurement of glomerular filtration rate

The measurement of GFR is one of the commonest assessments of renal function in clinical practice. It is measured by determining the clearance of a substance which is filtered by the glomerulus but not reabsorbed or secreted by the renal tubule. The polyfructose inulin (MW 5000) is such a substance. Using the standard clearance formula:

$$C_{\text{IN}} = \frac{U_{\text{IN}}\,V}{P_{\text{IN}}} = 120 \text{ ml/min}$$

where C_{IN} = inulin clearance in ml/min
U_{IN} = inulin concentration in urine (mg/ml)
P_{IN} = inulin concentration in plasma (mg/ml)
V = urine volume (ml/min)

There are two major disadvantages to this technique. Firstly, as inulin does not occur naturally in the body, it is necessary to infuse inulin intravenously to achieve a steady plasma level. To overcome this, it is customary to measure creatinine clearance using plasma creatinine, a product of muscle metabolism. There is a slight diurnal variation of plasma creatinine levels and creatinine is secreted by the renal tubules at very low GFRs; however, creatinine clearance values are adequate for clinical practice and relate reasonably closely to inulin clearance.

The other disadvantage is the accuracy of timed urine collections. As with measurement of RPF, it is possible to use a radioactive-labelled substance to measure GFR. Chromium-labelled ethylene diamine tetracetic acid (^{51}Cr-EDTA) is injected intravenously, and the disappearance rate calculated from blood samples obtained at two and four hours after injection. This avoids urine collection, may be standardised for body surface area (as should all measurements of GFR), and may be used as an accurate reference method.

Filtration fraction

Although RPF is quite large, only a proportion is filtered and that proportion is called the filtration fraction (FF). It is derived as follows:

$$\text{FF} = \frac{\text{GFR}}{\text{RPF}} = \frac{C_{\text{IN}}}{C_{\text{PAH}}} = \frac{120 \text{ ml/min}}{600 \text{ ml/min}} = 0.2\ (20\%)$$

FF may alter as a result of autoregulation. For example, if RBF decreases there is an increase in efferent arteriolar vasoconstriction and FF increases in order to maintain glomerular filtration.

Tubular function

The role of the renal tubule is to modify the volume and composition of the glomerular filtrate according to the needs of the organism. This is an enormous task. 180 litres of filtrate are produced per day and it is necessary to reduce this volume by 99% to achieve a final 24-h urine volume of approximately 1.8 litres. Similarly, approximately 25 000 mmol of sodium are filtered per day, the vast majority of this being reabsorbed to provide a urinary output of 100 to 200 mmol/24 h. In addition, the kidney conserves other filtered substances that are essential for the maintenance of homeostasis, e.g. glucose, bicarbonate, phosphate, etc. The renal tubule is responsible also for excretion of waste products of ingestion or metabolism, e.g. potassium, urea, creatinine, etc. The final regulation of acid–base status and of the concentration or dilution of the urine are also performed along the renal tubule.

Although each nephron acts as a single unit, it is possible, for ease of understanding, to divide tubular function into the individual portions of the tubule, i.e. proximal tubule, loop of Henle, distal tubule and collecting tubule. In simple terms, the proximal tubule may be considered the 'bulk reabsorber' and the remainder, the 'fine regulator' (Fig. 4.2).

Proximal tubule

In many ways, the proximal tubule is considered the bulk reabsorber as it is responsible for reducing the volume of glomerular filtrate by 80%. Seventy per cent of sodium and chloride, 90% of calcium, bicarbonate and magnesium, and 100% of glucose, phosphate and amino acids are reabsorbed during their passage through the proximal tubule. The fluid entering the proximal tubule from Bowman's space has a composition similar to that of plasma except for the absence of protein (Table 4.1). As the reabsorptive process is isosmotic, the osmolality remains identical at the beginning and end of the proximal tubule (290 mosmol/kg). The main ion to be reabsorbed in terms of concentration, energy requirements and its effect on other reabsorptive processes is sodium.

Sodium reabsorption. Sodium is reabsorbed through the proximal tubular cell both passively and actively.

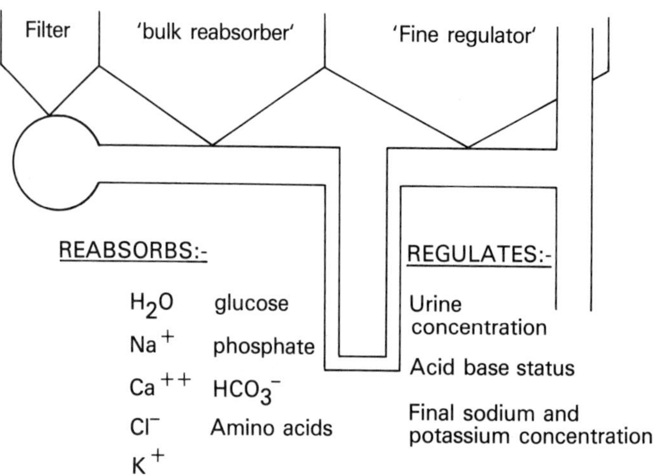

Fig. 4.2 Simple schema of tubular function.

Passive reabsorption. There are two forms of passive reabsorption for sodium:

1. Chemical. The intracellular sodium concentration in the proximal tubular cell is 30 mmol/litre. This is considerably less than the concentration of 140 mmol/litre in the tubular fluid. Sodium travels down the chemical gradient from the lumen to the cell.

2. Electrical. The potential difference within the tubular cell is −70 mV. This creates an electrical gradient for the positively charged sodium ions to travel from the lumen into the cell. Chloride, although negatively charged, travels with sodium in linked transport.

Active transport. Once sodium is within the cell it is pumped out (actively) in two directions. The first is into the intercellular space behind the so-called 'tight junction' (Fig. 4.3). This is an active energy-requiring pump which appears to be Na-K-ATPase independent. The effect of increased sodium concentration in the intercellular space is to increase the osmolality, and thus water passes from the cell into that space. The sodium and water within the intercellular space are then available for reabsorption by the peritubular capillary. In conditions of extracellular fluid expansion, the tight junction may open, and sodium flows together with water from the intercellular space into the tubular lumen (back flow).

There is a second sodium pump situated on the contraluminal surface of the tubular cell. This is an Na-K-ATPase-dependent pump which exchanges sodium for potassium. Potassium, however, is freely permeable through the cell wall and may diffuse passively out again into the peritubular space. Again, the sodium in the peritubular space is available for reabsorption into the peritubular capillary.

The movement of sodium, chloride and water into the peritubular capillary is governed by Starling's forces. The driving forces are hydrostatic pressure in the peritubular space and capillary oncotic pressure; the opposing forces are capillary hydrostatic pressure and oncotic pressure in the peritubular space. However, as peritubular space oncotic pressure is negligible, and the peritubular space hydrostatic pressure is small, the main

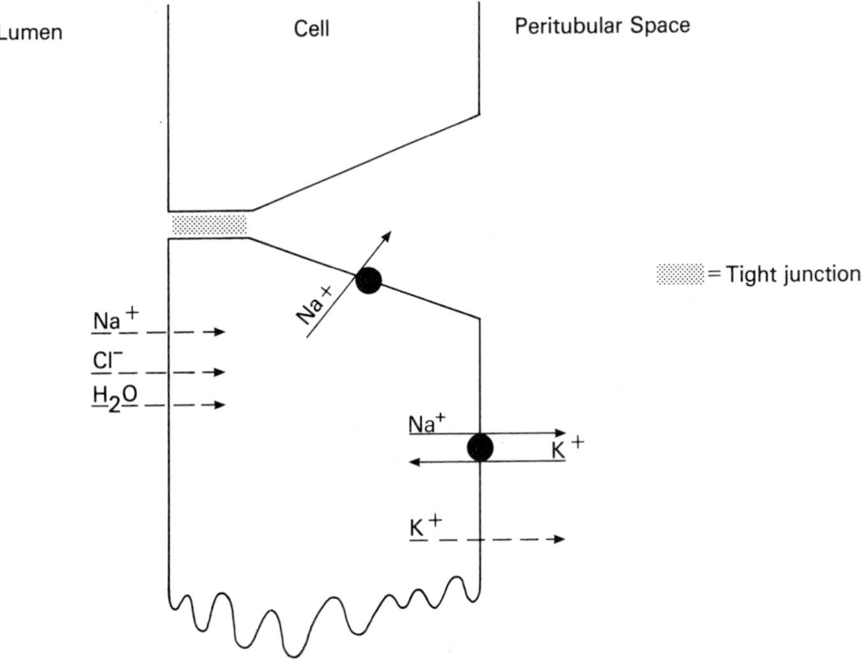

Fig. 4.3 Sodium transport through a proximal tubular cell.

controlling factor is peritubular oncotic pressure. The sodium, chloride and water which are not taken up into the peritubular capillary re-enter the tubular lumen via the tight junction, i.e. there is an increase in back flow.

Having described the mechanisms of sodium reabsorption within the proximal tubular cell it is necessary also to consider sodium reabsorption and excretion by the kidney as a whole. As previously stated, the daily fractional excretion of sodium (the amount of sodium excreted in the final urine relative to the filtered load of sodium) remains relatively constant at approximately 1–2%. Filtered load (expressed in mmol/min) is the product of GFR and plasma sodium concentration. However, the sodium intake varies, and various mechanisms are required to cope with states of relative hypo- and hypervolaemia. Three main mechanisms are responsible:

1. *Glomerulotubular balance*. Glomerular filtration rate remains relatively constant despite changes in systemic arterial pressure because of the autoregulatory mechanism. However, small changes in GFR produce large changes in the filtered load of sodium. When these occur, sodium reabsorption must alter in order to prevent large alterations in final sodium excretion. The anatomical arrangement of the peritubular capillaries, originating from the efferent arteriole, provides the ideal situation for a compensatory mechanism. When GFR decreases there is a decrease in filtration fraction. This reduces the normally occurring increase in peritubular capillary oncotic pressure which in turn decreases reabsorption of sodium, chloride and water from the peritubular space. Conversely, if GFR increases, there is an increase in filtration fraction, a greater increase in peritubular capillary oncotic pressure and enhanced reabsorption. This mechanism is known as 'glomerulotubular balance'.

2. *Aldosterone*. Aldosterone has its main site of action in the distal tubule and is considered later.

3. *Third factor*. It has been known for over 20 years that when blood of a volume-expanded animal is perfused into a normal animal, avoiding volume expansion in the recipient, there is a modest increase in fractional sodium excretion, despite unchanged renal haemodynamics. This phenomenon has been demonstrated in both isolated perfused kidneys and denervated kidneys and has led to the postulate that during volume expansion there is secretion of a so-called 'natriuretic factor' (see 'atrial natriuretic peptide', p. 74). The opposing view to the natriuretic factor is that all changes occurring during volume expansion may be explained by 'physical forces', e.g. changes in plasma proteins and therefore peritubular capillary oncotic pressure.

The possibility that redistribution of intrarenal blood flow exerts an influence on overall sodium balance has yet to be evaluated fully. It is known that in cardiac failure, when a state of positive sodium balance occurs from increased sodium reabsorption, blood flow is directed away from the short outer cortical nephrons (salt-losing) and directed to the longer juxtamedullary nephrons (salt-retaining). It is not known if a similar modified mechanism plays a significant role in daily sodium balance.

Rate-limited tubular transport

As shown in Figure 4.2, glucose, phosphate, bicarbonate and amino acids are reabsorbed almost totally in the proximal renal tubule. The mode of reabsorption differs from that described for sodium, chloride and water. The basic mechanism, as obtained in a titration study, is shown in Figure 4.4 using glucose as the example. During such a study the plasma glucose concentration is increased slowly, avoiding extracellular fluid volume expansion. Plasma and urinary glucose concentrations and GFR are measured. As the plasma glucose concentration increases, glucose appears in the urine when the point of the renal threshold for glucose has been reached. This occurs when the plasma glucose concentration is approximately 10 mmol/litre in man. The tubular reabsorption of glucose continues to increase with increments in plasma glucose concentration until a plateau is reached when no further increase in glucose reabsorption rate can be achieved despite an increase in the filtered load of glucose. At that point, the transport mechanisms for glucose reabsorption by the tubular cells have been saturated. Thereafter, glucose excretion increases in parallel

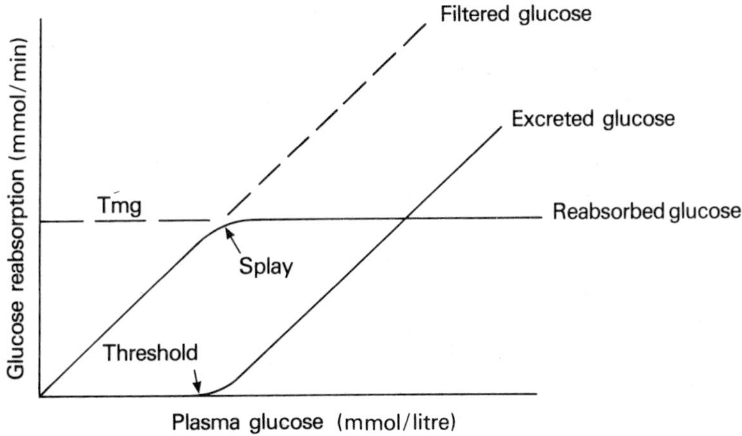

Fig. 4.4 The mechanism of glucose reabsorption in the proximal tubule.

with the filtered load of glucose as plasma glucose concentration increases. The 'plateau' at which maximal glucose reabsorption occurs is termed 'the tubular maximal reabsorption for glucose' (Tm_g). In man the value is 20 mmol/min. It should be noted from Figure 4.4 that the point at which glucose reabsorption reaches its maximum is not a fine 'cut off' but a small curve entitled 'splay'. Splay is caused by the heterogeneity of the nephron population in respect of glucose reabsorption. Some nephrons reabsorb maximally at a lower plasma glucose concentration than other nephrons within the kidney. A large splay is the cause of one type of renal glycosuria.

The same mechanism applies for phosphate reabsorption in the proximal tubule although this differs slightly from glucose in that the excretion of phosphate follows the filtered load more closely and the Tm for phosphate is much lower (0.125 mmol/min). The Tm for bicarbonate is approximately 3–3.5 mmol/min but may be altered by hydrogen ion secretion. There are five identified individual transport processes for the different groups of amino acids but their reabsorptive kinetics are similar to that of glucose. The reabsorption of sulphate in the proximal tubule follows a similar pattern. Many of the above substances share a cotransport system with sodium. It is known that when proximal tubular reabsorption of sodium decreases with an increased fractional excretion of sodium, Tm is decreased for glucose, phosphate and bicarbonate.

The mechanism of bicarbonate transport through the tubular cell (Fig. 4.5) is of particular importance because of its role in the renal regulation of acid-base balance. This mechanism may be summarised in three equations:

$$NaHCO_3 \rightleftharpoons Na^+ + HCO_3^- \qquad (1)$$

$$HCO_3^- + H^+ \rightleftharpoons H_2CO_3 \xrightleftharpoons[\text{ANHYDRASE}]{\text{CARBONIC}} H_2O + CO_2 \qquad (2)$$

$$H_2O + CO_2 \xrightleftharpoons[\text{ANHYDRASE}]{\text{CARBONIC}} H_2CO_3 \rightleftharpoons H^+ + HCO_3^- \qquad (3)$$

Bicarbonate enters the tubular lumen as sodium bicarbonate and dissociates into bicarbonate (a

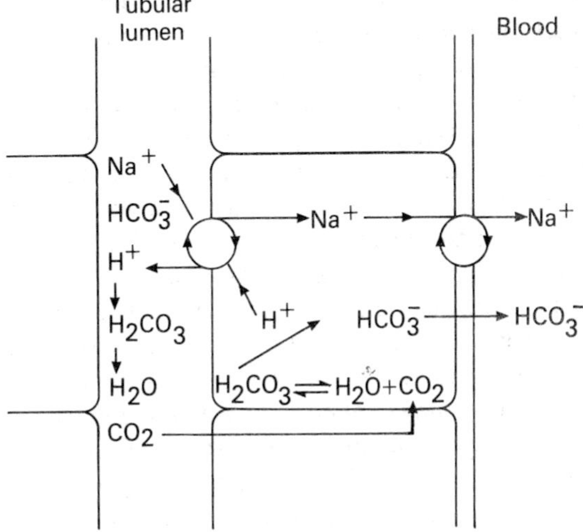

Fig. 4.5 Bicarbonate reabsorption in the proximal tubule.

relatively impermeable anion) and sodium (1). The sodium passes into the cell in exchange for a hydrogen ion. The hydrogen ion combines with bicarbonate in the tubular lumen to form carbonic acid. The enzyme carbonic anhydrase, present on the brush border of the proximal tubular cell, splits carbonic acid into carbon dioxide and water (2), both of which are freely permeable and enter the tubular cell. Here, intracellular carbonic anhydrase reforms carbonic acid which in turn dissociates into free hydrogen and bicarbonate ions (3). The bicarbonate ion passes through the basal cell membrane into the peritubular space and is available for reabsorption by the peritubular capillary. The hydrogen ion can be extruded from the cell in exchange for sodium and the cycle repeated. The enzyme carbonic anhydrase participates in both the dissociation and formation of carbonic acid depending on its site of action.

Another substance to be reabsorbed in the proximal tubule is uric acid. This is a small molecule which is filtered freely, and over 90% is reabsorbed in the proximal tubule. However, uric acid homeostasis is regulated by secretion of uric acid in the distal tubule. Another small molecule which is filtered freely is urea, and approximately 50% of the filtered load is reabsorbed passively in the proximal tubule, the remainder passing down into the distal tubule to participate in the osmolar regulatory mechanisms of the inner medulla.

In addition to hydrogen ions, some other substances such as organic acids and bases are secreted (i.e. moved from the peritubular capillary into the tubular lumen) in the proximal tubule. These include a number of drugs, e.g. penicillin, PAH. The secretory processes may be either active or passive and some have tubular maximal secretory capacities.

The loop of Henle, distal tubule and collecting tubule (Fig. 4.6)

The tubular fluid entering the loop of Henle is isosmotic and finally leaves the collecting duct as urine varying in volume, osmolality and composition according to the needs of the body. The fine

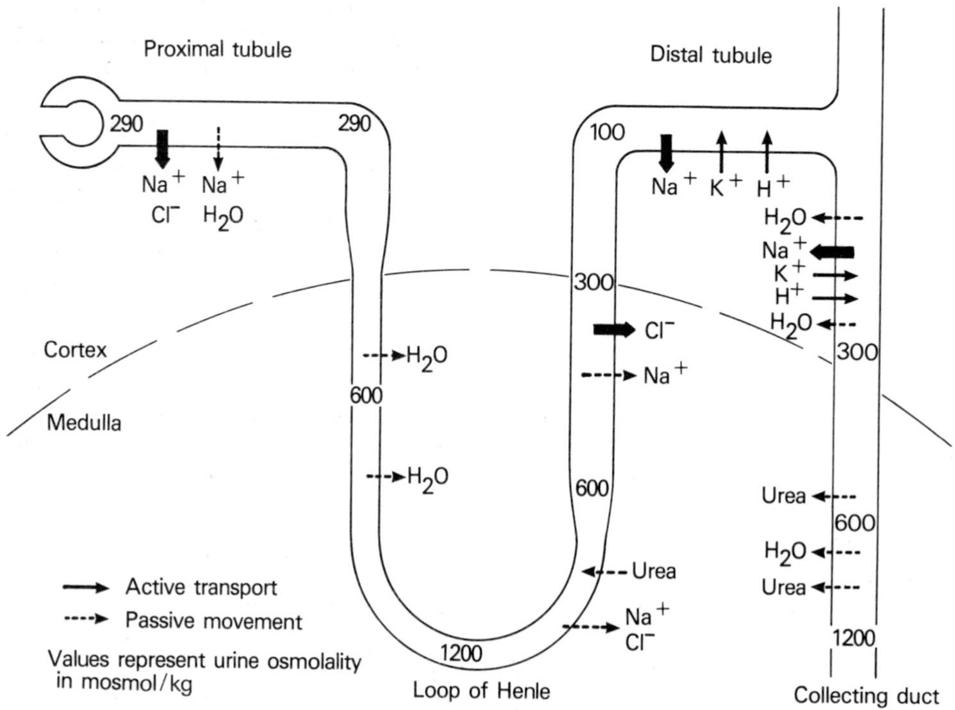

Fig. 4.6 Concentration of glomerular filtrate in the loop of Henle and collecting tubule.

regulatory mechanisms are situated in this portion of the nephron. The loops of Henle of the juxta-medullary nephrons dip deeply into the medulla whereas the collecting tubules of all nephrons pass through the medulla. There is an increase in osmolality from the cortex to the medulla; this is essential for the concentration and dilution of tubular fluid. The main mechanism for this is the counter-current multiplier situated in the loop of Henle (Fig. 4.6).

Counter-current mechanism

The loop of Henle consists of a thin descending limb, and a thin first part followed by thick upper part of the ascending limb. The volume of fluid entering the loop of Henle is approximately 15% of the glomerular filtrate and only one-third of this leaves the cortical part of the collecting tubule. The tubular fluid enters the loop with an osmolality of 290 mosmol/kg and leaves at 100 mosmol/kg. The loop is the active part (a counter-current multiplier) and the vasa recta surrounding the loop of Henle are the counter-current exchanger. Two main transport processes are responsible for the work of the counter-current mechanism:

1. *Sodium and water reabsorption*. The thick ascending part of the loop is impermeable to water but both sodium and chloride are transported into the interstitium. Although this is an active transport process there is much debate as to whether sodium or chloride is transported actively. Current opinion favours chloride, with sodium moving by a cotransport mechanism (see above). This results in an increase in the osmolality of the interstitium ranging from 300 mosmol/kg in the cortex to 1200 mosmol/kg at the tip of the loop. The descending limb is freely permeable to water, sodium and chloride, and all three move into the interstitium. Fluid enters the descending limb at an osmolality of 290 mosmol/kg and the osmolality increases slowly until it is equivalent to that at the tip of the loop, i.e. 1200 mosmol/kg. On passing up the ascending limb, sodium and chloride are removed but water is retained, and the osmolality decreases from 1200 to 100 mosmol/kg.

The vasa recta provide an important role in this osmolar transport. Although there is no active transport present in these vessels, water and solutes are freely permeable. The osmolality of blood entering the vasa recta is the same as that of the fluid entering the descending limb, i.e. 290 mosmol/kg and slowly increases to 1200 mosmol/kg as it passes down to the tip of the loop. This is achieved by the passage of water and solutes across its surface. The blood flow is significantly slower in the lower parts of the vasa recta, thus improving the efficiency of this exchange. As the vasa recta move from the medullary tip back towards the cortex, the same process occurs and the osmolality is returned to 290 mosmol/kg. As a consequence of the low flow rate in these vessels, oxygen content and energy requirements are markedly reduced.

2. *Urea recycling*. Urea, a waste product of protein metabolism, contributes up to 50% of the osmolality of the medullary interstitium. Because it is a small molecule it is filtered freely at the glomerulus and approximately half is reabsorbed during passage through the proximal tubule. As the tubular fluid passes down the descending limb the urea concentration is increased, firstly by the passage of water out of the descending limb, and secondly at the tip of the loop by the addition of urea, which moves freely from the medullary interstitium, an area of high urea concentration. The high concentration of urea at the tip of the medulla is achieved by the collecting tubule. The cortical part of the collecting tubule is impermeable to urea but permeable to water, resulting in an increase in urea concentration within the tubule. However, in the medullary portion of the collecting tubule, both water and urea pass into the interstitium. Hence, urea is recycled through the medulla and plays an important part in maintaining the high medullary osmolality essential for the counter-current mechanism.

Sodium-potassium exchange

More than 90% of filtered potassium is reabsorbed in the proximal tubule, and potassium which appears in the final urine is secreted in the distal tubule by a transport process coupled loosely to active sodium transport. As sodium is reabsorbed from the tubular lumen, a negative potential is created within the lumen which allows potassium to move passively down an electrochemical gradient. In this region, hydrogen ions are secreted also, and compete with potassium to a degree dependent on the acid–base status. The control of sodium reabsorption in the distal tubule is primarily hormonal and controlled probably via the renin–angiotensin system.

Renin–angiotensin system

The renin–angiotensin system is an important part of the complex mechanism responsible for controlling extracellular fluid volume, the other 'effector' parts being plasma proteins (vide supra) and osmolar control (vide infra). Renin is a proteolytic enzyme secreted from the juxtaglomerular apparatus situated in the afferent arteriole. The secretion of renin is a matter of some debate. It has been suggested that a baroreceptor mechanism situated in the afferent arteriole detects a decrease in renal blood flow and responds by increasing renin production. The alternative hypothesis is that changes in sodium concentration in the distal tubule are detected by the macula densa situated in the early part of the distal tubule, increases in sodium concentration causing an increase in renin secretion. However, there is conflicting evidence on this latter point. The renin acts on an α_2 plasma protein (angiotensinogen) and splits off a decapeptide, angiotensin I. A converting enzyme found both in plasma and various tissues of the body, including lung, converts angiotensin I to angiotensin II. This agent has three main actions. It is a potent vasopressor which may act on the glomerular arterioles and thereby contribute to glomerulotubular balance. It has a direct action on the brain, stimulating the thirst centre. Of most importance is its effect of stimulating secretion of aldosterone from the zona glomerulosa of the adrenal gland. Plasma aldosterone levels are affected also by the plasma potassium concentration, an increase in potassium reducing the aldosterone concentration. The converse occurs with plasma sodium concentration, i.e. a decrease in plasma sodium increases aldosterone. The main action of aldosterone is to increase sodium reabsorption in the distal tubule. Potassium and/or hydrogen ions are then secreted into the tubule in exchange for reabsorbed sodium. The renin–angiotensin system has its own feedback control, angiotensin II suppressing further secretion of renin.

Atrial natriuretic peptide (ANP)

In recent years, there has been great interest in a 28-amino acid peptide which is found in the atria of most mammalian species. The peptide is released in response to atrial stretching either by increased right or left atrial pressure or by an elevated central venous pressure. ANP has a dual effect on renal function. Firstly, it increases GFR by decreasing afferent arteriolar resistance and increasing efferent arteriolar resistance. Secondly, there are direct effects on tubular function, although these are more controversial. In essence, ANP produces a decrease in proximal tubular sodium reabsorption and an alteration in sodium handling in the ascending loop of Henle and in the inner medullary collecting tubule. The net effect of these alterations is a marked natriuresis accompanied by a diuresis with increased excretion of phosphate, magnesium, calcium and, to a lesser extent, potassium. In addition, ANP interacts with other renal hormones, decreasing renin and aldosterone secretion. Its final place in the control of extracellular fluid volume has yet to be established but it may occupy a pivotal role.

Renal regulation of acid–base balance

The distal tubule participates both qualitatively and quantitatively in acid–base control. As described previously the majority (up to 80%) of filtered bicarbonate is reabsorbed in the proximal tubule and the remainder by the distal tubule. The absorptive mechanism for bicarbonate reabsorption in the distal tubule is similar to that of the proximal tubule, namely the formation and dissociation of carbonic acid by the enzyme carbonic anhydrase. Conversely, although there is some hydrogen ion secretion in the proximal tubule, the bulk is secreted in the distal tubule.

Hydrogen ions are excreted in the final urine in

combination with either ammonia or phosphates. Approximately 60 mmol of hydrogen ions are excreted per day, of which two-thirds are combined with ammonia (NH_3) to form ammonium ion (NH_4^+) and one-third with sodium phosphate salts, often referred to as titratable acids (TA).

Ammonia (NH_3) is generated within the tubular cell mainly from the metabolism of the amino acid glutamine. When glutamine is converted to either glutamate or α-ketoglutarate, which enters the citric acid cycle, a free ammonia molecule is generated. This is freely permeable through the cell wall and passes down the concentration gradient into the tubular lumen. Here it combines with free hydrogen ions to form NH_4^+. This hydrophilic anion is unable to re-enter tubular cells and so is excreted in the urine.

The remaining one-third of hydrogen ions are excreted when combined with phosphate. Disodium hydrophosphate enters the distal tubule and dissociates. One sodium ion is reabsorbed, leaving a negatively charged molecule. The positive hydrogen ion in the tubular lumen combines to form sodium dihydrophosphate which is excreted in the final urine.

Hydrogen ions for both ammonium and TA formation come from intracellular dissociation of carbonic acid, and the net effect is the intracellular generation of a bicarbonate ion which passes through the basal border of the cell into the peritubular capillary. The amount of hydrogen ion secretion and bicarbonate regeneration depends predominantly on the acid–base status. The total hydrogen ion secretion may be expressed by the following formula:

$$\text{Total } H^+ \text{ excretion} = NH_4^+ \text{ excretion} + \text{TA excretion} - HCO_3^- \text{ excretion}$$

Osmolar regulation

By the time the glomerular filtrate enters the collecting tubule, its original volume has been reduced to 5% and when it leaves the collecting tubule it is reduced to 1%. Final urine volumes depend in part on the extracellular fluid volume and its regulation via sodium excretion, and in part on the regulation of plasma osmolality. The osmolar regulation system has a detector (osmoreceptors), a messenger (antidiuretic hormone ADH) and an effector (the collecting tubule).

The osmoreceptors situated in the hypothalamus detect changes in plasma osmolality, the major contribution being from plasma sodium. An increase in plasma osmolality stimulates the synthesis of ADH (vasopressin) in the supraoptic nuclei of the hypothalamus. The hormone is an octapeptide (8-arginine vasopressin) which passes along the nerve fibres to the posterior pituitary. After appropriate stimulation, the hormone is released from storage granules in the posterior pituitary and secreted into the systemic circulation. Its action on the peritubular cell membrane is to increase the permeability of water; this involves activation of the cylic 3′,5′-AMP system. Water is then reabsorbed from the collecting tubule and passes into the peritubular capillary to return the plasma osmolality to normal and reduce the urine volume. The reverse situation occurs if plasma osmolality decreases. ADH secretion ceases and the collecting tubule becomes impermeable to water; more water is excreted, urine volume increases and plasma osmolality increases towards normal levels. By this mechanism, it is possible that urine osmolality may vary from a hypotonic urine with a minimum value of approximately 60 mosmol/kg to a maximal value of 1200 to 1400 mosmol/kg. It should be noted that the final osmolality of hypertonic urine is equivalent to the tonicity at the tip of the renal medulla. ADH also increases the amount of urea reabsorbed in the cortical part of the collecting tubule, thereby contributing to the counter-current mechanism by increasing medullary tip osmolality.

It is possible to estimate the action of ADH by determining the amount of water excreted or reabsorbed compared with the amount of solutes excreted. Osmolar clearance (C_{osm}), an expression of solute excretion, is determined by using the standard clearance formula:

$$C_{osm} = \frac{U_{osm}\,V}{P_{osm}}$$

where U_{osm} = osmolar clearance in ml/min.
P_{osm} = plasma osmolality in mosmol/kg.
V = urine excretion rate in ml/min.

If urine is dilute, i.e. hypotonic, V is greater than C_{osm}. The difference is termed free water clearance (C_{H_2O}) and may be expressed as follows:

$$C_{H_2O} = V - C_{osm}$$

where C_{H_2O} = free water clearance in ml/min.

Conversely, if urine is concentrated, i.e. hypertonic, more water is reabsorbed and C_{osm} becomes greater than V. Free water clearance then becomes negative.

Another way of explaining negative free water clearance is to consider that water is being reabsorbed, i.e. solute-free water reabsorption, and may be expressed as follows:

$$V = C_{osm} - T^{c}_{H_2O}$$

$$\text{or, } T^{c}_{H_2O} = C_{osm} - V$$

where $T^{c}_{H_2O}$ = solute-free water reabsorption in ml/min.

By varying the amount of water reabsorbed in the collecting tubule and influencing the plasma sodium concentration it may be seen that osmolar regulation plays a vital part in controlling body fluid status. The two systems, i.e. osmolar regulation and volume regulation, are interrelated and in considering overall fluid balance it is not possible to dissociate the two.

In summary, the kidney plays a vital role in maintaining the 'milieu interieur'. It does so by variable adjustments of glomerular filtration rate, tubular reabsorption and secretion to produce a final urine which varies in volume, composition and acid–base status.

FURTHER READING

Bevan D R 1979 Renal function in anaesthesia and surgery. Academic Press, London

Davenport H W 1975 The ABC of acid-base chemistry, 6th edn. University of Chicago Press, Chicago

Lote C J 1987 Principles of renal physiology, 2nd edn. Croom Helm, London

5. Physiology of the nervous system

STRUCTURE AND FUNCTION

The function of the human nervous system is the acquisition of information from the external environment and its computation to produce an integrated response. The central nervous system (CNS) comprises the brain and spinal cord. The peripheral nervous system is composed of 43 pairs of nerves which contain afferent sensory fibres, conducting impulses to the central nervous system from the periphery, and efferent motor fibres conducting in the reverse direction. There are 10 000 000 000 neurones, each surrounded by neuroglial cells in the CNS. These cells are of two types:

1. Oligodendrocytes, which form myelin.
2. Microglia, which phagocytose degenerating neurones.

The physiology of the nervous system is related intimately to membrane physiology and cell excitation. Excitability results from specialisation of excitable cell membranes. The intracellular environment is controlled by cell membranes which exhibit selective permeability by virtue of membrane pumps. Excitable membranes undergo rapid reversible changes in permeability to some charged molecules or ions (i.e. to a specific stimulus). For example, at a pressure receptor the membrane ionic permeability alters as a response to mechanical deformation, and flow of ions occurs across the membrane.

A cell membrane is composed of lipids and protein (Fig. 5.1). Lipid forms the major part of the cell membrane, which may be considered as a lipid bilayer arranged such that a polar head is located on the outside of the cell membrane and 1–2 hydrocarbon chains, which are hydrophobic, constitute the inner part of the bilayer. Cell membrane proteins are composed of chains of amino acids with different side chains, either hydrophilic or hydrophobic, which by folding can 'hide' their hydrophobic amino acids on the interior.

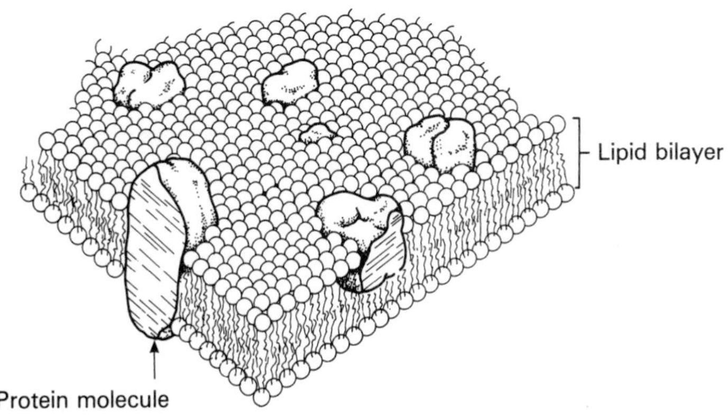

Fig. 5.1 Structure of the cell membrane.

A lipid bilayer is very *impermeable* to small ions; consequently, cell membrane permeability must reside in other structures, probably membrane proteins. The proteins confer specific ionic permeability on the membrane whilst only a small part of the membrane appears to be involved directly in ion flow.

Membrane protein as ion pump

Ion movement across a cell membrane occurs against the electrochemical gradient and is therefore active. Membrane proteins which achieve active transport are termed ion pumps. All cell membranes contain a sodium pump (Fig. 5.2). Ionic permeability is of two types:

1. Constant resting ionic permeability to ions including potassium (K^+) and chloride (Cl^-), which is not affected by physiological stimuli.
2. Non-constant permeability, which changes rapidly due to the action of a stimulus on an appropriate membrane protein.

Permeability is 'gated' by the stimulus. This is a feature characteristic of excitable membranes.

Several possibilities exist for the actual transport of an ion across the cell membrane. A protein may act as carrier and ferry the ion across, or it may span the bilayer and produce a pore (Fig. 5.3).

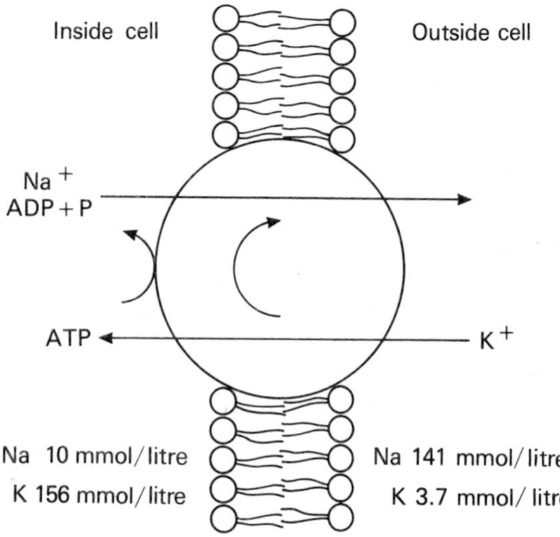

Fig. 5.2 The sodium pump.

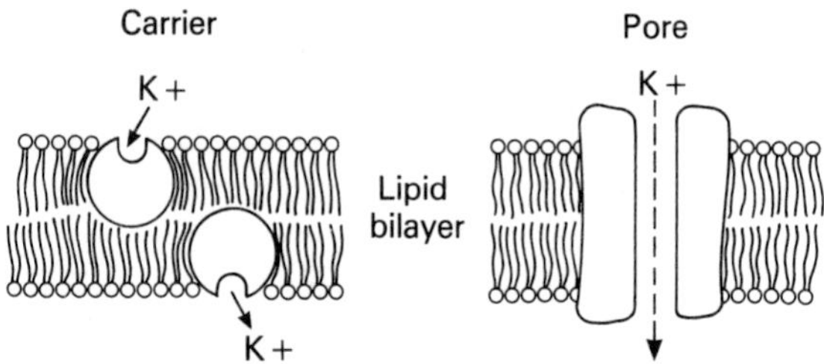

Fig. 5.3 Mechanisms of ion transport by proteins.

This latter mechanism produces much more rapid transport.

Electrochemical gradient

This is a measure of the force driving a specific ion into or out of the cell. It comprises an electrical component, which is the potential difference between the inside and outside of the cell (−60 mV). The chemical gradient is a simple concentration gradient. In certain conditions these two components may oppose and cancel each other out, at which point the ion is in electrochemical equilibrium across the membrane and the Nernst equation applies. This is dependent upon the unequal distribution of ions across membranes. If permeability to sodium (Na^+) and Cl^- are assumed to be zero at the resting potential of biological membranes, then

$$V = \frac{RT}{F} \log_e \frac{K_o^+}{K_i^+}$$

where:

V = potential difference
R = the gas constant
F = Faraday's constant
T = temperature
K_o^+ = concentration of K^+ in extracellular fluid
K_i^+ = concentration of K^+ in intracellular fluid

Nerve impulse and conduction

Characteristic changes in membrane potential on passage of a nerve impulse constitute an action potential. The passage of a stimulating current to this nerve axon produces first a stimulus artefact and then an action potential (Fig. 5.4).

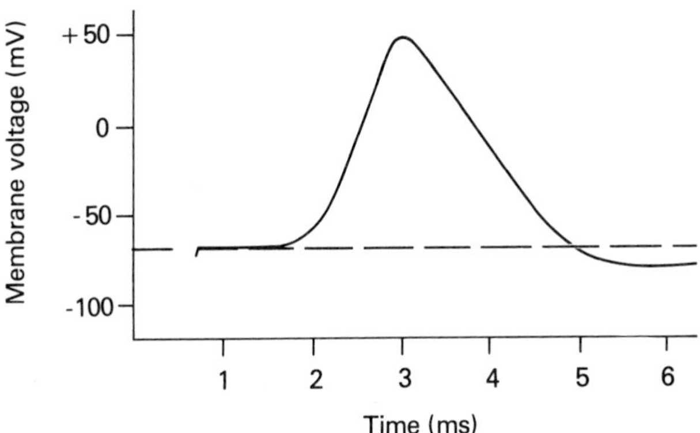

Fig. 5.4 The action potential.

Action potential. This is an all or none phenomenon. The least stimulus strength required to produce an action potential is termed the threshold stimulus. The transient reversal of the membrane potential propagates along an axon at constant velocity in a non-decremental manner. The refractory period is the period during which a second stimulating current does not elicit a second action potential. The absolute refractory period occurs immediately after the initial stimulus and lasts for approximately the same duration as the action potential itself. At this time, it is not possible to initiate a new impulse. Thereafter, the relative refractory period requires an increased threshold to initiate an impulse.

In the giant squid axon the resting membrane potential (−70 mV) is close to the Nernst potential for K^+ and results from selective permeability to K^+ in the axon membrane.

A change in resting potential is produced by changes in external and internal K^+ concentration.

The resting potential is the result of:

1. Ionic gradients produced by the sodium pump.
2. Selective permeability of the resting axon to K^+ with respect to Na^+.

As an action potential passes, the axon membrane becomes active and the membrane voltage is reversed from negative to positive. This corresponds to depolarisation with an overshoot to +40 mV. The action potential results from an increase in membrane *conductance* to Na^+, resulting in an increase in membrane potential towards the Nernst potential for Na^+. Thus, if the external Na^+ concentration decreases, the action potential becomes smaller in amplitude and eventually is reduced to zero. Selective block of Na^+ ion current can be produced experimentally with tetrodotoxin and of K^+ with tetraethylammonium. Such studies show that:

1. The sodium channel is opened rapidly by depolarisation of membrane voltage and closes slowly (inactivates) even if depolarisation is maintained. The open phase is always transient.
2. The potassium channel is opened slowly by depolarisation of the membrane and does not close during the short time scale of the action potential, i.e. there is late outward K^+ current whilst depolarisation is maintained.

A threshold stimulus produces an all-or-nothing response. The Na^+ channel is opened by membrane depolarisation; Na^+ ions pass through into the axon, to produce more depolarisation, thereby opening more channels and further increasing Na^+ ion influx and outward flux of K^+, which resists depolarisation. Na^+ channels do not open until the membrane voltage has changed by 20 mV from the resting potential. Inactivated Na^+ channels take a few milliseconds to become functional again and therefore are not opened again by immediate depolarisation. These are the underlying events of the refractory period. The increase in K^+ conductance always tends to increase K^+ ion current, which resists any change of membrane voltage away from the resting level.

Propagation of impulse (Fig. 5.5). Large axons have high conduction velocities. For fibres of a given diameter, conduction is increased greatly by myelination. Axons from 1 to 25 μm in diameter are myelinated; those less than 1 μm are non-myelinated. Nerve fibres have a structure akin to a shielded electrical cable, in other words a central conducting core with insulation and an external conducting area which is ECF. In vertebrate myelinated fibres, a Schwann cell lays down myelin in concentric layers. Between neighbouring segments of myelin there is a very narrow gap termed the node of Ranvier, which is less than 1 μm wide; here no obstacle exists between the axon membrane and the extracellular fluid. This accounts for conduction occurring in a saltatory manner. The myelin sheaths act as high-resistance barriers to current flow and excitation occurs only at the nodes of Ranvier. Thus, the impulse is propagated from node to node. The events are summarised in Table 5.1.

Table 5.1 Summary of nerve impulse propagation

1. Resting membrane has a low ionic permeability; therefore electrochemical gradients are not readily dissipated
2. Membrane contains a sodium pump which requires ATP for energy to create and maintain ion concentration gradients
3. The resting membrane is selectively permeable to K^+, so a resting potential of −70 mV is set up, which is close to the Nernst equilibrium potential for potassium
4. Two types of gated ion channel exist within the membrane, which are opened or closed by changes in the membrane voltage.

Repetitive stimulation of nerve fibres induces an increase in their size. This is the basis of experimental spinal cord stimulation techniques in the treatment of conditions such as chronic pain, and in patients with multiple sclerosis and bladder dysfunction.

The synapse

A synapse occurs where the membranes of two excitable cells are apposed closely and allows transmission of information. The transmitter is usually chemical, is released in a controlled amount by the cell, and diffuses rapidly to bind to a receptor site on the second cell, where it produces rapid changes in ion flux. Presynaptic fibres divide into numerous fine branches, producing presynaptic knobs. A single anterior horn cell may receive 30 000 knobs from a large number of axons. The presynaptic membrane releases transmitter from dense, spherical synaptic vesicles (50 nm diameter) into a synaptic cleft of some 20–25 nm to the postsynaptic membrane (Fig. 5.6).

Transmission of impulses across a synapse is strictly unidirectional (in a nerve it is bidirectional) and involves a time delay. In the spinal motor neurone this amounts to 0.4 ms. A knowledge of total delay in a reflex pathway is useful in determining the number of synapses involved. Synapses operate in a graded fashion which allows the neurone to carry out integration and sifting of

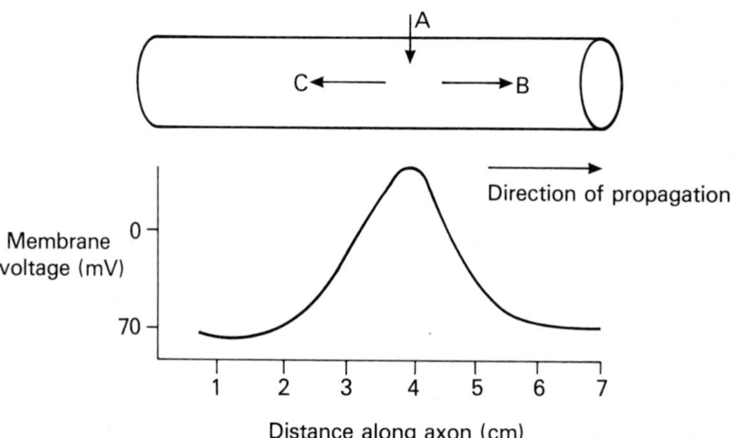

Fig. 5.5 Local circuit theory of impulse propagation. A = influx of Na^+ ions at active membrane. B, C = current flow. B propagates the impulse. C finds the membrane refractory.

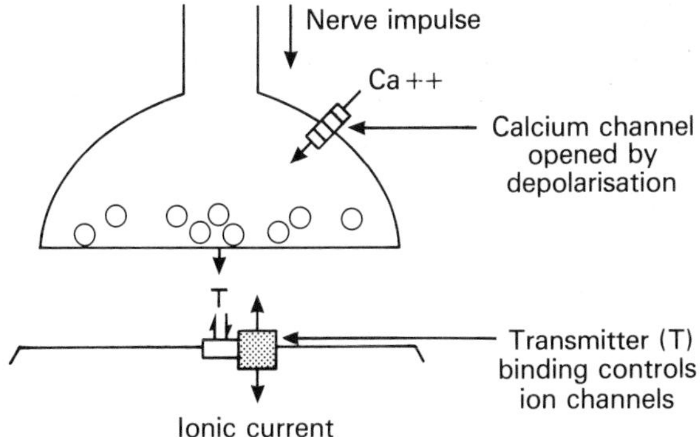

Fig. 5.6 Chemical synapse transmission.

information. Enzymes break down the transmitter released, thereby reducing its duration of action at the postsynaptic membrane.

Control of transmitter release

The arrival of an action potential produces depolarisation of the terminal membrane, which opens voltage-sensitive calcium (Ca^{2+}) ion channels, resulting in flux of Ca^{2+} into presynaptic areas. This in turn stimulates transient exocytosis of the transmitter into the synaptic gap, where it diffuses rapidly to specific protein binding sites (receptors) on the postsynaptic membrane. Ionic currents through these sites then alter the membrane potential of the postsynaptic cell in a direction determined by the ion selectivity of the channels concerned. Depolarisation causes excitation, and hyperpolarisation inhibition. When nerve terminal Ca^{2+} is increased, 100 vesicles are released within 1 ms. The postsynaptic membrane channels are gated by specific chemical stimuli. In the absence of nerve stimulation, miniature end-plate potentials (MEPP) may be recorded; these are produced by arrival of single transmitter vesicles. A propagative end-plate potential requires 100 transmitter vesicles. For example, at the neuromuscular junction 1 impulse produces 100 vesicles, each containing 50 000 molecules of acetylcholine (ACh). Of the 5 000 000 transmitter molecules released, only 100 000 open a postsynaptic channel, but this is sufficient to cause 10 000 000 000 Na^+ ions to enter muscle in 1 ms. Both excitatory and inhibitory postsynaptic potentials can be recorded intracellularly. Presynaptic inhibition may also occur from inhibitory terminals situated on excitatory presynaptic nerve endings; stimulation of these terminals reduces the amount of neurotransmitter released.

It is well known that antibiotics may interfere with neuromuscular conduction, often by decreasing end-plate transmitter. High concentrations of Mg^{2+} and some antibiotics decrease evoked release of ACh mainly by competition for Ca^{2+} binding sites on the nerve terminal. Postjunctional effects include receptor or end-plate ion channel blockade. There is considerable variability between antibiotics in their neuromuscular blocking mechanisms. Aminoglycosides, polymyxin and tetracyclines produce neuromuscular block by a combination of pre- and postjunctional effects.

Information processing by nerve networks shows:

1. Spatial summation. This occurs when stimulation of two afferent nerves together produces a response which neither alone can elicit. Both synapses may be excitatory for that particular nerve.
2. Temporal summation. Stimulation of the same nerve twice in rapid succession produces a response where a single stimulus elicits none.

There are also electrical synapses, e.g. in the retina, and synapses where transmitter release is controlled by graded depolarisations. There is, in fact, an immense variety of types of synapse between different classes of cell which use different transmitters and different polysynaptic channels.

Neurotransmitters

The number of putative central nervous system transmitters now exceeds 40. They comprise three main types (amino acids, monoamines and peptides), which are present in widely differing concentrations. This suggests that synaptic transmission is more complex than simple transfer of excitation or inhibition from presynaptic neurone to the postsynaptic cell. There is a great range of synaptic connections and the possibility of chemical coding exists. It is already known that axo-axonal synapses may regulate the amount of transmitter released from presynaptic terminals;

other inputs may trigger very long-lasting post-synaptic events (lasting for minutes) and therefore control the excitability of a target cell, rather than directly controlling its firing.

Fast chemical signalling in the central nervous system. This is the function of amino acid transmitters:

1. *γ-amino butyric acid (GABA).* This transmitter occurs in all regions of the brain and spinal cord, mainly in local inhibitory interneurones. GABA rapidly inhibits virtually all CNS neurones when applied locally by virtue of increased cell permeability to chloride ions, thereby stabilising the membrane potential at or near the chloride equilibrium level. Most of these responses are mediated by GABA receptors. GABA may be used by as many as one-third of all synapses in the mammalian brain.
2. *Glycine.* This amino acid predominates as the inhibitory transmitter in the spinal cord.
3. *L-Glutamate and L-aspartate.* These produce excitatory depolarisation by activating membrane sodium channels.

Diffuse regulatory systems: monoamines. These are associated with diffuse neural pathways, mainly in the brain stem. Much of the monoamine release may be at nonsynaptic sites.

Neuropeptides. Virtually all peptide hormones of the endocrine and neuroendocrine systems also exist in distinct systems of the central nervous system. Active peptides released from endocrine and neural tissue are called regulatory peptides. They are capable of producing an effect by acting as hormones, local regulators or neurotransmitters, or a combination of all these. Vasoactive intestinal peptide (VIP), which acts as a neurotransmitter, is one example. Enteric nerves containing peptides belong to a non-adrenergic, non-cholinergic subdivision of the autonomic nervous system. The spinal cord contains a very large number of regulatory peptides, including substance P, VIP, enkephalin and neuropeptide Y.

Membrane receptor function in anaesthesia

Most hormones and drugs produce effects by binding to cell recognition sites termed receptors. A receptor is an integral membrane protein which is recognised selectively by a precise hormone or neurotransmitter termed a ligand (Fig. 5.7). A ligand is an agonist if it activates a receptor to transduce a response, or an antagonist when the substance interacts with a receptor causing it to remain inactive and, by occupying the receptor, diminishes or aborts the effect of an agonist. The interaction between ligand and receptor is specific, reversible, saturable and a high-affinity binding process. Binding is followed by alterations in metabolic events within the cell, e.g. ion flux, which produce the characteristic physiological effect. Regulation of the concentration of receptors in the cell membrane constitutes an important mechanism of receptor regulation. A second is coupling to the effector mechanism.

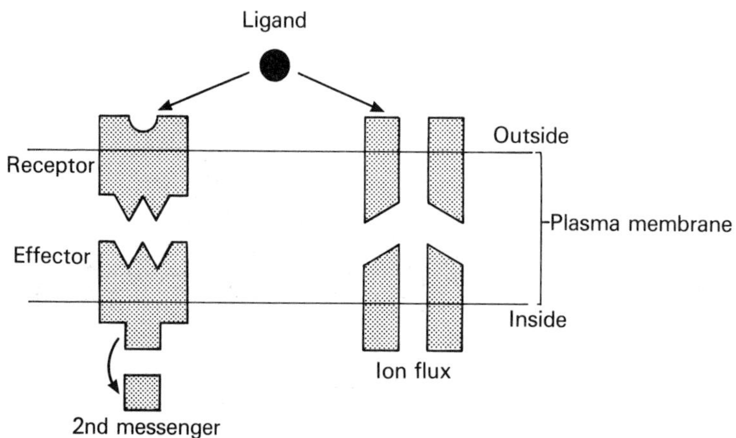

Fig. 5.7 Receptor–effector mechanisms: release of second messenger or promotion of ion flux.

Receptor types have been purified in recent years using affinity chromatography, photoaffinity labelling and radioligand techniques. Positron emission tomography allows quantitative imaging of muscarinic, cholinergic, opioid and benzodiazepine receptors. Radioactive tracer molecules (produced by a cyclotron) are incorporated into substrates such as glucose or into a drug, and become bound to receptors. Serial images can be obtained from different areas of the brain. Such techniques allow measurement of regional oxygen metabolism, permit better management in schizophrenia or drug addiction, assist the differential diagnosis of coma and are useful in cases of epilepsy if surgery is being considered.

Adrenergic receptors. Agonists at β-adrenoceptors in order of potency include: isoprenaline, adrenaline, noradrenaline and dopamine. β_1-Receptors are found in the heart and are equally sensitive to adrenaline and noradrenaline. β_2-Receptors are found in smooth muscle and are more sensitive to adrenaline than noradrenaline. The effects are mediated by intracellular cyclic AMP (cAMP), the second messenger, which activates protein kinases (Fig. 5.8). Thus the β-adrenergic agonist receptor complex diffuses laterally until it couples to adenylate cyclase (the effector molecule) which is then activated and catalyses synthesis of cAMP; this is hydrolysed subsequently by phosphodiesterase.

α-Adrenoceptors mediate control of smooth muscle in the vasculature of the uterus and gastrointestinal tract. The order of potency of agonists is: adrenaline, noradrenaline, isoprenaline. There are two classes of α-receptor (Fig. 5.9); α_1 are postsynaptic and mediate constriction

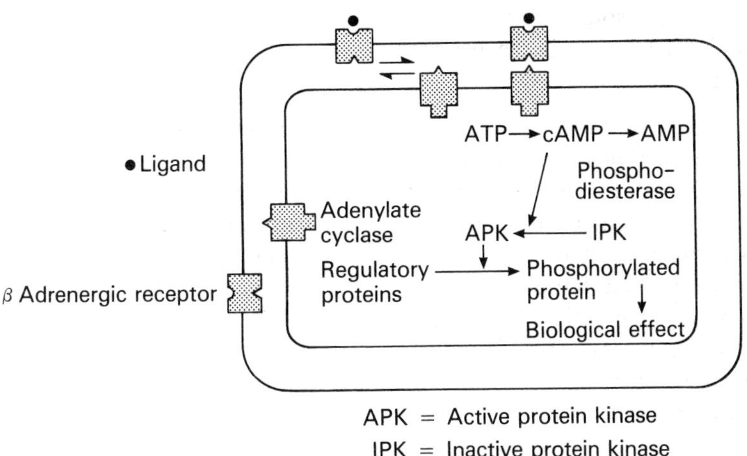

Fig. 5.8 β-Adrenergic receptor.

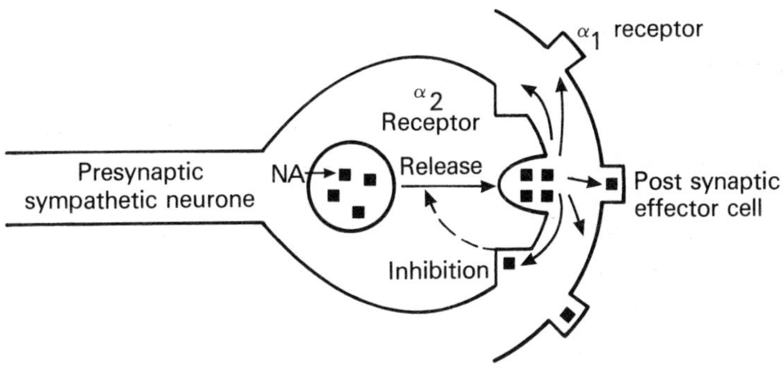

Fig. 5.9 Types of α-adrenergic receptors. NA = noradrenaline.

of smooth muscle. These are blocked selectively by prazosin and phenoxybenzamine. α_2-Receptors are presynaptic and mediate feedback inhibition by noradrenaline of further neurotransmitter release. These are blocked selectively by yohimbine. α_2-Receptors are found also on platelets where they mediate aggregation. Methoxamine and phenylephrine are selective α_1 agonists and clonidine is an α_2 agonist.

Within the CNS, adrenaline is found in small groups of cells in the pons and medulla which project to the hypothalamus and brain stem and to the nucleus tractus solitarius, which may be important in central arterial pressure control. Noradrenaline is found in all areas of the brain and spinal cord, with a high density in the hypothalamus.

Circulating plasma concentrations of noradrenaline are increased in patients with congestive cardiac failure and provide a guide to prognosis. Alpha and β-receptor agonists and antagonists are used widely in acute medicine.

Dopamine receptors. Dopamine receptors occur in basal ganglia, substantia nigra, corpus striatum and the limbic system. In the basal ganglia, dopamine is antagonistic to acetylcholine. Absence of dopamine is an important aetiological factor in Parkinsonism. In the hypothalamus, dopamine is concerned with release of prolactin. Dopamine suppresses prolactin secretion and dopamine antagonists, e.g. metoclopramide, increase hyperprolactinaemia.

A dopaminergic system connects the limbic cortex, basal ganglia and hypothalamus and is concerned with behaviour. This system is involved in the pathogenesis of schizophrenia (phenothiazines block dopamine receptors). Dopaminergic fibres are found in the chemoreceptor trigger zone; stimulation produces nausea and vomiting. Dopaminergic and sympathomimetic receptors have been identified in the coronary, renal, cerebral and mesenteric vessels. Dopamine receptors occur also on the presynaptic membrane of postganglionic sympathetic nerves and sympathetic ganglia where their physiological role is unclear.

Acetylcholine (ACh). This substance is found in motor neurones of the spinal cord and cranial nerve motor nuclei, where it acts as a *fast* chemical transmitter for neuromuscular transmission. In intrinsic pathways in the CNS, it probably acts as a modulator in basal ganglia, the hippocampus, and the diffuse ascending pathways to the cortex, and may represent what was known as the ascending reticular activating system. ACh probably plays an important part in cortical arousal and EEG changes of rapid eye movement (REM) sleep. The effects of ACh are terminated by hydrolysis by cholinesterase. Its peripheral effects may be classified into:

1. Muscarinic effects at postganglionic parasympathetic fibres.
2. Nicotinic effects at sympathetic and parasympathetic ganglia and the neuromuscular junction.

Muscarinic cholinergic receptors in the intestine stimulate electrolyte transport, whilst nicotinic agonists augment absorption. Tetrodotoxin is a potent neurotoxin which has been used experimentally to elucidate the interactions between neurotransmitters and nicotinic agonists. Muscarinic agonists alter electrolyte transport by acting directly on the enterocyte, whereas nicotinic agonists act indirectly by stimulating intermediary neurotransmitters. Such findings emphasise the increasing complexity of receptor and transmitter science.

Denervation of skeletal muscle enhances its sensitivity to ACh by development of a diffuse distribution of ACh receptors over postjunctional surfaces. Administration of suxamethonium in these circumstances results in severe hyperkalaemia.

Histamine receptors. H_1-receptors are responsible for contraction of smooth muscle (e.g. in the gut, and bronchi). H_2-receptors stimulate acid secretion by the stomach and increase heart rate. These effects are not prevented by H_1-antihistamines, but by H_2-receptor blockers, e.g. cimetidine and ranitidine. The vascular effects of histamine are mediated by both types of receptor. In some instances, H_1 and H_2 have opposing actions, e.g. H_1 produces pulmonary vasoconstriction, H_2 pulmonary vasodilatation. Both H_1 and H_2 and perhaps other receptors exist in the brain.

5-Hydroxytryptamine (5-HT, serotonin). This has been isolated from the brain stem, many forebrain sites and the dorsal horns of the spinal cord. It may represent one of the descending control pathways which modulate sensitivity of the spinal cord to pain input from the periphery, and therefore plays a key role in mediating analgesic actions of morphine and related opioid analgesics. In the forebrain, this system may be responsible for control of sleep and waking, central temperature regulation and control of aggressive behaviour.

Benzodiazepines. Although not endogenous substances, these drugs act at specific synapses in the CNS (including the spinal cord) at which GABA is the transmitter. Benzodiazepines selectively facilitate GABA action at synapses. Aminophylline may reverse diazepam sedation by its adenosine-blocking effect at GABA receptors. Adenosine is as potent a CNS depressant mediator as GABA, and may have an amplifying effect on the GABA receptor complex. Benzodiazepine antagonists are now available, e.g. flumazenil.

Neurotransmitters in disease

Increasingly, neurotransmitters are found to be concerned with disease states. *Anxiety* probably involves many neurotransmitters, e.g. GABA, serotonin, noradrenaline and dopamine. Benzodiazepines exert their effects via a GABA/benzodiazepine-receptor/chloride channel complex (Fig. 5.10), which may also mediate anxiety, and which is enclosed in the lipid bilayer of cell membranes. There are strong indications that central monoamine metabolism is disturbed in *endogenous depression*, and that the disturbance is causal.

Tricyclic antidepressants inhibit the presynaptic uptake of 5-HT and noradrenaline (Fig. 5.11). Research continues on the monoamine precursors, selective uptake inhibitors and postsynaptic agonists, and on the relationships between 5-HT, catecholamines and endocrine dysfunction.

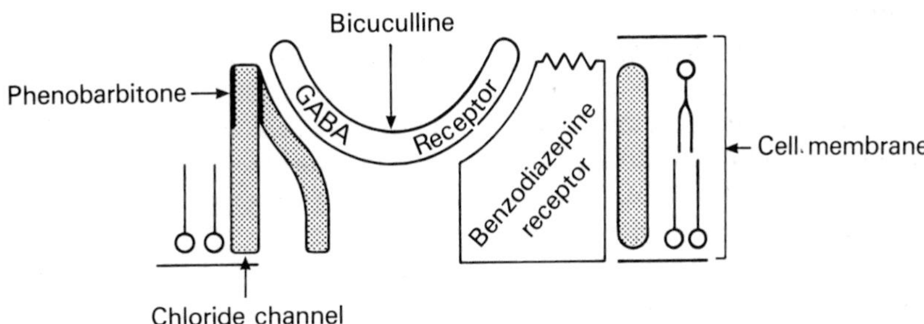

Fig. 5.10 GABA receptor, benzodiazepine receptor and chloride channel.

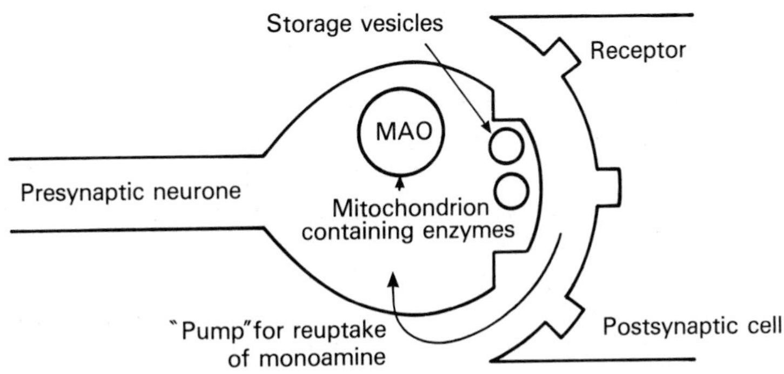

Fig. 5.11 Tricyclic antidepressants inhibit presynaptic uptake of 5-HT and noradrenaline. MAO = monoamine oxidase.

In patients with *affective disorders*, cholinergic receptor density is increased. All antidepressants facilitate synaptic activity of amines; however, tricyclic antidepressants block cholinergic receptors. The anticholinesterase physostigmine can relieve manic symptoms.

In *schizophrenia*, catecholamine activity may worsen symptoms. Neuroleptic drugs administered in small doses dramatically reverse amphetamine-induced psychoses; amphetamine induces schizophrenic exacerbations. This provides further support for the concept of a dopaminergic abnormality in schizophrenia. Some symptoms of schizophrenia are reduced by naloxone, suggesting that opioid peptides, e.g. enkephalins, are involved, although naloxone also blocks GABA receptors. The brain of patients who have died with *Alzheimer's disease* contains reduced concentrations of choline acetyltransferase, noradrenaline, GABA and somatostatin, although the most severe abnormality is a cholinergic deficit.

Epilepsy. A binding site for phenytoin, which interacts with the GABA/chloride inophore benzodiazepine complex and an endogenous compound which binds to this site have been isolated from the brain. It is thought that one or more components of the GABA inhibitory system may be concerned with maintenance of a normal state (Fig. 5.12). It may be that in epilepsy there is a lower threshold for seizure, but inhibitory systems within the brain terminate the seizure. Drugs which increase GABA in the CNS are useful in the control of epilepsy.

Hepatic encephalopathy. This may result from increased concentrations of false neurotransmitters such as octopamine and serotonin, which replace the normal dopamine and noradrenaline. GABA is produced in the gut by bacterial action on protein and may lead to coma by passing through the blood–brain barrier in liver failure. The number of binding sites for GABA, glycine and benzodiazepines on postsynaptic neurones is increased in acute liver failure; present data suggest that this mechanism is the most important contributor to hepatic encephalopathy. The benzodiazepine antagonists reverse hepatic encephalopathy temporarily. The hypersensitivity to benzodiazepines in patients with hepatic encephalopathy may be explained by an increase in the free drug concentration.

Asthma. In this condition, there is a reduced β-adrenergic, and increased cholinergic and α-adrenergic, responsiveness.

Generally, treatment of disease states with agonists produces alterations in receptor density and desensitisation, mediated probably via cyclic AMP. In the case of β-adrenergic receptors, this is effected by phosphorylation. Abrupt discontinuation of a β-blocking drug such as propranolol may produce hypersensitivity to catecholamines, and may precipitate angina or myocardial infarction.

Many intracellular events require release of a neurotransmitter, the action of which depends subsequently on activation of calmodulin by calcium binding.

There are huge numbers of circuits, transmit-

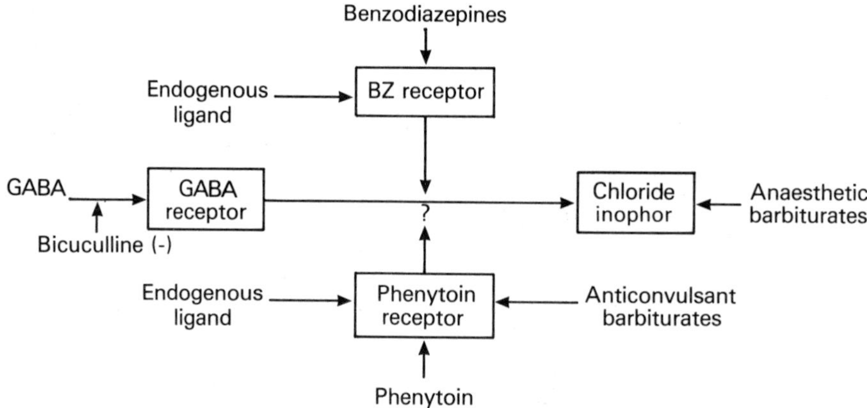

Fig. 5.12 Postulated receptor interactions in epilepsy. BZ = benzodiazepine.

ters and coupled reactions within the CNS. Several act simultaneously to produce coordinated CNS responses.

Classification of nerve fibres

In 1943 Gasser produced a classification of nerve fibres which remains valid today (Table 5.2).

The sensory system

Detection of mechanical stimuli

Peripheral receptors exist in excitable tissues. Skin receptors appreciate touch, cold, warmth and pain, and deeper receptors appreciate pressure and proprioception.

There are large numbers of different receptors and end-organs and although end-organs are specialised for one form of sensation, the quality of sensation does not depend on the type of stimulus arousing it. Information is transmitted to the central nervous system by varying the frequency and patterns of action potentials. There is often extensive branching of axons and a single fibre may be said to have a 'peripheral receptive field'.

Adaptation

A sustained, mechanical stimulus produces only a transient response, i.e. there is processing of information at receptor level, so that the brain is not informed constantly of an unchanging stimulus. Adaptation is said to be a function of the 'onion skin' of Pacinian corpuscles, where the accessory structure added to the nerve ending is visco-elastic and deformation of the surface has only a transient effect on the core of the corpuscle. Pacinian corpuscles can undergo hyperplasia and hypertrophy if there is a need for greater acuity of touch, as in blindness.

There is an electrical component of accommodation. A direct current applied to cause a sustained, artificial generator potential produces only a short burst of action potentials. Pacinian corpuscles show rapid adaptation so that steady state stimulus does not produce continuous activity. Conversely, muscle stretch receptors show less adaptation.

Mechanical transduction

This consists of transfer of a mechanical stimulus through accessory structures to the nerve terminal itself (Fig. 5.13). A graded electrical response is then produced equivalent to the generator or receptor potential, with initiation of an action potential.

A generator potential is produced by a mechanical stimulus and is a transient depolarisation of the nerve terminal membrane, independent of the ion channels. The potential appears to be created

Table 5.2 Classification of nerve fibres (Gasser 1943)

Description of nerve fibre	Group		Diameter (μm)	Conduction velocity (m/s)
Myelinated somatic	A	alpha	20	120
		beta		
		gamma		
		delta	3–4	6–30 (pain fibres)
		epsilon	2	5
Myelinated visceral (preganglionic autonomic)	B		<3	3–15
Unmyelinated somatic	C		<2	0.5–2 (pain fibres)

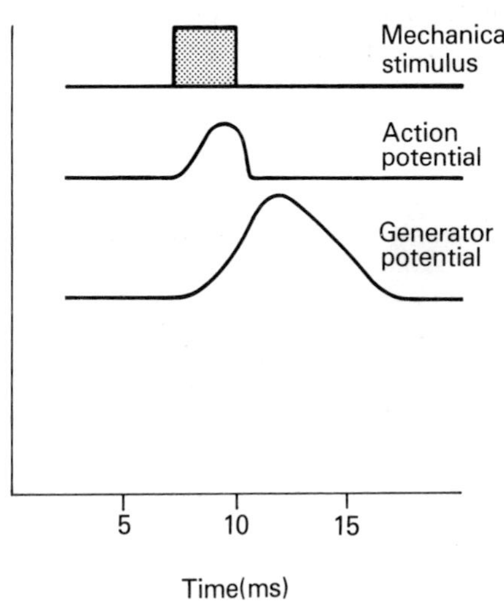

Fig. 5.13 Mechanical transduction.

by the nerve terminal itself and the important stimulus is distortion of the terminal.

Modalities of cutaneous sensation

There are four main modes of cutaneous sensation; touch, cold, warmth and pain.

Touch. Touch provides information on shape, texture and hardness of the object. Tactile sensation (Fig. 5.14) is distributed in a punctate fashion, with variability from day to day. The smallest pressure required to excite a sensation varies over the body surface. Touch spots are more frequent around hair follicles, the hair acting as a lever to transmit deformation to nerve endings around the shaft. Afferent fibres innervating these receptors have a large receptive field. Tactile sensation shows adaptation, localisation (which is also dependent on experience), discrimination between two points, and projection.

Temperature. Both warm spots and cold spots may be isolated on the skin. The latter are more numerous and there is daily variation in their distribution. This cutaneous sensation also shows adaptation. Sensitivity of the exposed skin varies with the area of the body, but at ordinary skin temperatures a temperature difference of 0.2°C can be detected by the forearms.

Pain. Pain registered by stimulation of the skin has a pricking, itching quality and is well localised. The pain threshold may be increased by one-third by distracting the subject's attention and reduced by half in sunburnt skin. The first sensation of pain arises abruptly and is carried by moderately large fibres, conducting impulses at 10 m/s. The second sensation is slower and of a burning nature, probably being carried by unmyelinated fibres.

Pain nerve endings are distributed in a punctate fashion independent of the end-organs concerned with touch and temperature. Further aspects of pain are considered separately later in this chapter.

Sensations from viscera and vessels travel in autonomic nerves and are often projected to a definite position on the surface of the body with the corresponding dermatome. This is relevant when considering referred pain (Fig. 5.15).

Spinal cord pathways

These may be divided into afferent (sensory), motor, cerebellar and autonomic.

Sensory afferent

Impulses arise in muscles, tendons, joints or skin. Dorsal root sensory ganglia and cranial nerve ganglia comprise primary neurones whose peripheral processes run with spinal nerves and whose central processes run into the cord. Some dorsal root fibres on entering the cord pass directly to motor neurones, constituting a monosynaptic reflex arc. Others synapse with cells in the dorsal horn of the grey matter and influence ventral horn

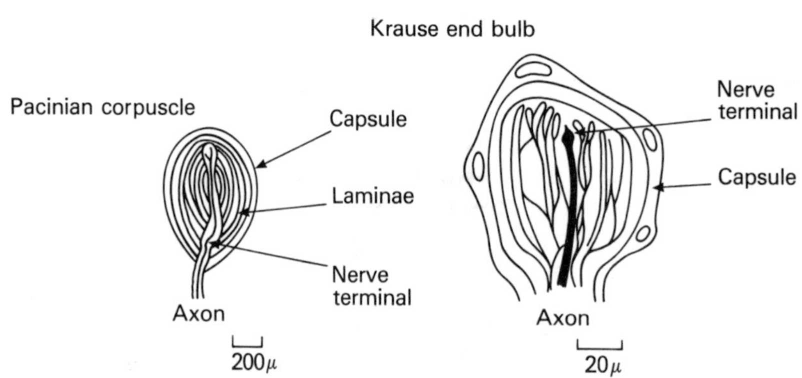

Fig. 5.14 Tactile receptors. Pacinian corpuscles are subcutaneous structures with receptive field 100 mm^2 which respond to vibration (40–600 Hz). Krause end bulbs are found in the dermis and respond to vibration (10–200 Hz) and movement from a field of 2 mm^2. They are concerned with spacial and intensity aspects of touch.

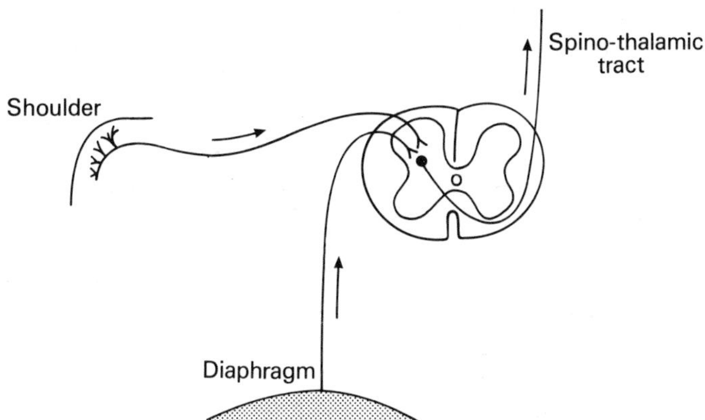

Fig. 5.15 Referred pain; irritation of the diaphragm is felt in the shoulder tip. Nerves from these areas synapse with common neurones in the spinal cord.

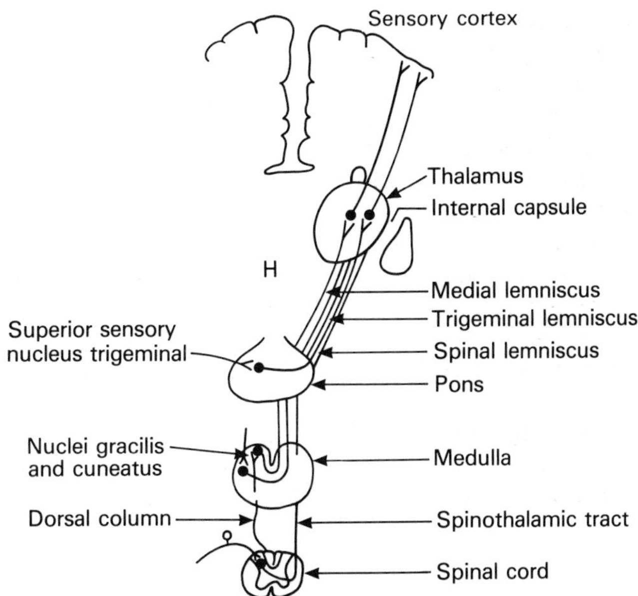

Fig. 5.16 Major somatic afferent, sensory pathways. H = hypothalamus.

cells by a reflex arc involving several neurones. The majority, however, form synapses with dorsal horn cells, cells in thoracic nuclei, the base of the dorsal horn or the nuclei gracilis and cuneatus (second order sensory neurones) (Fig. 5.16). These cross to the opposite side and end in the ventrolateral nucleus of the thalamus where they synapse with third order sensory neurones, the fibres of which pass through the posterior end of the internal capsule to the postcentral gyrus of the cerebral cortex. There are two major sensory systems:

1. The dorsal column–medial lemniscus system, which conducts proprioception, fine touch, vibration and some autonomic fibres.
2. The spinothalamic tract; crude touch and pressure are conducted along the anterior spinothalamic tract, and pain and temperature in the lateral spinothalamic tract.

Both the sensory systems decussate before they reach the sensory cortex. The dorsal column system decussates in the medulla and the lateral spinothalamic tract close to its site of entry in the cord.

Descending control of sensory pathways is by efferent nerves acting at synaptic junctions of the relay nuclei of the ascending pathways, e.g. the dorsal horn, dorsal column and thalamic nuclei. These may be either facilitatory or inhibitory.

In the medulla, the two spinothalamic tracts blend to form the spinal lemniscus which is closely associated with corresponding fibres from the fifth cranial nerve. The thalamus acts as a relay station for sensory pathways. Ultimately somatosensory impulses from one side of the body are represented on the contralateral cerebral cortex. Removal of the cerebral cortex results in the thalamus undertaking crude appreciation of sensation. The sensory cortex is responsible for perception of sensation including the full appreciation of pain. If this sensory gyrus is completely obliterated, there is impairment but no abolition of sensation, although agnosia and disturbance of body image occur (vide infra).

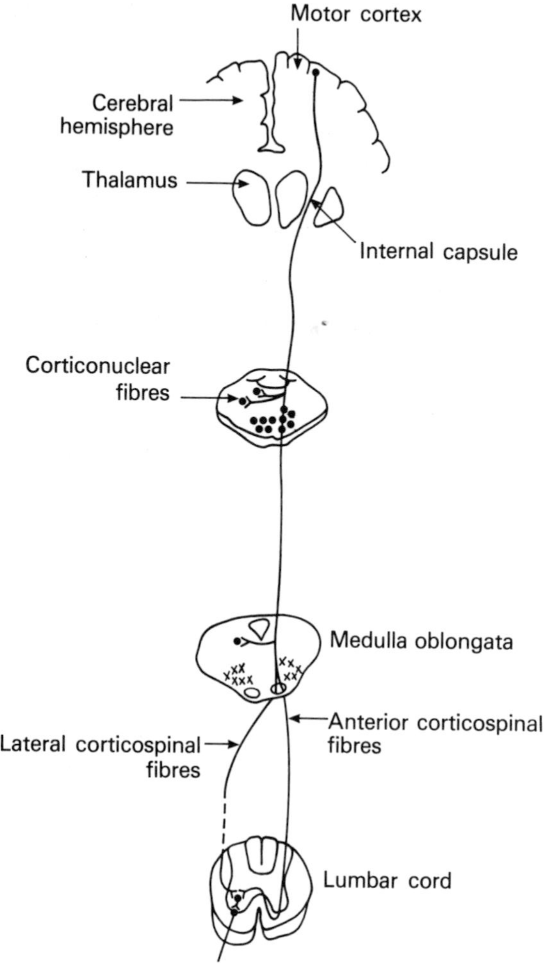

Fig. 5.17 The pyramidal tract.

Motor efferent

Lower motor neurones (LMNs) are anterior horn cells of the spinal cord grey matter and some cranial nerve nuclei whose axons innervate voluntary muscle.. Upper motor neurones run from the cortex or brain stem to LMNs and comprise the pyramidal and extrapyramidal tracts which are concerned with control of movement.

The pyramidal tract (Fig. 5.17) is so named because it forms the pyramid of the medulla. It originates mainly in the precentral gyrus of the cerebral cortex and runs first to cranial nerve nuclei (corticonuclear fibres) and then to the anterior columns of the spinal cord (corticospinal fibres). As these fibres descend from the cortex they traverse the internal capsule in an orderly arrangement. Most corticonuclear fibres cross the midline in the brain stem, terminating in the motor cranial nerve nuclei (cranial nerves III–VII, IX and X). Some uncrossed fibres remain and the tract continues through the pons in a dispersed fashion. Fibres become grouped together in a pyramid on the ventral aspect of the medulla oblongata. In the lower half of the medulla, 90% of fibres cross to the opposite side to descend in the posterior part of the lateral columns as the lateral pyramidal tract. A few fibres pass down on the same side in the anterior white column as the ventral pyramidal tract. A lesion of pyramidal fibres above the decussation produces a contralateral paralysis of voluntary muscles, impairing especially precise movements of the distal aspect of the limbs.

The extrapyramidal system is concerned chiefly with regulation of muscle tone, and influences posture and more stereotyped movements. It comprises a series of tracts connecting various areas of cerebral cortex, subcortical nuclei and brain stem nuclei. These tracts descend to the lower brain stem and spinal cord to influence LMNs through intermediate neurones.

Descending extrapyramidal tracts include the rubrobulbar and reticulospinal (Fig. 5.18). These accompany the pyramidal tracts to interneurones in the cord. Both systems influence the final, common pathways (LMNs) which are also influenced reflexly by sensory impulses.

The net result of extrapyramidal activity is inhibitory, so that lesions in the midbrain nuclei associated with this system may result in increased postural tone, and spasticity with uncontrolled tremors or movement. Two other descending pathways influence motor activity; the tectospinal and vestibulospinal tracts. These two tracts account for the influence of stimuli from the eye and the ear produced by movement.

Cerebellar pathways

Afferent and efferent pathways traverse via the cerebellar peduncles. The afferent pathways contain information from muscle spindles, Golgi tendon organs, and other proprioceptors, and reach the cerebellum in three main ascending pathways in each half of the spinal cord: the posterior and anterior spinocerebellar tracts and the posterior external arcuate fibres.

Efferent fibres from Purkinje cells in the cerebellar cortex ultimately traverse the superior cerebellar peduncles and cross to the opposite side in the lower half of the midbrain, ending mainly in the contralateral red nucleus. They project to the cerebral cortex, brain stem, reticular, vestibular and other nuclei.

Autonomic pathways

The sympathetic system (Fig. 5.19). This is a two-neurone system. Preganglionic sympathetic fibres have their cells of origin in the lateral horns of the grey matter in segments T1 to L2, and fibres leave the cord with motor nerves to voluntary muscle via the ventral nerve root. Preganglionic fibres run to the sympathetic trunk which lies a few centimetres from the vertebral column on each side from the level of the superior cervical ganglion down to the pelvis. Postganglionic fibres arise from these ganglia and usually join spinal nerves. Those to the head accompany the carotid artery. Sympathetic fibres to the gut do not relay in the sympathetic trunk, but in midline ganglia

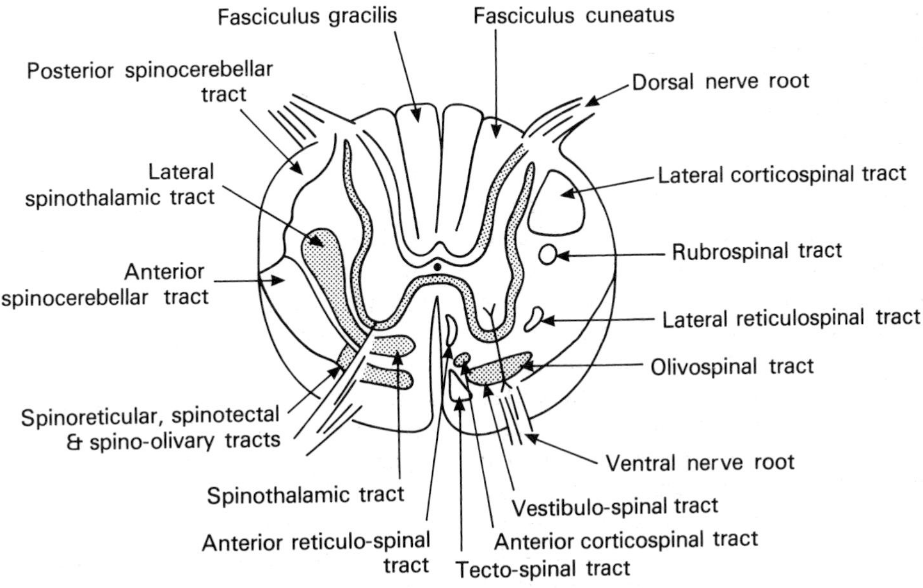

Fig. 5.18 Transverse section of the spinal cord to show major nerve tracts.

in front of the aorta (coeliac, superior and inferior mesenteric plexuses). The functions of the sympathetic nerves are described in Chapter 13, page 225.

Parasympathetic system (Fig. 5.20). This comprises a craniosacral outflow via cranial nerves III, VII, IX and X, and S2–4. The actions are described in Chapter 13, page 225, and Table 13.1.

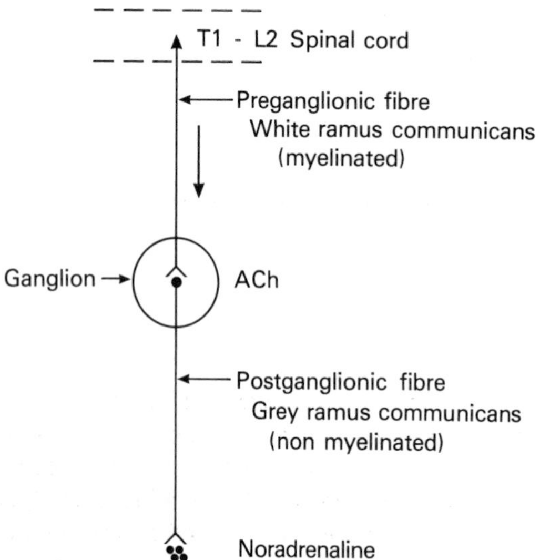

Fig. 5.19 Sympathetic nervous system. ACh = acetylcholine.

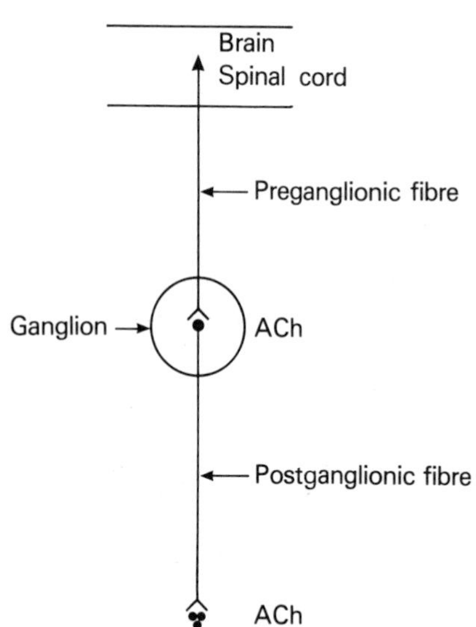

Fig. 5.20 Parasympathetic nervous system. ACh = acetylcholine.

Central representation. Integration of autonomic and somatic activity maintains stable internal conditions despite a changing environment. Central nervous system areas concerned with autonomic activity (Fig. 5.21) include nuclei in the hypothalamus around the third ventricle, particularly the supraoptic, paraventricular, dorsal and ventral medial hypothalamic, posterior hypothalamic and mamillary.

There is, therefore, close association with the frontal lobes and the posterior pituitary. The hippocampal circuit (hippocampus, fornix, mamillary body, anterior thalamic nuclei, cingulate gyrus, hippocampus) represents a continuous relationship between the cortex, thalamus, hypothalamus and hippocampus and is influenced by pathways ascending from the spinal cord and brain stem and descending from the cortex. This area is involved in emotional reactions which are often the result of somatic and emotional interactions (nausea, flushing) and with memory. The hypothalamus is also important in temperature regulation, the sleep/wake rhythm, and endocrine

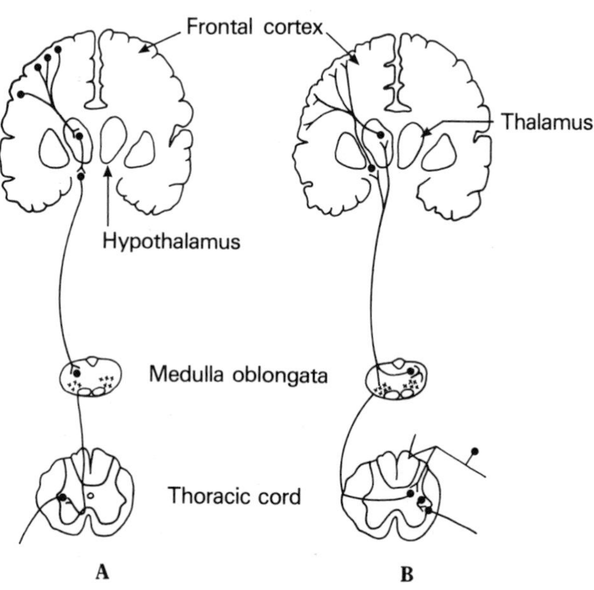

Fig. 5.21 Autonomic pathways between spinal cord and brain (not to scale) showing: (a) probable efferent autonomic pathways from brain to spinal cord; (b) probable afferent autonomic pathways from cord to brain.

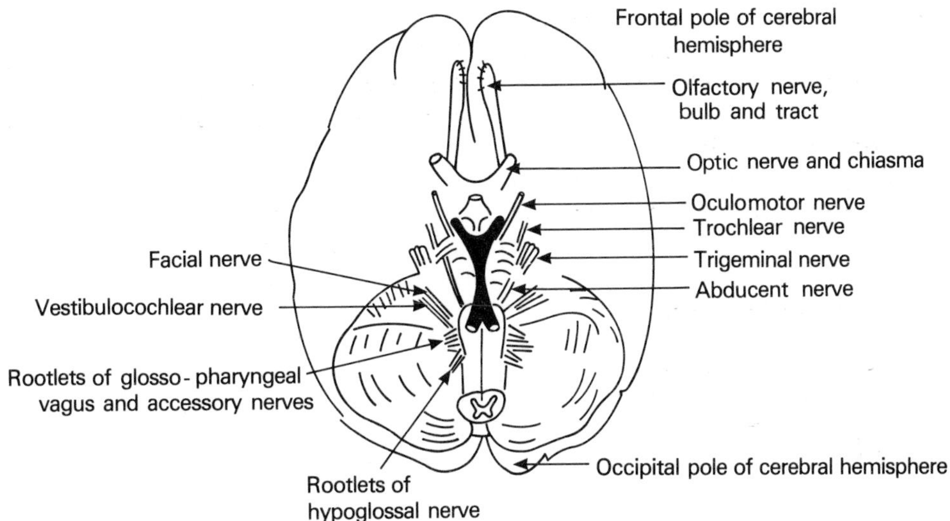

Fig. 5.22 Anatomical position of cranial nerves on base of brain.

and cardiovascular systems. Autonomic afferent fibres ascend through the cord and brain stem with somatosensory pathways to the hypothalamus, which acts as a relaying and redistributing centre from which impulses are projected onwards to the thalamus and frontal cortex.

Cranial nerves

These are situated on the base of the brain (Fig. 5.22). Cranial nerve I, the olfactory, is a special, visceral, afferent nerve, conveying impulses from the olfactory area of the nasal mucous membrane which traverses the cribriform plate of the ethmoid to the olfactory bulbs on the orbital surface of the frontal lobe.

Cranial nerve II, the optic nerve, is a special, sensory, afferent carrying visual impulses from the retina to the optic chiasma.

Cranial nerve III, the oculomotor, is a general, sensory, afferent and efferent nerve and constitutes the most important motor supply to extrinsic voluntary and intrinsic eye muscles.

The trochlear nerve (IV), is a general, sensory, afferent and efferent nerve and the only nerve to arise from the dorsal aspect of the brain stem. It supplies the superior oblique muscle.

Nerve V, the trigeminal nerve, is a general, sensory, afferent and special visceral efferent nerve, concerned with facial sensation. It also supplies the muscles of mastication. Its cutaneous distribution (Fig. 5.23) is of great clinical importance in the management of trigeminal neuralgia. This nerve may be involved together with cranial nerves VII and VIII in a tumour arising in the cerebellopontine angle, e.g. an acoustic neuroma.

The abducent nerve (VI), is a general, somatic, afferent and efferent nerve, supplying the lateral

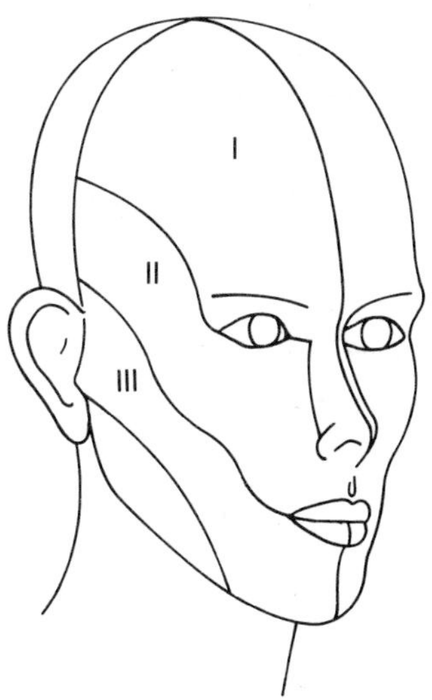

Fig. 5.23 Cutaneous divisions of the Vth nerve. I ophthalmic; II maxillary; III mandibular.

rectus muscle. It has the longest intracranial course and may be damaged in conditions which raise intracranial pressure.

Nerves III, IV and VI can be tested by comparing eye movements and examining for ptosis and diplopia.

Cranial nerve VII (facial) is a general and special visceral, afferent and efferent nerve, which provides the main motor nerve supply to the face.

Cranial nerve VIII, the auditory, is a special afferent nerve, concerned with hearing and equilibrium, which may be tested by audiometry and caloric testing.

The glossopharyngeal nerve (IX) is a general and special visceral, afferent and efferent nerve, which subserves one-third of taste and provides the motor supply to the pharynx.

Cranial nerve X, the vagus, is the major motor nerve to the viscera, palate and vocal cords and supplies most sensory modalities. Its function may be tested by examination of palatal movement, the voice and the ability to cough.

Nerve XI, the spinal accessory, is a general and special visceral efferent, which supplies the sternomastoid and the upper part of the trapezius muscle.

The hypoglossal nerve (XII) is a general, somatic afferent and efferent nerve which is motor to the tongue.

Because of the close proximity of the last four cranial nerves, they may be involved jointly in pathological lesions, producing a weak, hoarse voice, nasal speech, difficulty in swallowing and regurgitation with production of an aspiration pneumonia. This constitutes a bulbar palsy and the airway should be protected.

Brain stem and midbrain function

The functions of the brain stem have been highlighted in recent years by the concept of brain stem death. An understanding of the functions requires some knowledge of the anatomy of this area.

Medulla (Fig. 5.24)

1. Motor pathways are situated ventrally. Corticospinal fibres traverse the internal capsule via the genu. They are situated medially in the cerebral peduncle, crossing the midline to supply the relevant cranial nerves of the opposite side. The motor nucleus of V, controlling the muscles of mastication, derives only half its innervation from the opposite hemisphere, i.e. there is bilateral innervation. Nerve VII has similar innervation for the forehead muscles, but the muscles of the lower face are innervated mainly by crossed fibres.

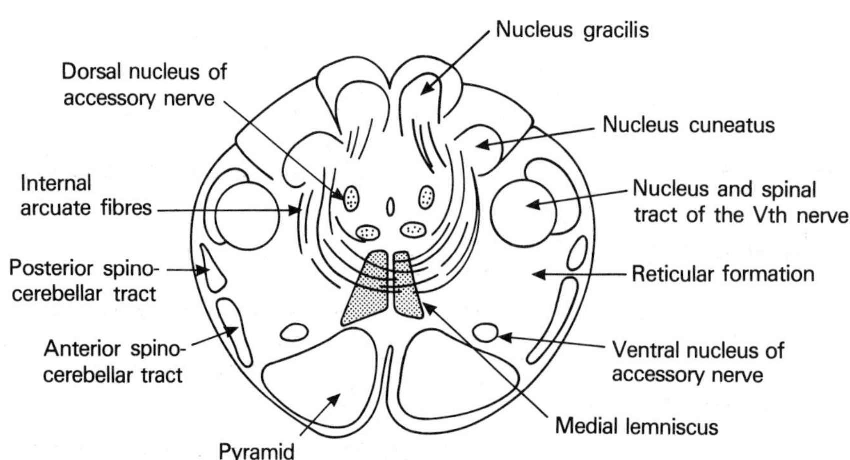

Fig. 5.24 Transverse section of medulla at level of sensory decussation.

Cranial nerve nuclei are situated in the dorsal areas of the medulla.

2. Sensory pathways constitute the intermediate layer of the brain stem. The gracile and cuneate nuclei are situated in the dorsal medulla. Spino-thalamic sensation is associated closely with descending sympathetic pathways.

The trigeminal sensory system is very complex. Information from one side of the face enters the brain stem in the fifth nerve at the level of the midpons. Fibres concerned with the corneal reflex and touch decussate to the opposite side. Pain and temperature fibres descend parallel to the descending nucleus of the fifth nerve, relay to the opposite side in the lower medulla and become the secondary ascending tract of the fifth nerve adjacent to the medial lemniscus.

3. The brain stem contains cranial nerve nuclei of cranial nerves III to XII.

4. Control of respiration, heart rate and blood pressure reside within the medulla; the so-called vital centres are concerned with the automatic reflex control of the heart, lungs and circulation. Afferent fibres originate in highly specialised visceral receptors, e.g. the carotid sinus and receptor cells within the medulla itself, which are responsive, for example, to Pa_{CO_2}. Groups of neurones in the floor of the fourth ventricle project downwards to synapse with anterior horn cells supplying the respiratory muscles. Control of swallowing, coughing and vomiting are also integrated in the medulla.

5. The fourth ventricle is situated within the brain stem.

Pons

A major feature of the pons is its peduncular connections. The medial lemniscus is the continuation upwards of the dorsal column sensory system.

Midbrain (Fig. 5.25)

This lies between the cerebrum and the pons. It contains the cerebral peduncles and the tectum. The cerebral aqueduct runs through the midbrain and connects the third and fourth ventricles. The tectum contains the colliculi, and receives some retinal fibres via the optic nerves, descending fibres from the optic cortex and ascending fibres from the cord. It is responsible for coordination of input from the auditory areas of the temporal cortex and cervical cord. The colliculi are also responsible for visual, auditory and vestibular reflexes.

The cerebral peduncles consist of a ventral aspect (which becomes continuous with the

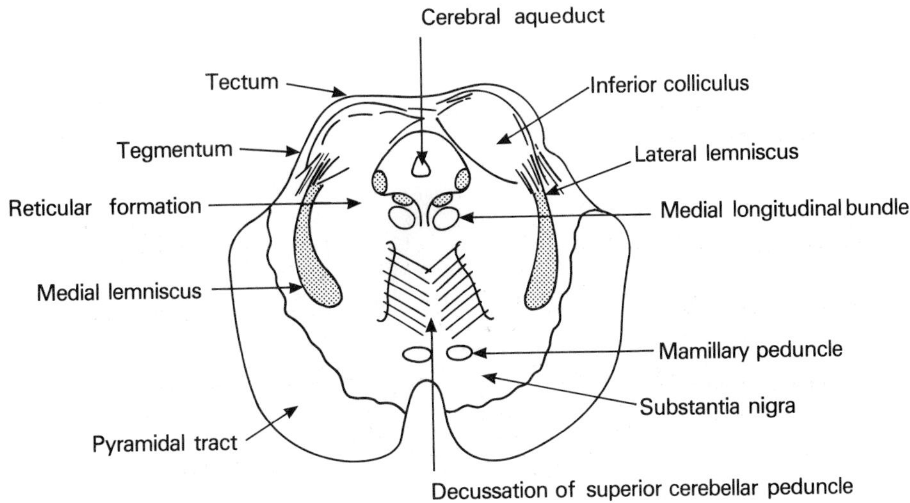

Fig. 5.25 Transverse section of midbrain at level of inferior colliculi.

internal capsule), the substantia nigra, and a dorsal tegmentum. The corticonuclear, corticospinal and corticopontine fibres traverse the ventral aspect. The peri-aqueductal grey matter contains nuclei of cranial nerves III and IV and the mesencephalic nucleus of V. The red nucleus, which is an important relay station in paths between cerebellum, corpus striatum and spinal cord, is situated in the tegmentum.

The reticular formation

This constitutes the central core of the brain stem, projecting widely to the limbic system and cortex with many ascending and descending connections. Stimulation activates the cortex, initiating an arousal reaction, i.e. this area is responsible for generating the capacity for consciousness. Attention and circadian rhythms are also dependent upon the correct functioning of the reticular formation.

Brain stem function tests

1. Activity of nerves II to XII may be tested individually to permit localisation of a lesion.

2. Transmission of all motor information occurs from the cortex to the spinal cord and all sensory information in the opposite direction. Although spinal reflexes may be active when the brain stem is destroyed there should be no abnormal posture, either decorticate (flexed forearms and extended legs) or decerebrate (extended hyperpronated forearms and extended legs), nor trismus.

3. Control of respiration. In the absence of brain stem activity there is apnoea. Loss of vasomotor control also occurs.

4. Brain stem reflexes:

(i) Oculocephalic. In the absence of brain stem function, when the head is rotated to one side and held there for 3–4 s and then rotated through 180° in the opposite direction, the head and eyes move together. In a patient with damaged cerebral hemispheres and an intact brain stem, there is deviation of the eyes to the opposite side as the head is rotated, followed by realignment of the eyes with the head.

(ii) Vestibulo-ocular. If the clear, external auditory canal is irrigated with ice-cold saline and the brain stem is intact, there is nystagmus. When the brain stem is totally destroyed there are no eye movements.

The cerebral cortex

The surface anatomy of the cerebral cortex with underlying functions is illustrated in Figure 5.26. The dominant hemisphere is that opposite the dominant hand in right-handed individuals, but variable in those who are left-handed. If the dominant hemisphere is destroyed early in life then the other may slowly but incompletely assume intellectual functions. The cerebral cortex

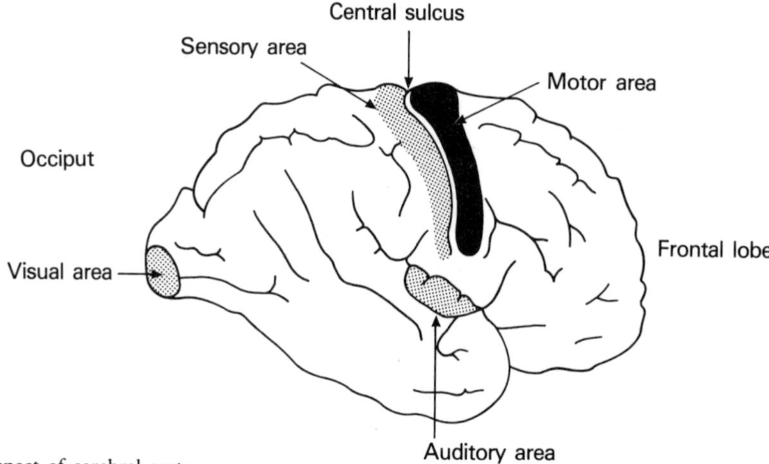

Fig. 5.26 Lateral aspect of cerebral cortex.

is concerned with higher intellectual functions: memory, learning and language. In the human, there are three major association areas:

1. Frontal, in front of the motor cortex.
2. Temporal, between the superior temporal gyrus and limbic cortex.
3. Parieto-occipital, between the sensory and visual cortex.

These areas have complex connections from the thalamus, to each other and to the deeper cortex.

Coning

Brain swelling may be evident anatomically as midline shift. Displacement may cause part of a cerebral hemisphere, usually the temporal lobe, to become impacted under the falx cerebri or tentorial hiatus. Any expanding supratentorial lesion, e.g. middle meningeal haemorrhage, forces the medial aspect of the temporal lobe into the tentorial hiatus. Compression of the cerebral peduncle and oculomotor nerve causes ipsilateral pupillary dilatation with contralateral hemiparesis. Later, brain stem compression produces apnoea.

An expanding posterior fossa lesion may push the cerebellum into the tentorial hiatus. Medullary coning from high intracranial pressure forces the medulla and cerebellar tonsil down into the foramen magnum, and is rapidly fatal because of compression of the respiratory and vasomotor centres.

Cerebrospinal fluid (CSF)

CSF is formed by secretory cells of the choroid plexus which project into the lateral and third ventricles (Fig. 5.27). CSF then flows via the third ventricle through the aqueduct and fourth ventricle to escape by two lateral foramina of Luschka and median foramen of Magendie into the subarachnoid space around the brain and spinal cord.

The total volume of CSF is approximately 140 ml in the adult; approximately 50% is intracranial, and the remainder occupies the spinal canal. CSF is produced at a rate of 0.3–0.5 ml/min. Production must match absorption to prevent an increase in pressure. Obstruction to the flow of CSF increases pressure, with dilatation of the ventricles upstream from the obstruction.

Resorption is mainly into the venous system via arachnoid villi, which are areas where the arachnoid invaginates into large venous sinuses. If the CSF pressure is less than venous pressure, the vacuoles collapse. Some CSF is also probably absorbed around spinal nerves into spinal veins and through the ependymal lining of the ventricles.

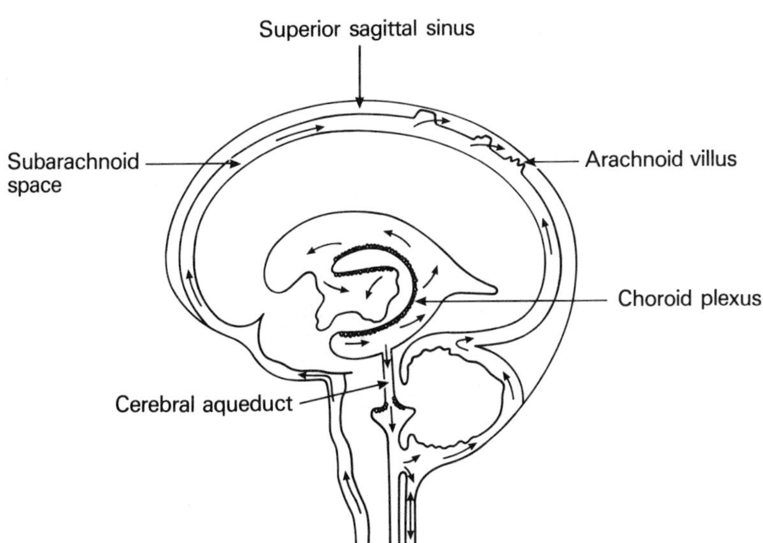

Fig. 5.27 The circulation of CSF.

CSF acts as a cushion between the skull and the brain. It may accommodate some change in brain volume by displacement into the lumbar region. In conditions producing cerebral atrophy there is an increase in CSF volume.

CSF is a clear, colourless liquid of specific gravity 1005, with less than 5 lymphocytes/mm^3 and pH 7.33 (Table 5.3). It is produced from plasma, probably by a combination of secretion and ultrafiltration. The high concentration of chloride arises because carbon dioxide passes into glial cells where, by the action of carbonic anhydrase, it is hydrated to carbonic acid (H_2CO_3). Resulting bicarbonate ions (HCO_3^-) are exchanged for chloride which passes into the CSF against a concentration gradient. CSF is slightly hypertonic; Na^+ and Mg^{2+} ions are transported actively into CSF. Lipophilic substances pass readily from blood to brain, but dissociated hydrophilic substances pass only very slowly.

The blood–brain barrier (Fig. 5.28) is composed of a lipid membrane of capillaries, the endothelial cells of which are joined by tight junctions around the entire periphery of each cell. Solutes at higher concentration in the ECF of the brain diffuse into CSF and are carried into blood at the arachnoid villi. Some substances are transported actively by cells of the choroid plexus from CSF into blood.

Electrophoresis of CSF proteins is now possible. CSF proteins are derived by filtration of plasma, from brain interstitial fluid and brain cells, and from cells of the CSF compartment itself.

These proteins may reflect abnormalities of the filtration mechanism, of barrier function, brain metabolism or activities of the CSF. Electrophoresis has clinical application for investigation of some neurological conditions, e.g. multiple sclerosis, Guillain-Barré syndrome and neurosyphilis.

Table 5.3 Composition of plasma and cerebrospinal fluid

	Plasma (mmol/litre)	Cerebrospinal fluid (mmol/litre)
Urea	2.5–6.5	2.0–7.0
Glucose (fasting)	3.0–5.0	2.5–4.5
Sodium	136–148	144–152
Potassium	3.8–5.0	2.0–3.0
Calcium	2.2–2.6	1.1–1.3
Chloride	95–105	123–128
Bicarbonate	24–32	24–32
Protein	60–80 g/litre	200–400 mg/litre

PAIN

Pain is a combination of severe discomfort, fear, autonomic changes, reflex activity and suffering. Peripheral nerve endings are stimulated by pressure, temperature and inflammatory substances such as prostaglandins, leukotrienes, peptides and amines.

Pain is transmitted by unmyelinated, peripheral, afferent fibres which terminate in the substantia gelatinosa of the dorsal horn (Fig. 5.29) and smaller, myelinated afferents which terminate in the nucleus proprius (lamina V). Spinothalamic fibres arise at this layer.

In 1952 Rexed showed that cells of the grey matter of the spinal cord are arranged in nine laminae, I to IX, from the dorsal to the ventral cord, the tenth lamina lying around the central zone. Lamina I comprises the marginal zone,

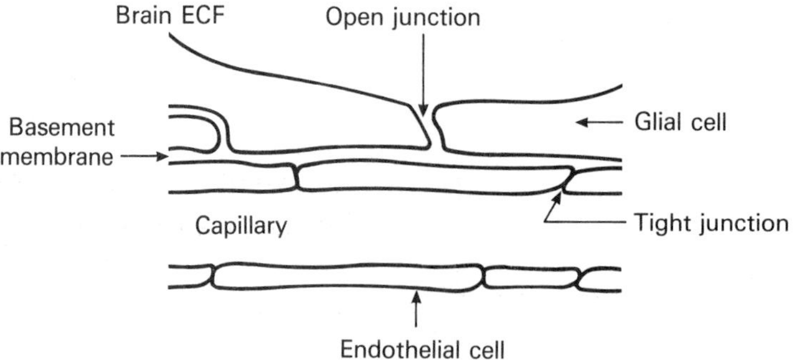

Fig. 5.28 Blood–brain barrier.

laminae II and III the substantia gelatinosa, and laminae IV, V and VI the nucleus proprius (Fig. 5.30). Small myelinated fibres activated by pin prick, and hot and cold receptors, terminate here. Laminae VII and VIII correspond to the nucleus intermedius, and give rise to spinoreticular fibres. Lamina IX is the ventral horn, and the output from this constitutes the ventral root.

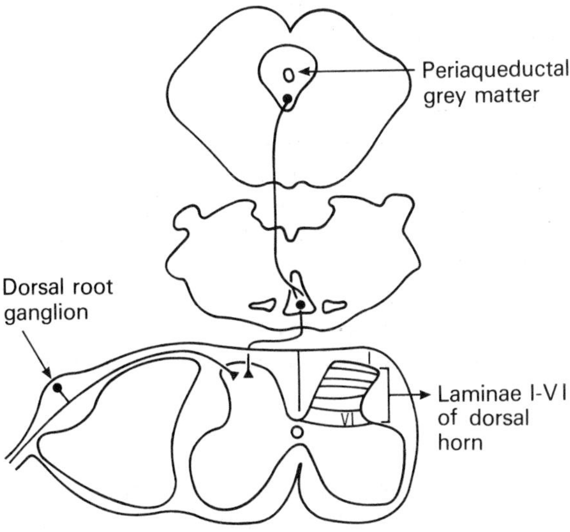

Fig. 5.29 Pain pathways.

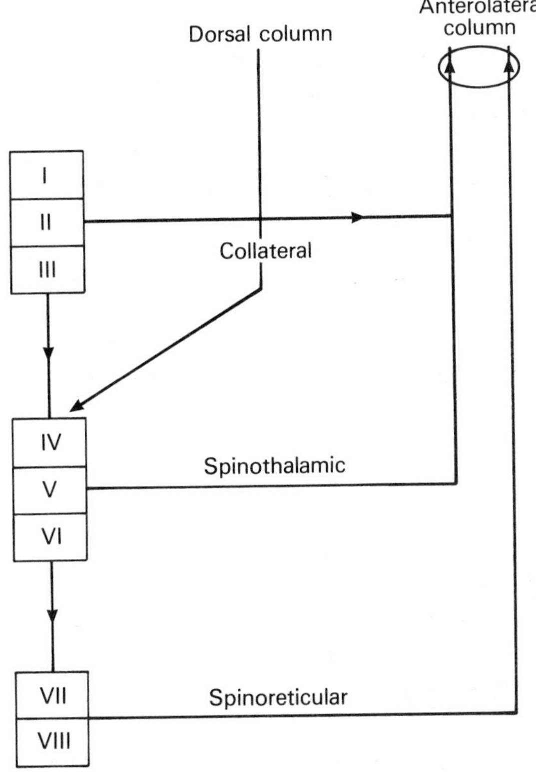

Fig. 5.30 Connections of Rexed laminae.

Gate control theory of pain

Nociceptive impulses activate:

1. Nerve fibres which stimulate the substantia gelatinosa and nucleus proprius.
2. Large myelinated axons of the dorsal column fibres.

Segmental collaterals from the dorsal column fibres synapse in lamina IV. These exert an inhibitory influence on transmission of impulses from the substantia gelatinosa, with a reduction in painful sensation. Descending impulses control sensory input by direct and indirect modulation at every level of the brain stem and spinal cord, including the dorsal horn of the cord where they form part of the gate control mechanism. It is known that pain may be suppressed by stress, hypnosis, electrical stimulation and trancelike euphoria.

The gate control theory of pain as illustrated in Figure 5.31, was developed originally by Melzack and Wall in 1965. They postulated that large diameter A fibres (Aα) and small diameter A fibres (Aδ) and C fibres are all activated during noxious stimulation of peripheral receptors. At cord level, a gate exists which, under specific circumstances, opens to permit pain stimuli to

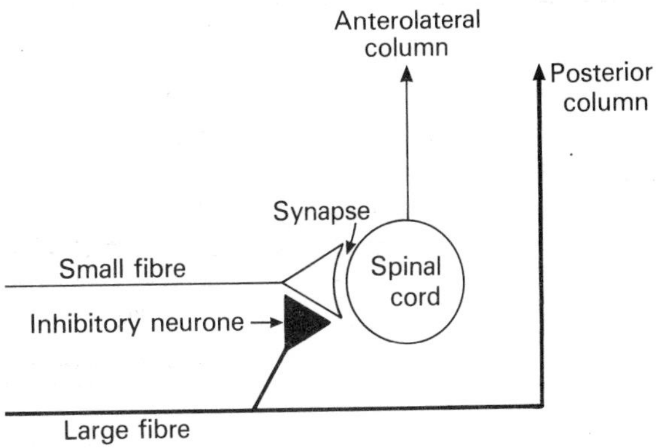

Fig. 5.31 Gate control mechanism.

pass through to higher centres. Small nerve fibre stimulation opens the gate, and large nerve fibre stimulation closes it by depression or facilitation of synaptic transmission. Two possible mechanisms of afferent synaptic inhibition have been described: (i) via a glycine transmitter site; (ii) via a GABA site with a longer latency.

In postherpetic neuralgia the pain results from loss of large fibres. In polyneuropathy, there is a relative increase in the small fibres without an increase in pain, i.e. selective inhibition of supraspinal origin, which can shut down transmission from nociceptors, leaving mechanoreceptor conduction almost unimpaired.

Endogenous opioids and pain

The opioid molecule is stereospecific, which supports the concept of specific binding sites. Sites of opioid receptors in the spinal cord include the marginal zone and substantia gelatinosa of the dorsal horn and the descending spinal trigeminal nucleus. At higher levels they are found in the palaeospinothalamic pain pathway and limbic system related to emotional behaviour. They are also found in the gut. In 1975 two related pentapeptides were isolated — methionine and leucine enkephalin. Met-enkephalin (methionine enkephalin) is formed by breakdown of pituitary β-lipotropin and is destroyed very rapidly. These features suggest its role as a neurotransmitter and, indeed, many enkephalin-containing neurones and nerve terminals are concentrated in laminae I and II of the dorsal horn.

There are several subclasses of opioid receptor, including μ, δ, and κ. The spinal distribution of μ opioid receptors parallels that of enkephalins. The μ receptors are those most likely to be associated with pain pathways. A descending projection from neurones of the peri-aqueductal grey matter is responsible for stimulus-produced analgesia and opioid analgesia, but these neurones do not project directly to the spinal cord. There is a possibility that there may be an excitatory neurotransmitter between the two, e.g. glutamate or aspartate. Evidence points, however, to enkephalin being the transmitter at the inhibitory synapse depicted in Figure 5.31 in the gate control mechanism of pain.

The most likely substance to be concerned with transmission of pain is substance P. Transmission from substance P-containing primary afferents is blocked by morphine or enkephalin and pretreatment with naloxone prevents this. The inhibitory enkephalinergic synapses are probably activated by segmental collaterals of large myelinated primary afferents of the dorsal columns, explaining the value of transcutaneous and dorsal column stimulation in pain relief. Lofentanil, a potent, long-acting opioid, has been used to evaluate the opioid-mediated control of substance P from primary afferents. Lofentanil inhibits release of substance P from both central and peripheral terminals of substance P-containing primary afferents. Descending control pathways in unmyelinated and serotoninergic neurones from the raphe nuclei are closely related anatomically to enkephalinergic neurones. It seems probable, therefore, that both systems are concerned with pain suppression. Deafferentation pain after spinal cord injury may be relieved by extradural administration of clonidine. This suggests that a noradrenergic system may be involved in transmission of pain. Intrathecal administration of midazolam depresses nociceptive sympathetic reflexes, an effect mediated perhaps through a non-opioid GABA mechanism.

Electrical stimulation of the brain, in particular the peri-aqueductal grey matter, releases endorphins which are the precursors of enkephalins, and it is well known that pain relief by acupuncture is antagonised by naloxone. Direct administration of small amounts of opioid peptide into the brain elicits a variety of behavioural responses, and neuropeptides may be neuromodulators rather than neurotransmitters. It is becoming apparent that neurones may secrete more than one biologically active substance, e.g. noradrenaline plus enkephalin. This leads to an increasing variety of chemically coded signals within CNS neurones. Chemical mediators such as prostaglandins seem to amplify pain transmission at the hypothalamic level.

The binding characteristics of opioid analgesics, such as receptor affinity and speed of binding, account for differences in analgesic properties and may explain 'sequential analgesia'. For example, the partial agonist buprenorphine possesses stronger affinity for the μ receptor than morphine, and with increasing dosage may initially reverse morphine-induced analgesia and ventilatory depression before causing these effects itself in high doses.

MECHANISMS OF GENERAL ANAESTHESIA

The underlying mechanism of general anaesthesia (a reversible loss of awareness and pain sensation) still awaits elucidation. Research is concentrated on the following questions:

1. What is the interaction of the anaesthetic agent with the receptor at molecular level?
2. What precisely is the disorder of cellular function produced by the anaesthetic?
3. What is the action of the anaesthetic at the synapse?
4. Which part of the neurone is affected, and in which part of the CNS?

The well-known correlation between anaesthetic potency and lipid solubility indicates that anaesthetics have a hydrophobic mechanism of action. Originally developed in 1901 by H. H. Meyer and E. Overton as the lipid solubility theory, this is illustrated in Figure 5.32 as the correlation of anaesthetic potency (MAC) with oil/gas partition coefficient. The oil/gas partition coefficient increases with decreasing temperature, and MAC decreases to maintain the constant relationship.

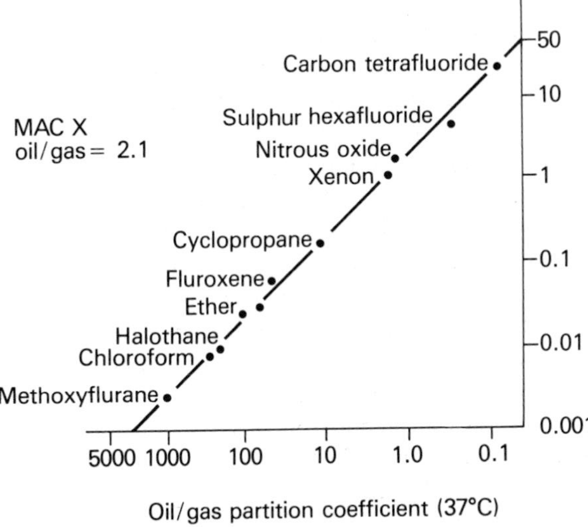

Fig. 5.32 Correlation of anaesthetic potency (MAC) with oil/gas partition coefficient. Standard deviations are omitted.

Against this is the aqueous theory of anaesthetic action suggested by the relationship between anaesthetic partial pressure and the composition pressure of the gas hydrates (clathrates) formed by the anaesthetics. It was suggested that anaesthetics affect water molecules in such a way as to reduce the conductance in the brain, perhaps by expanding the lipid membrane to occlude its microchannels. However, some potent volatile agents do not form clathrates under the relevant conditions. Some anaesthetics, e.g. fluorocarbons, do not fit this correlation and there is no mechanism for the additivity of anaesthetic potencies. Therefore the lipid region of the cell membrane or the hydrophobic region of protein molecules is most likely to be the site of a common anaesthetic mechanism.

Pressure reversal and the critical volume hypothesis

If mice are placed in a pressure chamber and anaesthetised with halothane, the addition of helium to the chamber to increase the pressure to 50 atmospheres allows the mice to wake up, although the partial pressures of halothane and oxygen are unaltered. In addition, high pressure reverses anaesthetic-induced depression of the evoked cortical response (see p. 106). The critical volume hypothesis proposes that there is a critical hydrophobic molecular site which is expanded by an anaesthetic and contracted by pressure. The percentage reduction in anaesthetic potency is related linearly to the total increase in pressure and the slope is the same for all agents. However, at very high pressures, this relationship no longer pertains and, in addition, not all agents behave in the same way at high pressure.

Anaesthetic action on the axonal membrane

Anaesthetics may block conduction by preventing channels opening, altering the ability to pass Na^+ or by favouring the inactive state. In addition, any agent which chronically depolarises a membrane favours the inactive state, preventing channels opening. However, K^+ channels may be blocked completely and an action potential may still be produced. Although relevant experimental evidence is lacking, anaesthetics might act by depolarising the membrane, thereby reducing the absolute magnitude of the action potential and favouring persistence of Na^+ channels in the inactive state. Volatile anaesthetic agents produce different effects on isolated neurones, suggesting a selective action which may involve multiple sites or mechanisms, or both.

Role of conduction block in anaesthesia

General anaesthetics may act by reducing synaptic transmission whilst the impulse in presynaptic terminals remains unimpaired. There are two possible mechanisms:

1. Anaesthetic agents may, by inducing chronic depolarisation, reduce the amount of transmitter release per impulse by a mechanism similar to presynaptic inhibition. This may be mediated by a specific effect of anaesthetics on Ca^{2+} entry.
2. Anaesthetics may interfere with the movement of the vesicle to, and its fusion with, the postsynaptic membrane.

Depression of the postsynaptic response

It is highly likely that this occurs in the anaesthetised patient. There is some evidence that anaesthetics may be selective for a specific type of synapse. For example, ketamine decreases synaptic transmission selectively at terminals of excitatory neurones, whereas Althesin and methohexitone enhance synaptic inhibition mediated by GABA. Such specific effects on particular synaptic processes do not support a common mechanism of anaesthesia.

In the invertebrates, volatile general anaesthetics preferentially depress excitatory rather than inhibitory transmission. Some analgesic properties of anaesthetics may be related to interactions with endorphin and enkephalin systems. Conductance changes to Na^+ can be detected at postsynaptic membranes and it seems likely that this neuronal function is altered by anaesthesia.

The critical volume hypothesis should permit temperature reversal of anaesthesia but this is difficult to test. Intravenous anaesthetics show considerable variation of pressure reversal between agents and this does not support the critical volume hypothesis for a single site of action for all anaesthetic agents. The concept, therefore, of a multisite expansion hypothesis has been developed by Halsey (1979).

Multisite expansion hypothesis

Much of this is controversial but the hypothesis may be summarised as follows:

1. General anaesthesia may be produced by the expansion of more than one molecular site; the sites may have different physical properties.
2. The physical properties of the molecular sites may be influenced by the presence of anaesthetics or pressure.
3. The molecular sites have a finite size and limited degree of occupancy.
4. Pressure need not necessarily act at the same site as the anaesthetic.
5. Molecular sites for anaesthesia are not perturbed by a decrease in temperature in a manner analagous to an increase in pressure.

Lipids in membranes move and rotate within the bilayer and influence the activity of proteins which control ionic and neurotransmitter fluxes. Perhaps the presence of a general anaesthetic in the membrane increases the movement of lipid and is associated with an increase in its volume. This might therefore effect conformational changes in the protein. The Na^+ channel protein requires an annulus of lipid in the more solid gel state to allow activity (i.e. the open state). Anaesthetics fluidise lipid, causing protein to relax into the inactive (closed channel) state. Other studies suggest that anaesthetic agents increase the thickness of the lipid bilayer so that the protein pore cannot expand the membrane adequately.

Protein change

Nuclear magnetic resonance studies of volatile agents on haemoglobin have provided the first evidence that anaesthetic agents interact with hydrophobic pockets within proteins at sites which appear to behave as bulk solvents. Conformational changes are then transmitted and detected in non-hydrophobic areas of the protein. Conformational changes specific to an individual anaesthetic have been observed in the same protein.

Sensory-motor modulation systems

Anaesthetic action on sensory-motor modulation systems switches off excitation and turns on inhibition such that messages between the periphery and brain are blocked mainly at thalamic level, with loss of motor control. Loss of consciousness occurs by a mechanism similar to an exaggerated sleep state. The number of synapses in such pathways is irrelevant but the degree of supraspinal modulation of postsynaptic membrane excitation is important.

General anaesthetics decrease the amplitude, and increase the latency, of evoked cortical responses.

Miscellaneous

It is well known that inhalational agents produce a dose-dependent toxic effect, e.g. depression of cell multiplication, mitotic abnormalities, reduced synthesis of DNA with perhaps mutagenic and carcinogenic effects. These may be related to anaesthetic mechanisms.

Other areas of study have included the effect of anaesthetic agents on the microtubules which give rigidity to cytoplasm. These are rings of protein molecules bound longitudinally. Cold and hydrostatic pressure both reversibly depolymerise these microtubular proteins, and produce narcosis. There remains the possibility that general anaesthetics reversibly depolymerise microtubular proteins by binding to nonpolar sites on globular proteins.

Proton pump leak theory

Anaesthetic agents increase leakiness in presynaptic vesicles; this reduces pH gradients, and in turn affects release and uptake of neurotransmitter. This concept is dependent primarily on intracellular pH. Cooling and high pressure reduce proton pump activity and neurotransmitter concentration. Anaesthetic effects of high concentrations of CO_2 (30%) in animals are not related to lipid solubility but to a direct action on intracellular pH. Complete anaesthesia occurs at a CSF pH of 6.7. Changes of ECF calcium concentration affect cell surface potential in a similar manner to addition of anaesthetic agents such as chloroform. It is possible therefore that modulation of surface potential by variation in ECF composition is important for the function of excitable cells.

Summary

Anaesthetics do expand one or more sites with hydrophobic solubility characteristics. Lipid and protein sites on the membrane, and synaptic transmission, are affected. The most susceptible function altered is the release and interaction of neurotransmitters, and the most vulnerable synapses are those in the ventrolateral thalamus.

NEUROPHYSIOLOGICAL INVESTIGATIONS

Background electrical activity of the brain may be recorded from the intact skull by scalp electrodes which may be unipolar or bipolar, the latter measuring the potential difference fluctuations between two electrodes. The electroencephalogram (Fig. 5.33) is a continuous recording of the immediate

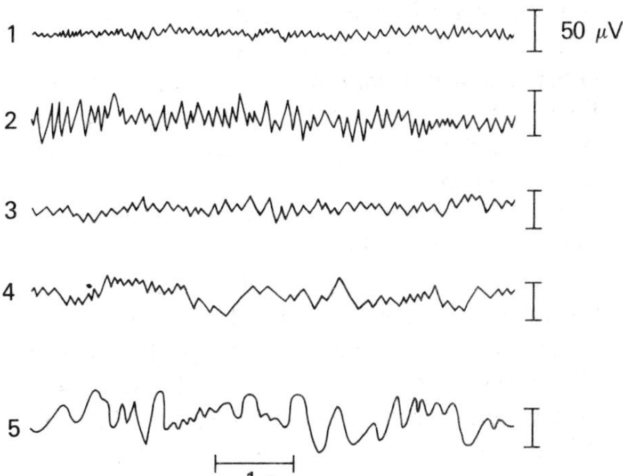

Fig. 5.33 EEG. 1: excited; 2: relaxed; 3: drowsy; 4: asleep; 5: deep sleep.

electrical responses from the underlying brain and represents excitatory and inhibitory postsynaptic potentials in the larger dendrites of neurones of the superficial cortex.

In the resting adult, with the mind wandering and eyes closed, the most prominent component is alpha rhythm, 8–13 Hz, 50 μV amplitude, recorded best in the parieto-occipital region. Beta activity is 18–30 Hz, of lower voltage, and is found mainly over the frontal region. Theta activity occurs in normal children at 4–7 Hz and is composed of large regular waves. Delta activity is very slow — less than 4 Hz. If the eyes are open, fast, irregular low voltage activity occurs with no dominant frequency. This is termed alpha block or desynchronisation, and occurs with any form of sensory stimulation.

Deep sleep induces large, irregular delta waves interspersed with alpha-like activity. Rapid eye movement (REM) or paradoxical sleep occurs with rapid, low voltage, irregular EEG activity, resembling arousal. Wakening during this period is associated with reports of dreaming. REM periods occur approximately every 50 min and occupy a total of 20% of the young adult's normal sleep time. They are associated with a marked reduction in skeletal muscle tone. Repeated awakening during REM sleep produces anxiety and irritability with an increased percentage of REM sleep in subsequent undisturbed nights.

Characteristic changes in the EEG occur in anaesthesia and other forms of coma. Increasing depth of anaesthesia with more potent agents produces slowing of the basic frequency of activity with a progressive increase in amplitude. Periods of iso-electricity appear, interspersed with bursts of activity. This is known as 'burst suppression'. With progressive depth of anaesthesia, there is increasing distance between bursts, resulting finally in an iso-electric line.

Characteristic changes with spike formation in the EEG occur during epilepsy. Hypoxaemia produces an acute increase in the amplitude of the EEG initially and then a marked reduction in amplitude with the appearance of slow waves as hypoxaemia worsens.

There are problems with using the EEG to monitor the brain continuously. These are related largely to the cumbersome equipment, problems of interpretation, and interference from other electrical equipment. The unprocessed EEG is still used by some anaesthetists in cerebrovascular surgery, including carotid artery surgery, as an indication of cerebral ischaemia, when it shows a good correlation with cerebral blood flow.

Processed EEG techniques

These offer no improvements in diagnostic sensitivity, but are simpler to use and clarify the display of information. Such techniques may be of limited value in evaluation of a complex situation, e.g. hypoxic changes occurring during hypothermia. There are numerous reports of the relationship between the processed EEG and anaesthetic depth indicating that small changes are detectable which would be missed in the absence of processing.

Cerebral function monitor (CFM)

This compresses all frequency and amplitude information in the EEG into a single value. It uses two parietal electrodes, the signal from which is passed through a wide-band frequency filter to remove frequencies of less than 2 Hz and more than 15 Hz (to reduce artefact and interference). The signal is amplified, rectified, integrated and compressed to produce a slow-running chart recording as a line, the height (above baseline) of which indicates total power (Fig. 5.34). Undulations reflect fluctuations in power from one moment to the next, upward movement indicating increased activity. The machine also monitors electrode impedance to detect artefacts from incorrect function of the electrodes.

Such a monitor requires supplementing at regular intervals by a full EEG because of the loss of information by processing. The main objection to the CFM is that the record is neither one of frequency nor amplitude but a mixture of the two. It does, however, permit continuous monitoring of electrical activity.

More recently, the cerebral function analysing monitor (CFAM) has become available. The CFAM produces a more detailed analysis of the EEG waveform and its frequency distribution (Fig. 5.35). Evoked potential computation is avail-

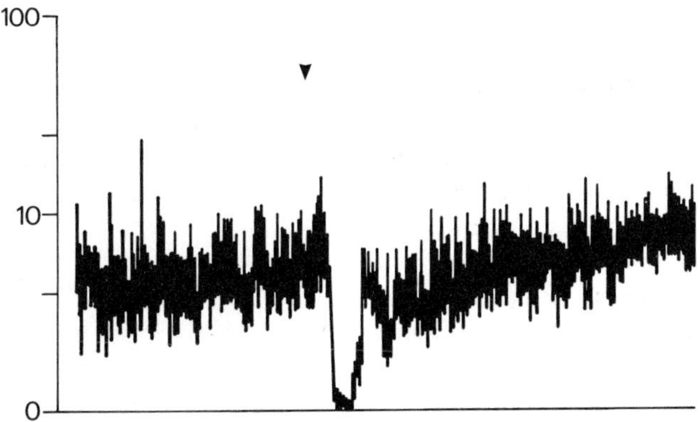

Fig. 5.34 Cerebral function monitor. This trace shows interruption of the circulation at the arrow, causing a transient absence of cerebral activity.

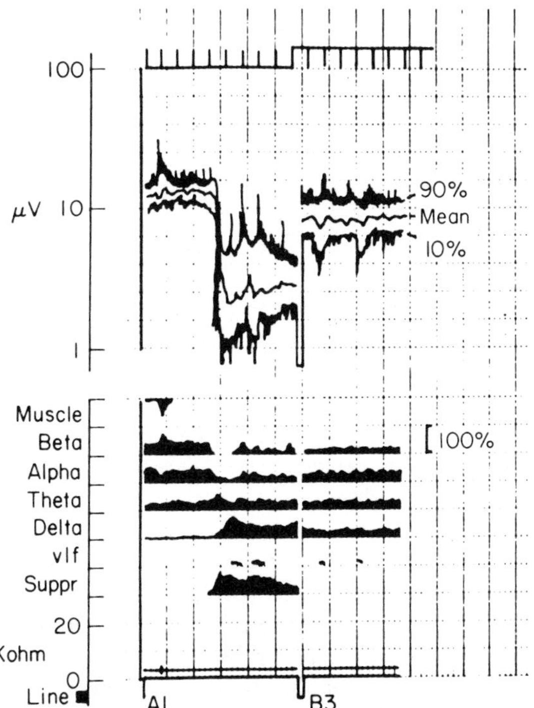

Fig. 5.35 Simulated trace from cerebral function analysing monitor, showing mean, 10th and 90th centiles of overall EEG amplitude distribution, and a display of relative distribution of activity in the beta, alpha, theta and delta frequency

able with the same machine. The percentage of weighted activity of the alpha, beta, theta and delta bands is displayed; this overcomes some of the objections to the loss of information which occurs with the standard CFM. Both muscle activity and electrode impedance are displayed continuously. Clinical experience is relatively limited, but anaesthetics such as nitrous oxide produce a significant reduction in amplitude and tendency towards lower frequencies on the CFAM.

Power spectrum analysis

This technique retains all information from the original EEG. Analysis of the EEG occurs as follows:

1. The EEG is digitised at frequent intervals known as epochs (2–16 s).
2. The epoch of data is subjected to Fourier analysis, separating the total EEG waveform into a number of component sine waves of different amplitudes, the sum of which is equal to the original wave form, i.e. conversion into a number of standard waves for easy comparison.
3. The power spectrum is calculated by squaring the amplitudes of each individual frequency component, and displayed for each epoch graphically, so that patterns may be identified by examination of a number of epochs in succession. If the epochs are short, i.e. 2–4 s, this constitutes almost a continuous monitor.

Advantages

1. All information is retained and small changes may be identified readily.

2. Each frequency band may be considered separately so that changes in one part of the spectrum cannot balance out changes elsewhere, as occurs with the CFM.

3. Generation of the power spectrum minimises baseline drift by converting all low-frequency components (0.05–0.50 Hz) to a single point.

4. Predictable changes may be detected, e.g. during halothane anaesthesia, there is less power at high frequencies and increased low frequency activity.

The currently available Berg analyser has the facility to switch from compressed data to raw data. It uses two pairs of electrodes and displays each hemisphere separately.

Display. A sophisticated, graphical display is essential because one of the main disadvantages of this technique is the vast amount of data generated (2000 data points per minute for each EEG channel processed). The printed output consists of a graph of relative power versus frequency at each epoch of the analysis (Fig. 5.36). Time is presented vertically to produce a three dimensional graph, with a hill and valley appearance. Hills constitute those frequencies making a large contribution and valleys occur at frequencies containing less power. The points behind the hill are not printed.

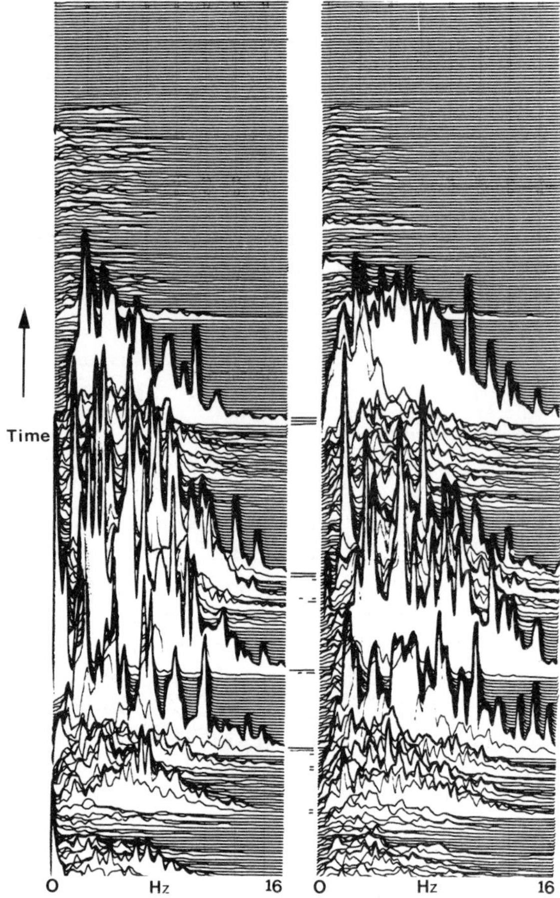

Fig. 5.36 Compressed spectral array. This trace shows fitting followed by electrical silence in a patient with meningoencephalitis.

Disadvantages

1. High-amplitude activity obscures subsequent lower amplitude activity at the same frequency.

2. Both time and power are displayed vertically and therefore output requires a two-dimensional XY plotter. Another technique for displaying power spectrum of the EEG uses density modulation, which produces a grey-scale display.

Power spectrum techniques can detect differences between the two hemispheres and monitor changes during cerebral sedation techniques. Such therapy may require reduction in EEG activity to the level of burst suppression or reduction of activity in the CFM to 5 μV.

The CFM is the simplest, automated, EEG processor for intra-operative use but is less sensitive than the multilead EEG for detection of focal ischaemia. It can discriminate between severe global cerebral ischaemia and hypoxia or hypotension, and to some extent indicates depth of anaesthesia. Gross anaesthetic overdose and severe global hypoperfusion are detectable. The CFM has proved useful in predicting the outcome of severe coma; patients with activity greater than 10 μV have survived whereas all those with less than 3 μV died.

Evoked potentials

Electrical events occurring in the cortex after stimulation of the sense organs may be detected by an exploring electrode over primary receiving areas for that particular sense. Evoked potential recordings constitute a non-invasive, objective, and repeatable supplement to clinical examination. Uses include assessment of functional integrity of specific cortical areas and pathways within the central nervous system. Visual, auditory and somatosensory evoked potentials are used widely in diagnosis. In order to detect the low amplitudes involved, an electronic averaging technique must be used to exclude the larger amplitude background electrical noise, composed largely of EEG activity, with some non-neuronal electrical activity. A plotter is also required. The signal varies with body size, position of the applied stimulus, conduction velocity of axons, number of synapses, location of neural generators of the evoked potential (EP) component, (i.e. either cortex or brain stem) and the presence of pathology.

Evoked potential recording is not yet a clinical tool for routine use, but subclinical lesions in multiple sclerosis may be detected by the combined use of auditory, visual and somatosensory EPs which show an abnormality in 80% of patients with a definite history of multiple sclerosis and in up to 50% of those without any sign of a brain stem lesion.

Clinical applications of evoked potentials

1. Multiple sclerosis. As demyelination increases, complete conduction block occurs at lower temperatures.
2. Other demyelinating diseases. In general, in demyelination, dissociation may occur of the EP peak latency and amplitude abnormalities. Latency prolongation with preservation of peak amplitude results from axon demyelination, but a reduction in peak amplitude occurs as more fibres die.
3. Intracranial tumours. EPs may be used in intraoperative monitoring of involvement of specific neural pathways. Auditory brain stem EPs have been used in the early diagnosis of posterior fossa tumours where there is an inverse relationship between operability and detectability for acoustic neuromas.
4. Head injury. Somatosensory EPs are sensitive to hypoxia and ischaemia. With a reduction in cerebral blood flow, there is a reduction in amplitude of somatosensory EPs, but the wave form is unchanged. Compressive lesions, e.g. subdural haematoma, increase the latency of the wave form. The number of wave peaks recognised in a finite period of time correlates well with outcome, but not with CAT scan findings (i.e. gives information on functional rather than anatomical lesions).
5. Disease of, and during surgery to, the spinal cord and brachial plexus.
6. Investigation of apnoea in preterm infants. Auditory brain stem EP conduction time is longer in babies with apnoea than in those without at similar post-conception ages, suggesting that apnoea may be related to neural function in the brain stem.

Central conduction time (CCT)

This is the time delay between an action potential generated in the brain stem and the first cortical potential recordable (normally less than 6.4 ms). Other times are also described, for example the dorsal column to cortex conduction time. CCT is independent of body size and peripheral nerve conduction velocity and is probably independent also of body temperature and barbiturate concentrations. Changes result from cortical dysfunction, abnormal synaptic delay in the thalamus or cortex (or both) and slowed axonal conduction. CCT at 10 and 35 days correlates well with outcome in head injury. Changes in brain electrical activity vary with cerebral blood flow, and CCT has been used as an index of reduction of cerebral blood flow in subarachnoid haemorrhage. It may be used also as a monitor of developing ischaemia in association with surgery for subarachnoid haemorrhage.

For prediction of outcome in severe head injury, multimodality EPs are more accurate than clinical neurological signs, or the Glasgow coma scale.

Nuclear magnetic resonance (NMR)

Nuclei of atoms with an odd number of protons or neutrons absorb or emit electromagnetic radiation when placed in a magnetic field. Hydrogen (protons), phosphorus ^{31}P, sodium ^{23}Na and carbon ^{13}C nuclei have been studied, ^{31}P spectroscopy is used to measure concentrations of ATP,

PCr and intracellular pH in muscle and neonatal brain metabolism. Repeated examinations, e.g. of tumour PCr, can indicate progression or remission of disease.

NMR imaging uses information on differences in relaxation times of nuclei. The contrast between grey and white matter in the brain is readily apparent, and excellent delineation is provided of pathologies such as demyelination and tumours in inaccessible sites. In the evaluation of lesions produced by multiple sclerosis or vascular lesions, findings are not pathognomonic but must be assessed, as with all ancillary investigation techniques, together with clinical signs. As with CAT scanning, contrast enhancement may be used. The hazards associated with NMR are discussed in Chapter 30.

Near-infrared spectrophotometry

Indices of cerebral oxygenation and haemodynamics may be quantified by this technique. Concentrations of oxygenated and reduced haemoglobin, oxidised cytochrome a_3 and total haemoglobin, together with cerebral blood volume and changes in cerebral blood flow, can be measured and displayed instantaneously. Striking changes have been observed in babies with cerebral oedema after birth trauma.

Some clinical aspects of neurophysiology may be investigated quantitatively, e.g. Glasgow coma scale (see p. 613). The increasing sophistication of peripheral nerve stimulators now makes it possible to monitor nerve conduction during neuromuscular blockade; this technique is discussed in Chapter 12. Electrodiagnostic procedures such as nerve conduction velocity and electromyography are useful investigations of neuromuscular disorders, but are beyond the scope of this chapter.

CEREBRAL CIRCULATION

The circle of Willis (Fig. 5.37) comprises an arterial circle at the base of the brain, supplied by the two internal carotid and two vertebral arteries. In man, there is almost no anastomosis between the internal and external carotid arteries but stenosis of one supplying vessel to the circle of Willis may be accommodated by an anastomotic collateral flow from other supplies. The branches of these four arteries communicate with each other over the surface of the cortex. Watershed areas between areas of major vessel supply are those most likely to suffer in hypoxia and ischaemia. Venous drainage is into sinuses which also receive CSF from arachnoid villi.

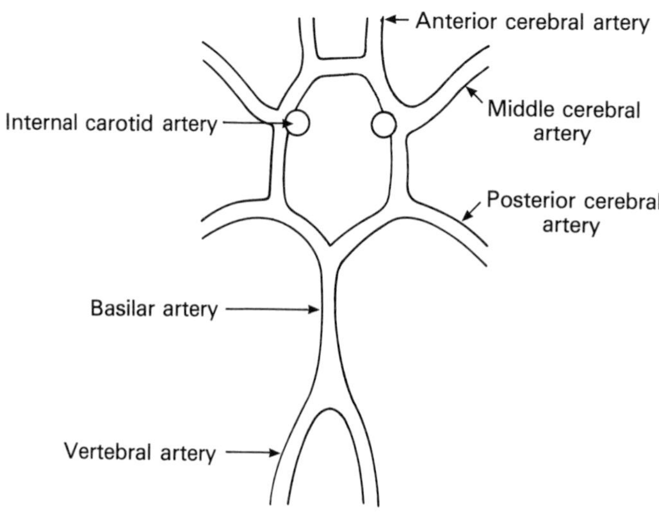

Fig. 5.37 The circle of Willis.

Cerebral blood flow

In dealing with the damaged brain, there are many circumstances in which it is important to obtain information on both global and regional blood flow. Autoregulation of cerebral blood flow and manipulation of intracranial pressure are discussed in Chapter 38, page 603. These two important aspects are therefore not considered further here.

FURTHER READING

Bell G H, Emsley-Smith D M 1980 In: Patterson C R (ed) Textbook of physiology, 10th edn. Churchill Livingstone, Edinburgh

Diuzewski A R, Halsey M J, Simmonds A C 1983 In: Baum H, Gergely J, Fauberg B L (eds) Molecular aspects of medicine 6. Pergamon Press, Oxford. p. 459

Greenburg R P, Ducker T P 1982 Evoked potentials in clinical neurosciences. Journal of Neurosurgery 56: 1

Hagbarth K-E 1983 Microelectric exploration of human nerves: physiological and clinical implications. Journal of the Royal Society of Medicine 76: 7

Hendry B 1981 Membrane physiology and cell excitation. Croom Helm, London

Larsson S J, Sauces A Jr, Ackman J J et al 1973 Noninvasive evaluation of head trauma patients. Surgery 74: 34

Levy W J, Shapiro H M, Maruchak G, Meathe E 1980 Automated EEG processing for intraoperative monitoring. Anesthesiology 53: 223

Lipton, Sampson 1979 Current topics in anaesthesia series no 2, Control of chronic pain. Arnold, London

Marshall B E 1981 Clinical implications of membrane receptor function in anesthesia. Anesthesiology 55: 160

McDowall G D 1976 Monitoring the brain. Anesthesiology 45: 117

Mitchell J D 1983 Nerve conduction studies and electromyography. Hospital Update 9: 443, 829

Wardley-Smith B, Halsey M J 1979 Recent molecular theories of anaesthesia. British Journal of Anaesthesia 51: 619

6. Maternal and neonatal physiology

The physiology of pregnancy and the neonatal period involves a 10-month period during which two (or more) individuals, the mother and the fetus/neonate, undergo more dramatic changes in the 'milieu interieur' than at any other time in their respective lives. The adjustments in maternal homeostasis which accompany the development of the products of conception frequently precede the demands which they appear to supply. The rapid change in maternal organ size and function during pregnancy is surpassed by the even more rapid regression to non-pregnant norms after delivery. The neonate then exhibits an independent anabolic capacity unequalled in any later period.

PREGNANCY

Cardiovascular system

Clinical examination in normal pregnancy may reveal evidence of slightly increased heart size and increased flow with a loud first heart sound, reduced splitting of the second sound and an early or mid-diastolic murmur at the left sternal border. The changed position of the heart alters the ECG axis; altered electrical complexes with more than the usual number of ectopic beats may be normal. Cardiac output, myocardial contractility, heart rate and stroke volume are increased; the increase in cardiac output (approximately 1.5 litres/min) starts in the first trimester, and is more marked in twin pregnancy. The arteriovenous oxygen content difference is reduced until the final month. When correlated with the reduced haemoglobin concentration in pregnancy, the oxygen flux (see Ch. 2) is little altered from the non-pregnant state by these combined effects.

Through the combined effects of reduced peripheral vascular tone and the formation of new vascular beds, peripheral resistance is decreased during pregnancy, particularly in the midtrimester, and returns towards normal at term. The effect on arterial pressure is offset partly by the increase in cardiac output during pregnancy. Pre-eclampsia is associated with increased peripheral resistance, reduced cardiac output and relative hypovolaemia.

As pregnancy progresses, venous pressure is raised particularly in the lower limbs, where oedema is seen in up to 40% of normotensive subjects. Central venous pressure may decrease dramatically in the supine position in late pregnancy, predominantly from mechanical obstruction of venous return by the gravid uterus with inadequate collateral circulation through vertebral and splanchnic venous channels. The decrease in venous return reduces cardiac output and, if compensatory vasoconstrictor reflexes are obtunded, e.g. during general anaesthesia or a spinal nerve block, may cause severe hypotension.

There is no change in pulmonary arterial pressure during pregnancy although pulmonary blood flow, and thus pulmonary vascularity on chest X-ray, are increased corresponding to the increase in cardiac output. Where raised pulmonary vascular resistance pre-exists, as in Eisenmenger's syndrome, pregnancy may lead to a rapid deterioration in the clinical state.

Although circulation time is not altered greatly in pregnancy, changes occur in regional distribution, with additional flow to uterus and placenta. The cardiovascular changes of pregnancy precede rather than follow formation of significant intervillous circulation. Renal blood flow rises to 400 ml/min above the non-pregnant level at the beginning of the second trimester and continues around this level until parturition. Increased skin blood flow results in subjective feelings of warmth and reduced heat tolerance although the increased peripheral blood flow is affected by posture and smoking. Capillary dilatation is demonstrable in pregnancy as is an increase in capillary numbers. Epistaxis and snoring in pregnancy coincide with nasal mucosal congestion and capillary dilatation. Breast engorgement and dilated veins on the breast surface may be part of the early signs of pregnancy. These multisystem changes reflect partly the increasing functional demands and contributions of maternal and fetal metabolism at this time. Exercise tolerance is reduced largely as a result of increased body mass.

In addition to the overall tendency to vasodilatation, some paradoxical responses occur where vasoconstriction would be expected normally. The pressor response to angiotensin is less than normal. Blocking the autonomic system may result in a dramatic decrease in systemic arterial pressure during pregnancy, suggesting a chronically active sympathetic tone.

Extradural nerve block is associated with increased venous capacity and decreased peripheral resistance in the lower limbs where pooling reduces venous return and effective circulating blood volume. Uterine contractions may mask the effective reduction in uterine perfusion by causing transient increases in systemic pressure as a result of iliac or aortic compression by the gravid uterus. In the hypertensive patient, uterine hypoperfusion may result from the combination of reduced circulating blood volume of pre-eclampsia and hypotension associated with an extradural block. In heart disease, e.g. mitral stenosis, the use of extradural anaesthesia with resultant reduced venous return helps to avoid pulmonary oedema, although cardiac output must be adequate to compensate for the effect of reduced peripheral resistance.

Respiratory system

Although some aspects of respiratory function have been studied inadequately in pregnancy because they necessitate invasive procedures or unrealistic demands on the pregnant woman, alterations in basic lung function throughout pregnancy have been well demonstrated.

In pregnancy, inspiratory capacity gradually increases by approximately 300 ml while residual and expiratory reserve volumes decrease by some 200–300 ml. As a result of a 200 ml increase in tidal volume and unchanged respiratory rate, the minute ventilation increases from approximately 7.5 litres/min to 10.5 litres/min in late pregnancy with a 30–40 ml/min increase in oxygen consumption. The main stimulation to overbreathing in pregnancy is a change in central respiratory control but mechanical factors contribute also. Forced expiratory volume remains at the normal 80–85% of vital capacity. Because of the greater reserve capacity of the respiratory system, significant functional deterioration is less common in pregnancy for respiratory than cardiovascular disease.

Arterial carbon dioxide tension is reduced, the change being most marked in early pregnancy in advance of the CO_2 transfer needs of the fetus. Breathlessness is a common complaint in pregnancy and relates more to changes in Pa_{CO_2} than in respiratory function; it is maximal up to 20 weeks' gestation. The low maternal Pa_{CO_2} allows transfer of CO_2 from fetal to maternal blood for excretion while maintaining fetal P_{CO_2} at a tolerable level. Arterial pH is maintained at 7.4 by reduced plasma bicarbonate and sodium concentrations.

Haematological system

The increased blood volume of pregnancy is seen from the first trimester and consists of increased red cell mass and, to a greater extent plasma volume, with consequent reduction in haemoglobin concentration despite a raised total haemoglobin content. The red cell concentration falls from approximately 4.2×10^{12}/litre to 3.7×10^{12}/litre in the third trimester. The lowest haemoglobin concentration (approximately 1.5 g/dl below non-pregnant levels in those with adequate iron intake) occurs at about 34 weeks' gestation.

There is an increased demand for iron in pregnancy to meet the maternal increase in red cell volume and the requirements of the fetus and placenta. Some 700–1400 mg are required for this total demand. Blood loss of 200–500 ml at delivery is equivalent to 100–250 mg iron, while subsequent breast feeding puts further demands on the mother's iron stores. The requirement for approximately 2.8 mg iron per day in early pregnancy, increasing to 6.6 mg per day in excess of normal needs, may be provided by maternal iron stores if the diet is adequate and absorption of dietary iron is maximal. Iron absorption increases in pregnancy from the normal 5–10% to 40% by late pregnancy. However, iron supplementation is recommended in many countries for the pregnant woman. The World Health Organisation recommends supplements of 30 to 60 mg iron per day to pregnant women with iron stores and 120 to 240 mg to women with no iron stores.

Folate requirements increase in pregnancy and the placenta transports folate actively to the fetus even when the mother is folate deficient. The first sign of folate deficiency is a low serum folate concentration, which precedes megaloblastic anaemia by several months. Because of the difficulty in confirming folate deficiency by laboratory means, poor haematological response to, or macrocytosis following, iron therapy should raise the suspicion of folate deficiency.

Increased folate intake should continue into the puerperium; signs of folate deficiency may appear first during breast feeding. A daily supplement of 300–500 mg of folate adequately covers the extra demands of pregnancy if the diet is suspect. Folate deficiency may be associated with abortion, fetal deformity, premature delivery and antepartum haemorrhage. The possible role of folate and vitamin deficiency at the time of conception in predisposing to neural tube defects in a susceptible group is now being investigated.

Vitamin B_{12} levels diminish during pregnancy especially in smokers, although maternal B_{12} stores are affected little. There is preferential transfer to the fetus. Deficiency of vitamin B_{12} is associated with subfertility or fetal death in utero. However, inadequate B_{12} intake is rare in all but strict vegans, who require supplementation at all times, including pregnancy.

The neutrophil count increases in pregnancy, related partly to oestrogenic stimulation, and reaches a plateau by 30 weeks. The peripheral white cell count may increase dramatically, even during uncomplicated labour. The lymphocyte count is affected little but function is suppressed, particularly with regard to cell-mediated immunity. Immunoglobulin and humoral immunity remain normal. These changes are thought to be crucial for the survival of the fetus although they result in decreased resistance to viral infection, to some bacteria and to malaria in susceptible populations. The platelet count shows a slight decrease in pregnancy.

Blood clotting and fibrinolysis alter during pregnancy as concentrations of factors VII, VIII, X and fibrinogen increase. The placenta plays a major role as a source of the specific lipoprotein thromboplastin, the action of which accelerates coagulation, bypassing the series of reactions involved in the contact system. Changes in coagulation factors are present from the third month. Low-grade coagulation may be demonstrated in the intervillous spaces of the placenta and walls of the spiral arteries. At placental separation, there is contraction of the myometrium and rapid closure of terminal spiral arteries, with a fibrin mesh covering the placental site.

Fibrinolysis in pregnancy is reduced until approximately 1 h after placental delivery, an inhibition thought to be mediated through the placenta while the increase in fibrin degradation products during labour may stem from the uterus. To accommodate the need for rapid coagulation following delivery, there is throughout pregnancy a state of hypercoagulability and a potential for thrombotic complications. Low-grade intravascular coagulation with altered clotting factor activity may occur in pre-eclampsia from 24 weeks. The coagulation changes, but not pre-eclampsia itself, may be counteracted by use of low-dose heparin.

Alimentary system

Increased appetite and thirst are common in pregnancy, as are food cravings and aversions, highly flavoured foods being favoured as taste threshold rises. The gums often swell and soften under the influence of oestrogen.

Gastro-oesophageal reflux and its symptoms occur more frequently as gastro-oesophageal sphincter pressure decreases. Gastric secretion diminishes in the first and second trimesters, increasing towards term. Gastric motility is reduced in pregnancy, particularly in labour or when opioid analgesics have been administered.

Small intestinal function shows changes compatible with increasing demand for nutrients such as iron and calcium. Gut motility is reduced and, with the angiotensin/aldosterone-induced increase in water and sodium absorption from the large intestine, constipation is a common complaint.

Liver function has been studied extensively in animals but less so in humans. Temporary cholestatic jaundice occurs in some women with increased bile viscosity and canalicular dilation; the changes reverse after parturition. Liver blood flow and carbohydrate metabolism alter little in pregnancy. Serum bilirubin concentration is moderately raised in up to 15% of pregnant women, and this causes pruritus in some. The smooth muscle of the gall bladder becomes hypotonic and bile is discharged less efficiently than normal.

Nutrition in pregnancy must supply adequate protein, fat and carbohydrate for growth of the products of conception and of the uterus. The increased maternal energy needs are balanced partly by reduced activity. An estimate of total nutrients of fetus and mother amassed over pregnancy is 1 kg protein and 3.5–4 kg fat which, with ongoing metabolic activity, approximates to an energy cost of 315–355 MJ (75–85 000 kcal). Energy is supplied by fat and carbohydrate, the latter mainly for the maternal brain and fetus, but with a small added requirement for structural material. Fat provides a fuel source apart from a small requirement for structural lipids and carrier substances. The new tissues laid down in the second half of pregnancy account for much of pregnancy's energy demands. Over the middle weeks maternal fat stores accumulate but in the final weeks before term the fetus, not the mother, stores fat. Overall, an extra 1 MJ (250 kcal) per day throughout pregnancy (or the equivalent in reduced energy expenditure) provide for increased demands. Calcium for the fetal skeleton includes approximately 30 g drawn from the maternal store. The general recommendation that an adequate mixed diet provides all the necessary nutrients for pregnancy appears to hold true, although iron and folate supplements are often advisable.

Plasma protein and albumin concentrations decrease in pregnancy; total lipid concentration, including phospholipids and non-esterified fatty acids, rises. Amino acids show cyclical changes during the menstrual cycle with a decrease after menstruation. Only glutamic acid and alanine/valine increase in concentration over the course of pregnancy. In general, vitamin concentrations change in pregnancy according to their type; fat-soluble vitamins increase with plasma fat concentrations while water-soluble vitamin concentrations decrease. Subclinical vitamin and mineral deficiencies are receiving attention currently in relation to a possible role in subfertility and a predisposition to neural tube defects (NTD). Emphasis is placed on preconception nutrition. Supplementation may be advisable both for replacement (e.g. zinc for smokers who eat a poor diet) and for therapy (e.g. high-dose vitamin supplements before and after conception for those at risk for NTD). The benefits of such dietary supplementation for the low-risk mother are unproven.

The needs for, and changes in, nutritional supplies during pregnancy cannot be estimated simply by measuring maternal plasma concentrations. There is a two-way exchange of metabolic products between mother and fetus and the homeostasis of pregnancy is only now being studied in detail.

Renal system

Renal blood flow and glomerular filtration rates rise in pregnancy. Renal glucose handling is altered in pregnancy, reflecting the increased GFR, changes in plasma volume, sodium and potassium reabsorption and possibly the action of sex steroid hormones. Mild to moderate glycosuria is common in the normal healthy pregnant woman. In pregnant diabetics, diabetic control must be based on blood glucose measurement.

Renal handling of bicarbonate is altered little in

pregnancy but there is a lower steady state plasma bicarbonate concentration and lower Pa_{CO_2}, i.e. a reduced buffer pool. Potassium is conserved progressively throughout pregnancy in order to supply the cellular needs of the developing fetus and maternal tissues. There is a relative resistance to action of mineralocorticoids during pregnancy. The altered water balance results in a reduced plasma osmolality. Because of the increased GFR, renal tubular reabsorption must increase in pregnancy, and there is increased aldosterone secretion.

Routine tests of renal function in pregnancy must be related to the pregnant norm. Serial creatinine clearances are useful and there are standards for urinary sediment findings in pregnancy. In the presence of renal disease, deteriorating renal function associated with hypertension is of grave significance.

Genital system

The corpus luteum of the ovary secretes progesterone which allows maintenance of early pregnancy prior to establishment of placental progesterone output, a function stimulated by human chorionic gonadotrophin (hCG) in association with luteinising hormone (LH).

The role of the uterus in pregnancy is to relax and contain the developing fetus and placenta with its associated tissues until the time of parturition when it must contract in a coordinated fashion to expel the uterine content. As pregnancy progresses, mild myometrial hypertrophy and possibly some hyperplasia occur.

Uterine activity progresses from high-frequency low-amplitude uncoordinated activity before 20 weeks, to lower-frequency, higher-amplitude contractions as term approaches. In the early months the uterus is insensitive to oxytocin. In contrast, prostaglandins E_2 and $F_{2\alpha}$ cause uterine contraction throughout pregnancy. The cervix softens and dilates during pregnancy to the end-point of full effacement and dilatation at delivery. The timing of cervical changes shows marked interindividual variation.

The factors controlling the onset of labour in the human remain uncertain despite intensive investigation. Pregnancy may continue to term and labour occur in women who have had oophorectomy or hypophysectomy during pregnancy. Fetal brain plays a part in the precise control of length of gestation; anencephalic pregnancies are often prolonged. In the sheep, the fetal pituitary and adrenal have a central role in initiating labour, but evidence for a similar mechanism in man is not conclusive. The changes in prostaglandin concentrations during labour have suggested their possible role in its induction and maintenance.

During labour itself, prostaglandin secretion is likely to be crucial, with fetal and maternal posterior pituitary hormones playing their part in the second stage. Local reflexes such as the stimulation of oxytocin and prostaglandin secretion by cervical dilatation, natural or artificial, may be affected by extradural anaesthesia. The uterus and cervix regress after parturition to near prepregnancy dimensions.

Endocrine system

Pituitary gland

The size of the pituitary gland increases in pregnancy with a dramatic increase in the number of prolactin-secreting cells and a decrease in growth hormone-secreting cells. The hormones of the pituitary show varying responses to pregnancy and lactation. Plasma prolactin concentrations increase progressively through pregnancy as secretion responds to oestrogen stimulation. The action of prolactin leads to changes in the mammary gland, may influence fetal fluid and electrolyte balance, and may have a role in maintaining calcium balance. After parturition, the concentration of prolactin declines but remains above non-pregnant concentrations to maintain lactation and prevent ovulation and conception during breastfeeding.

Growth hormone levels diminish during pregnancy and response to stimulation is reduced. ACTH, cortisol and metabolically inactive cortisone levels are higher than normal in pregnancy, possibly indicating a metabolic contribution from the placenta and fetus. Concentrations of thyrotrophin are altered little by pregnancy, although its effects may be mimicked weakly by hCG.

Antidiuretic hormone is not known to play a specific role in pregnancy. Pituitary tumour expansion during pregnancy may lead to diabetes insipidus which is usually temporary and need not compromise the pregnancy. Oxytocin is secreted during labour and exogenous oxytocin, particularly if administered intermittently, augments labour. Oxytocin is released during suckling, causing myometrial cell contraction and milk ejection, actions independent of vasopressin secretion.

Thyroid gland

Thyroxine and triiodothyronine have a primary role in cellular metabolism. Their secretion is controlled by thyroid stimulating hormone synthesised in the anterior pituitary in response to hypothalamic thyrotrophin releasing hormone which is secreted in the presence of low thyroid hormone concentrations. If iodine intake is borderline, the increased demand of pregnancy may stimulate compensatory follicular hyperplasia and goitre. Thyroxine binding globulin (TBG) concentration is raised in pregnancy; this is associated with increased T_4 and, in the last trimester, T_3. However, the free thyroxine index gives a result within, or at the upper end of, the normal range.

Clinical features of hyperthyroidism may occur in normal pregnancy as heat intolerance, tachycardia, emotional lability and goitre. However, when these features are combined with poor weight gain or lid lag they should raise the suspicion of hyperthyroidism, which, if untreated, carries a significant risk of perinatal mortality. Known autoimmune hyperthyroidism may remit in pregnancy with its relative immune suppression but is then likely to be exacerbated postpartum. If Graves' disease is associated with increased concentrations of long-acting thyroid stimulator (LATS), neonatal hyperthyroidism is likely and raised fetal heart rate may be recorded. Mild hypothyroidism is commoner than hyperthyroidism during pregnancy. Its diagnosis is important, carrying a risk, if untreated, of stillbirth or reduced infant IQ.

Placenta

The placenta forms a physical barrier between maternal and fetal tissues but contributes actively to the maintenance of pregnancy in both. The human placenta is of the syncytiotrophoblastic type, separating maternal and fetal tissue with a single cell matrix. Renin is secreted by the placenta and may have a role in regulating placental blood flow. Fibrin deposition on the placental villi is a common finding and may act in the immunological processes of pregnancy. The immune system is active in both mother and fetus yet is modified in such a way as to allow the fetus to develop within the mother without the expected stimulation of host rejection. The mechanism by which this occurs over nine months with subsequent return to normal immune responsiveness in both organisms is understood poorly. The mother may modify the antigenic activity of the fetus as the fetus may influence permanently the maternal response to its antigens.

The respiratory function of the placenta must ensure adequate oxygen transfer to the fetus and extraction for its own needs. Placental blood flow and the characteristics of adult and fetal blood allow these functions to be fulfilled. Because 2,3-diphosphoglycerate is less bound to fetal than adult haemoglobin there is less competition for oxygen binding sites. Fetal blood takes up oxygen more avidly than adult while maternal blood has reduced oxygen affinity. On reaching the tissues, the steep oxygen dissociation curve allows release of oxygen for a relatively small decrease in P_{O_2}.

Carbon dioxide diffuses readily from fetus to mother down the concentration gradient provided by the mother's hyperventilation. The placenta allows free diffusion of CO_2 from the fetus but buffers him from the effects of maternal acidosis. Carbon monoxide diffuses across the placenta and is taken up avidly by fetal haemoglobin causing reduced oxygen-carrying capacity and supply to the fetus; this is of importance if the mother smokes heavily in pregnancy.

Water diffuses freely among maternal and fetal tissues but net transfer is approximately 20–25 ml/day from mother to fetus. Any overhydration or dehydration of the mother affects the fetus in a similar way. Clinically this has occurred when women given low sodium fluids plus oxytocin in labour develop an antidiuresis with fetal and maternal hypo-osmolality and hyponatraemia leading to convulsions or death. Sodium and potassium exchange far in excess of the 6–7 g incorporated by the term fetus occurs during pregnancy.

The fetus is supplied with some 25–30 g glucose per day. The transfer is facilitated by diffusion stereospecific for D-glucose and there is a close correlation between maternal and fetal glucose levels. The placenta itself uses glucose for glycolytic and hexose monophosphate pathways. A small glycogen store occurs in the placenta, but its availability and purpose are uncertain.

Amino acids are transferred actively from mother to fetus with the highest amino acid levels in the placenta. Relative concentrations vary and some amino acids, e.g. glutamic acid, may play a carrier role. Only immunoglobulins are transferred as proteins to the fetus; these are mainly IgG, and may include abnormal antibodies such as those against platelets, leucocytes, red cells and long-acting thyroid stimulator (LATS).

Free fatty acids cross the placenta freely, the fetus synthesising lipids actively. Most lipids reflect maternal plasma levels but the concentration of arachidonic acid is higher in fetal plasma, possibly due to placental action on linoleic acid. Cholesterol transfers only slowly, most being synthesised by the fetoplacental unit.

Vitamins transfer by several methods, e.g. vitamin C crosses the placenta as dihydroascorbic acid and is converted to ascorbic acid which cannot recross the placenta. Folic acid occurs in different major forms in mother, placenta and fetus. Other water-soluble vitamins are thought to be transferred to the fetus in similar fashion.

Iron is transferred actively to the fetus with preferential placental uptake in situations of iron deficiency. Calcium, iodine and chromium are transported actively to the fetus, emphasising the danger of radio-iodine studies in pregnancy. Most toxic metals reach the fetus poorly but mercury and, to a lesser degree, lead may be transferred freely.

Viruses may cross to the fetus, especially cytomegalovirus (CMV), rubella, herpes simplex, varicella, variola, hepatitis B, enteroviruses, Echo, polio and sometimes HBSAg (large particles of surface antigen). Listeria, treponema, Group B streptococci, toxoplasma and, in some countries, malaria parasites are the most common bacterial pathogens to infect the fetus. The gestational age at which the fetus is exposed to teratogenic infection determines the extent to which he is likely to be affected. Viruses such as rubella and CMV which can disrupt development have their most profound effect in the first trimester while varicella is of greatest danger when it infects the late third trimester fetus. Pathogens such as group B β-haemolytic streptococci, HIV, herpes genitalis and chlamydia are acquired usually from the infected birth canal.

The placenta forms part of the fetoplacental unit and neither fetus nor placenta is complete as an endocrine organ. Placental steroids form part of a two-way traffic between mother and fetus. Its protein hormones appear to affect the mother while responding to fetal needs; human chorionic gonadotrophin (hCG), placental lactogen (hPL) and pregnancy-associated plasma proteins are described. The early appearance of hCG allows its detection to be used as a test for pregnancy; its role appears to be to stimulate ovarian and possibly placental steroidogenesis.

Progesterone is the major progestogen in pregnancy. Progesterone has an overall catabolic nitrogen-losing effect on maternal metabolism. Although progesterone levels in the fetus are higher than those in the mother, its fetal role is unclear.

THE NEONATE

Cardiovascular system

Fetal blood is oxygenated via the placenta from which venous blood flows through the umbilical vein with a P_{O_2} of 4 kPa. Approximately half of this flow bypasses the hepatic capillary system via the ductus venosus to the inferior vena cava and thence to the right (40%) and left (60%) atria, the latter by the streaming effect of the crista dividens and foramen ovale. Right atrial blood mixes with blood returning via the superior vena cava from the head and neck and with coronary sinus blood. At least 97% of blood from the superior vena cava enters the right ventricle and pulmonary artery while the left atrium and left ventricle receive better oxygenated umbilical vein blood and eject it through the ascending aorta, carotid and cerebral circulations to the head, neck and upper limbs. The less oxygenated right ventricular output supplies the lungs (10%) and, via the ductus arteriosus, the descending aorta. The high pulmonary vascular resistance, widely patent ductus arteriosus and low pressure placenta allow approximately half of total cardiac output to return to the placenta for oxygenation. Redistribution of blood flow in the fetus may occur in response to changes in demand.

During the early weeks of postnatal life there is a gradual readjustment of blood flow through the cardiac chambers and major vessels as supply matches the new demands. Initially the ventricles are of equal thickness, the pulmonary arteries are relatively small and the ductus arteriosus may be widely open or a large ductal diverticulum may be present. Cardiac output is relatively high in the neonate. The systolic arterial pressure of the term neonate is 70–90 mmHg. The normal preterm infant's arterial pressure is slightly lower.

Pulmonary vascular resistance is high in the fetus as a result of the low P_{O_2} in utero. The pulmonary vessels constrict in response to hypoxia, low pH and hypercapnia, dilating after birth when the P_{O_2} and pH rise and P_{CO_2} falls. Pulmonary expansion also adds to the effect of pulmonary vasodilatation. Pulmonary arterial pressure decreases dramatically over the first three days, then more slowly to reach adult levels by two weeks as thinning of the medial layer of the pulmonary vessels follows the early release of vasoconstrictor tone. Problems arise if pulmonary vascular resistance (PVR) remains high after birth, a situation which may accompany the hypoxia of lung disease or central hypoventilation, or as a primary disorder (persistent pulmonary hypertension). A left-to-right shunt defect (e.g. PDA, VSD) may lead to cardiac failure in the term infant after the first month when PVR has fallen. The onset of symptoms of congestive cardiac failure is often earlier in the preterm infant.

Autonomic responsiveness of the cardiovascular system may be demonstrated from an early stage of fetal development, although the balance of parasympathetic and sympathetic tone may change at different gestational ages. There may thus be unpredictable effects on the fetal heart rate of any autonomic stimulants or suppressors which cross the placenta after administration to the mother, e.g. to suppress labour or treat hypertension.

By full term, normal reflex control is present and significant baroreceptor function seems to be present in the premature infant. The specialised conducting tissues of the heart are present from early in the first trimester of pregnancy. By the time of delivery, the entire conducting system is fully formed. However, the neonatal myocardium has a limited capacity to compensate for a slow heart rate by increasing stroke volume. Thus, bradycardia causes a greater reduction in cardiac output than is usual in the adult.

The electrocardiogram differs markedly in the neonatal period from later infancy and childhood. Recording of V_4R is essential to allow interpretation of the childhood ECG. The QRS axis is normally right-sided at birth, approaching the adult left-sided pattern from the end of the neonatal period onwards. The T-wave changes rapidly after birth from upright to isoelectric or inverted in left chest leads while right chest leads show positive waves for the first 2–3 days. The changes in ECG complexes in the neonatal period are not explained fully by known anatomical changes, for dramatic haemodynamic changes occur mainly in the first two days.

Respiratory system

The fetus thrives at a P_{O_2} of 4 kPa, P_{CO_2} 6.5–7 kPa and pH 7.2. Irregular fetal breathing movements may be detected from the second trimester, becoming more vigorous and occupying longer periods as pregnancy advances. These movements appear to coincide with REM sleep; their significance is unknown but they are associated with movement of liquor and are vital for lung growth and development. They are affected by maternal smoking and may give some indication of fetal well-being.

At birth, the neonate must establish spontaneous pulmonary ventilation within seconds to maintain oxygenation. The stimuli to breathing appear to be sensory, involving touch, proprioception and the effects of cord occlusion. The readjustment of respiratory control which resets the sensors to maintain more 'adult' blood gas values involves changes in carotid chemoreceptor activity.

The importance of pulmonary surfactant in the establishment of normal respiration in the neonate is now accepted. The surface tension-lowering effect of surfactant reduces the work needed to re-expand the lung with inspiration. Levels of surfactant are low in the idiopathic respiratory distress syndrome (IRDS) and may diminish also after prolonged exposure to pure oxygen, or after such stresses as hypothermia or infection.

The stimulus to synthesis of surfactant is not known but its production by the fetus can be deduced from the study of amniotic fluid lipids. Attempts to hasten surfactant production by use of exogenous steroids given to the mother have not been consistently successful, although they may be effective in some cases if there is no maternal infection or hypertension and if they can be administered for 48 h before delivery. Use of continuous positive airways pressure to mimic the 'splinting' effect of surfactant may improve ventilatory function in IRDS. Recent trials have aimed to correct the respiratory abnormality by administration of artificial surfactant into the airway.

If the infant fails to establish spontaneous respiration at birth, the sequence of events leads from primary apnoea through gasping irregular respiration to the 'last gasp'; this is followed by secondary or terminal apnoea, when the heart continues to beat but spontaneous respiration will occur only after effective resuscitative intervention. Neonatal asphyxia may follow intra-uterine or intrapartum hypoxia, exposure to maternal opioids, acute blood loss, trauma (particularly intracranial injury) or massive aspiration. Hypoxaemia stimulates ventilation transiently in the neonate; in infants under two weeks hypoxaemia causes respiratory depression. The neonate may withstand hypoxaemia for longer than the adult but full cardiopulmonary resuscitation must be instituted promptly as the duration of hypoxaemia before delivery is seldom known. Heat loss, particularly from wet exposed skin, acidosis and hypoglycaemia, may exacerbate the neurological effects of asphyxia and should be corrected.

The gas-exchanging capacity of the lungs in utero is unknown but is likely to be small. Major gas exchange occurs via the placenta. The first breath requires a large negative intrathoracic pressure of -4 to -10 kPa with a volume of 30–40 ml. Thereafter compliance of the lungs increases and much smaller pressures are required. The tidal volume of a 3 kg infant is approximately 19 ml, his minute ventilation 530 ml/min and respiration rate 28/min. Total pulmonary resistance including airway and nasal resistance is approximately 2.7 kPa litre^{-1} s^{-1}, of which almost 50% results from nasal resistance, emphasising the importance of any nasal obstruction in the obligatory nose-breathing neonate. Lung tissue resistance is approximately 30% of total resistance.

Oxygen consumption in the neonate is approximately 7 ml min^{-1} kg^{-1} in a thermoneutral environment. CO_2 output is proportional to O_2 consumption, and depends on the respiratory quotient, which is low initially as brown fat is metabolised (0.7 on day 1 to 0.8 on day 7).

Ventilation perfusion ($\dot{V}/\dot{Q}$) mismatching in the neonate results from:

1. Perfusion of poorly ventilated lung (dead-space) assessed as 30% of each breath.
2. Poor perfusion of ventilated areas (venous admixture) or right to left shunting which decreases in the normal neonate from 24% at birth to 10% by the end of the first week. This shunt is increased when fetal channels including the foramen ovale or ductus arteriosus are open, a situation which is likely in hypoxaemia.

The neonatal Pa_{O_2} is approximately 10 kPa by 5 h, Pa_{CO_2} is normal by 20 min and pH by 24 h. Over the first two days, Pa_{CO_2} continues to decrease to approximately 4.5 kPa, then returns to normal, reflecting the respiratory compensation of the initial metabolic acidosis accompanying the elevated lactate levels at birth. The normal neonate has a slightly lower Pa_{O_2} than the adult but his haemoglobin is 97% saturated by day 2 as he has 60–70% HbF; this is replaced gradually with HbA over the first 3 months (Table 6.1).

Haematological system

The full term infant has a red cell count of 4.6–5.3 $\times$ 10^{12}/litre and a haemoglobin concentration of 13.7–20.2 g/dl, varying greatly with the extent of placental transfusion which may be up to one-third of neonatal blood volume. During the second month marrow activity, though present, is much reduced and is outstripped by the growing neonate's blood volume, resulting in a fall

Table 6.1 Effect of HbF on oxygen saturation (%) at pH 7.4 during the early months of life in a term infant. The normal S-shaped curve of oxygen dissociation is shifted to the left by HbF

Age	Oxygen tension (kPa)		
	4	7	10
Day 1	75–80	95	>95
Day 5	70–75	90–95	>95
3 weeks	65–70	90	>95
6–9 weeks	60–65	85–90	95
3–4 months	55–60	85	90–95
6 months	50–55	80–85	90–95
8–11 months	50	80	90–95

in haemoglobin concentration to approximately 11 g/dl by the ninth week; the fall in haematocrit is even greater because MCV decreases simultaneously, attaining the adult range by age 1 year. Supplementary haematinics do not prevent this 'physiological anaemia' but the preterm infant, who has foregone the normal accumulation of iron stores in the third trimester, may require supplementary iron in addition to vitamins, folic acid and in some cases vitamin E.

Various red cell antigens develop during fetal life, their perinatal importance being their potential for crossing the placenta and inducing an immune reaction in the mother. If the maternal antibody so formed is of the IgG class and in sufficient quantity it may cross to the fetus and induce significant haemolysis with the risks of hyperbilirubinaemia and anaemia before or after birth. This occurs with the Rhesus D antigen formed early in fetal life, other Rhesus antibodies being rare. In the 10% of Rhesus-negative pregnancies in which a sensitised mother carries a Rhesus-positive infant there is a 1 in 15–20 chance of that infant suffering haemolytic disease of the newborn. Sensitisation has usually occurred during an earlier pregnancy (recognised or not) or following transfusion of Rhesus-positive blood.

The administration of anti-D immunoglobulin to the Rhesus-negative mother after first exposure to Rhesus antigen (i.e. after delivery of a first D-positive infant or termination of a D-positive pregnancy) removes the circulating antigen, prevents or reduces the stimulation of the immune response and minimises the risk to the next Rhesus-positive fetus.

The ABO system antigens develop early but remain relatively ineffective as immune stimulants until after birth so that the risk of haemolytic disease of the newborn from ABO incompatibility is much less than that from Rhesus disease. In addition, much of the anti-A and anti-B antibody is IgM and therefore does not cross the placenta. The IgG form does cross and may cause neonatal haemolysis with early jaundice and subsequent anaemia. The other blood group antigens develop at different times and with varying antigenicity. The Kell antibody is a rare but well-recognised cause of haemolytic disease.

Maternal IgG crosses to the fetus from 32 weeks' gestation to provide passive immunity to the term neonate against many common infections. Maternal IgG concentrations decrease over the first 3 months as the neonate's active antibody synthesis becomes effective. The early months are a time of immature immune function. The extremely preterm infant suffers also from lack of maternal immunoglobulin transfer before birth, and is, in effect, immunocompromised with all the hazards that this implies.

At term, HbF constitutes some 80–90% of the total haemoglobin although γ-chain synthesis is already on the decline. This proportion falls rapidly during the first four months to approximately 10–15% as HbF-containing red cells leave the circulation. Adult β-chain HbA concentration rises as HbF falls, eventually constituting more than 90% of the total. The normal decrease in HbF and resultant change in oxygen-carrying capacity is hastened by transfusion with adult blood. The diagnosis of α-thalassaemia may be made from study of trophoblast aspirates in early pregnancy, but in the infant diagnosis is delayed until after completion of the normal decline in HbF.

The normal granulocyte count at term is approximately 8×10^9/litre with a wide range of normal (6–26). Lymphocytes appear in the blood at the tenth week of gestation and increase to approximately 4.0×10^9/litre by term (range 2–11). Although chemotaxis of granulo- and monocytes is less efficient in the healthy neonate, phagocytosis and killing are normal. Humoral factors (e.g. complement) are reduced especially in the preterm infant, while the stress of illness reduces granulocyte bactericidal activity.

Alimentary system

The functions of the gut include swallowing, digestion, absorption and onward propulsion of ingested nutrients. Swallowing occurs first at approximately the twelfth fetal week, increasing in frequency until, by the twenty-third week, approximately 5 ml kg^{-1} h^{-1} of amniotic fluid is swallowed. The coordination of swallowing involves tongue, palatal and pharyngeal muscles with the reflex response then allowing laryngeal elevation and glottic closure.

The oesophagus provides a transit route for swallowed material; absorption does not occur there although salivary amylase is already initiating digestion of starch. The lower oesophageal sphincter is variable in action in the neonate and may permit gastro-oesophageal reflux.

While gastric mixing involves all areas of the stomach, onward propulsion requires coordination of antral, pyloric, duodenal and thence intestinal activity. Rates of gastric emptying show marked individual variation in the newborn and may be slowed by any coexisting systemic illness, effects of some maternal drugs and extreme prematurity.

In common with the adult, the neonate absorbs fat as chylomicra after its digestion by pancreatic lipase, action of bile salts, hydrolysis and re-esterification. Although deranged exocrine pancreatic function affects fat absorption, this is rarely a significant problem in the neonate. Bile salt abnormalities may affect fat absorption with associated malabsorption of the fat-soluble vitamins A, D, E and K; these must therefore be supplemented parenterally if fat absorption is reduced. In the neonate, vitamin K deficiency may present as haemorrhagic disease of the newborn with spontaneous bleeding, usually into the gut, the renal tract or the central nervous system. This disorder occurs in wholly breast-fed infants because breast milk contains very much less vitamin K than the artificial formula feeds. A single dose of vitamin K given enterally or parenterally after birth prevents this potentially serious problem.

Water and electrolyte absorption is one of the major roles of the large intestine. Osmotic gradients play an important role in facilitated reabsorption of water and electrolytes and severe diarrhoea can result in the neonate from inappropriate use of hyperosmolar feeds. Colonic fluid absorption is associated with a prostaglandin-mediated mechanism.

Passage of meconium occurs normally within the first 24 h in the term infant. Delayed passage beyond 48 h or associated with abdominal distension raises the suspicion of Hirschsprung's disease. Meconium is an alkaline mixture of swallowed debris, desquamated cells and bile. Meconium staining of the amniotic fluid indicates fetal distress and an infant born from such an intra-uterine environment risks meconium aspiration. Rigorous aspiration of the oro- and nasopharynx before the first breath with direct aspiration of the trachea if necessary minimise the risk of the potentially life-threatening meconium aspiration syndrome which results from mechanical obstruction of airways and chemical pneumonitis.

Neonatal jaundice

Jaundice is common in the neonatal period. Up to half of all neonates become noticeably icteric. Pathological processes may explain the development of jaundice by excess haemoglobin breakdown, e.g. Rhesus disease, ABO incompatibility, red cell fragility in hereditary spherocytosis, red cell enzyme defects in glucose-6-phosphate dehydrogenase (G-6-PD) and pyruvate kinase deficiencies, systemic infection, polycythaemia following a large placental transfusion or resorption of extravasated blood caused by bruising at delivery. Much less commonly, metabolic or hepatic defects may give rise to jaundice. However, no specific cause for jaundice is identified in the majority of neonates and the label 'physiological jaundice' may be applied. This is thought to result from a combination of reduced red cell lifespan, increased haem breakdown and limited hepatic enzyme capacity for conjugation. The hyperbilirubinaemia is thus unconjugated, appears after the first 2 days, rises to a peak around day 4–5, then decreases over a similar period as the liver enzymes increase in activity.

The most significant risk of unconjugated hyperbilirubinaemia is deposition of bilirubin in the cells of the basal ganglia, midbrain and brain stem leading to kernicterus with later deafness, low IQ and dyskinetic cerebral palsy. There is no absolute level of bilirubin at which this occurs but levels of unconjugated bilirubin much above 350 μmol/litre in a well, full-term infant are avoided by use of exchange transfusion or phototherapy; the latter induces photodegradation of bilirubin in the skin to water-soluble products excreted in the urine. The risks of hyperbilirubinaemia are increased by coexisting hypothermia, hypoglycaemia, acidosis, dehydration and prematurity.

Drugs in the neonate may affect jaundice by displacing bilirubin from albumin (e.g. sulphonamides), by affecting hepatic enzyme activity (e.g. phenobarbitone) or by increasing red cell breakdown in the G-6-PD deficient subject.

Nervous system

Although development of the central and peripheral nervous systems occurs throughout gestation, a massive further growth in size and complexity occurs after birth. Myelination is achieved over the late fetal period and into the early months of life. Pathological processes in late pregnancy and the neonatal period may have much greater effects on the subsequent potential for development in the nervous system in comparison with systems whose basic structure is laid down in early gestation. The presence of so-called primitive reflexes is recognised at term but lack of integration of spinal and autonomic reflexes may result in an unpredictable response of the neonate to environmental stimuli. Thus, thermoregulation may be inefficient, causing rapid onset of hypothermia, and nasal occlusion may result in central apnoea rather than mouth breathing.

Renal system

Renal function in utero differs from that after birth in that the placenta regulates water and electrolyte transport until parturition. The fetal kidneys regulate production of amniotic fluid by producing large volumes of urine with a relatively low sodium concentration. Intra-uterine renal blood flow is low relative to postnatal values because of higher renal vascular resistance.

At birth the neonate continues to have a high urine flow rate with little sodium reabsorption over the early hours, although this increases after the first week. Neonatal plasma osmolarity is influenced profoundly by the osmolality of the mother's plasma and later by administered enteral and parenteral fluids; there is limited ability to handle water or solute loads. Renal bicarbonate handling shows a pattern of maturation reflecting changes in the neonatal capacity for handling sodium. Urine pH may therefore remain inappropriately high in the presence of acidaemia.

Endocrine system

Pituitary and adrenal glands

The adrenal cortex in the fetus functions as part of the so-called fetoplacental unit. Placental pregnenolone offers the fetal adrenal zone its required precursor for cortisol and corticosterone synthesis. As term approaches, the adult zone expands with the necessary 3-β-hydroxy-dehydrogenase for independent conversion of pregnenolone to progesterone.

The fetal pituitary is sensitive to feedback inhibition by excess maternal corticosteroids administered at high dose therapeutically or resulting from excessive maternal synthesis in Cushing's syndrome. Such infants are at risk of hypoadrenalism after delivery. Normally fetal pituitary ACTH stimulates the fetal and adult areas of the adrenal from the end of the first trimester. Growth hormone is secreted by the neonatal pituitary gland but at this stage it appears to affect insulin action and glucose metabolism rather than acting as a primary determinant of somatic growth.

Thyroid gland

Neonatal thyroxine concentration is very nearly equal to maternal levels with a rapid increase in thyroid activity associated with TSH secretion over the first 2 days, then a fall by 5 days. TSH levels are higher in cord than maternal blood, peak at 15–30 min after birth then fall to childhood levels by 2 to 3 days. This peak may be influenced by body and environmental temperature changes at delivery.

The thyroid hormones affect total energy expenditure, primary physiological functions including cardiac output, heart rate, glomerular filtration rate, renal plasma flow and water secretion, and CNS function. The hypothyroid neonate may be diagnosed clinically at birth or in the early weeks, or may be identified by high TSH levels on neonatal screening with no signs or symptoms, presumably with some residual thyroid responding to increased TSH stimulation. An ectopic or lingual thyroid may produce this biochemical picture. Early detection and treatment improves prognosis for development and growth.

Neonatal hyperthyroidism is rare but may occur in an infant whose mother has been hyperthyroid due to LATS action. The infant may be irritable, jaundiced with hepatosplenomegaly, thrombocytopenia, exomphalos, goitre and congestive cardiac failure. Signs may appear only after some days or weeks and, although treatment may be required to control symptoms, the disorder is self-limiting.

Endocrine pancreas

The normal term infant has a normal insulin response to ingested carbohydrate from birth. Blood glucose concentrations of neonates are often

Table 6.2 Some common drugs to be avoided in pregnancy

Drug	Adverse effect
β-Adrenoceptor blocking drugs (risk greatest if severely hypertensive)	Neonatal hypoglycaemia and bradycardia
Bethanidine Debrisoquine Guanethidine	Reduced uteroplacental perfusion due to postural hypotension
Captopril	May affect fetal neonatal blood pressure and renal function
Diazoxide	Inhibits uterine activity in labour. Prolonged use impairs glucose tolerance in neonate
Reserpine	Neonatal bradycardia, drowsiness and nasal stuffiness
Oral anticoagulants	Congenital malformations. Fetal and neonatal haemorrhage
Streptokinase/urokinase	Premature placental separation and possibly fetal haemorrhage

Table 6.2 (Cont'd)

Drug	Adverse effect
Barbiturates	Withdrawal effects in neonates
Benzodiazepines	Neonatal drowsiness, hypotonia, hypotension, hypoglycaemia
Phenothiazines	Neonatal extrapyramidal effects
Tricyclic antidepressants	Tachycardia, irritability, convulsions
Aspirin	Impaired platelet function. Kernicterus in jaundiced neonate. Possible effect on fetal ductus arteriosus and pulmonary artery pressure
Indomethacin, naproxen, etc.	May close fetal ductus and cause persistent neonatal pulmonary hypertension
Opioid analgesics	Long term — severe withdrawal. Short term — depress ventilation
Phenytoin	Congenital malformations, bleeding
Phenobarbitone	Congenital malformations
Aminoglycosides	Auditory nerve damage
Chloramphenicol	Blood dyscrasia (grey syndrome)
Sulphonamides (incl. cotrimoxazole)	Neonatal haemolysis. Displaces bilirubin increasing risk of kernicterus
Tetracyclines	Tooth discoloration
Trimethoprim	Folate antagonism
Primaquine	Neonatal haemolysis and methaemoglobinaemia
Antithyroid drugs	Neonatal goitre and hypothyroidism
Cytotoxic agents	Teratogenesis
Inhalational anaesthetics	Depress neonatal ventilation
Local anaesthetics	Large doses may depress neonatal ventilation and produce hypotonia, bradycardia
Prilocaine	Neonatal methaemoglobinaemia

lower than those of adults without causing apparent symptoms of hypoglycaemia, particularly in preterm infants. Treatment of hypoglycaemia is indicated if symptoms are present or if it is persistent despite feeding.

Pancreatic hypersecretion of glucagon and insulin with hypoglycaemia may occur in neonates with erythroblastosis fetalis, particularly if preterm. There are marked changes in glucagon levels although the details of these interactions are not yet fully understood. Infants of poorly controlled diabetics are also at risk of neonatal hypoglycaemia.

Parathyroid glands and calcitonin-producing cells in the thyroid

The fetus maintains higher serum concentrations of calcium and phosphorus than the mother as a result of an active placental transport system. Abnormalities of maternal calcium homeostasis may affect the fetus secondarily. Maternal parathyroid hormone does not cross the placenta to the fetus. The hypercalcaemic fetal norm is associated with high phosphate levels and high renal tubular reabsorption of phosphorus.

Drugs and the fetus

Metabolism of drugs by the neonate may be very different from that in the adult and may change rapidly as enzyme activity alters. As in any patient, the risks of drug therapy may outweigh potential benefits. Exposure of the fetus to drugs in early pregnancy may interfere with normal growth and differentiation, e.g. thalidomide, phenytoin, warfarin. Use of drugs in late pregnancy may produce postpartum effects; for example, sedation may result from administration of opioid analgesics to the mother, and profound hypotonia, hypotension and hypoglycaemia may follow administration of benzodiazepines, some of which have a half-life of several days in the neonate. Table 6.2 lists some common drugs which may produce adverse effects if administered during pregnancy.

FURTHER READING

Comline R S, Cross K W, Dawes G S, Nathanielsz P W 1975 Fetal and neonatal physiology. Proceedings of the Sir Joseph Barcroft Centenary Symposium. Cambridge University Press, Cambridge

Davis J A, Dobbing J 1981 Scientific foundations of paediatrics, 2nd edn. William Heinemann, London

Godfrey S, Baum J D 1979 Clinical paediatric physiology. Blackwell Scientific Publications, Oxford

Hytten F E, Chamberlain G 1980 Clinical physiology in obstetrics. Blackwell Scientific Publications, Oxford

Hytten F E, Leitch I 1971 The physiology of human pregnancy, 2nd edn. Blackwell Scientific Publications, Oxford

MacDonald R (ed) 1978 Scientific basis of obstetrics and gynaecology, 2nd edn. Churchill Livingstone, Edinburgh

Mirkin B L 1975 Perinatal pharmacology: placental transfer, fetal localisation and neonatal distribution of drugs. Anesthesiology 43: 156

Shearman R P (ed) 1979 Human reproductive physiology. Blackwell Scientific Publications, Oxford

Smith C A, Nelson N M (eds) 1976 The physiology of the newborn infant. Charles C Thomas, Springfield, Illinois

Stern L 1972 Drug interaction, part II: drugs, the newborn infant and the binding of bilirubin to albumin. Paediatrics 47: 916

7. Haematology

Surgery and anaesthesia make heavy demands on departments of haematology and blood transfusion. Consultation between the anaesthetist and haematologist should be frequent both in the operating theatre and intensive therapy unit if the provision of, for example, appropriate blood products and the correct investigation of the bleeding patient are to proceed smoothly and expeditiously.

ANAEMIA

Anaemia is present when the red cell mass (the erythron) is reduced below that which is normal for the patient's age and sex. There are many causes and these are classified conventionally as:

1. *Blood loss* which may be acute or chronic.
2. *Failure of erythropoiesis* resulting from, for example, inadequate supplies to the bone marrow of nutrients: iron, vitamin B_{12}, folate, some hormones or protein. Erythropoiesis may be impaired also by bone marrow infiltration in leukaemia or other malignant disease. Most chronic disorders produce what is termed secondary or symptomatic anaemia. This is seen in inflammation, infection and malignant disease (even when the marrow is not infiltrated). Secondary anaemias are seen commonly in rheumatoid arthritis, renal failure and chronic sepsis.
3. *Shortened red cell lifespan*. The haemolytic anaemias are subdivided into:
   a. inherited and congenital, e.g. hereditary spherocytosis, sickle cell anaemia and some red cell enzyme defects;
   b. acquired, e.g. autoimmune haemolytic anaemia, paroxysmal nocturnal haemoglobinuria and drug-induced haemolysis.

It is obvious that alternative classifications are possible, and also true that many forms of anaemia may be allocated to more than one category. Thus, chronic blood loss produces negative iron balance with eventual failure of erythropoiesis from iron deficiency. Pernicious anaemia is an erythropoietic failure resulting from lack of correct digestion of vitamin B_{12}, but red cell precursors and mature red cells in this disease have a shortened lifespan.

Anaemia is demonstrated by the measurement of the amount of haemoglobin in a known volume of blood. Haemoglobin concentration is reported commonly as grams per decilitre (g/dl) but this unit is being replaced progressively by grams per litre (g/litre). Anaemia is said to be present in an adult male if the haemoglobin concentration is less than 13.5 g/dl (135 g/litre) and in an adult female if less than 11.5 g/dl (115 g/litre). In the first year of life the haemoglobin concentration decreases from 18–20 g/dl at birth to 9.5 g/dl at one month to attain levels at 12 months close to those of female adults. In pregnancy, haemoglobin levels should not decrease below 11.5 g/dl if iron and folate are taken as prescribed.

Modern electronic blood counting equipment provides accurate red cell indices in addition to haemoglobin estimation and provides guidance on the type of anaemia before resort to further investigation.

With the notable exception of acute blood loss, reduction in red cell mass is accompanied by an increase in plasma volume, thus preserving blood volume. The mechanism for this is not clear but it is one of the compensatory mechanisms adopted during anaemia of any duration. Of equal importance is a shift of the oxygen dissociation curve to the right through increased synthesis of 2,3-diphosphoglycerate (2,3-DPG) in the red cell via the Embden–Meyerhof pathway of anaerobic glycolysis and the Rapaport–Luebering shunt. Increases in 2,3-DPG render the haemoglobin molecule less avid for oxygen at any given partial pressure and improve tissue oxygenation. Two remaining compensatory mechanisms in anaemia are an increase in cardiac stroke volume and an increase in heart rate.

In acute blood loss, red cells and plasma are lost together, such that in the first few hours haemoglobin and haematocrit measurements change little and cannot be used to estimate blood loss. Surgeons have always attributed much importance to the haematocrit but in continued acute bleeding the haemoglobin and haematocrit move in parallel as haemodilution takes place, the reduction being complete by 24–48 h if transfusion is not carried out.

HAEMOGLOBINOPATHIES AND THALASSAEMIAS

The haemoglobinopathies and thalassaemias are a complex and diverse series of inherited abnormalities of globin chain synthesis. The thalassaemias are characterised by absent or reduced production of the affected globin chain whilst the other chains which make up the haemoglobin molecule are normal. In the haemoglobinopathies the affected chain, usually the β or α chain, has an amino acid substitution which, if it affects the structure or function of the haemoglobin molecule as a whole, may produce clinical effects.

β-Thalassaemia

β-Thalassaemia, in which β-globin chain synthesis is impaired, is classified into three clinical grades.

1. *β-Thalassaemia trait (thalassaemia minor)* is the heterozygous state and produces little clinical effect. There may be slight anaemia and the condition may be mistaken for iron deficiency. In pregnancy the haemoglobin level may decrease below the normal range.

2. *Thalassaemia intermedia*, as the name implies, is associated with more marked anaemia than thalassaemia trait and generally is caused by homozygosity of a less severe β-thalassaemia gene. Occasionally, patients may require transfusion.

3. *Thalassaemia major (Cooley's anaemia)* is the homozygous inheritance of a severe β-thalassaemia gene. No β-chains are produced, thus preventing the synthesis of adult haemoglobin. Without blood transfusion, the condition is generally fatal in the early years of childhood and even with regular transfusion support patients may not live beyond their early twenties as a result of iron overload. Long-term iron chelation therapy may prevent transfusional iron overload. Bone marrow transplantation may be considered.

α-Thalasseamia

α-Thalassaemia is a genetically variegate disorder which ranges in severity from fetal death in utero in the homozygous form to a mild hypochromic disorder in the heterozygous form. Patients with three of the four α-chain genes deleted suffer HbH disease of intermediate severity, and some require transfusion with red cells.

Haemoglobinopathies

More than 100 haemoglobin variants have been described but only one has significant global clinical impact — haemoglobin S. Ten per cent of patients of African extraction carry the S gene. It is also seen in Italy, Greece, Arabia and the Indian subcontinent. Haemoglobin S has valine substituted for glutamine in position 6 of the β-globin chain and this confers physical differences on the haemoglobin molecule with profound clinical consequences in homozygotes. Haemoglobin S becomes insoluble at oxygen tensions in the venous range (5–5.5 kPa) and crystallises, imposing a sickle-cell shape on the red cell. The sickled red cell is rigid and does not pass easily through capillaries, leading to occlusion, tissue infarction and the pain which is characteristic of clinical episodes known as crises. Red cell survival is reduced greatly and homozygous patients invariably have anaemia (6–10 g/dl) and jaundice. Heterozygotes are almost asymptomatic and their red cells sickle only when oxygen tensions are unphysiologically low (2 kPa). Sickle haemoglobin may be demonstrated rapidly in patients' blood using a commercial kit, e.g. Sickledex. The presence or absence of HbS should be established before anaesthesia in all patients of affected ethnic groups. It may be necessary to pretransfuse electively homozygotes with HbA or consider exchange transfusion to raise percentages of HbA compared with HbS. Clearly it is essential to maintain good oxygenation of the homozygous patient pre-, intra- and postoperatively and consideration should be given to oxygen therapy for 24 h after anaesthesia. Postoperative infarctive episodes may occur even with the most meticulous attention to detail. Sickling is enhanced by low blood pH, high red cell 2,3-DPG, stasis, dehydration and increased plasma osmolality.

HAEMOSTASIS AND FIBRINOLYSIS

The haemostatic mechanism

There are three principal components: platelets, coagulation and what may be termed limiting mechanisms including fibrinolysis. These may be altered individually or collectively in disease to produce haemostatic failure. Investigation of the bleeding patient should include all three components.

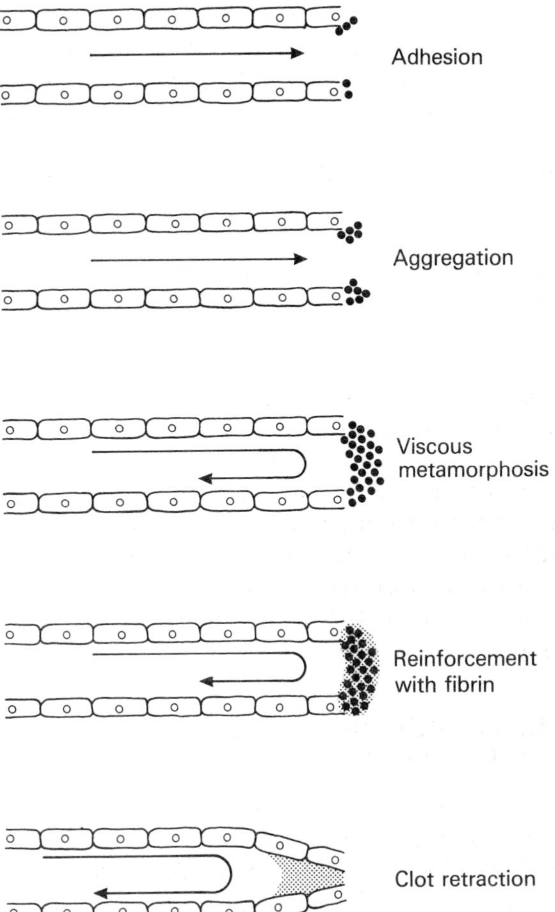

Fig. 7.1 Formation of a platelet plug.

Platelets

Primary haemostasis depends solely on the presence of adequate functional platelet numbers (Fig. 7.1). The normal whole-blood platelet count is $150–400 \times 10^9$/litre. The lower limit of 'normal' depends upon the method used for their quantitation but a platelet count below 100×10^9/litre is considered to be thrombocytopenia. The risk of haemostatic failure increases as the platelet count decreases and when levels below 30×10^9/litre are reached spontaneous bleeding may occur. Bleeding is precipitated if there is local pathology, e.g. peptic ulcer, or if there is a surgical wound. Thrombocytopenic bleeding occurs less at a particular platelet count if the low platelet numbers result from peripheral destruction with a functional bone marrow (e.g. autoimmune thrombocytopenia) than if platelet production is impaired, for example in bone marrow disorders (e.g. leukaemia or myeloma).

For adequate primary haemostasis the platelets should also function normally. In comparison to the rare inherited platelet functional disorders, drug-induced platelet metabolic damage occurs more commonly. Non-steroidal anti-inflammatory drugs (NSAIDs) impair prostaglandin synthetic pathways by inhibition of the enzyme cyclo-oxygenase. Aspirin (acetylsalicylic acid) is the prime example and its effect on measured in vitro function of platelets lasts up to 14 days. Other therapeutic agents affecting platelet function include sulphinpyrazone, dipyridamole and dextran. Drug-induced platelet dysfunction may cause bleeding in the face of adequate platelet numbers and patients should be encouraged to discontinue the drug, preferably 2 weeks before major surgery, particularly with respect to the NSAIDs.

Uraemia is accompanied by acquired platelet dysfunction which may be corrected by dialysis. Platelets in the myeloproliferative disorders including some leukaemias may function poorly.

Stored whole blood for transfusion contains few viable platelets; after storage for only 3 days, platelet recovery in vivo is only 20%. Thus, in massive transfusion (more than 10 units), platelet numbers decline progressively but rarely decrease below 50×10^9/litre even when twice the patient's blood volume has been transfused.

Platelet function in vivo is measured best by the bleeding time carried out by haematology staff according to strict methodology. This should not be undertaken unless platelet numbers have been shown to be normal, or bleeding is out of proportion to platelet numbers and coagulation is demonstrably normal. Careful examination of the patient reveals clues to thrombocytopenia: petechial purpura particularly below the knee, blood-filled blisters in the mouth and fundal haemorrhages. In the patient in theatre, oozing at the operation and venepuncture sites acts as an indicator. The strategy of platelet transfusion is described below.

Coagulation

The second phase of haemostasis involves the coagulation proteins (Table 7.1) which stabilise the haemostatic plug provided by the platelets. Central to this is the production of thrombin (Fig. 7.2) from prothrombin by the action of activated

Table 7.1 International nomenclature of clotting factors

Factor	Synonym
I	Fibrinogen
II	Prothrombin
III	Tissue thromboplastin
IV	Calcium ions
V	Labile factor
VI	Unassigned
VII	Stable factor
VIII	Antihaemophilic factor (AHF)
IX	Christmas factor
X	Stuart–Prower factor
XI	Plasma thromboplastin antecedent (PTA)
XII	Contact factor
XIII	Fibrin stabilising factor

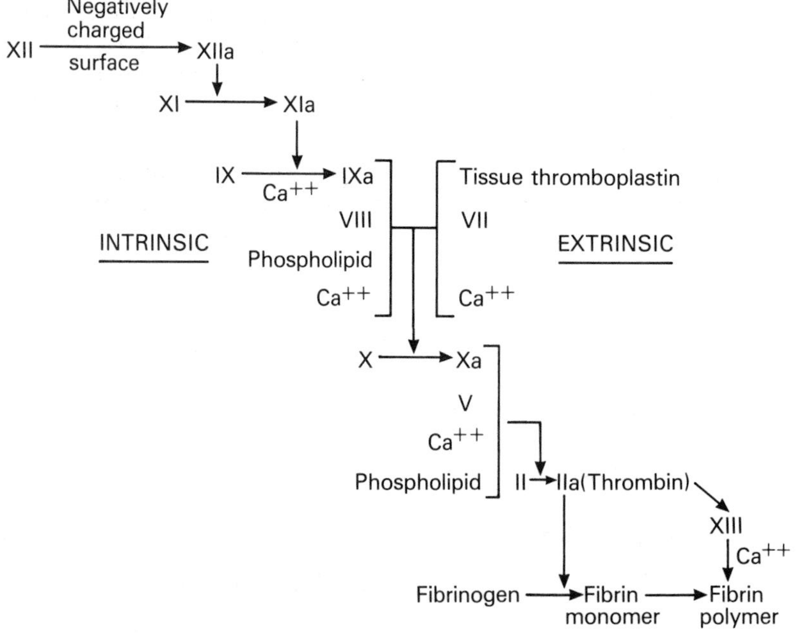

Fig. 7.2 Intrinsic and extrinsic coagulation pathways; 'a' indicates activation of the factor concerned. Phospholipid is provided by platelets and plasma.

factor X. Thrombin cleaves fibrinogen to form fibrin. Two pathways lead to the conversion of prothrombin and are composed of linked proteolytic enzymes which act first as substrates and then as activated enzymes. The first pathway is intrinsic (all components circulate in plasma). Its first component is the contact factor XII which requires an exposed subendothelial surface for its activation. A series of reactions involving coagulation factors and cofactors culminates in the prothrombin–thrombin reaction. Extrinsic coagulation joins the cascade at the pivotal factor X and requires tissue juices for its inception. Activated by thrombin, factor XIII stabilises the fibrin polymer by cross-linkages between amino acids in adjacent fibrin strands.

Limiting factors

The third set of reactions serves to inhibit the unbridled extension of thrombus and vessel occlusion. Firstly, as the vessel relaxes, returning blood flow dilutes activated clotting proteins and mechanically discourages extension of the plug. Vascular endothelial cells secrete prostacyclin, a powerful inhibitor of platelet aggregation. Circulating inhibitors neutralise clotting intermediates, the most important being antithrombin III.

The fibrinolytic system (Fig. 7.3) is also of great importance. Plasmin (the active enzyme of fibrinolysis) cleaves fibrin and fibrinogen and is derived from an inactive precursor, plasminogen. Activator of plasminogen is released from damaged endothelial cells and activated factor XII also converts plasminogen. Thus fibrinolysis has similar triggers to coagulation. The resulting fibrin fragments (fibrin degradation products, FDP) are both anticoagulant and interfere with fibrin polymerisation.

A new vitamin K-dependent inhibitor of coagulation (protein C) has been described recently. It is a proteolytic enzyme and is inhibited by warfarin. It exerts its anticoagulant properties by degradation of factor V and factor VIII.

The interaction of and balance between coagulation and fibrinolysis are essential in maintaining vessel integrity and patency after injury. Risk factors for venous thrombosis are well recognised; important among these is the hypercoagulability that follows surgery and anaesthesia. Surgeons are increasingly employing various prophylactic strategies to prevent this complication.

DISSEMINATED INTRAVASCULAR COAGULATION (DIC)

This is also referred to as *consumption coagulopathy*, which suggests the pathogenesis. Essentially, the process represents the inappropriate triggering of the coagulation cascade in flowing blood by specific disease processes. There is considerable variation in severity, ranging from the coagulopathy as the predominant clinical manifestation (with haemostatic failure) to merely a laboratory sign of the underlying disease with no clinical haemostatic lesion. Some possible causes are listed in Table 7.2.

The principal laboratory findings are produced by the consumption of platelets during intravascular coagulation with reduction of fibrinogen and

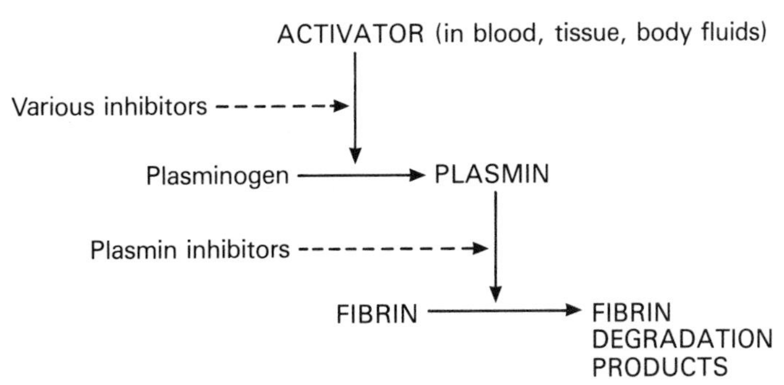

Fig. 7.3 The fibrinolytic system.

Table 7.2 Clinical associations of disseminated intravascular coagulation

Release of tissue thromboplastin	Eclampsia Placental abruption Fetal death in utero Amniotic fluid embolism Disseminated malignancy including acute leukaemia Head injury Burns
Infection	Malaria, Bacteria, especially Gram-negative Viruses
Miscellaneous	Incompatible blood transfusion Extracorporeal circulation Antigen–antibody complexes Fat embolism Pulmonary embolism Shock

elevation of FDP in the serum as secondary (physiological) fibrinolysis breaks down thrombus. Thrombocytopenia, hypofibrinogenaemia and elevation of serum FDP are thus the hallmarks of DIC. Scrutiny of the blood film may reveal red cell distortion or fragmentation if there is associated microangiopathy.

As the majority of clotting tests rely on the fibrinogen–fibrin reaction as the end-point, the prothrombin time, partial thromboplastin time and thrombin time are prolonged as a result of the anticoagulant effect of FDP and consumption of other coagulation factors (II, V, VIII). DIC which is associated with endotoxaemia and endothelial damage tends to have more profound thrombocytopenia. There is some suggestion that in severe DIC there is, in addition, an induced platelet functional defect. DIC is inevitable to some degree where there is tissue damage (particularly the brain), hypotension, shock and poor organ perfusion.

Variants of the syndrome (with similar laboratory findings) may occur with localised extravascular consumption (e.g. placental abruption) and localised intravascular consumption (e.g. thrombotic thrombocytopenic purpura). Occasionally, primary pathological firbinolysis (PF) occurs without the microthrombosis seen in DIC, e.g. in neoplasia. Laboratory tests are not dissimilar to DIC but the platelet count tends to be higher. Differentiation of the commoner DIC from the less common PF rests on a careful clinical assessment and informed interpretation of additional laboratory tests, which may require haematological advice.

The management of DIC depends on clinical rather than laboratory severity. Whatever the degree of DIC, the first principle is an attempt to alleviate the underlying cause. In septicaemia, the infection should be treated vigorously along conventional lines. In hypovolaemic shock with DIC, adequate blood volume expansion is required and in placental abruption the uterus requires emptying. After successful treatment, most patients with DIC settle spontaneously and only in those with significant and continuing coagulation failure is there a need to repair the haemostatic mechanism with blood products. The approach to each patient depends on clinical circumstances and laboratory results but measures may include the administration of fresh frozen plasma (FFP), cryoprecipitate (fibrinogen, factor VIII and fibronectin), platelets and heparin (rarely). Advice should be sought from the haematologist.

THE BLEEDING PATIENT

The anaesthetist and surgeon are confronted not infrequently with a patient who is known to have a pre-existing haemostatic defect and the haematologist is asked if the patient is either fit for surgery or can be rendered operable.

Inherited coagulation abnormalities

These comprise classical haemophilia (haemophilia A) arising from coagulation factor VIII deficiency, Christmas disease (haemophilia B) from deficiency of factor IX (and clinically identical to classical haemophilia) and von Willebrand's disease from absence of part of the factor VIII molecule. Other inherited coagulation factor deficiencies occur but are rare.

The bleeding manifestations in the haemophilias are related directly to the degree of deficiency. The patient with severe classical haemophilia, with coagulation factor VIII levels of less than 1%

(0.01 i.u./ml) of average normal, bleeds spontaneously particularly into joints. In those with higher levels (1 to 3% of average normal) spontaneous bleeding is less common. In those moderately affected (3–16%), spontaneous bleeding is uncommon. The least affected group (16–40%) may remain undiagnosed until late in life. However, any haemophiliac patient of whatever grade of severity bleeds excessively if challenged by trauma or by surgery and an occasional patient is diagnosed initially under those circumstances.

For surgery to proceed safely, the concentration of appropriate factor must be raised to, and maintained at, a haemostatic level. The manner in which this is achieved depends on the type of surgery envisaged, the native factor level in the plasma, the half-life of the factor concerned after infusion, the type of factor concentrate available and the number of days to healing (which in turn depends on the procedure which has been performed). With the availability of factor VIII and IX concentrates, surgery of any type may now be contemplated safely. Six per cent of severe haemophiliacs develop antibodies to factor VIII, making management much more difficult. Surgery of any type, however minor, should be carried out only in designated haemophilia centres which have the staff, technical facilities and experience to supervise the haemostatic management of such patients. In the emergency situation, recourse should be made to telephonic communication with the haematologist at the nearest designated centre.

Between one-third and two-thirds of previously treated haemophiliacs in the UK have antibody to human immunodeficiency virus (HIV) in their serum; the percentage in each haemophiliac population depends on geographical location and previous treatment policy. These infection rates are related to the previous use of contaminated blood products. Heat treatment of both National Health Service and commercial factor concentrates may have interrupted this trend.

The anticoagulated patient

A more commonly encountered problem is that of the orally anticoagulated patient who presents as an emergency requiring surgical intervention within a short time. Although major surgery may be carried out in the fully orally anticoagulated patient, surgeons are generally reluctant to proceed without at least partial reversal of anticoagulation.

The oral anticoagulant drug of choice in the United Kingdom is warfarin sodium, and maintenance doses range from 3 to 10 mg daily. This prolongs the prothrombin time to 2 to 4 times normal (the therapeutic range). Phytomenadione (vitamin K_1) may be used (orally, i.m. or i.v.) to reverse the warfarin lesion. Its effect is equally rapid by each route. It should be noted that if an excess is given, it renders the patient refractory to further warfarinisation for up to several weeks. The dose of vitamin K_1 in warfarin-induced haemorrhage or overdosage is 2.5 to 20 mg but in the therapeutically anticoagulated patient about to undergo surgery, doses as small as 0.5 to 1.0 mg may be sufficient. Reversal takes up to 12 h to be adequate and the affected vitamin K-dependent clotting factors II, VII, IX and X return to the plasma in order of their half-lives. If the planned surgical intervention cannot wait for the 12 h required, the vitamin K-dependent factors require replacement using blood products. The most widely available material is FFP. The material from three donations (approximately 540 ml) should be administered and the effect on prothrombin time measured. Meanwhile phytomenadione is given. FFP takes up to 20 min to thaw, so foresight is required. Further FFP may be given (group O and group A is available) if the desired effect is not obtained. Resort to freeze-dried preparations containing vitamin K-dependent factors is rarely necessary and is not recommended presently because of the dangers of triggering DIC.

In patients who are receiving permanent anticoagulation therapy, e.g. for atrial fibrillation or prosthetic cardiac valves, it is prudent to give prophylactic s.c. heparin during the period when warfarin is suspended in an attempt to prevent thromboembolic sequelae. The suggested dose is 5000 units of calcium heparin 8 to 12 hourly s.c. until warfarinisation is re-established. These sub-pharmacological doses of heparin do not induce bleeding during surgery. The use of a heparin assay ensures that therapeutic concentrations of plasma heparin are attained.

Liver disease

Hepatocellular disease (cirrhosis or acute liver failure) results in diminished synthesis of vitamin K-dependent clotting factors (II, VII, IX and X) and fibrinogen, producing a laboratory lesion similar to that resulting from oral anticoagulants. In addition, these patients may be thrombocytopenic and clear FDP from the plasma at a reduced rate. Recourse to vitamin K, FFP and platelet support may be required.

HEPARIN

Heparin is a potent, naturally occurring anticoagulant which is isolated commercially from animal intestinal mucous membranes. Bearing a strong negative charge, it interferes with the thrombin–fibrinogen reaction and potentiates the physiological antagonist of activated clotting factors, antithrombin III. It is given i.v. preferably continuously, at a dose of 24–48 000 units per 24 h (for deep vein thrombosis). It is possible that the administration of similar doses intermittently but subcutaneously may produce the plasma concentration of heparin required for treatment of deep venous thrombosis or pulmonary embolus. Its action is immediate and if given by bolus it has a half-life of only 40 to 80 min. It has now gained wide acceptance in some but not all forms of major surgery as a successful means of preventing postoperative deep vein thrombosis. For this indication, the dose by the s.c. route is 5000 units 8- or 12-hourly given for 7 to 10 days.

If a patient who is therapeutically heparinised requires emergency surgery, cessation of the infusion may suffice because of the short half-life of the drug. The laboratory test of choice to monitor adequacy of full heparinisation is the partial thromboplastin time with kaolin (PTTK or APTT) which should be 1.5 to 2.5 times prolonged compared to the control time. This desired ratio may differ between laboratories. Prior to emergency surgery in the heparinised patient, recourse to the PTTK may indicate that there is little risk of bleeding if the test is prolonged less than 1.5:1. Reversal of heparin in an emergency may be achieved using protamine sulphate given by slow i.v. injection at a dose of 1 mg per 100 units of heparin. Not more than 50 mg of protamine sulphate should be given because, in addition to side effects of flushing, bradycardia and hypotension, it is itself an anticoagulant.

PLATELET THERAPY

Unlike red cells, platelets have an inconveniently short shelf-life. Whereas red cells in citrate–phosphate dextrose with adenine have a safe storage life of 28 days, platelets in the same anticoagulant are only satisfactory when given to the recipient within 4 days of donation. This places obvious constraints on the supply of viable platelets to hospitals by transfusion centres. Platelets are supplied usually as concentrates, i.e. platelet-rich plasma (PRP) (produced by low *g* spun freshly donated blood) spun down again and much of the supernatant plasma removed. Platelet concentrates are stored at 22°C.

The indications for platelet transfusion remain controversial. In patients with e.g. acute leukaemia, who (because both of bone marrow disease and cytotoxic chemotherapy) are producing no endogenous platelets, the debate centres on the need for prophylactic versus therapeutic platelet transfusions. Because of rapid development of platelet antibodies, leukaemia centres are tending to limit prophylaxis to specific situations when the risk of haemorrhage is high, e.g. during serious infective episodes, and opting to treat other haemorrhagic episodes vigorously as they occur. Seventy per cent of patients develop platelet-destroying alloantibodies after repeated transfusions.

In surgical practice, as a general rule, significant bleeding should not occur if platelet numbers are greater than 100×10^9/litre. Below 30×10^9/litre, bleeding may be anticipated. Between 30 and 100×10^9/litre, operative and postoperative oozing depends on the nature of the surgical procedure and the aetiology of the thrombocytopenia.

In autoimmune thrombocytopenia (e.g. idiopathic thrombocytopenic purpura and Felty's syndrome) patients in whom medical treatment has failed may be referred for splenectomy with very low platelet counts. They do not require platelet transfusion for two reasons. Firstly, therapeutic platelets would be of short survival, being cleared by the same immune mechanism which is causing the patient's thrombocytopenia. Secondly, following the tying of the splenic pedicle, platelet counts may increase rapidly, ensuring adequate intra- and postoperative haemostasis. However, the local regional transfusion centre should be notified of the elective splenectomy in order that platelets might be furnished at relatively short notice if required.

If surgery is to be covered with platelet transfusions, the standard dose is 4 units per square metre of body surface, a unit being the platelets from a single donation. Currently, platelets are not cross-matched but where possible ABO and Rhesus-compatible platelets should be chosen. This dose may need to be given twice on the day of surgery and half of the first dose at least 60 min preoperatively. Further twice-daily doses on the first and succeeding postoperative days may be required and the need for further platelets should be assessed on the patient's progress and demonstration of normal coagulation proteins if haemostasis is not total. Satisfactory post-transfusion increments in the platelet count should be demonstrated if bleeding continues to be troublesome.

In DIC from any cause, platelet transfusions are rarely needed but should be given if platelet consumption has been documented as severe, and haemorrhage is a clinical problem. In the massively transfused patient with haemostatic failure, platelets may be required if thrombocytopenia is unusually low (less than 50×10^9/litre) and the coagulation mechanism is not judged to be at fault on laboratory testing.

BLOOD TRANSFUSION

The ABO blood groups first described in 1901 by Landsteiner and the Rhesus system described by Landsteiner and Weiner in 1940 together form the important blood group systems for those practising blood transfusion primarily at the bedside. However, there are many other clinically important blood group systems which are the more immediate concern of the blood transfusion laboratory staff. Problems relating to these groups are normally resolved by the laboratory before blood products are issued as compatible for use in the patient.

ABO groups

In the United Kingdom, 47% of persons are group O, 42% group A, 8% group B and 3% group AB. Patients, and thus donors, have these percentage distributions (Table 7.3). Proportions vary elsewhere in the world mainly from increased gene frequency of B. ABO blood group substances may be found also on leucocytes and platelets and 77% of persons secrete ABO blood group substances in body fluids. ABO antibodies are said to be naturally occurring, that is they are a constant feature of the system in all persons and do not arise as a result of exposure to A or B blood group substances at some time during life. Although A and B blood group substances appear in RBCs early in fetal development, the corresponding antibodies appear only after birth at 3–6 months of age and are present in greatest strength at the age of 10 years. After the early months of life, anti-A and anti-B are present invariably in the serum when the red cells lack the corresponding antigen. Table 7.3 shows the old rationale, now outmoded, for the designation of group O persons as 'universal donors', because they lack group A and B substances in their red cells, and persons of group AB as 'universal recipients' as their serum does not contain either anti-A or anti-B. ABO antibodies are predominantly IgM and thus do not cross the placenta. An occasional person, usually group O, may have 'immune' anti-A (or less

Table 7.3 Distribution of ABO blood groups in the United Kingdom, their red cell antigens and antibodies

	%	RBC antigen	Serum	
O	47	—	Anti-A	'Universal donor'
			Anti-B	
A	42	A	Anti-B	
B	8	B	Anti-A	
AB	3	A + B	—	'Universal recipient'

Rhesus D positive 85%
Rhesus D negative 15%

commonly anti-B), an IgG molecule capable of crossing the placenta and active at 37°C. Such persons are called 'dangerous' donors and are screened at transfusion centres. If pregnant with a group A (or B) fetus, ABO maternofetal incompatibility may ensue with haemolytic disease of the newborn.

Whenever possible, blood transfusion laboratories try to provide blood of the same ABO group as the recipient. If a patient of group AB requires an emergency transfusion of more than a few units, further AB units may be unavailable and A blood is used, being likely to be more plentiful than B. If ABO compatible blood is unavailable for a group B patient, group O is used with suitable preceding cross-matching tests.

ABO incompatible transfusion accidents are the most serious of the transfusion incompatibilities and have significant morbidity and mortality. Properly conducted routine cross-matching techniques detect such incompatibilities in vitro and they occur only if there has been an error of patient identification or sample identification. Most accidents of this type result from clerical errors.

Rhesus groups

Shortly after the discovery of the Rhesus groups it was recognised that some haemolytic transfusion reactions and haemolytic disease of the newborn (erythroblastosis fetalis) resulted from incompatibilities in this system. In bedside blood transfusion practice, the Rhesus D antigen is the most important of the Rhesus antigens and units of blood or blood products labelled Rhesus positive are D positive although they may also be positive for C and E antigens. Units labelled Rhesus negative lack all three antigens C, D and E and thus have the Rhesus phenotype cde/cde. The Rhesus factors are inherited in a 'packet', one from each parent, each 'packet' containing one of each pair of alleles C or c, D or d and E or e. The commonest genes are CDe (gene frequency 0.41) and cde (0.39) followed by cDE (0.14). The other genes are much less common.

Antibodies of clinical significance occur in the Rhesus system but these rarely occur naturally, i.e. they are formed as the result of exposure to Rhesus antigens which the patient does not possess naturally. The commonest circumstance is the bearing of a Rhesus positive fetus by a Rhesus negative woman. The most common antibody is anti-D and at least two pregnancies are required. Such antibodies are detected readily in cross-matching techniques but, if undetected, may result in an immediate transfusion reaction, or at best, impaired survival of the transfused cells.

Other blood groups

The known number of blood group antigens is increasing constantly, usually because of the discovery first of the corresponding antibody. Many are of little clinical significance. Ability to react at 37°C and specificity characterise those antibodies in recipient serum which necessitate the provision of red cells lacking the corresponding antigen. Of greatest importance are, in order of frequency, Kell, Duffy, Kidd, Ss and Lewis. Of all clinically significant alloantibodies, 83% are in the Rhesus system (Table 7.4).

Storage and preservation of blood

Until recently, blood for transfusion was collected into ACD (acid citrate dextrose solution containing trisodium citrate, citric acid and dextrose) which acted both as an anticoagulant and red cell preservative. This was superseded in some parts of the world in the 1970s by CPD (citrate phosphate dextrose) in which the addition of sodium dihydrogen phosphate raised the pH of the

Table 7.4 Percentage frequency of clinically important 37°C alloantibodies detected in recipients

Anti-D	61
Anti-C (± D)	11
Anti-E	7
Anti-Kell	6
Anti-c	4
Anti-Duffy	2.2
Anti-Kidd	0.9
Anti-e	0.5
Anti-Ss	0.04
Others (Lewis included)	7

solution and improved red cell survival in vivo. The duration of storage considered suitable with an anticoagulant is such that, on the last day of storage, 70% of red cells are recoverable in the circulation at 24 h after transfusion and subsequently have a normal survival pattern. In this context red cell survival is related to cellular levels of ATP. The addition of adenine to CPD assists maintenance of ATP levels and this preferred anticoagulant–preservative, known as CPD-A, enables the shelf life of stored blood to be increased to 28 days or even 35 days compared with 21 days for ACD and standard CPD. Storage of red cells for transfusion should be at 2 to 6°C in a blood bank refrigerator. Resort to other domestic-type refrigerators is hazardous because of the risk of inadequate thermostatic control leading to the possibility of freezing of blood and lysis of red cells on warming in the event of equipment failure. Ministry of Health-type insulated boxes maintain precooled red cells for transfusion at a satisfactory temperature, when used with ice inserts, for up to 24 h.

At appropriate storage temperatures, bacterial replication in blood is inhibited and red cell glycolysis is slowed with some preservation of 2,3-DPG levels. Red cell survival in vitro is thus preserved. The prime function of the erythrocyte is delivery of oxygen to the tissues and this is dependent on red cell levels of 2,3-DPG. In ACD, red cells lose 40% and 90% of 2,3-DPG at 1 and 2 weeks respectively with a resulting shift to the left of the oxygen dissociation curve. In CPD, 2,3-DPG is better maintained (20% loss at 2 weeks) but slightly less so in CPD-A. Whatever the storage medium, however, levels of 2,3-DPG return to normal in 6–24 h after transfusion.

Blood grouping and cross-matching tests

Elective grouping is now being undertaken more commonly using automated apparatus suited to large batches. This process may take up to half a day. In the emergency situation, if the patient's group is not known it can be ascertained using a tile within 5–10 min of receipt of the samples.

There is incomplete agreement as to what constitutes the ideal cross-matching test system to ensure compatibility between donor red cells and patient's serum. Essential components include a test at room temperature to detect the important ABO incompatibilities between donor and patient and two or more tests at 37°C to detect Rhesus and other alloantibodies in the patient's serum which would result in a transfusion reaction and reduced red cell survival. The clinically important antibodies are shown in Table 7.4. The introduction of low ionic strength saline (LISS) to replace ordinary saline as a red cell suspension medium has resulted in incubation times being greatly reduced and an acceptable 30 min cross-match is now a reality.

Trends towards the elective screening of all patients' sera for irregular antibodies simultaneously with automated grouping may soon obviate the need for any cross-matching technique. This would ensure that once a patient had been shown to be free of alloantibodies to blood group antigens, blood of appropriate ABO and Rhesus group would simply be selected and given without matching (and the resultant time delays).

Red cell concentrates ('packed cells', plasma-reduced cells)

In the UK, regional transfusion centres issue a minority of units as whole blood and an increasing proportion is distributed as red cell concentrates. Some red cell concentrates are suspended in plasma. These are produced by the removal of 150–200 ml of citrated plasma from the final donated volume of 510 ml (450 ml blood + 60 ml of CPD-A anticoagulant–preservative). This fresh, platelet-rich plasma is used for production of platelet concentrates and as raw material for blood product manufacture. An increasing proportion of donations has a much greater percentage of plasma removed and replaced by a preservative solution as a suspension medium. The additive used in the UK is SAGM (saline, adenine, glucose, mannitol). Both types of red cell concentrate are produced in sterile closed plastic blood-bag systems and have the same shelf-life as whole blood.

Cryoprecipitate is manufactured from some freshly donated units for the treatment of haemophilia A, and results in a unit of whole blood with an almost normal amount of plasma but labelled 'cryoprecipitate poor'.

Many hospital blood-bank laboratories now provide the first 2 units of blood for surgery as red cell concentrates. These have a high haematocrit and are more viscous than whole blood. The volume of red cell concentrates is 380–410 ml.

Donations of blood in the UK have been tested for HIV antibody since October 1985. Future developments may include the manufacture of artificial blood in the form of oxygen-carrying plasma volume expander solutions.

Transfusion reactions

In addition to the haemolytic transfusion reactions referred to above there are other types of reaction which may interfere with the completion of transfusion of blood or blood products. About 2% of all transfusions are followed by some form of reaction and three-quarters of these are febrile reactions. These latter result from antibodies to white cells in the HLA system. Such reactions may be accompanied by rigors, hypotension, dyspnoea, occasionally cyanosis, nausea and vomiting. It is worth remembering that the symptoms and signs of any form of transfusion reaction may be obscured or abolished by general anaesthesia. Fever after platelet transfusion in patients with platelet alloantibodies is less common but platelet preparations are always contaminated by white cells. Prevention of reactions to white cells includes the transfusion of buffy coat-poor blood, washing of red cells or the use of white cell filters at the bedside.

Milder anaphylactic reactions are associated frequently with urticaria (weals or hives) and very occasionally with flushing, dyspnoea and hypotension and are thought to result from reaction between IgA in the transfused blood and anti-IgA in the recipient. Less commonly, other antibodies may be implicated in an atopic subject.

Non-immunological reactions to stored blood include induced hypothermia from transfusion of large volumes of cold blood and citrate toxicity in similar circumstances. Other consequences are air embolism, transfusion of particulate matter from transfusion equipment and reactions to cellular debris in blood, for example 'postperfusion' lung. Some complications of blood transfusion are listed in Table 7.5.

Table 7.5 Complications of blood transfusion

Transmission of disease, e.g. viral hepatitis, syphilis, malaria, HIV
Bacterial contamination
Pyrogenic reactions
Incompatibility reactions
Haemolytic reactions
Allergic reactions
Citrate toxicity
Hypothermia
Hyperkalaemia
Metabolic acidosis
Circulatory overload
Air embolism
Microaggregate embolism

Plasma volume expanders

In acute hypovolaemia plasma volume expanders are frequently used while blood is being prepared. Transfusion is often started with electrolyte solutions but continued with volume expanders.

Three non-human source materials are in use.

Gelatins

In these preparations, bovine gelatin is modified to produce an average molecular weight of 30 000–35 000. The two available products, polygeline (Haemaccel) and succinylated gelatin (Gelofusine), have a pH, colloid osmotic pressure and viscosity similar to those of plasma. Their half-lives are approximately 4 h. They have a shelf-life at ambient temperatures of up to 8 years. Occasionally, rapid infusion, particularly in a normovolaemic patient, may result in the release of vasoactive substances which cause a rash, hypotension and tachycardia; these may be managed by antihistamines and/or hydrocortisone, and the infusion should be discontinued. Gelatin solutions do not interfere with blood grouping or cross-matching and renal function is not impaired.

The two preparations differ in their electrolyte content. Polygeline must not be allowed to mix with citrated blood products as it has a high calcium content (6.25 mmol/litre). Gelofusine contains little potassium (0.4 mmol/litre). No more than 1–1.5 litres of gelatin solution should be transfused before whole blood is available.

Dextrans

Dextran 70 injection BP (6% dextran) is most frequently employed in 5% glucose or in 0.9% saline. The average molecular weight of the material is 70 000. Dextrans should not be administered to patients with renal impairment, severe congestive heart failure or thrombocytopenia. The dextrans are believed to interfere with the haemostatic mechanism if transfused in large quantity and cause difficulty with grouping and cross-matching tests in the laboratory by promotion of rouleaux. No acutely haemorrhagic patient should receive more than 1.5 litres and, as unpredictable anaphylactic reactions may occur with erythema, bronchospasm, urticaria and hypotension, the patient should be observed carefully during the first few minutes of the infusion. If such a reaction occurs, the infusion should be stopped immediately and resuscitation measures instituted.

Hetastarch (hydroxyethyl starch)

This plasma volume expander, available in the UK under the proprietary name Hespan, is an artificial colloid derived from amylopectin, and closely resembles glycogen. Its average molecular weight is 450 000 and its infusion results in an expansion of plasma volume slightly in excess of the volume infused. Plasma volume expansion is maintained for at least 24 h. Contraindications and side effects are similar to those of Dextran 70. No more than 1 litre should be given.

Human albumin solution

This material, known previously as plasma protein fraction, is prepared from donor plasma both by the Blood Products Laboratory of the National Blood Transfusion Service and by the pharmaceutical industry. It contains protein (principally albumin), 45 g/litre in saline. It is heat-treated and present evidence suggests that this inactivates hepatitis-producing agents. It has a 3-year shelf-life (away from light). It is remarkably free from adverse effects.

The Blood Products Laboratory material remains in short supply and hospitals frequently supplement stocks from commercial sources.

The relative prices of these volume expanders (October 1988) for one unit to hospital pharmacies are: succinylated gelatin £3.30; polygeline £2.88; dextran 70 in saline £5.64; hetastarch £18.27; and commercial human albumin £33.50.

FURTHER READING

Bloom A L, Thomas D P 1987 Haemostasis and thrombosis. Churchill Livingstone, Edinburgh

Hardisty R M, Weatherall D J (eds) 1982 Blood and its disorders, 2nd edn. Blackwell Scientific Publications, Oxford

Herxheimer A (ed) 1987 Plasma substitutes. Drug and Therapeutics Bulletin 25: 10, 37

Hoffbrand A V, Pettit J E 1989 Essential haematology, 3rd edn. Blackwell Scientific Publications, Oxford

Mollison P L 1987 Blood transfusion in clinical medicine, 8th edn. Blackwell Scientific Publications, Oxford

Retz L D, Swisher S M N (eds) 1981 Clinical practice of blood transfusion. Churchill Livingstone, Edinburgh

Serjeant G R 1985 Sickle cell disease. Oxford University Press, Oxford

Weatherall D J, Clegg J B 1981 Thalassaemia syndromes, 3rd edn. Blackwell Scientific Publications, Edinburgh

8. Principles of general pharmacology and pharmacokinetics

Pharmacokinetics comprises the study and characterisation of the time course of drug absorption, distribution, metabolism and excretion in addition to the relationship of these processes to the time course of desirable and toxic effects of drugs. Pharmacodynamics comprises the study of the pharmacological effects of a drug determined by its action on specific receptors and the concentration of the drug at the receptor site. In simple terms this reduces to:

pharmacokinetics — what the body does to a drug
pharmacodynamics — what the drug does to the body (Fig. 8.1).

Recently, very sensitive, accurate and reproducible methods have become available for measuring drug concentrations in plasma. This has produced a remarkable increase in the number of pharmacokinetic studies. Many of these articles provide no data concerning the relationship between kinetic measurements and the pharmacological effects of the drug. Pharmacokinetics is a technique and not an end in itself. Clinical pharmacology is concerned with the biological effects of a drug. Thus in the selection of a drug for use, pharmacokinetics is of importance only if two or more drugs are available with very similar effects and toxicity.

However, pharmacokinetics generally and the study of drug absorption, distribution, metabolism and excretion have a great contribution to make in anaesthesia and clinical pharmacology.

PHARMACODYNAMICS — BASIC CONCEPTS OF DRUG ACTION

Drugs may exert their effect in one of three ways:

1. *Action dependent on chemical or physicochemical properties*. Some drugs act by combining with a small molecule or ion (e.g. neutralisation of gastric acid by antacids or chelation of ferrous ion

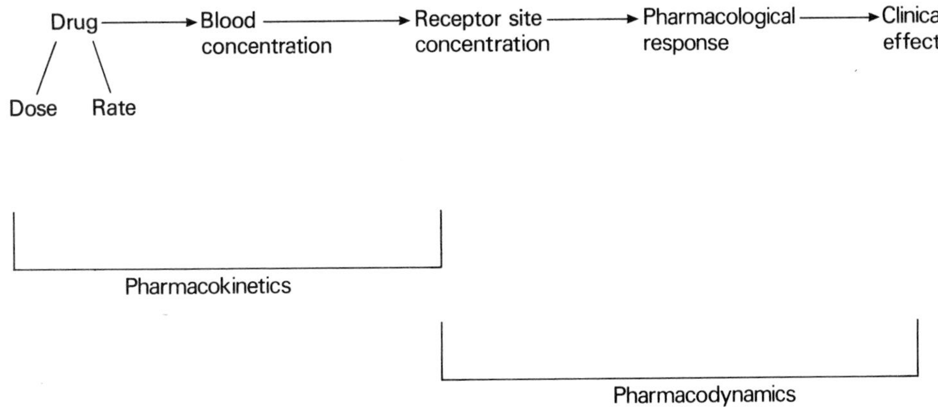

Fig. 8.1 Factors concerned in drug responses.

by desferrioxamine). Local anaesthetics and inhalational anaesthetics may produce non-specific changes in the lipid or protein components of nerve membranes and thus change the diameter of the pores that are concerned with ion transport and nerve conduction (see Ch. 5).

2. *Enzyme inhibition*. Many drugs act by inhibiting naturally occurring enzymes. They are often related chemically to natural substrates and may be metabolised by the enzyme system. Examples include allopurinol which inhibits xanthine oxidase and sulphanilamide which inhibits folate synthetase. Reversible enzyme inhibitors compete with natural substrates for enzymes and their action does not depend on the formation of stable chemical bonds. Their effects are usually of short duration. Edrophonium, neostigmine and pyridostigmine inhibit cholinesterase by formation of a covalent chemical bond resulting in carbamylation of the enzyme. The covalent bond is hydrolysed slowly and the enzyme is regenerated slowly.

Enzyme inhibition may be irreversible as a result of the formation of a stable chemical bond between enzyme and its inhibitor. Subsequent recovery from enzyme inhibition depends upon regeneration of the enzyme (e.g. monoamine oxidase inhibitors, organophosphorus insecticides). These drugs have a very long duration of action and may produce effects lasting for weeks.

3. *Receptors*. In most instances, drug action is produced by a physicochemical interaction between the drug and macromolecular components of tissues (receptors). These receptor sites are not readily identifiable physical entities but usually are related closely to tissue cells which mediate the effects. Normally they are areas of cell membranes. In some instances, 'second messengers' (e.g. cyclic AMP or calcium ions) may be released as a result of drug–receptor interaction and mediate the response to the drug.

Receptors are very sensitive to low concentrations of drug, and the magnitude of the response depends on the concentration of the free drug at the receptor site, which in turn depends on the dose and the continuing processes of drug absorption, distribution and elimination. Other normal characteristics of drug–receptor interactions include saturability, reversibility and specificity. The L-form of a stereo-isomer may be pharmacologically active while the D-form is inactive (e.g. opioid analgesics).

Relationship between drug dose and response

A drug response results from the reversible combination of drug and receptor, the magnitude of the response depending on the amount of drug–receptor complex formed. A drug which 'fits' the receptor well binds strongly and thus has a high *affinity* for the receptor. Pharmacological effect is related usually to drug dosage or concentration by a dose–response curve (Fig. 8.2). The shape of this curve reflects the extent of occupancy of receptor sites by the drug. The maximal response should correspond to occupancy of all receptor sites. However, if 'second messengers' are involved, they may be the limiting factor in the production of the maximal response. The relative affinity of a drug for a receptor may be defined as the concentration required to produce half the maximal response. In some instances, the magnitude of the pharmacological response may

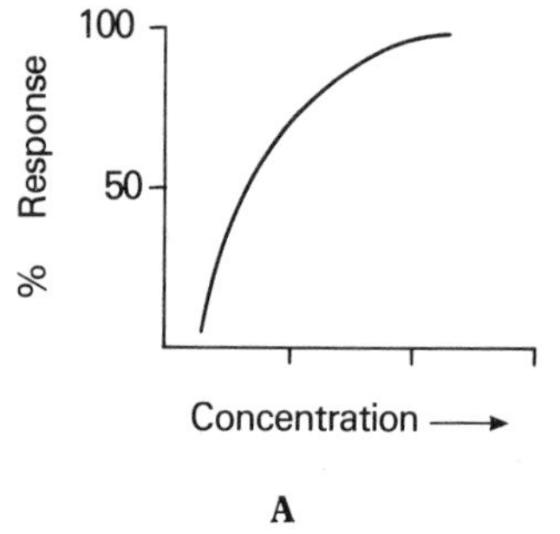

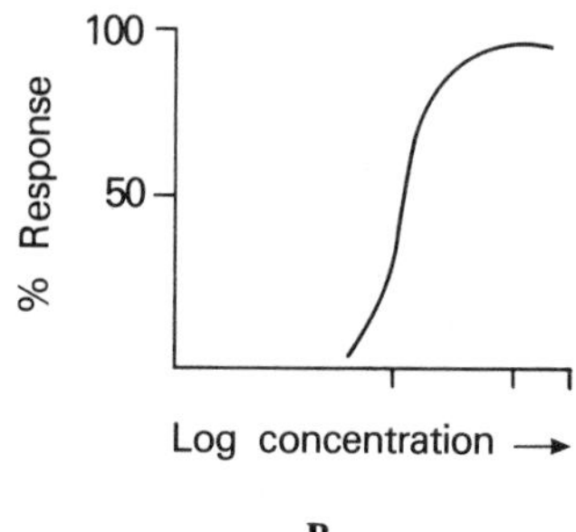

Fig. 8.2 The relationship between drug concentration and response. In (a) the concentration is plotted on a linear scale and the shape is hyperbolic. In (b) the concentration is plotted on a logarithmic scale and the shape is sigmoid.

not be related predictably to the proportion of receptors occupied by the drug. Very potent drugs may produce a maximal response when occupying a small proportion of the total population of receptors. The presence of these 'spare receptors' ensures that adequate pharmacological effects may be produced by relatively low concentrations of drug or transmitter. Spare receptors occur probably at the neuromuscular junction (e.g. only 25% of the receptor population is required to produce a maximum twitch response). Thus competitive antagonists, e.g. D-tubocurarine, may require to occupy a significant number of receptors before any effect is obvious on neuromuscular transmission.

In addition to the affinity of the drug for the receptor, the *intrinsic activity* of the drug is important. This may be defined as a measure of the maximal response that the drug can produce when given in very high concentrations. Thus, two similarly acting drugs with similar affinity for the receptor site but with different intrinsic activities require a different extent of receptor occupation to produce the same response. The drug with high intrinsic activity requires less receptor occupancy and thus a lower dose (Fig. 8.3).

Agonists, partial agonists and antagonists

A drug with high affinity and high intrinsic activity is termed an *agonist*. An agent with high affinity but no intrinsic activity is an *antagonist* because it prevents a drug that does have activity from interacting with the receptor site. *Partial agonists* are drugs which cannot produce a maximal response in spite of very high concentrations. Morphine, naloxone and buprenorphine are examples of agonist, antagonist and partial agonist respectively.

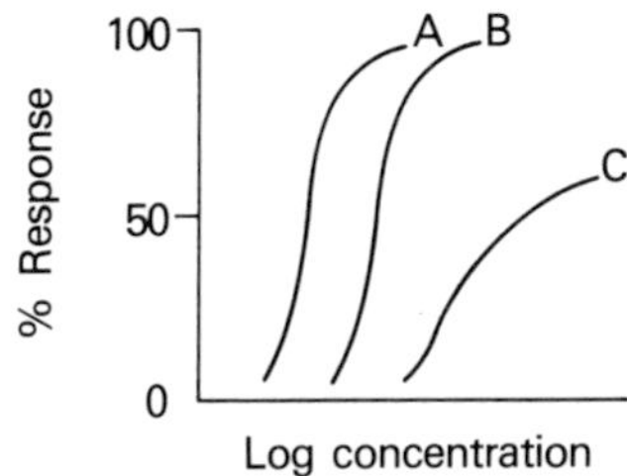

Fig. 8.3 Log concentration–response curves. A — agonist with high affinity for receptor. B — agonist with lower affinity than A but still achieving 100% response. C — partial agonist; this drug does not achieve a maximal response.

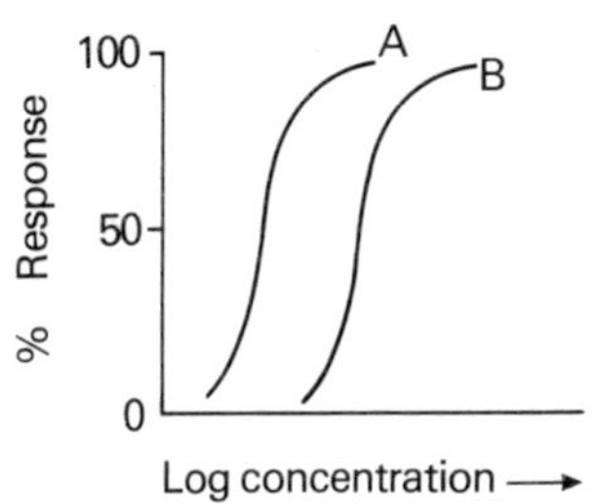

Fig. 8.4 Log concentration–response curves. A — agonist alone. B — agonist A in the presence of a competitive antagonist.

Antagonists are competitive if they combine *reversibly* with the same receptor as the agonist. Because of this reversibility, the maximal response to the agonist may still be obtained if the concentration of the agonist is high enough, i.e. the dose–response curve shifts to the right and is parallel to that of the agonist in the absence of the antagonist (Fig. 8.4). There are many examples (Table 8.1).

Antagonists are non-competitive if they *inactivate* the receptor. The effect is to reduce the intrinsic activity of the agonist without changing its affinity so that a maximal response cannot be obtained by increasing the concentration of the agonist (Fig. 8.5). This effect may be reversible or irreversible.

Non-competitive antagonists often have a long duration of action and their effects are usually unrelated to their plasma concentration. An example is phenoxybenzamine antagonism at α-adrenoceptors.

Table 8.1 Some examples of competitive antagonism

Drug	Drug or transmitter antagonised
Naloxone	Morphine and other opioids
Atropine	Acetylcholine (muscarinic)
D-Tubocurarine Pancuronium	Acetylcholine (neuromuscular junction)
Hexamethonium Trimetaphan	Acetylcholine (ganglia)
Propranolol	Adrenaline (β-receptors)
Cimetidine	Histamine (H_2-receptors)

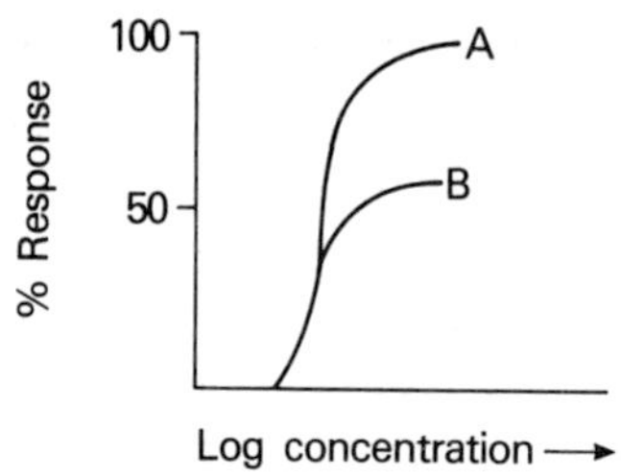

Fig. 8.5 Log concentration–response curves. A — agonist alone. B — agonist A in the presence of a non-competitive antagonist.

Desensitisation, tachyphylaxis and tolerance

Repeated or continuous use of drugs may lead to a progressive decrease in the observed response. This process may be called desensitisation, tachyphylaxis or tolerance. *Desensitisation* is a decrease in cellular sensitivity or responsiveness to the repeated use of a drug. Acute desensitisation occurs quickly and is reversible. This may be explained by receptors existing in the resting, activated and desensitised states. Chronic desensitisation occurs slowly and is less readily reversible. It may result from loss of receptors from effector cells (e.g. in myasthenia gravis or after chronic use of sympathomimetic bronchodilators in asthma). *Tachyphylaxis* is a rapid decrease in pharmacological response. One example is a drug which acts by releasing endogenous transmitters from nerve endings (e.g. ephedrine). The response to repeated doses declines rapidly because of transmitter exhaustion. *Tolerance* occurs classically with opioid analgesics. Larger and larger doses are required to produce a pharmacological response. It may result from altered responsiveness of cells of the central nervous system and this may be similar to chronic desensitisation. For barbiturates, induction of hepatic microsomal enzymes may play an important part.

DRUG ABSORPTION

Unless a drug is applied directly to its site of action (e.g. local anaesthetic drugs or antacids) or is given intravenously, it must be absorbed from the site of application before being carried in the circulation to its site of action.

Drugs may be given:

1. Via the gastrointestinal tract: oral, rectal, sublingual.
2. Parenterally: intramuscular, subcutaneous.
3. By inhalation.
4. Transdermally.

Oral administration

Most drugs are given orally and there are very many factors which influence the rate and the amount of drug absorbed (Table 8.2). In acute situations, e.g. analgesic, sedative or anti-arrhythmic therapy, the rate of absorption is more important than the amount of drug absorbed and delayed absorption may result in therapeutic failure. In chronic therapy, e.g. warfarin, digoxin or corticosteroid administration, the amount of drug absorbed is more important than the rate.

Table 8.2 Factors affecting drug absorption after oral administration

Factor	Notes
Drug characteristics	
Tablet disintegration Dissolution time	Solution is absorbed more rapidly than tablets
Chelation or formation of insoluble complex with another drug	e.g. Fe^{2+} and tetracycline
Patient characteristics	
pH	For some drugs, changes in pH change the solubility or the degree of ionisation
Gastric emptying rate	Usually the most important factor affecting rate of absorption. It is influenced by posture, drugs, food and disease
Intestinal transit time	Diarrhoea may decrease the amount of drug absorbed
'First-pass' metabolism	Occurs in the small intestine or the liver and reduces the amount of drug that reaches the systemic circulation
Gastrointestinal disease	e.g. Pyloric stenosis delays gastric emptying and drug absorption

There are four possible mechanisms of absorption:

1. *Passive diffusion.* This is by far the most important process. The drug must be in solution and be lipid-soluble (i.e. unionised). Absorption occurs because of a concentration gradient across the small intestinal mucosa. Theoretically, acidic drugs, e.g. aspirin, should be absorbed better in the stomach where the pH is low and the drug is unionised, but in practice, because the gastric mucosa has a small surface area compared with the small intestine, it is absorbed better in the small bowel. Almost all drugs are absorbed by passive diffusion in the small intestine and the rate of gastric emptying is an important rate-limiting factor.

2. *Active transport.* This mechanism is highly specific and requires energy expenditure. Some amino acids, sugars and vitamins are absorbed by this mechanism. Methyldopa and L-dopa may be absorbed by this process.

3. *Filtration through pores.* These pores are so small that only compounds with a molecular weight less than 100 can be absorbed. This is unimportant for drug absorption.

4. *Pinocytosis.* Some macromolecules may be absorbed by this mechanism but it is unimportant for drug absorption.

Drugs including lignocaine, glyceryl trinitrate, propranolol and opioid analgesics undergo extensive 'first-pass' metabolism. This tends to inactivate the drug before it reaches the systemic circulation. Thus the intravenous dose is much smaller than an oral dose and pharmacological effects after oral administration may be unpredictable.

Sublingual administration of a drug avoids the phenomenon of 'first-pass' metabolism because the drug is absorbed directly into the systemic circulation. Variation in absorption occurs if a varying amount of the drug is swallowed with saliva.

Rectal administration is popular in some cultures. Part of a dose of drug given rectally is absorbed systemically and part into the portal circulation. Thus absorption may vary. However, this route avoids gastric irritation, e.g. with aspirin administration by mouth.

Intramuscular and subcutaneous administration

Drugs may be administered parenterally because they are destroyed in the stomach (e.g. benzylpenicillin), absorbed poorly from the gut (e.g. gentamicin or quaternary amines), or have significant 'first-pass' metabolism (e.g. opioid analgesics). However, intramuscular administration does not guarantee rapid or complete absorption. Diazepam is absorbed more rapidly and predictably after oral administration than after intramuscular injection.

The major factor affecting absorption is regional blood flow; the better the perfusion, the faster the absorption. Reduced cardiac output may result in delayed absorption. Water solubility of the drug is also a major determinant of the rate and the completeness of absorption. The drug should be sufficiently water-soluble at physiological pH to remain in solution in the interstitium of the muscle until absorption occurs. Drugs including diazepam, phenytoin and digoxin may precipitate at the site of injection and absorption is slow and erratic.

Inhalation

Drugs given by inhalation usually have a rapid onset of action because there is an extremely large epithelial surface available for absorption. Many anaesthetic agents are given by this route.

General anaesthesia occurs when the partial pressure (tension) of agent in the central nervous system (which is assumed to be related to that in the alveoli) is sufficiently great to induce loss of consciousness. The factors which affect alveolar concentration are shown in Table 8.3. The three

Table 8.3 Factors affecting rate of absorption of inhalational anaesthetics

1. Apparatus
    - deadspace
    - solubility of drug in rubber
    - concentration of drug
2. Alveolar ventilation
3. Uptake of agent into blood
    - cardiac output
    - solubility of drug in blood
    - ventilation/perfusion
    - tissue uptake

major factors are alveolar ventilation, drug uptake and concentration. Ventilation raises the alveolar concentration by bringing anaesthetic into the lungs and uptake decreases alveolar concentration by removing the agent.

Factors which determine the uptake of the agent by blood are solubility, cardiac output and the concentration gradient between alveoli and venous blood. The higher the solubility of the anaesthetic agent *in blood* the greater the uptake and the more slowly are the necessary alveolar concentrations (and thus anaesthesia) achieved. Less soluble agents have a more rapid onset of anaesthesia. The same is true in reverse on withdrawing anaesthesia; less soluble agents are eliminated from the body more rapidly.

Increased cardiac output increases uptake from the alveoli and slows the onset of anaesthesia. Conversely, shock reduces uptake and accelerates the onset of anaesthesia or may lead to overdosage, especially with more soluble agents (Fig. 8.6).

The concentration gradient between the alveoli and blood is maximum at the beginning of induction of anaesthesia and is zero at equilibrium.

The inspired concentration of the anaesthetic agent influences the rate at which alveolar concentration rises (concentration effect). A higher inspired concentration results in a more rapid approach of alveolar concentration to the inspired concentration (Fig. 8.6).

Changes in ventilation have a small effect on the less soluble anaesthetics, e.g. nitrous oxide, cyclo-

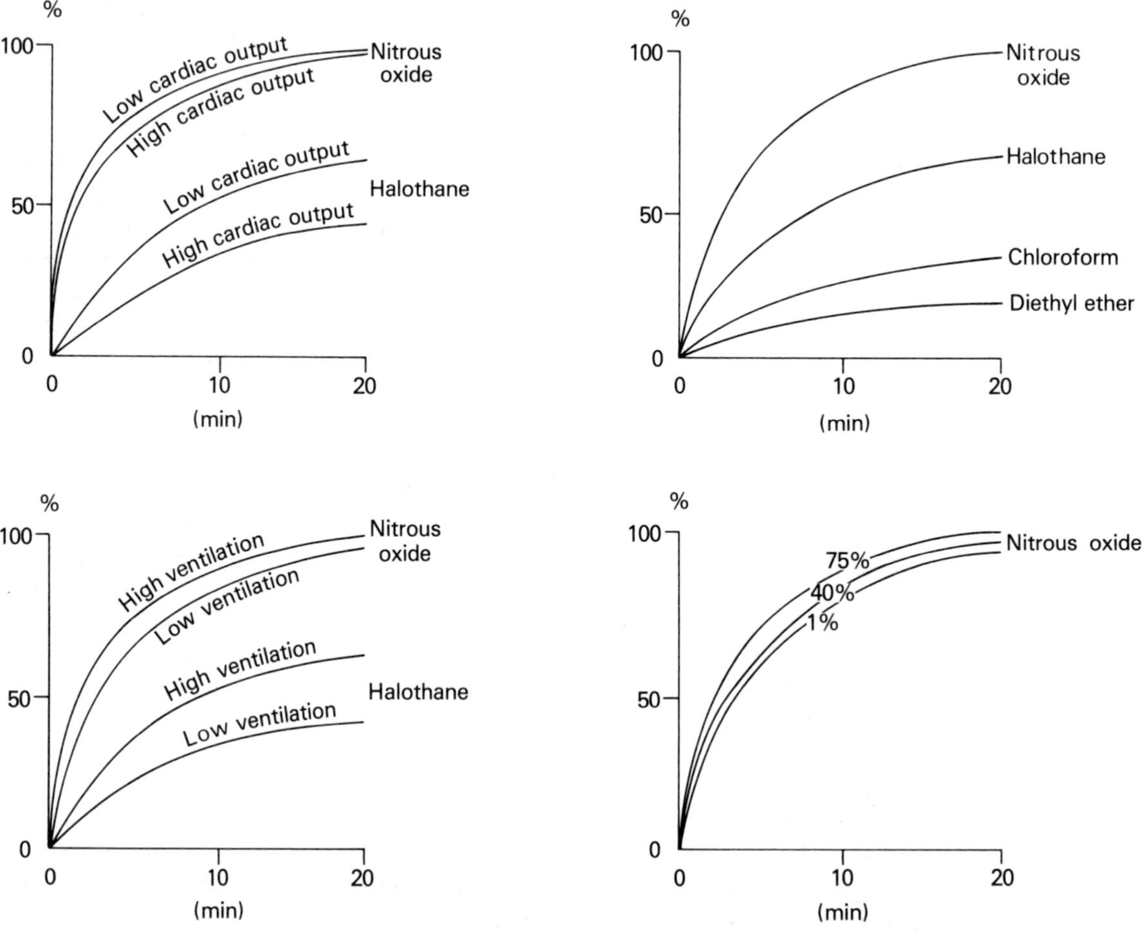

Fig. 8.6 Factors affecting the rate of uptake of volatile anaesthetic agents. On the *y* axis, the alveolar concentration of the gas is expressed as a percentage of the inspired concentration.

propane or enflurane, but they have a profound effect on the very soluble agents, e.g. ether, methoxyflurane or chloroform. Doubling ventilation may almost double the alveolar concentration for the soluble agents.

Ventilation/perfusion abnormalities affect less soluble agents more than soluble agents. In one lung anaesthesia, doubling the ventilation to one lung doubles the alveolar partial pressure of the soluble agent in that lung. This compensates for the unventilated lung. No such compensation occurs with less soluble agents.

The anaesthetic system may influence the uptake of agents. If it is large then changes occur slowly. If the agent is soluble in rubber (e.g. halothane), concentrations rise more slowly at induction. In practice, therefore, high concentrations of anaesthetic agents are given at induction of anaesthesia followed by a rapid reduction to maintenance inspired concentrations. This mirrors the high initial uptake which reduces rapidly in 5 to 15 min. Uptake continues to decrease at a much slower rate.

After total body equilibration, elimination of anaesthetics occurs as an inversion of uptake. The output of less soluble agents is high initially and declines rapidly to a lower level. The output of soluble agents is high initially but decreases gradually over a period of time. Recovery parallels this output and is rapid with less soluble agents and slow with soluble agents. Increasing alveolar ventilation accelerates recovery while depressed ventilation slows recovery.

Transdermal absorption

Most drugs are well absorbed when applied to the skin surface and up to 10 mg of drug can be administered by this route in 24 h. Examples are hyoscine for travel sickness and glyceryl trinitrate for angina.

DISTRIBUTION

Drug distribution throughout the body depends largely on physicochemical properties (e.g. lipid solubility and protein binding) and blood flow. Ionised water-soluble drugs, e.g. penicillin or myoneural blocking drugs, cannot penetrate cell membranes readily and therefore have a small apparent volume of distribution. Lipid-soluble drugs have a large volume of distribution and are distributed widely in tissues.

Plasma protein binding

Drug distribution may be affected by reversible binding to plasma proteins (e.g. albumin, α_1-acid glycoprotein or globulin) because only the unbound fraction is available immediately for diffusion into tissues. Protein binding is primarily a method for the rapid distribution of drugs from their site of absorption to their site of action. The binding of highly lipid-soluble drugs (e.g. thiopentone) is essential for transport in plasma because of their low solubility in plasma water. During perfusion of the tissues, the concentration of unbound drug in plasma decreases and the protein-bound drug dissociates.

Protein binding is of relevance only if drugs are more than 80% bound. Two drugs may compete with each other for the same binding site and thus increase the free concentration of one or both agents. Enhancement of the therapeutic effect may occur (e.g. aspirin displaces warfarin from its protein-binding sites and increases its anticoagulant effect). Binding to plasma proteins may be decreased in renal or hepatic disease.

Blood–brain barrier

Ionised drugs (e.g. myoneural blocking drugs) do not cross the blood–brain barrier and drugs which are extensively protein-bound (e.g. warfarin) cross in very small amounts. Drugs with a high molecular weight do not cross readily. In contrast, low molecular weight, lipid-soluble drugs cross into the brain rapidly.

Placenta

Low molecular weight, lipid-soluble drugs are transferred readily across the placenta. Thus all sedative drugs used in anaesthesia cross into the fetus. Some metabolites of these drugs which are active may then accumulate in the fetus and result in neonatal depression (e.g. desmethyldiazepam, norpethidine).

Intravenous anaesthetic agents

After intravenous administration, anaesthetic agents (e.g. thiopentone) induce sleep in one arm–brain circulation time because the brain has a rich blood supply and because the drug is lipid-soluble and crosses the blood–brain barrier rapidly. All tissues with a rich blood supply (vessel-rich group: brain, heart, kidney, glands and gastrointestinal tract) achieve high concentrations of drug very rapidly. As the plasma concentration decreases by distribution, the drug leaves these tissues and is distributed to other tissues which have not yet achieved equilibrium because of a poorer blood supply (muscle group and then fat group). Because of this distribution, the drug leaves the brain, the drug effect wears off and the patient awakens. At the time of recovery from the drug's effects, virtually no drug has been metabolised in the body. Thus thiopentone, in common with almost all anaesthetic agents; has a short duration of action because of its rapid distribution throughout the body.

If thiopentone is given repeatedly to maintain anaesthesia, its duration of action becomes more prolonged with each injection. After four or five administrations, recovery from the drug no longer occurs because of distribution but is delayed until metabolism reduces the blood concentration. This is a very much slower process and the effects of the drug may be prolonged and unpredictable with repeated administration.

METABOLISM

Most drugs are lipid-soluble and therefore cannot be excreted unchanged in the urine or bile. They must undergo a process of biotransformation known as metabolism. The main purpose of metabolism is to make the drug more water-soluble so that it can be excreted. It results usually in inactivation of the drug.

Some drugs used in anaesthesia are esters and are hydrolysed in the plasma by cholinesterase. Their breakdown is very rapid (e.g. procaine, suxamethonium). For some drugs a significant amount is metabolised in the kidney (dopamine), bowel mucosa (isoprenaline) or lung (prilocaine). However, the liver is the major site of drug metabolism in man. Drugs may undergo phase 1 or phase 2 reactions or both. Phase 1 reactions are simple chemical reactions including oxidation, reduction, hydroxylation or acetylation. Phase 2 reactions are conjugations with glucuronide, sulphate or glycine. Both reactions make the drug more water-soluble.

Drugs which undergo phase 1 reactions include benzodiazepines, barbiturates, halothane, rifampicin, anticonvulsants and corticosteroids. Many of the reactions are catalysed by a group of non-specific enzymes in the endoplasmic reticulum (known as hepatic microsomal enzymes) or the mixed function oxidase system which includes the enzyme cytochrome P450. The most important of the phase 2 reactions is glucuronidation, which depends also on the enzyme systems in the endoplasmic reticulum.

Enzyme induction

Drugs which are substrates for the mixed function oxidase system have the capacity to enhance the enzyme system with the consequence that they and other drugs which share this route of metabolism are metabolised more rapidly. This results in a very profound change in metabolising capacity, which reaches a maximum after 1–2 weeks of therapy. Drugs which are known to induce enzymes include phenobarbitone, phenytoin, carbamazepine, rifampicin, griseofulvin, inhalational anaesthetics and alcohol. Drugs whose effects are reduced or abolished by this increase in metabolism include the oral contraceptive pill, warfarin and anticonvulsants. All these drugs have a long duration of action which terminates because of drug metabolism. Drugs which are given as a single bolus intravenous injection and the effects of which diminish normally because of distribution (e.g. thiopentone, diazepam, morphine) are not affected by enzyme induction unless they are given repeatedly. Sometimes, phase 1 metabolism does not result in inactivation of the drug and the metabolites of a drug are active pharmacologically. Examples of this phenomenon include diazepam, pethidine, chlorpromazine, lignocaine, chloral hydrate and trichloroethylene. For other drugs, the metabolites may be toxic (e.g. halothane, paracetamol, methoxyflurane). In these instances, enzyme induction may enhance drug activity or toxicity. A few drugs have phase 2 metabolites which are active pharmacologically, e.g. morphine-6-glucuronide.

Enzyme inhibition

Some drugs may inhibit hepatic microsomal enzymes in a competitive or non-competitive manner (e.g. tolbutamide, cimetidine, phenylbutazone, chloramphenicol). Other drugs compete for an enzyme system, e.g. plasma cholinesterase (suxamethonium) or monoamine oxidase. The net result is usually a prolongation of drug action.

EXCRETION

Relatively few drugs are water-soluble and therefore excreted unchanged by the kidney. However, almost all metabolites are eventually eliminated from the body in urine or bile. Small amounts appear in saliva or milk. Compounds with a low molecular weight are excreted in urine and drugs with a larger molecular weight (e.g. tubocurarine) appear in the bile.

Renal excretion

The processes involved in renal excretion include:

1. Glomerular filtration.
2. Active tubular reabsorption.
3. Passive reabsorption.
4. Active secretion.

Glomerular filtration

All non-bound drug is filtered at the glomerulus. As the glomerular perfusion time is much longer than the drug–protein dissociation time, a significant amount of protein-bound drug may be filtered also.

Active tubular reabsorption

Some ions and physiological compounds (e.g. lithium, amino acids and glucose) are reabsorbed in the proximal tubule by an active process. This is relatively unimportant for drugs.

Passive reabsorption

The reabsorption of water along the nephron results in a reduction of urine flow from 125 ml/min at the glomerulus to 1 ml/min in the collecting duct. This concentration of non-reabsorbed solute in the lumen by a factor of 125:1 encourages passive diffusion of lipid-soluble drugs across the tubules to be reabsorbed in the blood stream.

Most drugs are weak acids or weak bases and thus exist in both ionised and un-ionised forms at physiological pH. Consequently, the pH of the luminal fluid alters the proportion of the drug that is un-ionised and therefore absorbed passively from the tubules. Acidification of the urine results in ionisation of basic drugs and thus enhances excretion by reducing the amount reabsorbed. Ephedrine, fenfluramine and amphetamine excretion is enhanced by acidification of the urine. Conversely, alkalinisation of the urine results in enhanced excretion of acidic drugs such as aspirin and phenobarbitone. Alkalinisation of the urine is often induced in aspirin poisoning in an attempt to increase the rate of renal excretion.

Active secretion

This is the usual mechanism by which the kidney excretes drugs. Proximal tubular secretion results in the elimination of penicillins, aminoglycosides, antibiotics, digoxin and neuromuscular blocking drugs. This process requires energy and it acts against a concentration gradient. Protein-binding of drugs does not inhibit it and drugs may compete with each other for the process (e.g. probenecid and penicillin).

Biliary excretion

Biliary excretion is the major route of elimination for water-soluble compounds of high molecular weight (400–500). Drugs or their metabolites are eliminated from the liver cells usually by active transport. The mechanism is similar to that described for active renal tubular secretion. Radiographic dyes, penicillins and neuromuscular blocking drugs are secreted into bile. In particular, monoquaternary ammonium compounds (e.g. D-tubocurarine) are eliminated more rapidly than bisquaternary ammonium compounds (e.g. dimethyltubocurarine.)

Some compounds eliminated as the glucuronide in the bile are hydrolysed within the lumen of the bowel and are then reabsorbed. This is known as enterohepatic circulation.

PHARMACOKINETICS

One-compartment model

Many processes in pharmacology may be described satisfactorily by 'first order' kinetics — the rate of change of concentrations or of transfer between compartments is proportional to the drug concentration in each compartment. For example, if plasma concentrations of drug are plotted against time (Fig. 8.7a), a single exponential curve is obtained. If the logarithm of the concentration is plotted against time, a straight line results (Fig. 8.7b).

If the natural logarithm is used, the slope of the line is K, the rate constant for the system. If the logarithm to base 10 is used:

$$K = \text{slope} \times 2.3$$

K has the units of reciprocal time and represents the proportion of drug eliminated from the system in unit time. Thus $K = 0.1/\text{h}$ means that 10% of the drug is removed from the system each hour. The half-life ($T_{\frac{1}{2}}$) is defined as the time required for the concentration of drug to decline by 50%. It is related inversely to K thus:

$$T_{\frac{1}{2}} = \frac{0.693}{K}$$

The total apparent volume of distribution (V) of the compartment may be calculated from the equation:

$$V = \frac{\text{dose}}{\text{concentration at time 0}} = \frac{D}{C_0}$$

The clearance (Cl) of a drug is the volume of plasma that is cleared of the drug in unit time. Total body clearance represents the sum of all clearances (renal, hepatic, pulmonary etc.).

It follows from the definitions given above that

$$\frac{\text{clearance}}{\text{volume of distribution}} = K$$

i.e.

$$\frac{Cl}{V} = K$$

By substitution,

$$T_{\frac{1}{2}} = \frac{0.693 \times V}{Cl}$$

Although this one-compartment model approximates to the clinical situation some time after intravenous administration of a drug (when distribution is complete and only elimination processes need to be considered) a model with two compart-

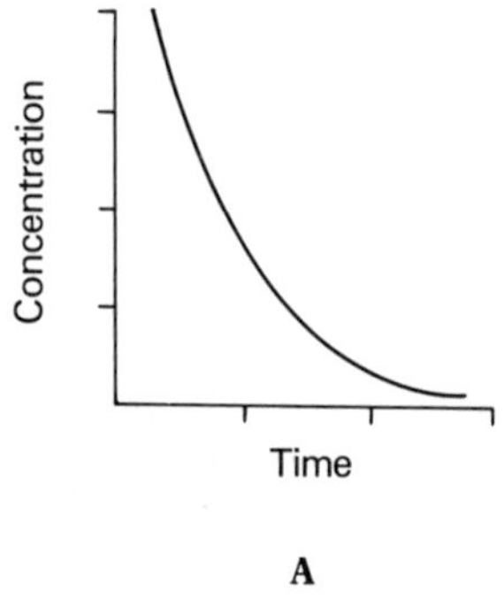

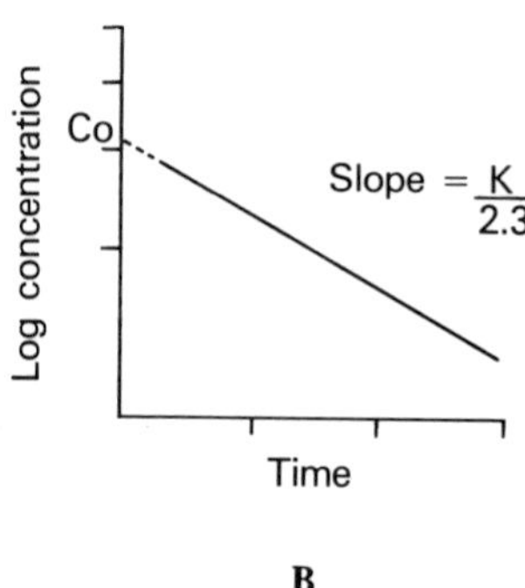

A B

Fig. 8.7 A one-compartment model — monoexponential decline in plasma concentration. (a) Linear scale. (b) Logarithm (to the base 10) scale. C_0 = concentration at time 0.

ments provides a more adequate description of plasma concentrations after intravenous injection of a drug.

Two-compartment model

This approximation assumes that the body may be resolved into a central compartment of small apparent volume and a peripheral compartment of larger volume. The compartment do not necessarily correspond to specific anatomical entities. The decrease in plasma concentration of many drugs after intravenous injection is consistent with this concept and comprises a biexponential decline. An initial rapid decline (resulting from drug distribution) is followed by a slower phase (drug elimination) (Fig. 8.8). Hybrid values for volume of distribution (V_β) and the slow half-time ($T_{\frac{1}{2}\beta}$) may be calculated as described for the one-compartment model. By subtraction of an extrapolation of the β slope from the data points, similar calculations may be performed for the rapid phase (Fig. 8.8).

Total body clearance (Cl) may be calculated from the equation:

$$Cl = \frac{\text{dose}}{AUC \text{ from } t = 0 \text{ to } t = \infty}$$

(AUC = the area under the plasma concentration time curve).

Intravenous infusion

Constant-rate intravenous infusion results in gradually increasing plasma concentrations until steady state concentrations are achieved. At steady state:

amount of drug in = amount of drug out

i.e., infusion rate = plasma concentration × clearance

$$I = C_{ss} \times Cl$$

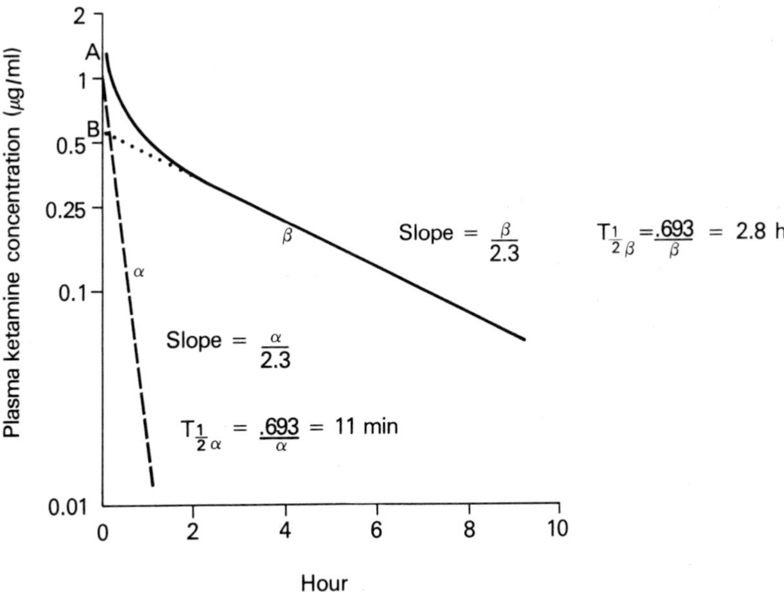

Fig. 8.8 A two-compartment model. The biexponential decline in plasma ketamine concentration (after i.v. injection of 2 mg/kg) is represented by the solid line. By extrapolating the β slope back to the y axis and subtracting the values on the line from the measured concentration at each time point, the α slope is obtained. The β and α slopes meet the y axis at B and A respectively. The equation that fits the data best is:

$$C_t = Ae^{-\alpha t} + Be^{-\beta t}$$

where C_t = concentration at time t.

Table 8.4 Mechanisms of drug interactions

	Example	Effect
1. Pharmaceutical incompatibility	Thiopentone and suxamethonium	Precipitate
2. Interference with drug absorption	Opioid analgesics and orally administered drugs	Delayed absorption
3. Changes in drug distribution (e.g. displacement from plasma protein binding sites)	Aspirin and warfarin	Bleeding
4. Competition at receptor sites	Adrenaline and propranolol	Antagonism
5. Change in hepatic metabolism		
a enzyme induction	Phenobarbitone and warfarin	Reduced effect of warfarin
b enzyme inhibition	Cimetidine and many other drugs	Prolonged effect
c changes in liver blood flow	Halothane and ketamine	Delayed elimination of ketamine
6. Interference with excretion		
a. renal	Probenecid and penicillin	High penicillin concentration
b. biliary	—	—
7. Antagonism or potentiation by drugs acting on the same physiological system or at the same time	Alcohol and barbiturates	Potentiation
8. Changes in fluid and electrolyte balance	Diuretics and digoxin	Digoxin toxicity
9. Miscellaneous		
a. monoamine oxidase inhibition	—	—
b. antagonism of antibiotics	—	—

From the start of infusion, half the steady state plasma concentration is achieved in one half-life of the drug. After infusion of a duration equal to four times the half-life, concentrations are within 10% of the eventual steady state concentration.

Oral administration

When the drug reaches the mucosa of the small intestine and absorption rate (assumed to be a first order process also) is greater than elimination rate, plasma concentrations rise. When the amount of drug at the absorption site is sufficiently reduced so that elimination rate exceeds absorption rate, plasma concentrations decrease with time.

The bioavailability of a drug is the extent of its absorption. It is calculated usually by comparing the areas under the plasma concentration-time curves (*AUC*) after oral and intravenous administration of the same dose of the drug and expressing the former as a percentage of the latter. Drugs with a high 'first-pass' metabolism have a low bioavailability.

Drug interactions

In modern therapeutic and anaesthetic practice, polypharmacy is the rule and drug interactions are likely. A classification with examples is given in Table 8.4

FURTHER READING

Curry S 1977 Drug disposition and pharmacokinetics, 2nd edn. Blackwell Scientific Publications, Oxford

Dollery C T 1973 Pharmacokinetics — master or servant. European Journal of Clinical Pharmacology 6: 1

Eger E I 1981 Uptake, distribution and elimination of inhaled anaesthetics. In: Scurr C, Feldman S (eds) Scientific foundations of anaesthesia, 3rd edn. Heinemann, London
Gibaldi M 1977 Biopharmaceutics and clinical pharmacokinetics, 2nd edn. Lea & Febiger, Philadelphia
Greenblatt D J, Koch-Weser J 1975 Clinical pharmacokinetics. New England Journal of Medicine 702: 964
Meffin P J, Birkett D J, Wing L M H 1979 Fundamentals of clinical pharmacology 2. How drugs act. Current Therapeutics 20: 87
Prescott L F 1980 Clinically important drug interactions. In: Avery G S (ed) Drug treatment, 2nd edn. Churchill Livingstone, Edinburgh
Tognoni G, Bellantuono C, Bonati M, et al 1980 Clinical relevance of pharmacokinetics. Clinical Pharmacokinetics 5: 105
Tucker G T 1979 Drug metabolism. British Journal of Anaesthesia 51: 603

9. Inhalational anaesthetic agents

Volatile and gaseous anaesthetic agents remain popular for maintenance of anaesthesia and, under some circumstances, for induction of anaesthesia. In many situations, it is appropriate to use a mixture of 66% N_2O in oxygen and a small concentration of a volatile agent to maintain anaesthesia, although for reasons discussed below there are occasions when an anaesthetist might wish actively to avoid the use of nitrous oxide.

Because pharmacological and pharmacokinetic properties of agents are related usually to physical properties, some knowledge of the older anaesthetic drugs which are no longer used may still be expected of the trainee anaesthetist. For example, comparison of the physical properties of a series of agents is helpful in understanding the uptake and distribution of an inhaled anaesthetic (see Ch. 8). Consequently, this chapter includes a description of agents which are no longer in current anaesthetic practice; these are referred to as the agents of largely historical interest. Ether occupies a special role in anaesthesia; its flammable nature has led to its abandonment in anaesthetic practice in Western countries, but it is used occasionally in emergency situations and it remains an agent of widespread use in underdeveloped countries; for this reason it is described under the title 'Agents in occasional use'.

PROPERTIES OF THE IDEAL INHALATIONAL ANAESTHETIC AGENT

1. It should have a pleasant odour, be non-irritant to the respiratory tract and allow a pleasant and rapid induction of anaesthesia.
2. It should possess a low blood/gas solubility, which permits rapid induction of and rapid recovery from anaesthesia.
3. It should be chemically stable in storage, and should not interact with the material of anaesthetic circuits or with soda lime.
4. It should be neither flammable nor explosive.
5. It should be capable of producing unconsciousness with analgesia and preferably some degree of muscle relaxation.
6. It should be sufficiently potent to allow the use of high inspired oxygen concentrations when necessary.
7. It should not be metabolised in the body, should be non-toxic and should not provoke allergic reactions.
8. It should produce minimal depression of the cardiovascular and respiratory systems and should not interact with other drugs used commonly during anaesthesia, e.g. pressor agents or catecholamines.
9. It should be completely inert and eliminated completely and rapidly in an unchanged form via the lungs.

None of the inhalational anaesthetic agents either of historical interest or in current use approaches the standards required of the ideal agent.

Minimum alveolar anaesthetic concentration

MAC is the minimum alveolar concentration of an anaesthetic at 1 atmosphere absolute that prevents movement of 50% of the population to a standard stimulus. Anaesthesia is related to the partial pressure of an inhalational agent in brain rather than its percentage concentration in alveoli, but the term MAC has gained widespread acceptance as an index of anaesthetic potency as it is measured. It can be applied to all inhalational anaesthetics and it permits comparison of different agents. However, it represents only one point on a dose–response curve; 1 MAC of one agent is equivalent in anaesthetic potency to 1 MAC of another, but it does not follow that the agents are equipotent at 2 MAC. Nevertheless, in general terms, 0.5 MAC of one agent in combination with 0.5 MAC of another approximates to 1 MAC in total.

The MAC values for the anaesthetic agents quoted in Appendix II on page 723 were determined experimentally in humans (volunteers) breathing a mixture of the agent in oxygen. MAC values vary under the following circumstances:

1. MAC is reduced in the presence of premedication agents.
2. MAC is reduced in the presence of nitrous oxide.
3. MAC may change in some disease states, e.g. an increase in thyrotoxicosis and a decrease in myxoedema.
4. MAC is increased in the presence of pyrexia.
5. Sympathoadrenal stimulation induced, for example, by hypercapnia is associated with an increase in MAC. Thus, estimation of MAC in an individual requires stabilisation of factors such as the end-tidal CO_2 concentration.
6. MAC decreases with advancing age. MAC is higher in infants and neonates than in adults and declines with advancing years. For halothane, MAC is almost 1.1% in the neonate, 0.95% in the infant, 0.9% at 1–2 years, 0.75% at 40 years and 0.65% at 80 years.
7. Drugs which affect release of CNS neurotransmitters affect MAC. MAC values are increased in the presence of ephedrine, amphetamine, or iproniazid and decreased by reserpine, methyldopa; pancuronium and clonidine.
8. MAC changes with atmospheric pressure, as anaesthetic potency is related to partial pressure. For example, MAC for enflurane is 1.68% (1.66 kPa) at a pressure of 1 atmosphere absolute (ata), but 0.84% (still 1.66 kPa) at 2 ata.

Individual anaesthetic agents

Physical and pharmacological properties of the inhalational anaesthetic agents are summarised in Appendix II. (p. 723). The structural formulae of the agents discussed in this chapter are shown in Table 9.1.

AGENTS OF MAINLY HISTORICAL INTEREST

Ethyl chloride

Ethyl chloride is a clear fluid with an ethereal odour. It has a boiling point of 12.5°C and thus forms a vapour at room temperature. It is contained normally in closed bottles as a liquid which vaporises on release.

The vapour is explosive in air at concentrations between 3.8% and 15.4%, and is slightly irritant to the respiratory tract. It is a potent anaesthetic and was used in the past on an open mask for rapid induction of anaesthesia before maintenance with diethyl ether. Because of the ease of producing overdosage with apnoea and cardiovascular depression, it is no longer used.

Ethyl chloride is still in occasional use for producing cooling of the skin ('refrigeration anaesthesia'). A spray is directed on to the skin, causing local cooling to −20°C with production of fine water crystals over the treated area. An incision is made quickly through the cold skin, which remains painless when cold but becomes painful rapidly with warming.

Ethylene

Ethylene is a colourless non-irritant gas with a lower blood/gas solubility than that of any agent in common use (0.14, compared with 0.47 for nitrous oxide). Because of this property, it induces anaesthesia very rapidly. It causes slightly more muscle relaxation than nitrous oxide, but it is highly explosive.

Divinyl ether

Divinyl ether is a colourless non-irritant liquid with a low stability and high volatility. It was mixed with ethyl alcohol 4% (in order to reduce

Table 9.1 Structural formulae of inhalational anaesthetic agents

A. *Ethers*

Diethyl ether

$$\begin{array}{ccccccccccccc} & & \mathrm{H} & & \mathrm{H} & & & & \mathrm{H} & & \mathrm{H} & & \\ & & | & & | & & & & | & & | & & \\ \mathrm{H} & — & \mathrm{C} & — & \mathrm{C} & — & \mathrm{O} & — & \mathrm{C} & — & \mathrm{C} & — & \mathrm{H} \\ & & | & & | & & & & | & & | & & \\ & & \mathrm{H} & & \mathrm{H} & & & & \mathrm{H} & & \mathrm{H} & & \end{array}$$

Divinyl ether

$$\begin{array}{ccccccccccccc} \mathrm{H} & \diagdown & & & & & & & & & & \diagup & \mathrm{H} \\ & & \mathrm{C} & = & \mathrm{C} & — & \mathrm{O} & — & \mathrm{C} & = & \mathrm{C} & & \\ \mathrm{H} & \diagup & & & | & & & & | & & & \diagdown & \mathrm{H} \\ & & & & \mathrm{H} & & & & \mathrm{H} & & & & \end{array}$$

Methoxyflurane

$$\begin{array}{ccccccccccc} & & \mathrm{Cl} & & \mathrm{F} & & & & \mathrm{H} & & \\ & & | & & | & & & & | & & \\ \mathrm{H} & — & \mathrm{C} & — & \mathrm{C} & — & \mathrm{O} & — & \mathrm{C} & — & \mathrm{H} \\ & & | & & | & & & & | & & \\ & & \mathrm{Cl} & & \mathrm{F} & & & & \mathrm{H} & & \end{array}$$

Enflurane

$$\begin{array}{ccccccccccc} & & \mathrm{Cl} & & \mathrm{F} & & & & \mathrm{F} & & \\ & & | & & | & & & & | & & \\ \mathrm{H} & — & \mathrm{C} & — & \mathrm{C} & — & \mathrm{O} & — & \mathrm{C} & — & \mathrm{H} \\ & & | & & | & & & & | & & \\ & & \mathrm{F} & & \mathrm{F} & & & & \mathrm{F} & & \end{array}$$

Isoflurane

$$\begin{array}{ccccccccccc} & & \mathrm{F} & & \mathrm{H} & & & & \mathrm{F} & & \\ & & | & & | & & & & | & & \\ \mathrm{F} & — & \mathrm{C} & — & \mathrm{C} & — & \mathrm{O} & — & \mathrm{C} & — & \mathrm{H} \\ & & | & & | & & & & | & & \\ & & \mathrm{F} & & \mathrm{Cl} & & & & \mathrm{F} & & \end{array}$$

B. *Halogenated hydrocarbons*

Halothane

$$\begin{array}{ccccccc} & & \mathrm{F} & & \mathrm{Br} & & \\ & & | & & | & & \\ \mathrm{F} & — & \mathrm{C} & — & \mathrm{C} & — & \mathrm{H} \\ & & | & & | & & \\ & & \mathrm{F} & & \mathrm{Cl} & & \end{array}$$

Trichloroethylene

$$\begin{array}{ccccccc} \mathrm{Cl} & \diagdown & & & & \diagup & \mathrm{Cl} \\ & & \mathrm{C} & = & \mathrm{C} & & \\ \mathrm{Cl} & \diagup & & & & \diagdown & \mathrm{H} \end{array}$$

Table 9.1 (Cont'd)

Chloroform	$CHCl_3$ (Cl—C(Cl)(Cl)—H)
Ethyl chloride	$H_2C{=}CHCl$
C. *Hydrocarbons*	
Cyclopropane	$(CH_2)_3$ (ring of three CH_2)
Ethylene	$H_2C{=}CH_2$

the volatility) and an anti-oxidant (phenyl α-naphthylamine) in a commercial product termed 'Vinesthene'.

Divinyl ether is similar in some respects to diethyl ether, but did not achieve great popularity, probably because of its greater cost. However, a mixture of diethyl ether 75% and divinyl ether 25% (Vinesthene Anaesthetic Mixture) had a vogue for some time.

Chloroform

Chloroform is a colourless transparent fluid with a sweet-smelling odour. It is decomposed in light to phosgene, which is highly toxic, and it is therefore stored in dark bottles. Although the agent is no longer used for anaesthesia, it is used widely in biochemical laboratories as a solvent for extraction procedures.

In many respects, administration of anaesthesia with chloroform is similar to that with halothane. Induction of anaesthesia is smooth because the vapour is pleasant to inhale. The potency of chloroform is similar to that of halothane (MAC 0.5% for chloroform, 0.75% for halothane), with a similar oil/gas solubility coefficient. However, the blood/gas solubility differs markedly (chloroform 8.4, halothane 2.3) and therefore induction of anaesthesia is slower with chloroform (see Ch. 8).

In common with other anaesthetic agents, chloroform is a potent depressant of ventilation but the major reasons for its withdrawal from anaesthetic practice relate to actions on the heart and liver. In addition to depression of myocardial contractility and conduction, marked sensitisation of the myocardium to adrenaline occurs with predisposition to development of ventricular fibrillation during induction of anaesthesia. Chloroform is a direct hepatic toxin, causing central hepatic necrosis in a dose-related manner. Toxic effects occur also in the kidneys and other organs.

Methoxyflurane

Methoxyflurane is a clear, almost colourless, volatile liquid with a characteristic fruity odour. It is non-corrosive and compatible with soda lime. It has a very low saturated vapour pressure (3 kPa, 23 mmHg at 20°C) but a high blood/gas solubility coefficient of 13 and therefore the rate of induction of anaesthesia is extremely slow. In contrast, the oil/gas solubility is very high and consequently the drug has one of the lowest MAC values (see p. 723). It is non-flammable under ordinary conditions, but burns in oxygen at higher temperatures and concentrations.

In common with most agents it depresses ventilation in a dose-related manner; it also depresses the cardiovascular system, causing hypotension as a result of a reduction in cardiac output with little change in peripheral resistance. It does not sensitise the heart to the effects of exogenous catecholamines. It has little effect on the neuromuscular junction.

The major reasons for the loss of popularity of methoxyflurane were that the rate of induction of anaesthesia and recovery from anaesthesia are extremely slow and the agent is toxic to the kidneys. A significant quantity of an inhaled dose (50–70%) is metabolised to oxalic acid, fluoride ion, carbon dioxide, dichloroacetic acid and methoxyfluroacetic acid. Two of these metabolites (particularly fluoride) are responsible for the occurrence of 'high-output renal failure', in which the distal convoluted tubule becomes insensitive to the effects of ADH. Concentrations of fluoride ion reach a peak between the second and fourth post-anaesthetic days, resulting in renal toxicity in a small proportion of patients. It is recommended that the total dose of methoxyflurane is restricted to less than 2 MAC hours, in order to maintain serum fluoride ion concentrations below toxic levels.

Because of its good analgesic properties, 0.35% methoxyflurane in air was used for analgesia in childbirth by drawover vaporiser (Cardiff inhaler). This apparatus is no longer approved by the Central Midwives Board.

Trichloroethylene

Trichloroethylene is a colourless liquid, but the anaesthetic preparation is coloured with waxoline blue to prevent confusion with chloroform. It contains 0.01% thymol to retard decomposition.

On exposure to heat or sunlight, trichloroethylene is converted into hydrochloric acid and phosgene. It must not be used with soda lime because:

1. Heat decomposes trichloroethylene with the formation of phosgene and hydrochloric acid.
2. Heat in the presence of alkali converts tricholoroethylene into hydrochloric acid and dichloroacetylene, the latter combining with oxygen to form carbon monoxide and phosgene.

The drug is highly soluble in blood and relatively involatile. Consequently, induction of anaesthesia and recovery are prolonged. However, in common with methoxyflurane, it possesses a high oil/water solubility and a low MAC value.

Because of its low saturated vapour pressure, it is difficult to administer trichloroethylene in useful concentrations and the drug is therefore described frequently (incorrectly) as a weak anaesthetic. It is moderately irritant to the respiratory tract but tends to cause shallow rapid ventilation as a result of stimulation of stretch receptors in the lung. Because the level of anaesthesia is rarely deep with trichloroethylene, there is little depression of arterial pressure or cardiac output but arrhythmias are common. The incidence of arrhythmia is increased by the exogenous administration of adrenaline.

Trichloroethylene has little effect on the neuromuscular junction. Its use is associated with a high incidence of postoperative nausea and vomiting.

On its own, trichloroethylene was used rarely as an anaesthetic agent because it was difficult to achieve an adequate depth of anaesthesia as a result of the involatility and high blood/gas solubility of the agent. However, it was used frequently to supplement balanced nitrous oxide/oxygen/relaxant techniques and perhaps achieved greatest popularity in obstetric anaesthesia, where it was administered in a concentration of 0.35–0.5% in air, using the Emotril or Tecota drawover inhalers. Approval for use of these techniques was withdrawn by the Central Midwives Board in 1983.

Cyclopropane

Cyclopropane is a colourless gas with a characteristic pleasant sweet smell. It is stored as a liquefied gas in orange-coloured metal cylinders at a pressure of 5 bar at 15°C. Thus, the cylinder does not require a reducing valve on the anaesthetic machine. As with nitrous oxide, the pressure in the cylinder provides no indication of the volume of gas remaining. Cyclopropane has been virtually abandoned in all anaesthetic practice as it forms a highly explosive mixture with oxygen and nitrous oxide throughout the anaesthetic range of concentrations, and in air at concentrations between 3 and 10%.

Because of its relatively low blood/gas solubility coefficient, induction of anaesthesia and recovery are very rapid and it is possible to induce anaesthesia within several breaths. Cyclopropane is non-irritant to the respiratory tract but it is a very powerful depressant of ventilation and leads to carbon dioxide retention. The sympathoadrenal stimulation produced by hypercapnia, together with surgical stimulation, helps to maintain the patient's arterial pressure during surgery. However, on restoration of normocapnia and cessation of surgical stimulus during emergence there may be a profound decrease in arterial pressure because of previously masked relative hypovolaemia. This is referred to as 'cyclopropane shock'. In addition, the drug is itself a direct depressant of myocardial contractility and causes a high incidence of arrhythmias.

Cyclopropane was particularly popular until recent years for induction of anaesthesia in the shocked patient, using a closed circle system with CO_2 absorber.

AGENTS IN OCCASIONAL USE

Diethyl ether

Diethyl ether is a colourless, highly volatile liquid with a characteristic smell. In air it forms a mixture which burns with a blue flame; in oxygen-enriched mixtures, it forms an explosive combination. In air, the flammability range of ether is 1.9–48% but in oxygen the range is 2.0–82%. Characteristically, because ether is denser than air, ether vapour pools on the floor of the anaesthetic room and if ignited forms a blue flame which may cause an explosion if it reaches a rich source of oxygen.

Diethyl ether is manufactured by heating a mixture of ethyl alcohol and concentrated sulphuric acid to 130°C in a still with a constant flow of alcohol. The resulting vapour contains a mixture of ether, alcohol and water. Any sulphur dioxide is removed by sodium hydroxide and the ether and alcohol are separated by fractionation. Ether is dried using calcium chloride, and distilled.

Ether is decomposed by air, light and heat, the most important products being acetaldehyde and ether peroxide. Decomposition is retarded in the presence of copper or hydroquinone, and the drug should be stored in a cool environment in opaque containers.

Uptake and distribution

Ether has a relatively high blood/gas solubility coefficient of 12 and thus the rate of equilibration of alveolar with inspired concentrations is slow. In addition, ether is irritant to the respiratory tract and so the inspired concentration must be increased slowly. The net effect is that induction of anaesthesia is prolonged; recovery is also slow. Inspired concentrations may be raised gradually to 20% for induction of anaesthesia.

Central nervous system

In common with all general anaesthetic agents, there is depression of the cortex, resulting in loss of higher inhibitions initially, followed by depression. Because induction of anaesthesia with ether is so slow, the classical stages of anaesthesia are seen; these are described in detail on page 353 and Figure 20.2.

Depression of the respiratory centre precedes that of the vasomotor centre. Ether anaesthesia is associated with stimulation of the sympatho-adrenal system and increased levels of circulating catecholamines which offset the direct myocardial depressant effect of the drug.

Respiratory system

Ether is irritant to the respiratory tract and provokes coughing, breath-holding and profuse secretions from all mucus-secreting glands, including the salivary glands and those of the bronchial and respiratory tracts. Premedication with atropine or hyoscine is therefore essential.

Ether stimulates ventilation, and minute volume is maintained with increasing depth of anaesthesia until surgical anaesthesia is achieved; thereafter, there is a gradual diminution in alveolar ventilation as plane 4 of stage 3 is approached (Fig. 20.2). Arterial carbon dioxide tensions of approximately 4 kPa occur commonly during ether anaesthesia; Pa_{CO_2} does not increase above normal until alveolar ether concentrations of 6% are reached. Respiratory stimulation caused by ether is a result of:

1. Direct stimulation of the respiratory centre.
2. Stimulation of receptors in the respiratory tract.
3. Stimulation of pulmonary stretch receptors.
4. Stimulation of extrapulmonary stretch receptors.
5. Occasionally, the development of metabolic acidosis.

Laryngeal spasm is not uncommon during induction with ether, but during established anaesthesia there is dilation of the bronchi and bronchioles; at one time, the drug was recommended for treatment of bronchospasm.

Cardiovascular system

In vitro, ether is a direct myocardial depressant, but during light planes of clinical anaesthesia there is usually little change in cardiac ouput, arterial pressure or peripheral resistance. However, in patients who are receiving β-blocking or ganglion blocking drugs, or in combination with subarachnoid or extradural anaesthesia, the indirect sympathoadrenal stimulant effects of ether are obviated and myocardial depression may become clinically evident. In deep planes of anaesthesia, cardiac output decreases as a result of myocardial depression.

Cardiac arrhythmias occur rarely with ether and there is no sensitisation of the myocardium to circulating catecholamines. It is therefore safe to use ether on occasions when surgeons infiltrate with local anaesthetic solutions containing adrenaline.

Alimentary system

Salivary and gastric secretions are increased during light anaesthesia but decreased during deep anaesthesia. Smooth muscle of the intestine is depressed in proportion to the blood concentration of ether. Ether causes a very high incidence of postoperative nausea and vomiting by two mechanisms:

1. Solution in saliva which is swallowed and causes irritation to the stomach.
2. Stimulation of the vomiting centre.

Skeletal muscle

Ether relaxes skeletal muscle by two mechanisms:

1. Depression of spinal reflexes.
2. Blockade of the motor end-plates by a post-junctional mechanism similar, but not identical, to that of *d*-tubocurarine. Thus, ether potentiates the effects of non-depolarising muscle relaxants.

Uterus and placenta

The pregnant uterus is not affected during light anaesthesia but relaxation occurs during deep anaesthesia. Placental transmission causes depression of the fetus.

Metabolism

At least 15% of ether is metabolised to carbon dioxide and water; approximately 4% of ether is metabolised in the liver to acetaldehyde and ethanol.

Ether stimulates gluconeogenesis and therefore causes hyperglycaemia. In patients whose glycogen stores are impaired, ketone bodies may be formed with consequent metabolic acidosis.

Clinical use of ether

Ether has a much higher therapeutic ratio than the three modern volatile agents (halothane, enflurane and isoflurane), and is therefore safer for administration in the hands of unskilled individuals, or from an uncalibrated vaporiser. Because of its high blood/gas solubility coefficient and irritant properties to the respiratory tract, induction of anaesthesia is very slow.

Administration of ether is undertaken usually using an anaesthetic breathing system with a non-calibrated vaporiser (Boyle's bottle), or calibrated vaporiser (the EMO, which may be used as a drawover or as a plenum vaporiser). It may be used safely in a closed circuit with soda lime absorption. Occasionally, ether is administered using a Schimmelbusch mask.

Vapour strengths of up to 20% are required for induction; light anaesthesia can be maintained with 3–5% and deep anaesthesia with 5–6% inspired concentrations.

The latent heat of vaporisation of ether is 374 J/g (cf. halothane, 147 J/g) and it is necessary to avoid significant cooling, which diminishes the rate of vaporisation. Thus, ether vaporisers are designed to reduce cooling (e.g. the use of a large water jacket as in the EMO apparatus).

Ether should not be used in patients with diabetes mellitus or severe liver disease. Its use is inadvisable in patients with fever, particularly in children, as such patients may develop convulsions.

AGENTS IN COMMON CLINICAL USE

In Western countries, it is customary to use one of the three modern volatile anaesthetic agents, halothane, enflurane or isoflurane, vaporised in a mixture of nitrous oxide in oxygen. In recent years, the use of halothane has declined, particularly in North America, because of medicolegal pressure relating to the very rare occurrence of hepatotoxicity. Whilst this concern is less acute in Europe there is a clear trend to avoidance of repeated halothane anaesthesia. Apart from this problem, the selection of one of these three agents is based frequently upon relatively small differences in physical and pharmacological properties.

The following account of these agents, with a comparison of their pharmacological properties, may tend to exaggerate the differences between them. However, an equally satisfactory anaesthetic may be administered in the majority of patients with any of the three agents.

Halothane

Halothane (2-bromo-2-chloro-1,1,1-trifluoroethane) was synthesised in 1951 and introduced into clinical practice in the UK in 1956. It is a colourless liquid with a relatively pleasant smell. It is decomposed by light. The addition of 0.01% thymol and storage in amber-coloured bottles renders it stable. Although it is decomposed by soda lime, it may be used safely with this mixture. It corrodes metals in vaporisers and breathing systems. In the presence of moisture it corrodes aluminium, tin, lead, magnesium and alloys. It should be stored in a closed container away from light and heat.

Uptake and distribution

Halothane has a relatively low blood/gas solubility coefficient of 2.5 and thus induction of anaesthesia is relatively rapid. However, it may take at least 30 min for the alveolar inspired concentration to reach 50% of the inspired concentration (Fig. 9.1); this is slower than for enflurane or isoflurane. As with all the volatile agents, it is customary to use the technique of 'over-pressure' and induce halothane anaesthesia with concentrations 2–3 times higher than the MAC value (0.75%); the inspired concentration is reduced when a stable level of anaesthesia has been achieved.

Metabolism

Approximately 20% of halothane is metabolised in the liver, usually by oxidative pathways. The end products are excreted in the urine. The major metabolites are bromine, chlorine, trifluoroacetic acid and trifluoroacetylethanol amide.

A small proportion of halothane may undergo reductive metabolism, particularly in the presence

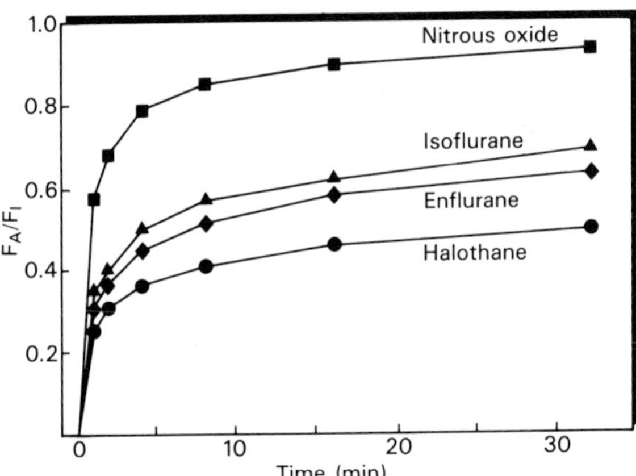

Fig. 9.1 Ratio of alveolar (F_A) to inspired (F_I) fractional concentrations of nitrous oxide, isoflurane, enflurane and halothane in the first 10 min of anaesthesia. The plot of F_A/F_I expresses the rapidity with which alveolar concentration equilibrates with inspired concentration. It is most rapid for agents with a low blood/gas partition coefficient.

of hypoxaemia and when the hepatic microsomal enzymes have been stimulated by enzyme-inducing agents such as phenobarbitone. Reductive metabolism may result in the formation of reactive metabolites and fluoride, although normally serum fluoride ion concentrations are considerably lower than those likely to induce renal dysfunction.

Respiratory system

Halothane is non-irritant and pleasant to breathe during induction of anaesthesia. There is rapid loss of pharyngeal and laryngeal reflexes, and inhibition of salivary and bronchial secretions. In the unpremedicated subject, halothane anaesthesia is associated with an increase in ventilatory rate and reduction in tidal volume. Pa_{CO_2} increases as the depth of halothane anaesthesia increases.

Halothane causes a dose-dependent decrease in mucociliary function which may persist for several hours after anaesthesia. This may contribute to postoperative sputum retention.

Halothane antagonises bronchospasm and reduces airway resistance in patients with bronchoconstriction, possibly by central inhibition of reflex bronchoconstriction and relaxation of bronchial smooth muscle. It has been suggested that halothane exerts a β-mimetic effect on bronchial muscle.

Cardiovascular system

Halothane is a potent depressant of myocardial contractility and myocardial metabolic activity as a result of inhibition of glucose uptake by myocardial cells. During controlled ventilation, halothane anaesthesia is associated with dose-related depression of cardiac output (by decrease in myocardial contractility) with little effect on peripheral resistance. Thus, there is a reduction in arterial pressure and an increase in right atrial pressure. In spontaneously breathing patients, some of these effects may be offset by a small increase in Pa_{CO_2} which leads to a reduction in systemic vascular resistance and a shift in cardiac output back towards baseline values as a result of indirect sympathoadrenal stimulation.

The hypotensive effect of halothane is augmented by a reduction in heart rate, which commonly accompanies halothane anaesthesia. Antagonism of the bradycardia by administration of atropine frequently leads to an increase in arterial pressure.

The reduction in myocardial contractility is associated with reductions in myocardial oxygen demand and coronary blood flow. Provided that undue elevations in left ventricular diastolic pressure and undue hypotension do not occur, halothane may be advantageous in patients with coronary artery disease because of the reduced oxygen demand caused by a low heart rate and decreased contractility.

The depressant effects of halothane on cardiac output are augmented in the presence of β-blockade.

Arrhythmias are very common during halothane anaesthesia and far more frequent than with either enflurane or isoflurane. Arrhythmias are produced by:

1. Increased myocardial excitability augmented by the presence of hypercapnia, hypoxaemia or increased circulating catecholamines.
2. Bradycardia caused by central vagal stimulation.

During local infiltration with adrenaline-containing local anaesthetic solutions, multifocal ventricular extrasystoles and sinus tachycardia have been observed and cardiac arrest has been reported. Thus, caution should be exercised when these solutions are used. The following recommendations have been made:

1. Avoid hypoxaemia and hypercapnia.
2. Avoid concentrations of adrenaline greater than 1 in 100 000.
3. Avoid a dosage in adults exceeding 10 ml of 1 in 100 000 adrenaline in 10 min or 30 ml/h.

Gastrointestinal tract

Gastrointestinal motility is inhibited. Postoperative nausea and vomiting are seldom severe.

Uterus

Halothane relaxes uterine muscle and may cause postpartum haemorrhage. It is said that a concentration of less than 0.5% is not associated with increased blood loss during anaesthesia for Caesarean section, but this concentration causes increased blood loss during therapeutic abortion.

Skeletal muscle

Halothane causes skeletal muscle relaxation and potentiates non-depolarising relaxants. Postoperatively, shivering is common; this increases oxygen requirements and results in hypoxaemia unless oxygen is administered.

Halothane-associated hepatic dysfunction

On extremely rare occasions the administration of halothane may be associated with the production of hepatic dysfunction. The exact cause of this dysfunction is not known; theories include the production of toxic metabolites. It is thought that the products of reductive metabolic pathways are more toxic than those produced by oxidation. This theory is supported by the fact that the risk of postoperative liver dysfunction is increased in the presence of:

1. Obesity, which results in increased tissue hypoxia and greater storage capacity for halothane.
2. Hypoxaemia.
3. A short interval between administrations of the drug.
4. Enzyme induction produced by drugs, e.g. phenobarbitone or phenytoin.

Toxicity after halothane anaesthesia has been a source of great controversy in recent years, largely because the diagnosis is dependent on exclusion of all other possible causes of hepatotoxicity. The recent demonstration of antibodies to halothane metabolites may help to clarify the situation.

As a result of this concern, the Committee on Safety of Medicines has made the following recommendations in respect of halothane anaesthesia:

1. A careful anaesthetic history should be taken to determine previous exposure and any previous reaction to halothane.
2. Repeated exposure to halothane within a period of 3 months should be avoided unless there are overriding clinical circumstances.
3. A history of unexplained jaundice or pyrexia after previous exposure to halothane is an absolute contraindication to its future use in that patient.

The incidence of halothane hepatotoxicity in paediatric practice is extremely low, although there have been case reports in children. Nevertheless, halothane remains the drug of choice for paediatric anaesthesia, in preference to enflurane or isoflurane.

In summary, halothane is a very useful inhalational anaesthetic agent. Its main advantages are:

1. Rapid, smooth induction.
2. Minimal stimulation of salivary and bronchial secretions; prior administration of atropine is unnecessary.
3. Bronchodilation.
4. Muscle relaxation.
5. Relatively rapid recovery.

The disadvantages are:

1. Poor analgesia.
2. Arrhythmias.

3. Postoperative shivering.
4. Possibility of liver toxicity, especially with repeated administrations.

Enflurane

Enflurane (2-chloro-1,1,2-trifluoroethyl difluoromethyl ether) was synthesised in 1963 and first evaluated clinically in 1966. It was introduced into clinical practice in the USA in 1971.

Physical properties

Enflurane is a clear, colourless, volatile anaesthetic agent with a pleasant ethereal smell. It is non-flammable in clinical concentrations, stable with soda lime and metals and does not require preservatives.

Uptake and distribution

Enflurane has a low blood/gas solubility coefficient of 1.9, resulting in rapid equilibration between alveolar and inspired partial pressures. Thus, induction of anaesthesia and recovery from anaesthesia are rapid (Fig. 9.1).

Metabolism

Approximately 2.5% of the absorbed dose is metabolised, predominantly to fluoride. In common with other ether anaesthetic agents (diethyl ether and isoflurane), the presence of the ether bond imparts stability to the molecule.

Defluorination of enflurane is increased in patients treated with isoniazid, but not with a classical enzyme-inducing agent such as phenobarbitone. Serum fluoride ion concentrations are greater after administration of enflurane to obese patients. To date, extensive studies have failed to demonstrate that the serum concentrations of fluoride ion reach toxic levels after enflurane anaesthesia.

Respiratory system

Enflurane is non-irritant and does not increase salivary or bronchial secretions; thus inhalational induction is relatively pleasant and rapid.

In common with all other volatile anaesthetic agents, enflurane causes a dose-dependent depression of alveolar ventilation with a reduction in tidal volume and an increase in ventilatory rate in the unpremedicated subject.

Cardiovascular system

Enflurane causes dose-dependent depression of myocardial contractility, leading to a reduction in cardiac output. In association with a small reduction in systemic vascular resistance, this leads to a dose-dependent reduction in arterial pressure. Because enflurane (unlike halothane) has no central vagal effects, hypotension leads to reflex tachycardia.

Enflurane anaesthesia is associated with a much smaller incidence of arrhythmias than halothane and much less sensitisation of the myocardium to catecholamines, either endogenous or exogenous.

Uterus

Enflurane relaxes uterine muscle in a dose-related manner.

Central nervous system

Enflurane produces a dose-dependent depression of EEG activity, but at moderate to high concentrations (more than 3%) it produces epileptiform paroxysmal spike activity and burst suppression. These are accentuated by hypocapnia. Twitching of the face and arm muscles may be seen occasionally. Enflurane should be avoided in the epileptic patient.

Muscle relaxation

Enflurane produces dose-dependent muscle relaxation with potentiation of non-depolarising neuromuscular blocking drugs to a greater extent than that produced by halothane.

Hepatotoxicity

There have been several case reports of jaundice attributable to the use of enflurane.

In summary, enflurane is a useful alternative agent to halothane. Its main advantages are:

1. Rapid induction and recovery.
2. Little biotransformation, and therefore little risk of hepatic dysfunction.
3. Muscle relaxation.
4. Low incidence of arrhythmias, even in the presence of high circulating catecholamine concentrations.

Its disadvantages are:

1. Relatively high cost.
2. Seizure activity on EEG.

Isoflurane

Isoflurane (1-chloro-2,2,2-trifluoroethyl difluoromethyl ether) is an isomer of enflurane and was synthesised in 1965. Clinical studies were undertaken in 1970, but because of early laboratory reports of carcinogenesis (which were not confirmed subsequently) it was not approved by the Food and Drug Administration in the United States until 1980.

Physical properties

Isoflurane is a colourless, volatile liquid with a slightly pungent odour. It is stable and does not react with metal or other substances and does not require preservatives. It is non-flammable in clinical concentrations.

Uptake and distribution

Isoflurane is the least soluble of the modern inhalational agents and thus alveolar concentrations equilibrate more rapidly with inspired concentrations. The alveolar (or arterial) partial pressure of isoflurane increases to 50% of the inspired partial pressure within 4–8 min, and to 60% by 15 min (Fig. 9.1). However, the rate of induction is limited by the pungency of the vapour and clinically may be no faster than that which can be achieved with halothane. The incidence of coughing or breath-holding on induction is significantly greater with isoflurane than with halothane.

Metabolism

Approximately 0.17% of the absorbed dose is metabolised. Metabolism takes place predominantly in the form of oxidation to produce difluromethanol and trifluroacetic acid; the former breaks down to formic acid and fluoride. Because of the minimal metabolism, only very small concentrations of serum fluoride ions are found, even after prolonged administration. The minimal metabolism renders hepatic and renal toxicity most unlikely.

Respiratory system

In common with halothane and enflurane, isoflurane causes dose-dependent depression of ventilation; there is a decrease in tidal volume but an increase in ventilatory rate in the absence of opioid drugs.

Cardiovascular system

In vitro, isoflurane is a myocardial depressant but in clinical use there is less depression of cardiac output than with halothane or enflurane. Systemic hypotension occurs predominantly as a result of reduction in systemic vascular resistance. Arrhythmias are uncommon and there is little sensitisation of the myocardium to catecholamines.

In addition to dilating systemic arterioles, isoflurane causes coronary vasodilatation. There has been some controversy recently regarding the safety of isoflurane in patients with coronary artery disease because of the possibility that the coronary steal syndrome may be induced; dilatation in normal coronary arteries offers a low resistance to flow, and may reduce perfusion through stenosed vessels. It has been shown that isoflurane affects small arterioles (which makes steal a theoretical possibility), but the effect seems to occur only in end-tidal concentrations in excess of 0.5%. Production of myocardial ischaemia in clinical practice may be produced by a large number of factors in addition to coronary vasodilatation, including tachycardia, hypotension, increase in left ventricular end-diastolic pressure and reduced ventricular compliance. Attention should be directed to these factors before a diagnosis of isoflurane-induced coronary steal is considered.

Uterus

Isoflurane has an effect on the pregnant uterus similar to that of halothane and enflurane.

Central nervous system

Low concentrations of isoflurane do not cause any change in cerebral blood flow at normocapnia. In this respect, the drug is superior to enflurane and halothane, both of which cause cerebral vasodilatation. However, higher inspired concentrations of isoflurane cause vasodilatation and increase cerebral blood flow. It does not cause seizure activity on the EEG.

Muscle relaxation

Isoflurane causes dose-dependent depression of neuromuscular transmission with potentiation of non-depolarising neuromuscular blocking drugs.

The advantages of isoflurane are:

1. Rapid induction and recovery.
2. Minimal biotransformation with little risk of hepatic or renal toxicity.
3. Cardiovascular stability.
4. Muscle relaxation.

Its disadvantages are:

1. High cost.
2. A pungent odour which makes inhalational induction relatively unpleasant, particularly in children, and which inhibits the rate of induction of anaesthesia.
3. Coronary vasodilatation with the possibility of coronary steal syndrome at high inspired concentrations.

Comparison of halothane, enflurane and isoflurane

Pharmacokinetics

The rate of equilibration of alveolar with inspired concentrations is related to blood/gas solubility. The rate of uptake of isoflurane is faster than that of enflurane and considerably faster than that of halothane, although much slower than that of nitrous oxide (Fig. 9.1). However, rate of induction of anaesthesia with isoflurane may be reduced because of the pungent odour compared with the more pleasant odours of halothane and enflurane.

On recovery from anaesthesia, the rate of elimination of isoflurane is faster than that of halothane or enflurane. Although it is possible using sensitive tests of psychomotor performance to demonstrate that recovery from isoflurane anaesthesia is faster than from enflurane anaesthesia (which in turn is faster than from halothane anaesthesia), tests of 'street fitness' reveal that there are no significant differences in recovery among the three agents. Recovery from these three agents to a state at which it is possible to respond to questions is in the range of 10–15 min after discontinuing administration of the volatile agent after 1–2 h of anaesthesia. More prolonged anaesthetic time prolongs the rate of recovery because of greater saturation of tissues.

Respiratory system

In unstimulated volunteers, enflurane causes greater ventilatory depression than isoflurane, which in turn causes greater depression of ventilation than halothane (Fig. 9.2). Nitrous oxide does not cause hypercapnia. Thus a reduction in inspired volatile anaesthetic concentration permitted by addition of nitrous oxide is associated with less

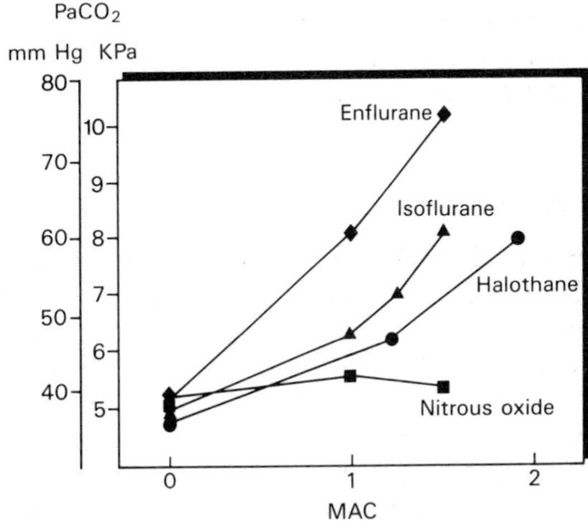

Fig. 9.2 Effects on Pa_{CO_2} of enflurane, isoflurane, halothane or nitrous oxide at equivalent MAC during spontaneous ventilation by healthy volunteers. (Nitrous oxide was administered in a hyperbaric chamber.)

ventilatory depression. In addition, surgical stimulation is responsible for considerable antagonism of ventilatory depression during anaesthesia and Pa_{CO_2} does not reach the values shown in Figure 9.2 during surgery.

With all three agents, depression of ventilation is associated with depression of whole body oxygen consumption and carbon dioxide production.

During surgery, an anaesthetic technique comprising spontaneous breathing of nitrous oxide/oxygen supplemented with halothane or isoflurane (inspired concentrations approximating to 1–1.5 MAC in total) results often in a Pa_{CO_2} value in the range 5.3–6.7 kPa (40–50 mmHg).

Cardiovascular system

In vitro studies have revealed that all three agents cause depression of contractility of isolated cardiac muscle. The effects of isoflurane and halothane are similar, and greater than that of enflurane.

However, isoflurane causes relatively little depression of cardiac output in vivo whilst enflurane causes the most (Fig. 9.3); the reduction in cardiac output is produced predominantly by a decrease in stroke volume. At normocapnia, halothane has no effect on peripheral resistance, whilst isoflurane causes the greatest degree of peripheral vasodilatation (Fig. 9.4). Consequently, all three agents cause hypotension in the order enflurane > isoflurane > halothane (Fig. 9.5). With the former two agents, there is a tendency for reflex compensatory tachycardia, but this is not manifest with halothane because of its direct vagal stimulatory properties. Halothane and enflurane cause a greater increase in right atrial pressure than does isoflurane.

The data in Figures 9.3–9.5 were derived from studies in volunteers, who were not subjected to

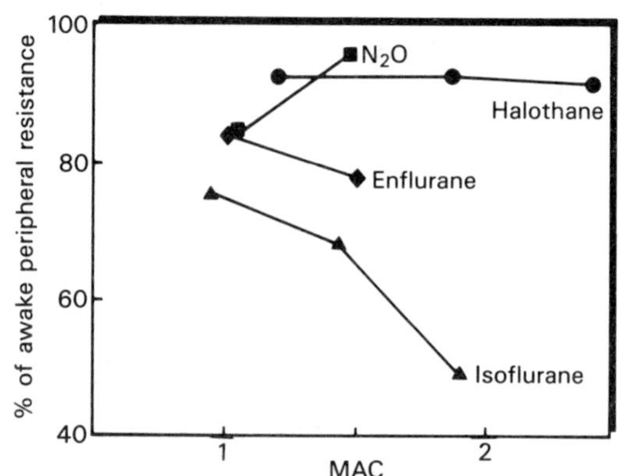

Fig. 9.4 Comparative effects of nitrous oxide, halothane, enflurane and isoflurane on peripheral vascular resistance in healthy volunteers.

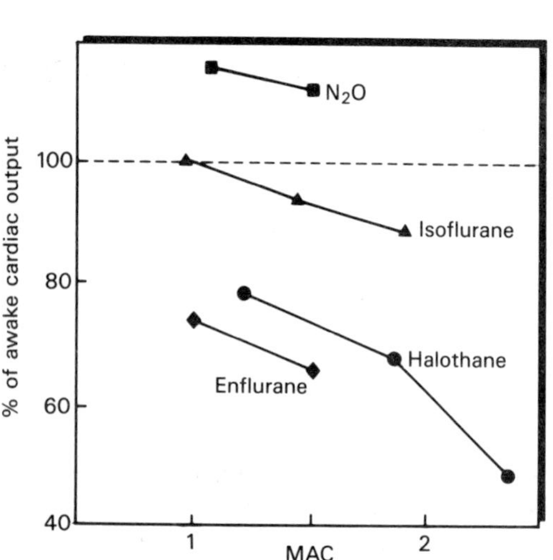

Fig. 9.3 Comparative effects of nitrous oxide, isoflurane, halothane and enflurane in healthy volunteers.

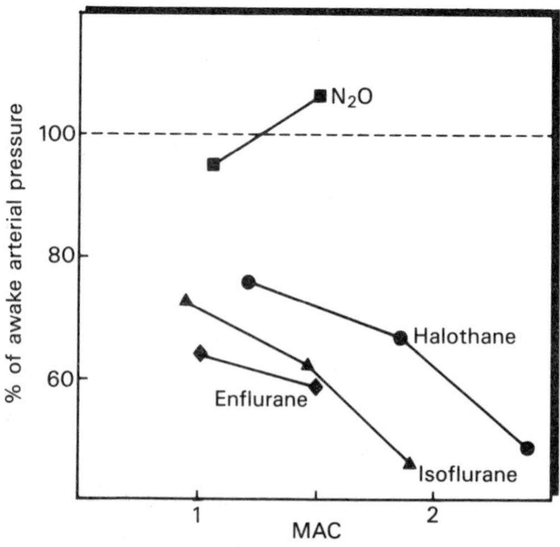

Fig. 9.5 Comparative effects of nitrous oxide, halothane, isoflurane and enflurane on arterial pressure in healthy volunteers.

surgical stimulation and in whom artificial ventilation was used to achieve normocapnia.

Some of the cardiovascular effects of these volatile agents are antagonised by the addition of nitrous oxide. In addition, during spontaneous ventilation, the modest hypercapnia which occurs with all three agents also offsets some of the changes. With enflurane and isoflurane, for example, cardiac output may be increased compared with pre-anaesthesia levels, although there is little effect on systemic arterial pressure. The effects of enflurane and isoflurane on right atrial pressure are reduced considerably during spontaneous ventilation; indeed, there may be little change. In contrast, the right atrial pressure remains elevated in the presence of hypercapnia during halothane anaesthesia.

Arrhythmias

Arrhythmias are common during halothane, but not during enflurane or isoflurane, anaesthesia.

After exogenous administration of adrenaline, stability of heart rhythm is greatest in patients anaesthetised with isoflurane, less with enflurane and least with halothane (Fig. 9.6).

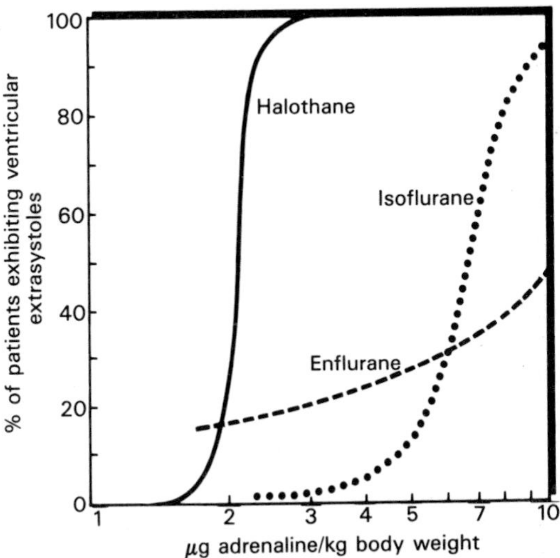

Fig. 9.6 Cumulative plots representing dose of adrenaline required to induce ventricular extrasystoles in normocapnic patients receiving 1.25 MAC of halothane, isoflurane or enflurane.

Neuromuscular junction

All three agents cause relaxation sufficient to perform lower abdominal surgery in thin subjects. In addition, however, there is potentiation of non-depolarising muscle relaxants. In this respect, isoflurane and enflurane are similar and cause markedly greater potentiation than that produced by halothane.

A comparison of other characteristics of the three agents is shown in Table 9.2.

Table 9.2 Comparison of modern volatile anaesthetic agents

	Halothane	Enflurane	Isoflurane
Molecular weight	197	184.5	184.5
Boiling point (°C)	50	56	49
Blood/gas partition coefficient	2.5	1.9	1.4
Oil/gas partition coefficient	220	98	97
MAC (in O_2)	0.75	1.68	1.15
Preservative	0.01% thymol	none	none
Percentage metabolised	20	2.4	0.17
Effect on EEG	depression	seizure activity	depression
Neuromuscular relaxation	moderate	strong	strong
Approximate cost (250 ml)	£10.50	£35.30	£83.75

NEW VOLATILE ANAESTHETIC AGENTS

Sevoflurane

```
          F
          |
     F —  C — F     H
          |         |
     H —  C — O  —  C — F
          |         |
     F —  C — F     H
          |
          F
```

Sevoflurane is a methyl propyl ether which was isolated in the early 1970s and first used in humans in 1981. The drug is now manufactured and used in Japan but is not available in the United Kingdom.

It is non-flammable and has a pleasant smell, a blood-gas partition coefficient of 0.6, an oil-gas partition coefficient of 55 and a MAC value of approximately 2.0%. The agent does not appear to be stable in soda lime. It undergoes biotransformation producing a mean peak fluoride ion concentration of 22 mmol/litre after 60 min of anaesthesia at 1 MAC. It does not sensitise the myocardium to catecholamines and it appears to have relatively little effect on the cardiovascular and respiratory systems.

Its physical properties suggest that it may be useful for gaseous induction of anaesthesia in children.

Desflurane (**I 653**)

```
     F     F           F
     |     |           |
F —  C  —  C  —  O  —  C  — F
     |     |           |
     F     H           H
```

This drug was first used in humans in 1988. The structure of the compound differs from isoflurane only in the substitution of fluorine for chlorine.

The drug has a blood–gas partition coefficient of 0.42 and an oil–gas partition coefficient of 18.7. Because it has a boiling point of 23.5°C it cannot be used with conventional vaporisers. It contains no preservative and is stable with soda lime. It has an ethereal but much less pungent odour than isoflurane. It undergoes minimal biodegradation and does not sensitise the myocardium to catecholamines.

Preliminary studies in volunteers suggest that it has very little effect on the cardiovascular or respiratory systems other than slight increases in respiratory rate and end-tidal CO_2, and mild hypotension.

The uptake and elimination of desflurane are virtually identical to those of nitrous oxide and the drug therefore has theoretical advantage over the conventional volatile anaesthetic agents.

ANAESTHETIC GASES

Nitrous oxide (N_2O)

Manufacture

Nitrous oxide is prepared commercially by heating ammonium nitrate to a temperature of 245–270°C. Various impurities are produced in this process, including ammonia, nitric acid, nitrogen, nitric oxide and nitrogen dioxide.

After cooling, ammonia and nitric acid are reconstituted to ammonium nitrate, which is returned to the beginning of the process. The remaining gases then pass through a series of scrubbers. The purified gases are compressed and dried in an aluminium dryer. The resultant gases are expanded in a liquefier, with the nitrogen escaping as gas. Nitrous oxide is then evaporated, compressed and passed through another aluminium dryer before being stored in cylinders.

The higher oxides of nitrogen dissolve in water to form nitrous and nitric acids. These substances are toxic and produce methaemoglobinaemia and pulmonary oedema if inhaled. In the past, there have been several reports of death occurring during anaesthesia as a result of the inhalation of nitrous oxide contaminated with higher oxides of nitrogen.

Storage

Nitrous oxide is stored in compressed form as a liquid in cylinders at a pressure of 50 bar (5000 kPa; 750 lb/in^2). In the UK, the cylinders are painted blue.

Because the cylinder contains liquid and vapour, the total quantity of nitrous oxide contained in a cylinder can be ascertained only by weighing. Thus, the cylinder weights, full and empty, are stamped on the shoulder. Nitrous oxide cylinders should be kept in a vertical position during use so that the liquid phase remains at the bottom of the cylinder. During continuous use, the cylinder may cool as a result of the latent heat of vaporisation of liquid anaesthetic and ice may form on the lower part of the cylinder.

Physical properties

Nitrous oxide is a sweet-smelling, non-irritant colourless gas, with a molecular weight of 44, boiling point −88°C, critical temperature 36.5°C and critical pressure 72.6 bar.

Nitrous oxide is not flammable but it supports combustion of fuels in the absence of oxygen.

Pharmacology

Nitrous oxide is frequently said to be a good analgesic but a weak anaesthetic. The latter refers to the fact that its MAC value is 105%. This value was calculated theoretically from its low oil/water solubility coefficient of 3.2 and has been confirmed experimentally in volunteers anaesthetised in a pressure chamber compressed to 2 atmospheres absolute (ata), where the MAC value was found to be 55% N_2O.

As it is essential to administer a minimum FI_{O_2} of 0.3, nitrous oxide alone is insufficient to produce an adequate depth of anaesthesia in all but the most seriously ill patient; therefore, nitrous oxide is used usually in combination with other agents. When using nitrous oxide in a relaxant technique, the inspired gas mixture should be supplemented with a low concentration of a volatile agent to minimise the possibility of awareness which may occur if nitrous oxide anaesthesia is supplemented only by the administration of opioids.

Of the anaesthetic agents in current clinical use, nitrous oxide has the lowest blood/gas solubility coefficient (0.47 at 37°C) and therefore the rate of equilibration of alveolar with inspired concentrations is very fast (Fig. 9.1).

Because of the low solubility, a change in alveolar ventilation has less effect on the rate of uptake than occurs with the more soluble agents such as halothane and ether (Fig. 9.7). Similarly, changes in cardiac output have less effect with nitrous oxide (Fig. 9.8). Nitrous oxide does not undergo metabolism in the body and is excreted unchanged.

The concentration effect

The inspired concentration of nitrous oxide affects its rate of equilibration; the higher the inspired concentration the faster is the rate of equilibration between alveolar and inspired concentrations. Nitrous oxide is more soluble in blood than nitrogen. Thus, the volume of nitrous oxide

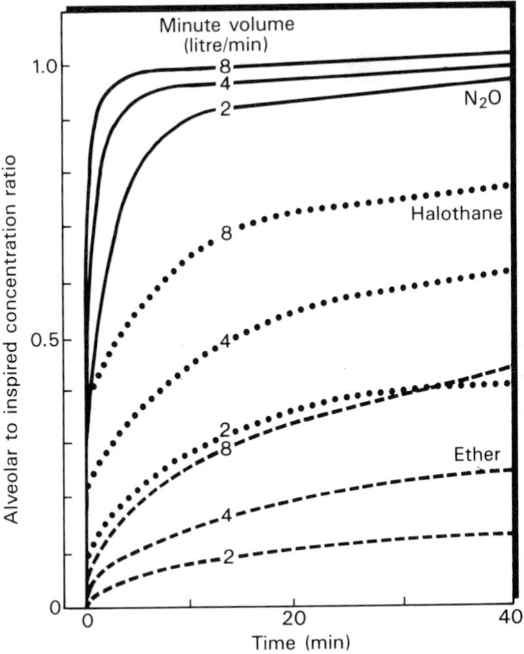

Fig. 9.7 Influence of minute volume on the rate of equilibration between alveolar and inspired concentrations of nitrous oxide, halothane and ether. The effects of ventilation are more marked on the agents with higher blood/gas solubility coefficients.

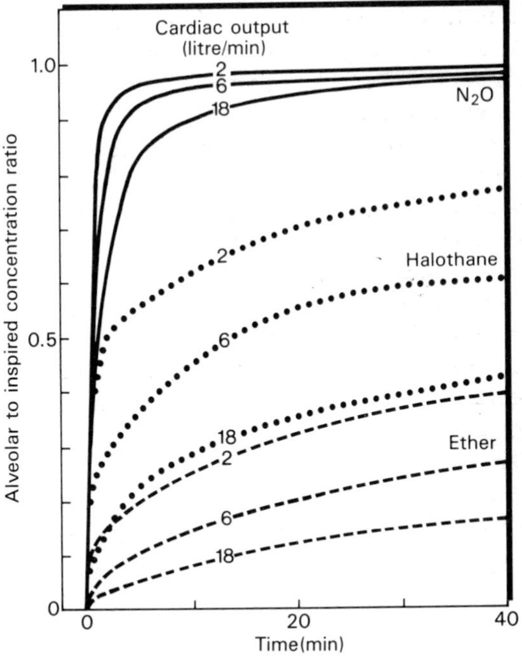

Fig. 9.8 Influence of cardiac output on the rate of equilibration between alveolar and inspired concentrations of nitrous oxide, halothane and ether. The effects of cardiac output are more marked on the agents with higher blood/gas solubility coefficients.

entering pulmonary capillary blood from the alveolus is greater than the volume of nitrogen moving in the opposite direction. As a result, the total volume of gas in the alveolus diminishes and the fractional concentrations of the remaining gases increase. This has two consequences:

1. The higher the inspired concentration of nitrous oxide, the greater is the concentrating effect on the nitrous oxide remaining in the alveolus.
2. At high inspired concentrations of nitrous oxide, the reduction in alveolar gas volume causes an increase in $P\text{A}_{CO_2}$. Equilibration with pulmonary capillary blood results in an increase in Pa_{CO_2}.

The result of the concentration effect on equilibration of nitrous oxide is illustrated in Figure 9.9.

The second gas effect

When nitrous oxide is administered in a high concentration with a second anaesthetic agent, e.g. halothane, the reduction in gas volume in the alveoli caused by absorption of nitrous oxide increases the alveolar concentration of halothane, thereby augmenting the rate of equilibration with inspired gas. This is illustrated in the lower part of Figure 9.9. The second gas effect results also in small increases in Pa_{O_2} and Pa_{CO_2}.

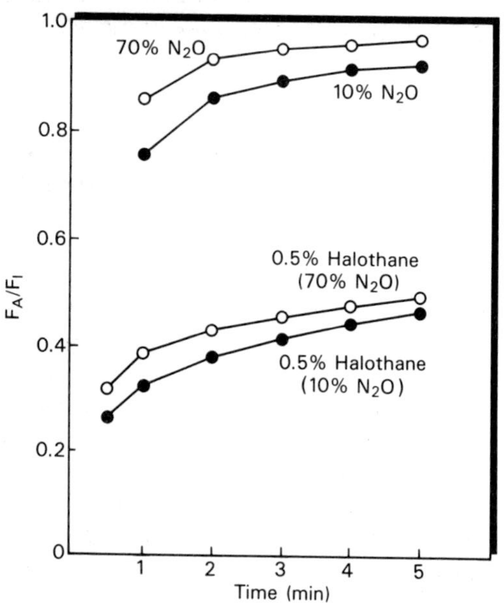

Fig. 9.9 The concentration and second gas effects. High concentrations of nitrous oxide increase the rate of increase of F_A/F_I ratio for nitrous oxide (the concentration effect) and for a volatile agent administered with nitrous oxide (the second gas effect). See text for details.

Side effects of nitrous oxide

1. *Diffusion hypoxia*. At the end of an anaesthetic, when the inspired gas mixture is changed from nitrous oxide/oxygen to nitrogen/oxygen, hypoxaemia may occur as the volume of nitrous oxide diffusing from mixed venous blood into the alveolus is greater than the volume of nitrogen taken up from the alveolus into pulmonary capillary blood (the opposite of the concentration effect). Thus, the concentration of gases in the alveolus is diluted by nitrous oxide, leading to a reduction in $P\text{A}_{O_2}$ and $P\text{A}_{CO_2}$. In the healthy individual, diffusion hypoxia is relatively transient, but may last for up to 10 min at the end of anaesthesia; the extent of reduction in Pa_{O_2} may be of the order of 0.5–1.5 kPa. Administration of oxygen during this period is advisable.

2. *Effect on closed gas spaces*. When blood containing nitrous oxide equilibrates with closed air-containing spaces inside the body, the volume of nitrous oxide that diffuses into the cavity exceeds the volume of nitrogen diffusing out. Thus, in compliant spaces such as the bowel lumen or the pleural or peritoneal cavities, there is an increase in volume of the space. If the space cannot expand (e.g. sinuses, middle ear) there is an increase in pressure. In the middle ear, this may cause problems with surgery on the tympanic membrane. When nitrous oxide is administered in a concentration of 75%, the volume of a cavity may increase to as much as 3–4 times the original volume within 30 min. If an air embolus occurs in a patient who is breathing nitrous oxide, equilibration with the gas bubble leads to expansion of the embolus within seconds; the volume of the embolus may double within a very short period of time.

3. *Cardiovascular depression*. Nitrous oxide is a direct myocardial depressant but in the normal individual this effect is antagonised by indirectly mediated sympathoadrenal stimulation (effects

similar to those produced by carbon dioxide). Thus, healthy patients exhibit little change in the cardiovascular system during nitrous oxide anaesthesia. However, in patients with pre-existing high levels of sympathoadrenal activity and poor myocardial contractility, the administration of nitrous oxide may cause a reduction in cardiac output and arterial pressure. For this reason (in addition to avoidance of the risk of doubling the size of air emboli) nitrous oxide is avoided in some centres during anaesthesia for cardiac surgery.

4. *Toxicity.* Nitrous oxide affects vitamin B_{12} synthesis by inhibiting the enzyme methionine synthetase. This effect is of importance if the duration of nitrous oxide anaesthesia exceeds 8 h. Nitrous oxide interferes also with folic acid metabolism and impairs synthesis of DNA; prolonged exposure may cause agranulocytosis and bone marrow aplasia. Exposure of patients to nitrous oxide for 6 h or longer may result in megaloblastic anaemia. Occupational exposure to nitrous oxide may result in myeloneuropathy. This condition is similar to subacute combined degeneration of the spinal cord, and has been reported in some dentists and also in individuals addicted to inhalation of nitrous oxide.

5. *Teratogenic changes.* Teratogenic changes have been observed in pregnant rats exposed to nitrous oxide for prolonged periods. There is no evidence that similar effects occur in man, but it has been suggested that nitrous oxide should be avoided in early pregnancy; however, this is not a generally held view at the present time.

OTHER GASES USED DURING ANAESTHESIA

Oxygen

Manufacture

Oxygen is manufactured commercially by fractional distillation of liquid air. Before liquefaction of air, carbon dioxide is removed and liquid oxygen and nitrogen separated by means of their different boiling points (oxygen −183°C, nitrogen −195°C).

Oxygen is supplied in cylinders at a pressure of 137 bar (approximately 2000 lb/in^2) at 15°C. The cylinders are painted black with a white shoulder.

Many institutions use piped oxygen and this is supplied either by a bank of oxygen cylinders, ensuring a continuous supply, or as liquid oxygen. Premises using in excess of 150 000 litres of oxygen per week find the latter more economical. The pressure of oxygen in a hospital pipeline is approximately 4 bar (60 lb/in^2), which is the same as the pressure distal to the reducing valves of gas cylinders attached to anaesthetic machines.

Oxygen is tasteless, colourless and odourless, with a specific gravity of 1.105 and a molecular weight of 32. At atmospheric pressure it liquefies at −183°C but at 50 atmospheres the liquefaction temperature increases to −119°C.

Oxygen supports combustion, although the gas itself is not flammable.

Oxygen concentrators

Oxygen concentrators produce oxygen from ambient air by absorption of nitrogen onto some types of alumina silicates. Oxygen concentrators are useful both in hospitals and in long-term domestic use in remote areas, in developing countries and in military surgery. The gas produced by oxygen concentrators contains small quantities of inert gases (e.g. argon) which are harmless.

Physiological effects

The physiological aspects of oxygen are discussed in Chapter 2 and the clinical uses in Chapter 24.

Adverse effects of oxygen

1. *Fire.* Oxygen supports combustion of fuels. An increase in the concentration of oxygen from 21% up to 100% causes a progressive increase in the rate of combustion with the production of either conflagrations or explosions with appropriate fuels (see Ch. 16).

2. *Cardiovascular depression.* An increase in Pa_{O_2} leads to direct vasoconstriction, which occurs in peripheral vasculature and also in the cerebral, coronary, hepatic and renal circulations. This effect is not manifest at a Pa_{O_2} of less than 30 kPa and assumes clinical importance only at hyperbaric pressures of oxygen. Hyperbaric pressures of oxygen also cause direct myocardial depression.

In patients with severe cardiovascular disease, elevation of Pa_{O_2} from the normal physiological range to 80 kPa may produce clinically evident cardiovascular depression.

3. *Absorption atelectasis*. Because oxygen is highly soluble in blood, the use of 100% oxygen as the inspired gas may lead to absorption atelectasis in lung units distal to the site of airway closure. Absorption collapse may occur in as short a time as 6 min with 100% oxygen, and 60 min with 85% oxygen. Thus, even small concentrations of nitrogen exert an important splinting effect and this accounts for current avoidance of 100% oxygen in estimation of pulmonary shunt ratio (Q_s/Q_t) in patients with lung pathology, in whom a greater degree of airway closure would result in greater areas of alveolar atelectasis. Absorption atelectasis has been demonstrated in volunteers breathing 100% oxygen at FRC; atelectasis is evident on chest radiography for a period of at least 24 h after exposure.

4. *CO_2 narcosis*. In patients with chronic bronchitis and chronic CO_2 retention, there may be loss of sensitivity of the central chemoreceptors and some dependence of ventilation on drive from the peripheral chemoreceptors that respond to oxygen. Administration of a high F_{IO_2} to such a patient may cause loss of peripheral chemoreceptor drive with the subsequent development of ventilatory failure.

5. *Pulmonary oxygen toxicity*. Chronic inhalation of a high inspired concentration of oxygen may result in the condition termed pulmonary oxygen toxicity (Lorrain–Smith effect), which is manifest by hyaline membranes, thickening of the interlobular and alveolar septa by oedema and fibroplastic proliferation. The clinical and radiological appearance of these changes is almost identical to that of the adult respiratory distress syndrome. The biochemical mechanisms underlying pulmonary oxygen toxicity probably include:

a. Oxidation of SH groups on essential enzymes such as co-enzyme A.
b. Peroxidation of lipids; the resulting lipid peroxides inhibit the function of the cell.
c. Inhibition of the pathway of reversed electron transport, possibly by inhibition of iron and SH-containing flavoproteins.

These changes lead to loss of synthesis of pulmonary surfactant, encouraging the development of absorption collapse and alveolar oedema. The onset of oxygen-induced lung pathology occurs after approximately 30 h exposure to a P_{IO_2} of 100 kPa.

6. *Central nervous system oxygen toxicity*. Convulsions, similar to those of grand mal epilepsy, occur during exposure to hyperbaric pressures of oxygen.

7. *Retrolental fibroplasia*. Retrolental fibroplasia (RLF) is the result of oxygen-induced retinal vasoconstriction, with obliteration of the most immature retinal vessels and subsequent new vessel formation at the site of damage in the form of a proliferative retinopathy. Leakage of intravascular fluid leads to vitreoretinal adhesions and even retinal detachment. Retrolental fibroplasia occurs in infants exposed to hyperoxia in the paediatric intensive care unit and is related not to the F_{IO_2} per se, but to an elevated retinal artery P_{O_2}. It is not known what the threshold of Pa_{O_2} is for the development of retinal damage, but an umbilical arterial P_{O_2} of 8–12 kPa (60–90 mmHg) is associated with a very low incidence of RLF and no signs of systemic hypoxia. It should be stressed, however, that there are many factors involved in the development of RLF in addition to arterial hyperoxia.

8. *Depressed haemopoiesis*. Long-term exposure to elevated F_{IO_2} leads to depresion of haemopoiesis and anaemia.

Carbon dioxide

Carbon dioxide is a colourless gas with a pungent odour. It has a molecular weight of 44, a critical temperature of 31°C and a critical pressure of 73.8 bar.

Carbon dioxide is obtained commercially from four sources:

1. As a byproduct of fermentation in brewing of beer.
2. As a byproduct of the manufacture of hydrogen.
3. By heating magnesium and calcium carbonate in the presence of their oxides.
4. As a combustion gas from burning fuel.

Carbon dioxide is supplied in a liquid state in grey cylinders at a pressure of 50 bar. The filling ratio (see p. 272) is 0.75 and the liquid phase occupies approximately 90–95% of the cylinder capacity.

Physiological data

The physiological aspects of CO_2 are dealt with predominantly in Chapter 2. Variations in cardiovascular state induced by alterations in Pa_{CO_2} may be similar to those induced by pain or lightness of anaesthesia and the differential diagnosis is described in Table 24.2. The cardiovascular effects of CO_2 are summarised in Table 9.3.

Table 9.3 Cardiovascular effects of CO_2

Arterial pressure Cardiac output Heart rate	Biphasic response. Progressive increase in these variables with increase in Pa_{CO_2} up to approximately 10 kPa as a result of indirect sympathetic stimulation. At very high Pa_{CO_2}, these variables decrease as a result of myocardial depression
Skin Coronary circulation Cerebral circulation Gastrointestinal circulation	Dilatation with hypercapnia Constriction with hypocapnia

Uses of carbon dioxide in anaesthesia

1. During inhalational induction of anaesthesia, carbon dioxide may be used to stimulate ventilation after a heavy opioid premedication. Care should be taken to avoid undue hypercapnia.

2. To produce hyperventilation in order to facilitate blind nasal intubation.

3. To increase cerebral blood flow during carotid artery surgery. This is an area of some controversy, as hypercapnia may induce 'stealing' of blood away from an ischaemic area of brain. Many anaesthetists prefer to maintain normocapnia during this surgical procedure.

4 To assist in reinstitution of spontaneous ventilation after a period of artificial hyperventilation.

The use of carbon dioxide in anaesthetic practice has declined as appreciation of its disadvantages has increased and as a result of the introduction of i.v. induction agents and relaxant anaesthetic techniques. In many countries, CO_2 is not available on anaesthetic machines.

FURTHER READING

Eger E I 1974 Anaesthetic uptake and action. Williams & Wilkins, Baltimore

Prys-Roberts C (Ed) 1980 The circulation in anaesthesia. Blackwell Scientific Publications, Oxford

Jones R M (1989). Inhalational and intravenous anaesthetic agents. In: Nimmo W S, Smith G (eds) Anaesthesia. Blackwell Scientific Publications, Oxford.

10. Intravenous anaesthetic agents

General anaesthesia may be produced by many drugs which depress the central nervous system, including sedatives, tranquillisers and hypnotic agents. However, for some drugs the doses required to produce surgical anaesthesia are so large that cardiovascular and respiratory depression may occur commonly, and recovery is delayed for hours or even days. Only a few drugs are suitable for use routinely to produce anaesthesia after i.v. injection.

Intravenous anaesthetic agents are used commonly to induce anaesthesia, as induction is usually more rapid and smoother than that associated with inhalational agents. In some circumstances, i.v. anaesthetics are used also for maintenance, either alone or in combination with nitrous oxide; they may be administered as repeated bolus doses or by continuous i.v. infusion. Other uses include sedation during regional anaesthesia, sedation in ITU and treatment of status epilepticus.

Properties of the ideal intravenous anaesthetic agent

1. Rapid onset. This is achieved by an agent which is mainly un-ionised at blood pH and which is highly soluble in lipid; these properties permit penetration of the blood–brain barrier.
2. Rapid recovery. Early recovery of consciousness is produced usually by rapid redistribution of the drug from the brain into other well-perfused tissues, particularly muscle. The plasma concentration of the drug decreases, and the drug diffuses out of the brain along a concentration gradient. The quality of the later recovery period is related more to the rate of metabolism of the drug; drugs with slow metabolism are associated with a more prolonged 'hangover' effect and accumulate if used in repeated doses or by infusion for maintenance of anaesthesia.
3. Analgesia at subanaesthetic concentrations.
4. Minimal cardiovascular and respiratory depression.
5. No emetic effects.
6. No excitatory phenomena (e.g. coughing, hiccup, involuntary movement) on induction.
7. No emergence phenomena (e.g. nightmares).
8. No interaction with neuromuscular blocking drugs.
9. No pain on injection.
10. No venous sequelae.
11. Safe if injected inadvertently into an artery.
12. No toxic effects on other organs.
13. No release of histamine.
14. No hypersensitivity reactions.
15. Water-soluble formulation.
16. Long shelf-life.
17. No stimulation of porphyria.

None of the agents available at present meets all these requirements. Features of the commonly used i.v. anaesthetic agents are compared in Table 10.1.

A classification of i.v. anaesthetic drugs is shown in Table 10.2.

Pharmacokinetics of i.v. anaesthetic drugs

After i.v. administration of a drug, there is an immediate rapid increase in plasma concentration followed by a slower decline. Anaesthesia is produced by diffusion of drug from arterial blood across the blood–brain barrier into brain. The rate

Table 10.1 Main properties of intravenous anaesthetics

	Thiopentone	Methohexitone	Propofol	Ketamine	Etomidate
Physical properties					
Water-soluble	+	+	−	+	+*
Stable in solution	−	−	+	+	+
Long shelf-life	−	−	+	+	+
Pain on i.v. injection	−	+	++	−	++
Non-irritant on s.c. injection	−	±	+	+	
Painful on arterial injection	+	+	−		
No sequelae from intra-arterial injection	−	±	+		
Low incidence of venous thrombosis	+	+	−	+	−
Effects on body					
Rapid onset	+	+	+	−	+
Recovery due to:					
redistribution	+	+	+	+	
detoxification		+	+		
Cumulation	++	+	−	−	−
Induction:					
excitatory effects	−	++	+	+	+++
respiratory complications	−	+	+	−	−
Cardiovascular:					
hypotension	+	+	++	−	+
Analgesic	−	−	−	++	−
Antanalgesic	+	+	−	−	?
Interaction with relaxants	−	−	−	−	−
Postop. vomiting	−	−	−	++	+
Emergence delirium	−	−	−	++	−
Safe in porphyria	−	−	+	+	−

* Aqueous solution not commercially available.

Table 10.2 Classification of i.v. anaesthetics

Rapidly acting (primary induction) agents
1. Barbiturates: methohexitone
   Thiobarbiturates: thiopentone, thiamylal
2. Imidazole compounds: etomidate*
3. Sterically hindered alkyl phenols: propofol

W (Steroids: Althesin, minaxolone)
W (Eugenols: propanidid)

Slower acting (basal narcotic) agents
4. Ketamine
5. Benzodiazepines: diazepam, flunitrazepam, midazolam
6. Large-dose opioids: fentanyl, alfentanil, sufentanil
7. Neurolept combination: opioid + neuroleptic

* Limited use as infusion; W = withdrawn from market.

of transfer into brain, and therefore the anaesthetic effect, is regulated by:

1. Protein binding. Only unbound drug is free to cross the blood–brain barrier. Protein binding may be reduced by low plasma protein concentrations or displacement by other drugs, resulting in higher concentrations of free drug and an exaggerated anaesthetic effect. Protein binding is affected also by changes in blood pH. Thus, hyperventilation decreases protein binding and increases anaesthetic effect.

2. Blood flow to brain. Reduced cerebral blood flow (CBF), e.g. carotid artery stenosis, results in reduced delivery of drug to brain. However, if CBF is reduced because of low cardiac output, initial blood concentrations are higher than normal after i.v. administration, and the anaesthetic effect may be delayed but enhanced.

3. Extracellular pH and pK_a of the drug. Only the non-ionised fraction of the drug penetrates the lipid blood–brain barrier; thus, the potency of the drug depends on the degree of ionisation at the pH of extracellular fluid and the pK_a of the drug.

4. The relative solubilities of the drug in lipid and water. High lipid solubility enhances transfer into the brain.

5. Speed of injection. Rapid i.v. administration results in high initial concentrations of drug. This

increases speed of induction, and also the extent of cardiovascular and respiratory side effects.

In general, any factor which increases the blood concentration of free drug, e.g reduced protein binding or low cardiac output, also increases the intensity of side effects.

Distribution to other tissues

The anaesthetic effect of all i.v. anaesthetic drugs in current use is terminated predominantly by distribution to other tissues. Figure 10.1 shows this distribution for thiopentone. The percentage of the injected dose in each of four body compartments as time elapses is shown after i.v. injection. A large proportion of the drug is distributed initially into the well-perfused organs (termed the vessel-rich group, or viscera: predominantly brain, liver and kidneys). Distribution into muscle (lean) is slower because of its low lipid content, but is quantitatively important because of its relatively good blood supply and large mass. Despite their high lipid solubility, i.v. anaesthetic drugs distribute slowly to adipose tissue (fat) because of its poor blood supply. Fat contributes little to the initial redistribution or termination of action of i.v. anaesthetic agents, but fat depots contain a large proportion of the injected dose of thiopentone at 90 min, and 65–75% of the total remaining in the body at 24 h. There is also a small amount of redistribution to areas with a very poor blood supply, e.g. bone. Table 10.3 indicates some of the properties of the body compartments in respect of the distribution of i.v. anaesthetic agents.

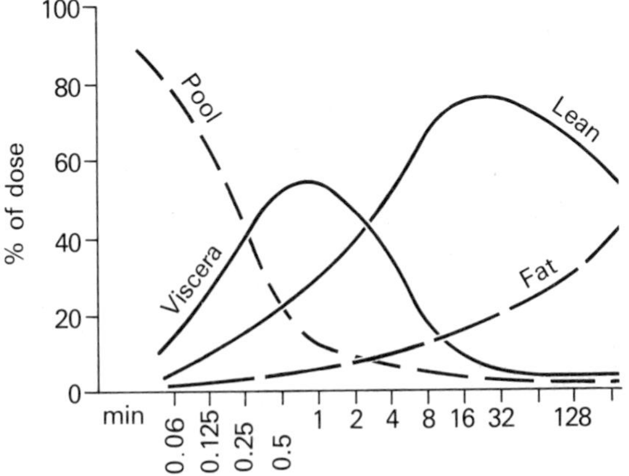

Fig. 10.1 Distribution of thiopentone after i.v. bolus administration.

Table 10.3 Factors influencing the distribution of thiopentone in the body

	Viscera	Muscle	Fat	Others
Relative blood flow	Rich	Good	Poor	Very poor
Blood flow (litre/min)	4.5	1.1	0.32	0.08
Tissue volume (litre) (A)	6	33	15	13
Tissue/blood partition coefficient (B)	1.5	1.5	11.0	1.5
Potential capacity (litre) (A × B)	9	50	160	20
Time constant (capacity/flow) (min)	2	45	500	250

After a single i.v. dose, the concentration of drug in blood decreases as distribution occurs into viscera, and particularly muscle. Drug diffuses from the brain into blood along the changing concentration gradient, and recovery of consciousness occurs. Metabolism of most i.v. anaesthetic drugs occurs predominantly in the liver; if metabolism is rapid (indicated by a short elimination half-life), it may contribute to some extent to the recovery of consciousness. However, because of the large distribution volume of i.v. anaesthetic drugs, total elimination takes many hours, or in some instances, days. A small proportion of drug may be excreted unchanged in the urine; the amount depends on the degree of ionisation and the pH of urine.

BARBITURATES

Amylobarbitone and pentobarbitone were used i.v. to induce anaesthesia in the late 1920s, but their actions were unpredictable and recovery was prolonged. Manipulation of the barbituric acid ring (Fig. 10.2) enabled a short duration of action to be achieved by:

1. Substitution of a sulphur atom for oxygen at position 2.
2. Substitution of a methyl group at position 1; this also confers potential convulsive activity and increases the incidence of excitatory phenomena.

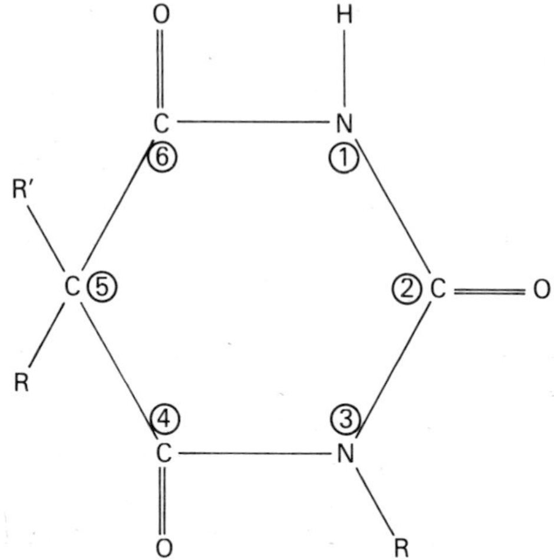

Fig. 10.2 Structure of barbiturate ring.

An increased number of carbon atoms in the side chains at position 5 increases the potency of the agent. The presence of an aromatic nucleus in an alkyl group at position 5 produces compounds with convulsant properties; direct substitution with a phenyl group confers anticonvulsant activity.

The anaesthetically active barbiturates are classified chemically into four groups (Table 10.4). The methylated oxybarbiturate hexobarbitone was moderately successful as an i.v. anaesthetic agent, but was superseded by the development in 1932 of thiopentone. Thiopentone remains the most commonly used i.v. anaesthetic agent throughout the world. Its pharmacology is therefore described fully in this chapter. Many of its effects are shared by other i.v. anaesthetic agents and consequently the pharmacology of these drugs is described more briefly.

Thiopentone sodium

Chemical structure

Sodium 5-ethyl-5-(1-methylbutyl)-2-thiobarbiturate.

Physical properties and presentation

Thiopentone sodium, the sulphur analogue of pentobarbitone, is a yellowish powder with a bitter taste and a faint smell of garlic. It is stored in nitrogen to prevent chemical reaction with atmospheric carbon dioxide, and mixed with 6% anhydrous sodium carbonate to increase its solubility in water. It is available in single-dose ampoules of 500 mg or multidose bottles which contain 2.5 g, and is dissolved in distilled water to produce a 2.5% (25 mg/ml) solution with a pH of 10.8; this solution is slightly hypotonic. Freshly prepared solution may be kept for 24 h. The oil/water partition coefficient of thiopentone is 4.7, and the pK_a 7.6.

Pharmacology

Central nervous system. Thiopentone produces anaesthesia usually in less than 30 s after i.v. injection, although there may be some delay in patients with a low cardiac output. There is progressive depression of the CNS, including

Table 10.4 Relation of chemical grouping to clinical action of barbiturates

Group	Substituents Position (1)	Position (2)	Group characteristics when given i.v.
Oxybarbiturates	H	O	Delay in onset of action depending on 5 and 5′ side chain. Useful as basal hypnotics. Prolonged action
Methyl barbiturates	CH_3	O	Usually rapidly acting with fairly rapid recovery. High incidence of excitatory phenomena
Thiobarbiturates	H	S	Rapidly acting, usually smooth onset of sleep and fairly prompt recovery
Methyl thiobarbiturates	CH_3	S	Rapid onset of action and very rapid recovery but with so high an incidence of excitatory phenomena as to preclude use in clinical practice

spinal cord reflexes. The hypnotic action of thiopentone is potent, but its analgesic effect is poor, and surgical anaesthesia is difficult to achieve unless large doses are used; these are associated with cardiorespiratory depression. Cerebral metabolic rate is reduced, and there are secondary decreases in cerebral blood flow, cerebral blood volume and intracranial pressure. Recovery of consciousness occurs at a higher blood concentration if a large dose is given, or if the drug is injected rapidly; this has been attributed to 'acute tolerance', but may represent only altered redistribution. Consciousness is regained usually in 5–10 min. At subanaesthetic blood concentrations (i.e. at low doses, or during recovery), thiopentone has an antanalgesic effect, and reduces the pain threshold; this may result in restlessness in the postoperative period. Thiopentone is a very potent anticonvulsant.

Sympathetic nervous system activity is depressed to a greater extent than parasympathetic; this may result occasionally in bradycardia. However, it is more usual for tachycardia to develop after induction of anaesthesia partly because of baroreceptor inhibition caused by modest hypotension and partly because of loss of vagal tone which may predominate normally in young healthy adults.

Cardiovascular system. Myocardial contractility is depressed and peripheral vasodilatation occurs, particularly when large doses are administered or if injection is rapid. Arterial pressure decreases, and profound hypotension may occur in the patient with hypovolaemia or cardiac disease. Heart rate may decrease, but there is often a reflex tachycardia (vide supra).

Respiratory system. Ventilatory drive is decreased by thiopentone as a result of reduced sensitivity of the respiratory centre to carbon dioxide. A short period of apnoea is common, preceded frequently by a few deep breaths. Respiratory depression is influenced by premedication, and is more pronounced if opioids have been administered; assisted or controlled ventilation may be required. When spontaneous ventilation is resumed, ventilatory rate and tidal volume are usually lower than normal, but they increase in response to surgical stimulation. There is an increase in bronchial muscle tone, although frank bronchospasm is uncommon.

Laryngeal spasm may be precipitated by surgical stimulation or the presence of secretions, blood or foreign bodies (e.g. an oropharyngeal airway) in the region of the pharynx or larynx. Thiopentone is less satisfactory in this respect than most other anaesthetic agents, and appears to depress the parasympathetic laryngeal reflex arc to a lesser extent than other areas of the CNS.

Skeletal muscle. Skeletal muscle tone is reduced at high blood concentrations, partly as a result of suppression of spinal cord reflexes. There is no significant direct effect on the neuromuscular junction. When thiopentone is used as the sole anaesthetic agent, there is poor muscle relaxation and movement in response to surgical stimulation is common.

Uterus and placenta. There is little effect on resting uterine tone, but uterine contractions are suppressed at high doses. Thiopentone crosses the placenta readily, although fetal blood concentrations do not reach the same levels as those observed in the mother.

Eye. Intraocular pressure is reduced by approximately 40%. The pupil dilates first, and then constricts; the light reflex remains present until surgical anaesthesia has been attained. The corneal, conjunctival, eyelash and eyelid reflexes are abolished.

Hepatorenal function. The functions of the liver and kidneys are impaired transiently after administration of thiopentone. Hepatic microsomal enzymes are induced and this may increase the metabolism and elimination of other drugs.

Pharmacokinetics

Blood concentrations of thiopentone increase rapidly after i.v. administration. Between 75 and 85% of the drug is bound to protein, mostly albumin; thus, more free drug is available if plasma protein concentrations are reduced by malnutrition or disease. Protein binding is affected by pH, and is decreased by alkalaemia; thus concentration of free drug is increased during hyperventilation. Some drugs, e.g. phenylbutazone, occupy the same binding sites, and protein binding of thiopentone may be reduced in their presence.

Thiopentone diffuses readily into the CNS because of its lipid solubility and predominantly un-ionised state (61%) at body pH. Consciousness returns when brain concentration decreases to a threshold value, dependent on the individual patient, the dose of drug and its rate of administration, but at this time nearly all of the injected dose is still present in the body.

Metabolism of thiopentone occurs predominantly in the liver, and the metabolites are excreted by the kidneys; a small proportion is excreted unchanged in the urine. The terminal elimination half-life is approximately 11.5 h. Metabolism is a zero-order process; 10–15% of the remaining drug is metabolised each hour. Thus, up to 30% of the original dose may remain in the body at 24 h. Consequently, a 'hangover' effect is common; in addition, further doses of thiopentone administered within 1–2 days may result in cumulation. Elimination is impaired in the elderly. In obese patients, dosage should be based on an estimate of lean body mass, as distribution to fat is slow. However, elimination may be delayed in obese patients because of increased retention of the drug by adipose tissue.

Dosage and administration

Thiopentone is administered i.v. as a 2.5% solution; although some anaesthetists use a 5% solution, this increases the likelihood of serious complications and is *not* recommended. A small volume, e.g. 2 ml in adults, should be administered initially; the patient should be asked if any pain is experienced in case of inadvertent intra-arterial injection (see below) before the remainder of the induction dose is given.

The dose required to produce anaesthesia varies, and the response of each patient must be assessed carefully; cardiovascular depression is exaggerated if excessive doses are given. In healthy adults, an initial dose of 4 mg/kg should be administered over 15–20 s; if loss of the eyelash reflex does not occur within 30 s, supplementary doses of 50–100 mg should be given. In young children, a dose of 6 mg/kg is usually necessary. Elderly patients require smaller doses (2.5–3 mg/kg) than young adults.

Induction is usually smooth, and may be preceded by a taste of garlic. Side effects are related to peak blood concentrations, and in patients in whom cardiovascular depression may occur the drug should be administered more slowly; in very frail patients, as little as 50 mg may be sufficient to induce sleep.

No other drug should be mixed with thiopentone. Muscle relaxants should *not* be given until it is certain that anaesthesia has been induced. The i.v. cannula should be flushed with saline before vecuronium or atracurium is administered, to obviate precipitation.

Supplementary doses of 25–100 mg may be given to augment nitrous oxide/oxygen anaesthesia during short surgical procedures. However, recovery may be prolonged considerably if large total doses are used (>10 mg/kg).

Thiopentone in a 5 or 10% solution may be administered rectally to induce basal narcosis in children. A dose of 44 mg/kg induces sleep in 10–15 min. This technique may be used to sedate uncooperative children before anaesthesia. However, there may be loss of airway control, and the child must be supervised by skilled staff.

Adverse effects

1. *Hypotension*. The risk is increased if excessive doses are used, or if thiopentone is administered to hypovolaemic, shocked, or previously hypertensive patients. Hypotension is minimised by administering the drug slowly. Thiopentone should not be administered to patients in the sitting position.

2. *Respiratory depression*. The risk is increased if excessive doses are used, or if opioid drugs have been administered. Facilities must be available to provide artificial ventilation.

3. *Tissue necrosis*. Local necrosis may follow perivenous injection. Median nerve damage may occur after extravasation in the antecubital fossa, and this site is not recommended. If perivenous injection occurs, the needle should be left in place, and hyaluronidase injected. Tissue damage is worse if the 5% solution is used.

4. *Intra-arterial injection*. This is usually the result of inadvertent injection into the brachial

artery or an aberrant ulnar artery in the antecubital fossa (see Ch. 1). The patient complains usually of intense, burning pain, and this is an indication to stop injecting the drug immediately. The foream and hand may become blanched, and blisters may appear distally. Intra-arterial thiopentone causes profound constriction of the artery accompanied by local release of noradrenaline. In addition, crystals of thiopentone form in arterioles. In combination with thrombosis caused by endarteritis, ATP release from damaged red cells and aggregation of platelets, these result in emboli and may cause ischaemia or gangrene in parts of the forearm, hand or fingers.

The needle should be left in the artery and a vasodilator (e.g. papaverine 20 mg) administered. Stellate ganglion or brachial plexus block may reduce arterial spasm. Heparin should be given i.v. and oral anticoagulants should be prescribed after operation.

The risk of ischaemic damage after intra-arterial injection is much greater if a 5% solution of thiopentone is used.

5. *Laryngeal spasm.* The causes have been discussed above.

6. *Bronchospasm.* This is unusual, but may be precipitated in asthmatic patients.

7. *Allergic reactions.* These range from cutaneous rashes to severe or fatal anaphylactic or anaphylactoid reactions with cardiovascular collapse. Severe reactions are rare (approximately 1 in 14–20 000). Hypersensitivity reactions to drugs administered during anaesthesia are discussed on pages 190 and 418.

8. *Thrombophlebitis.* This is relatively uncommon (Table 10.5) unless the 5% solution is used.

Table 10.5 Percentage incidences of pain on injection and thrombophlebitis after i.v. administration of anaesthetic drugs into a large vein in the antecubital fossa or a small vein in the dorsum of the hand or wrist

	Pain		Thrombophlebitis	
Agent	Large	Small	Large	Small
Saline 0.9%	0	0	0	0
Thiopentone 2.5%	0	12	1	0
Methohexitone 1%	8	21	0	0
Propofol	10	40	0	0
Etomidate	8	80	15	20

Indications

1. Induction of anaesthesia.
2. Maintenance of anaesthesia. Thiopentone is suitable only for short procedures because cumulation occurs with repeated doses.
3. Basal narcosis by rectal administration.
4. Treatment of status epilepticus.
5. Reduction of intracranial pressure (see Ch. 38).

Absolute contraindications

1. *Airway obstruction.* Intravenous anaesthesia should not be employed if there is anticipated difficulty in maintaining an adequate airway, e.g. epiglottitis, oral or pharyngeal tumours.
2. *Porphyria.* Barbiturates may precipitate lower motor neurone paralysis or severe cardiovascular collapse in patients with porphyria.
3. *Previous hypersensitivity reaction.*

Precautions

Special care is needed when thiopentone is administered in the following circumstances.

1. *Cardiovascular disease.* Patients with hypovolaemia, myocardial disease, cardiac valvular stenosis or constrictive pericarditis are particularly sensitive to the hypotensive effects of thiopentone. However, if the drug is administered with extreme caution, it is probably no more hazardous than other i.v. anaesthetic agents. Myocardial depression may be severe in patients with a right-to-left intracardiac shunt because of high coronary artery concentrations of thiopentone.
2. *Severe hepatic disease.* Reduced protein binding results in higher concentrations of free drug. Metabolism may be impaired, but this has little effect on early recovery. A normal dose may be administered, but very slowly.
3. *Renal disease.* In chronic renal failure, protein binding is reduced, but elimination is unaltered. A normal dose may be administered, but very slowly.
4. *Muscle disease.* Respiratory depression is exaggerated in patients with myasthenia gravis or dystrophia myotonica.

5. *Reduced metabolic rate.* Patients with myxoedema are exquisitely sensitive to the effects of thiopentone.

6. *Obstetrics.* An adequate dose must be given to ensure that the mother is anaesthetised. However, excessive doses may result in respiratory or cardiovascular depression in the fetus, particularly if the interval between induction and delivery is short.

7. *Outpatient anaesthesia.* Early recovery is slow in comparison with other agents. This is seldom important unless rapid return of airway reflexes is essential, e.g. after oral or dental surgery. However, slow elimination of thiopentone may result in persistent drowsiness for 24–36 h, and this impairs the ability to drive or use machinery. There is also potentiation of the effect of alcohol or sedative drugs ingested during that period. It is preferable to use a drug with more rapid elimination for patients who are ambulant within a few hours.

8. *Adrenocortical insufficiency.*

9. *Extremes of age.*

10. *Asthma.*

Methohexitone sodium

Chemical structure

Sodium α-*dl*-5-allyl-l-methyl-5-(1-methyl-2-pentynyl) barbiturate.

Physical properties and presentation

Methohexitone has two asymmetrical carbon atoms, and therefore four isomers. The α-*dl* isomers are clinically useful. The drug is presented as a white powder mixed with 6% anhydrous sodium carbonate, and is readily soluble in distilled water. The resulting 1% (10 mg/ml) solution has a pH of 11.1 and pK_a of 7.9. Single-dose vials of 100 mg and multidose bottles containing 500 mg or 2.5 g are available. Although the solution is chemically stable for up to 6 weeks, the manufacturers recommend that it should not be stored for longer than 24 h because it contains no antibacterial preservative.

Pharmacology

Central nervous system. Unconsciousness is induced usually in 15–30 s. Recovery is more rapid with methohexitone than thiopentone, and occurs after 2–3 min; it is caused predominantly by redistribution. Drowsiness may persist for several hours until blood concentrations are decreased further by metabolism. Epileptiform activity has been demonstrated by EEG in epileptic patients. However, in sufficient doses, methohexitone acts as an anticonvulsant.

Cardiovascular system. In general, there is less hypotension in otherwise healthy patients than occurs after thiopentone; the decrease in arterial pressure is mediated predominantly by vasodilatation. Heart rate may increase slightly because of a decrease in baroreceptor activity. The cardiovascular effects are more pronounced in patients with cardiac disease or hypovolaemia.

Respiratory system. Moderate hypoventilation occurs. There may be a short period of apnoea after i.v. injection.

Pharmacokinetics

A greater proportion of methohexitone than thiopentone is in the non-ionised state at body pH (approximately 75%), although the drug is less lipid-soluble than the thiobarbiturate. Binding to plasma protein occurs to a similar degree. Clearance from plasma is higher than that of thiopentone, and the elimination half-life is considerably shorter (approximately 4 h). Thus, cumulation is less likely to occur after repeated doses.

Dosage and administration

Methohexitone is administered i.v. in a dose of 1–1.5 mg/kg to induce anaesthesia in healthy young adult patients; smaller doses are required in the elderly and infirm.

Methohexitone has been used by the i.m. route in a dose of 6.6 mg/kg, or rectally (20–25 mg/kg), to provide heavy preoperative sedation in children. Administration by these routes may result in unconsciousness and loss of airway reflexes, and patients must be supervised closely by trained staff.

Adverse effects

1. *Cardiovascular and respiratory depression*. This is probably less than that associated with thiopentone.
2. *Excitatory phenomena* during induction, including dyskinetic muscle movements, coughing and hiccups. Muscle movements are reduced by administration of an opioid; the incidence of cough and hiccups is reduced by premedication with an anticholinergic agent. The incidence of excitatory effects is dose-related.
3. *Epileptiform activity* on EEG in epileptic subjects.
4. *Pain on injection* (Table 10.5).
5. *Tissue damage* after perivenous injection is rare with 1% solution.
6. *Intra-arterial injection* can cause gangrene, but the risk with 1% solution is considerably less than with 2.5% thiopentone.
7. *Allergic reactions* occur, but are uncommon.
8. *Thrombophlebitis* is a rare complication.

Indications

Induction of anaesthesia, particularly when a rapid recovery is desirable. Methohexitone is used commonly as the anaesthetic agent for electroconvulsive therapy (ECT), and for induction of anaesthesia for outpatient dental and other minor procedures.

Absolute contraindications

These are the same as for thiopentone.

Precautions

These are similar to the precautions listed for thiopentone. However, methohexitone is a suitable agent for outpatients. It should not be used to induce anaesthesia in patients who are known to be epileptic.

Thiamylal sodium

This is the sulphur analogue of quinalbarbitone. It is slightly more potent than thiopentone, but otherwise almost identical in its properties. It is not available in the United Kingdom, but is used in some other countries.

NON-BARBITURATE I.V. ANAESTHETIC AGENTS

Propofol

This phenol derivative was identified as a potentially useful intravenous anaesthetic agent in 1980, and became available commercially in 1986. Currently, an induction dose of propofol is approximately 5 times more expensive than thiopentone.

Chemical structure

2,6-Di-isopropylphenol.

Physical properties and presentation

Propofol is extremely lipid-soluble, but almost insoluble in water. The drug was formulated initially in Cremophor EL. However, a number of other drugs formulated in this solubilising agent were associated with release of histamine, and an unacceptably high incidence of anaphylactoid reactions. Consequently, propofol was reformulated in a white, aqueous emulsion containing soyabean oil and purified egg phosphatide. Ampoules of the drug contain 200 mg of propofol in 20 ml (10 mg/ml).

Pharmacology

Central nervous system. Anaesthesia is induced within 10–30 s after i.v. administration in otherwise healthy young adults. There is a delay in disappearance of the eyelash reflex, used normally as a sign of unconsciousness after administration of barbiturate anaesthetic agents. Overdosage of propofol may result if this clinical sign is used; loss of verbal contact is a better end-point. EEG frequency decreases, and amplitude increases. Propofol reduces the duration of seizures induced by ECT in man. In 1989, the CSM drew attention to reports of convulsions following the use of propofol and recommended that caution should be exercised in administration of propofol to epileptic patients. Normally cerebral metabolic rate, cerebral blood flow and intracranial pressure are reduced.

Recovery of consciousness is rapid, and there is a minimal 'hangover' effect even in the immediate postanaesthetic period.

Cardiovascular system. In healthy patients, arterial pressure decreases to a greater degree after induction of anaesthesia with propofol than with thiopentone; the reduction results mostly from vasodilatation, although cardiac output decreases slightly. In some patients, large decreases (>40%) occur. The degree of hypotension is reduced by decreasing the rate of administration of the drug. The pressor response to tracheal intubation is attenuated to a greater degree by propofol than thiopentone. Heart rate increases slightly after induction of anaesthesia with propofol.

Respiratory system. After induction, apnoea occurs more commonly, and for a longer duration, than after thiopentone. During infusion of propofol, tidal volume is lower, and respiratory rate higher, than in the conscious state. There is decreased ventilatory response to carbon dioxide. As with other agents, ventilatory depression is more marked if opioids are administered.

Propofol has no effect on bronchial muscle tone and laryngospasm is particularly uncommon.

Skeletal muscle. Tone is reduced, but movements may occur in response to surgical stimulation.

Gastrointestinal system. Propofol has no effect on gastrointestinal motility in animals.

Uterus and placenta. Little is known of the effects of propofol on uterine tone or of its placental transfer.

Hepatorenal. There is a transient decrease in renal function, but the impairment is less than that associated with thiopentone. Hepatic blood flow is decreased by the reductions in arterial pressure and cardiac output. Liver function tests are not deranged after infusion of propofol for 24 h.

Endocrine. Plasma concentrations of cortisol are decreased after administration of propofol, but a normal response occurs to administration of Synacthen.

Pharmacokinetics

In common with other i.v. anaesthetic drugs, propofol is distributed rapidly, and blood concentrations decline exponentially. Clearance of the drug from plasma is greater than would be expected if the drug was metabolised only in the liver, and it is suspected that extrahepatic sites of metabolism exist. The kidneys excrete the metabolites of propofol (mainly glucuronides); only 0.3% of the administered dose of propofol is excreted unchanged. The elimination half-life of propofol is 3–4.8 h. The distribution and clearance of propofol are altered by the concomitant administration of fentanyl. Elimination of propofol remains relatively constant even after infusions lasting several days.

Dosage and administration

In healthy, unpremedicated adults, a dose of 2–2.5 mg/kg is required to induce anaesthesia. The dose should be reduced in the elderly; an initial dose of 1.25 mg/kg is appropriate, with subsequent additional doses of 10 mg until consciousness is lost. In children, a dose of 3–3.5 mg/kg is usually required. Cardiovascular side effects are reduced if the drug is injected slowly. Lower doses are required for induction in premedicated patients. Sedation during regional analgesia or endoscopy can be achieved with doses of 50–150 μg kg^{-1} h^{-1}. Doses of up to 250 μg kg^{-1} h^{-1} are required to supplement nitrous oxide/oxygen for surgical anaesthesia, although these may be reduced substantially if an opioid drug is administered. The average infusion rate is approximately 50 μg kg^{-1} h^{-1} in conjunction with a slow infusion of morphine (2 mg/h) for patients in ITU.

Adverse effects

1. *Cardiovascular depression.* This is greater than that associated with barbiturates, and is

likely to cause profound hypotension in hypovolaemic or previously hypertensive patients and in those with cardiac disease.

2. *Respiratory depression.* Apnoea is more common and of longer duration than after barbiturate administration.

3. *Excitatory phenomena.* These are more frequent than with thiopentone, but less than with methohexitone.

4. *Pain on injection.* This occurs in up to 40% of patients (Table 10.5). The incidence is reduced if a large vein is used, or a small dose (10 mg) of lignocaine is injected shortly before propofol.

5. *Allergic reactions.* Skin rashes occur occasionally. A small number of more severe reactions have been reported.

Indications

1. *Induction of anaesthesia.* Propofol is indicated particularly when rapid early recovery of consciousness is required. Two hours after anaesthesia, there is no difference in psychomotor function between patients who have received propofol and those given thiopentone or methohexitone, but the former complain of less drowsiness in the ensuing 12 h. The rapid recovery characteristics are lost if induction is followed by maintenance with inhalational agents for longer than 10–15 min. Theoretically the nature of recovery from propofol may increase the risks of awareness during tracheal intubation after the administration of non-depolarising muscle relaxants.

2. *Sedation during surgery.* Propofol has been used successfully for sedation during regional analgesic techniques, and during endoscopy. Control of the airway may be lost at any time, and patients must be supervised continuously by an anaesthetist.

3. *Total i.v. anaesthesia* (vide infra). Propofol appears to be the most suitable of the agents currently available. Recovery time is increased after infusion of propofol compared with that after a single bolus dose, but cumulation is significantly less than with the barbiturates.

4. *Sedation in ITU.* Propofol has been used successfully to sedate patients for several days in ITU. The level of sedation is controlled easily, and recovery is rapid (usually <30 min). However, data from controlled trials are limited.

Absolute contraindications

Airway obstruction and known hypersensitivity to the drug are probably the only contraindications. It is thought that propofol is safe in porphyric patients.

Precautions

These are similar to those listed for thiopentone. The side effects of propofol make it less suitable than thiopentone or methohexitone for patients with existing cardiovascular compromise. Propofol may be more suitable than thiopentone for outpatient anaesthesia, but its use does not obviate the need for an adequate period of recovery before discharge.

Etomidate

This carboxylated imidazole compound was introduced in 1972.

Chemical structure

D-Ethyl-1-(α-methylbenzyl)-imidazole-5-carboxylate.

Physical characteristics and presentation

Etomidate is soluble but unstable in water. It is presented as a clear aqueous solution containing 35% propylene glycol. Ampoules contain 20 mg of etomidate in 10 ml (2 mg/ml). The pH of the solution is 8.1.

Pharmacology

Etomidate is a rapidly acting general anaesthetic agent with a short duration of action (2–3 min) resulting predominantly from redistribution, although it is eliminated rapidly from the body. In healthy patients, it produces less cardiovascular depression than thiopentone; however, there is little evidence that this occurs if the cardiovascular system is compromised. Large doses may produce tachycardia. Respiratory depression is less than that with other agents.

Etomidate depresses the synthesis of cortisol by the adrenal gland, and impairs the response to ACTH. Long-term infusions of the drug in ITU have resulted in increased infection and mortality, related probably to reduced immunological competence. Its effects on the adrenal gland occur also after a single bolus dose, and last for several hours.

Pharmacokinetics

Etomidate redistributes rapidly in the body. Approximately 76% is bound to protein. It is metabolised in the plasma and liver, mainly by esterase hydrolysis, and the metabolites are excreted in the urine; 2% is excreted unchanged. The terminal elimination half-life is approximately 75 min. There is little cumulation when repeated doses are given. The distribution and clearance of etomidate may be altered by the concomitant administration of fentanyl.

Dosage and administration

An average dose of 0.3 mg/kg i.v. induces anaesthesia. The drug should be administered into a large vein to reduce the incidence of pain on injection.

Adverse effects

1. *Suppression of synthesis of cortisol.* See above.
2. *Excitatory phenomena.* Moderate or severe involuntary movements occur in up to 40% of patients during induction of anaesthesia. This incidence is reduced in patients premedicated with an opioid. Cough and hiccups occur in up to 10% of patients.
3. *Pain on injection.* This occurs in up to 80% of patients if a small vein is used, but in less than 10% when the drug is injected into a large vein in the antecubital fossa (Table 10.5). The incidence is reduced by prior injection of lignocaine 10 mg.
4. *Nausea and vomiting.* The incidence of nausea and vomiting is approximately 30%. This is very much higher than after barbiturates or propofol.
5. *Emergence phenomena.* The incidence of severe restlessness and delirium during recovery is greater with etomidate than barbiturates or propofol.
6. *Venous thrombosis* is more common than with other agents.

Indications

There are very few positive indications for etomidate. It is suitable for outpatient anaesthesia, but has been superseded by propofol.

Absolute contraindications

1. Airway obstruction.
2. Porphyria.
3. Adrenal insufficiency.
4. Long-term infusion.

Precautions

These are similar to the precautions listed for thiopentone. Etomidate is suitable for outpatient anaesthesia. However, the incidence of excitatory phenomena is unacceptably high unless an opioid is administered; this delays recovery and is unsuitable for most outpatients.

Ketamine hydrochloride

This is a phencyclidine derivative and was introduced in 1965. It differs from other i.v. anaesthetic agents in many respects, and produces 'dissociative anaesthesia' rather than generalised depression of the CNS.

Chemical structure

2-(*o*-Chlorophenyl)-2-(methylamino)-cyclohexanone hydrochloride.

Physical characteristics and presentation

Ketamine is soluble in water and is presented as solutions of 10 mg/ml containing sodium chloride to produce isotonicity, and 50 or 100 mg/ml in multidose vials which contain 0.1 mg/ml benzethonium chloride as preservative. The pH of the solutions is 3.5–5.5. The pK_a of ketamine is 7.5.

Pharmacology

Central nervous system. Ketamine is extremely lipid-soluble. After i.v. injection, it induces anaesthesia in 30–60 s. A single i.v. dose produces unconsciousness for 10–15 min. Ketamine is also effective within 3–4 min after i.m. injection, and has a duration of action of 15–25 min. It is a potent somatic analgesic at subanaesthetic blood concentrations. Amnesia often persists for up to 1 h after recovery of consciousness. Induction of anaesthesia is smooth, but emergence delirium may occur, with restlessness, disorientation and agitation. Vivid and often unpleasant nightmares or hallucinations may occur during recovery and for up to 24 h. The incidences of emergence delirium and hallucinations are reduced by avoidance of verbal and tactile stimulation during the recovery period, or by concomitant administration of opioids, butyrophenones, benzodiazepines or physostigmine; however, unpleasant dreams may persist. Nightmares are reported less commonly by children and elderly patients.

The EEG changes associated with ketamine are unlike those seen with other i.v. anaesthetics, and consist of loss of alpha rhythm and predominant theta activity. Cerebral metabolic rate is increased in several regions of the brain, and cerebral blood flow, cerebral blood volume and intracranial pressure increase.

Cardiovascular system. Arterial pressure increases by up to 25%, and heart rate by approximately 20%. Cardiac output may rise, and myocardial oxygen consumption increases; the positive inotropic effect may be related to increased calcium influx modulated by cyclic AMP. There is increased myocardial sensitivity to adrenaline. Sympathetic stimulation of the peripheral circulation is decreased, resulting in vasodilatation in tissues innervated predominantly by α-adrenergic receptors, and vasoconstriction in those with β-receptors.

Respiratory system. Transient apnoea may occur after i.v. injection, but ventilation is well maintained thereafter, and may increase slightly, unless high doses are given. Pharyngeal and laryngeal reflexes and a patent airway are maintained well in comparison with other i.v. agents; however, their presence cannot be guaranteed, and normal precautions must be taken to protect the airway and prevent aspiration. Bronchial muscle is dilated.

Skeletal muscle. Muscle tone is usually increased. Spontaneous movements may occur, but reflex movement in response to surgery is uncommon.

Gastrointestinal system. Salivation is increased.

Uterus and placenta. Ketamine crosses the placenta readily. Fetal concentrations are approximately equal to those in the mother.

The eye. Intraocular pressure increases, although this effect is often transient. Eye movements often persist during surgical anaesthesia.

Pharmacokinetics

Only approximately 12% of ketamine is bound to protein. The initial peak concentration after i.v. injection decreases as the drug is distributed, but this occurs more slowly than with other i.v. anaesthetic agents. Metabolism occurs predominantly in the liver by demethylation and hydroxylation of the cyclohexanone ring; among the metabolites is norketamine, which is pharmacologically active. Approximately 80% of the injected dose is excreted renally as glucuronides; only 2.5% is excreted unchanged. The elimination half-life is approximately 2.5 h. Distribution and elimination are slower if halothane, benzodiazepines or barbiturates are administered concurrently.

After i.m. injection, peak concentrations are achieved after approximately 20 min.

Dosage and administration

Induction of anaesthesia is achieved with an average dose of 2 mg/kg i.v.; larger doses may be required in some patients, and smaller doses in the elderly or shocked patient. In all cases, the drug should be administered slowly. Additional doses of 1–1.5 mg/kg are required every 5–10 min. Between 8 and 10 mg/kg is used i.m. A dose of 0.25–0.5 mg/kg, or an infusion of 50 μg kg^{-1} min^{-1}, may be used to produce analgesia without loss of consciousness.

Adverse effects

1. *Emergence delirium, nightmares and hallucinations.*

2. *Hypertension and tachycardia.* This may be harmful in previously hypertensive patients and in those with ischaemic heart disease.

3. *Prolonged recovery.*

4. *Salivation.* Anticholinergic premedication is essential.

5. *Increased intracranial pressure.*

6. *Allergic reactions.* Skin rashes have been reported.

Indications

1. *The high-risk patient.* Ketamine is useful in the shocked patient. Arterial pressure may decrease if hypovolaemia is present, and the drug must be given cautiously. These patients are usually sedated heavily in the postoperative period, and the risk of nightmares is therefore minimised.

2. *Paediatric anaesthesia.* Children undergoing minor surgery, investigations (e.g. cardiac catheterisation), ophthalmic examinations or radiotherapy may be managed successfully with ketamine administered either i.m. or i.v.

3. *Difficult locations.* Ketamine has been used successfully at the site of accidents, and for analgesia and anaesthesia in casualties of war.

4. *Analgesia and sedation.* The analgesic action of ketamine may be employed when wound dressings are changed, or while positioning patients with pain before performing regional anaesthesia (e.g. fractured neck of femur). Ketamine has been used to sedate asthmatic patients in ITU.

5. *Developing countries.* Ketamine is used extensively in countries where anaesthetic equipment and trained staff are in short supply.

Absolute contraindications

1. *Airway obstruction.* Although the airway is maintained better with ketamine than other agents, its patency cannot be guaranteed. Inhalational agents should be used for induction of anaesthesia if airway obstruction is anticipated.

2. *Raised intracranial pressure.*

Precautions

1. *Cardiovascular disease.* Ketamine is unsuitable for patients with pre-existing hypertension, ischaemic heart disease or severe cardiac decompensation.

2. *Repeated administration.* Because of the prolonged recovery period, ketamine is not the most suitable drug for frequent procedures, e.g. prolonged courses of radiotherapy, as it disrupts sleep and eating patterns.

3. *Visceral stimulation.* Ketamine suppresses poorly the response to visceral stimulation; supplementation, e.g. with an opioid, is indicated if visceral stimulation is anticipated.

4. *Outpatient anaesthesia.* The prolonged recovery period and emergence phenomena make ketamine unsuitable for adult outpatients.

Other drugs

Benzodiazepines and opioids may also be used to induce general anaesthesia. However, very large doses are required, and recovery is prolonged. Their use is confined to specialist areas, e.g. cardiac anaesthesia. The pharmacology of these drugs is described in Chapter 11.

TOTAL I.V. ANAESTHESIA

This technique is popular with a small number of anaesthetists. It is used in situations where it is desirable to avoid nitrous oxide (see Ch. 9). However, it is employed also to supplement nitrous oxide in place of a volatile anaesthetic agent.

Drugs used for total i.v. anaesthesia (TIVA) must be metabolised and eliminated rapidly in order to prevent accumulation of the drug or active metabolites. At present, only propofol is appropriate for TIVA; the barbiturates are eliminated slowly and etomidate is associated with depression of cortisol synthesis. The quality of anaesthesia is not ideal, and opioid and muscle relaxant drugs are often administered concurrently.

The major problem associated with TIVA is prediction of the correct dose of drug. In general, a bolus dose or high infusion rate must be administered initially to achieve an adequate blood concentration, and then a slower maintenance infusion rate must be selected. The concentration of drug required to produce anaesthesia varies among patients, as is the case with inhalational agents. However, the distribution and elimination of i.v. drugs are much more variable and unpredictable than those of inhalational anaesthetics. The concept of a minimum infusion rate (MIR) which produces loss of motor response to surgical stimulation in 50% of patients (i.e. the ED_{50}) has been developed, and is equivalent to MAC for inhalational anaesthetic drugs. However, the variability among patients of distribution and elimination of i.v. agents results in a considerable number of patients requiring doses which may be associated with cardiovascular and respiratory depression if movement during surgery is to be prevented. There is also a risk in the paralysed patient that an insufficient dose of drug may be administered to ensure unconsciousness.

Indications for TIVA

1. *Short surgical procedures*. Intravenous agents may be administered as repeated boluses or by infusion.
2. *Cardiac surgery*.
3. *Neurosurgery*.
4. *Prolonged surgery*. Nitrous oxide depresses bone marrow function if administered for longer than 8 h.

Disadvantages

1. Variable and unpredictable dosage.
2. Expensive apparatus required.
3. High incidence of movement during surgery unless used to supplement nitrous oxide.
4. Risk of awareness in paralysed patients if inadequate doses administered.

DRUGS OF HISTORICAL INTEREST

Hexobarbitone

This methylated oxybarbiturate was introduced in 1932, and was the first i.v. anaesthetic agent to be used successfully. Its duration of action was intermediate between those of thiopentone and methohexitone, but there was a high incidence of excitatory phenomena during induction.

Propanidid

This agent was derived from eugenol (oil of cloves), and was used first in 1964. Its duration of action was exceedingly short, as it was metabolised very rapidly by plasma cholinesterase. There were high incidences of nausea, vomiting and muscle movements. It was solubilised in Cremophor EL (polyoxylated castor oil), and was associated with an unacceptable incidence of severe anaphylactoid reactions.

γ-Hydroxybutyric acid

Anaesthesia of slow onset and recovery was produced by this agent, which is related chemically to the neurotransmitter γ-aminobutyric acid. It was introduced in 1962. It is still used for basal sedation in some European countries.

Althesin

This drug, a mixture of two steroids (alphaxalone and alphadolone), was very similar to propofol in its anaesthetic profile, but was metabolised even more rapidly. It was introduced in 1972. In common with propanidid, it was solubilised in Cremophor EL, and an unacceptable number of adverse reactions was reported.

ADVERSE REACTIONS TO I.V. ANAESTHETIC AGENTS

These may take the form of pain on injection, venous thrombosis, involuntary muscle movement, hiccup, hypotension and postoperative delirium. All of these reactions may be modified by the anaesthetic technique.

Hypersensitivity reactions, which resemble the effects of histamine release, are more rare and less predictable. Other vasoactive agents may be released also. Reactions to i.v. anaesthetic agents are caused usually by one of the following mechanisms:

1. *Type I hypersensitivity response*. The drug interacts with specific IgE antibodies, which are often bound to the surface of mast cells; these become degranulated and release histamine and other vasoactive amines.

2. *Classical complement-mediated reaction.* The classical complement pathway may be activated by Type II (cell surface antigen) or Type III (immune complex formation) hypersensitivity reactions. IgG or IgM antibodies are involved.

3. *Alternate complement pathway activation.* Preformed antibodies to an antigen are not necessary for activation of this pathway; thus, these reactions may occur without prior exposure to the drug.

4. *Direct pharmacological effects of the drug.* These 'anaphylactoid' reactions result from a direct effect on mast cells and basophils. There may be local cutaneous signs only. In more severe reactions there are signs of systemic release of histamine.

Clinical features

In a severe hypersensitivity reaction, a flush may develop over the upper half of the body. There is usually hypotension, which may be profound. Cutaneous and glottic oedema may develop, and may result in hypovolaemia because of loss of fluid from the circulation. Bronchospasm occurs in less than 50% of instances. Rarely, abdominal pain and vomiting may occur.

Predisposing factors

1. *Age.* In general, adverse reactions are less common in children than in adults.

2. *Pregnancy.* There is an increased incidence of adverse reactions in pregnancy.

3. *Gender.* There is probably no difference between the incidence of reactions in men and that in non-pregnant women.

4. *Atopy.* There may be an increased incidence of Type IV (delayed hypersensitivity) reactions in non-atopic individuals, and a higher incidence of Type I reactions in those with a history of extrinsic asthma, hay fever or penicillin allergy.

5. *Previous exposure.* Previous exposure to the drug, or to a drug with similar constituents, exerts a much greater influence on the incidence of reactions than does a history of atopy.

6. *Solvents.* Cremophor EL, which was used as a solvent for a number of i.v. anaesthetic agents, was associated with a high incidence of hypersensitivity reactions.

Incidence

The incidences of hypersensitivity reactions associated with i.v. anaesthetic agents are shown in Table 10.6.

Table 10.6 Incidences of adverse reactions to i.v. anaesthetic agents

Drug	Incidence
Thiopentone	1:14 000–1:20 000
Methohexitone	1:1600–1:7000
Althesin	1:400–1:11 000
Propanidid	1:500–1:17 000
Etomidate	1:450 000
Propofol	1:100 000 (estimated)

Treatment

This is summarised in Table 10.7.

Table 10.7 Management of allergic reactions

Aims:
1. Correct arterial hypoxaemia
2. Restore intravascular fluid volume
3. Inhibit further release of chemical mediators

Routine:
- *Airway*
- *Added inspired oxygen*
- *Adrenaline* (either intravenous or intramuscular, depending on the severity of the reaction). 0.5 ml of 1:1000. If the main problem is cardiovascular collapse, metaraminol may be effective; less likely to cause ventricular arrhythmias
- *Fluids:* both crystalloids (normal saline or Hartmann's solution) and colloids. The former may be ineffective in some cases.
- *Bronchodilators* if there is bronchospasm (e.g. aminophylline, 250–500 mg i.v.). If adverse reaction occurs during anaesthesia, consider use of halothane, ether or ketamine for the relief of bronchoconstriction
- *Intermittent positive pressure ventilation:* if there is pulmonary oedema
- *Use of inotropes to support the circulation*, and *antiarrhythmic drugs*

No data to show a beneficial effect of steroids in acute allergic anaphylactic reactions
No agent affects the gastrointestinal symptoms
Isoprenaline may worsen arterial hypoxaemia, by increasing deadspace
Antihistamines may be useful in angioneurotic oedema

Consider cerebral resuscitation if prolonged period of arrest, hypotension or arterial hypoxaemia (e.g. mannitol, IPPV with mild hypocapnia)

FURTHER READING

Nimmo W S, Smith G (eds) 1989 Anaesthesia. Blackwell Scientific Publications, Oxford

Saidman L J 1974 Uptake, distribution and elimination of barbiturates. In: Eger E I (ed) Anesthetic uptake and action. Williams & Wilkins, Baltimore

Sear J W 1983 General kinetic and dynamic principles and their application to continuous infusion anaesthesia. Anaesthesia 38 (supplement), 10–25

Sear J W 1987 Adverse effects of drugs given by injection. In: Taylor T H, Major E (eds) Hazards and complications of anaesthesia. Churchill Livingstone, Edinburgh

Vickers M D, Schnieden H, Wood-Smith F G 1984 Drugs in anaesthetic practice, 6th edn. Butterworths, London

11. Drugs used to supplement anaesthesia

ANALGESICS

Opioids

The opioid analgesics are drugs which act on specific receptors in the CNS. Most of those in clinical use have analgesic properties. The opioids are sometimes termed 'narcotics', but this implies physical dependence, and this term should be avoided as it may not occur with some of the newer opioid analgesics. The term 'opiate' suggests that the drug is derived from opium; however, many compounds used in anaesthetic practice are synthetic or semisynthetic and therefore this term should usually be avoided.

Drugs such as morphine, which bind to opioid receptors and produce dose-dependent agonist effects, are termed opioid agonists. Naloxone binds to opioid receptors also, antagonising the effects of morphine, and is termed an opioid antagonist. The term opioid agonist–antagonist is applied to drugs such as nalbuphine which possess agonist effects at one receptor type and antagonist effects at another. As the dose–response relationships differ at each receptor type, biphasic clinical effects may be observed, e.g. antagonism of opioid-induced analgesia at low doses and analgesia at high doses. The partial opioid agonists, e.g. buprenorphine, produce morphine-like effects in low concentrations, but the agonist effect reaches a plateau and increased doses have no further effect. Table 11.1 contains a classification of some commonly used opioids.

Table 11.1 Classification of commonly used opioids

Opioid agonists
1. Natural opium alkaloids
Morphine
Codeine
2. Semisynthetic opium alkaloid
Diamorphine
3. Synthetic opioids
Pethidine
Fentanyl
Alfentanil
Sufentanil
Partial opioid agonists
Buprenorphine
Meptazinol
Opioid agonist/antagonists
Pentazocine
Nalbuphine
Opioid antagonist
Naloxone

Opioid receptors

Opioids act on specific receptors which are distributed throughout the CNS and are the site of action of a series of endogenous polypeptides (the endorphins and enkephalins); these possess analgesic properties similar to those of exogenous opioids. The enkephalins are found in high concentrations in central grey matter of the brain stem and areas of the spinal cord; β-endorphin is structurally a much larger molecule with a longer duration of action, and is present in high concentrations in the pituitary.

Experimental evidence suggests that there are a large number of opioid receptors. At least five have been identified: μ (mu), κ (kappa), σ (sigma), δ (delta) and ϵ (epsilon). Table 11.2 lists the effects produced by stimulation of the first three of these receptors. Recently, the μ receptors have been subdivided into μ_1 (mediating ventilatory depression) and μ_2. The σ receptor mediates stimulation of

Table 11.2 Effects of pharmacological stimulation of the three major types of opioid receptor

Effect	mu	kappa	sigma
Analgesia	Yes	Yes	No
Ventilation	Depression	Depression	Stimulation
Behaviour	Euphoria	Sedation	Dysphoria
Pupil	Miosis	Mydriasis	Mydriasis
Physical dependence	Yes	No	No

Table 11.3 Effects of some opioid drugs on the three major types of opioid receptor

Drug	mu	kappa	sigma
Morphine	Agonist	Agonist	No activity
Buprenorphine	Partial agonist	No activity	No activity
Meptazinol	Partial agonist	No activity	No activity
Nalorphine	Antagonist	Partial agonist	Agonist
Pentazocine	Antagonist	Partial agonist	Agonist
Nalbuphine	Antagonist	Partial agonist	Agonist
Naloxone	Antagonist	Antagonist	Antagonist

ventilation. The effects of some opioid drugs on the three main receptor types are shown in Table 11.3. In theory, drugs with partial agonist effects at the μ receptor, or those with mixed agonist and antagonist actions, might be able to produce analgesia equivalent to that of morphine but with less depression of ventilation. However, none of the agents developed to date have achieved this goal.

Pharmacokinetics and pharmacodynamics

Although the pattern of receptor occupancy determines the clinical effects of some opioids, the differences between the actions of the μ agonists result largely from pharmacokinetic and pharmacodynamic factors. The principles of drug distribution are described in Chapter 8. The initial distribution of opioids into CNS is related to the degree of ionisation of the drug in blood and to the lipid solubility of the un-ionised portion. Drugs which are poorly soluble in lipid, e.g. morphine, reach the receptors more slowly than lipid-soluble agents, e.g. fentanyl. Thus, a lipid-insoluble drug has a slow onset of action; CNS concentrations decay slowly as drug is eliminated from the body by metabolism and excretion. In contrast, a lipid-soluble opioid with a short distribution half-life acts rapidly, because the drug transfers readily into CNS along a high initial blood–brain concentration gradient. The duration of action is short because brain and blood concentrations decrease after redistribution of the drug to other vessel-rich tissues. However, if a large dose is given, the effect of the drug declines only when blood concentrations decrease as a result of elimination; the duration of action is related usually to the elimination half-life of the drug. Hepatic extraction of opioids is reduced during general anaesthesia, because of reduced hepatic blood flow and impaired hepatic clearance.

Another factor which influences clinical action is the presence of active metabolites. The most significant of these is morphine-6-glucuronide, which is a more potent μ agonist than morphine itself. Although the water-soluble metabolites of morphine are normally excreted fairly rapidly, they are known to accumulate in patients with renal insufficiency, and may result in a prolonged duration of action. Opioid metabolites are present in high concentrations after oral administration as a result of first-pass metabolism.

The following factors must be considered in order to minimise the risk of postoperative ventilatory depression when determining the appropriate dose of an opioid for intraoperative use:

1. *Age*. There is increased sensitivity to opioids in the elderly.
2. *Duration of surgery*. The anticipated duration of action of the opioid selected should match the duration of surgery.
3. *Other depressant drugs*. Anaesthetic and sedative agents which depress ventilation may have additive effects with opioids.
4. *Pulmonary disease*. The respiratory depressant actions of opioids may precipitate ventilatory failure; special care is required in patients with chronic obstructive airways disease. The antitussive action of opioids may impair postoperative clearance of pulmonary or bronchial secretions. Obese patients, or those with other conditions which restrict pulmonary expansion, e.g. severe kyphosis, may develop ventilatory insufficiency when given opioids.

5. *Endocrine abnormalities*. There is increased opioid sensitivity in hypothyroidism and Addison's disease.

6. *Hepatic disease*. There may be increased sensitivity to some opioids, particularly in cirrhosis and infective hepatitis, because of reduced drug metabolism.

7. *Intracranial pathology*. Administration of opioids interferes with assessment of conscious level, and may increase intracranial pressure because of hypercapnia.

8. *Miscellaneous*. There is increased sensitivity in patients who are debilitated and in those suffering from advanced malignancy or chronic infection.

Contrary to popular opinion, dose–response relationships for opioids are not related to body weight in adults.

Morphine

Although it is possible to synthesise morphine, it is produced commercially from the dried juices of seed capsules of the poppy *Papaver somniferum*. Morphine is a tertiary amine and a weak base. It is more water-soluble than most other opioids used in anaesthetic practice. Although morphine has a number of undesirable side effects, it is an excellent analgesic and represents the 'gold standard' against which all other opioids are judged. The drug is presented usually as morphine sulphate; 10 mg morphine sulphate contains approximately 8.5 mg anhydrous morphine.

Actions

The actions of morphine may be classified as central and peripheral (Table 11.4); it possesses both depressant and stimulant effects on the CNS.

Table 11.4 Summary of actions and side effects of morphine

Central
Depressant
Analgesia
Sedation
Depression of cough reflex
Depression of respiratory centre
Depression of metabolic rate (hypothermia)
Depression of vasomotor centre
Excitatory
Euphoria, hallucinations
Convulsions (in very high dosage)
Miosis (stimulation of oculomotor centre)
Vomiting, Nausea } (stimulation of chemoreceptor trigger zone)
Bradycardia (vagal stimulation)
Release of ADH and other pituitary hormones
Peripheral
Increase in smooth muscle tone
Histamine release
Bronchospasm
Hypotension
Erythema
Sensation of warmth, flushing

Analgesia

All types of pain are relieved. However, morphine is more effective against dull and continuous than sharp and intermittent pain. The pain threshold is elevated, and the psychological and emotional components of pain (see Ch. 25) diminished. These effects are augmented by a sensation of euphoria and drowsiness which, as the dose is increased, progresses to sleep and eventually to an anaesthetic state characterised by decreased reflex irritability and profound ventilatory depression.

Respiratory system

Depression of ventilation occurs as a result of direct depression of the medullary respiratory centre. The carbon dioxide response curve is shifted to the right and the slope is reduced (Fig. 11.1). Both ventilatory rate and tidal volume decrease within 2–5 min after i.v. injection, and more slowly after i.m. administration.

Depression of the cough reflex occurs after administration of morphine and its derivatives.

Cardiovascular system

There is little effect on arterial pressure in normal supine individuals. However, hypotension may occur in patients with a decreased blood volume or to whom drugs with vasodilator properties (e.g. phenothiazines) have been administered, as morphine may cause peripheral arteriolar and venous dilatation as a result of central depression

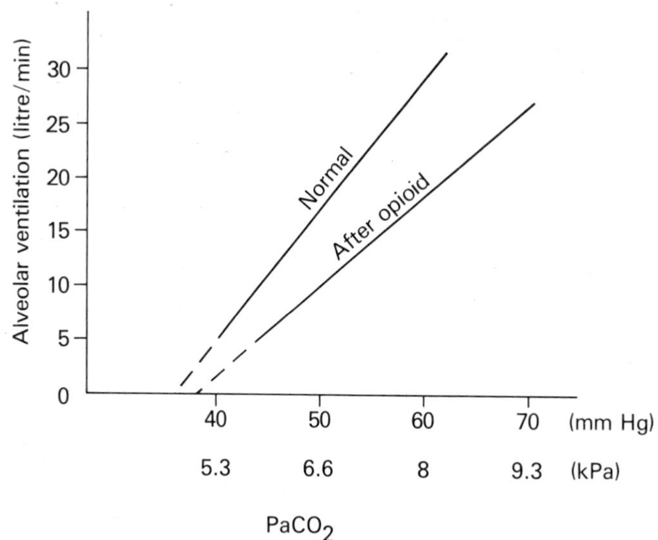

Fig. 11.1 The ventilatory response to arterial P_{CO_2} in the normal individual and after administration of morphine. Note that the response curve is not only shifted to the right but that its slope is decreased also.

of the vasomotor centre, reduction in vasoconstrictor tone and release of histamine.

Bradycardia occurs occasionally as a result of stimulation of the vagal centre.

Gastrointestinal system

Nausea and vomiting. These symptoms are distressing and unpleasant, and represent one of the most common complaints after operation. Morphine stimulates the chemoreceptor trigger zone in the floor of the fourth ventricle; it may cause nausea with or without vomiting some hours after administration, persisting for 6–8 h. This side effect appears to be related to a dopamine-like effect; drugs with dopamine-blocking actions, e.g. butyrophenones and phenothiazines, are effective antiemetics in opioid-induced vomiting. However, there is also a vestibular component to morphine-induced vomiting, and ambulant patients are more likely to suffer from this side effect. The emetic effects of morphine are similar to those of other opioids administered in equianalgesic doses.

Gastrointestinal motility. Morphine causes reduced peristalsis, but increased non-peristaltic contractility, in the gastrointestinal system. Gastric emptying is delayed, and this may contribute to vomiting. Absorption of orally administered drugs is impaired and constipation is common. Increased non-peristaltic bowel contractility may contribute to dehiscence of large bowel anastomoses. Smooth muscle contraction is increased in the sphincter of Oddi, the ureter and the bladder sphincter. Morphine should be avoided in biliary and renal colic. Occasionally, it may produce biliary pain if given as a premedicant to patients scheduled to undergo cholecystectomy.

Miosis

This results from stimulation of the Edinger–Westphal nucleus of the oculomotor centre. Pupillary constriction may interfere with assessment of depth of anaesthesia.

Other actions

Histamine release. This is responsible for the flush and sensation of warmth which follow i.v. injection, and for erythema at or near the site of injection. Bronchospasm occurs occasionally, and morphine should not be administered to asthmatic patients.

Endocrine effects. These include release of ADH from the anterior pituitary, and inhibition of release of ACTH, FSH and LH. These actions resemble those of endogenous opioids.

Metabolic. Large doses of morphine may contribute to hypothermia by decreasing muscle activity and basal metabolic rate, and by increasing heat loss through vasodilatation.

Distribution and elimination

After i.v. injection, 35% of morphine is bound to protein. The remainder is distributed with a half-life of 20–25 min (Table 11.5). Plasma concentrations depend subsequently on metabolism, redistribution back into the vascular compartment, excretion and possibly enterohepatic recirculation. Metabolism occurs predominantly in the liver; the drug is inactivated by dealkylation, oxidation and conjugation with glucuronide. The elimination half-life of morphine is 2–4 h. However, one of the two major metabolites, morphine-6-glucuronide, is active and is present in high concentrations. Consequently, the clinical effect of morphine may exceed that expected from the elimination half-life, particularly in patients who have impaired renal function and who are unable to excrete the water-soluble metabolites normally.

Morphine crosses the placental barrier and may depress neonatal ventilation profoundly.

Dosage and administration

After i.v. administration, analgesia reaches a peak after 15–20 min. Failure to appreciate this delay in onset of action may result in over-dosage if incremental doses are given frequently. The dose of morphine selected for intraoperative use depends on the type of premedication, anticipated duration of surgery and general health of the patient. In a healthy adult, a single bolus dose of 10–15 mg i.v., or administration of incremental doses of 2–5 mg at 20-min intervals, is appropriate.

In the postoperative period, morphine is administered usually by the i.m. route, in a dose of 5–20 mg; the peak effect occurs 60–90 min after administration, but there is great variation between individual patients. The duration of action after either i.v. or i.m. injection is 3–4 h. An i.v. infusion of morphine is used occasionally after operation. A dose of 1–2 mg/h is usually appropriate, but must be adjusted according to the individual patient's response. Intravenous infusions of opioid must be administered *only* in a high-dependency or intensive therapy unit, because of the risk of ventilatory depression.

Oral morphine is used in the treatment of chronic pain. The bioavailability of oral morphine is only 20–30% because of first-pass metabolism in the gut wall and liver, and thus higher doses are required. However, the concentration of morphine-6-glucuronide is also higher than after i.v. or i.m. administration. Thus, oral morphine is effective in a dose of 20–40 mg. Morphine should not be administered orally in the early postoperative period, as gastric emptying is impaired.

Table 11.5 Physical and pharmacokinetic data relating to some common opioid drugs. V_{ss}, volume of distribution at steady state; $T_{\frac{1}{2}\alpha}$, distribution half-life; $T_{\frac{1}{2}\beta}$, elimination half-life; Cl, clearance. Lipid solubility is expressed as octanol:water partition coefficient. Pharmacokinetic parameters are average values in adults; there is wide interindividual variability

Drug	V_{ss} (litres)	$T_{\frac{1}{2}\alpha}$ (min)	$T_{\frac{1}{2}\beta}$ (h)	Cl (litres/min)	Lipid solubility
Morphine	200	25	3.5	1.2	1.4
Methadone	420	10	36	0.15	116
Pethidine	250	8	3.5	0.8	40
Fentanyl	375	3	4	1.0	810
Alfentanil	36	2	1.5	0.3	130
Sufentanil	98	1	2.5	0.75	1800

Diamorphine

Diamorphine (diacetylmorphine) is a semisynthetic morphine derivative with similar actions and side effects. It is approximately twice as potent as morphine, and has a more rapid onset of action because of greater lipid solubility. Diamorphine undergoes rapid deacetylation, first to monoacetylmorphine (an active opioid) and then very rapidly to morphine. It is said to produce more euphoric and antitussive actions, and to cause less respiratory depression, nausea and vomiting, than morphine; these claims have not been substantiated in clinical trials. Diamorphine may be regarded as a pro-drug for the active metabolites monoacetylmorphine and morphine. It is administered usually in a dose of 5–10 mg i.m. (reduced by 50% in elderly patients).

Papaveretum

This is a partially purified extract of opium, and contains 50% anhydrous morphine. The remainder comprises other alkaloids (principally codeine, thebaine, narcotine and papaverine) with a mixture of analgesic and smooth muscle effects. Consequently, papaveretum causes less spasm of smooth muscle than morphine alone. Papaveretum 20 mg is equipotent with morphine 12.5 mg in respect of analgesia, but there is a greater degree of sedation and possibly of ventilatory depression. The average dose for a healthy adult is 15–20 mg i.m.

Pethidine

Pethidine is a synthetic opioid with an analgesic potency approximately one-tenth that of morphine. It has mild cholinergic effects and relaxes smooth muscle. It produces sedation but little euphoria. Ventilatory depression is similar in degree to that produced by morphine in equipotent doses, but pethidine has no specific action on the cough reflex.

Unlike morphine, pethidine possesses mild quinidine-like actions which may reduce myocardial excitability and the incidence of ventricular arrhythmias. This may be related to the local anaesthetic action of pethidine. Arterial pressure is normally unaffected, but hypotension may occur in the hypovolaemic patient as a result of venous and arterial dilatation.

Pethidine tends to relax the tone of smooth muscle in the gastrointestinal tract; it may relieve spasm, but reduces motility. The incidence of nausea and vomiting is similar to, or slightly greater than, that associated with morphine.

Pethidine produces less release of histamine than morphine, and is preferable for asthmatic patients.

Pethidine may be used in a dose of 25–50 mg i.v. or 100–150 mg i.m. in the healthy adult. Its duration of action is 2–3 h. It crosses the placenta and may cause ventilatory depression in the fetus; however, this is of shorter duration than that resulting from morphine. One of its metabolites, norpethidine, causes hyperexcitability and convulsions; norpethidine may accumulate if large doses of pethidine are given to patients with renal insufficiency.

Convulsions, coma and hypertensive crises have been reported after administration of pethidine to patients taking monoamine oxidase inhibitors.

Buprenorphine

This is a synthetic analgesic derived from the opium alkaloid thebaine, and is closely related structurally to morphine. It is a partial agonist at the μ receptor; thus, there is a 'ceiling' to its analgesic action. Buprenorphine has a low potential for physical dependence and addiction, and is not subject at present to controlled drug regulations. It has a delayed onset of action and, although its elimination half-life is 2–4.5 h, its duration of action is prolonged (6–8 h) because of slow dissociation from the μ receptor. It is a potent agent; buprenorphine 0.4 mg is equianalgesic with morphine 10 mg.

Euphoria and dysphoria occur infrequently, but there are high incidences of sedation, drowsiness and vomiting. Ventilatory depression may be of slow onset and prolonged duration; there is a 'ceiling' to the ventilatory depression induced by buprenorphine in animals, but it is not clear if this occurs in man. Ventilatory depression may be difficult to reverse even with large doses of naloxone; it is probably preferable to use a non-specific ventilatory stimulant, e.g. doxapram.

A dose of 0.3–0.6 mg i.v. or i.m. is appropriate for an adult. A sublingual tablet is available in a dose of 0.2 mg. A dose of 0.2–0.4 mg is effective after major surgery, although parenteral buprenorphine may be required initially because of the slow onset of analgesia. Buprenorphine undergoes a high degree of first-pass metabolism and has a low bioavailability if administered orally. Consequently, inactivation of a sublingual tablet occurs if it is swallowed; however, another sublingual tablet may be administered, as only a small percentage of buprenorphine is absorbed from the swallowed tablet and the risk of overdosage is small.

Buprenorphine displaces other opioid agonists from the μ receptor, and may antagonise analgesia induced previously by, for example, morphine. Consequently, if buprenorphine is to be used for provision of postoperative analgesia, it should be employed also during anaesthesia if an intraoperative analgesic is required.

Fentanyl

Fentanyl is a synthetic opioid related structurally to pethidine. Its analgesic potency is approximately 100 times that of morphine. It is very lipid-soluble, and reaches opioid receptors very rapidly. Thus, its onset of action occurs in 1–2 min. After a single dose, its duration of action is limited to 20–30 min by redistribution, but in high doses, or after infusion, its effects may last for 2–5 h and are terminated by elimination of the drug; in the elderly, its actions may last for up to 9 h.

Respiratory system

Doses in excess of 50 μg in combination with anaesthetic drugs may result in depression of ventilation for several minutes. Large doses, or infusion of fentanyl, should be used only if IPPV is planned.

Delayed ventilatory depression may occur after a bolus i.v. dose. This may be related to sequestration in gastric juice, and subsequent absorption from the small intestine; this phenomenon occurs with most opioids, but peaks in blood concentration are reflected rapidly by an increase in the CNS effects of fentanyl because of its high lipid solubility.

Cardiovascular system

Fentanyl has little effect. A small reduction in arterial pressure may occur, and heart rate may decrease because of vagal stimulation.

Other effects

Sedation is relatively poor in comparison with that produced by morphine or pethidine. The incidence of nausea and vomiting is similar to that associated with other opioids.

Chest wall rigidity may occur after large doses of fentanyl, making artificial ventilation of the lungs difficult.

Fentanyl causes little release of histamine.

Spasm of the sphincter of Oddi has occurred after moderate doses of fentanyl, mimicking the presence of a gallstone on intraoperative cholangiography.

Dosage

Fentanyl is used most commonly as an analgesic supplement during anaesthesia. Doses of 50–100 μg may be given i.v. to the spontaneously breathing patient. Larger doses (200–800 μg i.v.) are appropriate when IPPV is used; the dose selected is determined by the anticipated duration of surgery. Fentanyl has been used in very high doses, e.g. 50 μg/kg, for major surgery in order to avoid the use of volatile anaesthetic agents. These large doses may suppress totally the metabolic effects of anaesthesia and surgery (increased plasma concentrations of glucose, cortisol, GH, ACTH, etc.). However, the duration of action is very prolonged and patients may require IPPV for some hours after operation; even if spontaneous ventilation appears adequate, observation is required in the ITU for 24 h postoperatively.

Alfentanil

This synthetic derivative of fentanyl has a high lipid solubility, and acts within one arm–brain circulation time after i.v. administration. It has a small volume of distribution and short elimination half-life, and therefore has a short duration of action even after large doses. Consequently, it is more suitable for continuous i.v. infusion during surgery than fentanyl, as postoperative depression of ventilation is less likely.

Alfentanil depresses the cardiovascular system to a greater extent than fentanyl, particularly in the elderly and in patients of ASA classes III or IV.

Depression of ventilation is common for some minutes after administration of alfentanil, and the drug should be administered only if equipment is available for IPPV.

Doses approaching 500 μg of alfentanil may be given to patients who are breathing spontaneously; the duration of action is only 5–10 min. An initial bolus dose followed by a continuous infusion (30–60 μg/min) is appropriate for patients receiving IPPV.

Phenoperidine

This opioid is another synthetic pethidine derivative, and is approximately 10 times more potent than morphine. It is lipid-soluble, and thus has a rapid onset of action. Its duration of action is 1–2 h in young adults, but is significantly longer in the elderly. Phenoperidine causes greater systemic hypotension than other opioids.

A dose of 1–3 mg is appropriate during anaesthesia, depending on the duration of surgery. It should be used only in patients receiving IPPV.

Other opioids

Several other opioids are used occasionally during anaesthesia.

Levorphanol

This drug is 4–5 times more potent than morphine and has a long duration of action (6–8 h). It causes less sedation, nausea and vomiting than morphine. The dose is 1–2 mg i.v. Its prolonged action provides satisfactory analgesia extending into the postoperative period, but administration of other opioids in the early postoperative period may result in ventilatory depression.

Sufentanil

This drug is related to fentanyl, and is 600–700 times more potent than morphine. It is highly lipid-soluble and has a more rapid onset of action than fentanyl; its duration of action is slightly shorter. It is a suitable alternative to fentanyl for intraoperative use, in a dose of 5–10 μg for the spontaneously breathing patient and 25–30 μg in those receiving IPPV. However, it has a very high therapeutic index, and doses of 10–30 μg/kg have been used to produce hypnosis and analgesia during surgery.

Meptazinol

This agent possesses analgesic properties similar to those of pethidine, but is claimed to produce a low risk of ventilatory depression. Its use is associated with a high incidence of nausea and vomiting.

Methadone

Methadone is equipotent with morphine, but has a long elimination half-life (35 h) because of limited capacity of the liver to metabolise the drug. Analgesia lasts for approximately 20 h.

Nalbuphine

This is a synthetic agonist–antagonist opioid related to naloxone. It possesses a 'ceiling' effect in respect of ventilatory depression, but its analgesic effects are also restricted. It has a potency 0.5–0.75 times that of morphine. Nalbuphine reduces cardiac work, but has a minimal effect on arterial pressure or heart rate.

Spinal opioids (see also p. 456)

It was demonstrated in 1976 that opioid receptors exist in the spinal cord, and that analgesia results if these are blocked locally by administration of opioid drugs. Many subsequent studies have confirmed that administration of opioids by either the subarachnoid or extradural route produces analgesia without the cardiovascular side effects that result from spinal administration of local anaesthetic drugs. Unfortunately, few well-controlled studies have been conducted to define the optimum drug and site of injection, or to compare the quality of analgesia provided with that resulting from other forms of pain relief.

Almost all opioids have been administered by one or both of the spinal routes. In general, drugs which are poorly lipid-soluble may be given in smaller doses (relative to the systemic dose) than more lipid-soluble agents (Table 11.5), and thus produce fewer side effects attributable to high circulating concentrations of drug; they also have a longer duration of action. However, a higher proportion of the less lipid-soluble drug remains in CSF and may result in a greater degree of spread of analgesia. This occurs because diffusion within the CSF, and circulation of the CSF itself, carry the drug to segments of the spinal cord away

Table 11.6 Doses and durations of action of intrathecal and extradural opioids

Drug	Route	Dose (mg)	Onset (min)	Typical duration (h)
Morphine	Subarachnoid	0.1–0.5	15–20	17–24
	Extradural	5–10	25–30	12–18
Pethidine	Extradural	30–100	5–10	6–8
Methadone	Extradural	5	12	7–8
Hydromorphone	Extradural	1	13	6–11
Diamorphine	Extradural	5	5	10–14
Fentanyl	Extradural	0.1	5	3–4
Sufentanil	Extradural	0.05	8	5
Buprenorphine	Extradural	0.3	12	6

from the site of injection; this increases the risk of opioid reaching the brain stem, where it may cause ventilatory depression some hours after administration ('delayed ventilatory depression').

Spinal opioids are useful after major surgery when there are no contraindications to the use of subarachnoid or extradural techniques (see Ch. 26). Bolus administration through an extradural catheter results in analgesia for 6–12 h, and continuous infusions have also been used to provide uninterrupted pain relief. Intrathecal administration of opioids results in analgesia for longer periods with a much smaller dose (Table 11.6). The duration of analgesia, and the incidence and magnitude of side effects, are dose-related.

Side effects

1. *Ventilatory depression*. The incidence is highest with lipid-insoluble drugs, e.g. morphine, but is a potential risk with *any* opioid administered by the spinal route. It may occur up to 12 h after administration. It is more likely to occur in older patients, or if systemic opioids have also been administered. Ventilatory rate is not a reliable indicator of opioid-induced ventilatory depression, and patients who have received spinal opioids *must* be nursed in a high-dependency or intensive care unit, or ventilation monitored with an electronic device, for at least 12 h after the last dose of opioid.

2. *Urinary retention*. This occurs in approximately 90% of men. It is commoner after intrathecal than extradural administration.

3. *Pruritus*. Itching occurs in 70–80% of patients who receive extradural morphine, although it causes distress in only 5–10%. It is less common when other opioids are used.

4. *Nausea and vomiting*. These complications are probably no commoner after spinal administration than after systemic injection.

At present, the use of spinal opioids cannot be considered as a routine method of providing postoperative analgesia because of the high incidence of side effects and the requirement for close nursing supervision.

Opioid antagonists

These drugs act as competitive antagonists at opioid receptor sites both in the CNS and peripheral tissues. Some of the antagonists also possess intrinsic agonist activity, and have different affinities for different receptor types. Thus, they may behave as competitive antagonists at one site but agonists at another. Naloxone is the only drug with pure antagonist activity at all identified opioid receptors.

Naloxone

This opioid antagonist is related structurally to oxymorphone. It is well tolerated and rarely causes any side effect. It acts within 1 min of i.v. injection and has a duration of action of approximately 30 min. This relatively short duration may result in return of ventilatory depression induced by an opioid of longer action. Consequently, patients should be monitored carefully for an appropriate period after its use.

All the CNS effects of opioids administered systemically are antagonised by naloxone, including analgesia. In low doses, naloxone antagonises opioid-induced ventilatory depression and excessive sedation without affecting pain relief. Thus, the drug should be titrated slowly against the clinical effect to avoid the emergence of excessive pain. Analgesia produced by administration of spinal opioids is antagonised only by very large doses of naloxone. Arterial pressure may increase after administration of naloxone, but this results usually from reduction in the degree of sedation or emergence of pain, rather than a direct effect. Naloxone is effective in relieving opioid-induced spasm of the sphincter of Oddi.

Ventilatory depression caused by buprenorphine is relatively resistant to reversal by naloxone because of the very high affinity of buprenorphine for the μ receptor. Naloxone is ineffective in reversing sedation or ventilatory depression induced by non-opioid drugs, e.g barbiturates or benzodiazepines.

Naloxone is the drug of choice in antagonising opioid-induced ventilatory depression in the neonate.

The average dose of naloxone for adults is 200–400 μg i.v.; this should be administered in increments of 50–100 μg; supplementary doses may be required after 20–30 min.

Other opioid antagonists

Nalorphine. This drug is related to morphine. It antagonises the effects of morphine at the μ receptor, but has agonist activity at other sites.

Levallorphan. This agent is related to levorphanol, and in common with nalorphine possesses agonist and antagonist activity at different opioid receptors.

Both of these agents have been superseded by naloxone, and are no longer available in the UK.

NON-OPIOID ANALGESICS

These drugs may be useful after minor surgery and are used to provide analgesia during the later recovery period after major surgery. They are employed also to supplement opioid analgesia after some types of operation. The non-steroidal anti-inflammatory drugs (NSAIDs) are generally more effective than the other non-opioid analgesics after surgery or trauma because of their anti-inflammatory properties.

Non-steroidal anti-inflammatory drugs

NSAIDs produce analgesia by a peripheral effect, and are effective in pain of low to moderate intensity. By reducing the activity of the enzyme cyclo-oxygenase they inhibit the synthesis and release of prostaglandins, prostacyclins and thromboxane, which sensitise pain receptors to mechanical stimulation or to other pain mediators. The drugs differ in their precise actions on cyclo-oxygenase, and in their spectrum of activity as analgesic, antipyretic and anti-inflammatory agents.

Prostaglandins are synthesised by the gastric mucosa; their inhibition by NSAIDs may result in gastric erosions or ulceration. In addition, chronic use leads occasionally to renal papillary necrosis and chronic interstitial nephritis.

The principal uses of the NSAIDs are for treatment of minor ailments and chronic musculoskeletal pain. However, some drugs of this type have been used successfully to provide analgesia after surgery or in association with trauma.

Acetylsalicylic acid

Aspirin is used for the moderate pain which persists 3–4 days after major surgery. A parenteral form of the drug has been used in limited trials to provide analgesia in the early postoperative period. Aspirin is also in widespread use as an antipyretic. The relatively high incidence of gastric side effects after oral administration is reduced by the use of soluble aspirin. The drug may be administered also by the rectal route.

Indomethacin

This has been used in combination with opioids to treat pain after thoracotomy or orthopaedic surgery and in patients with fractured ribs. Because of gastrointestinal side effects and delayed gastric emptying resulting from opioid administration, it is usually most appropriate to administer indomethacin by the rectal route.

Diclofenac

This NSAID may be administered orally, rectally or i.m. It is claimed that its use reduces the dosage of opioid required after abdominal surgery, but this has not been substantiated.

Paracetamol

This is an analgesic and antipyretic agent which does not possess the anti-inflammatory properties of the NSAIDs. However, it is effective in treatment of mild to moderate postoperative pain, and has the major advantage that it does not cause gastrointestinal side effects.

BENZODIAZEPINES

These drugs are used primarily as sedatives and hypnotics, although in large doses anaesthesia is induced. In addition, they produce mild muscle relaxation and possess anticonvulsant properties.

Site and mode of action

The benzodiazepines affect polysynaptic pathways within the spinal cord and brain, particularly in the midbrain reticular formation (affecting wakefulness) and the amygdala area of the limbic system (a relay for the expression of emotion, and therefore affecting anxiety).

The mechanism of action is related to stimulation of the activity of the inhibitory transmitter γ-aminobutyric acid (GABA), causing presynaptic inhibition within these areas.

Central nervous system

Sedation. There is a progressive, dose-dependent transition from sedation through hypnosis to unconsciousness. In large doses, anaesthesia is induced, but there is wide interindividual variability in the dose required, and the onset of unconsciousness is slow. In lower doses, benzodiazepines reduce the MAC value of inhalational anaesthetics (see p. 154). Diazepam may induce transient analgesia after i.v. injection, but other benzodiazepines possess no analgesic properties.

Amnesia. Dose-related anterograde amnesia occurs after administration of diazepam as a result of effects on the early consolidation phase of memory processing. Although it has been claimed that some benzodiazepines induce retrograde amnesia (i.e. for events before administration), this has not been demonstrated.

Anxiolysis. Benzodiazepines are effective in alleviating acute and chronic anxiety states and are prescribed widely for this purpose. This action makes these drugs useful as premedicants in anaesthetic practice.

Anticonvulsant effect. Most benzodiazepines possess anticonvulsant properties. They do not affect the seizure focus, but prevent subcortical spread of seizure activity. Diazepam and clonazepam are useful by i.v. injection for the management of status epilepticus; clobazam is used orally as an adjunct to chronic anticonvulsant therapy.

Respiratory system

Large i.v. doses of benzodiazepines produce depression of ventilation. There is direct depression of ventilatory drive in response to both hypoxaemia and hypercapnia, and a slight decrease in ventilatory muscle activity. Severe ventilatory depression may occur in the elderly or debilitated patient after i.v. administration. Airway obstruction may occur if consciousness is impaired. Clinically significant decreases in oxygen saturation occur during upper gastrointestinal endoscopy when i.v. benzodiazepines are used for sedation.

Cardiovascular system

Large doses of benzodiazepines decrease cardiac output and systemic arterial pressure, particularly if given in combination with opioids, and a reflex tachycardia occurs commonly. Hypotension is more likely in the hypovolaemic patient. Benzodiazepines potentiate the effects of ganglion-blocking agents and other drugs used to induce hypotension.

Muscle relaxation

Benzodiazepines produce relaxation of smooth muscle by depression of polysynaptic transmission in the brain and spinal cord, and by mild depression of motor nerve and muscle function. This effect is useful in tetanus and in spastic conditions. The muscle relaxation produced is inadequate for surgery, and there is no significant potentiation of depolarising or non-depolarising neuromuscular blockers at the neuromuscular junction. However, the central effects of benzodiazepines may reduce requirements for neuromuscular blocking agents.

Other effects

Transfer occurs rapidly across the placenta and this may cause neonatal depression. Chronic administration of benzodiazepines may result in physical and psychological dependence.

Indications for the use of benzodiazepines in anaesthetic practice

1. *Premedication*. Diazepam, temazepam and lorazepam are used commonly by the oral route for premedication; these drugs may be administered also as hypnotics at night. Midazolam is also suitable as a premedicant agent by the i.m. route.
2. *Endoscopy*. Diazepam or midazolam administered i.v. provides satisfactory sedation and amnesia during gastrointestinal or tracheobronchial endoscopy. Patients should be fasted, as laryngeal reflexes may be lost. Airway obstruction and ventilatory depression may occur, and supplemental oxygen should be administered.
3. *Dentistry*. Diazepam or midazolam may be administered i.v. in small doses to produce sedation and cooperation in anxious patients during minor dental procedures undertaken using local anaesthesia. Temazepam administered orally 1 h before the procedure is a useful alternative.
4. *Cardioversion*. Diazepam or midazolam have been used to induce sedation and amnesia for this procedure, but recovery is slow.
5. *Sedation in the ITU*. Diazepam, lorazepam and midazolam may be administered i.v. to induce sedation and amnesia in patients who require IPPV in the ITU. Analgesics should be administered if the patient is in pain. The major disadvantage of benzodiazepines in the critically ill is prolonged sedation resulting from accumulation of the drug or its metabolites.
6. *Supplementation of anaesthesia*. Benzodiazepines are used occasionally to induce anaesthesia in patients undergoing cardiac surgery. They are used in some centres to supplement balanced anaesthesia during other procedures. It has been claimed that their amnesic effect reduces the incidence of awareness during general anaesthesia. However, there is no evidence that this is true and the drugs should *not* be used primarily for this purpose.

Adverse effects

1. Residual drowsiness, impairment of mental functions, dysarthria and ataxia.
2. Ventilatory depression after i.v. administration.
3. Muscle weakness, headache, nausea and vomiting, vertigo, joint and chest pains may occur occasionally.

The incidence of these effects is higher in elderly or debilitated patients unless a reduced dose is given.

Diazepam

This benzodiazepine is relatively lipid-soluble and water-insoluble. Absorption is slow, erratic and incomplete after i.m. administration and the drug should only be administered orally or by the i.v. route. Diazepam is available for i.v. administration either as a viscous solution containing organic solvents (propylene glycol, ethanol and sodium benzoate in benzoic acid) or as an emulsion in lipid (Diazemuls); both preparations contain diazepam 5 mg/ml. The drug is available for oral use as tablets or syrup. The drug can be administered also by the rectal route.

Diazepam is effective within 30–45 min after oral administration, and has a duration of action of at least 4–6 h. It induces sedation within

Table 11.7 Elimination half-lives of four commonly used benzodiazepines

	Half-life (h)	Active metabolites	Half-life (h) of metabolites
Diazepam	36	Yes	100
Midazolam	2	No	—
Temazepam	8	No	—
Lorazepam	15	No	—

1–2 min after a bolus i.v. dose. The elimination half-life is extremely long (20–90 h; Table 11.7); this results partly from enterohepatic recirculation. In addition, one of its metabolites, *N*-desmethyl diazepam, is pharmacologically active, and has a longer half-life.

Dosage

1. *Premedication.* 10–15 mg orally (1–5 mg in children).
2. *Sedation.* 0.15–0.20 mg/kg by slow i.v. injection. The dose should be reduced by 50% in elderly patients.
3. *Intensive care.* Bolus doses of 0.1–0.2 mg/kg. Because of the prolonged half-life, there is no indication for infusion of diazepam. In tetanus, a dose of up to 5 mg/kg may be required daily.
4. *Status epilepticus.* 0.2–0.3 mg/kg i.v. over 5 min, repeated if necessary after 30–60 min.

Precautions and adverse effects

Patients should be instructed in writing concerning the dangers of taking alcohol, of driving or of operating machinery within 24 h.

Intravenous administration of diazepam causes a high incidence of thrombophlebitis (50–60%). This complication is obviated by the use of Diazemuls.

Midazolam

This is a water-soluble benzodiazepine which has almost replaced diazepam as an i.v. sedative. It is not recommended as an anticonvulsant. It is presented in 2-ml ampoules containing 5 mg/ml, but it is preferable to use the alternative, more dilute formulation of 2 mg/ml (5-ml ampoules) for i.v. injection, as the dose may be titrated more accurately.

Midazolam has a slightly more rapid onset of action than diazepam after i.v. injection, and a shorter duration of action; the elimination half-life is 1.5–2.5 h. Its metabolites are inactive. Metabolism is reduced in some critically ill patients; this results in prolonged elimination half-life (up to 21 h) and greatly delayed recovery of consciousness.

Dosage

1. *Sedation.* 2.5–7.5 mg (0.035–0.105 mg/kg) i.v. in the adult, with a maximum of 2.5 mg in elderly patients. The midazolam:diazepam potency ratio is between 1.5:1 and 2:1. A number of fatalities have resulted from the use of midazolam as an i.v. sedative when given in the same dose range as that recommended for diazepam. Midazolam *must* be administered slowly; the onset of its clinical effect may be delayed, and there is a danger of overdosage if the drug is given rapidly without waiting to assess its effects.
2. *Premedication.* 5 mg i.m. (2.5 mg in the elderly).
3. *Intensive care.* Bolus dose of 5–10 mg i.v. followed by i.v. infusion; requirements vary widely from 1 to 20 mg/h. Infusions should not be maintained in high doses, as cumulation is likely.

Advantages

Midazolam has a shorter duration of action than diazepam and residual mental impairment is less marked. It is associated with a low incidence of thrombophlebitis.

Disadvantages

In common with diazepam, it may induce ventilatory depression, especially in elderly patients. Cardiovascular depression may occur in the hypovolaemic patient. Recovery is prolonged in some critically ill patients.

Other benzodiazepines

Temazepam

This is a short-acting benzodiazepine which produces little hangover effect. It is a useful premedicant which induces hypnosis and anxiolysis when given in a dose of 20 mg orally 1 h before surgery. In a dose of 30 mg it is as effective as i.v. midazolam in producing sedation and anxiolysis in patients undergoing dental procedures.

Lorazepam

This has a long duration of action (half-life 10–20 h). Its use as a premedicant in doses of 2–5 mg is associated usually with amnesia lasting several hours.

Flumazenil

Flumazenil antagonises the central effects of benzodiazepine agonists by competing for occupancy of benzodiazepine receptors. In very high doses it has slight agonist properties, and may have mild direct inverse agonist effects at lower doses. The drug is metabolised in the liver, and its elimination half-life is less than 1 h.

All the central effects of benzodiazepine agonists are antagonised by flumazenil; performance in psychometric tests is restored to normal and amnesia is attenuated. EEG studies indicate that antagonism starts within 1 min. The duration of action is dose-dependent; after small but effective doses, amnesia and sedation may return within 30 min.

Indications

1. *Antagonism of sedation*. Inadvertent overdosage, or undue sensitivity to the effects of benzodiazepine agonists, may be antagonised by flumazenil. However, sedation may recur and the patient must be observed carefully for several hours. The routine use of flumazenil to antagonise residual effects of i.v. sedation is not recommended. Prolonged sedation resulting from accumulation of benzodiazepines in the critically ill patient is usually reversible with flumazenil. However, sedation and ventilatory depression are likely to recur unless repeated doses of flumazenil are administered or a continuous infusion instituted. It may be more appropriate to sedate patients in the ITU using a drug with a short elimination half-life rather than antagonising a long-acting benzodiazepine with a short-acting antagonist.

2. *Self-poisoning*. Deliberate overdosage with benzodiazepines may result in prolonged unconsciousness and ventilatory depression, with subsequent development of pulmonary atelectasis and infection. Flumazenil restores consciousness, but repeated doses, or a continuous infusion, are necessary until plasma concentrations of the agonist have diminished.

Precautions

Flumazenil may induce withdrawal symptoms in patients who have received benzodiazepines for long periods.

BUTYROPHENONES

These drugs share many properties, and some structural similarities, with the phenothiazines. Their principal use in anaesthesia is as neuroleptic agents. Neurolepsis is a drug-induced state of suppressed spontaneous movements, but intact spinal and central reflexes. There is a lack of initiative, disinterest in the environment, little display of emotion and a limited range of affect. Intellectual function remains intact.

Neuroleptanalgesia is the term used to describe the combined use of a neuroleptic agent with a potent analgesic, usually fentanyl. Large doses may induce profound ventilatory depression while preserving consciousness. A state may be induced in which the patient is hypoxaemic and cyanosed, but remains conscious and responds to orders to breathe (a state that has been likened to 'Ondine's curse'). This combination of neuroleptic and opioid drugs is used in moderate dosage to provide sedation during minor surgical procedures, usually as a supplement to a local anaesthetic block, e.g. during ophthalmic surgery.

Neuroleptanaesthesia is the term employed to describe the use of larger doses to supplement nitrous oxide anaesthesia. This technique is used in some centres for neurosurgical and cardiac procedures.

In addition to their effect on behaviour, the butyrophenones are powerful antiemetics. They antagonise dopamine-mediated synaptic transmission in the CNS, probably by occupation of GABA receptors. This is thought to be the major mechanism by which their therapeutic actions are mediated. The basal ganglia are rich in dopamine-mediated synapses, and the major side effect of the butyrophenones is the production of dyskinetic involuntary (extrapyramidal) movements. The incidence of extrapyramidal movements is reduced if butyrophenones are administered in combination with an opioid.

The butyrophenones have no specific analgesic action, but may prolong the duration of action of opioids.

Droperidol

This is the most widely used butyrophenone in anaesthetic practice. When administered alone, it produces a tranquil and placid appearance in the patient. However, patients may complain subsequently of unpleasant sensations of mental restlessness and agitation; these are avoided by administering an opioid or benzodiazepine simultaneously.

The onset of action of droperidol starts within 3–10 min of i.v. injection and its duration may exceed 12 h. Most of the injected dose is metabolised in the liver and reduced doses are required in patients with hepatic disease. Approximately 10% of the drug is excreted unchanged in the urine.

Cardiovascular system

Droperidol possesses mild α-blocking actions which may cause a reduction in arterial pressure. This occurs seldom after oral or i.m. administration, but may result in significant hypotension after i.v. injection, particularly if hypovolaemia is present. Droperidol has some effect in protecting the heart against catecholamine-induced arrhythmias.

Central nervous system

Droperidol causes mild cerebral vasoconstriction and a reduction in CSF pressure. Its neuroleptic properties occur within a few minutes of i.v. administration and may persist for 6–12 h. Thus, there may be re-emergence of unpleasant subjective sensations if the drug is given in conjunction with a short-acting opioid. Extrapyramidal side effects may occur 24 h or more after administration. If severe, these may be treated with procyclidine; promethazine (12.5 mg i.v. + 12.5 mg i.m.) is usually effective if symptoms are mild. Although droperidol possesses little intrinsic sedative activity, it may potentiate anaesthetic or sedative drugs and result in delayed recovery of consciousness.

Other effects

Total body oxygen consumption is reduced. There is little effect on ventilation.

Indications

1. *Premedication.* 1.25–2.5 mg orally or i.m., in conjunction with a benzodiazepine or opioid. There is some evidence that doses in excess of 2.5 mg do not produce more effective antiemesis. Doses exceeding 5 mg should not be used as the effects of the drug are prolonged but sedation is not improved.
2. *Neuroleptanalgesia/anaesthesia.* Up to 10 mg i.v. with fentanyl. A mixture of fentanyl and droperidol (Thalamonal) is available, and contains fentanyl 50 μg/ml and droperidol 2.5 mg/ml.

Haloperidol

This drug is used less commonly in anaesthesia. Its effects are similar to those of droperidol, but it has a more prolonged duration of action (up to 24 h), and has virtually no α-adrenergic activity. It causes a high incidence of extrapyramidal side effects.

PHENOTHIAZINES

These agents are less potent neuroleptic drugs than the butyrophenones. Their principal use in anaesthesia is in the prevention and treatment of nausea and vomiting. In common with the butyrophenones, the phenothiazines have a specific action on the chemoreceptor trigger zone, and in large doses exert a direct depressant effect on the vomiting centre (see Ch. 14). In addition, some members of the group possess sedative properties, and are useful for premedication. Their major side effects are also similar to those of the butyrophenones: extrapyramidal movements, hypotension produced by α-receptor blockade and central depression of sympathetic activity.

Chlorpromazine

This phenothiazine is used widely in psychiatric practice, but some of its actions are useful in anaesthesia. It has sedative actions, and has been used for premedication and to calm manic or disturbed patients in the ITU. It may be used i.v. in small doses to produce α-receptor blockade. Thermoregulation is depressed, and shivering reduced; this property, together with the vasodilatation induced by α-blockade, resulted in its use as an adjuvant during active cooling to induce hypothermia for neurosurgery. It is also an antiemetic.

Jaundice occurs in 0.5% of patients who receive chlorpromazine, and is independent of dose or duration of treatment.

Dosage

1. *Premedication.* 25–50 mg i.m. 1 h before operation.
2. *Vasodilatation.* Increments of 2.5 mg i.v. after dilution (25 mg in 10–20 ml).

Promethazine

This drug has more marked antihistamine (H_1) properties than other phenothiazines. In addition, it has an atropine-like action, producing bronchodilation and a reduction of oral and bronchial secretions. There is a spasmolytic action on the gastrointestinal tract. Its sedative action is greater than that of chlorpromazine.

The principal use of promethazine in anaesthesia is as a premedicant, usually in combination with an opioid. The combination of promethazine 25 mg and pethidine 50–100 mg i.m. is suitable especially for asthmatic or bronchitic patients.

Phenothiazines used in the treatment of nausea and vomiting are discussed on page 242.

VENTILATORY STIMULANTS

These drugs have a limited role in the treatment of ventilatory failure in patients with chronic obstructive airways disease or in those with residual drowsiness or sedation after anaesthesia. They act by stimulating medullary centres and by an effect on peripheral chemoreceptors. They are effective only when administered i.v., and have a short duration of action. All these drugs are non-specific CNS stimulants which may produce cerebral arousal, clonic movements and convulsions. In very high doses, cortical and medullary depression occur and result in ventilatory failure and cardiovascular collapse.

The use of ventilatory stimulants in patients with chronic obstructive airways disease is controversial. Although minute volume is increased, the stimulation of muscle activity also increases oxygen consumption and carbon dioxide production. However, clearance of secretions may be improved.

Doxapram

This drug is the most specific of the analeptic drugs in its ability to stimulate ventilation without development of other signs of CNS stimulation. Tidal volume, and to a lesser extent ventilatory rate, increase for approximately 5 min after a slow bolus dose of 1–1.5 mg/kg i.v. If a satisfactory effect is achieved, doxapram should be administered by infusion at a rate of 0.5–4 mg/min and titrated against effect. Side effects include coughing, nausea, vomiting, restlessness, hypertension, tachycardia, cardiac arrhythmias and muscle rigidity.

It has been claimed that a single bolus dose of doxapram in the early postoperative period reduces the incidence of pulmonary complications after abdominal surgery, but this has not been substantiated.

Nikethamide

This drug increases the sensitivity of the medulla to carbon dioxide. Because of its toxic effects (tremor, convulsions), it should not be given by infusion. However, a dose of 0.5–1 g produces arousal and increased ventilation for approximately 2 min, during which time the patient is encouraged to cough vigorously. The use of this drug has reduced substantially since the introduction of doxapram.

FURTHER READING

Feldman S A, Scurr C F, Paton W 1987 Drugs in anaesthesia: mechanisms of action. Edward Arnold, London

Goodman-Gilman A, Goodman L S, Gilman A (eds) 1985 The pharmacological basis of therapeutics, 7th edn. Macmillan, New York

Rogers H J, Spector R G, Trounce J R 1985 A textbook of clinical pharmacology. Hodder & Stoughton, London

Vickers M D, Schneiden H, Ward-Smith F G 1984 Drugs in anaesthetic practice, 6th edn. Butterworths, London

12. Neuromuscular blockade

Anaesthetists use neuromuscular blocking drugs to abolish skeletal muscle contractions which may occur as reflex responses to painful stimuli or to tracheal intubation, and also to abolish or reduce skeletal muscle tone which may hinder access to a surgical field or make artificial ventilation difficult. These requirements may be produced by other means, e.g. deep general anaesthesia, or local anaesthetic blocks which affect the specific motor nerves involved. However, the former method is accompanied usually by undesirable side effects whilst local anaesthetic techniques are time-consuming and may not be appropriate. The introduction of tubocurarine in 1942 produced an expansion in anaesthetic techniques and the number of neuromuscular blocking drugs available at present is considerable.

PHYSIOLOGY OF NEUROMUSCULAR TRANSMISSION

Skeletal muscle rarely contracts in the absence of activity in the motor nerve supplying it. An exception is the contracture seen sometimes in patients with malignant hyperthermia. The link between nerve activity and muscle contraction was shown by Claud Bernard in his demonstration in 1857 that curare acts somewhere between the nerve and the muscle and in 1936 Sir Henry Dale established that acetylcholine is the transmitter involved.

The whole process whereby a nerve action potential leads to a contraction of the myosin and actin filaments in the muscle is complex. The stages are summarised in Table 12.1.

Table 12.1 Mechanism of neuromuscular transmission

Nerve action potential
↓
Depolarisation of nerve terminal
↓
Ca^{2+} entry
↓
Acetylcholine release
↓
Combination with acetylcholine receptor
↓
Increase in end-plate permeability
↓
Muscle action potential
↓
Ca^{2+} entry
↓
Actin-myosin interaction
↓
Contraction

The following description is necessarily simplified: a detailed account may be found in Katz (1966), Bowman (1980) and Bowman & Rand (1980).

Release of acetylcholine by a nerve impulse

The nerve impulse arises in cells in the ventral horns of the spinal cord and the equivalent cells in the brain for the cranial nerves. Each impulse travels down the nerve axon as a wave of depolarisation, jumping in myelinated nerves from one node of Ranvier to the next (see Ch. 5). At its termination, each nerve fibre divides and may supply between 4 and 300 muscle fibres. The junction between nerve and muscle is termed the neuromuscular junction (Fig. 12.1).

The nerve action potential invades all the nerve terminals and depolarisation occurs as a transient initial increase in permeability to sodium ions followed by an increase in potassium permeability.

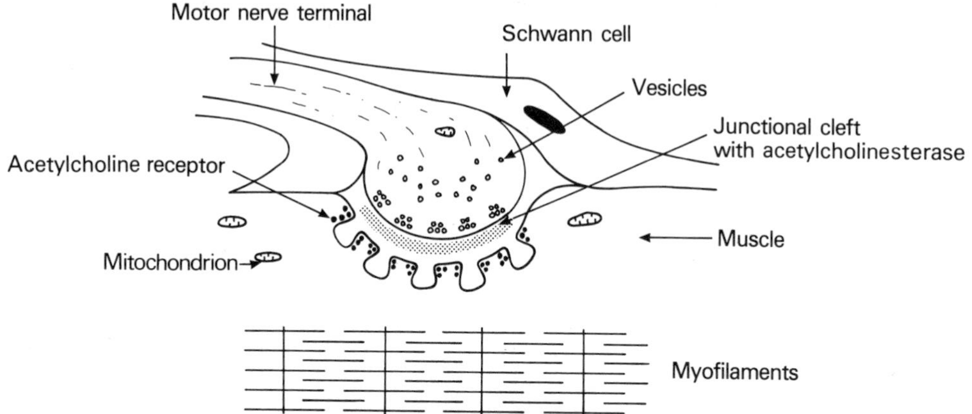

Fig. 12.1 Diagram of the neuromuscular junction.

In addition, there is an increase in calcium permeability. An increase in intracellular Ca^{2+} concentration occurs and is essential for the next step — the release of acetylcholine. Low extracellular $[Ca^{2+}]$ leads to less release of acetylcholine. High magnesium concentrations antagonise entry of calcium and reduce the release of acetylcholine.

The central role of acetylcholine

Acetylcholine as the transmitter is the key to neuromuscular transmission. In skeletal muscle, the electrical forces produced by the nerve action potential are too weak to initiate a muscle action potential. Acetylcholine acts as a chemical amplifier to ensure transmission. It is synthesised, stored and released from the nerve terminal, diffuses across the junction to combine with a specific receptor and is destroyed finally by a specific enzyme.

Synthesis. Acetylcholine is synthesised in the cytoplasm of the nerve terminal from choline and acetyl coenzyme A under the control of a specific enzyme, choline acetyltransferase. Choline is taken up by a carrier system in the nerve terminal membrane from the amount present in the cleft both by diffusion from plasma and by breakdown of acetylcholine. Acetylcoenzyme A is generated initially in the mitochondria. Blocking drugs similar to acetylcholine (e.g. hemicholinium-3) are taken up into the cell in place of choline and may produce myoneural block by depleting the nerve terminal of acetylcholine.

Storage. Whilst there is some free acetylcholine present in the nerve terminal, the majority is packed into vesicles. Each vesicle is spherical with a bilayer wall. The concentration of acetylcholine in the vesicle greatly exceeds that in the cytoplasm. Whilst vesicles are present throughout the nerve terminal, many are concentrated in specific zones opposite the folds on the muscle side of the junction. The vesicles are formed from membrane material synthesised originally perhaps in the cell body but also recycled from the terminal membrane following exocytosis.

Release of acetylcholine. Acetylcholine is released from the nerve terminal in one of two ways. Although some is released from the cytoplasm of the nerve, release from vesicles is most important physiologically.

Some acetylcholine is released spontaneously. The effects can be detected as low-voltage depolarisations of the muscle membrane — termed *miniature end-plate potentials* (MEPPs) — but these are insufficient to generate a muscle action potential. They occur randomly but are approximately equal in size. Each one corresponds with the release of the contents of one vesicle from the nerve terminal. Release occurs as a result of exocytosis with the vesicle membrane fusing with that at the terminal.

Depolarisation produced by a nerve action potential and subsequent entry of calcium ion leads to a release of the contents of two to three hundred vesicles synchronously. This larger amount diffuses across the synaptic cleft and produces an *end-plate potential* (EPP) in the adjacent muscle membrane.

The *acetylcholine receptor* is a specific protein present in maximum concentration on the crests of the folds opposite the local clustering of vesicles in the nerve terminal. It consists of a number of subunits. Acetylcholine binds to specific points of the receptor and initiates a chain of events. Firstly there is a change in the shape of the receptor molecule; this affects the shape of a protein in the membrane which acts as a channel through the membrane — an ionophore. Normally the channel is closed. When influenced by the union of acetylcholine with its receptor, it opens for approximately 1 ms, during which time sodium ions flood into the muscle cell and potassium ions pass out. The normal resting muscle membrane potential (about –70 mV) is produced as a result of a relative impermeability to sodium ions and a relative permeability to potassium. The changes in permeability lead to a reduction in the transmembrane voltage; this depolarisation changes the potential to about –15 mV. Normally, however, the depolarisation sets up local currents in the muscle membrane and produces a spreading depolarisation. Muscle membrane is similar to all excitable membranes and excitation produces a wave of depolarisation spreading along the fibre by opening selective channels for sodium ions. These ionophores are opened electrically whereas those at the end-plate are driven chemically.

Destruction of acetylcholine. The acetylcholine released by the nerve impulse or spontaneously is destroyed by acetylcholinesterase present in the synaptic cleft. The enzyme is extremely efficient and virtually all the acetylcholine is metabolised before the ionophore has relaxed back into its normally closed state. The choline released may re-enter the nerve and be used for further synthesis of acetylcholine.

Muscle excitation-contraction coupling

If an end-plate potential depolarises the adjacent muscle membrane sufficiently, a muscle action potential is generated which spreads to each end of the muscle. The spread is accompanied by an inward spread down into the T-tubule system and results in a release of calcium ions from the sarcoplasmic reticulum. In turn, this activates myosin ATPase, which results in the creation of force in the cross-bridges linking the thick myosin and thin actin filaments. Muscle shortening or force generation or both occur. The calcium release is transitory and calcium is taken up actively again into the sarcoplasmic reticulum and mitochondria. When the normal low intracellular calcium ion concentration is achieved, muscle relaxation occurs. The muscle action potential lasts approximately 1 to 2 ms; the contraction evoked by a single *twitch* lasts about 100–200 ms.

Effect of repetitive nerve stimulation

The events described so far show how one nerve impulse may generate one muscle twitch. However, effective muscle contraction usually requires a combination of activity in many muscle fibres and repetitive activity to generate sustained tension. This latter is a *tetanic* contraction. A single nerve action potential leads to the release of more than enough acetylcholine to produce an end-plate potential of sufficient size to generate a muscle action potential. Only approximately 20% of the released acetylcholine is needed to generate the muscle action potential.

In order to tetanise muscle, it is necessary that nerve and muscle action potentials occur fast enough to abolish the fade of tension seen with a single twitch. The rates needed vary from muscle to muscle but are normally of the order of 25 Hz. Rates of up to 200 Hz produce sustained contractions; each nerve impulse evokes a muscle action potential. The amount of acetylcholine released by each nerve impulse in such a train is not the same. The first impulse releases most and then there is a decrement to a new steady level. With the release of the contents of the vesicles near the junction, a transport process comes into play to bring up new vesicles; time is required to re-form and fill the old vesicles. However, the decrement that occurs is not sufficient to reduce the total amount of acetylcholine released per nerve impulse to an amount below the threshold required to generate an action potential.

This is the traditionally accepted view of the cause of the decrement in end-plate potentials seen during tetanus. Not all workers accept this explanation, which has been derived largely from experiments in muscles paralysed partially or totally with a curare-like drug. An alternative hypothesis suggests the presence of additional acetylcholine receptors on the nerve terminal. Some of the acetylcholine released acts on these and produces an increased mobilisation of vesicles and hence improved release of acetylcholine on the next impulse (a type of positive feedback). Curare-like drugs act not only on the postjunctional but also on the prejunctional receptors and destroy this feedback. Consequently, less acetylcholine is released on each impulse at the start of a tetanic train. A decrement occurs until the level of release matches the level of delivery of vesicles to the nerve terminal.

A second phenomenon occurs with tetanic rates of stimulation. During the tetanus there is a decrement in rate of release of acetylcholine. Immediately after the tetanus, single nerve impulses release a greater amount of acetylcholine than before as more vesicles discharge than normally. The exact mechanism is uncertain; it may involve a hyperpolarisation of the nerve terminal by the tetanic train of stimuli or an effect on intracellular calcium.

Both phenomena are important when normal transmission is impaired, especially by curare-like drugs.

PHARMACOLOGY OF NEUROMUSCULAR BLOCK

Neuromuscular block may be produced by a variety of mechanisms. Only two are used therapeutically, but anaesthetists may be involved in resuscitation and intensive care of victims of other toxins. A brief classification of the types of block is contained in Table 12.2.

Table 12.2 Classification of types of neuromuscular block

Drugs preventing acetylcholine synthesis:
hemicholiniums.

Prevention of acetylcholine release:
botulinum toxin
high magnesium concentration

Depletion of acetylcholine stores:
black widow spider venom
funnel-web spider venom
β-bungarotoxin
tetanus toxin

Block of acetylcholine receptors:
α-bungarotoxin
non-depolarising relaxants
depolarising relaxants
myasthenia gravis.

Block of cholinesterase:
reversal agents, e.g. neostigmine, edrophonium
organophosphorus compounds

Non-depolarising acetylcholine antagonists

These drugs (of which tubocurarine was the first to be used clinically) act by combining with the postjunctional acetylcholine receptors without stimulation. Their actions may be overcome by increasing the acetylcholine concentration: thus they are competitive blockers.

The characteristics of a non-depolarising block are:

1. The block appears without any preceding stimulation.
2. During a partial block a train of nerve impulses (which normally produces a sustained tetanus) shows an initial contraction which fades.
3. Following a tetanic train of stimuli, single shocks lead to a temporary increase in the strength of the muscle twitch. This is termed post-tetanic potentiation, or facilitation or decurarisation.
4. The block is antagonised by drugs which mimic the action of acetylcholine (e.g. suxamethonium) or by drugs producing an increased local concentration of acetylcholine (anticholinesterases).

Two explanations of tetanic fade have been mentioned already. There is a third possibility. Experimentally, it can be shown that tubocurarine acts not only on the postjunctional receptor but may slip into an open ionophore to produce a block of ionic conductance. Obviously the channel in the ionophore has to be opened; this requires some acetylcholine–receptor interaction. Thus channel blocking becomes apparent during intense use and shows tetanic fade. It is uncertain if this mechanism occurs in humans in physiological conditions.

Depolarising drugs

Whilst the actions of drugs such as tubocurarine are relatively easy to explain, those of suxamethonium and decamethonium are less so. These drugs mimic the action of acetylcholine and result in an initial depolarisation and brief muscle contraction seen clinically as muscle fasciculations. The drugs are not destroyed by the cholinesterase present at the neuromuscular junction and the depolarisation persists. However, it is unable to trigger any more muscle action potentials at the zone of muscle membrane adjacent to the end-plate. There is a persistent current flowing into the end-plate which does not trigger the explosive increase in sodium conductance necessary to fire the muscle action potential. A similar finding occurs if acetylcholine is kept at a high concentration by using large doses of anticholinesterases. Depolarisation block is characterised by:

1. An initial period of muscle fasciculation.
2. An absence of tetanic fade during partial block.
3. An absence of post-tetanic facilitation.
4. Anticholinesterases may make the block more intense.

With prolonged administration, the characteristics of depolarisation block change and come to resemble those seen with non-depolarising agents. In particular, tetanic fade and post-tetanic facilitation develop gradually. The explanation of this altered pattern is by no means certain. It may be that the drugs *desensitise* the receptors and, in effect, reduce their numbers; or it may be a result of a prejunctional action. On occasion, this type of block may be antagonised by an anticholinesterase. Unfortunately this is not always so, and the block may be intensified. The safest therapy is to maintain anaesthesia and artificial ventilation and to wait. Testing with a nerve stimulator helps to determine when recovery has occurred.

CLINICAL PHARMACOLOGY OF NEUROMUSCULAR BLOCKING DRUGS

Non-depolarising drugs

Six non-depolarising drugs are available currently in the United Kingdom. In order of introduction, they are tubocurarine, gallamine, alcuronium, pancuronium, atracurium and vecuronium. Each produces the characteristic block described already, but they differ in potency, in duration of action and in side effects.

All the drugs are ionised and water-soluble and contain at least two charged nitrogen atoms. Most have two quaternary nitrogen groups. Tubocurarine and vecuronium have only one but they possess a second tertiary nitrogen group which at physiological pH attracts a hydrogen ion — thus they have two charged nitrogen atoms..

Table 12.3 summarises the doses used normally to initiate full neuromuscular block, and the average expected duration of effect; duration of effect is dose-related. Being charged water-soluble compounds, it may be expected that they should have volumes of distribution similar to the ECF volume. Because some bind to plasma proteins and other constituents of the body, some have higher volumes of distribution. Water-soluble charged molecules are excreted by the kidney;

Table 12.3 Dosage and pharmacokinetics of non-depolarising drugs

Drug	Tubocurarine	Gallamine	Alcuronium	Atracurium	Vecuronium	Pancuronium
Initial dose (mg/kg)	0.25–0.5	1–2	0.15–0.3	0.3–0.5	0.05–0.1	0.05–0.1
Duration of effect (min)	30–60	15–25	20–40	20–25	15–25	20–30
Maintenance dose (mg/kg)	0.1	0.5	0.1	0.15	0.015	0.015
Duration (min)	20–30	20–30	20–30	20	15	30
Volume of distribution, Vd_{ss}(1/kg)	0.61	0.24	0.32	0.16	0.27	0.31
Clearance (ml min^{-1} kg^{-1})	2.9	1.2	1.4	5.5	5.1	1.8
$T_{\frac{1}{2}}$ (min)	170	160	200	20	55	116

thus the clearance values of these drugs are of the same order as glomerular filtration rate. Some clearances are greater, and liver uptake and biliary excretion play a part in eliminating tubocurarine, pancuronium and vecuronium. Renal failure and impaired liver perfusion and function impair the excretion of these drugs. Atracurium is unique in that its elimination is not dependent on hepatic or renal function (vide infra). Table 12.3 summarises the volumes of distribution, clearances and elimination half-lives. It shows also the size of incremental doses used commonly to maintain paralysis and the expected duration of effect of these doses.

The onset of block with these drugs depends on the dose used. With all drugs, if a dose is used which does not produce complete paralysis, it may take some 3–5 min to produce a maximal effect. Shorter onset times are seen with larger doses but with the penalty of prolonged recovery.

The duration of block with all drugs is variable. Coefficients of variation of 25% or more are usual even when doses are standardised for body mass. Factors increasing the duration include:

1. Poor renal function — especially in the elderly.
2. Pre-existing liver disease.
3. The use of inhalational anaesthetics, especially enflurane and diethyl ether. Halothane has a lesser potentiating effect.
4. The use of suxamethonium to facilitate tracheal intubation.
5. Pre-existing disease, especially myasthenia gravis and the myasthenic syndrome associated classically with carcinoma of the bronchus.
6. Hypokalaemia.
7. Acidosis may delay recovery; it is not clear if this is a direct action or an effect on excretion.

Side effects

The choice of a particular non-depolarising drug is often influenced by the side effects produced. Table 12.4 lists the common ones. It may be necessary to avoid the use of some of the drugs in some patients, but the side effects can be useful. For example, the combination of ganglion block and histamine release with tubocurarine produces hypotension. This may help in producing a bloodless field. In contrast, when it is necessary to maintain arterial pressure, pancuronium is a better choice with its mild sympathomimetic effect. Vecuronium and atracurium were selected for introduction as agents devoid of significant cardiovascular action at doses which produce complete neuromuscular block.

In addition to these effects it is probable that all these drugs can initiate an anaphylactoid reaction featuring skin rashes, bronchospasm, laryngeal oedema and hypotension. The anaesthetist must have available all the necessary equipment and drugs to cope with this life-threatening response.

Dosage

The degree of paralysis and duration of effect of non-depolarising neuromuscular blockers are dose-dependent. An initial dose at the upper end of the range shown in Table 12.3 produces profound paralysis, and may be used to facilitate tracheal intubation; doses at the lower end of the range result in sufficient relaxation for most surgical procedures if tracheal intubation has been performed after administration of suxamethonium. Maintenance doses should be approximately 25% of the initial dose, although a larger maintenance dose of atracurium is necessary because of its rapid metabolism.

Table 12.4 Side effects of non-depolarising drugs

Drug	Tubocurarine	Gallamine	Alcuronium	Atracurium	Vecuronium	Pancuronium
Histamine release	++		+	+	–	
Ganglion blockade	++				–	–
Vagal blockade		++		–	–	+
Sympathomimetic action				–	–	+

Curare (D-tubocurarine)

Curare was the first neuromuscular blocking drug to be introduced into anaesthetic practice (in 1942). It is a monoquaternary alkaloid obtained from the plant *Chondrodendron tomentosum*. After i.v. injection, it is bound to albumin. A dose of 0.5 mg/kg produces profound paralysis in approximately 3 min; a smaller dose is sufficient for surgical procedures if tracheal intubation has been performed after administration of suxamethonium. The duration of action is 30–60 min.

Curare causes ganglion blockade, which results in a dose-related reduction in arterial pressure; this is potentiated by cardiodepressant anaesthetic drugs. Hypotension produced by curare may be useful in reducing surgical bleeding (see Ch. 37), but is potentially dangerous in elderly patients and in those with ischaemic heart disease. Histamine is released in some patients, and may reduce arterial pressure further; bronchospasm may result also. Larger than normal doses are required in patients with hepatic disease.

Gallamine

This drug has a shorter duration of action than curare. It crosses the placenta more readily, and is contraindicated in obstetric practice. Gallamine causes a tachycardia by an atropine-like vagal blockade and possibly by direct β-adrenergic receptor stimulation. Consequently, it is an inappropriate drug in patients with a pre-existing tachycardia and in those with ischaemic heart disease.

Approximately 80% of gallamine is excreted by the kidney. The remainder is metabolised in the liver, but one of the water-soluble metabolites is an active neuromuscular blocking agent. Consequently, the duration of action of gallamine may be prolonged excessively in the presence of renal dysfunction or failure.

Alcuronium

Alcuronium is derived from the alkaloid toxiferin. It deteriorates if exposed to air or sunlight, and is stored in dark brown ampoules. Its onset of action is slightly more rapid than that of curare, and its duration of action a little shorter. It causes a moderate decrease in arterial pressure. Alcuronium is bound to serum albumin, and smaller doses are required in the presence of hypoalbuminaemia. Histamine release may occur occasionally. It is an excellent drug for procedures that are expected to last more than 30 min, provided that moderate hypotension is not contraindicated.

Pancuronium

This is a bisquaternary aminosteroid with no hormonal activity. It has a relatively long duration of action. Approximately 30% of the drug is excreted by the kidney, and it should not be used in the presence of renal failure. It is bound predominantly to globulin in plasma. Pancuronium causes release of noradrenaline, and this may result in a moderate increase in heart rate and arterial pressure. Although myocardial stimulation may be useful in the hypotensive patient, the tachycardia induced by pancuronium may be undesirable if the heart rate is already elevated (e.g. hypovolaemia, septic shock), and also in the patient with ischaemic or valvular heart disease.

Vecuronium

This drug is also a steroid, with the structure modified to produce a shorter duration of action than that of pancuronium. A solution of vecuronium is stable for only approximately 24 h, and the drug is presented as a white powder which is dissolved in water (2 mg/ml) immediately before use. Vecuronium acts rapidly (within 2 min) and has a duration of action of approximately 20 min. Restoration of neuromuscular function is more rapid than with the older agents when the effects of the drug begin to wear off. Consequently, it may be preferable to infuse vecuronium during a long procedure, adjusting the rate according to assessment of neuromuscular function by a nerve stimulator (vide infra).

Vecuronium is devoid of cardiovascular actions, and is one of the two agents of choice when cardiovascular stability is required. It is metabolised in the liver to inactive products and may be used safely in patients with renal failure. Its duration of action may be prolonged in the presence of hepatic dysfunction.

Atracurium

This agent has attracted particular interest because of the mechanism of its elimination. Atracurium degrades spontaneously by a process termed 'Hofmann degradation' and alkaline ester hydrolysis. The rate of degradation is influenced by pH and temperature; in normothermic man, the elimination half-life is approximately 20 min. Thus, unlike all other non-depolarising relaxants, the elimination of atracurium does not depend on hepatic or renal function. The principal metabolite, laudanosine, has a very prolonged half-life and may cause CNS effects, including convulsions, in animals; however, no such occurrences have been reported in man, even after very prolonged use. Ampoules of atracurium should be stored in a refrigerator to reduce the rate of degradation of the molecule.

In most patients, atracurium has virtually no effect on arterial pressure or heart rate. However, histamine is released in some patients, and may cause flushing and hypotension; the incidence is reduced if the drug is administered slowly (over 60–90 s).

When recovery from neuromuscular blockade starts, it proceeds rapidly. Thus, an infusion technique is preferable if prolonged surgery is contemplated. Neuromuscular function should be assessed. The average infusion rate is 0.5 mg kg^{-1} h^{-1}.

Atracurium is the drug of choice in patients with severe hepatic or renal disease. It is indicated also if cardiovascular stability is required, although the possibility of histamine release should be borne in mind. It may be the most appropriate agent when neuromuscular blockade is required in patients who require intensive therapy.

Pipecuronium

This is a new agent which may be made available in the United Kingdom. It is an analogue of pancuronium. Approximately 40% of the drug is excreted by the kidneys. It has very little effect on the cardiovascular system. The dose is 0.5 mg/kg.

Depolarising drugs

Suxamethonium, suxethonium and decamethonium are the three depolarising agents available currently. Of these, suxamethonium is the most popular. Suxamethonium is available as a solution and some deterioration occurs if it is not stored at 4°C. Suxethonium is very similar and is available as a powder.

Dosage of suxamethonium

Tracheal intubation is usually carried out easily after an i.v. injection of 1 mg/kg. The drug may be given by i.m. injection in double these doses. Neonates also appear to need a somewhat greater dose.

In adults, 1 mg/kg produces apnoea which usually lasts approximately 5 min. Complete recovery of hand muscle paralysis takes another 5 min.

Paralysis may be maintained using further bolus i.v. injections of 0.25–0.5 mg/kg or using a continuous infusion with a solution of 1 or 2 mg/ml. The rate of infusion should be adjusted by monitoring its effect by means of a nerve stimulator. Tachyphylaxis occurs commonly and the character of the block changes gradually from that associated normally with depolarising drugs to the pattern seen with competitive agents ('desensitisation block'). The first signs of a change may occur as early as 10 min following the initial injection.

Metabolism of suxamethonium

The ester links in the molecule are vulnerable and metabolism is catalysed by the enzyme plasma cholinesterase. Normally, this is present in sufficient concentration to ensure a half-life of approximately 4 min for suxamethonium. The production of the enzyme is controlled genetically and five variants of the enzyme are known.

Patients homozygous for atypical enzymes do not destroy suxamethonium. These patients are sensitive to the effects of the drug and a normal dose may result in respiratory paralysis for 2 h or more. Recovery is associated with a desensitisation block. Treatment is based on artificial ventilation and maintenance of anaesthesia until recovery occurs. Subsequently, the patient and the family should be investigated to determine the nature and extent of the abnormality. Susceptible patients should carry a warning card to help prevent subsequent mishaps.

Low concentrations of normal plasma cholinesterase are found also in patients undergoing plasmapheresis, in those using ecothiopate eye drops and in those with terminal liver cell failure. The normal half-life of plasma cholinesterase is approximately 2 weeks.

Side effects and dangers of suxamethonium

The muscle relaxation produced by suxamethonium is profound, of rapid onset and, usually, ephemeral. No other neuromuscular blocking drug matches these desirable properties and the drug is still in common use despite considerable disadvantages from the following side effects.

Malignant hyperthermia. Suxamethonium is the most potent triggering agent to induce malignant hyperthermia in susceptible subjects (see p. 417).

Hyperkalaemia. The depolarisation produced by suxamethonium leads to movement of potassium from the intracellular to the extracellular space. Some patients may exhibit a very large potassium flux and develop dangerous increases in serum potassium concentration. The following groups are susceptible:

1. Patients with severe burns.
2. Patients with extensive muscle damage.
3. Paraplegic patients.
4. Patients with a peripheral neuropathy.

The patients in the first three groups develop the problem gradually. There is no problem immediately after an injury; susceptibility develops one week later. Patients with hyperkalaemia and renal failure are less at risk unless they have peripheral neuropathy.

Arrhythmias. A bradycardia, which may lead to cardiac arrest, is common, especially in children given repeated i.v. injections. The slowing is usually maximal after the third or fourth injection. Atropine should be used before administering multiple doses of suxamethonium.

Muscle pain. Patients, especially young, ambulant women, may develop severe muscle pains on the day after receiving suxamethonium. The fasciculations may produce tearing of muscle fibres and local small haemorrhages. Up to 50% of patients experience pains after suxamethonium administration. The incidence is reduced if a small dose of a non-depolarising drug is given (e.g. gallamine 20 mg) 1–2 min before the suxamethonium. As many of the non-depolarising drugs have some protective action against depolarising drugs the dose of suxamethonium may need to be increased by 30–50%; pancuronium, having a mild anticholinesterase action, is an exception.

Intraocular (and intracranial) pressure. Suxamethonium causes a transient increase in intraocular and, to a lesser extent, intracranial pressure. Part of this effect results from increases in arterial and venous pressures. There is also prolonged contracture of the extraocular muscles. This effect is important if intraocular pressure is raised or if there is an open injury to the eye as it may result in loss of intraocular contents. If the use of suxamethonium cannot be avoided, pretreatment with a small dose of a non-depolarising drug attenuates the risk of extrusion of ocular contents.

Anaphylactoid reactions have been reported and may prove fatal. Patients claiming to be sensitive to suxamethonium should be assessed to see if they have atypical cholinesterase as opposed to drug allergy.

Myotonia. Patients develop a contracture with suxamethonium.

Decamethonium

This produces a longer duration of effect than an equipotent dose of suxamethonium. The block commences with a depolarisation pattern and transforms slowly to the non-depolarising pattern. It has little effect on the cardiovascular system. A dose of 4–6 mg is suggested for adults, with a maximum dose of 10 mg.

Anticholinesterase drugs and reversal of block

The actions of non-depolarising neuromuscular blocking drugs normally are, and those of depolarising drugs given over a long period may be, antagonised by increasing the local concentration of acetylcholine at the end-plate. Three anticholinesterase drugs are used clinically: edrophonium, neostigmine and pyridostigmine. Neostigmine is the most potent and a dose of 30 to 50 μg/kg is usually sufficient. Pyridostigmine is used in a dose of 0.1–0.2 mg/kg. Edrophonium in a dose of 0.5 to 1 mg/kg is also effective and of sufficient duration of action not to lead to a loss of action before the concentration of blocker has decreased to a safe level.

In attempting to antagonise a non-depolarising block, it should be remembered that the more intense the paralysis, the slower is the onset of action of the anticholinesterase. It may be impossible to reverse a block within the first few minutes after administration of the neuromuscular blocker, especially if atracurium has been used.

Non-depolarising block may not be reversed by administration of an anticholinesterase drug if caused, or contributed to, by acid-base or electrolyte abnormalities or by aminoglycoside antibiotics.

Neostigmine

This anticholinesterase is used most commonly to antagonise the effects of non-depolarising neuromuscular blockers. It stimulates all cholinergic synapses, including autonomic ganglia and postganglionic parasympathetic nerve endings. The parasympathetic (muscarinic) effects predominate and result in bradycardia, intestinal peristalsis and spasm, bronchial and salivary secretions, contraction of the bladder and occasionally bronchospasm. These effects are counteracted by the administration of atropine (15–20 μg/kg) or glycopyrronium (10 μg/kg) either immediately before, or with, neostigmine.

The maximum effect on the neuromuscular junction does not occur until 3–5 min after administration of neostigmine. Its duration of action is 20–30 min; if significant concentrations of neuromuscular blocker remain in the circulation after this time (e.g. in renal failure), muscle power may deteriorate and a further dose of neostigmine may be necessary.

Normally, a dose of 2.5 mg is used in the adult (50–80 μg/kg in the child), but additional increments may be given carefully up to a total dose of 5 mg.

The effect of neostigmine on the bowel has been implicated as a cause of disruption of intestinal anastomoses. In large doses, neostigmine may induce neuromuscular blockade by increasing the concentration of acetylcholine at the neuromuscular junction. Approximately 50% of neostigmine is excreted by the kidney and its duration of action is prolonged in patients with renal insufficiency.

Edrophonium

This agent has a more rapid onset of action than neostigmine; atropine or glycopyrronium should be given approximately 1 min before edrophonium to prevent muscarinic effects. The muscarinic effects may be less severe than those associated with neostigmine administration. The duration of action of edrophonium 10 mg is approximately 10 min, and further doses are required if neuromuscular blockade returns. However, larger doses (50–70 mg) result in a more prolonged duration of action. A dose of 0.5–1 mg/kg is recommended for reversal of neuromuscular blockade.

Pyridostigmine

This drug has a slower onset and more prolonged duration of action than neostigmine. Its muscarinic effects are claimed to be less severe. A dose of 0.1–0.2 mg/kg (given with atropine or glycopyrronium) is satisfactory for reversal of neuromuscular blockade.

ASSESSMENT OF NEUROMUSCULAR BLOCK

At the end of any anaesthetic during which neuromuscular blocking drugs are used, the anaesthetist must be certain that there is no residual block before discharging the patient to the recovery room. Consequently, the assessment of the nature and degree of block is vital.

Clinical assessment

It is relatively easy to ask a conscious patient to produce a tetanic contraction of a muscle group. Lifting the head above a pillow for 5 s, ability to cough, protruding the tongue, or sustaining a hand grip are examples of readily available methods (Table 12.5). Measurements available include monitoring of tidal and minute volumes and vital capacity. The last is preferable as many patients, even when partially paralysed, have enough muscle power to maintain a normal minute volume. In unconscious patients, the presence of adequate tidal and minute volumes or a normal arterial carbon dioxide tension does not necessarily indicate that recovery is complete. It is useful to examine the pattern of breathing; partially paralysed patients often have an uncoordinated pattern with the diaphragm contracting but the intercostal muscles paralysed, resulting in a see-saw pattern of breathing (paradoxical respiration).

Nerve stimulators

The use of an electrical nerve stimulator should ensure that no patient is left partially paralysed without adequate ventilatory support.

The nerve stimulator uses an electrical pulse to depolarise all motor nerve fibres in a peripheral nerve. Acetylcholine is released at all the nerve terminals to produce maximum depolarisation at the muscle receptors (supramaximal stimulation). The evoked muscle response may be observed visually by the anaesthetist, palpated, or recorded as either the electrical activity (EMG) or the force produced (force transducer). The electrical pulses may be delivered as single shocks, as a sequence of high-frequency pulses to evoke a tetanic contraction or as trains at lower frequencies.

Table 12.5 Clinical assessment of adequacy of neuromuscular transmission

1. Grip strength	subjective
2. Adequate cough	subjective
3. Ability of the patient to sustain a head lift for at least 5 s	
4. Ability to produce a vital capacity of at least 10 ml/kg body weight	

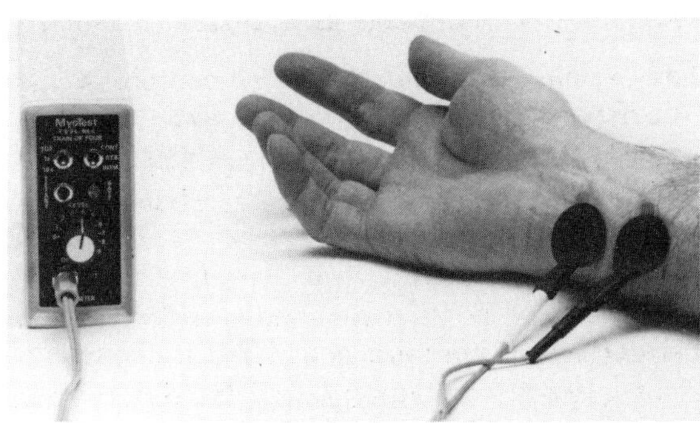

Fig. 12.2 The Myotest nerve stimulator.

Figure 12.2 shows a commercial instrument for delivering single twitches and trains of four.

Parameters for stimulators

In order to depolarise the nerve fibres, it is essential to apply an adequate current for a sufficient period of time. Using stimuli applied through the skin, a current of up to 50 mA may be needed for between 0.2 and 1.0 ms. This requires a voltage of the order of 50–300 V. The current passed is unlikely to cause any adverse cardiac effects.

Extending the duration of the pulse to longer than 2 ms may produce a double activation of the nerve because there is an 'off' effect when the duration exceeds the refractory period of the fibres.

Motor nerve fibres, being of the largest size, are the easiest to excite electrically. In conscious patients it is possible usually to evoke muscle contraction without undue pain. Tetanic stimulation rates are often an exception to this.

Patterns of stimulation

The correct use of a nerve stimulator should enable the anaesthetist to determine if neuromuscular transmission is normal, totally blocked or partially blocked. If partially blocked it is possible to estimate the type and degree of block. Three patterns of stimulation are useful and the effects may be observed visually (Fig. 12.3) or recorded on a chart recorder using a force transducer attached to the thumb (Fig. 12.4).

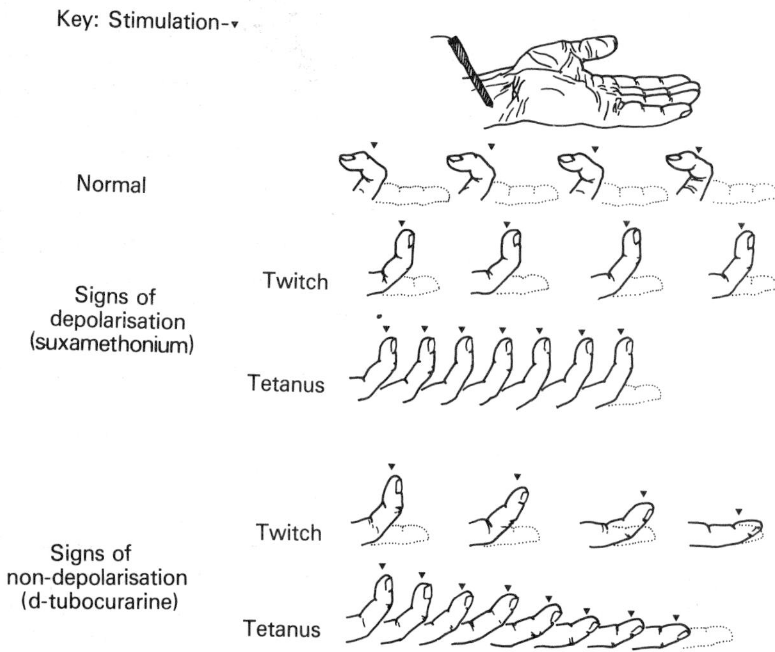

Fig. 12.3 Effects of single twitch and tetanic stimulation assessed by observation of finger movement.

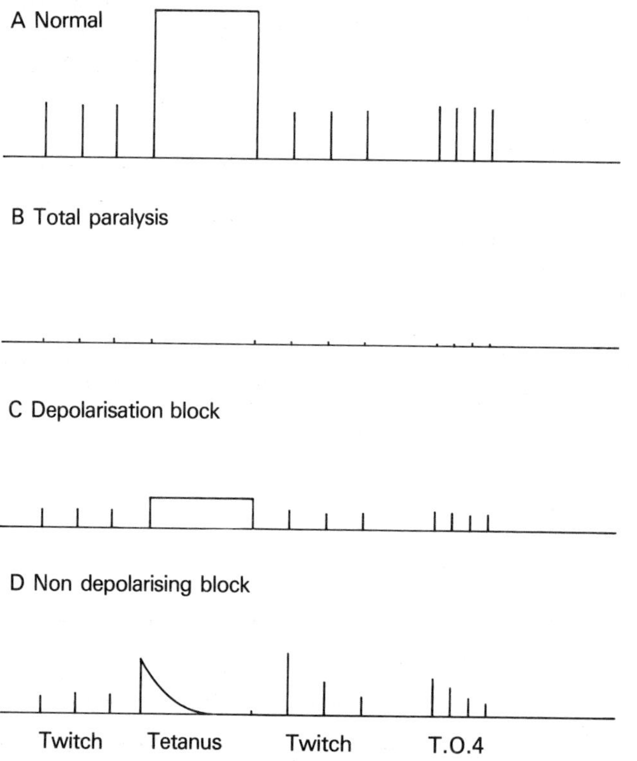

Fig. 12.4 Effects of single twitch, tetanus and train-of-four (T.O.4) assessed by a force transducer recording contraction of the adductor pollicis muscle.

1. *Twitch–tetanus–twitch*. A train of single shocks given at a rate of not more than 1 every 3 s is followed by a tetanic train (at 50 Hz or more) for 3 s and the train of single shocks is repeated. Four basic patterns of response are seen (Fig. 12.5).

  a. *Normal response*: twitch response followed by a strong sustained tetanic contraction and no potentiation of the post-tetanic twitches as compared with the pretetanic twitches.
  b. *Total block*. No responses.
  c. *Partial depolarising block*. The twitch responses are weak followed by a weak but sustained tetanic contraction. There is no post-tetanic potentiation.
  d. *Partial non-depolarising block*. The initial twitch responses are weak, the tetanic train evokes a contraction which fades rapidly and the post-tetanic twitches are markedly potentiated compared with the pretetanic twitches. A similar pattern is seen in myasthenia gravis.

2. *Train-of-four*. The continued use of the twitch–tetanus–twitch sequence is not advisable in routine monitoring. Continual high-frequency stimulation leads to some local reversal of block and in conscious subjects it is painful. However, the pattern of fade is seen at much lower stimulation frequencies without producing excessive local reversal. The train-of-four technique (Fig. 12.4) uses four stimuli given at 0.5 s intervals. It may be repeated every 10 s without significant loss of information. The results are interpreted in the same way as is the response to a tetanic burst.

The train-of-four ratio is calculated as the ratio of the force generated by the fourth contraction compared with the force of the first contraction; a force transducer is required. As transducers are not used widely, the train-of-four count is of more clinical relevance (Table 12.6). As recovery from total paralysis occurs, the first response seen is a twitch response with the first stimulus, then a response also to the second; later still the third and finally the fourth appear. The number of stimuli which evoke contractions is the train-of-four count. The lower the count the more paralysed is the patient. The higher the count the more easily a non-depolarising block is antagonised. Abdominal surgery using a thiopentone–opioid–relaxant sequence is possible usually with train-of-four counts of one or two (Table 12.6 and Fig. 12.5).

3. *Post-tetanic twitch count*. Frequently the stimulation patterns described produce no response. If a non-depolarising blocking drug has been used, one further test is possible. The nerve is stimulated at a frequency of 1 Hz, and subsequently a tetanic train at 50 Hz is applied for 5 s followed by stimulation at 1 Hz. The number of post-tetanic stimuli which evoke potentiated and detectable twitches is counted. There are usually about 12 to 20 before the train-of-four count detects the

Table 12.6 The train-of-four count

No. of twitches present (count)	Extent of block
1, 2, 3	75%
1, 2	80%
1	90%
None	100%

Note: The normal working range during anaesthesia is usually 75–95% block (see Fig. 12.5) with non-depolarising blockers.

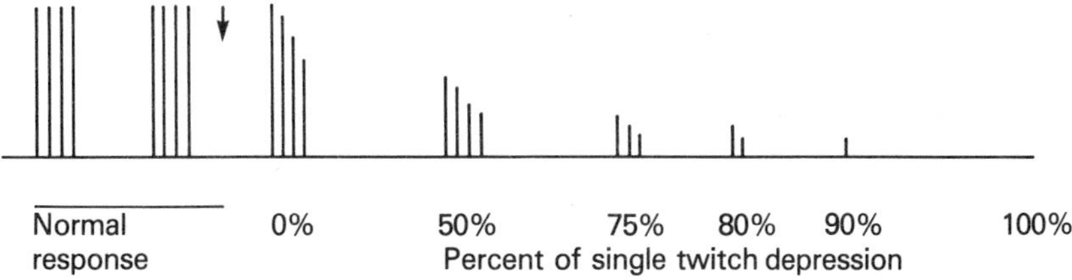

Fig. 12.5 Train-of-four (T.O.4) stimulation observed with a transducer and recorder permitting assessment of both T.O.4 count (Table 12.6) and T.O.4 ratio. The T.O.4 ratio is the ratio of the height of the 4th to the 1st twitch. A ratio greater than 70% indicates adequate neuromuscular transmission following non-depolarising blockers. The T.O.4 is more sensitive than single twitches: a T.O.4 count of two corresponds to 80% blockade of a single twitch response.

first response. Reversal of block is usually easy if the post-tetanic count is more than 10. (N.B. The absence of any response to a train-of-four does not necessarily imply that a block cannot be reversed easily.)

The first pattern of twitch–tetanus–twitch is useful for diagnosing block and the other two patterns help in the clinical administration of neuromuscular blocking drugs.

The successful use of nerve stimulators demands knowledge of the anatomical position of motor nerves. The ulnar at the elbow and the median and ulnar at the wrist are accessible, as are the facial nerve and the lateral popliteal nerve. With surface electrodes, it is useful to clean the skin thoroughly with a degreasing agent and apply a conductive jelly electrode.

Clinical use of nerve stimulation

It can be argued that a peripheral nerve stimulator should be used in every patient when blocking drugs are used in order to detect abnormal responses and to act as a guide to the need for incremental doses. A stimulator is particularly useful in the following situations:

1. When prolonged anaesthesia is undertaken.
2. In patients with renal or hepatic dysfunction.
3. In patients with known sensitivities.
4. When infusion techniques are used.
5. Where there is doubt regarding antagonism of block.
6. When new drugs are being investigated.
7. In patients with myasthenia or myasthenic syndromes.
8. In the ICU to assess any residual block and especially if it is necessary to make a diagnosis of brain death.

Evoked electromyography (EEMG)

This technique is a convenient but expensive alternative to the use of muscle contraction in assessing neuromuscular blockade. If an electrical stimulus is applied over a motor nerve, a compound action potential may be detected by a recording electrode positioned over the muscle. A computerised device is available for measurement of EEMG in anaesthesia. This produces a display of the height of the evoked response as a percentage of the control response (before administration of the neuromuscular blocking drug), and computes the train-of-four ratio automatically. Although the EEMG does not equate precisely with the force of contraction evoked by electrical stimulation, it is easy to use and has been employed extensively as a research tool.

FURTHER READING

Bowman W C 1980 Pharmacology of neuromuscular function. John Wright & Sons, Bristol

Bowman W C, Rand M J 1980 Textbook of pharmacology, 2nd edn. Blackwell Scientific Publications, Oxford

Katz B 1966 Nerve, muscle and synapse. McGraw-Hill, New York

Katz R L (ed) 1975 Monographs in anesthesiology, vol 3: muscle relaxants. Excerpta Medica, Amsterdam

Zaimis E 1976 Neuromuscular junction: handbook of experimental pharmacology, vol 42. Springer Verlag, New York

13. Drugs affecting the autonomic nervous system

THE AUTONOMIC NERVOUS SYSTEM

The term autonomic nervous system (ANS) refers to the nervous and humoral mechanisms which modify the function of the 'autonomous' or 'automatic' organs. These organs or functions include heart rate and force of contraction, calibre of blood vessels, contraction and relaxation of smooth muscle in gut, bladder and bronchi, visual accommodation and pupillary size, and secretion from exocrine and other glands. The ANS may be subdivided into two separate entities, the parasympathetic and sympathetic systems, on the basis of anatomical and pharmacological criteria. In order to understand the action of drugs on the ANS it is necessary initially to review these subdivisions briefly.

Parasympathetic system

The neuronal components of the parasympathetic system arise from cell bodies of the motor nuclei of the cranial nerves, III, VII, IX and X in the brain stem, and from the sacral segments of the spinal cord. The preganglionic fibres run almost to the organ innervated and synapse in ganglia within the organ, giving rise to postganglionic fibres which innervate the relevant tissues. The ganglion cells may be well organised as in the myenteric plexus of the intestine or diffuse as in the bladder or blood vessels. The chemical transmitter both at pre- and postganglionic synapses is acetylcholine (ACh). The neurotransmitter is stored in the presynaptic terminal in agranular vesicles, released by neuronal depolarisation, and acts at specific receptor sites on the postsynaptic terminal. Its activity is terminated by diffusion from the site of action and more specifically by degradation by acetylcholinesterase.

Based upon the actions of the alkaloids muscarine and nicotine, the specific receptor sites within the parasympathetic nervous system have been subdivided pharmacologically. Thus, the actions of ACh at the postganglionic neuroeffector site are mimicked by muscarine and are termed muscarinic, whereas preganglionic transmission is termed nicotinic. ACh is also the transmitter substance released from voluntary nerve endings at the neuromuscular junction. The receptor sites in this situation are also nicotinic; the pharmacology of drugs acting at this site is described in Chapter 12. Although it is possible to modify transmission at the preganglionic (nicotinic) site, drugs active at this site (ganglion-blocking drugs) are now rarely used clinically and we shall concentrate primarily in this chapter on drugs active at the postganglionic muscarinic site.

Sympathetic nervous system

The preganglionic fibres of the sympathetic nervous system arise in the cell bodies in the lateral horn of the spinal cord associated with spinal segments T1 to L2, the so called 'thoracolumbar' outflow. The first synapse occurs shortly after leaving the spinal cord in the sympathetic ganglionic chain, and gives rise to postganglionic fibres which innervate the effector organs. ACh is the transmitter, via a nicotinic receptor, at the preganglionic synapse (as in the parasympathetic ganglia). The adrenal medulla is innervated by preganglionic fibres from the thoracolumbar outflow, activation of which stimulates, via nicotinic ACh receptors, the release of adrenaline from this gland. At the postganglionic sympathetic endings, chemical transmission is mediated by noradrenaline, which is present in the presynaptic terminals as well as the adrenal medulla. Adrenaline is found in only insignificant amounts in the nerve endings and is released primarily as a circulating hormone from the adrenal medulla. Adrenaline and noradrenaline are composed of a basic ring structure with –OH groups in the 3 and 4 positions in relationship to a side chain ending in an amine subgroup (Fig. 13.1). Both catecholamines are synthesised from the essential amino acid phenylalanine via a number of steps including the production of dopamine, which may act as a precursor for both adrenaline and noradrenaline when administered exogenously (vide infra). The action of noradrenaline released from granules in the presynaptic terminals is terminated by diffusion from the site of action, reuptake back into the presynaptic nerve ending, and metabolism locally by the enzyme catechol-*o*-methyltransferase.

The actions of the catecholamines are mediated by specific postsynaptic cell surface receptors. Pharmacological subdivision of these receptors was first suggested by Ahlquist in 1948 into two groups (α and β) based upon the effects of adrenaline at peripheral sympathetic sites. These were originally termed excitatory and inhibitory receptors, respectively, because of their general tendency to produce those effects when stimulated, but as many exceptions to this general rule have been found, they are now referred to solely as α- and β-adrenoceptors. Since Ahlquist's original observations, further subdivision of both these receptor systems has been proposed on both functional and anatomical grounds. Thus, β-adrenoceptor-mediated events in the heart (β_1 effects; increase in force and rate of contraction) have been differentiated from those producing smooth muscle relaxation in bronchi and blood vessels (β_2 effects). Similarly, α-adrenoceptor-mediated postsynaptic events (e.g. vasoconstriction) have been termed α_1 effects to differentiate them from the feedback inhibition by noradrenaline of its own release from the presynaptic terminals mediated via an α_2-adrenoceptor on the presynaptic membrane. These various subdivisions are summarised in Table 13.1.

On the basis of more recent detailed pharmacological studies, it has become apparent that this

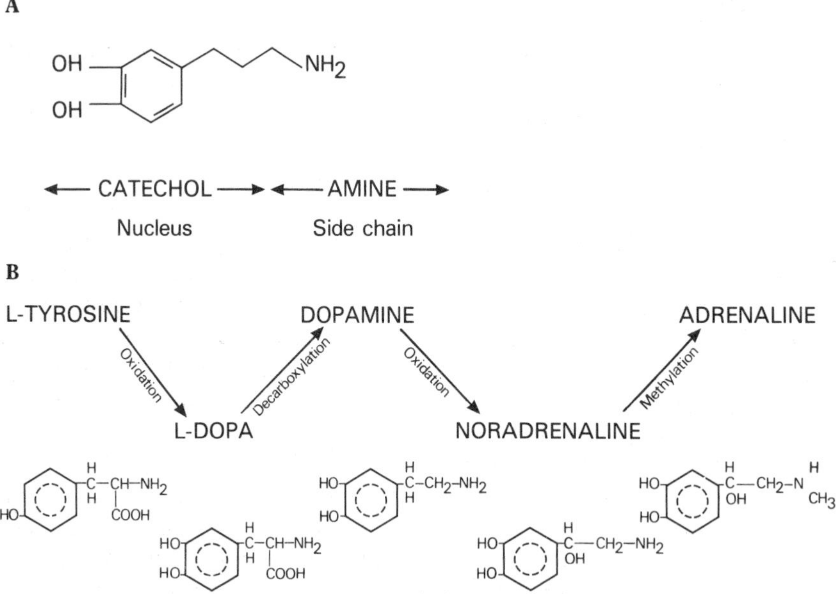

Fig. 13.1 (a) Standard molecular structure of catecholamines, composed of a 'catechol ring' with –OH substitution in the 3 and 4 positions relative to the 'amine side chain'. (b) Intermediate metabolism of naturally occurring catecholamines from the essential amino acid L-tyrosine.

Table 13.1 Responses of major effector organs to autonomic nerve impulses

Organ	Receptor subtype	Adrenergic	Cholinergic
Heart	β_1 (?β_2)	↑ Heart rate ↑ Force of contraction ↑ Automaticity and conduction velocity	↓ Heart rate ↓ Force of contraction ↓ Conduction velocity
Arteries	α_1 (?α_2) β_2	Constriction Dilatation	Dilatation
Veins	α_1 (?α_2) β_2	Constriction ++ Dilatation +	
Lung			
bronchial muscles	β_2	Relaxation +	Contraction ++
bronchial glands	?	(? Inhibition)	Stimulation +
GI tract			
motility	β_2 (?α_2)	Decrease	Increase +++
sphincters	α	Contraction	Relaxation
Kidney	β_2	Renin secretion	
Bladder			
detrusor	β_2	Relaxation	Contraction +++
sphincter	α	Contraction	Relaxation ++
Liver	β_2, α	Glycogenolysis ++ Gluconeogenesis +	? Glycogen synthesis
Uterus	β_2, α	Pregnant contraction (α) Non-pregnant relaxation (β)	

anatomical subdivision of the adrenoceptor subtypes is an oversimplification. Thus, most organs and tissues contain both β_1- and β_2-adrenoceptors, which may even subserve the same function. Differentiation of β-adrenoceptor subtypes is now based more directly on the hierarchical potencies of various catecholamine agonists (isoprenaline, adrenaline and noradrenaline) and assessed on the basis of the functional or biochemical response of adrenoceptors in different tissues. Thus, at β_2-adrenoceptors, isoprenaline is more potent than adrenaline, which is more potent than noradrenaline. In contrast, adrenaline and noradrenaline are equipotent at β_1-adrenoceptors. It seems probable that postsynpatic β_1-adrenoceptors in tissues are associated closely with the noradrenergic neurone and respond to released noradrenaline, whereas β_2-adrenoceptors are at sites distant to the nerve terminals and are controlled principally by circulating adrenaline. In addition, it is now well established that α_1- and α_2-adrenoceptors exist postsynaptically and subserve the function of vasoconstriction of resistance vessels which control arterial pressure and tissue perfusion.

However, for the purposes of general discussion of drugs acting on the sympathetic nervous system, the original anatomical subdivisions will be used and important departures from this scheme indicated where relevant. The important actions of the subdivisions of the ANS on various effector organs are summarised in Table 13.1.

Second messenger systems

Stimulation of catecholamine receptors on the extracellular surface of the cell membrane leads to activation of intracellular events by the generation of so-called second messengers. Thus, stimulation of the β-adrenoceptor leads, via coupling to the enzyme adenylate cyclase, to the generation of intracellular cyclic adenosine monophosphate (cAMP). Cyclic AMP in turn, via activation of intracellular enzyme pathways, produces the associated alteration in cell function (e.g. increased force of cardiac muscle contraction, liver glycogenolysis, bronchial smooth muscle relaxation). The concentration of intracellular cAMP is modulated also by the enzyme phosphodiesterase, which breaks down cAMP to its inactive form. Thus, the balance between production and degradation of cAMP is an important regulatory system for cell function. This somewhat simplified scheme is illustrated in Figure 13.2. The mechanism of transduction of the signal from the β-adrenoceptors across the cell membrane to the enzyme adenylate cyclase is incompletely understood, but almost certainly involves specialised intramembranous proteins that interact with guanine nucleotides.

Since β-adrenoceptor stimulation increases production of cAMP, its association with the enzyme adenylate cyclase is termed 'positive coupling'. The converse, receptor activation leading to reduction of intracellular cAMP, is termed 'negative coupling' to adenylate cyclase and this results from stimulation of the α_2-adrenoceptor (Fig. 13.2). An example of this 'negative coupling' is seen in α-adrenoceptor-mediated platelet aggregation, which is associated with a reduction in platelet cAMP content. The complex interactions between inhibitory (α_2) and stimulatory (β_1 and β_2) effects on cAMP in a single cell are still incompletely understood.

The α_1-adrenoceptor does not affect cAMP levels within the cell directly. Activation of this receptor produces changes in membrane transfer of Ca^{2+} and in intracellular calcium binding which lead, for example, to smooth muscle contraction. The mechanism whereby the α_1-adrenoceptor alters transmembrane ionic flux is related probably to receptor-activated changes in membrane phospholipid content and the modulation of calcium channels.

DRUG EFFECTS ON THE SYMPATHETIC NERVOUS SYSTEM

Drugs which partially or completely mimic the effects of sympathetic nerve stimulation or adrenal medullary discharge are termed sympathomimetic. A wide variety of drugs has sympathomimetic

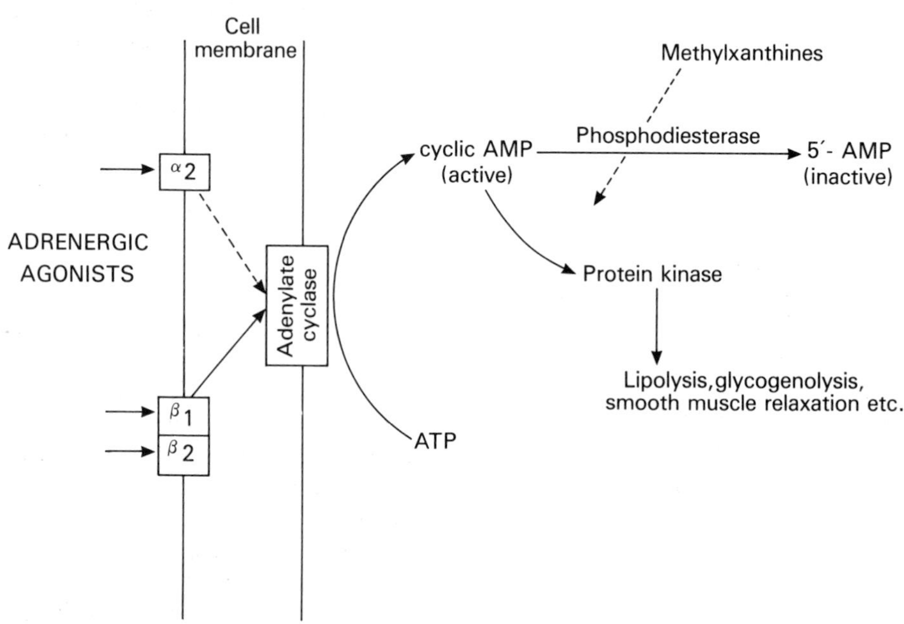

Fig. 13.2 Relationship between adrenergic agonists and the production of cyclic AMP. Binding of agonist to the adrenoceptors on the cell surface membrane activates either stimulation (→β_1, β_2) or inhibition (⇢ α_2) of the enzyme adenylate cyclase which catalyses the conversion of ATP to cyclic AMP and is, in turn, inactivated by the intracellular enzyme, phosphodiesterase. Cyclic AMP interacts with cytoplasmic protein kinase to initiate various cell functions.

activity, and they may be classified into drugs which act:

1. Directly on the adrenoceptor, e.g. the catecholamines adrenaline, noradrenaline and isoprenaline.
2. Indirectly, causing release of noradrenaline from the adrenergic nerve ending, e.g. amphetamine, ephedrine.
3. By both mechanisms, e.g. dopamine.

The major clinical effects of these drugs are produced via α- or β-adrenoceptors or both (dopamine also acts via dopamine receptors — vide infra), and can be classified as follows.

Cardiovascular effects

Blood vessel calibre

Contraction and relaxation of smooth muscle in the blood vessel walls determine the calibre of the lumen and thus resistance to blood flow. Contraction of the smooth muscle produces vasoconstriction and increased peripheral resistance and is mediated via α-adrenoceptor stimulation. This comprises the normal physiological noradrenergic vasoconstrictor tone in the blood vessels. Conversely, relaxation of arterial smooth muscle produces vasodilatation via activation of β_2-adrenoceptors and is mediated physiologically by circulating adrenaline.

Cardiac contraction

Stimulation of the force and rate of cardiac contraction (inotropic and chronotropic effects respectively) is mediated via β-adrenoceptors in the heart muscle stimulated physiologically by both adrenaline and noradrenaline. Although the β_1-adrenoceptor is associated classically with this activity, recent functional and biochemical studies have indicated a role also for the β_2-adrenoceptors which are present in cardiac cells in these actions of sympathomimetic drugs.

Cardiac output

The overall effect of catecholamines on cardiac output depends on the interaction between effects on cardiac rate and contractility and changes in peripheral vascular resistance. Thus, adrenaline and isoprenaline increase cardiac output via positive inotropism coupled with peripheral vasodilatation. However, noradrenaline, particularly in high dosage, may reduce cardiac output by intense vasoconstriction despite an equally effective action on cardiac contractility.

Arterial pressure

The effects on arterial pressure depend on the balance of cardiac output and peripheral resistance and vary with the effects of different sympathomimetic agents. Drugs which increase peripheral resistance in addition to cardiac contractility are most effective in increasing arterial pressure, but this may be at the expense of intense and possibly damaging vasoconstriction.

Non-vascular smooth muscle

In general, non-vascular smooth muscle is relaxed by sympathomimetic drugs. This effect is generalised and mediated by the β_2-adrenoceptor. Thus, bladder wall smooth muscle and, more importantly, uterine smooth muscle may be relaxed by these drugs. The latter effect is more pronounced in the oestrogen-dominated uterus and sympathomimetic agents are used to reduce uterine contractility in threatened premature labour. Most important, however, is bronchodilation; drugs specifically active at β_2-adrenoceptors (β_2-agonists) are potent bronchodilators (see Chapter 14), in addition to possessing vasodilating properties.

Metabolic effects

The metabolic effects of sympathetic nervous stimulation are related to effects on glucose and lipid metabolism. Insulin release is partially under sympathetic control and is stimulated via activation of a β_2-adrenoceptor. Likewise, adrenaline-induced glycogenolysis in both the liver and muscles is β_2-adrenoceptor-mediated. Thus, the physiological response to adrenaline release includes an increase in insulin release and provision of sufficient substrate for its action.

Stimulation of β_2-adrenoceptors on adipocytes induces mobilisation and release of free fatty acids and results in increased blood concentrations.

Type 1 hypersensitivity

The release of mediators of anaphylaxis (histamine, SRS-A) from mast cells is inhibited by drugs which cause an increase in mast cell cyclic AMP levels, including some sympathomimetic compounds active via the β_2-adrenoceptor on the mast cell surface. This effect may be relevant to the use of these drugs in acute asthma, and particularly anaphylaxis.

DRUGS ACTING ON THE SYMPATHETIC NERVOUS SYSTEM

We shall consider the most commonly used sympathomimetic agents in relationship to this classification of actions and to their most common clinical usage in shock, hypotension and cardiac failure. The use of β-agonists as bronchodilators is discussed in Chapter 14.

Catecholamines

This group comprises naturally occurring and synthetic compounds which have a common molecular configuration based upon the catechol nucleus and amine side chain illustrated in Figure 13.1. Their effects are produced by interaction at specific catecholamine receptors (α, β and dopamine).

Adrenaline

Adrenaline has both α- and β-adrenergic effects. It is used mainly as a bronchodilator and in the treatment of acute allergic (anaphylactic) reactions. Except in emergency situations, i.v. injection is avoided because of the risk of inducing cardiac arrhythmias. Subcutaneous administration produces local vasoconstriction and a 'smoothed-out' effect by slowing absorption.

Adrenaline may be used by aerosol inhalation in bronchial asthma but its use in this context has been superseded largely by the newer β_2-agonists (Chapter 14). Intravenous adrenaline is used in cardiac arrest to provoke ventricular fibrillation if asystole has occurred, so that electrical defibrillation can be initiated. There has been considerable interest in the administration of adrenaline by the tracheal route in emergency situations. Although apparently successful in animal models, absorption from the lungs in human cardiac arrest is limited and this route is not recommended.

The effects of adrenaline on arterial pressure and cardiac output are dependent on dose; although both α- and β-adrenoceptors are stimulated, β_2 vasodilatory effects are most sensitive. Thus, in large doses, direct stimulatory effects on cardiac output plus potent vasoconstriction (particularly in precapillary resistance vessels of skin, mucosa and kidney), produce a rapid increase in systolic arterial pressure. Diastolic pressure is affected less because of β_2 vasodilatation in muscle beds (the characteristic physiological redistribution of the circulation associated with adrenaline) and therefore pulse pressure widens. In low dosage, adrenaline may produce no overall effect on arterial pressure or a slight decrease with an increase in cardiac output.

Noradrenaline

In contrast to adrenaline, noradrenaline acts almost exclusively on α-adrenoceptors, although it is less potent at these receptor sites than adrenaline. Infusions of all doses of noradrenaline increase both systolic and diastolic arterial pressure by vasoconstriction of arteriolar and venous smooth muscle. Despite some stimulatory effects on cardiac contraction, the intense vasoconstriction leads either to no change or a decrease in cardiac output at the cost of increased myocardial oxygen demand. In high dosage the universal vasopressor effect reduces renal blood flow and glomerular filtration rate.

The problems of induction of cardiac arrhythmias, adverse effects on renal function and intense vasoconstriction (leading to ischaemia in the periphery) have limited the clinical use of this agent in hypotension and shock.

Isoprenaline

Isoprenaline has virtually no activity at α-adrenoceptors. Its main actions are via β-adrenoceptors in the heart, smooth muscle of bronchi, skeletal muscle vasculature and the gut. Intravenous infusion reduces peripheral resistance mainly in skeletal muscle but also in renal and mesenteric vascular beds. Cardiac output is raised by an increase in venous return to the heart, combined with the positive inotropic and chronotropic actions of the drug. This may result in an increase in systolic arterial pressure.

Bronchial smooth muscle is relaxed and this effect, combined with other β_2 effects on release of mast cell mediators, has led to its widespread use in asthma, although newer specific β_2-agonists are probably preferable because of less cardiac stimulation.

Isoprenaline is absorbed unreliably by sublingual or oral routes and is administered usually by i.v. infusion or aerosol. As a direct cardiac stimulant, its most important use is in increasing the rate of cardiac contraction in heart block by direct chronotropic action on the subsidiary pacemaker; this is usually an interim measure following acute myocardial infarction before insertion of a temporary pacing wire. Its use as a positive inotropic agent in septicaemic and cardiogenic shock has been superseded by newer agents.

Dopamine

Dopamine stimulates both α- and β-adrenoceptors in addition to specific dopamine receptors in renal and mesenteric arteries. The balance of agonist properties exhibited by dopamine is related closely to dosage. It is administered only by the i.v. route.

Dopamine has a direct positive inotropic action on the myocardium via β-adrenoceptors and also by release of noradrenaline from noradrenergic nerve terminals. In low dosage (2–5 $\mu g\ kg^{-1}\ min^{-1}$) the major effects of dopamine are reduction of regional arterial resistance in renal and mesenteric vascular beds by an action on specific dopamine receptors. The result is an increase in renal blood flow, glomerular filtration rate and sodium excretion. Slightly higher doses (5–10 $\mu g\ kg^{-1}\ min^{-1}$) lead to increasing direct inotropic action with little or no peripheral vasoconstrictor effects. This combination of increased cardiac output and renal vasodilatation is useful particularly in the management of cardiogenic, traumatic, septic and hypovolaemic shock, where excessive use of direct sympathomimetics associated with a major increase in physiological sympathetic activity may lead to severe compromise of renal blood flow and peripheral circulation. At these low and intermediate doses, direct cardiac chronotropic action is usually minimal, and tachyarrhythmias are less common than with other sympathomimetics. At these doses, dopamine increases systolic and pulse pressures, and has little effect on, or slightly increases, diastolic arterial pressure. Total peripheral resistance is usually unchanged.

In higher dosage ($> 15\ \mu g\ kg^{-1}\ min^{-1}$), dopamine produces pronounced α-adrenoceptor activity, with direct vasoconstriction and increased cardiac stimulation (simulating infusions of noradrenaline). In general, therefore, these higher dose rates should be avoided. Occasionally the combination of a direct acting vasodilator (e.g. sodium nitroprusside) and high-dose dopamine may be of use in cardiogenic shock, although results are generally not encouraging.

The half-life of dopamine is very short and therefore its effects are controlled readily by alteration of infusion rate.

Dobutamine

Dobutamine resembles dopamine chemically, but is primarily a β_1-agonist with little or no indirect activity. It has less β_2-agonist action than isoprenaline and no action at specific dopamine receptors. Dobutamine appears to be relatively more effective in enhancing cardiac contractile force than in increasing heart rate. Its effects on increasing sinus node automaticity, atrial and ventricular conduction velocity and enhancing A-V nodal conduction are less than those of isoprenaline. Recent experimental work in both animals and man indicates that dobutamine may exert some of its 'specific' inotropic action via myocardial α_1-adrenoceptors. This is suggested by inhibition of the increase in cardiac output by α-adrenergic blocking agents and the relative selectivity of the active stereoisomer of dobutamine for α-agonist effects in animal models.

Infusion of dobutamine at rates ranging from 2.5 to 15 $\mu g\ kg^{-1}\ min^{-1}$ produces a progressive increase in cardiac output. This is associated with increased systolic arterial pressure, as peripheral resistance does not decrease initially. A decrease in pulmonary artery wedge pressure occurs also, indicating reduced diastolic filling pressure of the left ventricle. Urine output and sodium excretion are increased, presumably secondarily to the improvement in cardiovascular status, as the drug has no direct effect on renal vascular resistance.

As the effects of dobutamine on heart rate and systolic arterial pressure are minimal in comparison with other catecholamines, oxygen demands on the myocardium may be increased to a lesser degree. Thus, dobutamine appears theoretically to have some advantages over other catecholamines for improving myocardial function in heart failure when peripheral resistance and heart rate are high; in this circumstance, combination with vasodilator drugs may increase efficacy.

Non-catecholamines

This group of drugs includes a large number of synthetic amines which have a wide variety of clinical actions mimicking those of the catecholamines in different combinations. These drugs may have direct actions at adrenergic receptors or may produce effects by causing release of catecholamines after first being taken up into sympathetic nerve terminals.

Those compounds which cause release of catecholamines (e.g. amphetamine, ephedrine) have considerable effects within the CNS and their use has been superseded largely by newer drugs with more specific and less unpredictable actions.

Compounds with a direct action at adrenergic receptors may affect α- or β-adrenoceptors selectively. Drugs with selective α-adrenoceptor effects are potent vasoconstrictor, e.g. phenylephrine, methoxamine. Their actions on the cardiovascular system are similar to those of noradrenaline, with its associated problems (vide supra). Phenylephrine is now used mostly as a nasal decongestant, a mydriatic or as a local vasoconstrictor in solutions of local anaesthetics. Absorption of phenylephrine from mucous membranes may occasionally produce systemic side effects. Drugs with a direct action at β-adrenoceptors have wider clinical use and will be considered in a little more detail.

Selective β_2-agonists

Compounds in this group include the drugs salbutamol, terbutaline, fenoterol and rimiterol. Because of their relative specificity for β_2-adrenoceptors these drugs relax smooth muscle of bronchi, uterus and vasculature whilst having much less stimulant effect on the heart than isoprenaline. However, these drugs are only partial agonists and their maximal stimulant activity even at β_2-adrenoceptors is less than that of isoprenaline.

The selective β_2-agonists are most widely used in the treatment of bronchospasm (see Ch. 14), thereby avoiding the direct and possibly toxic effects of isoprenaline on the heart. High dosage of these drugs by oral, i.v. or inhalational routes may still produce tachyarrhythmias and tremor.

The effects of these drugs on the cardiovascular system have been of interest recently in the treatment of cardiac failure. Intravenous administration of salbutamol decreases systemic vascular resistance and left ventricular filling pressure as a result of peripheral vasodilatation. There is a consequent increase in cardiac output in patients with cardiac decompensation. In moderate doses (13 μg/min) the changes in systemic arterial pressure and heart rate are small. These indirect positive inotropic effects are supplemented by direct action of salbutamol on cardiac function probably via β_2-adrenoceptors, which are present in cardiac muscle. In high doses, salbutamol is less selective and also has some stimulant activity on cardiac β_1-adrenoceptors which may limit its use because of tachycardia. Hypotension and reflex tachycardia produced by vasodilatation may also offset the advantages of decreasing myocardial work load. For these reasons, salbutamol may be less useful in cardiogenic shock than dopamine or dobutamine.

Selective β_1 agonists

Drugs with selective β_1 partial agonist properties have been developed from the group of β-adrenoceptor antagonists with intrinsic sympathomimetic (partial agonist) activity (vide infra). Enhancing the intrinsic activity of the β-blocking drugs produces compounds which, in low dosage, have stimulant activity at the β-adrenoceptor equivalent to approximately 40–50% of that of isoprenaline. In higher dosage, however, the agonist effect reaches a plateau and the resulting action of the drug on the heart rate is less than that of isoprenaline. In theory, drugs of this class would be useful for their positive inotropic effect, with no peripheral vasoconstrictor action, and a less direct chronotropic action on the heart than the catecholamines. Two experimental compounds in this group (with a chemical formula similar to practolol) have been investigated in man. The first, prenalterol, was considered originally to have pure β_1 effects, but also stimulates β_2-adrenoceptors in higher doses, possibly producing some vasodilatation. This pharmacological profile may be favourable in a drug for use in cardiac failure, i.e. positive inotropism (β_1) combined with afterload reduction (β_2 vasodilatation).

Unfortunately, prenalterol has been withdrawn because of possible carcinogenicity. The second preparation, xamaterol, possesses approximately 45% of the agonist activity of isoprenaline at β_1-adrenoceptors but no direct β_2 effects. It is under trial at present in patients with chronic heart failure.

In practice, use of these drugs in cardiac failure should be limited to situations of mild to moderate failure with low sympathetic drive. When high sympathetic activity is present, these drugs may exhibit the β-blocking activity expected of a partial agonist and thus worsen the clinical condition.

β-adrenoceptor antagonists

In general, the β-adrenoceptor antagonists (β-blockers) are similar structurally to the β-agonists, e.g. isoprenaline. However, alteration in molecular structure (primarily in the catechol ring) has produced compounds which do not activate adenylate cyclase and the second messenger system despite binding avidly to the β-adrenoceptor. These compounds possess high affinity for the receptor but little or no intrinsic activity and therefore inhibit competitively the effects of the naturally occurring catecholamines.

There is now a wide variety of β-blockers available for clinical use and choice of the appropriate agent is made more difficult. However, the general properties of these drugs are best reviewed collectively.

Pharmacodynamic properties of β-blockers

The properties of individual drugs are summarised in Table 13.2.

The relative potency of the β-blocking drugs is less important than their relative ability to antagonise selectively effects mediated by the β-adrenoceptor subtypes. Compounds are available which block preferentially either β_1- or β_2-adrenoceptors, although in clinical practice the β_1 or so-called 'cardioselective' drugs are more

Table 13.2 Pharmacological properties of β-adrenoceptor blockers

Drug	β-Blockade potency ratio; propranolol = 1	Approx. equiv. oral doses	Relative cardioselectivity	Partial agonist activity	Membrane stabilising effect
Acebutolol	0.3	100 mg	±	+	+
Atenolol	1	50 mg	+	0	0
Betaxolol	4	10 mg	+	–	–
Metoprolol	1	50 mg	+	0	±
Nadolol	2–4	20 mg	0	0	0
Oxprenolol	0.5–1	40–60 mg	0	++	+
Pindolol	6	5 mg	0	+++	+
Propranolol	1	40 mg	0	0	++
Sotalol	0.3	100 mg	0	0	0
Timolol	6	5 mg	0	±	0

important. However, β_1 selectivity is only a relative property and these drugs antagonise β_2 effects in higher doses. Practolol was the first drug to be developed with clinically useful cardioselectivity. More recent drugs are less cardioselective, e.g. atenolol, metoprolol and acebutolol. The clinical importance of cardioselectivity will be considered later.

Intrinsic sympathomimetic activity. The first drug shown to be capable of blocking β-adrenoceptors was dichloroisoprenaline. This compound has a very similar structure to isoprenaline, differing only in the substitution of two chlorine atoms for the —OH groups in the catechol ring. Because of this close similarity, it has some stimulant or agonist activity at the β-adrenoceptor, equivalent approximately to 50% of that of isoprenaline, i.e. it exhibits partial agonist or intrinsic sympathomimetic activity (ISA). This stimulant effect is apparent at low levels of sympathetic activity, but at high levels of sympathetic discharge blockade of endogenously released catecholamines is the major clinical effect. The clinical significance of ISA is largely theoretical, but may be of some practical importance as discussed later.

Membrane stabilising activity. Some β-blockers have a quinidine-like action on nerve and cardiac conducting tissue. This can be demonstrated in vivo as a stabilising effect on the cardiac action potential, reducing the slope of phase 4 noticeably, and thus decreasing excitability and automaticity of the myocardium (see Ch. 14). The membrane stabilising activity is thought to have little clinical significance generally, since it occurs at drug concentrations very much higher than those achieved ordinarily in plasma after usual therapeutic doses.

Pharmacokinetic properties of β-blockers

The pharmacokinetic properties of β-blockers are summarised in Table 13.3. All β-blockers are weak bases and most are well absorbed to produce peak plasma concentrations 1–3 h after oral administration. The effect of food is to delay the rate rather than reduce the extent of absorption. This is unlikely to have any important effect on chronic equilibrium concentrations of the drugs in plasma. An important characteristic of the highly metabolised β-blockers (e.g. propranolol) is their tendency to be affected by first pass through the liver. This reduces the bioavailability of the drugs, but this is offset by the fact that the 4-hydroxylated metabolites so formed are also active. The first-pass metabolism also tends to become saturated, so that proportionately higher plasma concentrations of the parent drug are achieved at higher oral doses. This adds an important complication to pharmacokinetic studies of these drugs,

Table 13.3 Pharmacokinetic properties of β-adrenoceptor blockers

	Half-life (h)	Volume of Distribution (litre/kg)	Bioavailability (%)	% Unchanged in urine	Is first-pass effect significant?	Active metabolites
Acebutolol	8	3.0	50*	35*	Yes	Yes
Atenolol	6–9	0.7	40	95	No	No
Betaxolol	12–16	—	90	90	No	No
Metoprolol	3–4	5.6	50	3	Yes	No
Nadolol	14–24	—	35	100	No	No
Oxprenolol	2	1.2	40	50	Yes	Yes
Pindolol	3–4	2.0	100	40	No	No
Propranolol	2–4	3.6	30	Under 1	Yes	Yes
Sotalol	5–13	2.4	100	75	No	No
Timolol	4	1.6	75	10	Yes	No

*includes active metabolites

which should include measurement of pharmacological effect to be useful. The first-pass effect is also a source of wide interindividual variation in plasma concentrations achieved from the same dose. Other highly metabolised β-blockers, metoprolol and acebutolol, also produce active metabolites.

Atenolol, nadolol, practolol, and sotalol are excreted largely unchanged in the urine and so are little affected by impairment of liver function. All β-blockers are distributed widely throughout the body and concentrations are present in the central nervous system. This is true particularly for the more lipid-soluble molecules (e.g. propranolol). Distribution is rapid over 5–30 min, so that after oral administration the β-blockers can be fitted to a one-compartment pharmacokinetic model, the distribution phase being of little clinical importance.

Most β-blockers have a half-life of 2–4 h. The less lipid-soluble drugs atenolol and practolol have longer half lives of 6–9 and 9–12 h respectively and nadolol has the longest (24 h). Although propranolol depends less on the kidney for elimination than other β-blockers, the possible accumulation of active metabolites, which are excreted renally, should be considered when these drugs are used in patients with renal failure. The plasma concentrations of unchanged propranolol are increased in uraemia.

Interindividual variation in plasma concentrations is less with drugs excreted renally than those primarily metabolised. The plasma concentration–response relationship also shows individual variation, possibly as a result of differences in level of sympathetic tone. β-Blockers have a flat dose–response curve, so that large changes in plasma concentration may give rise to only a small change in degree of β-blockade. Differences in the formation of active metabolites amongst highly metabolised β-blockers further complicates plasma concentration–response relationships.

Cardiovascular effects of β-blockers

Antiarrhythmic activity. Although the mechanism of antiarrhythmic action of β-blockers is unknown, it appears to be a property inherent in β-blockade itself, i.e. antagonism of catecholamine effects on the cardiac action potential and muscle contractility. The result is a slowing of rate of discharge from the sinus and any ectopic pacemaker, and slowing of conduction and increased refractoriness of the AV node. β-Blockers also retard conduction in anomalous pathways of the heart. The membrane stabilising properties do not appear relevant to the clinical antiarrhythmic effect. Most β-blockers have comparable antiarrhythmic properties in adequate dosage; choice is based therefore on tolerance to adverse effects. Sotalol has been shown to exhibit type III antiarrhythmic activity (see Ch. 14) and may have a more specific action in treatment of cardiac arrhythmias, in particular supraventricular tachycardia.

Negative inotropism. The action of catecholamine agonists on the force of contraction of cardiac muscle is antagonised by β-blockade. The resulting negative inotropic effect is of little significance in normal hearts but may be disastrous if increased sympathetic tone is supporting the 'failing' heart. In theory, compounds with ISA have less negative inotropism by virtue of their partial agonist activity. However, this putative benefit is of no practical use in cardiac failure when higher than normal sympathetic drive is present.

Antianginal activity. Angina pectoris occurs when oxygen demand exceeds supply. The oxygen demand of the left ventricle depends on contractility, heart rate and the pressure within the ventricle during systole. The reduction in heart rate caused by β-blockade results in a decrease in cardiac work, which reduces oxygen demand. A slower heart rate also permits longer diastolic filling time and this allows greater coronary perfusion. β-Blockade also reduces exercise-induced increases in arterial pressure, velocity of cardiac contraction and oxygen consumption at any work load.

All β-blockers, irrespective of other pharmacological properties, produce some degree of increased capacity for cardiac work in angina patients. They all limit the increase in heart rate during exercise but they differ in their effects on the heart at rest. Those with ISA have less effect on the resting heart rate; this is of benefit particularly in patients with an existing low heart rate as it reduces the risk of atrioventricular conduction disturbance. However, ISA may theoretically increase the metabolic demand of the myocardium. In practice, drugs without ISA may be more effective in patients with angina at rest or at very low levels of exercise.

Antihypertensive effect. β-Blockers are effective in controlling the arterial pressure of many hypertensive patients. The mechanism of action has not been elucidated fully but it is probable that some of the following are involved.

1. *A direct effect on the cardiovascular system.* This includes a reduction in cardiac output which correlates with a reduction in heart rate and some decrease in myocardial contractility. The significance of the reduction in heart rate is unclear, as β-blockers reduce cardiac output at rest and during exercise in paced hearts. After long-term oral treatment with β-blockers, cardiac output tends to return to pretreatment values.

2. *A reduction in sympathetic nervous activity.* This may be mediated by an action of β-blockers in the hypothalamus, altering central control of sympathetic tone. However, different drugs vary widely in their lipophilicity and consequent central nervous system penetration, but have similar effects on arterial pressure control. Thus, the significance of the central action of these drugs is uncertain.

3. *An effect on plasma renin concentrations.* β-blockers have variable effects on resting and orthostatic release of renin. The non-selective drugs propranolol and timolol cause the greatest reduction, while drugs with ISA (oxprenolol, pindolol) or β_1-selectivity are less effective. In addition, no correlation has been found between renin-lowering effect and antihypertensive activity of these drugs or with dosage of β-blocker used.

4. *An effect on peripheral resistance.* β-Blockade does not reduce peripheral resistance directly and may even cause an increase by allowing unopposed α-stimulation. As the vasodilating effect of catecholamines on skeletal muscle is β_2-mediated, unopposed α-stimulation would be expected to be less with cardioselective drugs or with those which possess ISA. However, cardioselectivity decreases with dosage and since hypertensive patients often require a large dose of β-blocker, little real advantage is offered. Drugs with ISA may not increase peripheral resistance as much as those without.

5. *The membrane stabilising effect.* This was considered of possible importance when early studies indicated that the antihypertensive effect of propranolol resembled that of quinidine. However, all β-blockers appear to reduce arterial pressure regardless of the presence of a membrane stabilising effect.

The full hypotensive effect of β-blockers is not achieved until about two weeks after the start of treatment, indicating the involvement of several mechanisms. Possibly, readjustment of cardiovascular reflexes, both central and peripheral, is an important contributory factor to the chronic antihypertensive effect. Arterial pressure reduction begins within an hour of administration of a β-blocker, but several days may elapse before the plateau is reached. During chronic administration, the hypotensive effects of β-blockers last longer than the pharmacological half-life, so that single daily dosage is adequate therapeutically.

In contrast, however, there is a more direct relationship between plasma concentration and cardiac β-blockade, so that to achieve adequate antianginal effect plasma concentrations must be maintained throughout the 24 h. To achieve this in single daily dosage, either the long-half-life drugs (e.g. atenolol, nadolol) or slow-release preparations (e.g. oxprenolol-SR, propranolol-LA, metoprolol-SR) are required. Regardless of pharmacological profile, all β-blockers are equally effective as hypotensive drugs at rest and during exercise. Patients unresponsive to one β-blocker are generally unresponsive to all.

Secondary prevention of myocardial infarction

It is now well established that a reduction of approximately 25% in mortality during the first 2 years after myocardial infarction is possible if continuous β-blockade is provided. This is possible only in patients without contraindications to these drugs, e.g. cardiac failure, asthma. The exact mechanism of this effect is uncertain but it is related probably to antagonism of catecholamine effects on cardiac β-receptors. Most β-blockers are thought to be effective, although the best clinical trial evidence relates to timolol, propranolol and metoprolol; drugs with ISA may be less effective. β-Blocker therapy started within hours of the onset of symptoms may achieve a reduction in infarct size. However, this early intervention does not improve long-term survival beyond the improvement achieved by chronic oral treatment.

Adverse reactions to β-blocking drugs

These can be classified into:

A. Reactions resulting from β-blockade

1. Induction of bronchospasm in patients who rely on sympathetically mediated bronchodilation (β_2), e.g. asthmatics, chronic bronchitics.

2. Precipitation of heart failure in patients with compromised cardiac function. Co-administration with other drugs affecting cardiac contractility (e.g. verapamil, disopyramide, quinidine) is potentially hazardous.

3. Production of cold extremities or worsening symptoms of Raynaud's phenomenon and peripheral vascular disease.

4. Impairment of cardiovascular and metabolic responses to insulin-induced hypoglycaemia in diabetics; reduced cardiovascular response (tachycardia — β_1) and hepatic glycogenolysis (β_2).

5. Increased muscle fatigue, resulting possibly from blockade of β_2-mediated vasodilatation in muscles during exercise.

6. A withdrawal phenomenon may occur after abrupt cessation of long-term β-blocker antianginal therapy. This may take the form of rebound tachycardia, worsening angina, or precipitation of myocardial infarction.

B. Idiosyncratic reactions

1. Central nervous system effects occur with some β-blockers, including nightmares, hallucinations, insomnia and depression. These effects are more common with the lipophilic drugs which cross the blood–brain barrier most readily (e.g. propranolol, acebutolol, oxprenolol and metoprolol).

2. Oculomucocutaneous syndrome was recognised in association with practolol therapy. It affects the eye, mucous and serous membranes. There is no firm evidence that any other β-blockers may provoke a similar reaction. Practolol is no longer available.

Theoretically, cardioselective (β_1-selective) drugs are less likely to aggravate bronchospasm in asthmatics, but as their selectivity is only relative, high doses still interact with bronchial β_2-adrenoceptors and therefore should not be considered safe. Similarly, β-blockers with ISA are promoted wrongly as safer in patients with mild cardiac failure, since at the higher levels of sympathetic activity seen in these patients the presence of small amounts of partial agonist activity are of no significance.

α-Adrenoceptor antagonists

α-Adrenoceptor antagonists (α-blockers) are used mainly as vasodilators and as urethral smooth muscle relaxants. Their use has been limited because of the widespread effects of α-adrenoceptor blockade on the sympathetic nervous system; these may produce a number of undesirable effects (e.g. postural hypotension, nasal stuffiness, diarrhoea, constipation, abdominal discomfort and inhibition of ejaculation). α-Adrenoceptor blocking drugs still have a role in the preoperative management of phaeochromocytoma although their use in other acute hypertensive situations has been replaced by directly acting vasodilators, e.g. sodium nitroprusside (see Ch. 14). The α-blockers bind selectively to the α subclass of adrenoceptor and inhibit catecholamine action at these sites. Drugs in this group may bind covalently (i.e. irreversibly) to the receptor (e.g. phenoxybenzamine) or, as with the β-blockers, in a competitive reversible manner (e.g. phentolamine).

Differences in the relative abilities of the α-blockers to antagonise effects at the two subtypes of α-adrenoceptor have led to the following classification:

1. Non-selective agents (block equally α_1 and α_2), e.g. phentolamine, tolazoline.
2. α_1-Selective, e.g. prazosin, indoramin, phenoxybenzamine.
3. α_2-Selective, e.g. yohimbine.

Only classes (1) and (2) are relevant presently in clinical practice. α-Blockers produce a decrease in peripheral vascular resistance and an increase in venous capacity resulting from blockade of noradrenergic vaso- and venoconstrictor tone.

The antihypertensive action may be combined synergistically with β-blockade in order to prevent reflex sympathetic tachycardia, consequent upon vasodilatation. Prazosin and indoramin are the most commonly used agents in this class and in comparison with direct acting vasodilators (hydralazine) and the non-selective α-blockers (phentolamine) reflex tachycardia and postural hypotension are less common. The mechanism of these changes is not completely understood, but may involve a difference in the proportions of α_1- and postsynaptic α_2-adrenoceptors in the arterial and venous smooth muscle. Thus, prazosin and indoramin may produce a more balanced effect on venous and arterial circulations. An alternative explanation is that non-selective α-antagonists block the feedback inhibition of noradrenaline on its own release at presynaptic α_2-adrenoceptors, thus encouraging increased chronotropic action of neuronally released noradrenaline at cardiac β-adrenoceptors. Non-selective α-blockers produce more postural hypotension and more reflex tachycardia, and there is a greater tendency for tolerance to develop to their therapeutic effects.

In common with other vasodilators, α-blockers may have indirect positive inotropic actions as a result of reduction in afterload and preload. Prazosin has been used for this effect as it produces balanced vaso- and venodilatation; consequently there is less likelihood of reflex tachycardia. Unfortunately the effects of prazosin in cardiac failure are limited by the development of tachyphylaxis after a few months, and it is being superseded by other agents.

Labetalol is an oral and parenteral antihypertensive agent with both an α_1-blocking and a β-blocking action. In acute use, it may produce a prompt reduction in arterial pressure, suggesting that its α-blocking action predominates. Its β-blocking action may be the more important property during chronic administration. It has been used successfully in the preoperative management of phaeochromocytoma.

DRUG EFFECTS ON THE PARASYMPATHETIC NERVOUS SYSTEM

Stimulation of both the cholinergic synapses in ganglia and, more importantly, the postganglionic muscarinic cholinergic receptors, affects chiefly the following systems.

Cardiovascular system

Acetylcholine has three primary effects on the cardiovascular system — vasodilatation, decrease in cardiac rate (negative chronotropic effect) and a decrease in the force of cardiac contraction (negative inotropic effect). The cardiac effects are characteristic of vagal overactivity and blocked by postganglionic muscarinic antagonists (e.g. atropine). These pure effects are often obscured in the whole organism by a number of factors, in particular the release of catecholamines by ACh from cardiac and extracardiac tissues, and the dampening of direct effects by baroreceptor and other reflexes.

Gastrointestinal system

All compounds acting on the parasympathetic nervous system are capable of producing increased tone, amplitude of contractions and peristaltic activity of the alimentary tract in addition to enhanced secretory activity. This may cause nausea, belching, vomiting, cramps and defaecation.

Urinary tract

Drug effects increase ureteral peristalsis, contract the detrusor muscle of the bladder and increase maximal voiding pressure, thus encouraging micturition.

Bronchial tree

Bronchoconstriction is produced in addition to increased mucus secretion. These effects may be a problem in asthmatic and allergic subjects in whom cholinergic drugs should be used with caution. Induction of bronchospasm by reflex cholinergic (vagal) effects in some asthmatics has led to the use of anticholinergics as bronchodilators (see Ch. 14).

Eye

Miosis and spasm of the ciliary muscle occur, so that the eye is accommodated for near vision. Intraocular pressure decreases as a result of increased reabsorption of intraocular fluids.

DRUGS ACTING ON THE PARASYMPATHETIC NERVOUS SYSTEM

The major drugs in use which act on the parasympathetic nervous system are parasympathetic agonists (e.g. bethanechol and the anticholinesterases, neostigmine and pyridostigmine) and muscarinic antagonists (e.g. atropine and propantheline).

Parasympathetic agonists

Bethanechol is used as a stimulant of the smooth muscle of the gastrointestinal tract and bladder. It is given subcutaneously or orally in postoperative abdominal distension and urinary retention. Bethanechol has mainly muscarinic activity at parasympathetic nerve terminals, an action which lasts several hours, as the drug is not hydrolysed by acetylcholinesterase. Bethanechol has also been used to prevent gastro-oesophageal reflux. Generally it has little effect on the cardiovascular system, although atrial fibrillation can be precipitated in hyperthyroid patients. Bradycardia may also aggravate ischaemic heart disease. Flushing, sweating and excessive salivation are predictable adverse effects which necessitate careful dosage selection. Bethanechol is contraindicated in patients with active peptic ulcer or obstructive airways disease.

Anticholinesterase agents (e.g. neostigmine, pyridostigmine) decrease the breakdown of released ACh and exert a parasympathomimetic effect in addition to an action on skeletal neuromuscular junctions. Their use in anaesthesia to reverse the neuromuscular blockade of non-depolarising muscle relaxants is discussed in Chapter 12. The action on the autonomic nervous system tends to appear at low doses. Anticholinesterases may be used to increase gastrointestinal and bladder smooth muscle tone in a similar way to bethanechol. Their other uses include the symptomatic management of myasthenia gravis, where pyridostigmine is a useful, relatively long-acting agent. Topical anticholinesterases are also used in ophthalmology as miotic agents.

Physostigmine differs from neostigmine and pyridostigmine in being capable of crossing into the central nervous system, producing excitation. Physostigmine has been used to arouse patients from drug-induced coma, particularly that following poisoning with anticholinergic agents, ketamine, diazepam or tricyclic antidepressants, which have anticholinergic effects. This is potentially hazardous with the last class of drug as physostigmine can induce convulsions and may exacerbate any cardiac bradyarrhythmias associated with direct toxicity of the tricyclic group.

Parasympathetic antagonists

Parasympathetic antagonists act by blockade of the muscarinic ACh receptor. They are either tertiary or quaternary amine compounds, which differ in their ability to cross biological membranes. Tertiary amines, e.g. atropine and hyoscine, may affect central acetylcholine receptors and may produce sedative or stimulatory effects. Similar antimuscarinic drugs, e.g. benztropine and procyclidine, are useful anti-Parkinsonian agents because of their predominant central action.

Many other parasympathetic antagonists which have been developed are quaternary amines, which are less likely to produce central effects but which also tend to be absorbed poorly after oral administration.

Atropine. The muscarinic-blocking action of atropine affects a wide range of parasympathetic autonomic nervous functions, depending upon dosage. Salivary secretion, micturition, heart rate and visual accommodation are impaired (in that order). Central nervous system effects (sedation or excitation) are possible, but uncommon at usual therapeutic doses in medical conditions. In anaesthesia, central effects may be more common, resulting in the 'central anticholinergic crisis' described in Chapter 24. Hyoscine crosses into the brain more readily and frequently produces confusion, sedation and ataxia. Hyoscine is also used as an antiemetic.

Atropine is administered subcutaneously or i.v. to counteract bradycardia in the presence of hypotension, or to prevent bradycardia associated with vagal stimulation or the use of anticholinesterase agents. Adverse cardiac effects of atropine include an increase in cardiac work and ventricular arrhythmias. Occasionally after subcutaneous administration, atropine may produce a transient slowing of heart rate, thought to be mediated by a central action. Atropine is also used to block salivary and respiratory secretions in anaesthetic premedication (see Ch. 19, p. 346).

Glycopyrronium bromide. This is a quaternary amine which has similar anticholinergic actions to atropine. It is used for its antisecretory and gastrointestinal actions. Some other quaternary amines, e.g. propantheline and dicyclomine, have a mainly peripheral parasympathetic antagonist action and are used as gastrointestinal and urinary antispasmodics. The extent to which these two agents reduce gastric acidity is limited by their lack of effect on acid secretion and the need to avoid doses which produce undesirable effects such as dry mouth and visual disturbances. Anticholinergic agents also delay gastric emptying, a disadvantage in peptic ulcer disease. Pirenzepine is an anticholinergic which has been developed recently to be rather more selective for receptor sites in the gastric mucosa. In general anticholinergic agents have little if any role in the treatment of peptic ulcer disease because of the advent of histamine H_2-antagonists. (See p. 245.)

Ipratropium is useful topically as an anticholinergic bronchodilator aerosol.

FURTHER READING

Breckenridge A 1983 Which beta-blocker? British Medical Journal 286:1085

Goodman-Gilman A, Goodman L S, Gilman A (eds) 1985 The pharmacological basis of therapeutics, 7th edn. Macmillan, New York

Gross F 1982 The place of alpha-adrenoceptor and beta-adrenoceptor blockade in the treatment of hypertension. British Journal of Clinical Pharmacology 13 (suppl): 5S

Heinsimer J A, Lefkowitz R J 1982 Adrenergic receptors: biochemistry, regulation, molecular mechanism and clinical implications. Journal of Laboratory and Clinical Medicine 100: 641

McDevitt D G 1979 Adrenoceptor blocking drugs: clinical pharmacology and therapeutic use. Drugs 17: 267

Motulsky H J, Insel P A 1982 Adrenergic receptors in man. New England Journal of Medicine 307: 18

Nelson H S 1982 Beta-adrenergic agonists. Chest 82 (suppl): 34S

Opie L H 1980 Drugs and the heart: 5 digitalis and sympathomimetic stimulants. Lancet 1: 912

Prichard B N C 1982 Propranolol and beta-adrenoceptor blocking drugs in the treatment of hypertension. British Journal of Clinical Pharmacology 13: 51

Taylor S H 1981 Vasodilators and alpha-adrenoceptor antagonists in hypertension and heart failure. British Journal of Clinical Pharmacology 12 (suppl 1): 27S

14. Miscellaneous drugs of importance in anaesthesia

DRUGS AFFFECTING THE GASTROINTESTINAL TRACT

Antacid or histamine H_2-antagonist therapy is used empirically to prevent bleeding from stress ulceration. H_2-antagonists are effective as prophylaxis against bleeding after severe head injury and erosive bleeding secondary to fulminant liver failure and after renal transplantation. In general, high doses are required, with adjustment according to measurement of gastric pH. Cimetidine does not prevent the occurrence of mucosal lesions but affects only the incidence of haemorrhage. Any effect on overall outcome in these patients has yet to be demonstrated. In stress ulcers, cimetidine is less effective in preventing bleeding than hourly, high-dose antacids. H_2-antagonists may be used preoperatively (1.25–2 h orally, 1 h parenterally) to prevent pulmonary acid aspiration syndrome in elective Caesarean section. In the treatment of acute upper gastrointestinal haemorrhage histamine, H_2-receptor antagonists do not affect the incidence of rebleeding.

Antacids

Antacids raise gastric pH and facilitate ulcer healing only when given in large doses equivalent to around 200 ml daily of a typical magnesium–aluminium preparation. In vitro neutralising capacity varies according to titration technique used and does not correlate with ability to relieve ulcer pain. Antacid mixtures containing local anaesthetics, barbiturates or anticholinergic agents have no proven advantages and are potentially harmful. Calcium-containing antacids should also be avoided since they can cause rebound hyperacidity and hypercalcaemia.

Magnesium compounds can produce diarrhoea whereas aluminium antacids tend to produce constipation. Particulate antacids may cause pneumonitis if aspirated and do not mix efficiently with gastric contents. Sodium citrate is preferred when preoperative antacid therapy is indicated for patients at risk of pulmonary aspiration of gastric fluid.

The high sodium content of some antacid mixtures should be taken into account when antacids are used in patients with cardiovascular or renal disease. Antacids may affect the absorption of drugs including tetracyclines, iron, ketoconazole, diflunisal, chlorpromazine, prednisone and (in high doses) cimetidine and ranitidine. Various other drugs may also be affected, so it is advisable to separate all oral medication from high dose antacid therapy by 1–2 h.

Histamine H_2-receptor antagonists

Basal and stimulated gastric acid secretion is mediated by the action of locally secreted histamine on gastric parietal cells. The receptors involved are H_2-receptors which are responsible also for the effect of histamine in increasing heart rate and counteracting uterine contraction. These actions of histamine are unaffected by traditional antihistamines which act on the other elements of the histamine receptor population (H_1-receptors) which are present in bronchi, arteries and gut.

The H_2-receptor antagonists, cimetidine, ranitidine and famotidine, reduce acid content and volume of gastric secretions. This effect varies with dose and correlates with plasma concentrations of the drugs. Both compounds are effective in healing gastric and duodenal ulcers when given for 4–6 weeks in a twice-daily regimen or in a single (nocturnal) daily dose. Their use in single courses of treatment does not affect the high relapse rate of peptic ulcer disease.

Cimetidine and ranitidine do not appear to produce a rebound hypersecretory state after discontinuation and early reports of acute perforation after a course of treatment probably reflect the tendency for peptic ulcers to revert to their former state of activity.

A variety of adverse effects has been observed with cimetidine. Central nervous system toxicity in elderly and seriously ill patients has led to various, quickly reversible manifestations, e.g. confusion, agitation, psychosis, seizures and decreased consciousness. Pre-existing renal or hepatic impairment have been implicated. Cardiovascular toxicity, including bradycardia, hypotension and asystole, has been reported after rapid i.v. injection but no ECG effects have been found during continuous infusions.

Endocrine effects of long-term use include gynaecomastia, oligospermia and impotence. A range of drug interactions is known to occur as a consequence of the ability of cimetidine to inhibit drug metabolism. Of particular importance is the need to monitor the effects of drugs including anticonvulsants, aminophylline/theophylline, warfarin and lignocaine, which carry a high risk of toxicity. Dosage of these drugs may need to be reduced by 50% or more. Other drugs which may be affected include benzodiazepines, chlormethiazole, propranolol, morphine and quinidine.

Ranitidine in therapeutic doses seems free of an inhibitory effect on drug metabolism and any endocrine actions, but is capable of producing CNS disturbances.

Antiemetics

Antiemetics are used frequently during the postoperative period. Inhibition of nausea and vomiting may be achieved by drugs which depress the vomiting centre (antihistamine/anticholinergic agents), by drugs which depress the chemoreceptor trigger zone (e.g. phenothiazines, metoclopramide) and by drugs which increase gastrointestinal motility (e.g. metoclopramide, domperidone).

Antihistamines

These agents are most useful in vestibular disorders and are thought to act mainly through an anticholinergic action which blocks stimulation of the vomiting centre by impulses from the vestibular nuclei. Drugs which possess antihistamine properties and which are used to treat perioperative vomiting include the phenothiazine promethazine (see p. 208) and the piperazine derivative cyclizine. Cyclizine is the most effective and least toxic of the piperazines. In opioid-induced vomiting, it is as effective as perphenazine, and extrapyramidal effects are rare. It causes some drowsiness and a dry mouth. The adult dose is 50 mg i.m.

Phenothiazines

These are the most useful antiemetic agents in the postoperative period. Their action is mediated probably by blockade of dopamine receptors in the chemoreceptor trigger zone. The phenothiazines are more effective in the treatment of nausea and vomiting produced by opioids than by cytotoxic drugs or motion sickness. Sedation (antihistamine and anticholinergic actions), hypotension (α-adrenoceptor blockade) and dystonic reactions (dopamine receptor blockade) are the major adverse effects. Sedation and hypotension are most frequent with chlorpromazine. Drugs based on the piperazine ring (perphenazine, prochlorperazine, thiethylperazine and trifluoperazine) are the most potent antiemetics, but also produce the highest incidence of extrapyramidal side effects, especially if given repeatedly. Acute dystonic reactions involving eyes, head and neck are more likely to occur in children and the elderly. Phenothiazines may lower the seizure threshold and therefore should be used with caution in epileptic patients. In common with all antiemetics, phenothiazines are more effective for prophylaxis than for treatment.

Perphenazine is the most effective phenothiazine antiemetic. It is usually administered i.m. in the postoperative period, in a dose of 2.5–5 mg. The duration of risk of extrapyramidal side effects exceeds that of its antiemetic actions. Cumulation, with an increased risk of dystonic movements, may occur if the drug is given more frequently than 6-hourly.

Prochlorperazine has less sedative effect than perphenazine. The usual i.m. adult dose is 12.5 mg.

Metoclopramide

In common with the phenothiazines, metoclopramide is a dopamine receptor antagonist which acts directly on the chemoreceptor trigger zone and the vomiting centre. It is effective in emesis induced by radiotherapy, and has been used in very high doses (10 mg/kg) to relieve sickness caused by cancer chemotherapy. Although it counteracts opioid-induced nausea and vomiting, it is less effective than the phenothiazines in relieving postoperative emesis.

Metoclopramide increases the tone of the lower oesophageal sphincter (see p. 530), and increases gastric and intestinal motility. The peripheral actions of metoclopramide are understood poorly but it appears to mimic the effect of acetylcholine in addition to its dopamine receptor blockade. It has virtually no sedative activity, but may induce excitement and restlessness after i.v. administration and in large doses can cause extrapyramidal effects; these are related to dopamine receptor blockade and respond to diazepam or to an anticholinergic anti-Parkinsonian agent, e.g. benztropine. Toxic effects of metoclopramide may be mistaken occasionally for idiopathic Parkinsonism.

The normal adult dose of metoclopramide is 10 mg i.m. or i.v., but this should be reduced in the presence of moderate or severe renal impairment.

Domperidone

This is a benzimidazole derivative, and is not related chemically to the phenothiazines. It acts at the chemoreceptor trigger zone and the vomiting centre, and increases the tone of the lower oesophageal sphincter and gastrointestinal motility. Cardiac arrhythmias and extrapyramidal reactions have been reported after i.v. use and the parenteral formulation of the drug has been withdrawn. It may be given orally or rectally to treat emesis induced by cytotoxic drugs, but is relatively ineffective in opioid-induced or postoperative vomiting.

BRONCHODILATORS

Aminophylline is the most widely used bronchodilator in acute bronchospasm. However, its perioperative use is controversial since individual reports of cardiac arrhythmias during anaesthesia indicate that patients under anaesthesia may be more sensitive to its toxic effects.

Xanthine bronchodilators

Theophylline and its more water-soluble ethylene diamine salt, aminophylline, are reliable bronchodilators for acute bronchospasm. Other xanthine derivatives including acepifylline, diprophylline, etamiphylline and proxyphylline have no advantages and are either too short-acting or are poorly absorbed orally.

Xanthines relax smooth muscle producing bronchodilation, a lowering of systemic vascular resistance and a reduction in left ventricular end-diastolic pressure. Venous pooling occurs and this is beneficial in acute pulmonary oedema of cardiac failure. Chronotropic and inotropic effects on the heart in addition to a direct action on renal tubules produces diuresis. The smooth muscle and cardiac effects of xanthines are produced, in part, by inhibition of phosphodiesterase, the enzyme responsible for degradation of cyclic adenosine monophosphate (cAMP) within the muscle cell. Potentiation of the effects of catecholamines and calcium is thought also to be involved. In this way, the pharmacological action of xanthines mimics β-adrenoceptor stimulation (see Ch. 13, p. 230). The therapeutic and toxic effects of xanthines in combination with β-agonists are additive.

Xanthines also cause stimulation of the central nervous system. Stimulation of the respiratory centre is exploited in the treatment of neonatal apnoea and Cheyne–Stokes respiration. CNS stimulation in high doses also produces nausea, vomiting, restlessness, irritability and convulsions. In acute situations, aminophylline should be administered i.v., since the pH (9.4) precludes the i.m. route and rectal administration is unreliable. Caution should be exercised in the i.v. use of aminophylline because the narrow therapeutic dose range requires attention to selection of dosage and rate of administration. Rapid injection of aminophylline produces high peak blood concentrations which may exceed the therapeutic range of 10–20 mg/litre during the first 15 min or so after administration, with the risk of convulsions, tachycardia, nausea and vomiting. Aminophylline should be given i.v. over at least 10–15 min to allow complete distribution of the drug throughout the body during this period.

Variations in dosage requirements arise from variations in metabolism of theophylline, resulting from age, disease and smoking habits. In otherwise healthy adults (non-smokers) the half-life of theophylline is 7–9 h, whilst the half-life is 4–5 h amongst smokers. In premature infants and patients with severe cirrhosis the half-life is approximately 20–30 h, whereas in children (aged 1–15 years) the half-life is approximately 3–4 h.

Since aminophylline is normally metabolised rapidly, maintenance treatment is best provided by a continuous i.v. infusion following a standard loading dose of approximately 5 mg/kg. The initial loading dose should be halved if the patient has been taking oral aminophylline/theophylline regularly. The previously recommended adult maintenance infusion rate (0.9 mg kg^{-1} h^{-1}) has been associated with fatalities from seizures. The initial maintenance dosage should be approximately 0.5–0.6 mg kg^{-1} h^{-1} and, wherever possible, should be adjusted by measurement of plasma concentration. It is important to appreciate that seizures may not be preceded by other warning symptoms (e.g. nausea). Patients also receiving cimetidine may require up to 50% reduction in maintenance dose (vide supra). Therapeutic benefit can be expected at plasma concentrations of 5–15 mg/litre, with little added benefit above this range and at the cost of greatly increased toxicity above 20 mg/litre. Other drugs (e.g. corticosteroids) should not be added to the infusion fluid. Aminophylline should not be given via a central venous catheter because of its cardiotoxicity.

Theophylline may be given orally in the salt form (choline theophyllinate), three times daily, or as a slow-release preparation twice daily. In view of the need to adjust dosage individually, oral formulations of combination products of theophylline/aminophylline (with, for example, sympathomimetics) should be avoided.

β-Adrenoceptor agonists

β-Adrenoceptor agonists are based chemically on isoprenaline and structural modification has produced relatively long-acting compounds, many of which are effective orally and most of which are selective to non-cardiac (β_2) receptors in therapeutic doses.

The pharmacological profiles of selective β_2-adrenoceptor agonists are identical, differing only in duration of action. β_2-Adrenoceptor agonists are popular when administered by self-propelled aerosol. Salbutamol and terbutaline can be given also by injection, by nebuliser and orally. Fenoterol, rimiterol and reproterol are available also for aerosol administration. The majority of β_2-agonists act for 5–7 h after inhalation, except for rimiterol which lasts for only approximately 2 h. Orciprenaline is a non-selective agent. Although these agonists produce less cardiac effects than isoprenaline or orciprenaline, tachycardia may occur after i.v. administration or after high-dose nebuliser therapy. The cardiac effects may result partly from reduction in systemic vascular resistance. Other signs of toxicity include tremor, headache and dizziness. These side effects are seen also during oral administration. Measurable tolerance to the therapeutic effects of long-term systemic therapy has been demonstrated and is supported by clinical impression.

The relatively small doses used in aerosol inhaler or powder insufflation (100–500 μg per metered dose) do not usually produce systemic effects. Careful attention should be paid to dosage of β_2 agonists administered via nebuliser, since the amounts of drug delivered (2.5–10 mg) are markedly greater than those given by aerosol. Drug absorbed by the lung avoids first-pass metabolism in the liver and is therefore analogous to parenteral administration. An optimum initial dose of salbutamol or terbutaline by nebuliser is 2.5–5 mg. Apart from convenience of administration, nebuliser therapy is no more effective than aerosol inhalation.

Faulty technique of aerosol administration is a common cause of poor control of chronic obstructive airways disease. Various alternative devices including an automatically triggered aerosol (rimiterol 'Autohaler'), a powder insufflation (salbutamol 'Rotahaler') and extended aerosol mouth-pieces (terbutaline 'Spacer' and 'Nebuhaler'; salbutamol 'Volumatic') are available.

Intravenous salbutamol or terbutaline are as effective as aminophylline in acute asthma. Intravenous aminophylline offers the advantage of theoretical (but unproven) synergy with inhaled β_2-agonist.

Ipratropium bromide

Ipratropium is an anticholinergic bronchodilator which may be given either by aerosol or nebuliser. It acts by blocking bronchoconstriction via cholinergic receptors and so decreases intracellular ionic calcium and cyclic guanosine monophosphate, an intracellular mediator of bronchoconstriction. Its effects occur within 15 min and peak slowly between 1–2 h. It has been found to be less effective than β_2-adrenoceptor agonists in asthmatic subjects but seems effective in chronic bronchitis. There is no evidence of systemic toxicity with inhaled ipratropium and the drug does not impair clearance of sputum. Ipratropium may have an additive bronchodilator action in combination with β_2-agonists or aminophylline in some patients.

DRUGS ACTING ON THE CARDIOVASCULAR SYSTEM

Diuretics

The management of oedema may require a planned approach to the use of diuretics, demanding an appreciation of the limitations of individual agents and the value of combining diuretics which have different sites and mechanisms of action.

Diuretics affect sodium reabsorption at four sites in the renal tubule (Fig. 14.1).

1. The proximal tubule, where blockade of active sodium reabsorption is of limited use as a

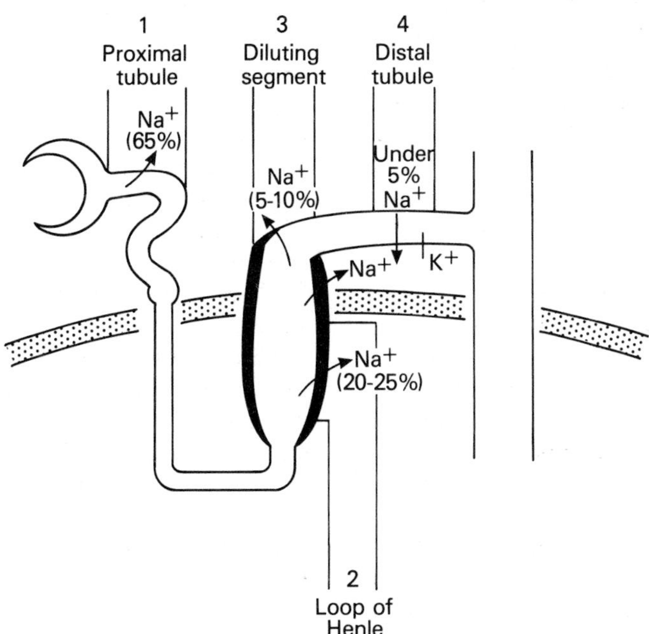

Fig. 14.1 Sites of action of diuretics. Percentages indicate the proportion of intraluminal sodium which is absorbed at different sites in the nephron.

result of development of compensatory mechanisms distally.

2. The ascending loop of Henle; action at this site produces a brisk, potentially large diuresis even at low glomerular filtration rates.

3. The diluting segment; action at this site produces a moderate diuresis.

4. The distal tubule, where blockade of sodium-potassium exchange leads to a mild diuresis and conservation of potassium.

The pharmacological properties of diuretics are indicated in Table 14.1.

High-potency diuretics are useful in left ventricular failure. After i.v. administration, the immediate beneficial effect of frusemide results partly from an increase in venous capacitance and decrease in preload. Rapid diuresis may worsen electrolyte imbalance in hepatic ascites. Spironolactone is particularly beneficial where secondary hyperaldosteronism contributes to the oedema (e.g. hepatic or cardiac failure). Potassium-retaining diuretics are potentially hazardous in the presence of declining renal function, when combined with potassium supplementation or when given with an angiotensin converting enzyme (ACE) inhibitor. When a combination of diuretics is necessary, the objective should be to use maximum tolerable effective doses of each agent.

Cardiac glycosides

Digoxin and other cardiac glycosides improve cardiac output by an inotropic action on myocardial contractility, whilst their ability to suppress

Table 14.1 Commonly used diuretics

Diuretic	Site(s) of action	Route	Onset	Duration (h)	Notes
High potency					
Frusemide	2	oral i.v.	30 min 5 min	4–6 2	Effective at low GFR. Produce hyperuricaemia, hyperglycaemia, hypokalaemia and hypomagnesaemia. Calcium excretion is increased. May cause hearing loss, tinnitus or vertigo after high doses i.v. (especially if too rapid), very high doses orally, in uraemia, or if combined with aminoglycosides
Bumetanide	2				
Ethacrynic acid	2				
Medium potency					
Thiazides	1 + 3	oral	2 h	6–12 (some longer)	Ineffective at GFR less than 20 ml/min. Maximum diuresis achieved after small increases in dose. Additive effect with high-potency diuretics. Produce hyperuricaemia, hyperglycaemia, hypokalaemia and hypomagnesaemia.
Mefruside	1 + 3	oral	2 h	12	
Metolazone	1 + 3	oral	2 h	12–24	Calcium excretion is reduced. Effective at GFR less than 20 ml/min. Synergy with high-potency diuretics. Diuresis can be profound, caution with initial dose
Low potency					
Spironolactone	4	oral	12 h	24	Acts by aldosterone inhibition. In absence of loading dose maximum effect takes 3 days
Potassium canrenoate		i.v.	12 h	24	I.v. form is the active metabolite (canrenone). Potassium retaining. Avoid in renal failure
Amiloride	4	oral	2 h	10	Independent of aldosterone. Potentially nephrotoxic. Potassium retaining. Avoid in renal failure
Triamterene	4	oral	2 h	12–16	
Actezolamide	1	oral i.v./i.m.	2 h	12	Inhibits carbonic anhydrase. Metabolic acidosis during first weeks leads to tolerance through Na^+–H^+ exchange. Synergy with high-potency diuretics

atrioventricular conduction is useful in controlling the ventricular rate in supraventricular arrhythmias, particularly atrial fibrillation.

The cardiovascular response to cardiac glycosides is complicated by indirect actions. In the failing heart, a slowing of heart rate occurs, brought about mainly by the reduction in sympathetic tone which results from the increase in cardiac output. In addition there is a direct vagal stimulatory action of cardiac glycosides. Peripheral vasodilatation occurs also as sympathetic tone is diminished but there is no clinically relevant direct effect on peripheral vasculature. Although cardiac glycosides might be expected to increase cardiac work and therefore oxygen demand, the work of the failing heart is often reduced because of reduced heart rate and cardiac size.

The mechanism of action of cardiac glycosides is incompletely understood but stems from inhibition of the sodium-potassium active exchange at the myocardial cell membrane. There is an associated increase in ionic calcium within the cell, either because of release from intracellular stores or because of increased influx of calcium in exchange for sodium ions. The increased availability of intracellular ionised calcium enhances excitation–contraction coupling within myofibrils.

The ability of cardiac glycosides to suppress conduction in the AV node is the basis for their use in supraventricular arrhythmias. The improvement in cardiac output is therefore most marked in congestive heart failure in the presence of atrial fibrillation. The use of cardiac glycosides in acute left ventricular failure has been superseded gradually by vasodilators and sympathomimetics. The glycosides are of no use in cardiogenic shock and are best avoided after acute myocardial infarction. Any long-term benefit on congestive heart failure in sinus rhythm remains to be demonstrated fully, since in many patients cardiac glycosides can be discontinued without detriment.

There is increased sensitivity to digoxin and similar cardiac glycosides in the presence of hypokalaemia, hypomagnesaemia, hypercalcaemia, renal impairment, chronic pulmonary or heart disease, myxoedema, and hypoxaemia. There is decreased sensitivity in thyrotoxicosis. Quinidine, and to a lesser extent amiodarone and verapamil, tend to increase plasma digoxin concentrations. β-Blockers and verapamil have combined effects on the AV node. Digoxin should be administered cautiously i.v. in situations where AV conduction is already suppressed.

There are various manifestations of cardiac glycoside toxicity. Ventricular arrhythmias (particularly bigeminy and trigeminy) are the commonest. Supraventricular arrhythmias may occur, often with some degree of heart block. Other symptoms are rather unpredictable, and in chronic toxicity include fatigue, weakness of arms or legs, agitation, nightmares, various visual disturbances, anorexia, and nausea or abdominal pain. These symptoms may not precede cardiac toxicity. Therapeutic and toxic blood concentrations overlap, and plasma determinations are useful primarily to substantiate clinical impressions of digitalis toxicity. Treatment of serious arrhythmias involves careful administration of potassium chloride under ECG control (especially in the presence of heart block or renal impairment). Lignocaine or phenytoin are useful for ventricular arrhythmias, whilst β-blockade is useful in supraventricular arrhythmias. Cardioversion during cardiac glycoside therapy may produce ventricular arrhythmias.

Digoxin has a long half-life (approximately 36 h) which is sensitive to changes in renal function. In the absence of a loading dose, effective plasma concentrations (1–2 μg/litre) occur after approximately 5–7 days if renal function is unimpaired. For an acute response, a loading (digitalising) dose is required which should be based approximately on lean body weight. Selection of maintenance doses of digoxin should take into account the presence of renal impairment. Although the effect of an i.v. injection begins within 30–60 min, distribution into cardiac tissue takes place slowly over the first 6 h after oral or i.v. administration. The maximum response occurs 4–6 h after i.v. administration and digoxin measurements in blood samples taken before this 6-h period cannot be interpreted correctly. Intramuscular injections are painful and the drug is absorbed unreliably when given by this route.

Deslanoside has an onset of action beginning 10–30 min after i.v. administration and reaching a maximum after 1–2 h.

Digitoxin is less dependent upon renal function for its elimination. Its long half-life (4–6 days) is a disadvantage, as toxic effects are very persistent.

Vasodilators

Drugs which dilate arteries or veins are used alone or in conjunction with inotropic agents in the management of acute left ventricular failure. Arterial vasodilators are useful also in the treatment of acute hypertensive episodes and in the selective induction of controlled hypotension to reduce haemorrhage during surgery. Some vasodilators are used investigationally to reduce infarct size after myocardial infarction. The main agents are sodium nitroprusside and the nitrates (isosorbide dinitrate and glyceryl trinitrate). Hydralazine and diazoxide are also important parenteral vasodilators, whereas prazosin, minoxidil, captopril and enalapril are oral agents which have a place in the chronic management of left ventricular failure and as third-line agents in the treatment of hypertension. Calcium channel blockers also have a mainly arterial vasodilator action, including an effect on the coronary artery.

The use of vasodilators in left ventricular failure is based on their ability to reduce afterload and preload. In cardiac failure, a reflex increase in sympathetic tone creates an increase in systemic vascular resistance in the arterial bed. By lowering this resistance (afterload), the work and oxygen requirements of the heart are reduced. Those vasodilators which are capable of acting on the venous side of the circulation increase venous capacitance, reduce venous return to the heart and so decrease the left ventricular filling pressure (preload). Lowering the filling pressure in the left ventricle decreases the degree of stretch of myocardial fibres, improves myocardial contractility and cardiac output and reduces myocardial oxygen consumption for the same degree of external cardiac work performed.

Vasodilators may be classified into those which act directly on arterial smooth muscle (nitroprusside, nitrates, hydralazine, diazoxide, minoxidil, calcium channel blockers), and those which are neurohumoral antagonists (prazosin and other adrenoceptor antagonists, and ACE inhibitors). This distinction is important as the drugs in the first category have a clear, often sensitive, dose–response relationship which requires haemodynamic monitoring (preferably by invasive techniques), whereas those in the second category have a relatively long duration of action and their intensity of effect is less sensitive to changes in dosage.

Another useful way of comparing vasodilators is to consider on which side of the heart they act preferentially. Hydralazine and minoxidil act mainly on afterload. Nitroprusside, the α-adrenoceptor antagonists and ACE inhibitors have a balanced effect on both arteries and veins.

Sodium nitroprusside

Sodium nitroprusside has an immediate, short-lived effect (lasting only for a few minutes) which requires that it be given by continuous infusion. A smooth reduction in arterial pressure can be achieved by adjustment of the infusion rate. The nitroprusside ion is responsible for a direct action on vascular smooth muscle and it is metabolised by red cells to cyanide. Cyanide ions are detoxified by the liver and kidney to thiocyanate (requiring thiosulphate and vitamin B_{12}) which is excreted slowly in the urine.

Sodium nitroprusside produces a balanced reduction in afterload and preload. In larger doses (e.g. when used for hypotensive anaesthesia) its use leads to an increase in heart rate. There is an additive effect with other vasodilators. In medical practice nitroprusside is well tolerated and most symptoms are non-specific (e.g. drowsiness, perspiration, nausea, dizziness) and are associated with too rapid a decrease in arterial pressure.

The accumulation of cyanide and thiocyanate, with the risk of lactic acidosis, is a possibility but is rare in the absence of impaired renal or hepatic function or if total dosage does not exceed 1.5 mg/kg. Where therapy is high-dose or prolonged, plasma bicarbonate monitoring is indicated. Plasma cyanide or thiocyanate concentrations may also be monitored if the drug is used for more than two days. Thiocyanate is potentially neurotoxic and can cause hypothyroidism. Thiosulphate and a specially prepared high-dose infusion of hydroxocobalamin have been used to reverse cyanide toxicity. Nitroprusside is photodegraded, and infusion solutions should be protected from light.

The use of sodium nitroprusside (SNP) in hypotensive anaesthesia is considered in Chapter 37.

Nitrates

The organic nitrates, glyceryl trinitrate and isosorbide dinitrate, affect mainly preload and are most effective in relieving pulmonary congestion secondary to left ventricular failure. However, this selectivity of action decreases with dosage, so that a decrease in arterial pressure, tachycardia and headaches may occur. The nitrates have a short duration of action and may be given i.v. The infusion rate should be controlled carefully according to heart rate and haemodynamic effects. The action of nitrates in left ventricular failure is enhanced by agents, including hydralazine, which preferentially reduce afterload.

The nitrates are absorbed by rubber and plastics (especially PVC infusion bags), so they are best administered by syringe pump. Intravenous nitrates are used also in unstable angina. The therapeutic effects of nitrates in myocardial ischaemia result not only from preload reduction but also from counteraction of coronary vasospasm and redistribution of blood within the myocardium.

Hydralazine, diazoxide and minoxidil

These drugs are direct-acting arterial vasodilators. Their main action is to reduce afterload, with little or no effect on preload, and their main limitation is reflex tachycardia, although this is less prominent in patients with cardiac failure.

In hypertensives, the reduction in arterial pressure is limited by reflex sympathetic discharge which tends to increase cardiac output. Their antihypertensive action is limited also by a tendency to cause sodium and water retention by a direct renal mechanism and by activation of the renin-angiotensin system. Consequently, they are often more effective if combined with a β-adrenoceptor blocker and a diuretic.

Hydralazine is the most widely used direct vasodilator drug. Its half-life is short (approximately 2.5 h) but its antihypertensive effect is relatively prolonged, permitting twice-daily dosage.

Diazoxide is of limited use because of its unpredictable duration of action, which is unrelated to its short plasma half-life. The initial i.v. dose of diazoxide must be given rapidly for maximum effect. A cumulative effect on arterial pressure may make it difficult to control the action of repeated doses. Multiple doses of diazoxide cause fluid retention and hyperglycaemia.

Minoxidil is available for oral use only and it too has a long duration of action (12–24 h) which is unrelated to its plasma half-life.

Calcium channel blockers

Calcium channel blockers, such as nifedipine and verapamil, have been used as antianginal and, more recently, as antihypertensive agents. They antagonise coronary artery spasm and relax systemic vascular smooth muscle predominantly on the arterial side of the circulation. Verapamil is also a useful drug for the treatment of supraventricular arrhythmias (vide infra) since it shows some preference for the AV node, through which conduction is dependent upon intracellular calcium (as opposed to sodium) influx. The antihypertensive effects of calcium channel blockers have not yet been studied widely but they appear modest and, in the case of nifedipine at least, have been inconsistent.

Intracellular calcium ion availability is important in the conduction of the cardiac action potential and in electromechanical coupling within smooth muscle cells. Drugs which affect the permeability to calcium of the extracellular or intracellular membranes can influence the size of the cytoplasmic pool of calcium ions. This action reduces cardiac contractility (producing a negative inotropic effect) and decreases vascular tone. Calcium channel blockers differ in their selectivity for myocardial or arterial tissue, verapamil being rather more selective for cardiac muscle than nifedipine. Nifedipine presents less risk of reducing contractility and has no important effect on conduction through the AV node.

Nifedipine is more potent than verapamil as a systemic and coronary arterial vasodilator, making it the more effective antianginal agent. It is effective in countering coronary artery spasm, which is thought to be an important component of all forms of angina. The antianginal effect of nifedipine is additive with that of β-adrenergic blocking drugs and nitrates. The marked negative inotropic action of verapamil presents a potential hazard when used in conjunction with β-adrenergic blockers or other cardiodepressant drugs (including disopyramide and the volatile anaesthetic agents) in patients with limited cardiac reserve. However, the effects of these agents in individual patients is unpredictable since the failing left ventricle can benefit from reductions in afterload brought about by peripheral vasodilatation.

Side effects of nifedipine are related to its vasodilator action and include flushing, headaches, dizziness, tiredness and palpitations. Nifedipine may also cause ankle oedema which arises from peripheral vasodilatation unrelated to any cardiodepressant action of the drug. Nifedipine is available for oral administration only but a swift action in angina can be obtained by advising the patient to bite on the soft gelatin capsule placed in the mouth. The drug is absorbed fairly rapidly if the capsule is swallowed, particularly when the stomach is empty. The slow-release tablet formulation may be tolerated better as it is less likely to reduce arterial pressure acutely.

Other calcium channel blockers include nicardipine and diltiazem.

Other interesting properties of calcium channel blockers include inhibition of platelet aggregation, protection against bronchospasm, use in Raynaud's syndrome and improvements in lower oesophageal sphincter function.

α-Adrenoceptor antagonists

The pharmacology of α-adrenoceptor antagonists (e.g. phentolamine, phenoxybenzamine) has been discussed in Chapter 13, p. 237). These agents have a balanced effect on venous capacitance and systemic arterial resistance. The oral postsynaptic (α_1) blocking agent, prazosin, is a widely used vasodilator in chronic left ventricular failure. It tends to produce little if any increase in heart rate. Initial administration may cause a sudden decrease in arterial pressure and so prazosin should be given as a low first dose, preferably with the patient supine. Syncope is more likely if the patient is receiving nitrates concurrently. There is concern that the short-term benefits of prazosin in left ventricular failure may not be maintained during long-term therapy.

As with many of these drugs, the duration of vasodilator action of prazosin (approximately 12 h) does not correlate with its short half-life in plasma (3–4 h). The short-acting phentolamine and the long-acting phenoxybenzamine are other α-adrenoceptor blocking drugs which are used occasionally by the parenteral route as adjuncts in hypertension or left ventricular failure.

Angiotensin converting enzyme (ACE) inhibitors

The orally administered ACE inhibitors (captopril and enalapril) reduce both preload and afterload. Vasodilatation and a decrease in blood volume result from blockade of the renin-angiotensin-aldosterone sequence. Captopril has a more rapid onset and shorter duration of action (plasma half-life approximately 2 h) compared with enalapril (approximately 36 h). As both drugs may produce a profound initial hypotensive response, the first dose must be small, particularly in patients already receiving diuretics.

Enalapril is de-esterified in the liver into its active form, enalaprilat. Captopril, enalapril and their active metabolites accumulate in renal failure. ACE inhibitors tend to increase plasma urea and creatinine concentrations and may produce hyperkalaemia if administered with potassium-sparing diuretics. The effects on arterial pressure and renal function are more marked in the presence of hypovolaemia or bilateral renal artery stenosis.

Other adverse effects of ACE inhibitors include disturbances of taste and a dry cough. Hypersensitivity reactions, including proteinuria, are uncommon but their incidence is increased by the use of high doses and by the presence of renal impairment or connective tissue disease.

Antiarrhythmic agents

The aim of drug treatment of cardiac arrhythmias is either to prevent the emergence of a tachyarrhythmia or to terminate a run of tachycardia. A continuous arrhythmia may be controlled either by slowing the primary mechanism or, in the case of supraventricular arrhythmias, by reducing the proportion of impulses transmitted through the AV node and ventricular conducting system.

The emergence of ectopic pacemaker cells may be explained by the phenomenon of re-entry. Re-entrant arrhythmias arise from retrograde conduction along a branch of tissue in which anterograde conduction has been blocked by disease. When retrograde conduction is sufficiently slow, it can influence cells which have already discharged and repolarised, triggering a further action potential which is both premature and ectopic. A vicious circle can ensue such that these action potentials become self-sustaining (circus movements) leading to multiple ectopic beats, tachycardia or fibrillation.

The basis for treatment of specific arrhythmias has arisen largely from clinical experience. The known electrophysiological properties of antiarrhythmics have provided explanations for observed effects and, in particular, it has become clear that any drug with an antiarrhythmic action may itself provoke arrhythmias. Consequently, antiarrhythmic agents tend to be used rather more conservatively than in the past.

Antiarrhythmic agents may be classified empirically on the basis of their effectiveness in supraventricular tachycardias (e.g. digoxin, β-blockers and verapamil) or in ventricular arrhythmias (lignocaine, mexiletine, tocainide, phenytoin and bretylium). Many agents (disopyramide, amiodarone, quinidine and procainamide) are effective in both supraventricular and ventricular arrhythmias.

The cardiac action potential

Antiarrhythmic agents are classified conventionally according to their effects on the cardiac action potential (Fig. 14.2) which comprises five phases, each corresponding to a changing state of depolarisation of the myocardial cell.

The action potential is triggered by a slow intracellular leak of sodium ions (and calcium ions at the AV node) until a threshold point is reached when sudden rapid influx of sodium ions generates an impulse (phase 0). The action potential starts to reverse (phase 1), but is sustained whilst there is slower inward movement of calcium ions (phase 2). Efflux of potassium ions brings about repolarisation (phase 3) and the gradual termination of the action potential. Thereafter, re-equilibration of sodium and potassium takes place and the resting membrane potential is restored (phase 4).

There are three important components of the cardiac action potential which are amenable to pharmacological intervention.

1. The *automaticity* (tendency to spontaneous discharge) of cells may be reduced. This result can be achieved by reducing the rate of leakage of sodium (reducing the slope of phase 4), by

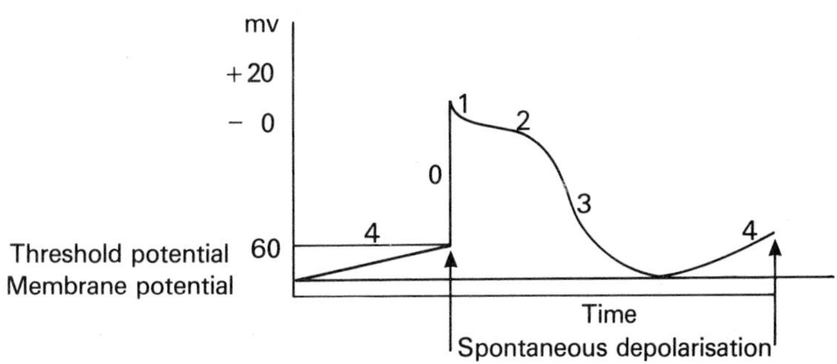

Fig. 14.2 The cardiac action potential.
Phase 0 — rapid depolarisation associated with fast Na^+ influx
1 — early repolarisation
2 — maintained depolarisation associated with slow Ca^{2+} influx
3 — repolarisation associated with K^+ efflux
4 — resting membrane potential; may have upward slope representing slow spontaneous depolarisation in automatic (pacemaker) tissues.

increasing the electronegativity of the resulting membrane potential or by decreasing the electronegativity of the threshold potential.

2. The speed of *conduction* of the action potential can be suppressed as indicated by a lowering of the height and slope of the phase 0 discharge. A reduction in the electronegativity of the membrane potential at the onset of phase 0 reduces both the amplitude and the slope of the phase 0 depolarisation. This situation occurs if the cell discharges before it has completely repolarised.

3. The *rate of repolarisation* may be reduced, which prolongs the refractory period of the discharging cell.

On the basis of these pharmacological effects, antiarrhythmic agents can be grouped into four classes (Table 14.2). Agents in class 1A antagonise primarily the fast influx of sodium ions and so reduce automaticity and conduction velocity, whilst prolonging the refractory period. Those in class 1B also affect automaticity in the same way, but they have much less effect on conduction velocity in usual therapeutic doses and they shorten the refractory period. β-blockers (class 2) depress automaticity but have no other specific effect on the action potential apart from reducing the effects of catecholamines (i.e. the increases in automaticity and conduction velocity in the sinus and AV node). Agents in class 3 lengthen the refractory period by prolonging the action potential. Verapamil (class 4) also prolongs the action potential in addition to depressing automaticity (especially in the AV node).

An appreciation of the general class of action of different antiarrhythmic agents enables the selection of a second agent to be made from a different class in the event of failure of a primary agent, or if there is need for combination therapy.

Table 14.2 Classification of antiarrhythmic agents

1 Membrane stabilisation	A Quinidine, procainamide, disopyramide B Lignocaine, mexiletine, tocainide, flecainide phenytoin
2 β-receptor blockade	All β-blockers
3 Prolongation of action potential	Amiodarone, bretylium, sotalol (also class 2)
4 Calcium channel blockade	Verapamil

Quinidine has now been superseded largely by newer agents including disopyramide. Intravenous administration may cause severe hypotension. Toxic effects may be dose-related or arise as drug idiosyncrasy. The most serious toxicity is depression of conduction and risk of ventricular fibrillation. Visual and auditory disturbances with vertigo and gastrointestinal symptoms are signs of toxicity. Skin reactions, thrombocytopenia and agranulocytosis may occur also. Quinidine enhances digoxin toxicity by doubling plasma concentrations. It also has an additive effect with hypotensive agents and drugs having cardiodepressant properties (e.g. disopyramide, β-blockers and calcium channel blockers).

Procainamide closely resembles quinidine in its effect on the heart. It may cause hypotension after i.v. administration. Its main application is as an oral antiarrhythmic, although therapy is limited by its short half-life (3 h) which necessitates frequent administration or the use of a sustained-release oral preparation. Procainamide is restricted usually to short-term use because of the risk of drug-induced systemic lupus erythematosus. Other manifestations of hypersensitivity include fever, rash, arthralgia and agranulocytosis.

Disopyramide has properties in common with both quinidine and lignocaine. It is useful in supraventricular tachycardias and as a second-line agent to lignocaine in ventricular arrhythmias. Its half-life (8 h) is prolonged in renal impairment and after myocardial infarction, necessitating dosage reduction. Side effects result mainly from the anticholinergic effect of the parent drug and a major metabolite, which can produce urinary retention and blurred vision. Disopyramide is markedly cardiodepressant, especially in combination with β-blockers, quinidine, procainamide or verapamil.

Lignocaine remains the first choice for ventricular arrhythmias. It has a short half-life of less than 2 h, although this is prolonged after myocardial infarction, in liver disease and during cimetidine treatment. The effect of a single loading dose may be brief as lignocaine distributes rapidly after an i.v. bolus, which may need to be repeated twice. A continuous infusion is used to maintain the effect, with the rate of infusion adjusted according to response. Close adjustment of the infusion rate is required to avoid toxicity (confusion, slurring of speech, numbness, dizziness and convulsions). The presence of heart failure, β-blockade or liver disease should be an indication to reduce maintenance dosage by half. A reduced loading dose is necessary also in heart failure. The presence of hypokalaemia is a common reason for failure of response to lignocaine.

Mexiletine is a longer-acting, orally effective, lignocaine analogue which has a half-life of 10 h. It shares lignocaine's low margin of safety, especially after i.v. administration when hypotension and bradycardia have been reported. Most frequent adverse effects involve the central nervous system and include tremors, nystagmus, confusion, speech disturbances, tinnitus, paraesthesiae and convulsions. Gastrointestinal effects are also common during oral treatment.

Tocainide is another lignocaine analogue which can be given orally or parenterally. It has a half-life of 13 h. Arrhythmias which do not respond to lignocaine are unlikely to respond to tocainide. Adverse effects resemble those of mexiletine.

Flecainide is another class I agent which may be administered orally or i.v. It differs from other drugs in this class by having little effect on the refractory period. Its half-life is 7–23 h, but this may be prolonged in renal failure.

Phenytoin is unique in that it accelerates intraventricular conduction and is particularly effective in controlling digitalis-induced ventricular arrhythmias.

β- *blockers* are used mainly in sinus and supraventricular tachycardias, especially those provoked by emotion or exercise. Their cardiodepressant effects are a disadvantage in the management of arrhythmias after acute myocardial infarction. For further discussion of the pharmacology of β-blockers see Chapter 13 (p. 233).

Amiodarone is a very effective agent against both supraventricular and ventricular arrhythmias. It has a long half-life (over 30 days) so that oral treatment should be started with a week of high doses to establish a therapeutic effect. Intravenous administration may cause bradycardia, hypotension (vasodilatation), heart block and thrombophlebitis. It must be diluted in an infusion of glucose. Long-term accumulation produces reversible microdeposits in the cornea which generally do not interfere with vision. Deposition in the skin produces photosensitivity and blue-grey discoloration. As amiodarone is an iodinated compound, it may disturb thyroid function tests and may produce clinical hyperthyroidism or, less commonly, hypothyroidism. Long-term treatment is associated with pulmonary fibrosis and hepatotoxicity. Amiodarone may increase blood concentrations of digoxin.

Bretylium is a quaternary ammonium compound which prevents noradrenaline uptake into sympathetic nerve endings. It has been used in recurrent life-threatening ventricular arrhythmias resistant to lignocaine or DC shock. It has a positive inotropic effect and usually causes an increase in arterial pressure during the first 24 h, followed by a decrease. It may cause bradycardia or asystole and may worsen ventricular arrhythmias transiently.

Verapamil is also a coronary and peripheral vasodilator which is useful in angina and hypertension and effective both orally and i.v. It is very effective in supraventricular tachycardias, in which it acts by depressing AV conduction and blocking re-entry mechanisms. Similarly, it controls the ventricular rate in atrial fibrillation. Intravenous administration may reduce arterial pressure (by vasodilatation) and caution is necessary in low-output states and in patients treated with negative inotropic agents, e.g. β-blockers, disopyramide, quinidine and procainamide.

DRUGS AFFECTING THE IMMUNE SYSTEM

The major drugs used in acute conditions involving the activation of immunological and inflammatory mechanisms are the corticosteroids and the antihistamines.

Corticosteroids

The corticosteroids have been advocated in a variety of acute life-threatening conditions, although few recommendations are supported by firm evidence of efficacy. Included in these conditions are bacteraemic and anaphylactic shock, adult respiratory distress syndrome, status asthmaticus and cerebral oedema.

Amongst the many complex actions of pharmacological doses of corticosteroids, those affecting the cellular and microvascular components of the inflammatory response are more relevant to any therapeutic benefit achieved in critically ill patients. These pharmacological effects seem to parallel the glucocorticoid properties of individual corticosteroids which are shown in Table 14.3.

The anti-inflammatory action of corticosteroids involves reduction in the permeability of capillaries to intravascular fluid, proteins and chemical mediators of the inflammatory process. The migration and phagocytosis of polymorphonuclear leucocytes is inhibited. In high doses, corticosteroids prevent tissue damage by stabilising lysosomal membranes; this reduces the extent of autolysis and hinders the perpetuation of the local inflammatory response. Corticosteroid administration leads to a relative lymphocytopenia which results from redistribution into the reticuloendothelial system and a cytolytic action affecting preferentially the T lymphocyte population. The action on B lymphocytes is less marked and antibody formation is reduced only by high doses.

High doses of steroids have a cardiac inotropic effect and they also reduce systemic and pulmonary vascular resistance. Capillary flow is increased and there is mobilisation of interstitial fluid and protein.

The use of corticosteroids in septic shock has gained theoretical support from the knowledge that the inflammatory process includes an early phase of vasodilatation and extensive capillary leakage which leads to hypovolaemia. β-Endorphin is probably also involved in vasodilatation and it is derived from the same precursor molecule as ACTH. Early administration of high-dose corticosteroids may conceivably affect both ACTH and β-endorphin release. However, the results of clinical studies carried out to date are controversial. There is no evidence for any beneficial effect of corticosteroids in cardiogenic shock.

An effect on pulmonary capillary leakage has formed the theoretical basis for the use of corticosteroids in the adult respiratory distress syndrome. Experimentally, steroids have been demonstrated to be beneficial in animal models of ARDS. It is likely that the drugs should be given early to be effective and this may be practical when respiratory distress is provoked by a specific event such as pulmonary aspiration. However, current evidence suggests that corticosteroids are of no benefit in adult respiratory distress syndrome and there is likely to be a greater risk of infection if steroids are used routinely.

In acute allergic emergencies, including status asthmaticus, the use of corticosteroids is empirical, hydrocortisone being used most commonly. Intensive corticosteroid therapy should be for as short a period as possible (ideally limited to within

Table 14.3 Glucocorticoid corticosteroids

	Equivalent dosage (mg)	Mean dose to suppress HPA* (mg/day)	Half-life in plasma (h)	Half-life of pharmacological effect** (h)
Hydrocortisone	20	15–30	1.5	8–12
Cortisone	25	20–35	1.5	8–12
Prednisolone	5	7.5–10	3+	18–36
Prednisone	5	7.5–10	3+	18–36
Methylprednisolone	4	7.5–10	3+	18–36
Dexamethasone	0.75	1–1.5	5+	36–54
Triamcinolone	4	7.5–10	3+	18–36
Betamethasone	0.6	1–1.5	5+	36–54

* HPA = hypothalamic-pituitary-adrenal axis
** Based on duration of suppression of HPA axis

48–72 h). In such instances, the dosage need not be tapered, or may be tapered quickly over the next 48–72 h, except in conditions (such as asthma) in which there may be a relapse unless dosage is reduced carefully. In asthma, a change to oral prednisolone should be undertaken when an adequate response has been obtained. Dosage can be tapered gradually over 1–2 weeks. There is no evidence that very high-dose potent steroids are more effective than conventional doses of hydrocortisone in acute allergy.

In cerebral oedema, corticosteroids (most commonly dexamethasone) have been used successfully to reduce raised intracranial pressure associated with cerebral tumours and symptomatic improvement can be obtained when oedema results from benign intracranial hypertension. In the case of head injury or stroke corticosteroids are of no benefit. In cerebral malaria steroid treatment is detrimental.

The potential hazards of corticosteroids argue against their use in indications where their effectiveness is in doubt. The most important risk is infection, as a consequence of the suppressed inflammatory response. Glucose intolerance and gastrointestinal haemorrhage are also risks to be considered, although an accurate assessment of their clinical importance is lacking. Effective antimicrobial cover is essential whenever corticosteroids are used in the critically ill.

Antihistamines

Although there are two distinct populations of histamine receptor (H_1 and H_2) the term antihistamines is used to refer to those drugs which block selectively histamine H_1-receptors found in the bronchi, arteries and gut. No compound currently in therapeutic use influences both H_1- and H_2-receptors.

Histamine is only one of many mediators which may be involved in acute allergic reactions. Some consequences of these substances (e.g. hypotension and bronchospasm) may be counteracted most effectively by adrenaline and other β-adrenoceptor agonists. Antihistamines (e.g. chlorpheniramine, promethazine) tend to have only a secondary role in the management of acute allergy. They are most effective against symptoms such as itch, oedema and urticaria. They are less effective against hypotension, and ineffective against bronchospasm, fever and arthralgia.

The most important adverse effect of antihistamines is sedation, although occasionally they may produce central nervous system stimulation (e.g. agitation or convulsions) especially in children. A new generation of antihistamines with less sedative properties, e.g. terfenadine, has been developed.

All antihistamines have anticholinergic effects which tend to dry mucosal secretions and may cause tachycardia.

FURTHER READING

Chernow B, Lake C R 1983 A pharmacologic approach to the critically ill patient. Williams & Wilkins, Baltimore

Feldman S A, Scurr C F, Paton W 1987 Drugs in anaesthesia: mechanisms of action. Edward Arnold, London

Goodman-Gilman A, Goodman L S, Gilman A (eds) 1985 The pharmacological basis of therapeutics, 7th edn. Macmillan, New York

Rogers H J, Spector R G, Trounce J R 1985 A textbook of clinical pharmacology. Hodder & Stoughton, London

Vickers M D, Schneiden H, Ward-Smith F G 1984 Drugs in anaesthetic practice, 6th edn. Butterworths, London

15. Local anaesthetic agents

Local anaesthetic drugs act by producing a reversible block to the transmission of peripheral nerve impulses. A reversible block may be produced also by physical factors including pressure and cold. Although nerve compression is of purely historical interest, cold (produced by the evaporation of ethyl chloride, the application of ice packs or use of the cryoprobe) still has a limited use.

Many types of drug have local anaesthetic actions (e.g. β-blockers and antihistamines), but all those known and used as local anaesthetics have originated from cocaine, the alkaloid found in the leaves of the South American bush *Erythroxylon coca*. Its local anaesthetic action was demonstrated first by Koller, an ophthalmic surgeon working in Vienna. Although most of the major local anaesthetic techniques were described within a few years of that discovery, the drug was not used widely other than as a topical agent because of its systemic toxicity, central nervous stimulant and addictive properties and tendency to produce allergic reactions.

The demonstration of the physical structure of cocaine as an ester of benzoic acid permitted the production of safer agents, all with the same general structure of an aromatic group joined to an amine by an intermediate chain (Fig. 15.1).

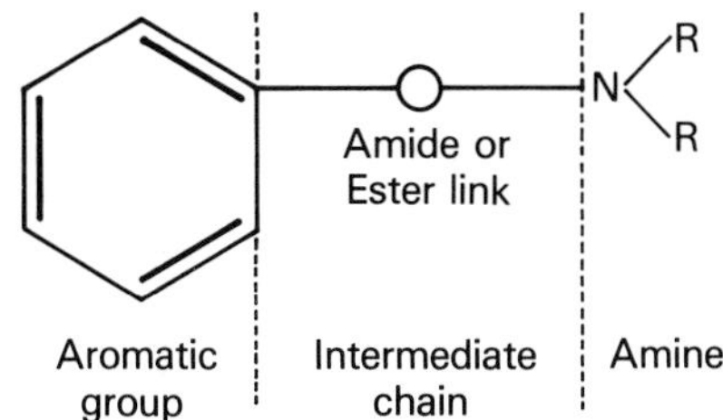

Fig. 15.1 General formula for local anaesthetic drugs.

Procaine, synthesised in 1904, was the first significant advance and it allowed wider use of local anaesthetic techniques. Many other drugs were introduced, but none displaced procaine as the standard until the synthesis of lignocaine in the 1940s. The intermediate chain in lignocaine contains an amide bond and this obviated many of the problems associated with the ester group present in the older drugs. The subsequent production of other amide agents with varying clinical profiles has greatly extended the scope of modern local anaesthesia.

The mode of action of local anaesthetics is by blocking membrane depolarisation in all excitable tissues. Since local anaesthetics are injected at their site of action, only peripheral nerve is usually exposed to concentrations high enough to have a significant effect. However, if sufficient drug reaches other organs via the circulation, more widespread effects occur.

MODE OF ACTION

Neural transmission (Fig. 15.2)

During the resting phase the interior of a peripheral nerve fibre has a potential difference of about −70 mV relative to the outside. When the nerve is stimulated there is a rapid increase in the membrane potential to approximately +20 mV, followed by an immediate restoration to the resting level. This depolarisation/repolarisation sequence lasts 1–2 ms and produces the familiar action potential associated with the passage of a nerve impulse.

The resting potential is the net result of several factors affecting the distribution of ions across the cell membrane. Electrochemical and concentration

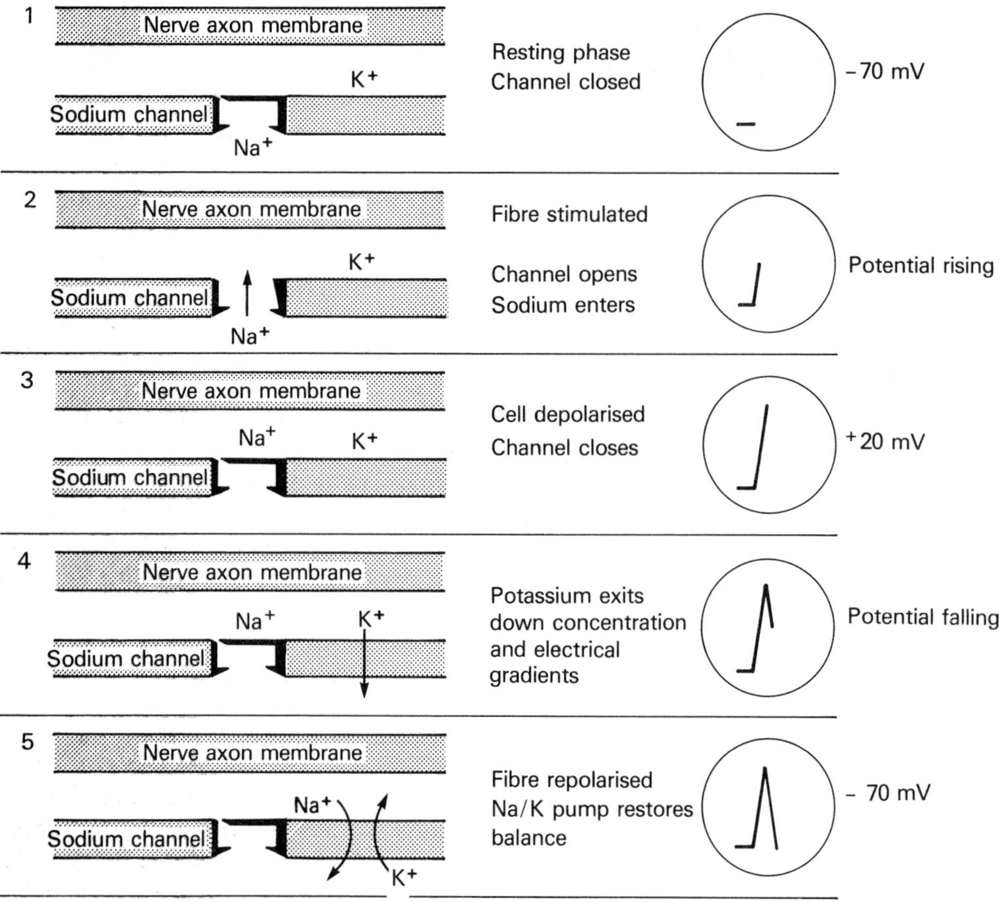

Fig. 15.2 Events occurring during transmission of a nerve impulse along an axon.

gradients modify ionic diffusion, which is adjusted further by the semipermeable nature of the membrane and the action of the sodium/potassium pump.

Depolarisation of the fibre is the result of a sudden increase in membrane permeability to sodium which can thus diffuse down both electrochemical and concentration gradients. Sodium ions enter the cell through large protein molecules in the membrane (known as channels), which are closed during the resting phase. Stimulation of the nerve changes the configuration of these protein molecules so that the channels open and allow positively charged sodium ions to enter the cell. This increases the membrane potential to approximately +20 mV, when the electrochemical and concentration gradients for sodium balance each other and the channels close. Both concentration and electrochemical gradients then favour movement of potassium out through the membrane until the resting potential is restored. Relative to the total amounts present, only small numbers of ions take part in this exchange and the sodium/potassium pump restores their distribution during the resting phase.

At sensory nerve endings, the initial opening of sodium channels is produced by the appropriate physiological stimulus, which may be chemically mediated in some instances. The impulse is transmitted along the axon because a local current flows between the depolarised segment of nerve (which has a positive charge) and the next segment (which has a negative charge). The voltage change associated with this current causes the configurational change in the sodium channels in the next segment, so that the action potential is propagated along the nerve.

Effect of local anaesthetic drugs (Fig. 15.3)

Local anaesthetics are usually injected in an acid solution as the hydrochloride salt (pH approximately 5). The tertiary amine group becomes quaternary and they are thus soluble in water and suitable for injection. Following injection, the pH increases as a result of buffering in the tissues and a proportion of the drug, determined by the pK, dissociates to release free base. As it is lipid-soluble, the free base is able to pass through the lipid cell membrane to the interior of the axon, where reionisation takes place. The reionised portion enters the sodium channels, and may be thought of simply as plugging them so that sodium ions cannot enter the cell. As a result, no action potential is generated or transmitted, and conduction blockade has occurred. Because it is the ionised form of drug that is active and re-ionisation has to take place intracellularly, individual drug pK has little effect on rate of onset of blockade.

In addition to diffusing into nerves at the site of injection, the drug also enters capillaries and is removed by the circulation. Eventually, tissue concentration decreases below that in the nerves and the drug diffuses out, so allowing restoration of normal function.

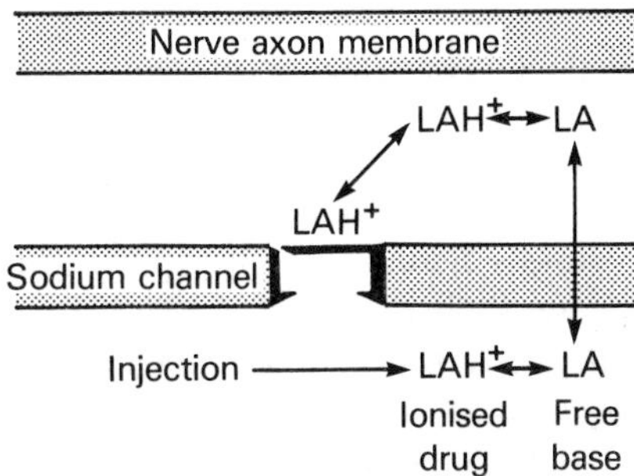

Fig. 15.3 Mode of action of a local anaesthetic drug. In order to penetrate the lipid cell membrane, the drug must be in free base form, while to effect a block reionisation must occur.

Systemic toxicity

If significant amounts of local anaesthetic drug reach the tissues of heart and brain they exert the same 'membrane stabilising' effect as on peripheral nerve, resulting in a progressive depression of function. The earliest feature of systemic toxicity is numbness or tingling of the tongue and circum-oral area; this is the result of a rich blood supply depositing enough drug to have an effect on the nerve endings. The patient may become light-headed, anxious, drowsy and/or complain of tinnitus. If concentrations continue to rise, consciousness is lost and this may be preceded or followed by convulsions.

Coma and apnoea may develop subsequently. Cardiovascular collapse may result from direct myocardial depression and vasodilatation, but more commonly it is a result of hypoxaemia secondary to apnoea.

Factors affecting toxicity

The most common cause of life-threatening systemic toxicity is an inadvertent intravascular injection, but it may result also from absolute overdosage. The changes in plasma concentration of drug following injection (Fig. 15.4) are dependent on the total dose administered, the rate of absorption, the pattern of distribution to other tissues and the rate of metabolism.

Absorption. Absorption from the site of injection depends on the blood flow; the higher the blood flow, the more rapid is the increase in plasma concentration, and the greater the resultant peak. Of the common sites of injection of large doses, the intercostal space has the highest blood supply, followed in turn by the extradural space, the brachial plexus and the sites of major lower limb nerve block. Absorption is slowest after infiltration anaesthesia.

Intravenous regional anaesthesia is a special case. If the tourniquet deflates immediately after drug injection, a large dose enters the circulation very rapidly. After 20 min of tourniquet application, sufficient drug has diffused out of the vessels into the tissues to result in the increase in systemic concentration being smaller than that following brachial plexus block.

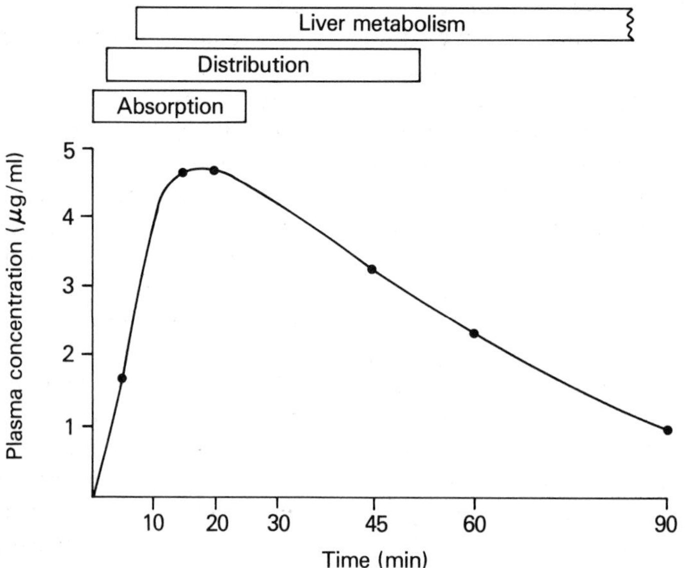

Fig. 15.4 Plasma concentration of lignocaine. Concentrations are shown after the injection into the lumbar extradural space of 400 mg of lignocaine without adrenaline. The injection was made at time zero and the phases of absorption, distribution and metabolism are indicated.

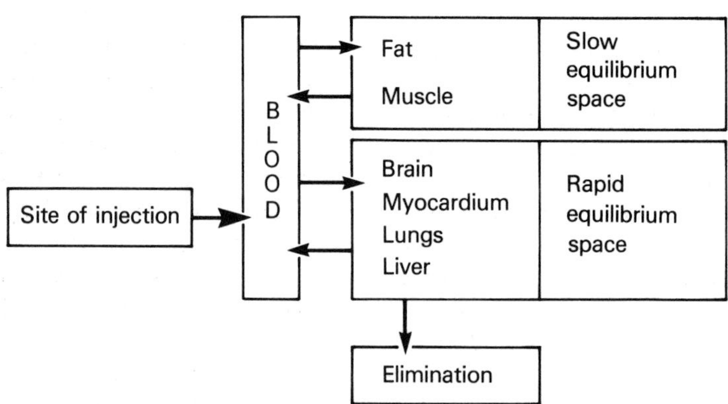

Fig. 15.5 Distribution of local anaesthetic drug after absorption from the site of injection.

Blood supply may be modified by the inherent vasoactive properties of the particular drug or by the addition of vasoconstrictors to the solution. Use of the latter permits the safe dose to be increased by 50–100%.

Distribution. (Fig. 15.5) After absorption, local anaesthetic drugs are distributed rapidly to, and taken up by, organs with a large blood supply and high affinity, e.g. brain, heart, liver and lungs. Muscle and fat, with low blood supplies, equilibrate more slowly, but the high affinity of fat for these drugs ensures that a large amount is taken up into adipose tissues. The lungs sequester (and possibly metabolise) local anaesthetic drugs, thereby preventing a large proportion of the injected dose from reaching the coronary and cerebral circulations.

Metabolism. In general, ester drugs are broken down so rapidly by plasma cholinesterase that systemic toxicity is unusual. Toxicity may occur with some of the slowly hydrolysed drugs or in patients with abnormal enzymes (cf. suxamethonium). The amides are metabolised by amidases located predominantly in the liver. Hepatocellular disease has to be severe before the rate of metabolism is slowed significantly, and in general the rate of disappearance of drug is dependent more upon liver blood flow. This has practical relevance to the use of lignocaine as an antiarrhythmic in cardiogenic shock, where liver blood flow is diminished.

Protein binding. Local anaesthetics are bound to plasma proteins to varying degrees. It is assumed sometimes that drugs with the greatest degrees of protein binding are less toxic because only a small fraction of the total amount in plasma is free to diffuse into the tissues and produce toxic effects. However, values for protein binding are obtained under laboratory conditions and probably bear little relationship to the dynamic situation that exists during the phase of rapid absorption. Furthermore, even if a drug is bound to protein, it is still available to diffuse into the tissues down a concentration gradient, as the bound portion is in equilibrium with that in solution in plasma. Thus, values for protein binding do not relate to acute toxicity of a drug.

Placental transfer. Much theoretical concern has been expressed about the mechanisms and effects of placental transfer of local anaesthetics administered to the mother during labour. Local anaesthetics cross the placenta as readily as other membranes, but their effects are of minimal significance when compared with those of conventional methods of analgesia and anaesthesia.

Fetal plasma protein may bind some drugs to a lesser extent than maternal protein so that *total* plasma concentration may be lower in the baby. It is claimed that such drugs are safer for the fetus. However, the concentration of *free* drug on each side of the placental membrane is the same and as a result tissue concentrations are more similar in mother and fetus than total plasma concentrations. The neonatal liver metabolises drugs slowly, but provided that delivery does not occur immediately after a toxic reaction, there should be little concern about effects on the baby.

Prevention of toxicity

The single most important factor in the prevention of toxicity is the avoidance of accidental intravascular injection. Careful aspiration tests are vital and should be repeated each time the needle is moved. However, a negative test is not an absolute guarantee, especially when a catheter technique is used. The initial injection of 2–3 ml of a solution that contains adrenaline (1 : 200 000) has been advocated; an increase in heart rate during the succeeding 1–2 min should indicate intravascular injection. However, adrenaline is not the safest of drugs and this method is no guarantee against subsequent migration of needle or cannula into a vessel.

An alternative is to repeat the aspiration test after each 5–10 ml of solution, and to inject slowly. The patient should be watched for early signs of toxicity so that the injection may be stopped before there are major sequelae. Particular care should be taken when performing head and neck blocks because a very small dose may produce a major reaction if injected into a carotid or vertebral artery.

Overdosage may be avoided by consideration of the behaviour of the various drugs after injection at the particular site. Most practical manuals indicate the appropriate drug and dosage for each block, and these recommendations should be followed. Maximum safe dosages (for use in any situation) are often quoted for local anaesthetics with and without vasoconstrictor, but such recommendations are not really helpful since they ignore variations caused by factors such as the site of injection, the patient's general condition and the concomitant use of a general anaesthetic. If the same total dose is used, variations in drug concentration have no effect on toxicity. In adults, body weight correlates poorly with the risk of toxicity and it is better to modify the dose on the basis of an informed assessment of the patient's general condition.

Treatment of toxicity

No matter how careful the anaesthetist is with regard to prevention, facilities for treatment must always be available. The airway is maintained and oxygen administered by facemask, using artificial ventilation if apnoea occurs. Convulsions may be controlled with small increments of either diazepam (2.5 mg) or thiopentone (50 mg). The latter is usually more readily available and acts more rapidly. Excessive doses should not be given to control convulsions, since cardiorespiratory depression may be exacerbated. If cardiovascular collapse occurs despite adequate oxygenation (and this is *rare*), it should be treated with an adrenergic drug with α and β properties, e.g. ephedrine in 5 mg increments.

Additional side effects

Local anaesthetics are remarkably free from side effects other than systemic toxicity which is an extension of pharmacological action. Complications of specific drugs are discussed later, but there are two general features.

Allergic reactions

Allergy to the esters was relatively common, particularly with procaine, and was caused by *para*-aminobenzoic acid produced on hydrolysis. Most reactions were dermal in personnel handling the drugs, but fatal anaphylaxis has been recorded. Allergy to the amides is extremely rare and most 'reactions' result from systemic toxicity, overdosage with vasoconstrictors, or are manifestations of anxiety. The occasional genuine allergic reaction is usually to a preservative in the solution rather than the drug itself.

Drug interactions

Interactions with other drugs do occur, although they rarely give rise to clinical problems. Therapy with anticholinesterases for myasthenia, or the concomitant administration of other drugs hydrolysed by plasma cholinesterase, increases the toxicity of the ester drugs, and competition for plasma protein binding sites may occur with the amides. Of more practical importance is that heavy sedation with anticonvulsants (e.g. benzodiazepines) may mask the early signs of toxicity. These drugs may even prevent convulsions, so that if a severe reaction does occur the patient may suddenly become deeply unconscious.

PHARMACOLOGY OF INDIVIDUAL DRUGS

The local anaesthetic drugs in current use vary in their clinical profile (stability, potency, duration, toxicity, etc.). These differences may be related to variations in physicochemical properties.

Local anaesthetic drug chemistry

As indicated above (Fig. 15.1) all the local anaesthetic drugs have a three-part structure, with either an ester or amide bond at the centre. The important effects of the nature of this linkage on the route of metabolism and allergenicity have been discussed. The ester drugs also have short shelf lives because they tend to hydrolyse spontaneously, especially on warming. The amides may be stored for long periods without loss of potency and are not heat-sensitive unless mixed with glucose to produce hyperbaric spinal solutions. As a general rule, solutions of amides in glucose and solutions of any ester may be heat-sterilised once, and should be used soon after autoclaving.

The aromatic end of the molecule determines fat solubility and the amine affects its water solubility. Addition of other organic groups to any part of the molecule increases lipid solubility, and therefore potency, since ability to penetrate the lipid cell membrane is increased. Duration of action increases in proportion to the extent of protein binding, which is also a property of the aromatic group. Sodium channels are formed from large protein molecules and drugs with longer durations of action bind to these proteins for longer periods.

The effects of a local anaesthetic drug on blood vessels also modify its profile. Cocaine is a vasoconstrictor, but most of the other agents produce some degree of vasodilatation, which tends to shorten duration of action and increase toxicity.

The effects of differences in molecular structure often interact in complex ways, but a simple example of a structure–activity relationship is the addition of a butyl group to mepivacaine to produce bupivacaine, which is four times as potent and significantly longer-acting. Alterations in structure also affect the rate, and the products, of metabolism.

Clinical factors affecting drug profile

Increasing the dose of a drug shortens its onset time and increases the duration of block. Dose may be increased by using either a higher concentration or a larger volume; a large volume of a dilute solution is usually more effective.

The site of injection also affects onset time and duration (in addition to potential toxicity). Onset is almost immediate after infiltration and is progressively delayed with subarachnoid, peripheral nerve and extradural blocks respectively. The slowest onset follows brachial plexus block. The dose required and the likely duration of action tend to increase in much the same order as for onset time.

Pregnancy and age are said to increase segmental spread of extradurals. For many blocks, young, fit, tall patients seem to require more drug, as do obese, alcoholic or anxious patients, the last perhaps because they react to any sensation from the operative area.

Individual drug properties

Only when all the above factors are taken into account may the properties of various drugs be compared. It is doubtful if, at *equipotent* concentrations, there are any real differences in speed of onset, but there are certainly variations in potency, duration and toxicity. The features of individual drugs are described below and in Table 15.1. Appropriate volumes and concentrations of local anaesthetic agents used commonly for specific blocks are detailed in Chapter 26.

Cocaine

Cocaine has no place in modern anaesthetic practice, although it is used in ENT surgery for its vasoconstrictor action. Because of its use as a drug of addiction, it is increasingly difficult to obtain cocaine legitimately at a reasonable price.

Benzocaine

This is an excellent topical agent of low toxicity. It does not ionise and therefore its use is limited to topical application. In addition, its mode of action cannot be explained according to the theory outlined above. Instead, it is thought that benzocaine diffuses into the cell membrane, but not into the cytoplasm, and either causes the membrane to expand in the same way as is suggested for general anaesthetics (see Chapter 5) or enters the sodium channel from the lipid phase of the membrane. Whichever is the case, the mechanism may also be relevant to the action of the other agents.

Procaine

The incidence of allergic problems, short shelf-life and brief duration of action of procaine have resulted in its infrequent use at the present time.

Chloroprocaine

This is a relatively new ester which is widely used in the USA. Its profile is very similar to procaine, from which it differs only by the addition of a chlorine atom (Table 15.1). As a result, it is hydrolysed four times as quickly by cholinesterase and seems to be less allergenic. It is claimed to have a more rapid onset than any other agent but this may relate to its very low toxicity, which permits the use of relatively larger doses. There has been some concern that chloroprocaine might be neurotoxic, because of a number of reports of paraplegia after its accidental intrathecal injection. However, the evidence suggests that it was the preservative in the solution that caused the problems and not the drug itself.

Amethocaine

This drug is relatively toxic for an ester because it is hydrolysed very slowly by cholinesterase. It is also very potent and is the standard drug in North America for subarachnoid anaesthesia.

Lignocaine

Having been used safely and effectively for every possible type of local anaesthetic procedure lignocaine is currently the standard agent. It has no unusual features and is also a standard antiarrhythmic.

Mepivacaine

This agent is very similar to lignocaine and seems to have neither advantages nor disadvantages in comparison.

Table 15.1 Features of individual local anaesthetics

Proper name / formula	% Equivalent concentration*	Relative duration*	Toxicity	pK	Partition coefficient	% protein bound	Main use by anaesthetists in the UK
COCAINE 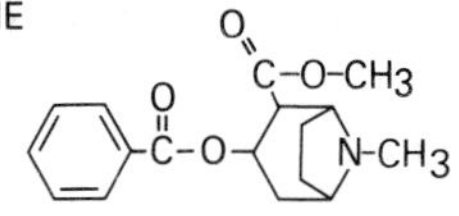	1	0.50	V. high	8.7	?	?	Nil
BENZOCAINE 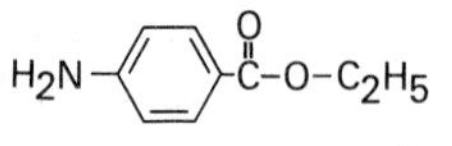	N/A	2	Low	2.9	?	?	Topical
PROCAINE 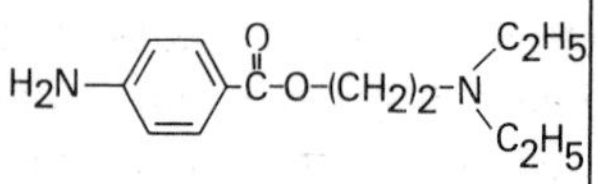	2	0.75	Low	8.9	0.6	5.8	Nil
CHLOROPROCAINE 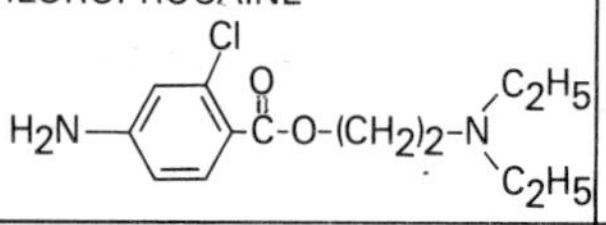	1	0.75	Low	9.1	1	?	Not available
AMETHOCAINE 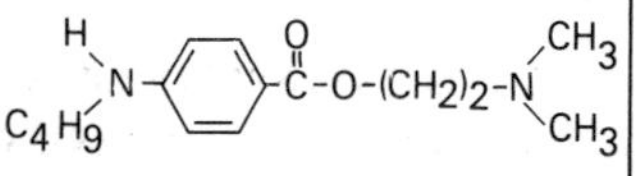	0.25	2	High	8.5	80	76	Topical
LIGNOCAINE 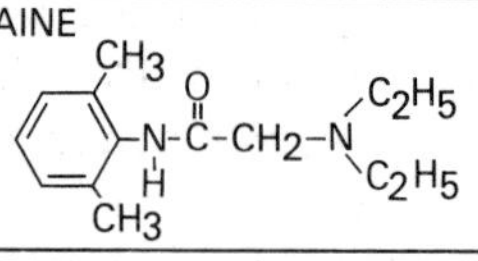	1	1	Medium	7.7	3	64	Infiltration Nerve block Extradural Topical (EMLA)
MEPIVACAINE 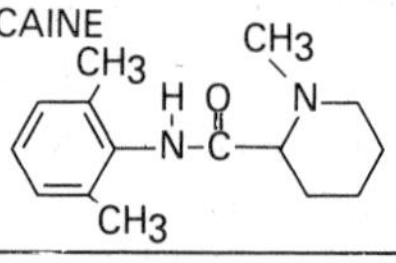	1	1	Medium	7.6	1	77	Not available
PRILOCAINE 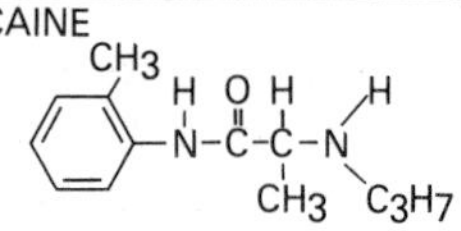	1	1.50	Low	7.7	1	55	Infiltration Nerve block IVRA Topical (EMLA)
BUPIVACAINE 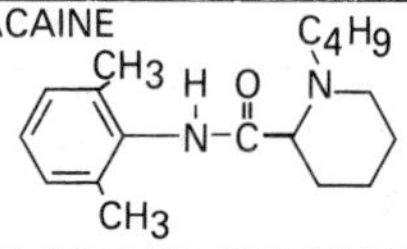	0.25	2-4	Medium	8.1	28	95	Extradural Spinal Nerve block
ETIDOCAINE 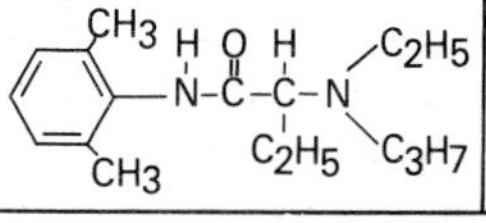	0.5	2-4	Medium	7.7	141	94	Not available

* Lignocaine = 1; N/A = not applicable — not used in solution;
? = information not available.
NB. All figures are approximations as there is some variation in published values.

Prilocaine

This is an underrated agent. It is equipotent to lignocaine, but has virtually no vasodilator action, is either metabolised or sequestered to a greater degree by the lungs, and is more rapidly metabolised by the liver. As a result, it is slightly longer-acting, considerably less toxic and is the drug of choice when the risk of toxicity is high. Metabolism produces *o*-toluidine, which reduces haemoglobin; thus, methaemoglobinaemia may occur but is rare unless the dose is considerably in excess of 600 mg. Cyanosis appears when 1.5 g/dl of haemoglobin are converted, and treatment with methylene blue (1 mg/kg) is effective immediately. Fetal haemoglobin is more sensitive, and prilocaine should not be used for extradural block during labour.

Cinchocaine

Cinchocaine was the first amide agent to be produced (two decades before lignocaine). It is very potent and toxic. Like amethocaine, it was used mainly for subarachnoid anaesthesia, but the drug is no longer available for clinical use.

Bupivacaine

The introduction of bupivacaine represented a significant advance in anaesthesia. Relative to potency, its acute CNS toxicity is only slightly less than that of lignocaine, but its longer duration of action reduces the need for repeated doses, and thus the risks of cumulative toxicity.

A number of deaths have occurred after the accidental i.v. administration of large doses of bupivacaine, and some concern has been expressed that this drug might have a more toxic effect on the myocardium than other local anaesthetic agents. There is some experimental evidence that this is so, but very large doses must be given rapidly and intravenously for the effect to be clinically apparent.

These events have stimulated interest in finding other long-acting agents which do not possess this cardiotoxic effect. *Ropivacaine* is similar chemically to bupivacaine (the butyl group attached to the amine is replaced by a propyl group) and shows some promise.

Etidocaine

This is an amide derived from lignocaine. It may be even longer-acting than bupivacaine and is of particular interest because it seems to produce a more profound effect on motor than sensory nerves; the reverse is probably true with other agents.

Additives

Many substances are added to local anaesthetics for pharmaceutical purposes. Sodium hydroxide and hydrochloric acid are used to adjust the pH, sodium chloride the tonicity, and glucose and water the baricity of solutions. Preservatives, e.g. methyl hydroxybenzoate, are added to multidose bottles and manufacturers recommend that these should not be used for subarachnoid or extradural block. Other additions are made for pharmacological reasons.

Vasoconstrictors

The addition of a vasoconstrictor to a solution of local anaesthetic drug slows the rate of absorption, reduces toxicity, prolongs duration and may result in a more profound block. These are all desirable effects, but vasoconstrictors are not used universally for several reasons. They are absolutely contraindicated for injection close to end-arteries (ring blocks of digits and penis) and in intravenous regional anaesthesia (IVRA) because of the risk of ischaemia.

There is also a theoretical risk that the use of vasoconstrictors may increase the risk of permanent neurological deficit by rendering nerve tissue ischaemic. While evidence is inconclusive, many anaesthetists feel that vasoconstrictors should not be used unless there is no alternative method of prolonging duration or reducing toxicity in the specific clinical situation.

Adrenaline is the most potent agent. It produces systemic toxicity, and should be used with particular care, if at all, in patients with cardiac disease. Even in healthy patients concentrations greater than 1:200 000 should not be used, and the maximum dose administered should not exceed 0.5 mg. Interactions with other sympathomimetic drugs, including tricyclic antidepressants, may occur especially when adrenergic drugs are used systemically to treat hypotension.

Felypressin is a safer drug although it causes pallor and may constrict the coronary circulation. It is available usually for dental use only.

Carbon dioxide

In order to speed the onset of blockade, some local anaesthetics have been produced as the carbonated salt, with carbon dioxide dissolved under pressure in the solution. The rationale for the use of these solutions is that after injection the carbon dioxide lowers intracellular pH and favours formation of more of the ionised active form of the drug. With blocks of slower onset there is good evidence that a significant improvement is obtained.

Dextrans

There have been many attempts to prolong duration of action by mixing local anaesthetics with high molecular weight dextrans. The results are inconclusive, but the very large dextrans may be effective, especially in combination with adrenaline. 'Macromolecules' may be formed between dextran and local anaesthetic so that the latter is held in the tissues for longer periods.

Hyaluronidase

For many years the enzyme hyaluronidase was added to local anaesthetics to aid spread by breaking down tissue barriers. There was little evidence that it had a significant effect and this practice has been abandoned.

Mixtures

Some practitioners deliberately mix different local anaesthetics together in an attempt to obtain the advantages of both. One such combination (sometimes referred to as 'compounding') is lignocaine and bupivacaine; the aim is to achieve the rapid onset of the former and the long duration of the latter with a single injection. Another advantage claimed for compounding two drugs is a decrease in toxicity. However, local anaesthetic drug toxicity is additive, so that the use of 'half a dose' of each of two drugs is of no benefit. If an ester is combined with an amide, toxicity may increase because the amide slows hydrolysis of the ester by inhibiting plasma cholinesterase. It is more appropriate to use a catheter technique, to initiate the block with a dose of lignocaine and to maintain it with a dose of bupivacaine as the effect of lignocaine starts to regress.

A more effective combination is the eutectic mixture of local anaesthetics (EMLA). This is a mixture of the base (un-ionised) forms of lignocaine and prilocaine in a cream formulation. It is a local anaesthetic preparation which penetrates intact skin with some reliability. It takes up to 1 h to become effective but is very useful in paediatric practice, especially in children who need repeated venepuncture. It may be of value for poor-risk patients undergoing skin grafting.

CHOICE OF LOCAL ANAESTHETIC AGENT

When using a local technique the anaesthetist has to decide upon the concentration, volume and nature of the agent to be used. For lignocaine (the relative potencies of other agents are shown in Table 15.1) concentrations required are:

skin infiltration IVRA	0.5%
minor nerve block	1.0%
brachial plexus sciatic/femoral	1.0–1.5%
extradural	1.5–2.0%
subarachnoid	2.0–5.0%

Higher concentrations than these may be used to produce more profound blocks of faster onset. The volumes required for specific techniques are described in Chapter 26 and the interrelationships that exist between patient status and the required amount of drug have been discussed above.

Ideally, several drugs of different potency, duration and toxicity should be available to permit a rational choice based upon the required dose, the particular risk of toxicity in that block and patient, and the likely duration of surgery. Often this is not possible, mainly for commercial reasons. For example, in the UK, lignocaine and bupivacaine are marketed in a full range of concentrations, but little else is available apart from the more dilute solutions of prilocaine. The availability of spinal anaesthetic solutions is particularly poor. For more peripheral blocks, lignocaine and bupivacaine may be used safely unless the risk of toxicity is relatively high (e.g. IVRA) when prilocaine is the drug of choice. When large volumes of more concentrated solutions are needed and the higher concentrations of prilocaine are not available, then one of the other agents should be used in combination with adrenaline.

FURTHER READING

Covino B G 1980 The mechanisms of local anaesthesia. In: Norman J, Whitman J G (eds) Topical reviews in anaesthesia. John Wright & Sons, Bristol

Covino B G, Vassallo H G 1976 Local anesthetics: mechanisms of action and clinical use. Grune & Stratton, New York

Henderson J J, Nimmo W S 1983 Practical regional anaesthesia. Blackwell Scientific Publications, Oxford

Stanton-Hicks M d'A (ed) 1978 Regional anesthesia: advances and selected topics. International Anesthesiology Clinics 16(4)

Wade A (ed) 1977 Martindale: the extra pharmacopoeia. The Pharmaceutical Press, London

Wildsmith J A W, Armitage E N 1987 Principles and practice of regional anaesthesia. Churchill Livingstone, Edinburgh

16. Basic physics for the anaesthetist

The application of physics in anaesthesia

A knowledge of simple physics is required in order to understand fully the function of many items of anaesthetic apparatus. This chapter is designed to emphasise the more elementary aspects of physical principles, and it is hoped that the reader will be stimulated to read some of the excellent books which are designed for anaesthetists and examine this topic in greater detail (see Further Reading). Sophisticated measurement techniques may be required for more complex types of anaesthesia, in the intensive therapy unit and during anaesthesia for severely ill patients, and an understanding of the principles involved in performing such measurements is required in the later stages of the anaesthetist's training.

This chapter does not describe all the physical principles which may be encountered in the early stages of anaesthetic training (e.g. magnetism and light), but concentrates on the more common applications, including pressure and flow in gases and liquids, electricity and electrical safety. However, it is necessary first to consider some basic definitions.

BASIC DEFINITIONS

It is now customary in medical practice to employ the International System (SI) of units. Common exceptions to the use of the SI system include measurement of arterial pressure and, to a lesser extent, gas pressure measurements. Arterial pressure is frequently measured using a mercury column and so 'mmHg' is retained. Pressures in gas cylinders are also referred to frequently in terms of the 'normal' atmospheric pressure of 760 mmHg; this is equal to 1.01 bar (or approximately 1 bar). Low pressures are expressed usually in the SI units of kPa whilst higher pressures are referred to in bar (100 kPa = 1 bar). The basic and derived units of the SI system are shown in Table 16.1.

The fundamental quantities in physics are mass, length and time.

Mass (m) is defined as the amount of matter in a body. The unit of mass is the kilogram (kg), for which the standard is a block of platinum held in a Physics Reference Laboratory.

Length (l) is defined as the distance between two points. The SI unit is the metre (m), which is defined as the distance occupied by a specified number of wavelengths of light.

Time (t) is measured in seconds. The reference standard for time is based on the frequency of resonation of the caesium atom.

From these basic definitions, several units of measurement may be derived.

Velocity is defined as the distance travelled per unit time:

$$\text{velocity } (v) = \frac{\text{distance}}{\text{time}} \text{ m/s}$$

Acceleration is defined as the rate of change of velocity:

$$\text{acceleration } (a) = \frac{\text{velocity}}{\text{time}} \text{ m/s}^2$$

Force is that which is required to give a mass acceleration:

$$\begin{aligned}\text{force} &= \text{mass} \times \text{acceleration}\\ &= ma\end{aligned}$$

Table 16.1 Physical quantities

Quantity	Definition	Symbol	SI Unit
Length	Unit of distance	l	metre (m)
Mass	Amount of matter	m	kilogram (kg)
Density	Mass per unit volume (m/v)	ρ	kg/m^3
Time		t	second (s)
Velocity	Distance per unit time (l/t)	v	m/s
Acceleration	Rate of change of velocity (v/t)	a	m/s^2
Force	Gives acceleration to a mass (ma)	F	newton (N) ($kg\ m\ s^{-2}$)
Weight	Force exerted by gravity on a mass (mg)	W	$kg \times 9.81\ m/s^2$
Pressure	Force per unit area (F/A)	P	N/m^2
Temperature	Tendency to gain or lose heat	T	kelvin (K) or degree Celsius (°C)
Work	Performed when a force moves an object (force × distance)	U	joule (J) (Nm)
Energy	Capacity for doing work (force × distance)	U	joule (J) (Nm)
Power	Rate of performing work (joules per second)	P	watt (W) (J/s)

The SI unit of force is the newton (N). 1 newton is the force required to give a mass of 1 kg an acceleration of 1 m/s^2:

$$1\ N = 1\ kg\ m\ s^{-2}$$

Weight is the force of the earth's attraction for a body. When a body falls freely under the influence of gravity, it accelerates at a rate of 9.81 m/s^2:

$$\begin{aligned} \text{weight} &= \text{mass} \times g \\ &= m \times g \\ &= m \times 9.81\ m/s^2 \end{aligned}$$

Momentum is defined as mass multiplied by velocity:

$$\text{momentum} = m \times v$$

Work is undertaken when a force moves an object:

$$\begin{aligned} \text{work} &= \text{force} \times \text{distance} \\ &= F \times l \\ &= U\ \text{Nm or joules (J)} \end{aligned}$$

Energy is the capacity for undertaking work. Thus it has the same units as those of work.

Power is the rate of doing work. The SI unit of power is the watt, which is equal to 1 J/s:

$$\begin{aligned} \text{power} &= \text{work per unit time} \\ &= \text{joules per second} \\ &= \text{watt (W)} \end{aligned}$$

Pressure is defined as force per unit area:

$$\begin{aligned} \text{pressure } (P) &= \frac{\text{force}}{\text{area}} \\ &= N/m^2 \\ &= \text{pascal (Pa)} \end{aligned}$$

As 1 Pa is a rather small unit, it is more common in medical practice to use the kilopascal (kPa).

FLUIDS

Substances may exist in solid, liquid or gaseous form. These forms or phases differ from each other according to the random movement of their constituent atoms or molecules. In solids, molecules oscillate about a fixed point, whereas in liquids the molecules possess higher velocities and move more freely and thus do not bear a constant relationship in space to other molecules. The molecules of gases also move freely, but to an even greater extent.

Both gases and liquids are termed fluids. Liquids are incompressible and at constant temperature occupy a fixed volume, conforming to the shape of a container; gases have no fixed volume but expand to occupy the total space of a container.

Heating a liquid increases the kinetic energy of its molecules, permitting some to escape from the surface into the vapour phase. Random loss of molecules with higher kinetic energies from a liquid occurs in the process of vaporisation. As these molecules possess higher kinetic states, this leads to a reduction in the energy state and cooling of the liquid.

Collision of randomly moving molecules in the gaseous phase with the walls of a container is responsible for the pressure exerted by a gas.

Gas pressures

There are three important laws which determine the behaviour of gases and which are important to anaesthetists.

Boyle's law states that, at constant temperature, the volume (V) of a given mass of gas varies inversely with its absolute pressure (P):

$$PV = \mathrm{k}_1$$

Charles' law states that, at constant pressure, the volume of a given mass of gas varies directly with its absolute temperature (T):

$$V = k_2T$$

The third gas law states that, at constant volume, the absolute pressure of a given mass of gas varies directly with its absolute temperature:

$$P = \mathrm{k}_3T$$

Combining these three gas laws:

$$PV = kT$$

or,

$$\frac{P_1V_1}{T_1} = \frac{P_2V_2}{T_2}$$

The behaviour of a mixture of gases in a container is described by *Dalton's law of partial pressures*. This states that, in a mixture of gases, the pressure exerted by each gas is the same as that which it would exert if it alone occupied the container.

Thus, in a cylinder of compressed air at a pressure of 100 bar, the pressure exerted by nitrogen is equal to 79 bar (as the fractional concentration of nitrogen is 0.79).

Avogadro's hypothesis

Avogadro's hypothesis states that equal volumes of gases at the same temperature and pressure contain equal numbers of molecules.

Avogadro's number is the number of molecules in one gram molecular weight of a substance and is equal to 6.022×10^{23}.

Under conditions of standard temperature and pressure, 1 gram molecular weight of any gas occupies a volume of 22.4 litres.

These data are useful in calculating, for example, the quantity of gas produced from liquid nitrous oxide. The molecular weight of nitrous oxide is 44. Thus, 44 g of N_2O occupy a volume of 22.4 litres at standard temperature and pressure (STP). If a full cylinder of N_2O contains 3.0 kg of liquid, then vaporisation of all the liquid would yield:

$$\frac{22.4 \times 3.0 \times 1000}{44} \text{ litres}$$

$$= 1527 \text{ litres at STP}$$

Critical temperature

The critical temperature of a substance is the temperature above which that substance cannot be liquefied by pressure, irrespective of its magnitude.

The critical temperature of oxygen is −118°C, that of nitrogen −147°C and that of air −141°C. Thus, at room temperature, cylinders of these substances contain gases. In contrast, the critical temperature of carbon dioxide is 31°C, and that of nitrous oxide 36.4°C. The critical pressures are 73.8 bar and 72.5 bar respectively; at higher pressures, cylinders of these substances contain a mixture of gas and liquid.

Clinical application of the gas laws

A 'full' cylinder of oxygen on an anaesthetic machine contains compressed gaseous oxygen at a pressure of 137 bar (2000 lb/in^2). If the cylinder of oxygen empties at constant temperature, the volume of gas contained is related linearly to its pressure (by Boyle's law). In practice, linearity is not followed because temperature falls as a result of adiabatic expansion of the compressed gas; the term adiabatic implies a change in the state of a gas without exchange of heat energy with its surroundings.

In contrast, the pressure in a cylinder of nitrous oxide remains relatively constant as the cylinder empties to the point at which liquid has totally vaporised. Subsequently, there is a linear decline in pressure proportional to the volume of gas remaining within the cylinder.

Filling ratio

The degree of filling of a nitrous oxide cylinder is expressed as the mass of nitrous oxide in the cylinder divided by the mass of water which the cylinder could hold. Normally, a cylinder of nitrous oxide is filled to a ratio of 0.67. This should not be confused with the volume of liquid nitrous oxide in a cylinder. A 'full' cylinder of nitrous oxide at room temperature is filled to the point at which approximately 90% of the interior of the cylinder is occupied by liquid, the remaining 10% being occupied by gaseous nitrous oxide. Incomplete filling of a cylinder is necessary, because thermally induced expansion of the liquid in a totally full cylinder may cause an explosion.

'Entonox'

Entonox is the trade name for a compressed gas mixture containing 50% oxygen and 50% nitrous oxide. The mixture is compressed into cylinders containing gas at a pressure of 137 bar (2000 lb/in^2). The nitrous oxide does not liquefy because the two gases in this mixture 'dissolve' in each other at high pressure. In other words, the presence of oxygen reduces the critical temperature of nitrous oxide. The critical temperature of the mixture is −7°C. Cooling of a cylinder of Entonox to a temperature below −7°C results in separation of liquid nitrous oxide. Use of such a cylinder results in oxygen-rich gas being emitted initially, followed by a hypoxic nitrous oxide rich gas. Consequently, it is recommended that when an Entonox cylinder may have been exposed to low temperatures, it should be stored horizontally for a period of not less than 24 h at a temperature of 5°C or above. In addition, the cylinder should be inverted several times before use.

Pressure notation in anaesthesia

Although the use of SI units of measurement is generally accepted in medicine, a variety of ways of expressing pressure is still used, reflecting custom and practice. Arterial pressure is still referred to universally in terms of mmHg because a column of mercury is one of the most common means of measurement of pressure, and is used also to calibrate electronic devices.

Similarly, measurement of central venous pressure is referred to customarily in cmH_2O.

Atmospheric pressure (P_B) exerts a pressure sufficient to support a column of mercury of height 760 mm (Fig. 16.1).

1 atmospheric pressure = 760 mmHg
= 1.01325 bar
= 750 torr
= 1 atmosphere absolute (ata)
= 14.7 lb/in^2
= 101.325 kPa

In considering pressure, it is necessary to indicate whether or not atmospheric pressure is taken into account. Thus, a diver working 10 m below the surface of the sea may be described as compressed to a depth of 1 atmosphere or working at a pressure of 2 atmospheres absolute (2 ata).

In order to avoid confusion when discussing compressed cylinders of gases, the term gauge pressure is used. This refers to the difference between the pressure of the contents of the cylinder and the ambient pressure. Thus, a full cylinder of oxygen has a gauge pressure of 137 bar, but the contents are at a pressure of 138 bar absolute.

Pressure relief valves

The Heidbrink valve is a common component of many anaesthesia breathing systems. In the Magill breathing system, the anaesthetist may vary the force in the spring(s), thereby controlling the pressure within the breathing system (Fig. 16.2). At equilibrium, the force exerted by the spring is equal to the force exerted by gas within the system:

$$\text{Force } (F) = \text{Gas pressure } (P) \times \text{Disc area } (a)$$

Modern anaesthesia systems contain a variety of pressure relief valves, in each of which the force is fixed so as to provide a gas escape mechanism when pressure reaches a preset level. Thus, an

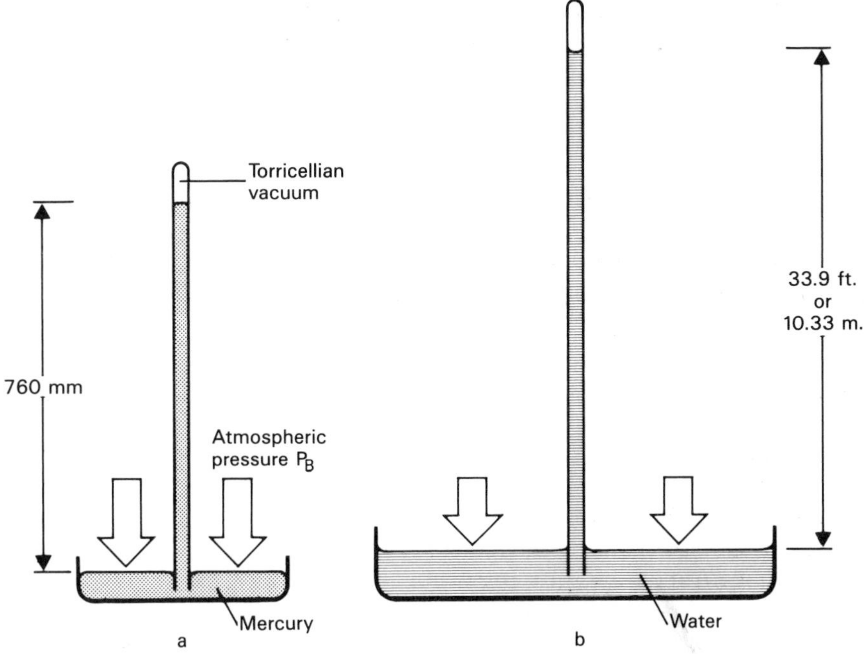

Fig. 16.1 The simple barometer described by Torricelli (a) filled with mercury (b) filled with water.

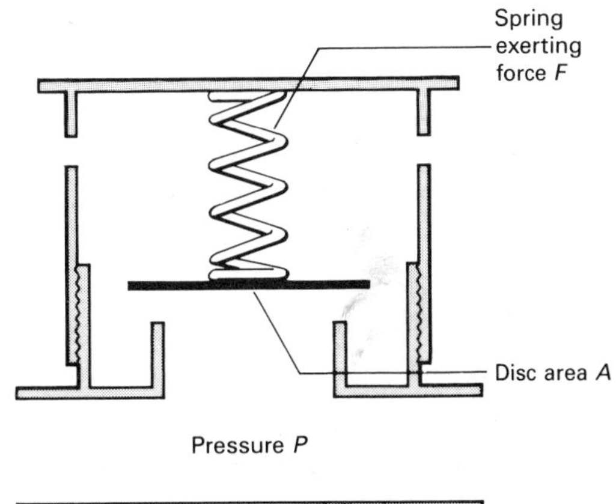

Fig. 16.2 A pressure relief valve.

anaesthetic machine may contain a pressure relief valve operating at 35 kPa, situated on the back bar of the machine between the vaporisers and the breathing system. Modern ventilators may contain a pressure relief valve set at 7 kPa. A much lower pressure is set in relief valves which form part of anaesthetic scavenging systems, and these may operate at pressures of 0.2–0.3 kPa.

Pressure-reducing valves (pressure regulators)

Pressure regulators have two important functions in anaesthetic machines:

1. They reduce high pressures of compressed gases to manageable levels (acting as pressure-reducing valves).
2. They minimise fluctuations in the pressure within an anaesthetic machine which would necessitate frequent manipulations of flowmeter controls.

Modern anaesthetic machines are designed to operate with an inlet gas supply at a pressure of 3–4 bar (usually 4 bar in the UK). Hospital pipeline supplies also operate at a pressure of 4 bar and therefore pressure regulators are not required between a hospital pipeline supply and an anaesthetic machine. In contrast, the contents of cylinders of all medical gases with the exception of cyclopropane (i.e. oxygen, nitrous oxide and carbon dioxide) are at much higher pressures. Thus, cylinders of these gases require a pressure-reducing valve between the cylinder and the flowmeter.

The principle on which the simplest type of pressure-reducing valve operates is shown in Figure 16.3. High-pressure gas enters through the valve and forces the flexible diaphragm upwards, tending to close the valve and prevent further ingress of gas from the high-pressure source.

If there is no tension in the spring, the relationship between the reduced pressure (p) and the high pressure (P) is very approximately equal to the ratio of the areas of the valve seating (a) and the diaphragm (A):

$$\frac{p}{P} = \frac{a}{A}$$

By tensing the spring, a force F is produced which offsets the closing effect of the valve. Thus, p may be increased by increasing the force in the spring.

Without the spring, the simple pressure regulator has the disadvantage that reduced pressure decreases proportionally with the decrease in cylinder pressure. The addition of a force from the spring considerably reduces but does not eliminate this problem, and in order to overcome it newer pressure regulators contain an extra closing spring.

The Adams valve (Fig. 16.4) is an early pressure regulator which is now obsolete, although it may still be seen on some older anaesthetic machines. The S60 M regulator (BOC) is a modern regulator used widely in the UK, and is illustrated in Figure 16.5. It should be noted that the high pressure tends to close the valve.

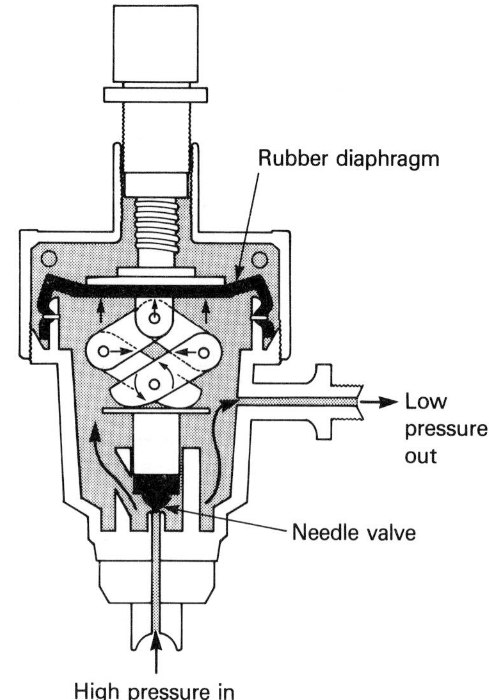

Fig. 16.4 The Adams pressure-regulating valve.

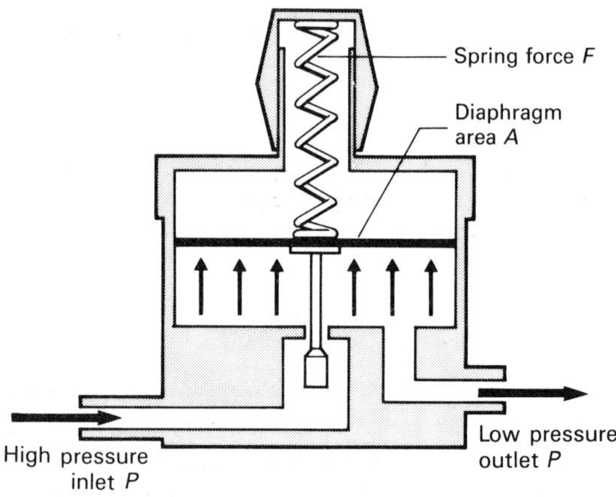

Fig. 16.3 A simple pressure-reducing valve.

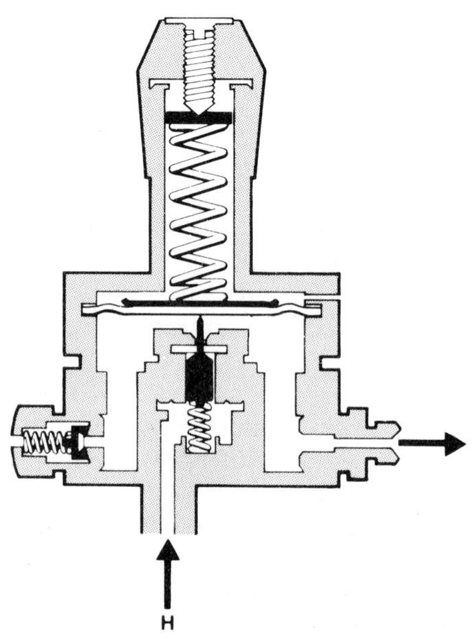

Fig. 16.5 A modern pressure-regulating valve: the S60 M regulator (BOC).

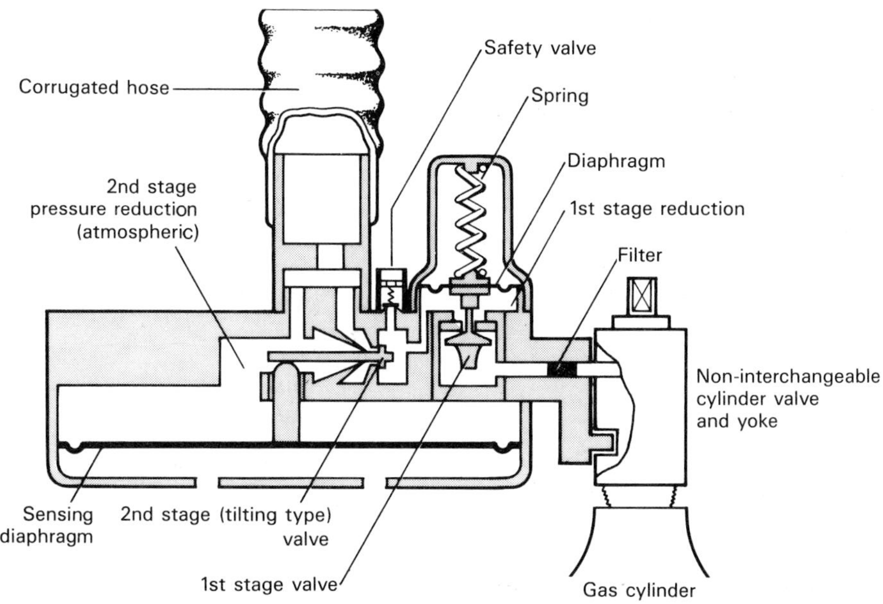

Fig. 16.6 The Entonox two-stage pressure demand regulator.

Pressure demand regulators

These are regulators in which gas flow occurs when an inspiratory effort is applied to the outlet port. The Entonox valve is a two-stage regulator and its mode of action is demonstrated in Figure 16.6.

Measurement of pressure in fluids

Gases

The simplest method of measuring pressure in gases is by the use of a manometer, illustrated in Figure 16.7. The manometer may be filled with water to measure low pressures; for measurement of larger pressures, the column is filled with mercury, which possesses a density 13.6 times greater than that of water. It is clear that liquid-filled manometers are not appropriate for measurement of either gas or liquid pressures in the majority of clinical situations.

In anaesthetic practice, pressures in gases may be measured by sensitive electrical pressure transducers similar to those used for measurement of intravascular pressures.

Pressure gauges on anaesthetic ventilators usually comprise a simple bellows type of aneroid gauge (Fig. 16.8) whilst high gas pressures (e.g. in medical gas cylinders) are measured using a type of Bourdon gauge (Fig. 16.9).

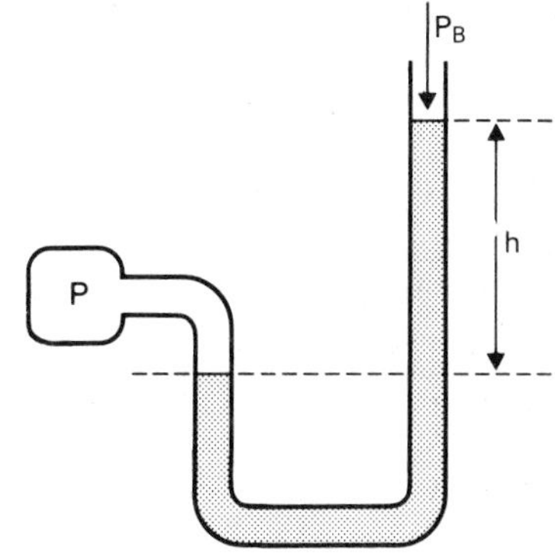

Fig. 16.7 A simple fluid-filled manometer for measurement of pressure *P*.

Liquids

In anaesthetic practice, measurement of pressures in liquids is required in assessment of the circulation. The simple manometer, filled with water, is used frequently for measurement of central venous pressure (see p. 372). Measurement of

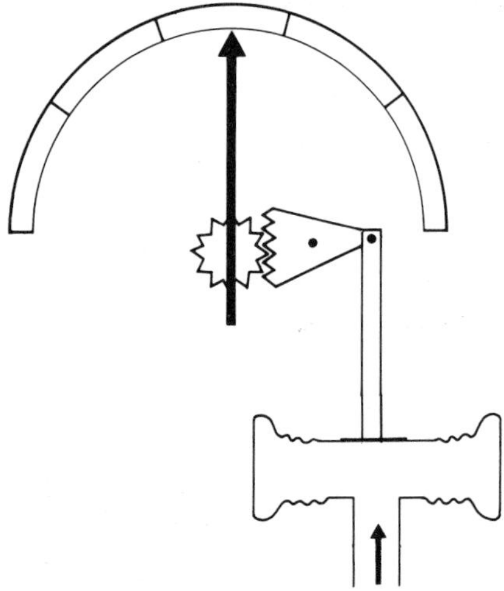

Fig. 16.8 A simple aneroid pressure gauge.

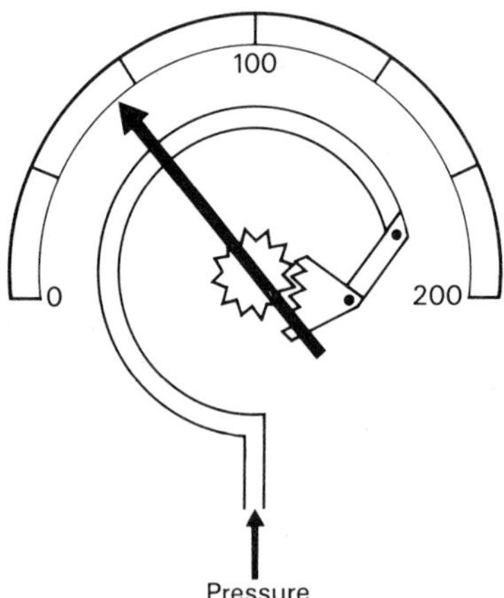

Fig. 16.9 A Bourdon type of pressure gauge. Increase in pressure tends to straighten the coiled metal tube.

arterial pressure is undertaken by a variety of different means including:

1. Sphygmomanometry. A pressure occlusion cuff is applied to the upper arm and the pressure raised until flow through the brachial artery ceases. The pressure within the cuff is measured by using either a simple mercury-filled manometer or an aneroid manometer. Flow beyond the cuff may be detected by:

(a) Palpation of the radial artery.
(b) Auscultation of the brachial artery.
(c) Application of a Doppler flowmeter over the radial artery (a method used principally in paediatric practice).
(d) By the use of finger plethysmography.
(e) By means of a special double cuff which is incorporated in a device termed the oscillotonometer.

2. Direct measurement of pressure by an electronic transducer connected through a fluid-filled column to a cannula sited in the arterial system.

These clinical methods of measuring arterial blood pressure are described in detail in Chapter 21.

Flow of fluids

Viscosity is defined as that property of a fluid which causes it to resist flow. The coefficient of viscosity (η) is defined as:

$$\eta = \frac{\text{force}}{\text{area}} \times \text{velocity gradient}$$

In this context, velocity gradient is equal to the difference between velocities of different fluid molecules divided by the distance between molecules (Fig. 16.10b). The units of the coefficient of viscosity are Pascal seconds.

Fluids which obey this formula are referred to as Newtonian fluids and η is a constant for each fluid. However, some biological fluids are non-Newtonian. A prime example is blood; viscosity changes with the rate of flow of blood (as a result of change in distribution of cells) and, in stored blood, with time (blood thickens on storage).

Viscosity of liquids diminishes with increase in temperature, whereas viscosity of a gas increases with increase in temperature.

Laminar flow

Laminar flow through a tube is illustrated in Figure 16.10b. In this situation, there is a smooth orderly flow of fluid such that molecules travel with the greatest velocity in the axial stream whilst the velocity of those in contact with the wall of the tube may be virtually zero. The linear velocity of axial flow may be twice the average linear velocity of flow.

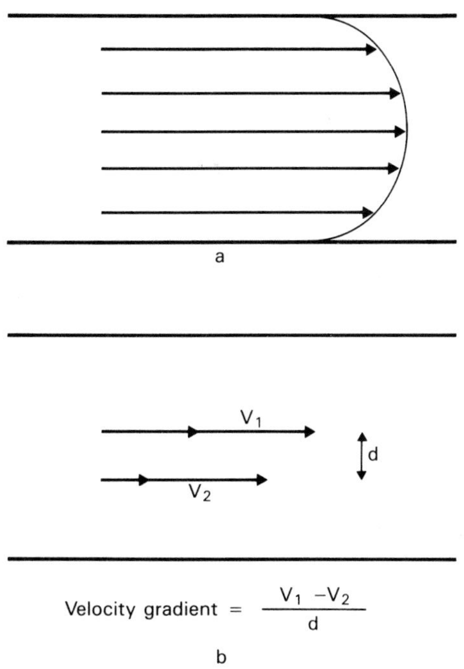

Fig. 16.10 (a) Diagrammatic illustration of laminar flow. (b) Velocity gradient.

In a tube, the factors determining flow are given by the Hagen–Poiseuille formula:

$$\dot{Q} = \frac{\pi P r^4}{8\eta l}$$

where Q= flow; P = pressure gradient along the tube; r = radius of the tube; η = viscosity of fluid; and l = length of the tube.

The Hagen–Poiseuille formula applies only to Newtonian fluids. In non-Newtonian fluids such as blood, increase in velocity of flow may alter viscosity because of variation in the dispersion of cells within plasma.

Turbulent flow

In turbulent flow, fluid no longer moves in orderly planes but swirls and eddies around in a haphazard manner as illustrated in Figure 16.11. Although viscosity affects laminar flow, it should be noted that this does not apply to turbulent flow, which is affected by changes in density.

It may be seen from Figure 16.12 that the relationship between pressure and flow is linear

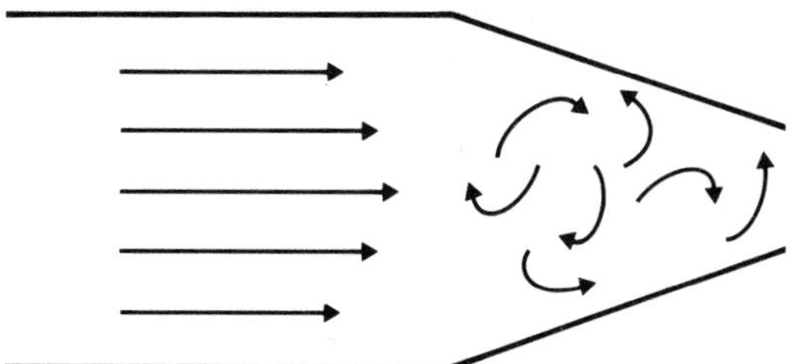

Fig. 16.11 Diagrammatic illustration of turbulent flow.

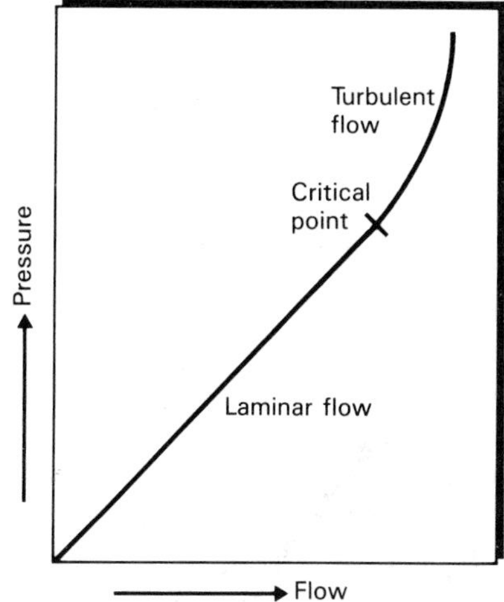

Fig. 16.12 The relationship between pressure and flow in a fluid is linear up to the critical point, above which flow becomes turbulent.

within certain limits. However, as velocity increases, a point is reached (the critical point, or critical velocity) at which the characteristics of flow change from laminar to turbulent. The critical point is dependent upon several factors which were investigated by the physicist Reynolds. The factors are related by the formula used for calculation of Reynolds' number:

$$\text{Reynolds' number} = \frac{v\rho r}{\eta}$$

where v = linear velocity; r = radius of tube; ρ = density; and η = viscosity.

Studies with cylindrical tubes have shown that if Reynolds' number exceeds 2000, flow is likely to be turbulent, whereas a Reynolds' number of less than 2000 is associated usually with laminar flow.

Flow of fluids through orifices

In an orifice, the diameter of the fluid pathway exceeds the length. The flow rate of a fluid through an orifice is dependent upon:

1. The square root of the pressure difference across the orifice.
2. The square of the diameter of the orifice.
3. The density of the fluid, as flow through an orifice inevitably involves some degree of turbulence.

Applications in anaesthetic practice

1. In upper respiratory tract obstruction of any severity, flow is inevitably turbulent; thus for the same respiratory effort, a lower tidal volume is achieved than when flow is laminar. The extent of turbulent flow may be reduced by reducing gas density; clinically it is common practice to administer oxygen-enriched helium rather than oxygen alone (the density of oxygen is 1.3 and that of helium is 0.16).
2. In anaesthetic breathing systems, a sudden change in diameter of tubing or irregularity of the wall may be responsible for a change from laminar to turbulent flow. Thus, tracheal and other breathing tubes should possess smooth internal surfaces, gradual bends, no constrictions and be of as large a diameter and as short a length as possible.
3. Resistance to breathing is much greater when a tracheal tube of small diameter is used (Fig. 16.13).

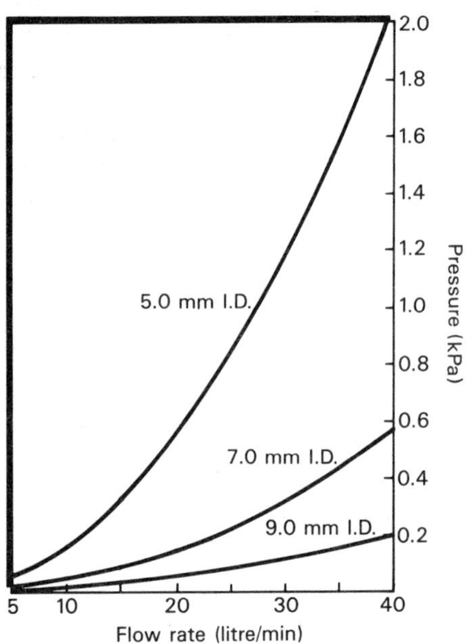

Fig. 16.13 Resistance to gas flow through tracheal tubes of different internal diameter (ID).

MEASUREMENT OF GAS VOLUMES

Spirometers

Spirometers may be classified as dry (e.g. the 'Vitalograph') or wet (e.g. the 'Benedict Roth' spirometer). Both the Vitalograph and Benedict Roth spirometers measure volumes of gases of the order of a few litres. Larger volumes of gases may be measured by the dry gas meter, an instrument used for measuring volumes in domestic gas supplies.

In anaesthesia, the Wright respirometer (see p. 377) is a convenient method of measuring gas volumes.

MEASUREMENT OF FLOW

Flowmeters

The principles of gas flow described above are used in the construction of anaesthetic flowmeters. There are two types of flowmeter: variable-orifice (constant-pressure) or fixed-orifice (variable-pressure).

Fixed-orifice flowmeters

The only common type of fixed-orifice meter used in anaesthetic practice comprises a Bourdon pressure gauge which measures the pressure through a small fixed orifice, beyond which the pressure varies little. Consequently, the flow rate is proportional to the pressure proximal to the fixed orifice and the pressure gauge may be calibrated in units of flow.

Variable-orifice flowmeters

These instruments may be either ball flowmeters or bobbin flowmeters, as illustrated in Figure

16.14. The commonest flowmeter used by the anaesthetist is the bobbin flowmeter, which is referred to frequently by the trade name of Rotameter. Readings are taken from the middle of the ball in a ball flowmeter, but from the top of the bobbin in a bobbin flowmeter.

In the Rotameter, the bobbin possesses small slots which cause it to rotate. Rotation reduces errors caused by friction between the walls of the tube and the bobbin. In order to reduce electrostatic charges and sticking of the bobbin, some modern flowmeter tubes are coated with a thin layer of tin oxide.

The pressure across the bobbin remains relatively constant, producing a force which is equal to the force of gravity on the bobbin. As the flow rate increases, the bobbin rises higher in the tube and the size of the annulus between the bobbin and the walls of the tube increases. At low flow rates, the narrow annular space between the bobbin and the wall mimics a tube. At high flow rates, the width of the annulus is large relative to the height of the bobbin, and the annular space forms an orifice. Thus at low flow rates, the viscosity of gas determines the position of the bobbin, whereas at higher rates the effect of density of the gas becomes more important. Consequently, flowmeters must be calibrated for individual gases.

The Wright peak flowmeter depends upon the variable-orifice principle.

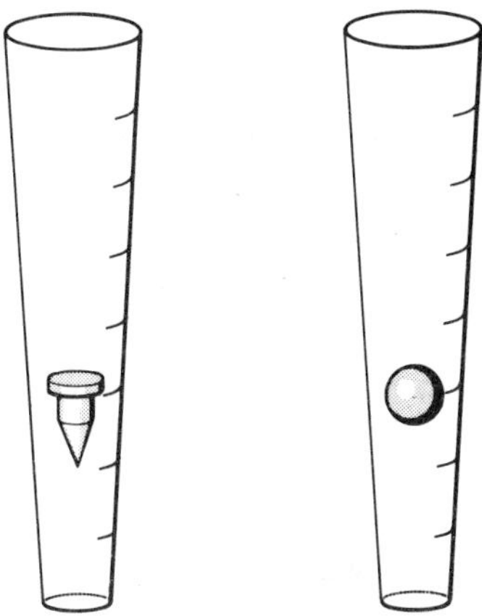

Fig. 16.14 The bobbin (left) and ball (right) flowmeters in exaggerated diagrammatic form to show tapering of tubes.

Pneumotachograph

The pneumotachograph is an instrument for measuring flow rate by sensing the pressure drop across a laminar resistance, i.e. a resistance through which laminar flow occurs.

The Fleisch pneumotachograph (Fig. 16.15) comprises a series of parallel tubes which generate laminar flow even at variable or high flow rates; the pressure change across the tubes is determined using a differential pressure transducer. The major problem with this device is condensation of water vapour; in order to prevent this, the laminar resistor may be surrounded by a heated coil. In addition, heating maintains a constant temperature which prevents errors caused by variations in gas viscosity.

Measurement of flow in liquids

Several methods exist for measurement of blood flow in the circulation.

1. *Limb plethysmography*. This simple technique for measuring blood flow in the limb entails temporary occlusion of venous outflow from the limb; the consequent increase in volume of the limb corresponds to arterial inflow. The increase in volume of the limb may be calculated either from volume displacement in a water container or from the increase in girth of the limb measured by a mercury-in-rubber strain gauge.

2. *The Fick principle*. This principle may be used for measurement of blood flow through a variety of organs, including heart, brain, liver and

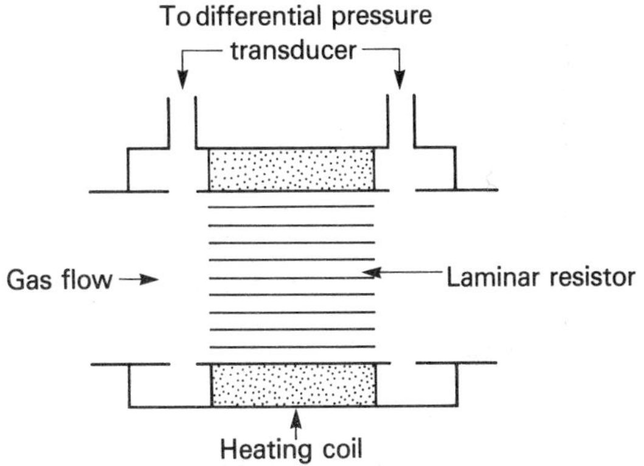

Fig. 16.15 The Fleisch pneumotachograph.

kidney. Total cardiac output may be measured by the use of the Fick principle as applied to the lung.

In essence, the principle states that the amount of substance or tracer taken up or given off by an organ in unit time is equal to the product of blood flow through the organ and the concentration difference of the substance across the organ:

$$\frac{\text{amount}}{\text{time}} = \text{flow} \times (\text{A} - \text{V}) \text{ content differences}$$

where A = arterial and V = venous.

Cardiac output ($\dot{Q}_t$) may be calculated by measuring oxygen consumption ($\dot{V}_{O_2}$) with a spirometer, and the oxygen contents of arterial (Ca_{O_2}) and mixed venous ($C\bar{v}_{O_2}$) blood samples drawn simultaneously from the radial artery and pulmonary artery. Then:

$$\dot{Q}_t = \frac{\dot{V}_{O_2}}{(Ca_{O_2} - Cv_{O_2})}$$

Typical values are:

$$5 \text{ litre/min} = \frac{250 \text{ ml/min}}{(20 - 15) \text{ ml/dl}}$$

3. *Electromagnetic flowmeter.* This instrument operates on the principle of electromagnetic induction. As blood (which is a conductor of electricity) moves through a magnetic field, an electric potential is induced which is proportional to the rate of movement of the blood. The potential is induced in a plane perpendicular to both the magnetic field and the direction of blood flow according to Faraday's left-hand rule (Fig. 16.16).

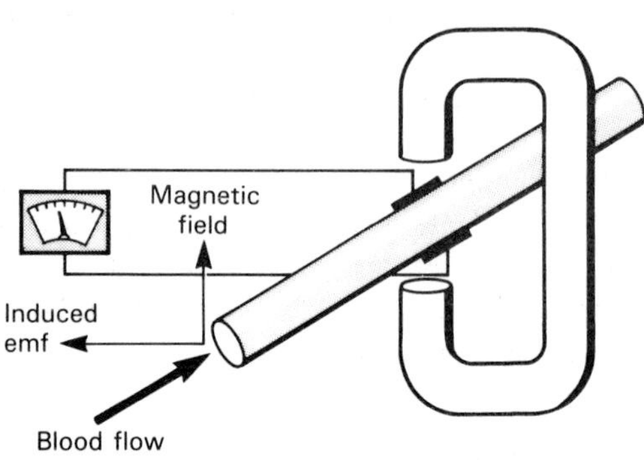

Fig. 16.16 Faraday's left-hand rule of electromagnetic induction in the principle underlying the electromagnetic flowmeter.

4. *Ultrasonic flowmeters.* These devices provide good qualitative but not quantitative information on flow.

5. *Dye-dilution and thermal dilution techniques.* These techniques are used clinically for measurement of cardiac output (see p. 374).

THE INJECTOR

The injector is frequently termed a Venturi, although the principles governing such an apparatus were formulated by Bernoulli in 1778, some 60 years earlier than Venturi. The principle is illustrated in Figure 16.17. As fluid passes through a constriction, there is an increase in velocity of the fluid; beyond the constriction, velocity decreases to the initial value. At point A, the energy in the fluid is both potential and kinetic, but at point B the amount of kinetic energy is much greater because of the increased velocity. As the total energy state must remain constant, potential energy is reduced at point B, and this is reflected by a reduction in pressure. Venturi's contribution to the injector lay in the design of the tube distal to the site of the constriction. For optimum performance, it is necessary for fluid flow to remain laminar in such a tube. In the Venturi tube, the pressure is least at the site of maximum constriction, and by gradual opening of the tube beyond the constriction a subatmospheric pressure may be induced distal to the constriction (Fig. 16.18).

The injector principle may be seen in anaesthetic practice in the following situations:

1. *Oxygen therapy.* Several types of Venturi oxygen masks are available which provide oxygen-

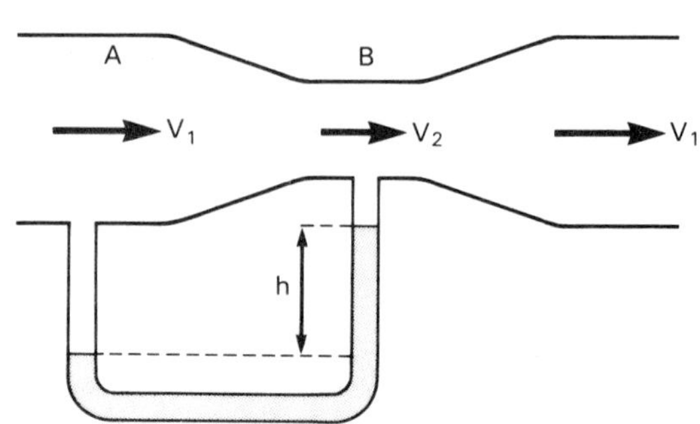

Fig. 16.17 The Bernoulli principle.

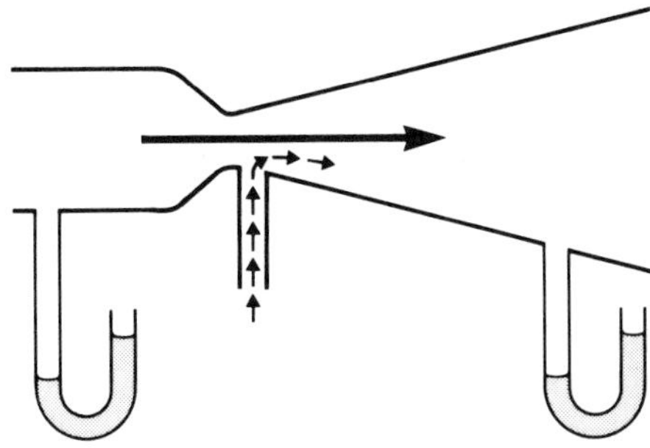

Fig. 16.18 Fluid entrainment by a Venturi injector.

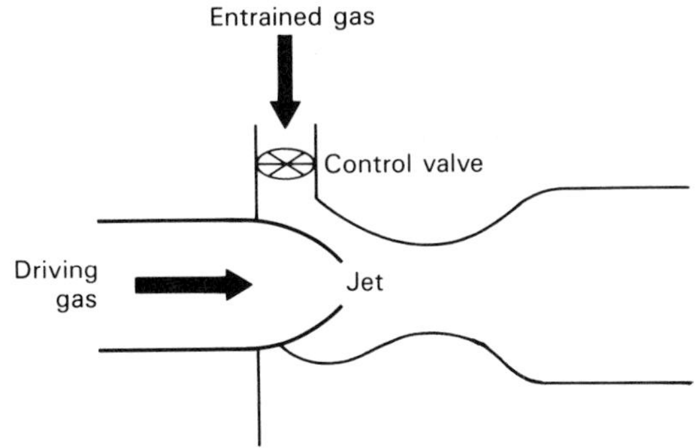

Fig. 16.19 A simple injector.

enriched air. With an appropriate flow of oxygen (usually exceeding 4 litres/min) there is a large degree of entrainment of air. This results in a total gas flow that exceeds the patient's peak inspiratory flow rate, thus ensuring that the inspired oxygen concentration remains constant, and it prevents an increase in apparatus deadspace which always accompanies the use of low-flow oxygen devices (see p. 433).

2. *Nebulisers.* These are used to entrain water from a reservoir. If the water inlet is suitably positioned, the entrained water may be broken up into a fine mist by the high gas velocity.

3. *Portable suction apparatus.*

4. *Oxygen tents.*

5. *As a driving gas in a ventilator* (Fig. 16.19).

The Coanda effect

The Coanda effect describes a phenomenon whereby gas flow through a tube with two Venturis tends to cling either to one side of the tube or to the other. The principle has been used in anaesthetic ventilators (termed fluidic ventilators), as the application of a small pressure distal to the restriction may enable gas flow to be switched from one side to another (Fig. 16.20).

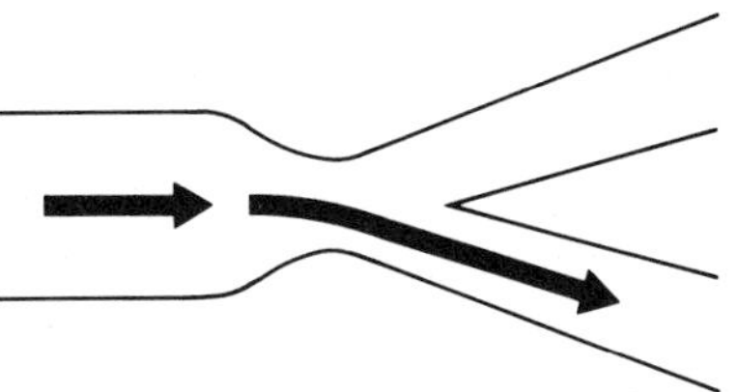

Fig. 16.20 The Coanda effect.

HEAT AND TEMPERATURE

Temperature is a measure of the tendency of an object to gain or lose heat. Heat is the energy which can be transferred from a body at a hotter temperature to one at a colder temperature.

Thermometry

In the SI system, the unit of temperature is the kelvin (K). The zero reference point on this scale is absolute zero (0 K or −273.15°C) and the upper point is the triple point of water (the temperature at which water exists simultaneously in solid, liquid and gaseous states); this corresponds to 273.16 K or 0.01°C.

Temperature is measured in clinical practice by one of the following techniques:

1. *Mercury in glass thermometer.*

2. *Thermistor.* This is a semiconductor which exhibits a reduction in electrical resistance with increase in temperature.

3. *Thermocouple.* This relies on the Seebeck effect. When two metal conductors are joined together to form a circuit, a potential difference is produced which is proportional to the difference in temperatures of the two junctions. In order to measure temperature, one junction has to be kept at a constant temperature.

Heat capacity

The heat capacity of a body is the amount of heat required to raise the temperature of the body by

1°C; in the SI nomenclature, heat capacity is measured in units of joules per kelvin.

Specific heat capacity

The specific heat capacity of a substance is the energy required to raise the temperature of 1 kg of a substance by 1 K. Thus:

heat capacity = mass × specific heat capacity

The specific heat capacity of different substances is of interest because anaesthetists are frequently concerned with maintenance of body temperature in unconscious patients.

Heat is lost from patients by the processes of:

1. Conduction.
2. Convection.
3. Radiation.
4. Evaporation.

The specific heat capacity of gases is up to 1000 times smaller than that of liquids. Consequently, humidification of inspired gases is a more important method of conserving heat than warming dry gases; in addition, the use of humidified gases minimises the very large energy loss produced by evaporation of fluid from the respiratory tract.

The skin of man acts as an almost perfect radiator; radiant losses in susceptible patients may be reduced by the use of reflective aluminium foil ('space blanket').

VAPORISATION AND VAPORISERS

In a liquid, molecules are in a state of continuous motion because of mutual attraction by Van der Waal's forces. Some molecules may develop velocities sufficient to escape from these forces, and if they are close to the surface of a liquid these molecules may escape to enter the vapour phase. Increasing the temperature of a liquid increases its kinetic energy and a greater number of molecules escape. As the faster moving molecules escape into the vapour phase, the net velocity of the remaining molecules reduces; thus the energy state and therefore temperature of the liquid phase are reduced. The amount of heat required to convert unit mass of liquid into a vapour without a change in temperature of the liquid is termed the heat of vaporisation.

In a closed vessel containing liquid and gas, a state of equilibrium is reached when the number of molecules escaping from the liquid is equal to the number of molecules re-entering the liquid phase. The vapour concentration is then said to be saturated at the specified temperature. Saturated vapour pressure of liquids is independent of the ambient pressure, but increases with increasing temperature.

The boiling point of a liquid is the temperature at which its saturated vapour pressure becomes equal to the ambient pressure. Thus, on the graph in Figure 16.21, the boiling point of each liquid at one atmosphere is the temperature at which its saturated vapour pressure is 101.3 kPa.

Vaporisers

Vaporisers may be classified into two types:

1. Drawover vaporisers.
2. Plenum vaporisers.

In the former type, gas is pulled through the vaporiser when the patient inspires, creating a subatmospheric pressure. In the latter type, gas is forced through the vaporiser by the pressure of the fresh gas supply. Consequently, the resistance to gas flow through a drawover vaporiser must be extremely small; the resistance of a plenum vaporiser may be high enough to prevent its use as a drawover vaporiser, although this is not necessarily so.

The principles of both devices are similar. If we consider the simplest form of vaporiser (Fig. 16.22), the concentration (C) of anaesthetic in the gas mixture emerging from the outlet port is dependent upon:

1. *The saturated vapour pressure* of the anaesthetic liquid in the vaporiser. Thus, a highly volatile agent such as diethyl ether is present in a much higher concentration than a less volatile agent (i.e. with a lower saturated vapour pressure) such as halothane.

2. The *temperature* of the liquid anaesthetic agent, as this determines its saturated vapour pressure.

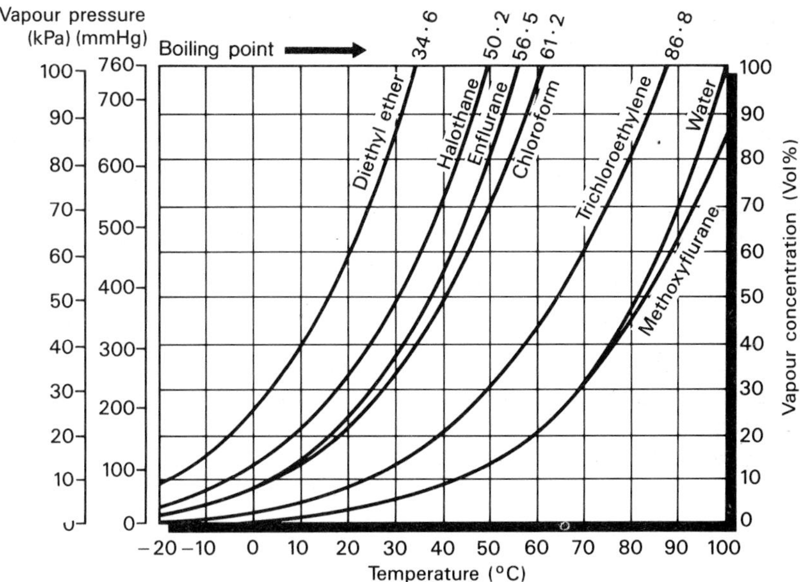

Fig. 16.21 Relationship between vapour pressure and temperature for different anaesthetic agents.

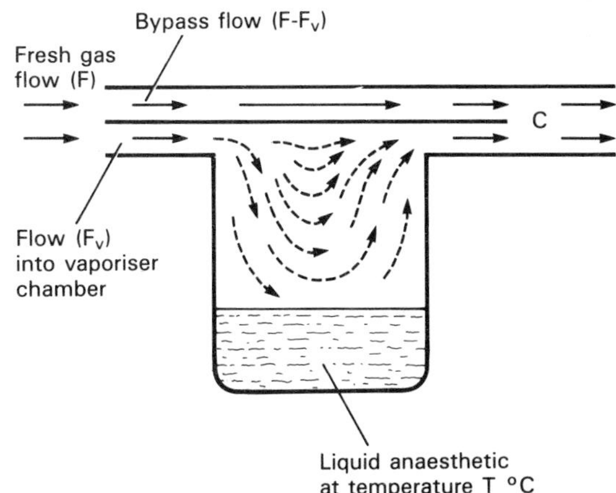

Fig. 16.22 A simple type of vaporiser.

3. The *splitting ratio*, i.e. the flow rate of gas through the vaporising chamber (F_v) in comparison with that through the bypass ($F - F_v$). Regulation of the splitting ratio is the usual mechanism whereby the anaesthetist controls the output concentration from a vaporiser.

4. The *surface area* of the anaesthetic agent in the vaporiser. If the surface area is relatively small during use, the flow of gas through the vaporising chamber may be too rapid to achieve complete saturation with anaesthetic molecules of the gas above the liquid.

5. *Duration of use.* As the liquid in the vaporising chamber evaporates, its temperature, and thus its saturated vapour pressure, decreases. This leads to a reduction in concentration of anaesthetic in the mixture leaving the exit port.

6. The *flow characteristics* through the vaporising chamber. In the simple vaporiser illustrated, gas passing through the vaporising chamber may fail to mix completely with vapour as a result of streaming because of poor design. This lack of mixing is flow-dependent.

Modern anaesthetic vaporisers overcome many of the problems described above. Maintenance of full saturation may be achieved by making available a large surface area for vaporisation. In the Tec series of vaporisers this is achieved by the use of wicks which draw up liquid anaesthetic and provide a very large surface area. Efficient vaporisation and prevention of streaming of gas through the vaporising chamber are achieved by ensuring that gas travels through a concentric helix which is bounded by the fabric wicks. Another method of ensuring full saturation is to bubble gas through liquid anaesthetic via a sintered disc. This method is used in the Halox vaporiser and in the Copper Kettle vaporiser, which is popular in the USA. In both these types of vaporiser the final concentration is determined by mixing a known flow of fresh gas with a measured flow of fully saturated vapour.

Temperature compensation

Temperature-compensated vaporisers possess a mechanism which produces an increase in flow through the vaporising chamber (i.e. an increased splitting ratio) as the temperature of liquid anaesthetic decreases. In the Tec vaporisers, a bimetallic strip controls (by bending) a valve which alters flow through the exit port of the vaporising chamber. In the EMO and Ohio vaporisers, a bellows mechanism is used to regulate the valve (by shortening with decreased temperature) whilst in the Drager Vapor 19 vaporisers a metal rod acts in a similar fashion.

In the Copper Kettle and Halox vaporisers, the temperature in the vaporiser is measured and the flow rate adjusted according to a calibration chart. In addition, reduction in temperature is minimised in the Copper Kettle vaporiser by the method of construction; this comprises a large mass of copper which provides a large heat capacity and efficient conduction of heat from the anaesthetic machine to which the vaporiser is attached.

Back pressure (pumping effect)

Some gas-driven mechanical ventilators (e.g. Manley) produce a considerable increase in pressure in the outlet port and back bar of the anaesthetic machine. This pressure is highest during the inspiratory phase of ventilation. If the simple vaporiser shown in Figure 16.2 is attached to the back bar, the increased pressure during inspiration compresses the gas in the vaporiser; some gas in the region of the outlet port of the vaporiser is forced back into the vaporising chamber, where more vapour is added to it. Subsequently, there is a temporary surge in anaesthetic concentration when the pressure decreases at the end of the inspiratory cycle.

This effect is minimal with efficient vaporisers (i.e. those which saturate gas fully in the vaporisation chamber) because gas in the outlet port is already saturated with vapour. However, when pressure reduces at the end of inspiration, some saturated gas passes retrogradely out of the inspiratory port and mixes with the bypass gas. Thus, a temporary increase in total vapour concentration may still occur in the gas supplied to the patient. Methods of overcoming this problem include:

1. Incorporation of a one-way valve in the outlet port.
2. Construction of a bypass chamber and vaporising chamber which are of equal volumes so that the gas in each is compressed or expanded equally.
3. Construction of a long inlet tube to the vaporising chamber so that retrograde flow from the vaporising chamber does not reach the bypass channel (as in the Mark 3 Tec vaporisers).

HUMIDITY AND HUMIDIFICATION

Absolute humidity is the mass of water vapour present in a given volume of gas. Relative humidity is the ratio of mass of water vapour in a given volume of gas to the mass required to saturate that volume of gas at the same temperature.

Relative humidity (RH) may be expressed as:

$$RH = \frac{\text{actual vapour pressure}}{\text{saturated vapour pressure}}$$

In normal practice, relative humidity may be measured using:

1. The *hair hygrometer*. This operates on the principle that a hair elongates if humidity increases; the hair length controls a pointer. This simple device may be mounted on a wall. It is reasonably accurate only in the range 15–85% relative humidity.
2. The *wet and dry bulb hygrometer*. The dry bulb measures the actual temperature, whereas the wet bulb measures a lower temperature as a result of the cooling effect of evaporation of water. The rate of vaporisation is related to the humidity of the ambient gas and the difference between the two temperatures is a measure of ambient humidity; the relative humidity is obtained from a set of tables.

3. *Regnault's hygrometer*. This consists of a thin silver tube containing ether and a thermometer to show the temperature of the ether. Air is pumped through the ether to produce evaporation, thereby cooling the silver tube. When gas in contact with the tube is saturated with water vapour it condenses as a mist on the bright silver. The temperature at which this takes place is known as the *dew point*, from which relative humidity is obtained from tables.

Humidification in the respiratory tract

Air drawn into the respiratory tract becomes fully saturated in the trachea at a temperature of 37°C. Under these conditions, the SVP of water is 6.3 kPa (47 mmHg); this represents a fractional concentration of 6.2%. The concentration of water is 44 mg/litre. At 21°C, saturated water vapour contains 2.4% water vapour or 18 mg/litre. Thus, there is a considerable capacity for patients to lose both water and heat when the lungs are ventilated with dry gases.

There are three means of humidifying inspired gas:

1. Heated humidifier (water vaporiser).
2. Nebuliser.
3. Condenser humidifier (also known as heat and moisture exchanging humidifier).

The hot water bath humidifier is a simple device for heating water to 45–60°C. These devices have several potential problems, including infection if the water temperature decreases below 45°C, scalding the patient if the temperature exceeds 60°C (these high temperatures may be employed to prevent growth of bacteria) and condensation of water in the inspiratory anaesthetic tubing. These devices are approximately 80% efficient.

Some nebulisers are based upon a Venturi system; a gas supply entrains water which is broken up into a large number of droplets. The ultrasonic nebuliser operates by dropping water on to a surface which is vibrated at a frequency of 2 MHz. This breaks up the water particles into extremely small droplets. The main problem with these nebulisers is the possibility that supersaturation of inspired gas may occur and the patient may be overloaded with water.

The condenser humidifier (or artificial nose), may consist of a simple wire mesh which is inserted between the tracheal tube and anaesthetic breathing system. More recently, humidifiers constructed of rolled corrugated paper have been introduced. These devices are approximately 70% efficient.

SOLUTION OF GASES

Henry's law states that, at a given temperature, the amount of a gas which dissolves in a liquid is directly proportional to the partial pressure of the gas in equilibrium with the liquid. If a liquid is heated and its temperature rises, the partial pressure of its vapour increases. As the total ambient pressure remains constant, the partial pressure of any dissolved gas must decrease.

It is customary to confine the term 'tension' to the partial pressure of a gas exerted by gas molecules in solution.

Solubility coefficients

The Bunsen solubility coefficient is the volume of gas which dissolves in unit volume of liquid at a given temperature when the gas in equilibrium with the liquid is at a pressure of one atmosphere.

The Ostwald solubility coefficient is the volume of gas which dissolves in unit volume of liquid at a given temperature. Thus, the Ostwald solubility coefficient is independent of pressure.

The partition coefficient is the ratio of the amount of substance in one phase compared with a second phase, each phase being of equal volume and in equilibrium. As with the Ostwald coefficient, it is necessary to define the temperature, but not the pressure. The partition coefficient may be applied to two liquids, but the Ostwald coefficient applies to partition between gas and liquid.

DIFFUSION AND OSMOSIS

If two different gases or liquids are separated in a container by an impermeable partition which is then removed, gradual mixing of the two different substances occurs as a result of the kinetic activity of each molecule. This is illustrated in Figure

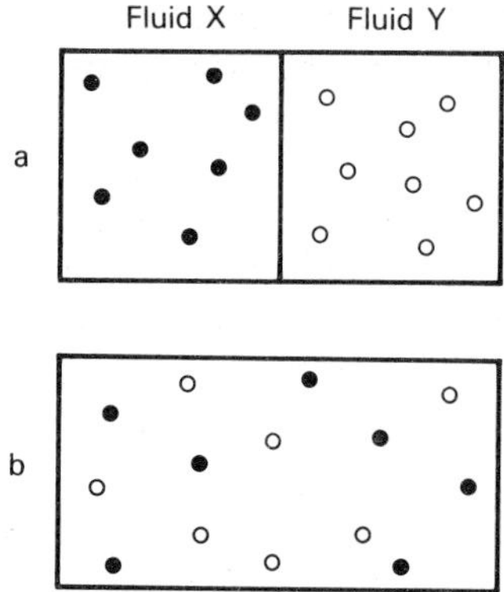

Fig. 16.23 Illustration of diffusion in fluids: (a) fluid X and Y separated by partition; (b) mixing of fluids after removal of partition.

16.23. The principle governing this process is described by Fick's law of diffusion, which states that the rate of diffusion of a substance across unit area is proportional to the concentration gradient. Graham's law (which applies to gases only) states that the rate of diffusion of a gas is inversely proportional to the square root of its molecular weight.

In the example shown in Figure 16.23b, the interface between fluids X and Y after removal of the partition would be the surface of the fluid. In biology, however, there is normally a membrane separating gases, or separating gas and liquids.

The rate of diffusion of gases may be affected by the nature of the membrane. In the lungs, the alveolar membrane is moist and may be regarded as a water film. Thus, diffusion of gases through the alveolar membrane is dependent not only on the properties of diffusion described above but also on the solubility of gas in the water film. As carbon dioxide is highly soluble compared with oxygen, it diffuses more rapidly across the alveolar membrane, despite the larger partial pressure gradient for oxygen.

Osmosis

In the examples given above, the membranes are permeable to all substances. However, in biology, membranes are frequently semipermeable, i.e. they allow the passage of some substances but are impermeable to others. This is illustrated in

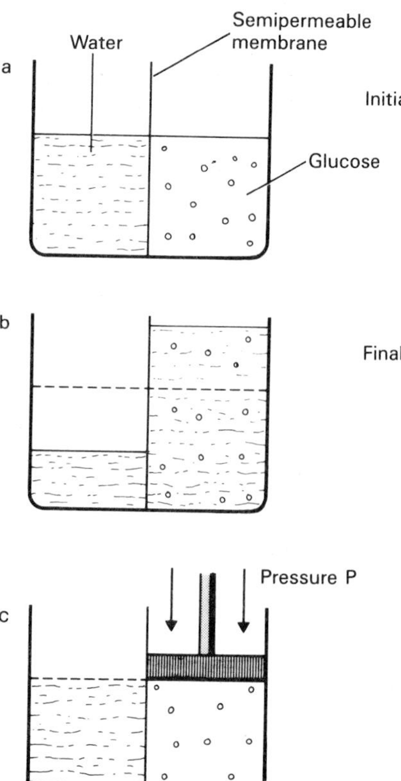

Fig. 16.24 Diagram to illustrate osmotic pressure: (a) water and glucose placed into two compartments separated by a semipermeable membrane; (b) at equilibrium, water has passed into the glucose compartment to balance osmotic pressure; (c) the magnitude of osmotic pressure of the glucose is denoted by a hydraulic pressure *P* applied to the glucose to prevent any movement of water into the glucose compartment.

Figure 16.24. In Figure 16.24a, initially equal volumes of water and glucose solution are separated by a semipermeable membrane. Water molecules pass freely through the membrane to dilute the glucose solution (Fig. 16.24b). By application of a hydrostatic pressure (Fig. 16.24c), the process of transfer of water molecules can be prevented; this pressure (*P*) is equal to the osmotic pressure exerted by the glucose solution.

Substances in dilute solution behave in accordance with the gas laws. Thus, 1 gram molecular weight of a dissolved substance occupying 22.4 litres of solvent exerts an osmotic pressure of 1 bar at 273 K. Dalton's law applies also; the total osmotic pressure of a mixture of solutes is equal to the sum of osmotic pressures exerted independently by each substance.

The osmotic pressure of a solution depends on the number of dissolved particles per litre. Thus, a molar solution of a substance which ionises into two particles exerts twice the osmotic pressure exerted by a molar solution of a non-ionising substance.

The term osmolarity refers to the osmotic pressure produced by all substances in a fluid. Thus, it is the sum of the individual molarities of each particle.

The term osmolality refers to the number of osmoles per kilogram of water or other solvent (whilst molarity refers to osmoles per litre of solution). Thus, osmolarity may vary slightly from osmolality as a result of changes in density due to the effect of temperature on volume, although in biological terms the difference is extremely small.

In the circulation, water and the majority of ions are freely permeable across the endothelial membrane, but plasma protein does not traverse into the interstitial fluid. The term oncotic pressure is used to describe the osmotic pressure exerted by the plasma proteins alone. Plasma oncotic pressure is relatively small (approximately 1 mosmol/litre) in relation to total osmotic pressure exerted by plasma (approximately 300 mosmol/litre).

ELECTRICAL SAFETY

The anaesthetist is in daily contact with a large amount of equipment which is powered by mains supply electricity; this includes monitoring equipment, some ventilators, suction apparatus, defibrillators and diathermy equipment.

Whilst a total understanding of this equipment and its mode of action may depend upon a detailed knowledge of electronics, the equipment can usually be used safely as a type of 'black box' (i.e. the inside of the box may be a mystery, but the anaesthetist must be familiar with the operating controls and the ways in which the apparatus may malfunction or, if a recording instrument, give rise to artefacts).

It is not possible in this brief chapter to provide a synopsis of the basic principles of electricity and electronics, but it is essential to stress some elements which have a bearing on the safety of both the patient and the anaesthetist in the operating theatre.

In the UK, the mains electricity is supplied at a voltage of 240 V with a frequency of 50 Hz, and in the USA at a voltage of 110 V and a frequency of 60 Hz. These voltages are potentially dangerous, although the danger is related predominantly to the current which flows through the patient:

$$\text{current } (I) = \frac{\text{voltage } (V)}{\text{resistance } (R)} \text{ (Ohm's law)}$$

When dealing with alternating current, it is necessary to use the term impedance in place of resistance, as impedance takes into account the presence of capacitors and resistors. Direct current cannot pass through capacitors; the resistance of a capacitor is inversely proportional to the frequency of an alternating current.

If an increasing electrical current at 50 Hz passes through the body, there is initially a tingling sensation at a current of 1 mA. Increase in the current produces increasing pain and muscle spasm until, at 80–100 mA, arrhythmias and ventricular fibrillation may occur.

The damage to tissue by alternating current is related also to the current density; a current passing through a small area is more dangerous than the same current passing through a much larger area. Other factors relating to the likelihood of ventricular fibrillation are the duration of passage of the current and its frequency. Radio frequencies (such as those used in diathermy) have no potential for fibrillating the heart.

It is clear from Ohm's law that the size of the current is dependent upon the size of the impedance to current flow. A common way of reducing the risk of a large current injuring the anaesthetist in the operating theatre is to wear antistatic shoes and to stand on the antistatic floor. This provides a high impedance (vide infra).

There are three classes of electrical insulation which are designed to minimise the risk of a patient or anaesthetist forming part of an electrical circuit between the live conductor of a piece of equipment and ground.

1. *Class I equipment.* The main supply lead has three cores (live, neutral and earth). The earth is

connected to all exposed conductive parts and in the event of a fault developing which short-circuits current to the casing of the equipment, current flows from the case to earth and blows a fuse.

2. *Class II equipment.* This has no protective earth. The power cable has only live and neutral conductors and these are 'double-insulated'. The casing is normally made of non-conductive material.

3. *Class III equipment.* This relies on a power supply at a very low voltage produced from a secondary transformer situated some distance away from the device. Potentials do not exceed 24 V AC or 50 V DC. Electric heating blankets, for example, are rendered safer in this way.

Isolation circuits

All modern patient-monitoring equipment uses an isolation transformer so that the patient is connected only to the secondary circuit of the transformer, which is not earthed. Thus, even if the patient makes contact between the live circuit of the secondary transformer and ground, no current is transmitted to ground.

Microshock

Mains electricity supplies may induce currents in other circuits or on cases of instruments. The resulting induced currents are termed leakage currents and may pass through either the patient or anaesthetist to ground. Although the currents are very small, they may present problems to patients with an intracardiac pacemaker, or a saline-filled intracardiac monitoring catheter.

The International Electrotechnical Commission has produced recommendations (adopted by the British Standards Institute) defining the levels of permitted leakage currents and patient currents from different types of electromedical equipment.

FIRES AND EXPLOSIONS

Although the use of inflammable anaesthetic agents has declined greatly over the last 2–3 decades, ether is still used commonly in many countries. In addition, other inflammable agents may be utilised in the operating theatre, e.g. alcohol for skin sterilisation. Thus the anaesthetist should have some understanding of the problems and risks of fire occurring in the operating theatre.

Fires are produced when fuels undergo combustion. A conflagration differs from a fire in having a more rapid and more violent rate of combustion. A fire becomes an explosion if the combustion is sufficiently rapid to cause pressure waves which in turn cause sound waves. If these pressure waves possess sufficient energy to ignite adjacent fuels, the combustion is extremely violent and termed a detonation.

Fires require three ingredients:

1. Fuel.
2. Oxygen or other substance capable of supporting combustion.
3. Source of ignition, i.e. a source of heat sufficient to raise the fuel temperature to its ignition temperature. This quantity of heat is termed the activation energy.

Fuels

The modern volatile anaesthetic agents (halothane, enflurane and isoflurane) are non-flammable and non-explosive at room temperature in either air or oxygen.

Oils and greases are petroleum-based, and form excellent fuels. In the presence of high pressures of oxygen, nitrous oxide or compressed air, these fuels may ignite spontaneously, an event termed dieseling (an analogy with the diesel engine). Thus oil or grease must not be used in compressed air, nitrous oxide or oxygen supplies.

Surgical spirit burns readily in air and the risk is increased in the presence of oxygen or nitrous oxide. Other non-anaesthetic inflammable substances include methane in the gut (which may be ignited by diathermy when the gut is opened), paper dressings and plastics found in the operating theatre suite.

Ether burns in air slowly with a blue flame but mixtures of nitrous oxide, oxygen and ether are always explosive. It has been suggested that if administration of ether is discontinued 5 min before exposure to a source of ignition, the patient's expired gas is unlikely to burn provided that an open circuit has been used after discontinuation of ether.

Cyclopropane is highly explosive when mixed with oxygen and the resulting mixture may be ignited by relatively low energies.

The stoichiometric concentration of a fuel and oxidising agent is the concentration at which all combustible vapour and agent are completely utilised. Thus the most violent reactions take place in stoichiometric mixtures, and as the concentration of the fuel moves away from the stoichiometric range the reaction gradually declines until a point is reached (the flammability limit) at which ignition does not occur.

The flammability range for ether is 2–82% in oxygen, 2–36% in air and 1.5–24% in nitrous oxide. The stoichiometric concentration of ether in oxygen is 14% and there is a risk of explosion with ether concentrations of approximately 12–40% in oxygen. In air, the stoichiometric concentration of ether is 3.4% and explosions do not occur.

Support of combustion

It should always be remembered that as the concentration of oxygen increases so does the likelihood of ignition of a fuel and the conversion of the reaction from fire to explosion.

Nitrous oxide supports combustion. During laparoscopy, there is a risk of perforation of the bowel and escape of methane or hydrogen into the peritoneal cavity. Consequently, the use of nitrous oxide to produce a pneumoperitoneum for this procedure is not recommended; carbon dioxide is to be preferred, as it does not support combustion (and in addition has a much greater solubility in blood than nitrous oxide, thereby diminishing the risk of gas embolism).

Sources of ignition

The two main sources of ignition in the operating theatre are static electricity and diathermy.

Static electricity

Static charges are produced on non-conductive material, such as rubber mattresses, plastic pillow cases and sheets, woollen blankets, nylon, terylene, hosiery garments, rubber tops of stools and non-conducting parts of anaesthetic machines and breathing systems.

Diathermy

Diathermy equipment has now become an essential element of most surgical practice. However, it should not be used in the presence of inflammable agents.

Other sources of ignition

1. Faulty electrical equipment.
2. Heat from endoscopes, thermocautery, lasers, etc.
3. Electric sparks from motor switches, X-ray machines, etc.

Prevention of static charges

Where possible, antistatic conducting material should be used in place of non-conductors. The resistance of antistatic material should be between 50 kΩ/cm and 10 MΩ/cm.

All material should be allowed to leak static charges through the floor of the operating theatre. However, if the conductivity of the floor is too high there is a risk of electrocution if an individual forms a contact between mains voltage and ground. Consequently, the floor of the operating theatre is designed to have a resistance of 25–50 kΩ when measured between two electrodes placed 1 m apart. This allows the gradual discharge of static electricity to earth. Personnel should wear conducting shoes, each with a resistance of between 0.1 and 1 MΩ.

Moisture encourages the leakage of static charges along surfaces to the floor. The risk of sparks from accumulated static electricity charges is reduced if the relative humidity of the atmosphere is kept above 50%.

FURTHER READING

Mushin W W, Jones P L 1987 Physics for the anaesthetist, 4th edn. Blackwell Scientific Publications, Oxford

Parbrook G D, Davis P D, Parbrook E O 1985 Basic physics and measurement in anaesthesia, 2nd edn. Heinemann, London

Sykes M K, Vickers M D, Hull C J 1981 Principles of clinical measurement, 2nd edn. Blackwell Scientific Publications, Oxford

17. Anaesthetic apparatus

It cannot be stressed too highly that anaesthetists should have a sound understanding and firm knowledge of the functioning of all anaesthetic equipment in common use. Although primary malfunction of equipment has not featured highly in surveys of anaesthetic-related morbidity and mortality, failure to understand the use of equipment features in these reports as a cause of morbidity and mortality. This is true especially of ventilators, where lack of knowledge regarding the function of equipment may result in a patient being subjected to the dangers of hypoxaemia and/or hypercapnia.

It is essential that the anaesthetist checks that all equipment is functioning correctly before he proceeds to anaesthetise patients. In some respects, the routine of testing anaesthetic equipment resembles the airline pilot's check list which is an essential preliminary to aircraft flight. Adverse events occur during anaesthesia with great rapidity, and faced with an imminent disaster the anaesthetist must be assured in advance that any equipment which he proposes to use is functioning correctly.

The purpose of this chapter is to describe briefly apparatus which is used in delivery of gases, from the sources of supply to the patient's lungs. Clearly, it is not possible to describe in detail equivalent models produced by all manufacturers. Consequently, this chapter concentrates only on principles and some equipment which is used commonly.

It is convenient to describe anaesthetic apparatus sequentially from the supply of gases to point of delivery to the patient. This sequence is shown in Table 17.1.

Table 17.1 Classification of anaesthetic equipment described in this chapter

Supply of gases
- from outside the operating theatre
- from cylinders within the operating theatre, together with the connections involved

The anaesthetic machine
- unions
- cylinders
- reducing valves
- flowmeters
- vaporisers

Safety features of the anaesthetic machine

Anaesthetic breathing systems

Ventilators

Apparatus used in scavenging waste anaesthetic gases

Apparatus used in interfacing the patient to the anaesthetic breathing system
- laryngoscopes
- anaesthetic masks and airways

Tracheal tubes

Accessory apparatus for the airway
- forceps
- laryngeal sprays
- bougies
- mouth gags
- stilletes
- catheter mounts

GAS SUPPLIES

Bulk supply of anaesthetic gases

In the majority of modern hospitals, piped medical gases and vacuum systems (PMGV) have been installed. These obviate the necessity for holding large numbers of cylinders in the operating theatre suite. Normally, only a few cylinders are kept in reserve, attached usually to the anaesthetic machine.

The advantages of the PMGV system are reductions in cost, in the necessity to transport cylinders and in accidents caused by cylinders becoming exhausted. However, there have been several well-publicised incidents in which anaesthetic morbidity or mortality has resulted from incorrect connections in piped medical gas supplies.

The PMGV services comprise five sections:

1. Bulk store.
2. Distribution pipelines in the hospital.
3. Terminal outlets, situated usually on the walls or ceilings of the operating theatre suite and other sites.
4. Flexible hoses connecting the terminal outlets to the anaesthetic machine.
5. Connections between flexible hoses and anaesthetic machines.

Responsibility for items 1–3 lies with the Engineering and Pharmacy Departments. Within the operating theatre, it is partly the anaesthetist's responsibility to check the correct functioning of items 4 and 5 (vide infra).

Bulk store

Oxygen

In small hospitals, oxygen may be supplied to the PMGV from a bank of several oxygen cylinders attached to a manifold. However, in larger hospitals, pipeline oxygen originates from a liquid oxygen store. Liquid oxygen is stored at a temperature of approximately −165°C at 10.5 bar in a giant Thermos flask — a vacuum insulated evaporator (VIE). Some heat passes from the environment through the insulating layer between the two shells of the flask, increasing the tendency to evaporation and elevation of pressure within the chamber. Pressure is maintained constant by transfer of gaseous oxygen into the pipeline system (via a warming device). However, if the pressure increases above 17 bar a safety valve opens and oxygen runs to waste. When the supply of oxygen resulting from the slow evaporation from the surface in the VIE is inadequate, the pressure decreases and a valve opens to allow liquid oxygen to pass into an evaporator, from which gas passes into the pipeline system.

Liquid oxygen plants are housed some distance away from hospital buildings because of the risk of fire. Even when a hospital possesses a liquid oxygen plant, it is still necessary to hold reserve banks of oxygen cylinders in case of supply failure.

Oxygen concentrators. Recently, oxygen concentrators have been used to supply hospitals and it is likely that the use of these devices will increase in future. The oxygen concentrator depends upon the ability of an artificial zeolight to entrap molecules of nitrogen. These devices cannot produce pure oxygen, but the concentration usually exceeds 90%; the remainder comprises nitrogen, argon and other inert gases. Small oxygen concentrators are provided for domiciliary use.

Nitrous oxide

Nitrous oxide and Entonox may be supplied from banks of cylinders connected to manifolds similar to those used for oxygen.

Medical compressed air

Compressed air is supplied from a bank of cylinders into the PMGV system. Air of medical quality is required, as industrial compressed air may contain fine particles of oil.

Piped medical vacuum

Piped medical vacuum is provided by large vacuum pumps which discharge via a filter and silencer to a suitable point, usually roof level, where gases are vented to atmosphere. Although concern has been expressed regarding the possibility of volatile anaesthetic agents dissolving in the lubricating oil of vacuum pumps and causing malfunction, this fear has not been substantiated.

Terminal outlets

There has been standardisation of terminal outlets in the United Kingdom since 1978, but there is no universal standard.

Seven types of terminal outlet are found commonly in the operating theatre. The terminals are colour-coded and also have non-interchangeable connections specific to each gas:

1. Vacuum (coloured yellow). A vacuum of at least 53 kPa (400 mmHg) should be maintained at the outlet, which should be able to take a free flow of air of at least 40 litres/min.
2. Compressed air (coloured white/black) at 4 bar. This is used for anaesthetic breathing systems and ventilators.
3. Air (coloured white/black) at 7 bar. This is to be used only for powering compressed air tools and is confined usually to the orthopaedic operating theatre.
4. Nitrous oxide (coloured blue) at 4 bar.
5. Oxygen (coloured white) at 4 bar.
6. Scavenging. There is a variety of scavenging outlets from the operating theatre. The passive systems are designed to accept a standard 30 mm connection.

Whenever a new pipeline system has been installed or servicing of an existing pipeline system has been undertaken, a designated member of the pharmacy staff should test the gas obtained from the sockets, using an oxygen analyser. Malfunction of an oxygen/air mixing device may result in entry of compressed air into the oxygen pipeline, rendering an anaesthetic mixture hypoxic. Because of this possibility, it has been advocated that oxygen analysers be used routinely during anaesthesia.

Gas supplies

Gas supplies to the anaesthetic machine should be checked at the beginning of each session to ensure that the gas which issues from the pipeline or cylinder is the same as that which passes through the appropriate flowmeter. This ensures that pipelines are not connected incorrectly. Both the machine in the operating theatre and that in the anaesthetic room should be checked. The following procedure has been recommended:

1. Check that the cylinders are in position, attached correctly to their yokes and switched off.
2. Open the oxygen and nitrous oxide flowmeter valves by 2–3 full turns and ensure that all others are closed. No flow should occur.
3. Turn on the oxygen cylinder. Check the oxygen gauge to ensure that sufficient oxygen is present in the cylinder. The oxygen flowmeter should be adjusted to provide a flow rate of 4 litres/min. If there is any flow in the nitrous oxide flowmeter, the machine should be rejected.
4. Turn on the nitrous oxide cylinder and check that the flowmeter registers a flow. If the oxygen flow changes, the machine should be rejected.
5. Set the oxygen failure device in operation, if it is not automatic.
6. Turn off the oxygen cylinder. Check that the oxygen bobbin falls completely to the bottom of the tube. Check that the oxygen failure device works. If the oxygen flowmeter registers any flow when the nitrous oxide only is turned on, the machine should be rejected.
7. Insert the probe into the wall connection for the oxygen supply. This should cancel the operation of the oxygen failure alarm. Apply a tug to ensure that it is connected correctly. Check the oxygen flowmeter, which should still show a flow rate of 4 litres/min.
8. Turn off the nitrous oxide cylinder. If the oxygen bobbin demonstrates any fall when nitrous oxide is turned off, the machine should be rejected.
9. Insert the nitrous oxide connection into the pipeline system and apply a tug. If there is any change in the position of the oxygen bobbin, the machine should be rejected.
10. Complete the check by occluding the outlet of the machine, and ensure that the pressure relief valve on the back bar operates.

CYLINDERS

Modern cylinders are constructed from molybdenum steel. They are checked at intervals by the manufacturer to ensure that they can withstand hydraulic pressures considerably in excess of those to which they are subjected in normal use. One cylinder in every 100 is cut into strips to test the metal for tensile strength, flattening impact and bend tests.

Medical gas cylinders are tested hydraulically every 5 years and the tests recorded by a mark stamped on the neck of the cylinder.

The cylinders are provided in a variety of sizes, and colour coded according to the gas supplied.

The cylinders comprise a body and a shoulder containing threads into which are fitted either a pin index valve block, a bull-nosed valve, or a handwheel valve.

The pin index system was devised to prevent interchangeability of cylinders of different gases. Pin index valves are provided for the smaller cylinders of oxygen and nitrous oxide (and also carbon dioxide and cyclopropane) which may be attached to anaesthetic machines. The pegs on the inlet connection slot into corresponding holes on the cylinder valve.

Full cylinders are supplied usually with a plastic dust cover in order to prevent contamination by dirt. This cover should not be removed until immediately before the cylinder is fitted to the anaesthetic machine. When fitting the cylinder to a machine, the yoke is positioned and tightened with the handle of the yoke spindle. After fitting, the cylinder should be opened to make sure that it is full and that there are no leaks at the gland nut or the pin index valve junction, caused for example by absence of, or damage to, the washer. The washer used is normally a Bodok seal which has a metal periphery designed to keep the seal in good condition for a long period.

Cylinder valves should be opened slowly to prevent sudden surges of pressure and should be closed with no more force than is necessary, otherwise the valve seating may be damaged.

The sealing material between the valve and the neck of the cylinder may be constructed of a fusable material which melts in the event of fire and allows the contents of the cylinder to escape around the threads of the joint.

The colour codes used for medical gas cylinders are shown in Table 17.2 and the cylinder sizes and capacities are shown in Table 17.3.

THE ANAESTHETIC MACHINE

The anaesthetic machine comprises:

1. A means of supplying gases either from attached cylinders or from piped medical supplies via appropriate unions on the machine.
2. Methods of measuring flow rate of gases.
3. Apparatus for vaporising volatile anaesthetic agents.
4. Breathing systems for delivery of gases and vapours from the machine to the patient.
5. Apparatus for scavenging anaesthetic gases in order to minimise environmental pollution.

Supply of gases

In the United Kingdom, gases are supplied at a pipeline pressure of 4 bar (400 kPa; 60 lb/in^2) and

Table 17.2 Medical gas cylinders

	Colour		Pressure at 15°C	
	Body	Shoulder	lbf/in^2	bar
Oxygen	Black	White	1987	137
Nitrous oxide	Blue	Blue	638	44
Cyclopropane	Orange	Orange	73	5
CO_2	Grey	Grey	725	50
Helium	Brown	Brown	1987	137
Air	Grey	White/black quarters	1987	137
O_2/helium	Black	White/brown quarters	1987	137
O_2/CO_2	Black	White/grey quarters	1987	137
N_2O/O_2 (Entonox)	Blue	White/blue quarters	1987	137

Table 17.3 Medical gas cylinder sizes and capacities

Cylinder size	A	B	C	D	E	F	G	J
Height (in)	10	10	14	18	31	34	49	57
Capacities (litres)								
Oxygen			170	340	680	1360	3400	6800
Nitrous oxide			450	900	1800	3600	9000	
Cyclopropane	90	180						
CO_2			450	900	1800			
Helium				300		1200		
Air							3200	6400
O_2/helium					600	1200		
O_2/CO_2						1360	3400	
Entonox							3200	6400

this pressure is transferred directly to the bank of flowmeters and back bar of the anaesthetic machine. With the exception of cyclopropane, the gas issuing from other medical gas cylinders is at a much higher pressure, necessitating the interposition of a pressure regulator between the cylinder and the bank of flowmeters. In some older anaesthetic machines (and in some other countries), the pressure in the pipelines of the anaesthetic machine may be 3 bar (300 kPa; 45 lb/in^2).

Pressure regulators

Pressure regulators are used on anaesthetic machines for three purposes:

1. To reduce the high pressure of gas in a cylinder to a safe working level.
2. To prevent damage to equipment on the anaesthetic machine, e.g. flow control valves.
3. As the contents of the cylinder are used, the pressure within the cylinder decreases and the regulating mechanism maintains a constant reduced pressure, obviating the necessity to make continuous adjustments to the flowmeter controls.

The principles underlying the operation of flowmeters are described in detail in Chapter 16.

The classical flow regulator for reducing valves is the Adams valve shown in Figure 16.4. Fins were incorporated originally on this valve to act as a radiator, in order to absorb heat; this was necessary to prevent malfunction of the valve produced by icing induced by the cooling effect of vaporisation of liquid nitrous oxide, as water vapour was present in small concentrations.

A modern anaesthetic reducing valve, the BOC S60M, is shown in Figure 16.5. Its mechanism of action will be clear from careful study of the diagram.

Flow restrictors

Pressure regulators are omitted usually when anaesthetic machines are supplied directly from a pipeline at a pressure of 4 bar. Changes in pipeline pressure would cause changes in flow rate, necessitating adjustment of the flow control valves. This is prevented by the use of a flow restrictor upstream of the flowmeter (flow restrictors are simply constrictions in the low-pressure circuit).

A different type of flow restrictor may be fitted also to the downstream end of the vaporisers to prevent back pressure effects (see Ch. 16). The absence of such a flow restrictor may be detected if a ventilator such as the Manley is employed, as this leads to fluctuations in the positions of the flowmeter bobbins during the respiratory cycle.

Pressure relief valves on regulators

Pressure relief valves are often fitted on the downstream side of regulators to allow escape of gas if the regulators were to fail (thereby causing a high output pressure). Relief valves are set usually at approximately 7 bar for regulators designed to give an output pressure of 4 bar.

Flowmeters

The principles of flowmeters are described in detail in Chapter 16.

Problems with flowmeters

1. *Non-vertical tube*. This causes a change in shape of the annulus and therefore variation in flow. If the bobbin touches the side of the tube, resulting friction causes an even more inaccurate reading.
2. *Static electricity*. This may cause inaccuracy (by as much as 35%) and sticking of the bobbin, especially at low flows. This may be reduced by coating the inside of the tube with a transparent film of gold or tin.
3. *Dirt*. Dirt on the bobbin may cause sticking or alteration in size of the annulus, and therefore inaccuracies.
4. *Back pressure*. Changes in accuracy may be produced by back pressure. For example, the Manley ventilator may exert a back pressure and depress the bobbin; there may be as much as 10% more gas flow than that indicated on the flowmeter. Similar problems may be produced by the insertion of any equipment which restricts flow downstream, e.g. Selectatec head, vaporiser.
5. *Leakage*. This results usually from defects in the top sealing washer of a rotameter.

It is unfortunate that in the United Kingdom the standard position of the flowmeters from left to right is oxygen, carbon dioxide, cyclopropane, nitrous oxide (if all four gases are supplied). On several recorded occasions, patients have suffered damage from hypoxia because of leakage of a broken flowmeter tube in this type of arrangement, as oxygen, being at the upstream end, passes out to atmosphere through any leak. This problem is reduced if the oxygen flowmeter is placed downstream (i.e. on the right-hand side of the bank of flowmeters) as is standard practice in the USA. In the UK, this problem is now avoided by designing the outlet from the oxygen flowmeter to enter the back bar distal to the outlets of other flowmeters.

On modern anaesthetic machines, the emergency oxygen flush lever is situated downstream from the vaporiser. This leads to dilution of the anaesthetic mixture with excess oxygen if the emergency oxygen tap is opened partially by mistake and results in the possibility of awareness. In addition, a much higher fresh gas flow is delivered than the anaesthetist has set on the flowmeter controls.

Quantiflex

The Quantiflex mixer flowmeter (Fig. 17.1) eliminates the possibility of reducing the oxygen supply inadvertently. One dial is set to the desired percentage of oxygen and the total flow rate adjusted independently. The percentage of oxygen

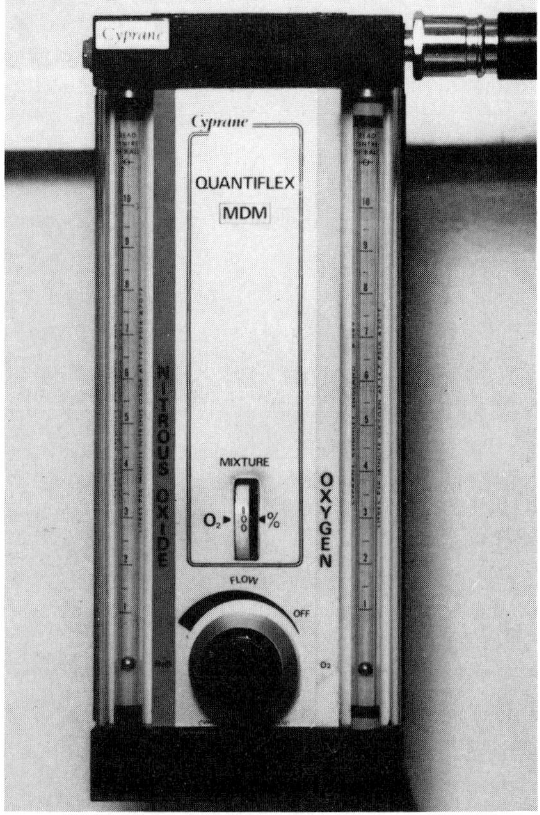

Fig. 17.1 A Quantiflex flowmeter. The required oxygen percentage is selected using the dial, and total flow of oxygen/nitrous oxide mixture adjusted using the black knob.

gas passes through a flowmeter to provide evidence of correct functioning of the linked valves. Both gases arrive via linked pressure-reducing regulators. The Quantiflex is useful in particular for varying the volume of fresh gas flow from moment to moment whilst keeping the proportions constant. In addition, the oxygen flowmeter is situated downstream of the nitrous oxide flowmeter.

Vaporisers

The principles of vaporisers have been described in detail in Chapter 16.

Modern vaporisers may be classified as:

1. *Plenum vaporisers*. These are intended for unidirectional gas flow, have a relatively high resistance to flow and are unsuitable for use either as drawover vaporisers or in a circle system. Examples include the 'Tec' type in which there is a variable bypass flow, and the Kettle type in which measured flows are used. Commonly used types of equipment are shown in Figures 17.2 to 17.6.

2. *Drawover vaporisers*. These have a very low resistance to gas flow and may be used in a circle system (e.g. Goldman vaporiser), for emergency use in the field (e.g. Oxford miniature vaporiser) or in underdeveloped countries (e.g. EMO vaporiser).

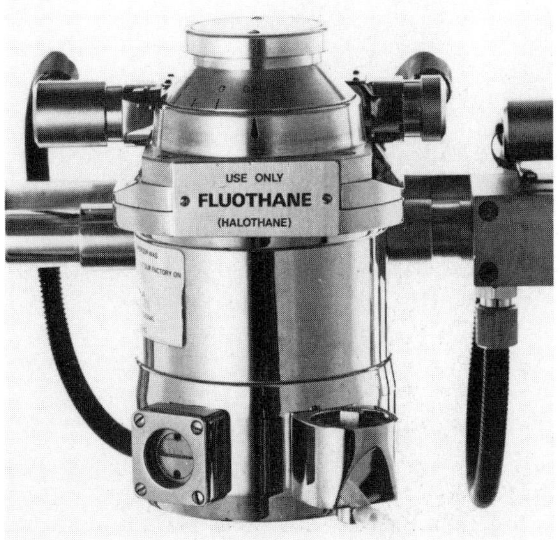

Fig. 17.2 A Mark 3 Tec flow- and temperature-compensated halothane vaporiser.

may be varied from 20% or 30% to 100%. Each

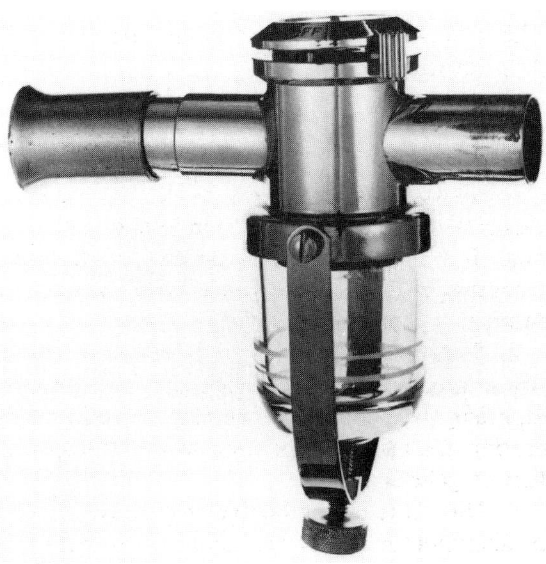

Fig. 17.3 The Goldman drawover vaporiser.

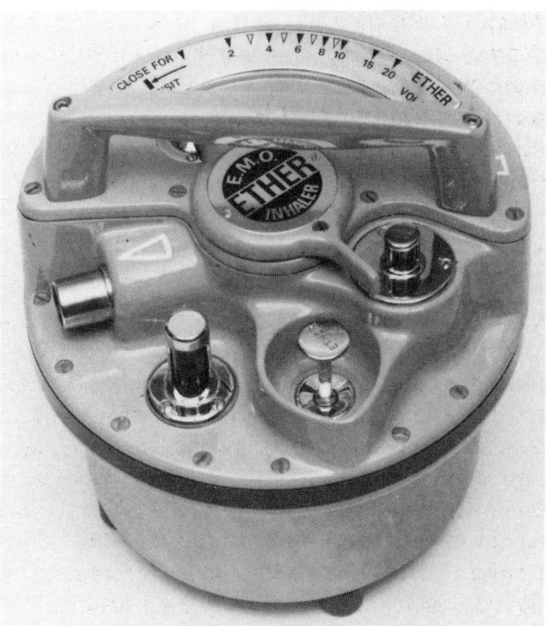

Fig. 17.4 The EMO (Epstein and Macintosh of Oxford) drawover ether vaporiser. A cutaway diagram is shown in Fig. 17.5.

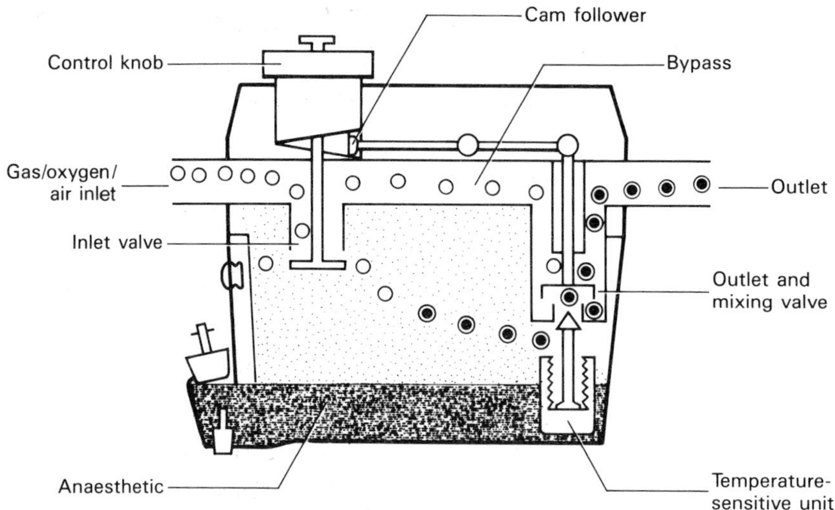

Fig. 17.5 Working principles of the EMO vaporiser. The water jacket provides a heat sink to reduce the decrease in temperature during vaporisation. Temperature compensation is provided by a valve operated by bellows filled with ether vapour. When the control lever is moved to the 'closed' position, the ether chamber is sealed to prevent spillage during transit.

A

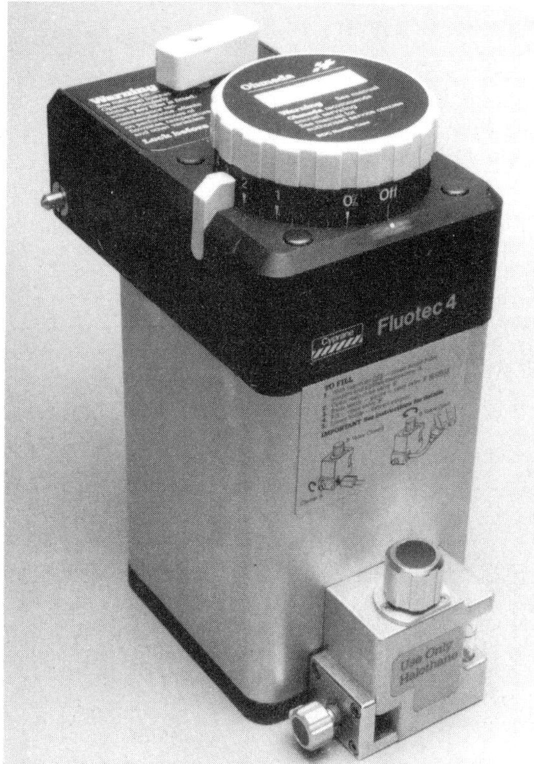

Fig. 17.6 (a) A Mark 4 Tec vaporiser. (b) Working principles. This vaporiser is in a different housing from the Mark 3 but it contains many of the same features and functions in the same way.

B

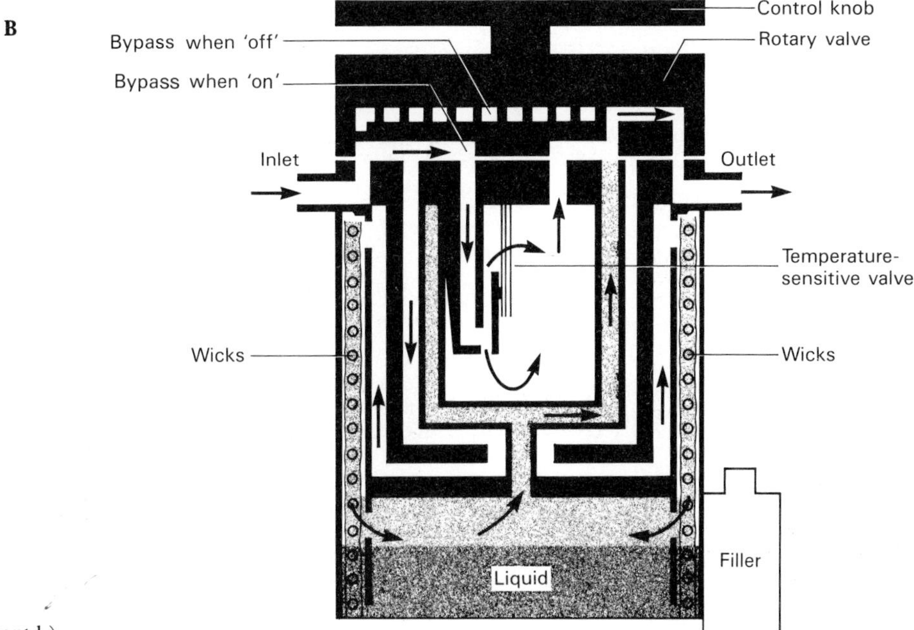

Fig. 17.6 (contd.)

Methods of temperature regulation include a bimetallic strip (Tec), bellows (EMO and Blease Universal vaporiser), and manual compensation (Drager Vapor and Copper Kettle).

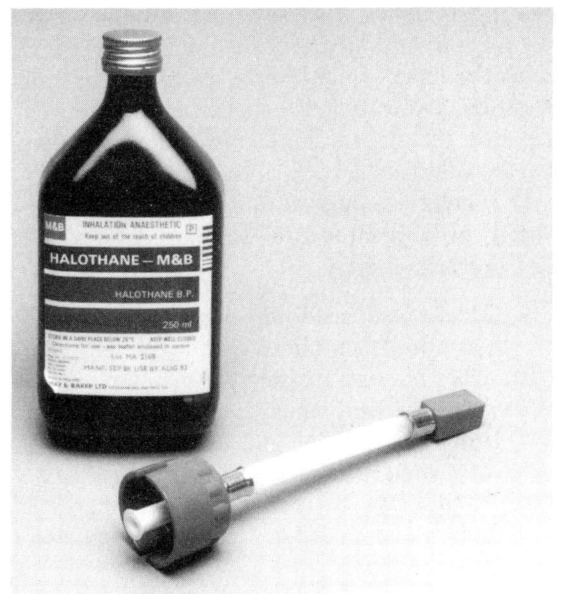

Fig. 17.7 An agent-specific connector for filling a vaporiser.

Anaesthetic-specific connections are available to link the supply bottle (container of liquid anaesthetic agent) to the appropriate vaporiser (Fig. 17.7). These connections reduce the extent of spillage (and thus atmospheric pollution) and also the likelihood of filling the vaporiser with an inappropriate liquid. In addition to being designed specifically for each liquid, the connections themselves may be colour-coded (e.g. purple for isoflurane, orange for enflurane and red for halothane).

Halothane contains a non-volatile stabilising agent (0.01% thymol) to prevent breakdown of the halothane by heat and ultraviolet light. Thymol is less volatile than halothane, and its concentration in the vaporiser increases as halothane is vaporised. If the vaporiser is used and refilled regularly, the concentration of thymol may become sufficiently high to impair vaporisation of halothane. In addition, very high concentrations may result in a significant degree of thymol vaporisation, which may be harmful to the patient. Consequently, it is recommended that halothane vaporisers be drained once every 2 weeks. Enflurane and isoflurane vaporisers require to be emptied at much less frequent intervals.

SAFETY FEATURES OF THE MODERN ANAESTHETIC MACHINE

1. Specificity of probes on flexible hoses between terminal outlets and connections with the anaesthetic machine.

2. Pin index system to prevent incorrect attachment of gas cylinders to anaesthetic machine.

3. Pressure relief valves on downstream side of regulators.

4. Flow restrictors on upstream side of flowmeters.

5. Arrangement of bank of flowmeters, such that oxygen flowmeter is on the right (i.e. downstream side).

6. Non-return valves. Sometimes a single regulator and contents meter is used both for cylinders in use and for the reserve cylinder. When one cylinder runs out, the presence of a non-return valve prevents the empty cylinder from being refilled by the reserve cylinder and also enables the empty cylinder to be removed and replaced without interrupting the supply of gas to the patient.

7. An oxygen bypass valve (emergency oxygen) delivers oxygen directly from a point upstream of the flowmeters to a point downstream of the vaporisers. When operated, the oxygen bypass should give a flow of at least 35 litres/min.

8. Mounting of vaporisers on the back bar. Temperature-compensated vaporisers should be mounted upstream because they contain wicks which absorb a considerable amount of anaesthetic agent. If two such vaporisers are mounted in series, the downstream vaporiser could become contaminated to a dangerous degree with the agent from the upstream vaporiser. It is preferable to have only one temperature-compensated calibrated vaporiser on the back bar. The Selectatec block (Fig. 17.8) enables vaporisers to be changed very quickly, provides versatility and removes the necessity to have more than one vaporiser on the back bar. A development has been a back bar carrying two Selectatec vaporisers but with a control which permits only one to be in use at any one time.

9. Pressure-linked flow controls. Some anaesthetic machines possess a device which switches off the supply of nitrous oxide automatically in the event of failure of the oxygen supply.

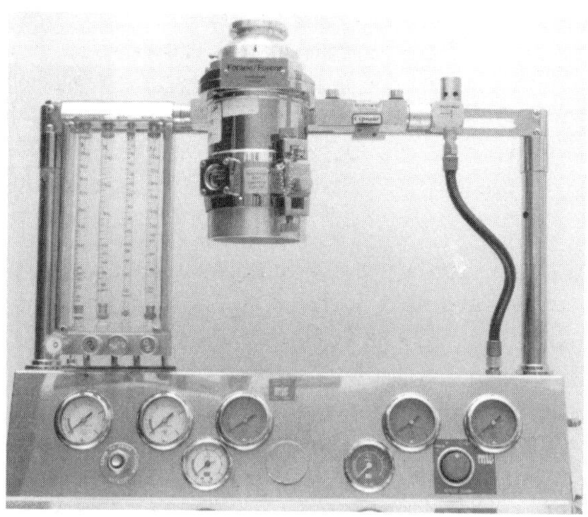

Fig. 17.8 A Selectatec block on the back bar of an anaesthetic machine. This permits the vaporiser to be changed rapidly without interrupting the flow of carrier gas to the patient.

10. A non-return valve situated downstream of the vaporisers prevents back pressure (e.g. when using a Manley ventilator) which may cause output of high concentrations of vapour.

11. A relief valve may be situated downstream of the vaporiser, opening at 34 kPa to prevent damage to the flowmeters or vaporisers if the outlet is obstructed.

12. A pressure relief valve set to blow off at a low pressure of 5 kPa may be fitted to prevent the patient's lungs from being damaged by high pressure. The presence of such a valve prevents the use of the machine with minute volume divider ventilators, such as the Manley.

13. Oxygen failure warning devices. There is a variety of oxygen failure warning devices. The ideal warning device:

(a) Does not depend on the pressure of any gas other than the oxygen itself.
(b) Does not use a battery or mains power.
(c) Gives a signal which is audible and of sufficient duration and volume and of distinctive character.
(d) Should give a warning of impending failure and a further warning that failure has occurred.
(e) Should interrupt the flow of all other gases when it comes into operation. The

breathing system should open to atmosphere, inspired oxygen concentration should be at least equal to that of air and accumulation of carbon dioxide should not occur. In addition, it should be impossible to resume anaesthesia until the oxygen supply has been restored.

14. The rubber reservoir bag in an anaesthetic breathing system is highly distensible and seldom reaches pressures exceeding 5 kPa.

BREATHING SYSTEMS

The delivery system which conducts anaesthetic gases from the machine to the patient is termed colloquially a 'circuit' but is described more accurately as a breathing system. Terms such as 'open circuits', 'semi-open circuits' or 'semi-closed circuits' should be avoided. The 'closed circuit', or circle system, is the only true circuit, as anaesthetic gases are recycled.

Adjustable pressure-limiting valve

Most breathing systems incorporate an adjustable pressure-limiting valve (spill valve; 'pop-off' valve; expiratory valve) which is designed to vent gas when there is a positive pressure within the system. During spontaneous ventilation, the valve opens when the patient generates a positive pressure within the system during expiration; during positive pressure ventilation, the valve is adjusted to produce a controlled leak during the inspiratory phase.

Several valves of this type are available. They comprise a light-weight disc (Fig. 17.9) which rests on a 'knife-edge' seating to minimise the area of contact and reduce the risk of adhesion resulting from surface tension of condensed water. The disc has a stem which acts as a guide to position the disc correctly. A light spring is incorporated in the valve so that the pressure required to open the valve may be adjusted. During spontaneous breathing, the tension of the spring is low so that the resistance to expiration is minimised. During controlled ventilation, the valve top is screwed down to increase the tension in the spring so that gas leaves the system at a higher pressure than during spontaneous ventilation.

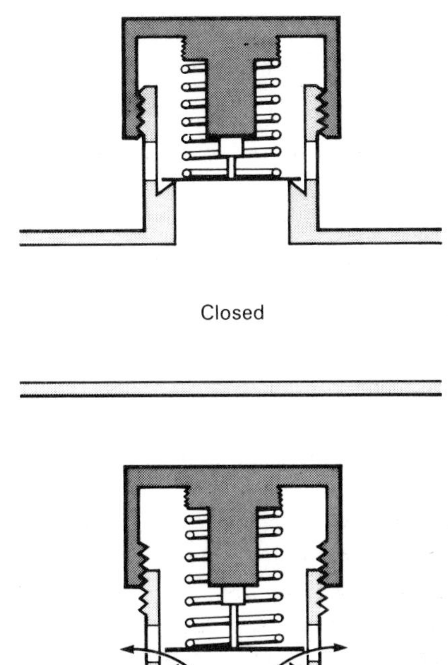

Fig. 17.9 Diagram of a spill valve. See text for details.

Classification of breathing systems

In 1954, Mapleson classified anaesthetic breathing systems into five types (Fig. 17.10); the Mapleson E system was modified subsequently by Rees, but is classified as the Mapleson F system. The systems differ considerably in their 'efficiency', which is measured in terms of the fresh gas flow rate required to prevent rebreathing of alveolar gas during ventilation.

Mapleson A systems

The most commonly used version is the Magill attachment. The corrugated hose should be of adequate length (usually approximately 110 cm). It is the most efficient system during spontaneous ventilation, but one of the least efficient when ventilation is controlled.

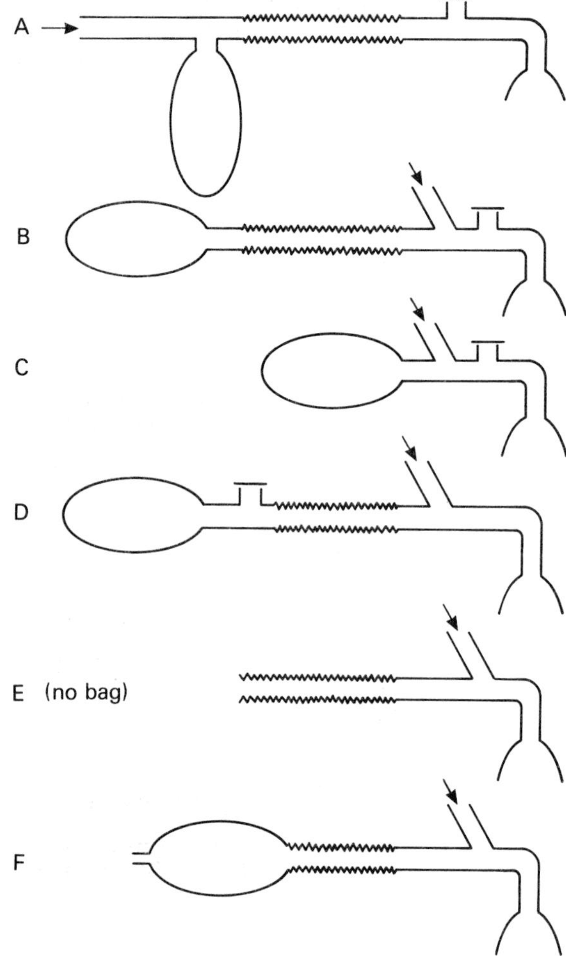

Fig. 17.10 Mapleson classification of anaesthetic breathing systems. The arrow indicates entry of fresh gas to the system.

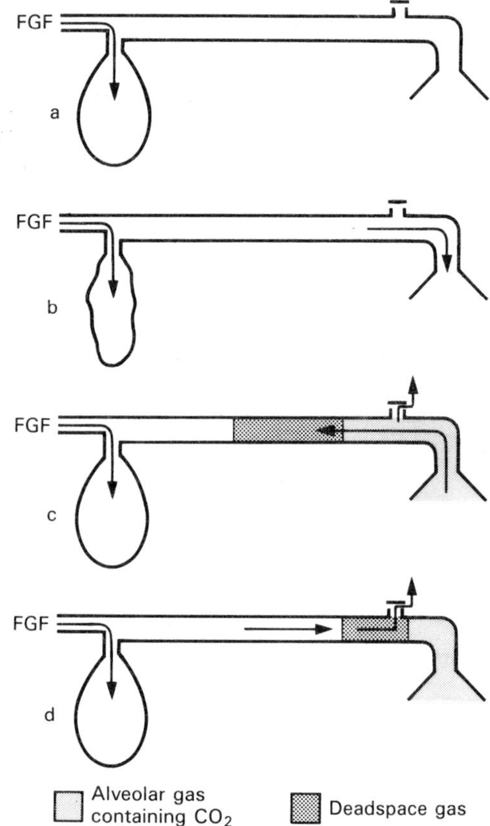

Fig. 17.11 Mode of action of Magill attachment during spontaneous ventilation. See text for details. FGF = fresh gas flow.

During spontaneous ventilation, there are three phases in the ventilatory cycle: inspiratory, expiratory and the expiratory pause. Gas is inhaled from the system during inspiration (Fig. 17.11b). During the initial part of expiration, the reservoir bag is not full, and thus the pressure in the system does not increase; exhaled gas (the initial portion of which is deadspace gas) passes along the corrugated tubing towards the bag (Fig. 17.11c), which is filled also by fresh gas from the anaesthetic machine. During the latter part of expiration, the bag becomes full, the pressure in the system increases and the spill valve opens, venting all subsequent exhaled gas to atmosphere. During the expiratory pause, continued flow of fresh gas from the machine pushes exhaled gas distally along the corrugated tube to be vented through the spill valve (Fig. 17.11d). Provided that the fresh gas flow rate is sufficiently high to vent all *alveolar* gas before the next inspiration, no rebreathing takes place from the corrugated tube. If the system is functioning correctly and no leaks are present, a fresh gas flow (FGF) rate equal to the patient's alveolar minute ventilation is sufficient to prevent rebreathing. In practice, a higher FGF is selected in order to compensate for leaks; the rate selected is usually equal to the patient's total minute volume (approximately 6 litres/min for a 70 kg adult).

The system increases deadspace to the extent of the volume of the anaesthetic facemask and angle-piece to the spill valve. The volume of this dead-space may amount to 100 ml or more for an adult facemask. Paediatric facemasks reduce the extent of deadspace but it remains too high to allow use of the system in infants or small children (less than 4 years of age).

The characteristics of the Mapleson A system are different during controlled ventilation (Fig. 17.12). At the end of inspiration (produced by the anaesthetist squeezing the reservoir bag), the bag is usually less than half full (vide infra). During expiration, deadspace and alveolar gas pass along the corrugated tube and are likely to reach the reservoir bag, which therefore contains some carbon dioxide (Fig. 17.12a). During inspiration, the valve does not open initially because its opening pressure has been increased by the anaesthetist in order to generate a sufficient pressure within the system to inflate the lungs. Thus, alveolar gas re-enters the patient's lungs, and is followed by a mixture of fresh, deadspace and alveolar gases (Fig. 17.12b). When the valve does open, it is this mixture which is vented (Fig. 17.12c). Consequently, fresh gas flow rate must be very high (at least three times alveolar minute volume) to prevent rebreathing. The volume of gas squeezed from the reservoir bag must be sufficient both to inflate the lungs and to vent gas from the system.

The major disadvantage of the Magill attachment during surgery is that the spill valve is attached close to the mask. This makes the system heavy, particularly when a scavenging system is used, and it is inconvenient if the valve is in this position during surgery of the head or neck. The Lack system (Fig. 17.13) is a modification of the

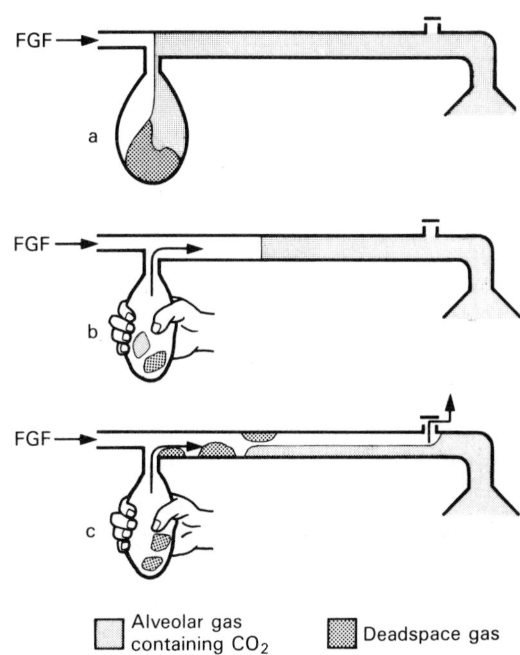

Fig. 17.12 Mode of action of Magill attachment during controlled ventilation. See text for details. FGF = fresh gas flow.

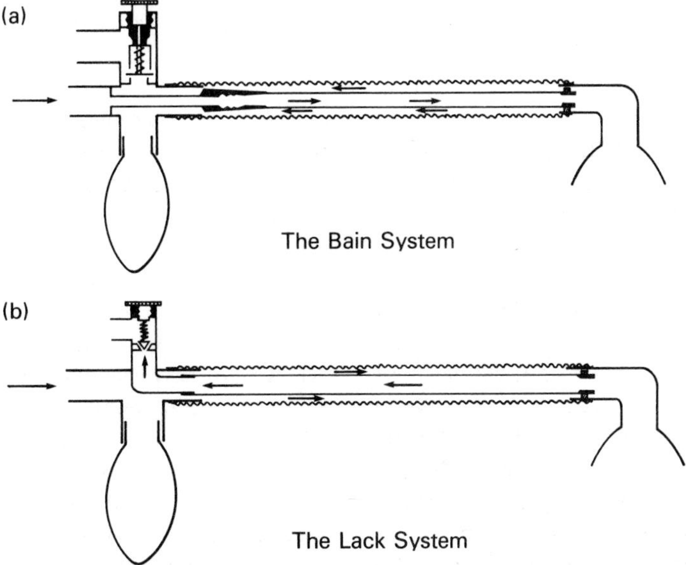

Fig. 17.13 Coaxial anaesthetic breathing systems. (a) Bain system (Mapleson D). (b) Lack system (Mapleson A).

Mapleson A system with a coaxial arrangement of tubing. This permits positioning of the spill valve at the proximal end of the system. The inner tube must be of sufficiently wide bore to allow the patient to exhale with minimal resistance. The Lack system is not quite as efficient as the Magill attachment.

Mapleson B and C systems

These systems cause mixing of alveolar and fresh gas during spontaneous or controlled ventilation. Very high FGF rates are required to prevent rebreathing. There is no clinical role for the Mapleson B system. The Mapleson C system is used in some hospitals to ventilate the lungs with oxygen during transport, but a self-inflating bag with a non-rebreathing valve is preferable.

Mapleson D system

The Mapleson D arrangement is inefficient during spontaneous breathing (Fig. 17.14). During expiration, exhaled gas and fresh gas mix in the corrugated tube and travel towards the reservoir bag (Fig. 17.14b). When the reservoir bag is full, the pressure in the system increases, the spill valve opens and a mixture of fresh and exhaled gas is vented; this includes the deadspace gas, which reaches the reservoir bag first (Fig. 17.14c). Although fresh gas pushes alveolar gas towards the valve during the expiratory pause, a mixture of alveolar and fresh gases is inhaled from the corrugated tube unless FGF rate is at least twice as great as the patient's minute volume (i.e. at least 12 litres/min in the adult); in some patients, a fresh gas flow rate of 250 ml kg^{-1} min^{-1} is required to prevent rebreathing.

However, the Mapleson D system is more efficient than the Mapleson A during controlled ventilation (Fig. 17.15), especially if an expiratory pause is incorporated into the ventilatory cycle. During expiration, the corrugated tubing and reservoir bag fill with a mixture of fresh and alveolar gas (Fig. 17.15a). Fresh gas fills the distal part of the corrugated tube during the expiratory pause (Fig. 17.15b). When the reservoir bag is squeezed, this fresh gas enters the lungs, and when the spill valve opens a mixture of fresh and alveolar gas is vented. The degree of rebreathing may thus be controlled by adjustment of the fresh gas flow rate, but this should always exceed the patient's minute volume.

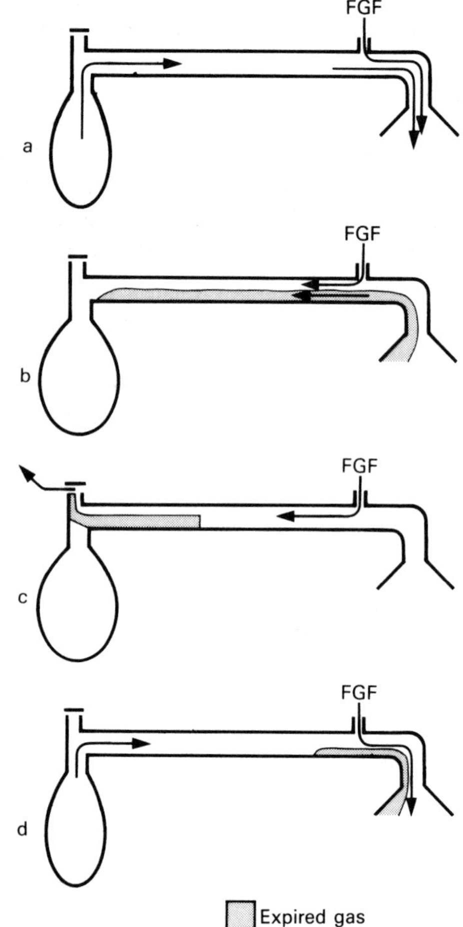

Fig. 17.14 Mode of action of Mapleson D breathing system during spontaneous ventilation. See text for details. FGF = fresh gas flow.

The Bain coaxial system (Fig. 17.13) is the most commonly used version of the Mapleson D system. FGF is supplied through a narrow inner tube. This tube may become disconnected, resulting in hypoxaemia and hypercapnia. Before use, the system should be tested by occluding the distal end of the inner tube transiently with a finger or the plunger of a 2-ml syringe; there should be a reduction in the flowmeter bobbin reading during occlusion, and an audible release of pressure when occlusion is discontinued. Movement of the reservoir bag during anaesthesia does *not* indicate that fresh gas is being delivered to the patient.

The Bain system may be used to ventilate the patient's lungs with some types of automatic ventilator (e.g. Penlon Nuffield 200). A 1-m length of corrugated tubing is interposed between the patient valve of the ventilator and the reservoir bag mount (Fig. 17.16); the spill valve *must* be closed completely. An appropriate tidal volume and ventilatory rate are selected on the ventilator, and anaesthetic gases are supplied to the Bain system. During inspiration, the gas from the ventilator pushes a mixture of anaesthetic and alveolar gas from the corrugated outer tube into the patient's lungs; during expiration, the ventilator gas and some of the alveolar gas are vented through the exhaust valve of the ventilator. The degree of rebreathing is regulated by the anaesthetic gas flow rate; a flow of 70–80 ml $kg^{-1} min^{-1}$ should result in normocapnia, and a flow of 100 ml kg^{-1} min^{-1} in moderate hypocapnia. A secure connection between the Bain system and the anaesthetic machine must be assured. If this connection is loose, a leak of fresh gas occurs; this causes rebreathing of ventilator gas, and results in awareness, hypoxaemia and hypercapnia.

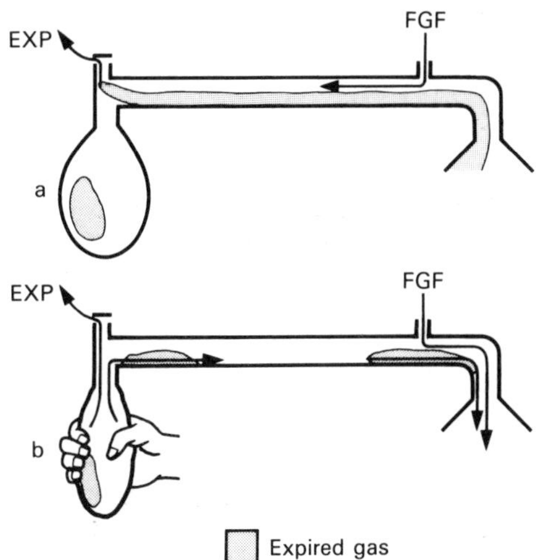

Fig. 17.15 Mode of action of Mapleson D breathing system during controlled ventilation. See text for details. FGF = fresh gas flow.

Mapleson E and F systems

The Mapleson E system, or Ayre's T-piece, has virtually no resistance to expiration and was used extensively in paediatric anaesthesia before the advantages of continuous positive airways pressure (CPAP) were recognised. It functions in a manner similar to the Mapleson D system in that the corrugated tube fills with a mixture of exhaled and fresh gas during expiration, and with fresh gas

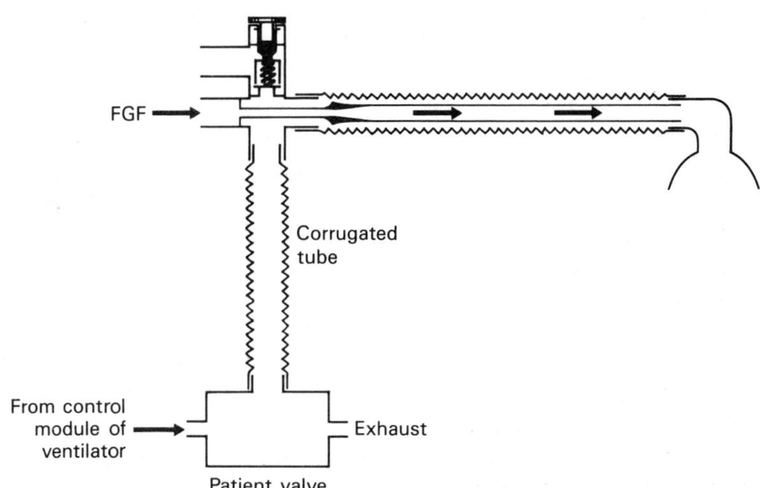

Fig. 17.16 The Bain system for controlled ventilation by a mechanical ventilator (e.g. Nuffield 200). A 1-m length of corrugated tubing with a capacity of at least 500 ml is required to prevent gas from the ventilator reaching the patient's lungs. Pa_{CO_2} is controlled by varying the fresh gas flow rate (FGF).

during the expiratory pause. Rebreathing is prevented if the FGF rate is 2.5–3 times the patient's minute volume. If the volume of the corrugated tube is less than the patient's tidal volume, some air may be inhaled at the end of inspiration; consequently, a fresh gas flow rate of at least 4 litres/min is recommended with a paediatric Mapleson E system.

During spontaneous ventilation, there is no indication of the presence, or the adequacy, of ventilation. It is possible to attach a visual indicator, such as a piece of tissue paper or a feather, at the end of the corrugated tube, but this is not very satisfactory.

IPPV may be applied by occluding the end of the corrugated tube with a finger; however, there is no way of assessing the pressure in the system, and there is a possibility of exposing the patient's lungs to excessive volumes and pressures.

The Mapleson F system, or Rees' modification of the.Ayre's T-piece, includes an open-ended bag attached to the end of the corrugated tube. This confers several advantages:

1. It provides visual evidence of breathing during spontaneous ventilation.
2. By occluding the open end of the bag temporarily, it is possible to confirm that fresh gas is entering the system.
3. It provides a degree of CPAP during spontaneous ventilation and PEEP during IPPV.
4. It provides a convenient method of assisting or controlling ventilation. The open end of the reservoir bag is occluded between the fourth and fifth fingers and the bag squeezed between the thumb and index finger; the fourth and fifth fingers are relaxed during expiration to allow gas to escape from the bag. It is possible with experience to assess (approximately) the inflation pressure and to detect changes in lung and chest wall compliance.

Drawover systems

Occasionally, it is necessary to administer anaesthesia at the scene of a major accident. If inhalational anaesthesia is required, it is necessary to use simple, portable equipment. The Triservice apparatus (Fig. 17.17) has been designed by the British armed forces for use in battle conditions. It comprises a self-inflating bag, a non-rebreathing valve (e.g. Ambu E, Rubens) which vents all expired gases to atmosphere, one or two Oxford Miniature Vaporisers (which have a low internal resistance), an oxygen supply and a length of corrugated tubing which serves as an oxygen reservoir. Either spontaneous or controlled ventilation may be employed using this apparatus.

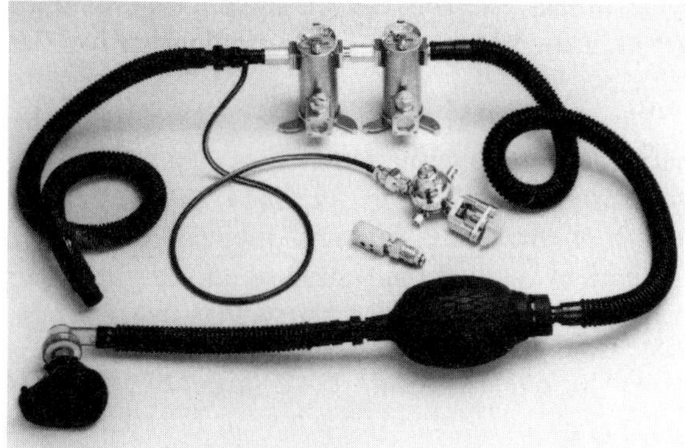

Fig. 17.17 The Triservice apparatus. See text for details.

Rebreathing systems

Anaesthetic breathing systems in which the same gases are rebreathed by the patient were designed originally to economise in the use of cyclopropane. In addition, they reduce the risk of atmospheric pollution and increase the humidity of inspired gases, thereby reducing heat loss from the patient. Rebreathing systems may be used as 'closed' systems, in which fresh gas is introduced only to replace oxygen and anaesthetic agents absorbed by the patient. More commonly, the system is used with a small leak through a spill valve and a fresh gas supply which exceeds basal oxygen requirements. Because rebreathing occurs, these systems must incorporate a means of absorbing carbon dioxide from exhaled alveolar gas.

Soda lime

Soda lime is the substance used most commonly for absorption of carbon dioxide in rebreathing

Table 17.4 Composition of soda lime

$Ca(OH)_2$	94%
NaOH	5%
KOH	1%
Silica	0.2%
Moisture content	14–19%

systems. The composition of soda lime is shown in Table 17.4. The major constituent is calcium hydroxide, but sodium and potassium hydroxides are present also. Absorption of carbon dioxide occurs by the following chemical reactions:

$$CO_2 + 2NaOH \rightarrow Na_2CO_3 + H_2O + \text{heat}$$
$$Na_2CO_3 + Ca(OH)_2 \rightarrow 2NaOH + CaCO_3$$

Water is required for efficient absorption. There is some water in soda lime, and more is added from the patient's expired gas and from the chemical reaction. The reaction generates heat and the temperature in the centre of a soda lime canister may exceed 60°C. Trichloroethylene degenerates at high temperatures, forming toxic substances including the neurotoxin dichloroacetylene; consequently, trichloroethylene must never be used in rebreathing systems which contain soda lime.

The size of soda lime granule is important. If granules are too large, the surface area for absorption is insufficient; if they are too small, the narrow space between granules results in a high resistance to breathing. Silica is added to soda lime to reduce the tendency of the granules to disintegrate into powder. In addition, soda lime contains an indicator which changes colour as the active constituents become exhausted. The rate at which soda lime becomes exhausted depends on the capacity of the canister, the fresh gas flow rate and the rate of carbon dioxide production. In a completely closed system, a standard 450-g canister becomes inefficient after approximately 2 h.

'To-and-fro' (Waters') system

This breathing system comprises a Mapleson C breathing system with a canister of soda lime interposed between the spill valve and reservoir bag (Fig. 17.18). The soda lime granules nearest the patient become exhausted first, increasing the deadspace of the system; in addition, the canister is positioned horizontally and gas may be channelled above the soda lime unless the canister is packed tightly. The system is cumbersome, and there is a risk that patients may inhale soda lime dust from the canister.

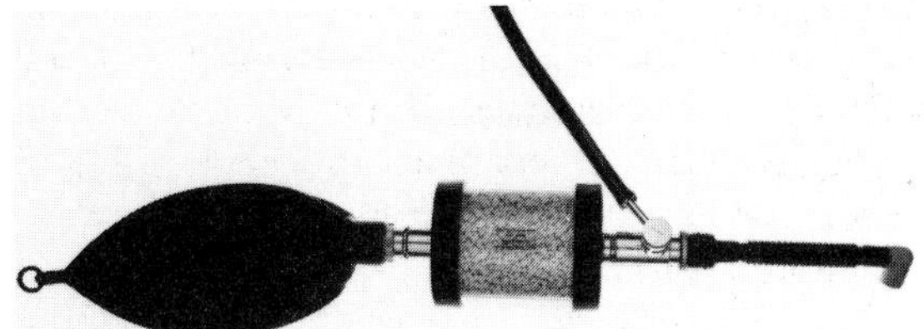

Fig. 17.18 Waters' anaesthetic breathing system, incorporating a canister of soda lime.

Circle system

This system has replaced the 'to-and-fro' system in most centres. The soda lime canister is mounted usually on the anaesthetic machine, and inspiratory and expiratory corrugated tubing conduct gas to and from the patient (Fig. 17.19). The system incorporates a reservoir bag and spill valve, and two low-resistance one-way valves to ensure unidirectional movement of gas. These valves are mounted normally in glass domes so that they may be observed to be functioning correctly. The spill valve may be mounted close to the patient or beside the absorber; during surgery to the head or neck, it is more convenient to use a valve near the absorber. Fresh gas enters the system between the absorber and the inspiratory tubing.

The soda lime canister is mounted vertically, and thus channelling of gas through unfilled areas is not possible. The canister cannot contribute to deadspace; consequently, a large canister may be used and the soda lime needs to be changed less often.

The major disadvantage of the circle system arises from its volume. If the system is filled with air initially, low flow rates of anaesthetic gases are diluted substantially and adequate concentrations cannot be achieved. Even if the system is primed

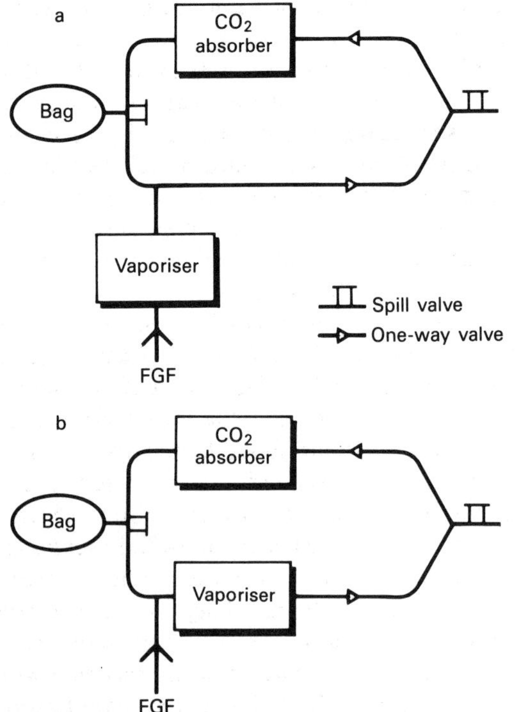

Fig. 17.19 Diagrammatic representation of circle system. (a) Vaporiser outside the circle (VOC). (b) Vaporiser inside the circle (VIC).

with a mixture of anaesthetic gases, the initial rapid uptake by the patient results in a marked decrease in concentrations of anaesthetic agents in the system, resulting in light anaesthesia. Consequently, it is necessary usually to provide a total fresh gas flow rate of 3–4 litres/min to the system initially. This flow rate may be reduced subsequently, but it must be remembered that dilution of fresh gas continues at low flow rates, and that rapid changes in depth of anaesthesia cannot be achieved.

Volatile anaesthetic agents may be delivered to a circle system in two ways:

1. *Vaporiser outside the circle* (*VOC*). If a standard vaporiser (e.g. Tec series) is used, it must be placed on the back bar of the anaesthetic machine because of its high internal resistance. If low FGF rates (<1 litre/min) are used, the change in concentration of volatile anaesthetic agent achieved in the circle system is very small because of dilution, even if the vaporiser is set to deliver a high concentration (Fig 17.20a), and it may be necessary to change FGF rate rather than the vaporiser setting to achieve a rapid change in depth of anaesthesia. The concentration of volatile

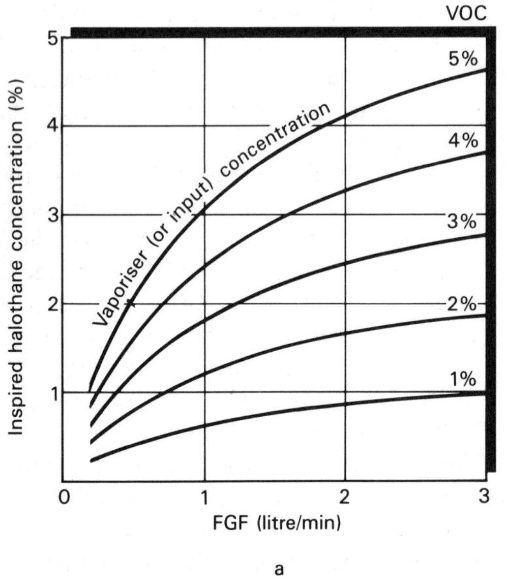

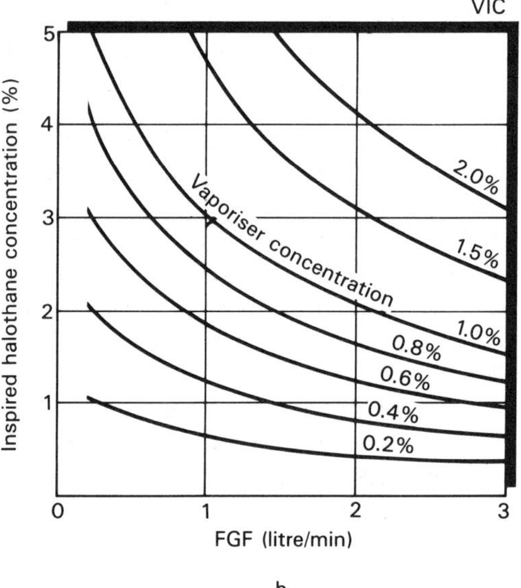

Fig. 17.20 Variation of inspired concentration of halothane with fresh gas flow rate. Total minute ventilation is 5 litres/min. (a) Vaporiser outside the circle (VOC); note that dilution of the fresh gas results in much lower concentrations in the circle system than the concentration set on the vaporiser unless fresh gas flow rate approaches 3 litres/min. (b) Vaporiser inside the circle (VIC); at low flow rates, lack of dilution of expired halothane concentrations, with additional halothane vaporised during each inspiration, results in inspired concentrations much higher than those set on the vaporiser. Even at a fresh gas flow rate of 3 litres/min, inspired concentration is approximately 50% higher than the vaporiser setting.

agent in the system depends on the patient's expired concentration (which is recycled), the rate of uptake by the patient (which decreases with time and is slower with agents of low blood/gas solubility coefficient), the concentration of agent supplied and the fresh gas flow rate.

2. *Vaporiser inside the circle (VIC)*. Drawover vaporisers with a low internal resistance (e.g. Goldman) may be placed within the circle system. During each inspiration, vapour is added to the inspired gas mixture. In contrast to a VOC system, the inspired concentration is higher at low FGF rates because the expired concentration is diluted to a lesser extent (Fig. 17.20b) and the vaporiser *adds* to the concentration present in the expired gas. Very high concentrations of volatile agent may be inspired if minute volume is large; this risk is greatest if IPPV is employed.

If FGF rate is low, the use of the circle system by the inexperienced anaesthetist may result either in inadequate anaesthesia or in severe cardiovascular and respiratory depression. In addition, a hypoxic gas mixture may be delivered if low flow rates of a nitrous oxide/oxygen mixture are supplied, because after 10–15 min oxygen is taken up in larger volumes than nitrous oxide. These difficulties may be overcome by monitoring the inspired concentrations of oxygen and volatile anaesthetic agent continuously (see Ch. 21). The trainee anaesthetist *must* be aware that:

1. It is inadvisable to use a VIC system unless inspired concentrations of anaesthetic agents are monitored continuously.
2. IPPV must *never* be used with a VIC system unless inspired concentrations of anaesthetic agents are monitored continuously, because of the risk of generating very high concentrations of volatile agent.
3. Nitrous oxide must *not* be used in any circle system if the total fresh gas flow rate is less than 1000 ml/min, unless inspired oxygen concentration is measured continuously.

VENTILATORS

Mechanical ventilation of the lung may be achieved by several mechanisms, including the generation of a negative pressure around the whole of the patient's body except the head and neck (cabinet ventilator or 'iron lung'), a negative pressure over the thorax and abdomen (cuirass ventilators) or a positive pressure over the thorax and abdomen (inflatable cuirass ventilators). However, during anaesthesia, and in the majority of patients who require mechanical ventilation in the intensive therapy unit, ventilation is achieved by the application of positive pressure to the lungs through a tracheal tube. Only this mode of ventilation is described here.

An enormous selection of ventilators exists and it is possible in this section to discuss only the principles involved in their use. Before using any ventilator, it is *essential* that the trainee understands its functions fully; failure to do so may result in the delivery of a hypoxic gas mixture, rebreathing of carbon dioxide and/or delivery of a mixture that contains no anaesthetic gases. If an unfamiliar ventilator is encountered, it may be helpful to use a 'dummy lung' (a small reservoir bag on the patient connection) and to discuss the capabilities and limitations of the machine with a senior colleague. In addition, the manufacturer's 'user handbook' may be consulted, or details may be obtained from a specialist book.

With simple ventilators, observation of the patient is the only means of assessing the adequacy of ventilation. Continuous clinical monitoring is essential when any ventilator is used, even those which incorporate sophisticated monitoring and warning devices. In addition to standard clinical monitoring systems attached to the patient (see Ch. 21), the minimum acceptable monitoring of ventilator function includes measurement of expired tidal volume, airway pressure and inspired oxygen concentration; in addition, a ventilator disconnection alarm should be incorporated in the system. Continuous monitoring of end-tidal carbon dioxide and inspired anaesthetic gas concentrations is desirable, but not always available. Pulse oximetry is recommended.

The incorporation of a humidifier in the inspiratory limb, or of a condenser humidifier at the connection with the tracheal tube, is essential in long-term ventilation in ITU. Bacterial filters may be desirable in patients with infected pulmonary secretions.

The principles of operation of ventilators are described best by considering each phase of the ventilatory cycle.

Inspiration

The pattern of volume change in the lung is determined by the characteristics of the ventilator. Ventilators may deliver a predetermined flow of gas (*flow generators*) or exert a predetermined pressure (*pressure generators*), although some machines produce a pattern which does not conform to either category. Most flow generators produce a constant flow of gas during inspiration, although a few generate a sinusoidal flow pattern if the ventilator bellows is driven via a crank, e.g.

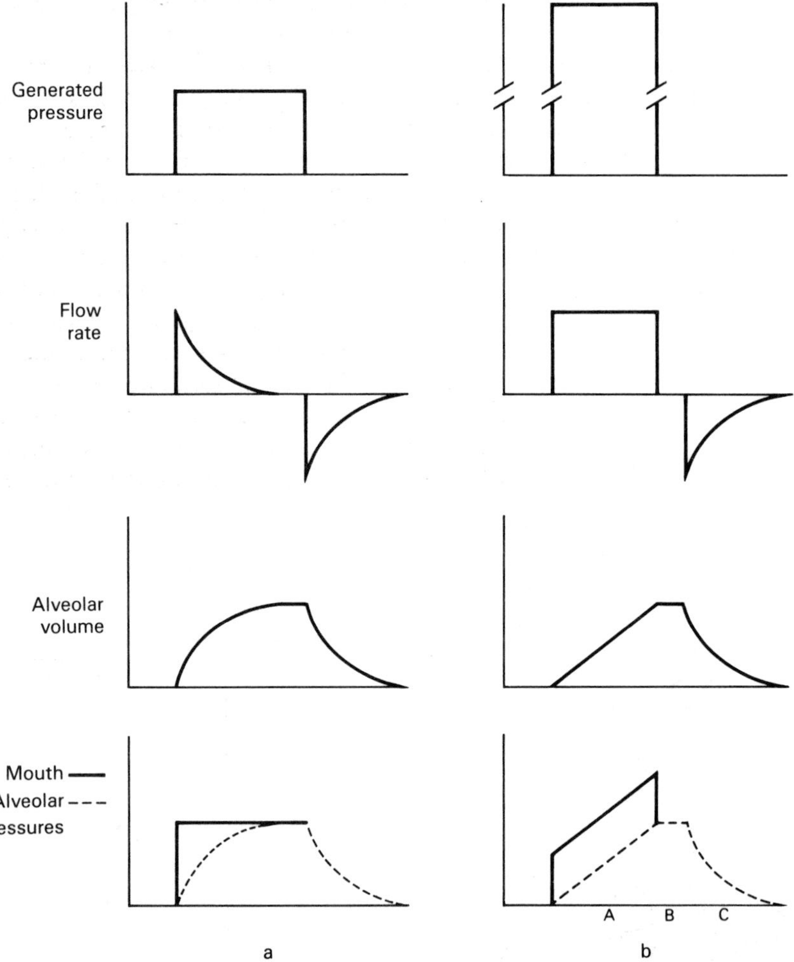

Fig. 17.21 Graphs of generated pressure, mouth (or tracheal tube) and alveolar pressures, flow rate and alveolar volume changes during inspiration and subsequent expiration produced by (a) a constant pressure generator, and (b) a constant flow generator. A constant pressure generator exerts a low (e.g. 1.5 kPa; 15 cm H_2O) pressure. At the start of inspiration, the pressure in the alveoli is zero. Gas flows rapidly into the alveoli at a rate determined by airways resistance resulting in rapid increases in alveolar volume and pressure. The mouth-alveolar pressure gradient decreases and flow rate, and consequently the rate of increase of alveolar volume and pressure, decrease also. When the alveolar pressure equals ventilator pressure, flow ceases.

A constant flow generator generates a very high internal pressure (e.g. 400 kPa) but has a high internal resistance to limit flow rate. The pressure gradient between machine and alveoli remains virtually constant throughout inspiration, and thus flow rate is constant. The increases in alveolar volume and (assuming constant compliance) pressure are linear. Because flow rate is constant, the pressure gradient between mouth and alveoli is constant throughout inspiration (A). Mouth pressure decreases to equal alveolar pressure during the inspiratory pause when flow ceases (B).

Gas flow out of the lung during expiration (C) is passive.

Cape–Waine ventilator. The characteristics of constant flow and constant pressure generators are shown in Figure 17.21.

Constant pressure generator. The East-Radcliffe ventilator is the only true pressure generator in common use. This machine contains a bellows with a capacity that greatly exceeds the normal tidal volume. The inspiratory pressure is generated by weights on top of the bellows. The bellows cease to empty when the pressure generated by the weights equals the pressure in the patient's alveoli. To a certain extent, the machine can compensate for leaks, as the bellows are large and continue to empty until a predetermined pressure has been achieved in the lungs. However, that pressure may be achieved after delivery to the lungs of different volumes of gas if the lung/chest wall compliance changes (Fig. 17.22). For example, if the patient is tipped head-down, compliance decreases and a smaller tidal volume is delivered (compliance = volume/pressure). If airways resistance increases, the flow rate of gas is decreased and the pressure in the lungs may not reach bellows pressure before the end of the inspiratory cycle; consequently, tidal volume decreases. Tidal volume is decreased also if a large leak develops.

Constant flow generator. Changes in resistance or compliance make little difference to the volume delivered (unless the ventilator is pressure-cycled; vide infra), although airway and alveolar pressures may change (Fig. 17.23). For example, decreased compliance results in delivery of a normal tidal volume; however, the rate of increase of alveolar pressure is greater than normal (i.e. the slope is greater) and airway pressure is correspondingly higher to maintain a gradient between the tracheal tube and the alveoli. If airway resistance increases, the pressure at the tracheal tube (and the gradient between tracheal tube and alveolar pressures) is higher than normal throughout inspiration, but alveolar pressure and the slopes of both pressure curves are normal. Constant flow generators do not compensate for leaks; the tidal volume delivered to the lungs decreases.

Some ventilators, e.g. Blease Brompton, generate a pressure rather higher than that required to inflate the lungs but not high enough to maintain

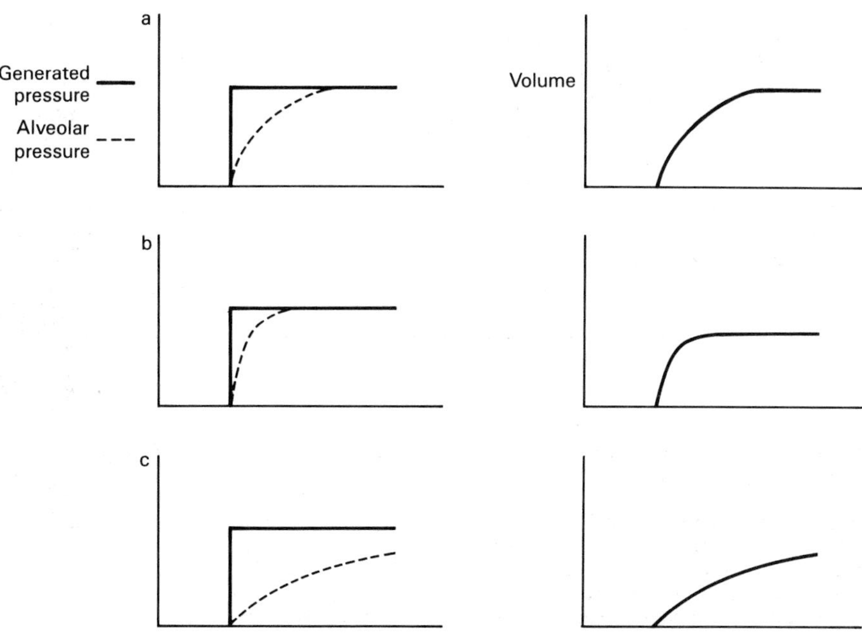

Fig. 17.22 Generated and alveolar pressures, and alveolar volume, during inspiration with a constant pressure generator. (a) Normal. (b) Decreased complicance. (c) Increased airway resistance. Note that both abnormalities reduce alveolar volume.

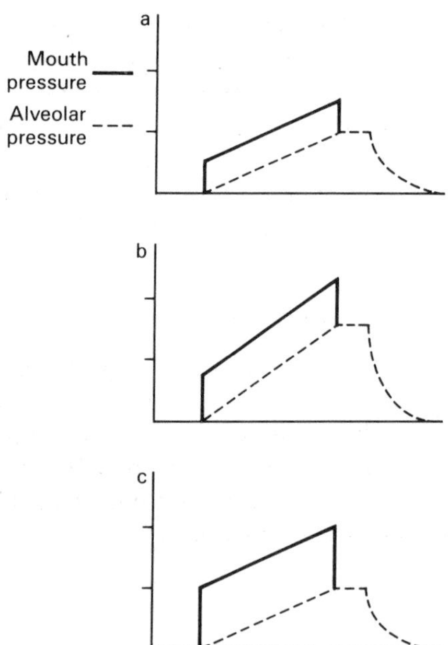

Fig. 17.23 Mouth and alveolar pressures during inspiration with a constant flow generator. (a) Normal. (b) Decreased compliance. (c) Increased airway resistance. Alveolar volume remains constant because flow rate is constant. Decreased compliance results in an increased rate of increase of alveolar pressure; mouth pressure also increases more steeply, but the gradient between mouth and alveolar pressures remains normal. Increased airway resistance increases the mouth–alveolar pressure gradient.

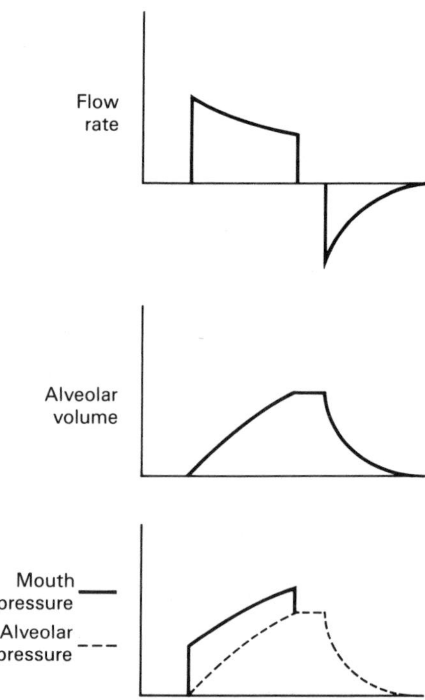

Fig. 17.24 Pressure, flow and alveolar volume characteristics during inspiration with a ventilator with a moderately high internal pressure (e.g. Blease Brompton). At higher bellows pressures, and in a patient with normal compliance and airway resistance, the characteristics approximate to those of a constant flow generator (Fig. 17.21). At low bellows pressures, if compliance decreases or if airway resistance increases, the pattern is similar to that of a constant pressure generator.

constant flow throughout inspiration. The flow, volume and pressure changes within the lung are shown in Figure 17.24.

Change from inspiration to expiration

This is termed 'cycling', and may be achieved in one of three ways:

1. *Volume-cycling*. The ventilator cycles into expiration whenever a predetermined tidal volume has been delivered. The duration of inspiration is determined by the inspiratory flow rate.

2. *Pressure-cycling*. The ventilator cycles into expiration when a preset *airway* pressure is achieved. This allows compensation for small leaks, but, in common with a constant pressure generator, a pressure-cycled ventilator delivers a different tidal volume if compliance or resistance changes. In addition, inspiratory time varies with changes in compliance and resistance.

3. *Time-cycling*. This is the method used most commonly by modern ventilators. The duration of inspiration is predetermined. With a constant flow generator, it may be desirable to preset a tidal volume; when this has been delivered, there is a short inspiratory pause (which improves gas distribution within the lung) before the inspiratory cycle ends. The use of this '*volume-preset*' mechanism must be differentiated from volume-cycling. When a constant pressure generator is time-cycled, the tidal volume delivered depends on the compliance and resistance of the lungs and on the pressure within the bellows.

Expiration

Usually, the patient is allowed to exhale to atmospheric pressure; flow rate decreases exponentially.

Subatmospheric pressure should not be used during expiration as it induces small airways closure and air-trapping. Positive end-expiratory pressure (PEEP) may be applied in some circumstances (see Ch. 42).

Change from expiration to inspiration

On most ventilators, this is achieved by time-cycling. However, it may be desirable occasionally to use pressure-cycling in response to a subatmospheric pressure generated by the patient's inspiratory effort.

Delivery of anaesthetic gas

Some ventilators deliver a minute volume determined by a preset tidal volume and rate. When used in anaesthesia, these machines must be supplied with a flow rate of anaesthetic gases which equals or exceeds the minute volume delivered or else air, or gas used to drive the ventilator, is entrained and delivered to the patient. A number of ventilators which are driven by the anaesthetic gas supply can deliver only that gas, and divide it into predetermined tidal volumes (*minute volume dividers*). Ventilators may be used to compress bellows in a separate system which contains anaesthetic gases ('bag-in-a-bottle'); it is possible to provide IPPV in a circle system in this way. Some devices may be used also to ventilate the patient through a Bain system (vide supra).

The characteristics of several common ventilators are summarised in Table 17.5.

High-frequency ventilation

This is discussed in Chapter 2. High-frequency jet ventilation is used during some operations on the larynx, trachea or lung and in a small number of patients in ITU. Gas exchange may be unpredictable and the technique should not be used by the trainee without supervision.

SCAVENGING

The possible adverse effects of pollution on staff in the operating theatre environment are discussed in Chapter 18. The principal sources of pollution by anaesthetic gases and vapours include:

1. Gas discharge from ventilators.
2. Expired gas vented from the spill valve of an anaesthetic breathing system.

Table 17.5 Classification of some common ventilators used during anaesthesia

Ventilator	Driven by	Cycling to expiration	Cycling to inspiration	Pressure/flow generator	Minute volume divider	Volume preset
Manley MP2, MN2, NO3	Anaesthetic gases	Time	Time	Pressure	Yes	Yes
Manley Pulmovent	Anaesthetic gases	Volume	Time	Flow	Yes	Yes
Blease Brompton	Anaesthetic gases	Volume or time	Time	Mixed	Yes	Yes
Philips AV1	Anaesthetic gases	Time (electrically operated valves)	Time (electrically operated valves)	Flow	Yes	No
Cape–Waine	Electric motor	Time	Time	Flow (sine wave)	Yes	No
East–Radcliffe	Electric motor	Time	Time	Pressure	No	No
Manley Servovent	Compressed air or oxygen	Volume	Time	Flow	No	Yes
Oxford	Compressed air or oxygen	Time	Time	Flow	No	Yes
Nuffield 200	Compressed air or oxygen	Time	Time	Flow	No	No
Servo 900	Anaesthetic gases	Time (electrically operated valves)	Time (electrically operated valves)	Flow (usually)	No	Yes

3. Leaks from equipment, e.g. from an ill-fitting facemask.
4. Gas exhaled by the patient after anaesthesia. This may occur in the operating theatre, corridors and recovery room.
5. Spillage during filling of vaporisers.

Although most attention has centred on removing gas from expiratory ports of breathing systems and ventilators, other methods of reducing pollution should be considered also:

1. *Reduced use of anaesthetic gases and vapours.* The use of the circle system reduces the potential for atmospheric pollution. The use of inhalational anaesthetics may be obviated totally by employing total intravenous anaesthesia (p. 188) or local anaesthetic techniques.
2. *Air conditioning.* Air conditioning units which produce a rapid change of air in the operating theatre reduce pollution substantially. However, some systems recycle air, and older operating theatres, dental surgeries and obstetric delivery suites may not be equipped with air conditioning.
3. *Care in filling vaporisers.* Great care should be taken not to spill volatile anaesthetic agents when vaporisers are filled. The use of agent-specific connections (see p. 298) reduces the risk of spillage. In some countries, vaporisers may be filled only in a portable fume cupboard.

Scavenging apparatus

Anaesthetic gases vented from the breathing system are removed by a collecting system. A variety of purpose-built scavenging spill valves is available; an example is shown in Figure 17.25.

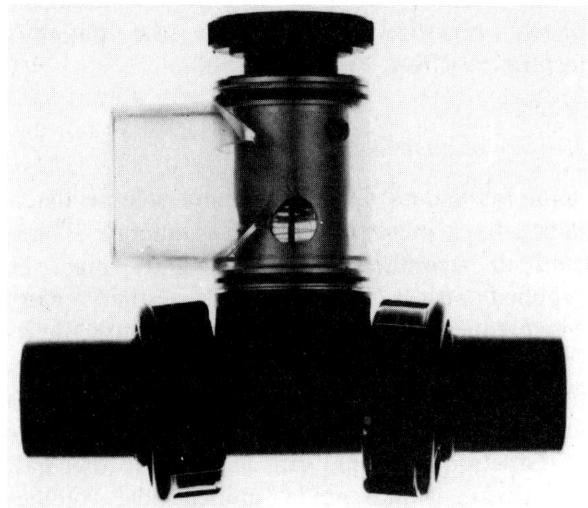

Fig. 17.25 An expiratory spill valve with scavenging attachment.

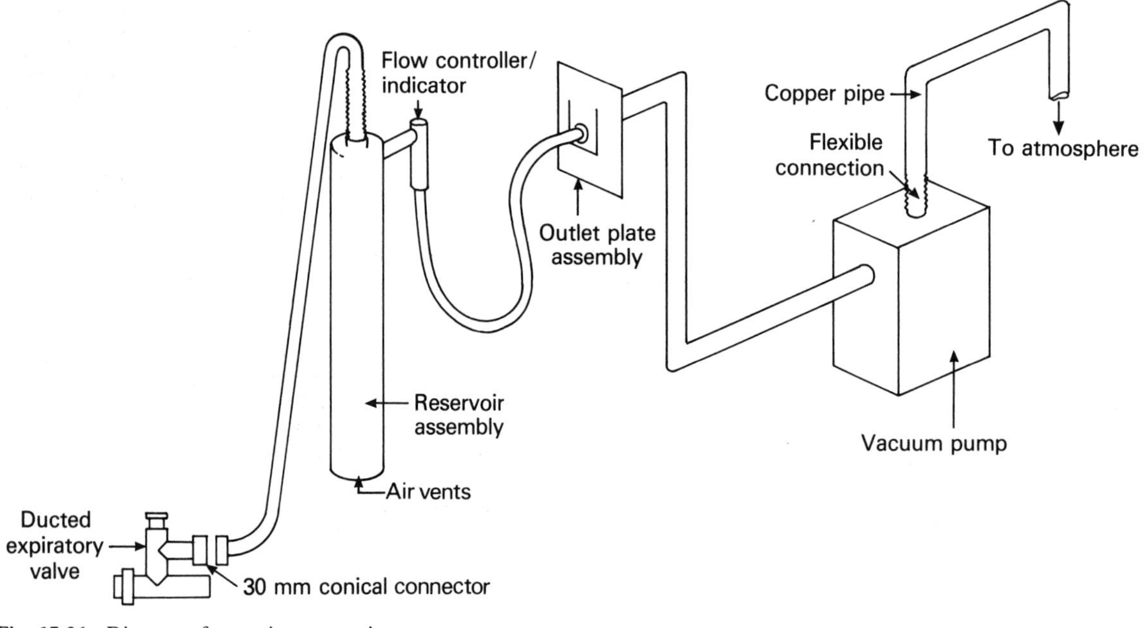

Fig. 17.26 Diagram of an active scavenging system.

Waste gases from ventilators are collected by attaching the scavenging system to the expiratory port of the ventilator. Connectors on scavenging systems have a diameter of 30 mm to ensure that inappropriate connections with anaesthetic apparatus cannot be made.

Disposal systems may be active, semi-active or passive.

Active systems

These employ apparatus to generate a negative pressure within the scavenging system which propels waste gases to the outside atmosphere. The system may be powered by a vacuum pump (Fig. 17.26) or a Venturi system (Fig. 17.27). The exhaust should be capable of accommodating 75 litres/min continuous flow with a peak of 130 litres/min. Usually, a reservoir system is used to permit high peak flow rates to be accommodated. In addition, there must be a pressure-limiting device within the system to prevent the application of negative pressure to the patient's lungs.

Semi-active systems

The waste gases may be conducted to the extraction side of the air-conditioning system, which generates a small negative pressure within the scavenging tubing. These systems have variable performance and efficiency.

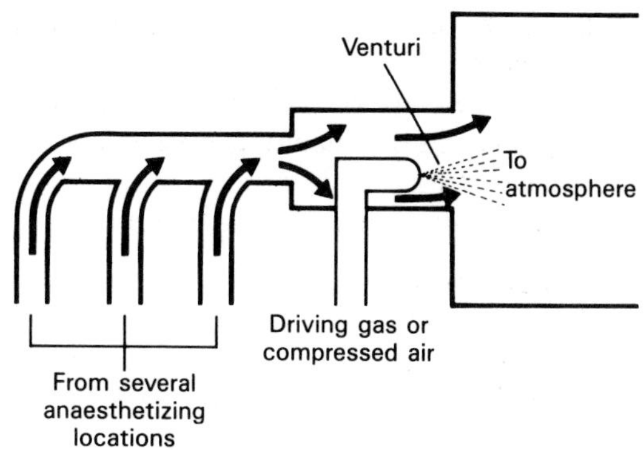

Fig. 17.27 Diagram of a Venturi system for active scavenging of anaesthetic gases.

Passive systems

These systems vent the expired gas to the outside atmosphere (Fig. 17.28). Gas movement is generated by the patient. Consequently, the total length of tubing must not be excessive, or resistance to expiration is high. The pressure within the system may be altered by wind conditions at the external terminal; on occasions, these may generate a

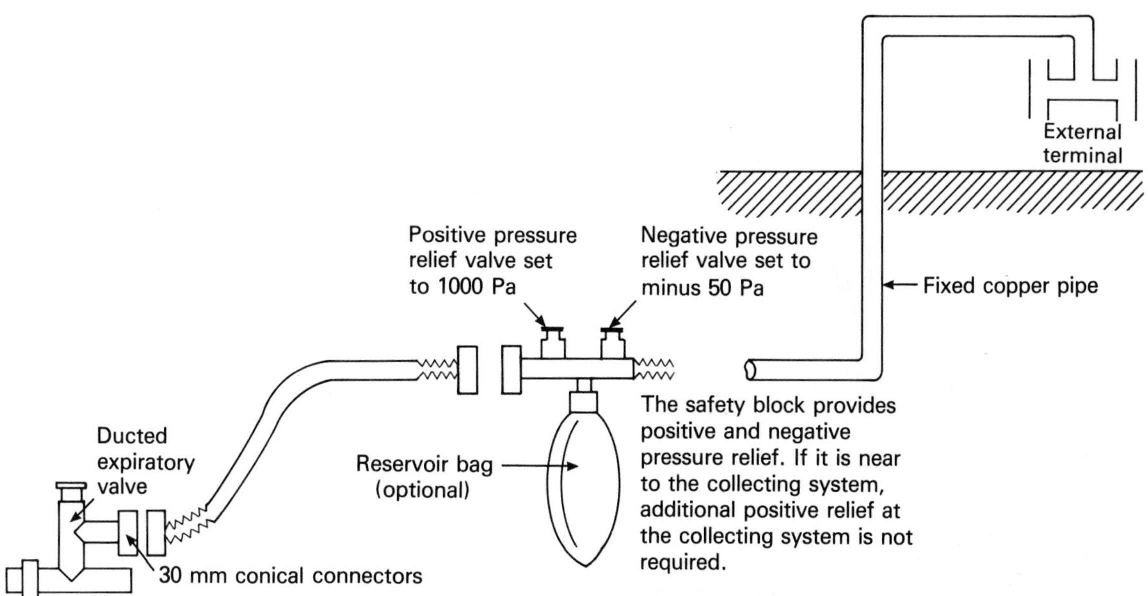

Fig. 17.28 Diagram of a passive scavenging system.

negative pressure, but may also generate high positive pressures. Each scavenging location should have a separate external terminal to prevent gases being vented into adjacent locations. Relief valves must be incorporated to prevent negative or high positive pressures within the system.

Irrespective of the type of disposal system, tubing used for scavenging must not be allowed to lie on the floor of the operating theatre as compression (e.g. by feet or by items of equipment) results in increased resistance to expiration and may generate dangerously high pressure within the patient's lungs.

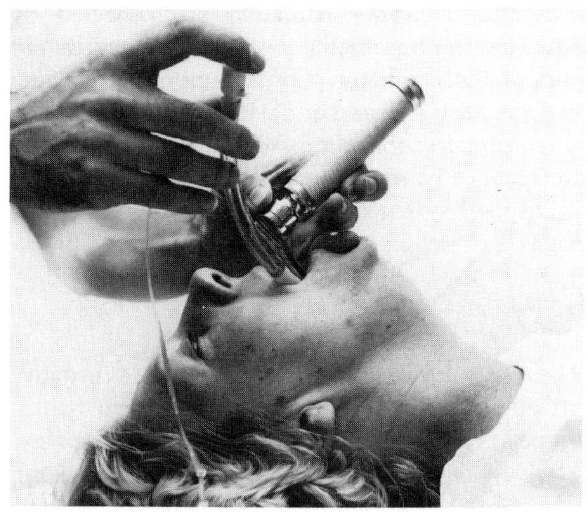

Fig. 17.30 Tracheal intubation using a curved-bladed laryngoscope.

LARYNGOSCOPES

Curved blade

The most commonly used adult laryngoscope blade is the Macintosh curved blade, which is manufactured in several sizes (Fig. 17.29). The handle is held firmly in the left hand (Fig. 17.30). The patient's neck should be flexed and the head extended. The mouth may be opened using the right forefinger, and the upper lip should be retracted using the right thumb so that the lip is not trapped between the laryngoscope blade and the teeth. It may be necessary also to retract the lower lip with the right middle finger.

The tip of the laryngoscope blade is advanced carefully over the surface of the tongue until it reaches the vallecula. The tip of the blade is rotated upwards, and the laryngoscope lifted along the axis of the handle to lift the larynx; the incisor teeth must not be used as a fulcrum to lever the tip of the blade upwards. When the arytenoids and posterior part of the cords are seen, gentle pressure on the larynx using the right thumb, or provided by an assistant, may help to improve the view.

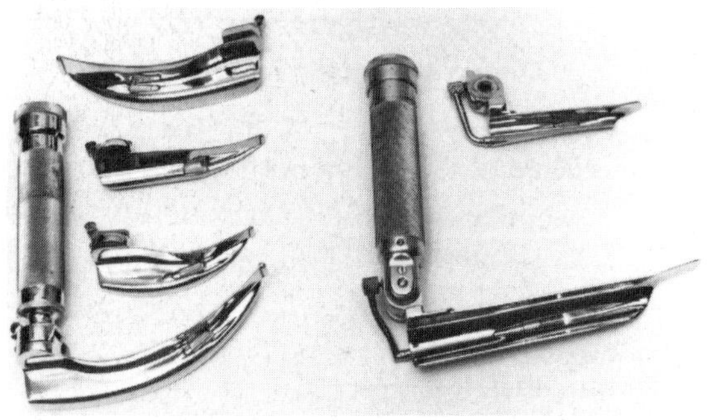

Fig. 17.29 Two laryngoscopes with a selection of blades. Left (from above downwards): Macintosh left-handed blade, Robertshaw blade, Macintosh infant blade and Macintosh adult blade. Right: Magill infant blade (above) and Magill adult blade (below).

Straight blade

The technique of laryngoscopy is slightly different when a straight blade (e.g. Magill) is used. Instead of placing the tip of the blade in the vallecula, it is advanced over the posterior border of the epiglottis, which is then lifted directly by the blade to provide a view of the larynx. This technique is useful particularly in babies, in whom the epiglottis is rather floppy and may obscure the view of the larynx if a curved blade is used. However, bruising of the epiglottis is more likely with a straight blade.

Most laryngoscopes are powered by batteries contained within the handle; these must be replaced regularly to prevent failure during laryngoscopy. On many laryngoscopes, the light source is a bulb which screws into a socket on the blade; a tight connection should be ensured before laryngoscopy is attempted. It is usual for the electrical circuit between the batteries and the bulb to be closed by a switch which operates automatically when the blade is opened. However, the electrical contacts of the switch may become corroded, causing a reduction in power or total failure. Because of these potential problems, it is important that the function of the laryngoscope is checked carefully before use. It is also wise to have a spare functioning laryngoscope and a variety of blades available.

TRACHEAL TUBES

Most tracheal tubes are constructed either of red rubber or plastic. Red rubber tubes are reusable, although they may start to show signs of deterioration after 2–3 years. Disposable plastic tubes are preferred in most centres as they eliminate the need to collect, clean, sterilise and check tubes after use. Plastic tubes are presented in a sterile pack, and should be cut to an appropriate length before use.

Tube size

In adults, there is little to be gained in the way of reduced resistance to breathing by selecting a tube larger than 8.0 mm internal diameter. However, it is common to use a tube of 9.0–9.5 mm internal diameter for male adults and 8.0–8.5 mm for females. Tubes of wide diameter may exert pressure on the laryngeal cords after insertion. Appropriate sizes of tracheal tubes for children are shown in Appendix V, p. 734.

Plain tubes

Uncuffed tubes are used in children. A cuff is unnecessary to secure an airtight fit if the correct diameter of tube is selected, because the narrowest part of the airway is in the trachea at the level of the cricoid cartilage. However, the larynx is the narrowest part of the airway in the adult, and a leak occurs if an uncuffed tube is used; in addition, there is a risk of aspiration of fluid from the pharynx into the trachea. However, nasotracheal intubation is less traumatic if an uncuffed tube is used. The incidence of sore throat is not influenced by the presence of a cuff on the tracheal tube.

Cuffed tubes

It is usual to use a cuffed tube whenever tracheal intubation is required in the adult. It is almost mandatory if IPPV is to be employed and is essential if there is a risk of blood, pus or gastric fluid entering the pharynx. Tracheal tubes with a streamlined cuff are available, and are suitable for nasotracheal intubation.

Cuff volume

A tube with a low-volume cuff (Fig. 17.31) may require inflation to a high pressure to effect a seal within the trachea. The pressure within a low-volume cuff does not necessarily relate to the pressure exerted by the cuff on the tracheal mucosa. However, a high pressure may be exerted if the cuff is overinflated. This may occur inadvertently during anaesthesia because nitrous oxide diffuses through some types of plastic. Some anaesthetists inflate the cuff with an oxygen/nitrous oxide mixture to obviate this problem. Alternatively, the cuff volume may be readjusted after 10–15 min of anaesthesia.

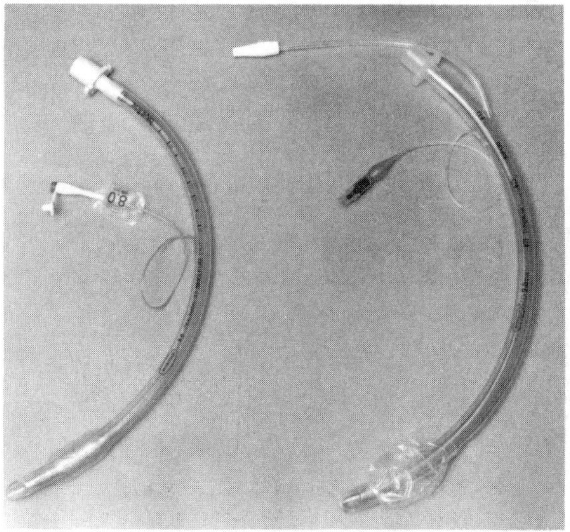

Fig. 17.31 Left: low-volume, high-pressure cuff. Right: high-volume, low-pressure ('floppy') cuff on tracheal tubes.

High-volume, low-pressure ('floppy') cuffs cover a larger area of tracheal wall and may effect a seal with less pressure exerted on the mucosa. However, they may cause more trauma during insertion and may become puckered in a relatively small trachea.

Herniation of an overinflated cuff may occlude the distal end of the tracheal tube and cause partial or total airway obstruction.

Shape of tube

In most centres, a curved tracheal tube is used. These should be cut to the correct length, and there is a risk of accidental intubation of a bronchus (usually the right main bronchus) if the tip is inserted too far. The Oxford tube is L-shaped, and the angle of the tube lies in the pharynx; the distal end is of a fixed length. It is claimed that the use of an Oxford tube reduces the risk of bronchial intubation. There may be less risk of an Oxford tube kinking if the head is flexed during surgery. However, an introducer is required to pass an Oxford tube through the larynx.

Some plastic tracheal tubes are pre-formed in shapes which either fit the pharyngeal contour or carry the proximal end of the tube away from the mouth (Fig. 17.32); the latter design is useful when surgery on the face or head is planned.

Specialised tubes

An armoured latex tube (Fig. 17.33) is useful if there is a danger of the tube kinking during surgery; a nylon spiral is incorporated in the wall of the tube and prevents obliteration of the lumen. Alternatively, a flexometallic tube, with a metal spiral in the wall, may be used. These tubes are very floppy, and a wire stilette is required for their insertion.

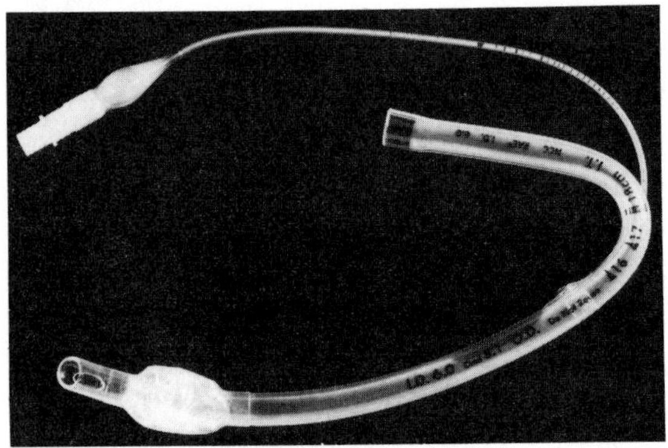

Fig. 17.32 A pre-formed disposable plastic tracheal tube.

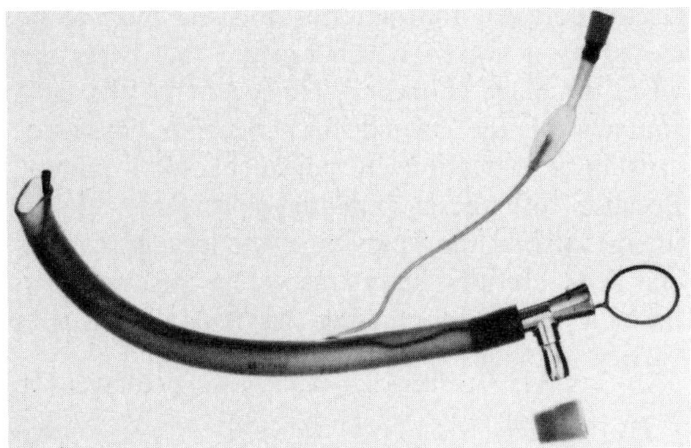

Fig. 17.33 Armoured latex cuffed tracheal tube, with stilette for introduction.

A flexible metal tube (Fig. 17.34) may be employed during procedures that require the use of lasers in the airway; plastic tubes may ignite if struck by the laser beam.

Connections

British standard connections with a 22-mm diameter taper are used in breathing systems. All modern adult tracheal tube connectors have a 15-mm diameter taper.

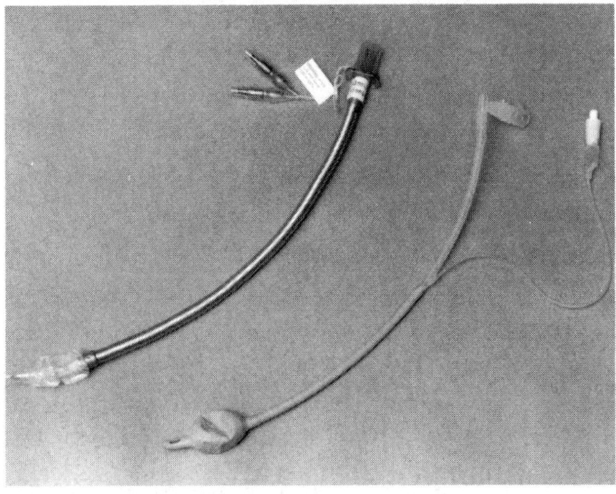

Fig. 17.34 Flexible metal tube and a metal-coated plastic tube suitable for use during laser surgery to the airway.

Tracheal tube connectors

Disposable 15-mm diameter connectors are provided with plastic disposable tubes; the diameter of the distal end is of an appropriate size to fit the internal diameter of the tube. A number of other connections (Fig. 17.35) may be used with plastic or rubber tracheal tubes. The Nosworthy connector is less bulky than the 15-mm disposable connector, and is used often in paediatric practice. The Magill connectors are useful particularly during surgery of the head or neck.

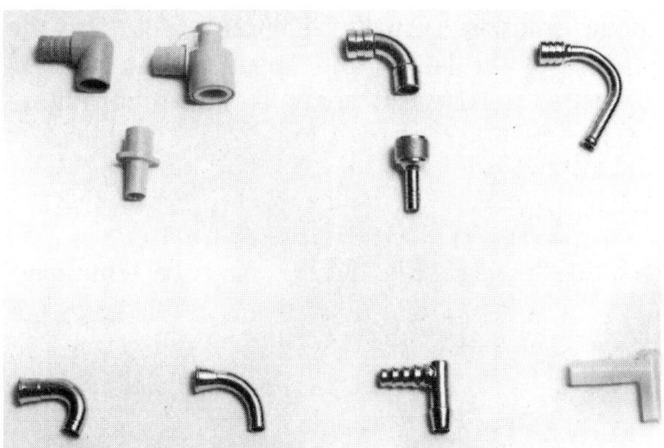

Fig. 17.35 A variety of tracheal tube connectors. From top left in clockwise rotation: Portex and Portex swivel with 15-mm tracheal tube connector, Nosworthy, Worcester, Cobbs, Rowbotham, Magill oral, Magill nasal.

The laryngeal mask

This recently introduced device consists of a shortened conventional silicone tracheal tube with an elliptical cuff, inflated through a pilot tube, attached to the distal end (Fig. 17.36). The cuff, which resembles a miniature face mask, has been designed to form a (relatively) airtight seal around the posterior perimeter of the larynx. A variety of sizes of cuff is available. The mask is inserted and the cuff inflated until no air leak is present; an introducer may be required to ensure that the epiglottis is in the correct position in relation to the proximal end of the cuff. The device is very effective in maintaining a patent airway in the spontaneously breathing patient. Positive pressure ventilation can be applied if necessary, but a conventional tracheal tube should be used if a technique employing muscle relaxants is planned. The mask is not suitable for patients who are at risk from regurgitation of gastric contents, or in whom pharyngeal soiling is anticipated.

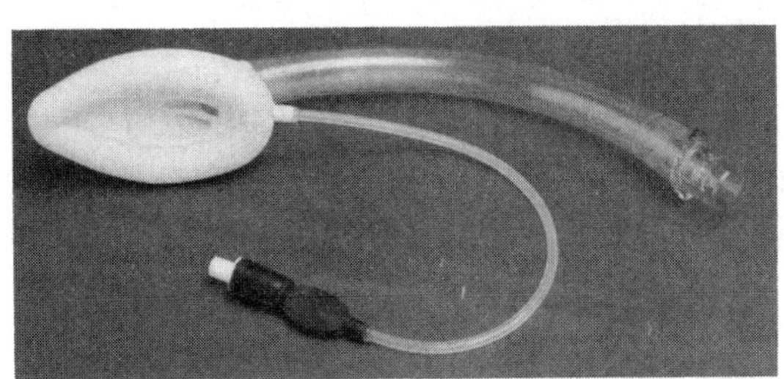

Fig. 17.36 Laryngeal mask.

OTHER APPARATUS

Face masks

These are designed to fit the face perfectly so that no leak of gas occurs, but without applying excessive pressure to the skin. An appropriate size of face mask must be selected to ensure a proper fit, but the smallest size possible should be used to minimise deadspace. Adult face masks have a 22 mm taper connection, and a 90° angle-piece is inserted usually between the mask and the anaesthetic breathing system.

A harness system (e.g. Clausen harness) is used by some anaesthetists to hold the mask on the face during surgery. However, airway obstruction may occur at any time and the excursion of the reservoir bag must be observed constantly.

Intubating forceps

The most commonly used intubating forceps is that designed by Magill (Fig. 17.37). The instru-

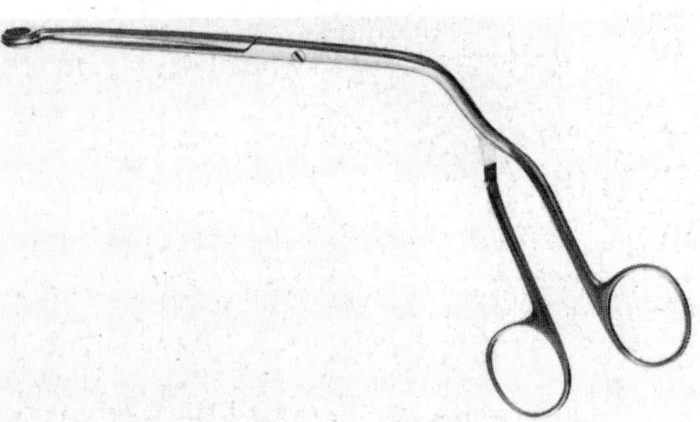

Fig. 17.37 Magill intubating forceps.

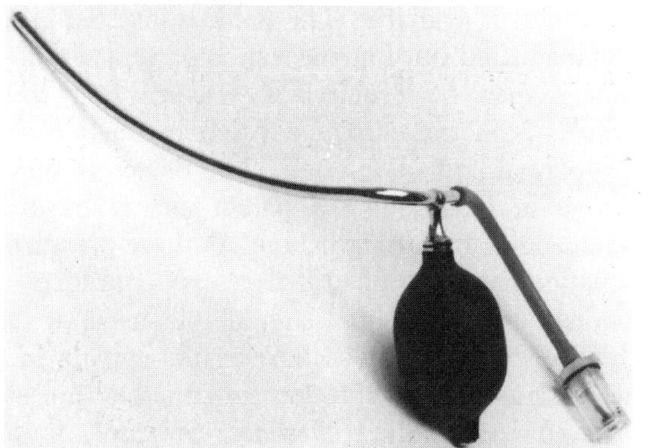

Fig. 17.38 Forrester laryngeal spray.

ment is employed to manipulate a nasotracheal or nasogastric tube through the oropharynx and into the correct position. A laryngoscope is used to obtain a view of the oropharynx.

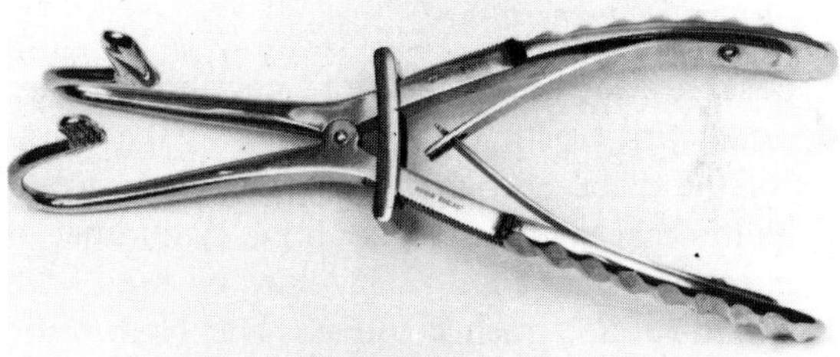

Fig. 17.39 Ferguson mouth gag.

Laryngeal spray

This is used to deposit a fine mist of local anaesthetic solution (usually lignocaine 4%) on the mucosa of the larynx and upper trachea. An example of a laryngeal spray is shown in Figure 17.38.

Mouth gag

A mouth gag (Fig. 17.39) may be employed

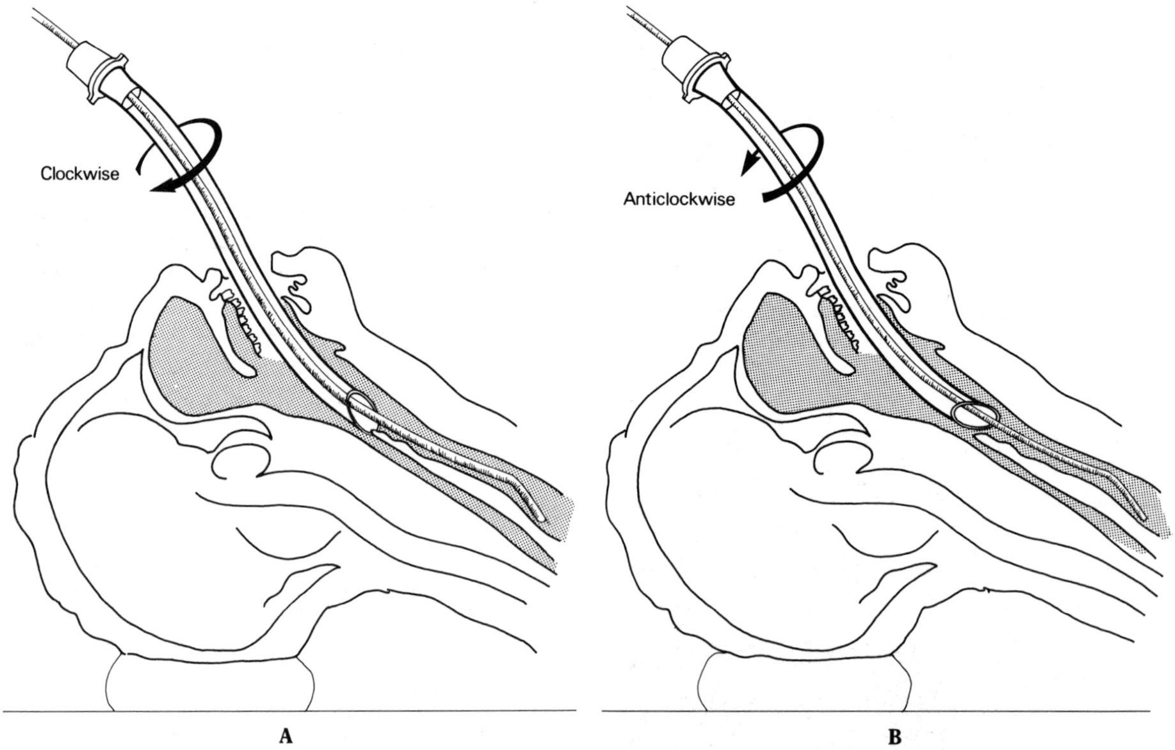

Fig. 17.40 A gum elastic bougie passed into the trachea. After insertion of the tracheal tube, clockwise rotation of the tube (A) may cause the tip to lodge against the aryepiglottic fold; anticlockwise rotation (B) permits the tube to slide past the fold into the trachea.

during dental anaesthesia, and is required occasionally to open the mouth in patients with trismus or if masseter spasm is present. It is positioned between the molar teeth and must be used with great care to avoid dental trauma.

Gum elastic bougie

If the larynx cannot be seen adequately during laryngoscopy, or if the tracheal tube cannot be manoeuvred into the laryngeal inlet, a gum elastic bougie may be used as an aid to tracheal intubation. The lubricated bougie is inserted into the trachea to act as a guide for the tracheal tube (Fig. 17.40). The tube should be rotated so that the bevel does not become lodged against the aryepiglottic fold.

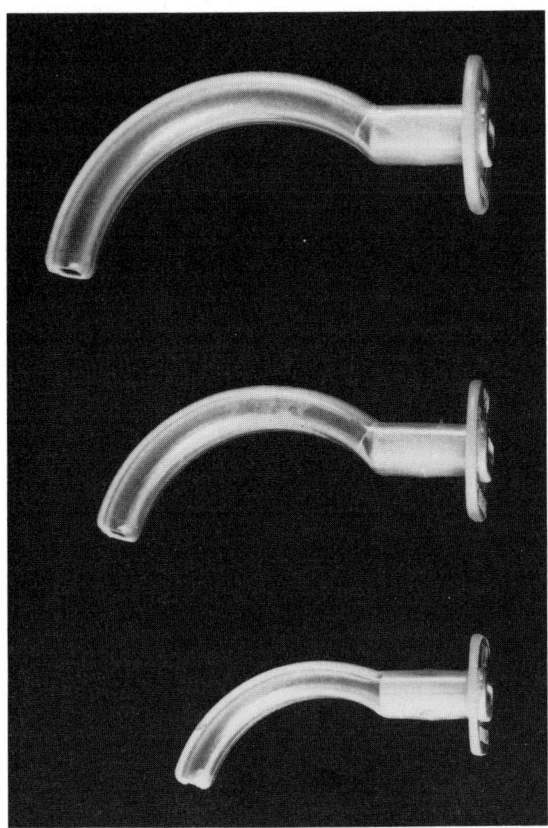

Fig. 17.41 Small, medium and large Guedel airways. Smaller sizes are available for use in infants and small children.

Stilettes

A malleable metal stilette may be used to adjust the degree of curvature of a tracheal tube as an aid to its insertion. The stilette must not protrude from the distal end of the tube.

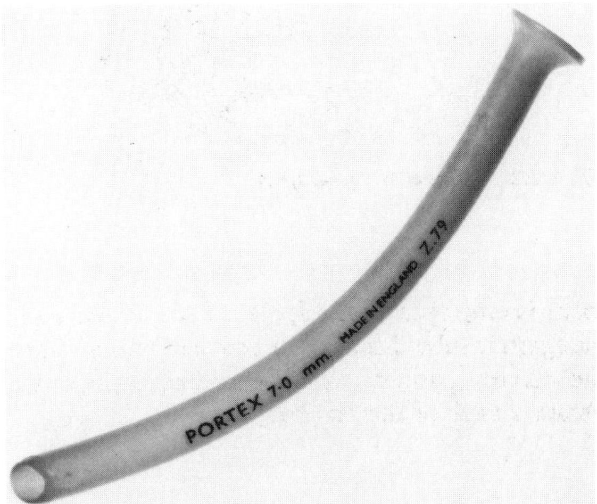

Fig. 17.42 Nasopharyngeal airway.

Airways

An *oropharyngeal* airway (Guedel airway; Fig. 17.41) may be required to prevent obstruction caused by the tongue or collapse of the pharynx in the unintubated patient. A *nasopharyngeal* airway (Fig. 17.42) is tolerated better during light anaesthesia and may be used also if it is difficult to insert an oropharyngeal airway, e.g. trismus.

FURTHER READING

Aldrete J A, Lowe H J, Virtue R W 1980 Low flow and closed system anesthesia. Grune & Stratton, New York

Mushin W W, Rendell-Baker L, Thompson P W, Mapleson W W 1980 Automatic ventilation of the lungs, 3rd edn. Blackwell Scientific Publications, Oxford

Scurr C, Feldman S 1983 Scientific foundations of anaesthesia, 3rd edn. Heinemann, London

Sykes M K, Hull C J, Vickers M D 1981 Principles of clinical measurement. Blackwell Scientific Publications, Oxford

Ward C S 1985 Anaesthetic equipment: physical principles and maintenance, 2nd edn. Baillière Tindall, London

18. The operating theatre environment

Until the middle of the nineteenth century, surgery was carried out in any convenient room, frequently one which was used for other purposes. Although the introduction of antisepsis resulted in the washing of instruments and operating table, the operating room itself was ignored as a source of infection. Operating rooms were designed with tiers of wooden benches around the operating table for spectators; thus the term 'operating theatre' was introduced. During the early part of the twentieth century, large windows were incorporated, as artificial light was relatively ineffective, and high ceilings were introduced to improve ventilation. Additional facilities became necessary for preparing and anaesthetising the patient, for sterilisation of instruments and for the surgeon and other theatre staff to change clothes and scrub up. In addition, the design of operating theatres changed, and smaller theatres were introduced to facilitate frequent cleaning.

A modern operating theatre incorporates the following design features:

1. Environmental controls of varying degrees of complexity, to reduce the risk of airborne infection.
2. Services for surgical and anaesthetic equipment.
3. An operating table on which the patient may be placed in the position required for surgery.
4. Artificial lighting appropriate for the requirements of both surgeon and anaesthetist.
5. Measures to ensure the safety of patient and staff.

In addition, provision should be made immediately adjacent to the operating theatre for anaesthetising the patient, preparing instruments, cleaning dirty instruments and for the surgeon to scrub up. There should also be separate areas for reception and recovery of patients. It is now common practice for each hospital to have a suite of theatres, rather than operating theatres close to each of the surgical wards. The use of theatre suites permits more flexible and efficient use of staff and resources.

THE OPERATING THEATRE SUITE

The number of operating theatres required is difficult to calculate, but approximates in most British cities to one for every 40 000 of the population served. Ideally, the operating theatre suite should be close to the surgical wards, and adjacent to, and on the same floor as, the accident and emergency department, intensive care unit, X-ray department, day-case ward and sterile supplies unit. It is logical for the anaesthetic department to be immediately adjacent to, or an integral part of, the operating theatre suite, although this seldom occurs in practice.

The main purpose of the operating theatre environment is to minimise the risk of transmission of infection to the patient from the air, the building or the staff. The operating theatre suite contains four zones of increasing degree of cleanliness (Table 18.1).

Transfer of patient

There is some evidence that anxiety in the surgical patient peaks as transfer from the ward to the operating theatre begins, and it is important that facilities for transfer minimise stress. A nurse from the ward usually accompanies the patient,

Table 18.1 Zones of cleanliness in the operating theatre suite

Outer zone
Hospital areas up to and including the reception area
Clean zone
The circulation area used by staff after they have changed, and the route taken by patients from the transfer bay to the anaesthetic room
Aseptic zone
Scrub-up and gowning area, anaesthetic room, theatre preparation room, operating room, exit bay
Disposal zone
Disposal area for waste products and soiled or used equipment and supplies

but it is customary for the ward nurse to leave the patient before anaesthesia has been induced.

On arrival at the reception area, the patient's identity and surgical procedure are checked. In a theatre suite, it may be necessary for patients to wait for some time in the reception area to prevent delays in the operating schedules. Consequently, adequate space should be provided for a number of beds, and there should be screens for patients who wish privacy. The staff in the reception area should include nurses. The decor should be cheerful, and the lighting subdued.

Transport should involve the minimum number of changes of trolley. A trolley is used commonly to transfer the patient to the operating theatre suite, but changes of trolley may be required to enter the clean area and also for transfer to the operating table after anaesthesia has been induced.

Alternatively, the patient's own bed may be taken to the operating theatre suite. If the patient is infirm or in severe pain, the bed may be taken to the anaesthetic room, and transfer delayed until after induction of anaesthesia, but this is appropriate only if the bed has the facility to be tipped head-down if necessary. In some hospitals, a single transfer is effected by transporting the patient to the theatre suite in bed, where the patient is moved on to the operating theatre table-top, which is mounted on a wheeled frame. After induction of anaesthesia, the table-top is wheeled into the theatre and the top attached to a fixed base, which allows it to be positioned for surgery.

There is no universal method of transferring patients from one trolley to another. This may be achieved by the use of canvas and poles, rollers or lifting the patient bodily.

All trolleys in the operating theatre suite should be equipped with oxygen, and this should be administered routinely to patients during transfer from theatre to the recovery room at the end of the procedure if general anaesthesia has been used.

Anaesthetic room

In many countries, the anaesthetic room has developed from a small annexe to the theatre to an integral part of the operating theatre suite. However, this is not universal, and in some parts of the world anaesthesia is induced in the operating theatre after the patient has been transferred on to the operating table. The main advantages of the anaesthetic room are:

1. The patient's anxiety may be reduced by avoiding the sights and sounds of the operating theatre. This is of special importance in children.
2. The equipment which may be necessary during induction of anaesthesia may be stored in a readily accessible form.
3. Time is saved by inducing anaesthesia while surgery is being completed on another patient. This is useful particularly if preparation is prolonged, e.g. performance of local anaesthetic blocks or establishment of invasive cardiovascular monitoring.

However, there are a number of disadvantages:

1. Anaesthetic and monitoring equipment must be duplicated, or moved to the operating theatre with the patient; this usually necessitates temporary disconnection from electrical or gas supplies.
2. Hazards are involved in transferring an unconscious patient from a trolley to the operating table.
3. Construction and maintenance of anaesthetic rooms are expensive.

Even in countries where anaesthetic rooms are used, it is customary to induce anaesthesia in the high-risk patient on the operating table, as the delay between onset of unconsciousness and the start of surgery must be kept to a minimum, e.g. emergency Caesarean section or severe haemorrhage.

The design of the anaesthetic room should allow easy access all round the patient's trolley, and should provide space for anaesthetic and monitoring equipment, and storage cupboards and shelves. The minimum floor area recommended by the Department of Health and Social Security (DHSS) in the UK is 17 m^2, but this is inadequate. A floor area of 21 m^2 is more appropriate. Piped gases and suction and electrical sockets are required near the head of the trolley. An anaesthetic machine, mechanical ventilator and monitoring system are also necessary. Cupboards must be available to store equipment and drugs, and worktops must be of sufficient size to allow syringes, needles, cannulae and drugs to be prepared. There should be a clock with a second hand.

Operating room

The operating room is designed around its centrally situated operating table with overhead lighting and ventilation systems. The ideal shape for the operating room is circular, but this is inefficient and most operating rooms are square or nearly square. In 1980, the Royal College of Surgeons suggested that the floor should be 625 ft^2 (approximately 58 m^2) in area, and no smaller than 484 ft^2 (approximately 45 m^2). Theatres for specialised surgery may require a larger area to accommodate bulky equipment.

Outlets for piped gases, and electrical sockets, must be positioned close to the head of the operating table; they are provided most conveniently by a boom or stalactite system. Electrical cables should not lie across the floor. The operating room should be of sufficient size to allow all types of surgery without moving the position of the head of the table; this location should be reached easily and without complex manoeuvres as the patient enters the theatre from the anaesthetic room.

Temperature, humidity and ventilation

The temperature in the operating theatre and anaesthetic room should be sufficiently high to minimise the risk of inducing hypothermia in the patient, but must be comfortable for theatre staff. The patient may develop hypothermia at an ambient temperature of less than 21°C. Temperatures of 22–24°C are usually acceptable in the operating room, with a relative humidity of 50–60%; a higher environmental temperature is required during surgery in the neonate or infant. Slightly lower temperature and humidity are acceptable in other parts of the theatre suite. Controls for temperature and humidity should be located within the operating theatre.

Heating and humidity are controlled usually by an air-conditioning and ventilation system, which provides an ambient pressure inside the operating room slightly higher than atmospheric. In general, air is introduced directly over the operating table, and leaves at the periphery through ducts positioned near floor level. In the area of the table, 400 air changes per hour are required to minimise the risk of airborne transmission of infection. More effective systems of ventilation, involving radial exponential air flow away from the operating table, or laminar flow, are used in some centres for some types of surgery, e.g. total hip replacement, in which infection is especially undesirable. High-flow systems may accelerate cooling of the patient.

Light

Daylight is not necessary in the operating theatre, although it is more pleasant for staff if there are windows in the theatre suite, e.g. in corridors and common rooms. A high level of illumination is required over the operating table, and ceiling-mounted lamps are standard; it is preferable if they can be positioned directly by the surgeon.

The intensity and colour temperature of general lighting is very important to the anaesthetist, as appreciation of skin colour is affected by the spectrum of the source of illumination. The spectrum provided by lighting tubes should be similar to that of daylight, with an emission temperature of 4000–5000 K. The colour of the decor should be neutral and uniform. The intensity of general illumination should be up to 325 lumens/m^2 in the operating theatre, and it should be diffuse to avoid glare. In the anaesthetic room and recovery area, a light intensity of approximately 220 lumen/m^2

is acceptable, but a spotlight should be available if increased illumination is required for specific procedures.

Safety in the operating theatre

Electrocution and gas explosions are the two main hazards to staff and patients in the operating theatre. In addition, there may be a risk to staff from pollution of the atmosphere with anaesthetic gases and vapours, and of contracting infection, particularly human immunodeficiency virus (HIV) or hepatitis B, from infected patients.

Electrical safety

Although some mention is made of electrical hazards in the operating theatre in Chapter 16, a detailed description is beyond the scope of this book, and the reader is referred to the article by Hull (1978). The electrical supply to the operating theatre and all electrical equipment connected to the patient incorporate design features which minimise the risk of electrical currents being transmitted through the patient to earth.

Explosions

The use of explosive anaesthetic gases and vapours has diminished greatly in recent years. However, cyclopropane and diethyl ether are still used occasionally. Ether burns in air, but forms an explosive mixture with oxygen; cyclopropane is explosive in both air and oxygen. An explosion may be initiated by a spark of very low energy (<1 μJ) or by contact with a temperature of 300°C or higher. The risk of explosion is highest within and close to the anaesthetic breathing system because of the presence of a high oxygen concentration. Beyond a distance of 10 cm from the breathing system, the oxygen concentration diminishes, and the risk is reduced.

The construction of anaesthetic apparatus is designed to minimise explosion hazards from generation of sparks caused by cumulation of static electricity. All rubber is conductive, so that electrical charges leak to earth, and non-conductive substances are treated with antistatic material. In most existing theatres, the operating theatre floor has a high but finite resistance, so that static charges leak to earth but electrocution risks are minimised. Theatre footwear is designed also to earth static charges. Sparks may be generated by clothing made of synthetic materials such as nylon. The risk of accumulation of static electricity on walls and equipment is reduced if the environmental humidity exceeds 70%. Diathermy must not be used if explosive anaesthetics are employed. However, the use of these agents is likely to cease in the United Kingdom, and many of the precautions, particularly the use of expensive antistatic flooring, is becoming unnecessary.

Atmospheric pollution

There has been considerable controversy regarding the risk to theatre staff from atmospheric pollution by anaesthetic gases and vapours. Earlier investigations suggested that theatre staff are more likely than other hospital personnel to suffer from hepatic and renal disease, to have non-specific neurological symptoms and for their children to have an increased risk of congenital abnormality. However, none of these problems has been substantiated.

There was more convincing evidence from the early studies that female staff who worked in the operating theatre during the early months of pregnancy suffered an increased incidence of spontaneous abortion. However, the most recent, comprehensive and only randomised prospective investigation (the MRC 10-year study) failed to demonstrate any increased health risk.

Trace concentrations of anaesthetic gases have been implicated in another area of concern, namely impairment of professional performance. Motor and intellectual performance was shown in an early laboratory study in volunteers to deteriorate in the presence of concentrations of nitrous oxide of 500 parts per million (ppm), with or without halothane 15 ppm. However, subsequent studies failed to confirm these findings, and the concensus of several studies is that concentrations of 8–12% nitrous oxide are required before significant impairment of performance occurs. Such concentrations might be inhaled if the anaesthetist is close to an unscavenged expiratory valve, or during inhalational induction of anaesthesia, but exceed those present in other areas of an adequately ventilated operating theatre.

Nevertheless, it is sensible to minimise atmospheric pollution in the operating theatre, and hospital regulations in both Western Europe and North America require the installation of anaesthetic gas scavenging systems in all areas in which anaesthesia is administered. In the USA, the National Institute of Occupational Safety and Hygiene (a federal regulatory body) dictates that environmental concentrations of anaesthetic gases should not exceed a value of 25 ppm of nitrous oxide and 2 ppm of volatile agent. Scavenging systems are described in Chapter 17.

Anaesthetic gases are not the only source of environmental pollution in the operating theatre; volatile skin-cleaning fluids and aerosol sprays, e.g. iodine or plastic skin dressing, should be used sensibly, and inhalation of vapours should be avoided.

Infection

The most serious types of acquired infection in operating theatre staff are HIV and hepatitis B, which may be contracted by contact with blood or body fluids from an infected patient. A number of health care workers have been infected in this way, either by a needle-stick injury, or through cuts and abrasions. The risk is believed to be extremely low, but the results of infection with these agents are devastating

Two thousand cases of hepatitis B are reported each year in the UK, although the true incidence is probably very much higher. Hepatitis B surface antigen persists for at least 6 months in 5–10% of infected individuals. The virus is highly infectious, and minute amounts of blood may transmit the disease. The Association of Anaesthetists of Great Britain and Ireland recommends that all anaesthetists should receive active immunisation against hepatitis B. A single dose of hepatitis B immunoglobulin combined with active immunisation is required immediately if an unprotected individual is inoculated with infected material.

The incidence of acquired immunodeficiency syndrome (AIDS) is doubling every 10 months. For every patient with fully developed AIDS, there are estimated to be five with a less severe form of the disease, and up to 50 asymptomatic carriers. At present, it is unclear what proportion of these will develop AIDS, but probably it may approach 100%. Thus, anaesthetists are likely to be exposed to an increasing number of patients who may transmit HIV; if the present rate of increase is maintained, there will be 3 000 000 HIV-positive individuals in the UK by the end of 1991. At present, compulsory screening of hospital patients for HIV is regarded as unacceptable. Consequently, precautions must be taken in patients who are believed to be at high risk of being HIV-positive; these include homosexual or bisexual men, haemophiliacs and sexual partners of high-risk patients. In some locations, e.g. California, it has been recommended that precautions should be taken with all patients.

The following precautions are recommended to reduce the risks of transmission of HIV; these are applicable also when patients with hepatitis B antigen are anaesthetised.

1. Needles should not be resheathed, or handed from one person to another.
2. All needles and other sharp objects should be disposed of in an appropriate tough disposal bin; cardboard bins are unsatisfactory.
3. Cuts or abrasions on the anaesthetist's hands should be covered with a waterproof dressing.
4. Gloves should be worn during performance of venepuncture or insertion of any intravascular cannula, and during tracheal intubation and extubation. A plastic apron, mask and eye protection should be worn if substantial spillage of blood is anticipated, e.g. during insertion of an arterial cannula.
5. If a needle-stick injury or contamination of a cut or abrasion occurs, bleeding should be encouraged and the skin washed thoroughly with soap and water.

Disposable equipment should be used where possible. Non-disposable equipment should be decontaminated with glutaraldehyde, washed with soap and water and left in glutaraldehyde for a further 3 h. Contaminated floors and surfaces should be washed with 1% hypochlorite solution. A filter should be placed between the tracheal tube and the anaesthetic breathing system.

Recovery room

A recovery room or ward is an essential requirement in the operating theatre environment. All patients require close surveillance in the immediate postoperative period, and for up to 24 h after major surgery.

The recovery room should be an integral part of the operating theatre suite, and should be located within the clean area. DHSS guidelines suggest that there should be 1.5 places in the recovery area for each operating theatre, although a greater number may be required if surgery with a high turnover, e.g. gynaecology or day-case surgery, is common. Each place requires a minimum floor area of approximately 10 m^2, and there must be sufficient space to move a patient without disturbing the remainder.

It is appropriate for most patients to lie on a trolley in the recovery room, but beds should be available for those who are likely to stay for more than 30–45 min, e.g. patients who have undergone major surgery, or ASA 3 or 4 patients who require even prolonged observation after minor surgery. Each place should have piped oxygen and suction outlets on the wall, with an oxygen flowmeter and suction apparatus attached to a wall rail. Lighting should conform to the same standards as apply to the operating theatre, and additional spotlights should be provided. It is not common practice in the UK to monitor the ECG in all patients in the recovery ward, although there are strong arguments for monitoring both ECG and oxygen saturation routinely. Most large recovery areas have two or three places which are equipped fully with piped nitrous oxide, a mechanical ventilator and complete cardiovascular monitoring facilities.

An anaesthetic machine, defibrillator and equipment and drugs for resuscitation should be available in the recovery room. Oxygen is administered usually by disposable facemask, but each place should have a self-inflating resuscitation bag and anaesthetic mask.

Drug cupboards and storage space for equipment should be provided and, in a large recovery area, several telephones are required. Nursing staff spend most of their time with the patient, but require a nursing station at which notes may be written and theatres and wards contacted by telephone. At least one nurse is required for each three bed spaces. At present, there is no specific training course in the UK for recovery room nurses. Student nurses receive only one week of training in this area.

In many hospitals, it is possible to provide supervision of patients in the recovery ward for up to 24 h after major surgery. This is highly desirable in the absence of a separate high-dependency unit, as intensive care facilities are often overwhelmed in large hospitals.

Clinical aspects of recovery room care are discussed in Chapter 24.

Other accommodation

Storage space is required for large items of equipment. In most modern operating theatre suites, instruments are sterilised in a separate department, which should be situated in close proximity. Access to blood gas analysis and measurement of serum electrolyte concentrations is essential, especially if major surgery is to be undertaken, and large operating theatre suites usually contain a small laboratory.

Staff accommodation includes changing rooms and rest rooms. There should be facilities for beverages and snacks. Offices are provided for the theatre supervisor and senior operating department assistants, and there should be a tutorial or seminar room for staff training. Some theatre suites incorporate an office for the anaesthetic department.

Other anaesthetising locations

The anaesthetist is often required to work in areas outside the operating theatre suite. Many hospitals have peripheral theatres for some types of surgery, e.g. a self-contained day-case unit. In addition, patients may require anaesthesia in the accident and emergency unit, the radiology and radiotherapy departments or, in some instances (e.g. paediatric oncology), the side room of a ward. In these circumstances, where conditions frequently are not ideal, it is essential that the same precautions are taken as in the operating theatre suite to ensure that the identity of the patient is checked, equipment is functioning correctly, skilled help for the anaesthetist is available and that recovery facilities and staff are satisfactory.

Ancillary staff

Skilled and dedicated help should be available to the anaesthetist at all times. In the majority of hospitals in the UK, this is provided by operating department assistants (ODAs), who undergo a 2-year training programme in recognised institutions and are required to sit examinations of the City and Guilds Institute. In some hospitals, 'anaesthetic nurses' assist the anaesthetist. It is important to differentiate between anaesthetic nurses and the nurse anaesthetists who are trained to deliver anaesthesia in some countries (e.g. CRNAs in the USA). The anaesthetic nurse performs essentially the same functions as the ODA. These include:

1. Preparation and preliminary checking of equipment. It should be stressed that this does not absolve the anaesthetist from the responsibility of checking the equipment fully before an operating list is started.
2. Alleviation of anxiety by reassurance and constant communication with the patient while awaiting anaesthesia.
3. The ODA or anaesthetic nurse is involved in checking the correct identity of the patient. However, it is the joint responsibility of the surgeon and anaesthetist to ensure that the appropriate procedure is undertaken on the correct patient, and this is one of the many reasons why the anaesthetist must see every patient preoperatively.
4. Preparation of intravenous infusions, cardiovascular monitoring transducers, etc.
5. Assistance during anaesthesia, particularly during induction, when special manoeuvres such as cricoid pressure may be required, and after transfer to the operating theatre to assist in re-establishment of monitoring.
6. Assistance in positioning the patient for local or regional blocks.
7. Assistance in obtaining drugs or equipment if complications arise during anaesthesia.
8. Assistance in the immediate postoperative period before the patient is transferred to the recovery room.

The ODA or anaesthetic nurse should never be left alone with an anaesthetised patient unless a dire emergency requires the anaesthetist's presence elsewhere.

THE MEDICOLEGAL ENVIRONMENT

The increasing volume of litigation instituted by patients in respect of alleged or actual injury arising from treatment is causing great concern within the medical profession. Insurance premiums for medical practice are escalating rapidly. Anaesthesia represents a high insurance risk, because anaesthetists manipulate the physiology of the cardiovascular and respiratory systems and administer potentially lethal drugs for reasons which are not primarily therapeutic; consequently, when a serious accident occurs, it may result in death or permanent neurological damage. In addition, even minor morbidity caused by anaesthesia or the anaesthetist may be regarded by the patient as unacceptable when it does not appear to be related to the primary illness.

Mortality associated with anaesthesia

The overwhelming majority of anaesthetics are uneventful. However, both surgery and anaesthesia carry a finite risk. Mortality is related usually to the extent of surgery and the preoperative condition of the patient (see Table 19.3). However, avoidable deaths occur. In 1982, Lunn and Mushin estimated that the risk of death attributable to anaesthesia alone was approximately 1 in 10 000. In a subsequent study of more than half a million operations (Confidential Enquiry into Perioperative Deaths; CEPOD), the overall death rate after anaesthesia and surgery was 0.7%. Anaesthesia alone was responsible for death in approximately 1 in 100 000 operations, but *contributed* to 14% of all deaths; in almost one-fifth of these deaths, avoidable errors occurred. Factors which contributed to death in these instances are listed in Table 18.2.

Table 18.2 Factors involved in deaths attributable in part to anaesthesia, in decreasing order of frequency (CEPOD report)

Failure to apply knowledge
Lack of care
Failure of organisation
Lack of experience
Lack of knowledge
Drug effect
Failure of equipment
Fatigue

Morbidity associated with anaesthesia

The incidence of major morbidity (causing permanent disability) related to anaesthesia is difficult to assess. Its causes are often similar to those associated with mortality. Table 18.3 lists the causes of death or cerebral damage reported to the Medical Defence Union between 1970 and 1982; Table 18.4 shows the detailed causes of the incidents resulting from errors in technique. Permanent disability may result also from spinal cord damage.

Other, albeit less serious, incidents may result in distress or physical injury to patients. Table 18.5 lists untoward events, other than death and cerebral damage, reported to the Medical Defence Union.

Critical incidents

These are incidents that could, or do, lead to death, permanent disability or prolongation of hospital stay. The majority of critical incidents in anaesthesia are detected before damage occurs; their incidence is 4–500 times greater than that of death attributable to anaesthesia. It has been estimated that a critical incident occurs on average once in every 80 anaesthetics. Analysis of the causes of critical incidents is valuable in indicating the potential causes of anaesthetic-related mortality and major morbidity. Human error is responsible for approximately 70% of critical incidents in anaesthesia; the commonest errors are shown in Table 18.6. Factors associated with critical incidents are shown in Table 18.7.

Minimising the risk

The most effective means of reducing the risk of an anaesthetic accident is to ensure that every aspect of anaesthetic management is conducted competently. Preoperative assessment (Ch. 19) is essential. In the anaesthetic room, the anaesthetist must check the identity of the patient before proceeding. The information contained in Tables 18.3–18.7 indicates areas of particular concern regarding intraoperative management. All anaesthetic equipment must be checked before use. The anaesthetist must understand the principles of all

Table 18.3 Causes of anaesthetic-related death or cerebral damage reported to the Medical Defence Union between 1970 and 1982

Mainly misadventure		Mainly error	
Coexisting disease	14%	Faulty technique	43%
Unknown	6%	Failure of postoperative care	9%
Drug sensitivity	5%	Drug overdosage	5%
Hypotension/blood loss	4%	Inadequate preoperative assessment	3%
Halothane-associated hepatic failure	3%	Drug error	1%
Hyperpyrexia	2%	Anaesthetist's failure	1%
Embolism	2%		

Table 18.4 Causes of anaesthetic-related death or cerebral damage reported to the Medical Defence Union and thought to be the result of errors in technique

Cause	% of total
Errors associated with tracheal intubation	31
Misuse of apparatus	23
Inhalation of gastric contents	14
Errors associated with induced hypotension	8
Hypoxia	4
Obstructed airway	4
Accidental pneumothorax/haemopericardium	4
Errors associated with extradural analgesia	3
Use of N_2O instead of O_2	2
Use of CO_2 instead of O_2	2
Errors associated with Bier's block	2
Underventilation	1
Use of halothane with adrenaline	1
Mismatched blood transfusion	<1
Vasovagal attack	<1

Table 18.5 Untoward anaesthetic-related events (other than death or cerebral damage) reported to the Medical Defence Union between 1970 and 1982

Event	% of total
Damage to teeth	52
Peripheral nerve damage	9
Extradural foreign bodies (needles, catheter tips)	7
Superficial thrombophlebitis and minor injuries (e.g. abrasions)	7
Awareness	7
Spinal cord damage	4
Pneumothoraces	3
Extravasation of injected drugs	2
Lacerations, falls from table	2
Impaired renal function (mismatched blood)	1
Burns	1
Other	5

the equipment used, especially mechanical ventilators. Drug doses must be calculated carefully and syringes labelled. After induction of anaesthesia, the correct placement of the tracheal tube must be confirmed on every occasion.

Table 18.6 Types of human error contributing to critical incidents during anaesthesia

Type of error	% of total
Wrong drug administered	24
Misuse of anaesthetic machine	22
Problem with airway management	16
Problem with breathing system	11
Fluid therapy mismanagement	5
I.v. infusion disconnection	6
Failure of monitoring	4
Others	12

Table 18.7 Associated factors producing critical incidents during anaesthesia, in decreasing order of frequency

Failure to check
First experience of procedure
Inadequate experience
Inattention/carelessness
Haste
Unfamiliarity
Visual restriction
Fatigue

Studies of critical incidents indicate that the time of highest risk is during maintenance of anaesthesia. For this reason, appropriate clinical and instrumental monitoring (see Ch. 21) must be used throughout anaesthesia. After operation, the anaesthetist is responsible for the patient until consciousness has returned and until the cardiovascular and respiratory systems are stable. He or she may be required to defend a decision to delegate the care of the patient to a nurse in the recovery room.

The following factors should be considered also:

1. *Awareness*. Patients may recall intraoperative events, and may experience pain and discomfort, if the doses or concentrations of anaesthetic drugs are insufficient (see p. 359). In high-risk groups, e.g. patients undergoing Caesarean section, it may be advisable to warn the patient of the possibility of awareness.

2. *Anaesthetic record.* A legible and comprehensive record must be made of every anaesthetic. The record should include details of preoperative findings, the doses and timing of all drugs administered during anaesthesia, frequent and regular recordings of cardiovascular and respiratory measurements, and notes regarding any untoward intraoperative event. This is an important document because it provides information which may assist other anaesthetists in the future and because a comprehensive record is *essential* in the event of medicolegal proceedings.

3. *Communication.* If a mishap occurs, failure on the part of the anaesthetist to communicate with the patient or relatives may arouse feelings of anger and suspicion. While no admission (or accusations) of liability should be made, an explanation should be offered. An interview with a patient or relatives in these circumstances requires skill and tact; the trainee should discuss the event with a consultant, and if possible, the consultant should be present at the interview. Any untoward event, or any complaint by a patient, should be reported promptly to the anaesthetist's defence society.

Each anaesthetic department should ensure that the channels of communication between trainees and consultants are clear, especially with regard to emergency procedures.

4. *Audit.* Standards of anaesthetic practice may be improved by identifying areas in which patient care has been suboptimal. Although case reports published in anaesthetic journals form a useful source of information, local meetings to discuss morbidity and mortality related to anaesthesia and surgery, together with critical incident analysis, should be convened regularly.

FURTHER READING

Aids and hepatitis B: guidelines for anaesthetists. 1988 Association of Anaesthetists of Great Britain and Ireland, London.

Buck N, Devlin H B, Lunn J N 1987 The report of a confidential enquiry into perioperative deaths. Nuffield Provincial Hospitals Trust, London

Cooper J B, Newbower R S, Kitz R J 1984 An analysis of major errors and equipment failure in anesthetic management: consideration for prevention and detection. Anesthesiology 60: 34

Drain C B, Christoph S S 1987 The recovery room, 2nd edn. W B Saunders, Philadelphia.

Hull C J 1978 Electrical hazards in the operating theatre. British Journal of Anaesthesia 50: 647

Johnston I D A, Hunter A R (eds) 1984 The design and utilization of operating theatres. Edward Arnold, London

Lunn J N, Mushin W W 1982 Mortality associated with anaesthesia. Nuffield Provincial Hospitals Trust, London

Smith G, Norman J (eds) 1987 A symposium on complications and medico-legal aspects of anaesthesia. British Journal of Anaesthesia 59: 813

Spence A A 1987 Environmental pollution by inhalation of anaesthetics. British Journal of Anaesthesia 59: 96

Taylor T H, Major E (eds) 1987 Hazards and complications of anaesthesia. Churchill Livingstone, Edinburgh

19. Preoperative assessment and premedication

Several of the large-scale epidemiological studies (e.g. the CEPOD study) have indicated that inadequate preoperative preparation of the patient may be a major contributory factor to the primary anaesthetic causes of perioperative mortality. It is therefore essential that the anaesthetist visits every patient in the ward before surgery to assess 'fitness for anaesthesia', as this function cannot be undertaken by surgical staff. Unfortunately, the anaesthetist is frequently under pressure to proceed with the planned operating theatre lists as he usually sees the patient on the ward only 1–2 days before the scheduled date for surgery, and cancellation would lead to inefficient use of operating theatre time and inconvenience for the patient. This problem may be obviated by the provision of anaesthetic outpatient assessment clinics, to which a patient is referred before an admission date is given. This allows the anaesthetist to plan optimum preparation of the patient for anaesthesia and surgery. Unfortunately, such anaesthetic assessment clinics are rare. Nevertheless, failure by the anaesthetist to perform a preoperative visit and assessment may be regarded as negligent if anaesthetic morbidity or mortality occur subsequently and therefore the anaesthetist *must* undertake a preoperative visit.

The purposes of the preoperative visit are to:

1. Establish rapport with the patient.
2. Obtain a history and perform a physical examination.
3. Order special investigations.
4. Assess the risks of anaesthesia and surgery and if necessary postpone or cancel the date of surgery.
5. Institute preoperative management.
6. Prescribe premedication and plan the anaesthetic management.

ESTABLISHMENT OF RAPPORT

The preoperative visit enables the patient to meet the doctor and discuss possible causes of anxiety regarding the anaesthetic or surgical management. The anaesthetist may explain in simple terms how the patient will be cared for during and after anaesthesia and the measures that will be taken to provide postoperative pain relief. The anaesthetist can also assure himself that the patient understands the proposed scope of surgery and that informed consent has been given for the proposed procedure.

HISTORY AND PHYSICAL EXAMINATION

Normally the patient has been clerked and examined by a house physician or house surgeon and the anaesthetist may concentrate on physiological systems of greatest relevance, e.g. the cardiovascular and respiratory systems.

Systematic evaluation of each system should be undertaken as described in most standard textbooks of medicine.

History

Direct questions should be asked about the following items of particular anaesthetic relevance:

1. A family history of hereditary conditions associated with anaesthetic problems, e.g. porphyria, malignant hyperpyrexia, hyper-

cholesterolaemia, haemophilia, cholinesterase abnormalities, dystrophia myotonica.

2. Diseases of the cardiovascular and respiratory systems are the most relevant in respect of fitness for anaesthesia. Specific questions should be addressed regarding exertional dyspnoea, paroxysmal nocturnal dyspnoea, orthopnoea, angina of effort, etc. It may be difficult to elicit a history of exertional dyspnoea if exercise is limited by arthritis, intermittent claudication, etc.

3. If relevant, enquiries should be made regarding possible pregnancy. The presence of pregnancy is a contraindication to elective surgery. In the early stages of pregnancy, anaesthetics are teratogenic (at least theoretically), but a more likely problem is the induction of spontaneous abortion. In late pregnancy, the patient presents risks of regurgitation and acid aspiration syndrome (see p. 548).

4. A history of previous anaesthesia should be sought and specific questions asked concerning drug allergy, postoperative nausea and vomiting, deep vein thrombosis or respiratory problems. If previous anaesthetic records are available, they should be inspected carefully; problems with tracheal intubation should be documented and the type of anaesthetic technique employed should be described in detail. The current recommendation of the Committee of Safety of Medicines is that halothane anaesthesia should not be repeated within 6 months of a previous halothane anaesthetic.

5. A history of allergies to drugs, plaster, rubber, etc. should be sought.

6. A history of HIV infection or jaundice, particularly viral hepatitis, has important implications for the patient and medical personnel (see p. 327).

Smoking

Deleterious effects of smoking include vascular disease of the peripheral, coronary and cerebral circulations, carcinoma of the lung and chronic bronchitis. It has been suggested recently that there are good theoretical reasons for advising all patients to cease cigarette smoking for at least 12 h prior to surgery.

The cardiovascular effects of smoking are caused by the action of nicotine on the sympathetic nervous system, producing tachycardia and hypertension. Furthermore, smoking causes an increase in coronary vascular resistance; cessation of smoking improves the symptoms of angina.

Cigarette smoke contains carbon monoxide, which converts haemoglobin to carboxyhaemoglobin. In heavy smokers, this may result in a reduction in available oxygen by as much as 25%. The half-life of carboxyhaemoglobin is short and therefore abstinence for 12 h leads to an increase in arterial oxygen content.

The effect of smoking on the respiratory tract leads to a sixfold increase in postoperative respiratory morbidity. It has been suggested that abstinence for 6 weeks results in reduced bronchoconstriction and mucus secretion in the tracheobronchial tree.

Alcohol

Regular alcohol intake leads to induction of liver enzymes and tolerance to anaesthetic drugs. Excessive alcohol intake causes both hepatic and cardiac damage. Delirium tremens may occur in alcoholics during the postoperative recovery phase as a result of withdrawal of the drug.

Drug history

It is essential that a complete history is obtained regarding concurrent medication. Many drugs interact with agents employed by the anaesthetist; the most important interactions are listed in Table 19.1.

In general terms, administration of most drugs should be continued up to and including the morning of operation, although some adjustment in dosage may be required (e.g. antihypertensives, insulin). Knowledge of the pharmacology of drug therapy is essential to permit the anaesthetist to adjust the dosage of anaesthetic agents appropriately and to avoid possibly dangerous interactions.

Some drugs should be discontinued preoperatively. The monoamine oxidase inhibitors should be withdrawn 2–3 weeks before surgery because of the risk of interactions with drugs used during anaesthesia; psychiatric advice may be required for the prescription of alternative antidepressant therapy. The oral contraceptive pill should be discontinued at least 6 weeks before elective

Table 19.1 Drug interactions in anaesthesia

Drug	Problems and interactions	Recommendations
Alcohol	*Acute intoxication* Effects of sedatives, opioids and anaesthetics enhanced *Chronic alcoholism* Tolerance to effect of these drugs as a result of enzyme induction	Continue with reduced dosage anaesthetic drugs Increased dosage usually required
Adrenaline	Arrhythmias with volatile anaesthetic agents halothane > enflurane > isoflurane	Do not exceed 1 μg/kg of adrenaline in the presence of halothane
Antibiotics (streptomycin, kanamycin, neomycin, polymyxin, bacitracin, colistin)	Some of these agents may produce neuromuscular block alone, and prolong the block produced by muscle relaxant	Caution using relaxant drugs. Monitor neuromuscular transmission May be antagonised with Ca^{2+}
Anticoagulants	Bleeding from nasotracheal intubation, i.m. injections and local anaesthetic injections Surgical haemorrhage	Avoid i.m. injections Control anticoagulant therapy as described on page 132 Avoid subarachnoid/extradural blocks
Anticholinesterases (ecothiopate eye drops, organophosphorus insecticides)	Inhibition of plasma cholinesterase causes potentiation of suxamethonium and antagonism of curare	Avoid suxamethonium
Anticonvulsants phenytoin phenobarbitone carbamazepine	All these drugs induce liver enzymes	May increase requirements for sedative/anaesthetic agents Avoid enflurane
Antihypertensives reserpine methyldopa guanethidine clonidine	Reserpine depletes noradrenaline stores	Hypotension with all anaesthetic agents, so reduce dosage. Clonidine may allow reduction in dosage of anaesthetics. Action of sympathomimetics increased by guanethidine
Antimitotic drugs cyclophosphamide thiotepa	Inhibit plasma cholinesterase	Caution with suxamethonium
β-Blockers — propranolol oxprenolol metoprolol atenolol, etc. timolol eyedrops — may be absorbed systemically	Negative inotropic effects additive with anaesthetic agents to cause exaggerated hypotension. Mask compensatory tachycardia	Monitor β-blockade therapy in perioperative period. Caution with dosage of all CVS-depressant drugs
Barbiturates	Long-term dosage induces liver enzymes and increases metabolism of many drugs	May need to increase dosage of induction agent and opioids
Benzodiazepines	Additive effect with many CNS-depressant drugs Additive effect with competitive muscle relaxants	Caution with induction agents and opioids. Curare potentiated. Suxamethonium antagonised
Ca^{2+} channel blockers		
verapamil	Depresses AV conduction and excitability. Interacts with volatile anaesthetic agents — bradyarrhythmias and decreased cardiac output	Caution with dosage of volatile anaesthetic agents
nifedipine diltiazem	Vasodilators and negative inotropes interact with volatile agents to produce hypotension. May augment action of competitive muscle relaxants	

Table 19.1 (Cont'd)

Drug	Problems and interactions	Recommendations
Contraceptive pill	Increased incidence of DVT. This risk does not exist with progesterone-only tablets	Discontinue o.c. for at least 6 weeks and cover with alternative contraceptive methods. Use low-dose heparin therapy if surgery is urgent and o.c. cannot be stopped.
Digoxin	Arrhythmias enhanced by calcium. Toxicity enhanced by hypokalaemia. Suxamethonium enhances toxicity. Danger of bradycardia	Avoid calcium. Check serum K^+. Caution in use of suxamethonium
Diuretics	May cause hypokalaemia which prolongs competitive neuromuscular block	Check K^+
Insulins	Hypoglycaemia augmented by subarachnoid and extradural anaesthesia and β-blocking drugs	Further recommendations given on page 668
Monoamine oxidase inhibitors (MAOI) phenelzine iproniazid tranylcypromine isocarboxazide	React with opioids — coma, twitching, CNS excitement → trauma. Severe hypertensive response to pressor agents	Adverse effects do not occur in all patients. Probably safest to withdraw drugs (takes 2–3 weeks) and utilise alternative antidepressants
Lithium	Potentiates non-depolarising relaxants	Discontinue 48–72 h before anaesthesia
L-Dopa	Risks of tachycardia and arrhythmias with halothane. Actions antagonised by droperidol. Augments hyperglycaemia in diabetes	Discontinue on day of operation
Magnesium	Potentiation of muscle relaxants	Caution with dosage
Phenothiazines	Interact with other hypotensive agents	Caution with dosage of all agents affecting CVS
Quinidine	I.v. quinidine may cause neuromuscular block, especially after suxamethonium	Caution with muscle relaxants
Steroids	Possible hypotension unless increased steroid cover is given	Avoid sympathomimetic amines because of danger of pressor responses
Sulphonamides	Potentiation of thiopentone	
Tricyclic antidepressants	Inhibit the metabolism of catecholamines → arrhythmias. Imipramine potentiates the CVS effects of adrenaline	

surgery because of the increased risk of venous thrombosis.

Physical examination

A full physical examination should be undertaken *and documented in the case records*. The examination should include all systems, even if not directly relevant to the operation. Even in an otherwise healthy individual presenting for relatively minor surgery, it is important to document the findings of full physical examination in case unexpected morbidity arises postoperatively, e.g. foot drop as a result of incorrect positioning on the operating theatre table, prolonged sensory anaesthesia following local anaesthetic techniques, etc.

In addition, the anaesthetist pays particular attention to assessment of the ease of tracheal intubation. The teeth should be inspected closely for the presence of caries, caps, loose teeth and particularly protruding upper incisors. The extent of mouth opening is assessed together with the degree of flexion of the cervical spine and extension of the atlanto-occipital joint. Features associated with difficulty in performing tracheal intubation are described on page 408.

SPECIAL INVESTIGATIONS

It is generally accepted that the clinical history and physical examination represent the best method of screening for the presence of disease. Routine laboratory tests in patients who are apparently healthy on clinical examination and history are invariably of little use and a waste of resources. Before ordering extensive investigations, the anaesthetist should ask himself the following questions:

1. Will this investigation yield information not revealed by physical examination?
2. Will the results of the investigation alter the management of the patient?

In order to reduce the volume of routine preoperative investigations, the following suggestions are made. It should be noted that these are guidelines only and should be modified according to the assessment obtained from the history and clinical examination.

Urine analysis

This should be performed on every patient. It is normally very inexpensive and may occasionally reveal an undiagnosed diabetic or the presence of urinary tract infection.

Haemoglobin concentration

Haemoglobin concentration should be measured in the following situations:

1. Males over 50 years of age.
2. All females.
3. Before major surgery.
4. When clinically indicated, e.g. history of blood loss, pallor, etc.
5. All Asian patients.

Urea and electrolyte concentrations

Serum urea and electrolyte concentrations are not required routinely in patients less than 50 years of age, but should be obtained in the following situations:

1. If there is a history of diarrhoea, vomiting or metabolic disease.
2. In the presence of renal or hepatic disease, diabetes or an abnormal nutritional state.
3. In patients receiving medication with diuretics, digoxin, antihypertensives, steroids or hypoglycaemic agents.

It is important to appreciate that patients who receive preoperative bowel preparation for colonic or rectal surgery may become dehydrated; intravenous fluid replacement may be required and electrolyte status should be monitored carefully.

Liver function tests

Liver function tests are required only in patients with:

1. Hepatic disease.
2. Abnormal nutritional state or metabolic disease.
3. A history of large intake of alcohol (>80 g/day).

Chest X-ray

A chest X-ray is not required routinely in patients below 60 years of age but should be obtained in the following situations:

1. If there is a history or physical signs of cardiac or respiratory disease.
2. If there may be metastases from carcinoma.
3. Before thoracic surgery.
4. In recent immigrants (who have not had a chest X-ray within the previous 12 months) from countries where tuberculosis is endemic.

Other X-rays

Cervical spine X-rays are required in all patients in whom there is anticipated difficulty with tracheal intubation, e.g. in the presence of rheumatoid arthritis. Thoracic inlet X-rays are required in patients with thyroid enlargement.

ECG

A 12-lead electrocardiogram should be obtained in the following situations:

1. If there is a history or physical signs of cardiac disease.
2. In the presence of hypertension.
3. In all patients over the age of 50 years.

Blood sugar concentration

Blood sugar measurement is required in patients receiving corticosteroid drugs and in those who have diabetes or vascular disease.

Sickle status

Patients whose ethnic origin or family history suggests that a haemoglobinopathy may be present should have haemoglobin concentration measured and haemoglobin electrophoresis undertaken. If such patients are scheduled for emergency surgery, a Sickledex test should be performed; if this is positive, haemoglobin electrophoresis should be undertaken as soon as possible but should not delay emergency surgery.

Pulmonary function tests

Peak expiratory flow rate, forced vital capacity and $FEV_{1.0}$ should be measured in all patients with severe dyspnoea on mild to moderate exertion.

Blood gas analysis

Arterial blood gas analysis is required in all patients with dyspnoea at rest and in patients scheduled for elective thoracotomy.

Coagulation tests

Coagulation tests (PTTK and INR) are required in patients who give a history of bleeding disorders, in patients receiving anticoagulant therapy and in those with liver disease.

RISK ASSESSMENT

Preoperative assessment of risk should embrace two broad questions:

1. Is the patient in optimum physical condition for anaesthesia?
2. Are the anticipated benefits of surgery greater than the anaesthetic and surgical risks produced by concurrent medical disease?

In principle, if there is any medical condition which may be improved, (e.g. pulmonary disease, hypertension, cardiac failure, chronic bronchitis, renal disease), surgery should be postponed and appropriate therapy instituted.

There has been great interest recently in quantifying factors preoperatively which correlate with the development of postoperative morbidity and mortality. Some accuracy is possible for populations of patients, but precision does not extend to accurate prediction of risk for an individual patient. Frequently, the decision to proceed can be made only by discussion between surgeon and anaesthetist.

Over a broad range of surgery and patient age, the overall mortality rate from surgery is of the order of 0.6%. This is many times greater than the overall mortality rate attributable to anaesthesia *per se* (approximately 1 in 10 000).

In many large-scale studies of mortality, common factors which have emerged as contributing to anaesthetic mortality include inadequate assessment of patients in the preoperative period, inadequate supervision and monitoring in the intraoperative period and inadequate postoperative supervision and management.

ASA grading

The ASA grading system (Table 19.2) was introduced originally as a simple description of the

Table 19.2 The ASA Physical Status Scale

Class I	A normally healthy individual
Class II	A patient with mild systemic disease
Class III	A patient with severe systemic disease that is not incapacitating
Class IV	A patient with incapacitating systemic disease that is a constant threat to life
Class V	A moribund patient who is not expected to survive 24 h with or without operation
Class E	Added as a suffix for emergency operation.

Table 19.3 Mortality rates after anaesthesia and surgery for each ASA physical status — emergency and elective cases

ASA rating	Mortality rate (%)
I	0.1
II	0.2
III	1.8
IV	7.8
V	9.4

physical state of a patient. Despite its apparent simplicity, it remains one of the few prospective descriptions of the patient which correlate with the risk of anaesthesia and surgery (Table 19.3). However, it does not embrace all aspects of anaesthetic risk, as there is no allowance for inclusion of many criteria such as age or difficulty in intubation. Nevertheless, it is extremely useful and should be applied to all patients who present for surgery.

Cardiovascular disease

Myocardial infarction

A large number of studies undertaken retrospectively in the 1970s demonstrated that the incidence of perioperative myocardial infarction (MI) was 0.1–0.4% in previously healthy patients, but 3.2–7.7% in patients who had suffered a previous MI. The majority of perioperative infarctions occur on the third day after surgery, and 50% are silent. The mortality associated with perioperative MI is 40–60%.

It is accepted generally that the development of perioperative reinfarction is related closely to the time interval between the first MI and surgery, and that an interval of 6 months or less is associated with the highest incidence of reinfarction. However, two recent studies have suggested that the rate of reinfarction and also cardiac death in patients with recent MI may be reduced greatly if patients are subjected to intensive invasive monitoring (radial artery cannulation and pulmonary artery catheterisation) and if heart rate and systemic arterial pressure are not allowed to fluctuate by more than 20% from preoperative values. In these studies, arrhythmias and tachycardia were treated immediately, and monitoring and treatment were continued in the ITU for 3–4 days after surgery. Unfortunately, it is not possible to monitor all patients for such a prolonged period of time in ITU and there are no data to identify which subgroup of patients requires more extensive monitoring or treatment than others. Consequently, it is still recommended that a myocardial infarction within 6 months of proposed surgery is a contraindication to elective anaesthesia and surgery, unless the risks of postponing surgery outweigh the likelihood of perioperative infarction.

Hypertension

There is some dispute as to whether or not arterial hypertension increases the risk of morbidity after anaesthesia and surgery. Arterial pressure increases with age, and on admission to the ward there is often some degree of hypertension associated with anxiety. The arterial pressure should therefore be measured at regular intervals in the preoperative period in order to assess the resting baseline level. The question then arises as to what constitutes hypertension. It is difficult to be precise on this point, but a number of authorities have formed the view that a diastolic pressure in excess of 110 mmHg is associated with an increased risk of myocardial ischaemia.

Gross hypertensive responses, with ECG evidence of ischaemia on some occasions, are likely to occur in response to noxious stimuli during anaesthesia in hypertensive patients, whether treated or not, if the preoperative diastolic pressure exceeds 110 mmHg. Episodes of marked hypertension, ischaemic ST changes on ECG and the combination of hypotension and tachycardia are associated with an increased incidence of postoperative myocardial infarction. It follows that patients should be prepared for surgery in such a way that these changes are less likely to occur. Thus, patients who present preoperatively with a diastolic arterial pressure in excess of 110 mmHg should receive antihypertensive treatment. As several days or weeks may be required to stabilise the cardiovascular system, surgery should be postponed for 2–3 weeks.

Multifactorial assessment of risk

Goldman and his colleagues have examined by multivariate analysis a number of risk factors in patients undergoing non-cardiac surgery and produced a risk index (Table 19.4) for the development of life-threatening cardiovascular complications in the perioperative period. The 'Goldman Cardiac Risk Index' has been shown in several studies to provide a reasonable prognostic indication of the risk of developing cardiac complications postoperatively.

Table 19.4 Goldman's index of cardiac risk in non-cardiac procedures

Risk factor	Points
3rd heart sound or jugular venous distension	11
MI in preceding 6 months	10
Rhythm other than sinus or premature atrial contractions	7
Abdominal, thoracic, or aortic operation	3
Age > 70 years	5
Important aortic stenosis	3
Emergency operation	4
Poor condition as defined by any one of:	3
Pa_{O_2} < 8 kPa Pa_{CO_2} > 6.5 kPa K^+ < 3.0 mmol/litre HCO_3^- < 20 mmol/litre urea >7.5 mmol/litre creatinine >270 μmol/litre SGOT abnormal chronic liver disease	

5 points or less— cardiac mortality 0.2%.
6–25 points — cardiac mortality 2%.
> 25 points — cardiac mortality 56%.

Pulmonary disease

Patients at risk of developing postoperative pulmonary complications include smokers, those with pre-existing lung disease, the obese, and those undergoing thoracic and abdominal surgery.

Unfortunately, sophisticated tests of pulmonary function (e.g. FRC, closing capacity, pulmonary diffusing capacity, etc.) are no more valuable in assessment of lung disease than simple spirometric tests, particularly vital capacity, forced vital capacity and $FEV_{1.0}$. Blood gas analysis is the most sensitive method of predicting the need for IPPV in the postoperative period.

Age

It is generally agreed that the elderly are subject to increased risks of anaesthesia and surgery. This is largely because of the association between many diseases of the cardiovascular or respiratory systems and age, and also because routine clinical evaluation often fails to detect cardiorespiratory dysfunction in geriatric patients.

Prediction of risk factors in general

Factors which are of greatest importance in predicting the development of postoperative morbidity and mortality include, in decreasing order of importance:

1. Clinical assessment — ASA greater than 3.
2. Cardiac failure.
3. Cardiac risk index.
4. Pulmonary disease.
5. Pulmonary abnormalities confirmed by X-ray.
6. ECG abnormalities.

Common causes for postponing surgery

1. *Acute upper respiratory tract infection* (common cold). Although many patients may admit to the presence of a cold, clarification of such an admission should be made. In general, the presence of nasal secretions, pyrexia or the unexpected presence of physical signs on clinical examination of the chest suggest that surgery should be post-

poned for a few weeks until the patient has recovered.

2. *Existing medical disease* (cardiac, respiratory, endocrine, etc.), which is not under optimum control (see Ch. 41).

3. *Emergency surgery for which the patient has not been resuscitated adequately*. Postponement may be necessary for only 1–2 h to permit restoration of circulating blood volume. This important principle may be breached if haemorrhage is extensive and continuous.

4. *Recent ingestion of food*. In general, anaesthesia for elective surgery should not be undertaken within 4–6 h of ingestion of food or liquids.

5. *Failure to obtain informed consent*. Informed consent for surgery should be obtained from all patients. Consent is invalid if obtained after the patient has received premedicant drugs. Consent from a parent or guardian is required if the patient is under 16 years of age in England or Wales, or under 14 years of age in Scotland. If parents or guardians cannot be contacted, consent may be obtained from a court of law or, in the case of emergency surgery, from a District Medical Officer.

6. *Drug therapy*. It is unwise to proceed to anaesthesia if the patient is receiving drug therapy which is not under optimum control.

PREOPERATIVE THERAPY

Having taken a full clinical history and performed a physical examination, reviewed the special investigations and decided that it is reasonable to proceed to anaesthesia and surgery, the anaesthetist should decide if further measures are required to prepare the patient satisfactorily. Some common problems are detailed below.

Respiratory disease

In patients with respiratory disease who are regarded as fit for surgery, chest physiotherapy should be started preoperatively. In addition, sputum should be obtained for bacteriological examination and culture to determine optimum antibiotic therapy in the event of postoperative chest infection.

Asthma

Chest physiotherapy should be started preoperatively. If severe asthma is present, instruction may be required in the use of appropriate bronchodilators, e.g. salbutamol by inhaler.

Cardiovascular disease

Subacute bacterial endocarditis

For those at risk of developing subacute bacterial endocarditis, prophylactic antibiotics are required, as described in Appendix IVd (p. 733).

Hypertension

In patients who are found to be hypertensive on admission, regular measurement of arterial pressure should be undertaken. Frequently, pressure declines as the initial anxiety of admission becomes attenuated. If the diastolic pressure decreases below 110 mmHg, it is reasonable to proceed with surgery. If diastolic pressure remains above 110 mmHg, surgery should be postponed and the patient referred to a physician. If the patient is a known hypertensive receiving therapy, adjustment of the dosage of antihypertensives may be required.

It is essential that antihypertensive therapy be continued throughout the postoperative period. Many β-blocking drugs have a relatively short half-life, and if a patient is receiving such therapy it may be preferable to change to a drug with a long duration of action, such as atenolol or nadolol. If bowel function is likely to remain disturbed for several days postoperatively, it may be necessary to use an i.v. infusion of atenolol 2–6 mg/h or labetalol 2.5–10 mg/h.

Diabetic management

See page 668.

Obstructive jaundice

This is associated with the hepatorenal syndrome and bleeding problems. To minimise the risk of renal failure, an i.v. infusion should be started on the night before surgery. Glucose 5% should be infused at a rate of 100 ml/h. In addition, mannitol 20 g should be given just before or at induction of anaesthesia. Vitamin K may be prescribed in a dose of 10 mg i.m. daily preoperatively, and postoperatively for 3 days.

Blood transfusion requests

Blood is an expensive commodity and blood transfusion carries very small but finite risks of incompatibility reactions and transmission of infection. Blood should therefore be used only if absolutely necessary. The object of transfusion is to ensure that the postoperative haemoglobin concentration does not decline to less than 10 g/dl. Thus the amount of blood ordered from the blood transfusion service depends upon both the patient's preoperative haemoglobin concentration and the extent of surgery.

Guidelines on the quantity of blood to request from the blood transfusion service are shown in Table 19.5.

PREMEDICATION

Premedication refers to the administration of drugs in the period 1–2 h before induction of anaesthesia. The objectives of premedication are to:

1. Allay anxiety and fear.
2. Reduce secretions.
3. Enhance the hypnotic effect of general anaesthetic agents.
4. Reduce postoperative nausea and vomiting.
5. Produce amnesia.
6. Reduce the volume and increase the pH of gastric contents.
7. Attenuate vagal reflexes.
8. Attenuate sympathoadrenal responses.

Relief from anxiety

Surgical patients have a high incidence of anxiety and there is a significant inverse relationship between anxiety and smoothness of induction of anaesthesia. Relief from anxiety is accomplished most effectively by non-pharmacological means, which may be termed psychotherapy. This is

Table 19.5 Guidelines for ordering blood for routine surgery

Group and screen only
- Amputation
- Bladder tumour: transurethral resection
- Cervical rib and thoracic inlet exploration
- Cholecystectomy and exploration of bile duct
- Colostomy, gastrostomy: closure or formation of
- Cone biopsy of cervix
- Embolectomy
- Femoral nail: removal of
- Glossectomy
- Hysterectomy
- Laminectomy
- Laparoscopy
- Laparotomy: planned exploratory
- Mastectomy: simple
- Mastoidectomy
- Mediastinoscopy
- Osteotomy: bone biospy
- Ovary: wedge resection
- Pacemaker: insertion of
- Palate: resection of
- Parathyroidectomy
- Pinning of long bone (planned)
- Prostatectomy: transurethral
- Salivary gland: dissection of
- Splenectomy
- Sympathectomy: abdominal
- Tonsillectomy
- Tracheostomy
- Tubal (Fallopian) surgery
- Ureters: reimplantation
- Vagotomy and pyloroplasty

Group, screen and cross-match one unit of blood
- Carotid or femoral endarterectomy
- Ovarian cystectomy
- Pinning fractured neck of femur

Group, screen and cross-match two units of blood
- Abdominoperineal resection
- Arthroplasty knee/shoulder
- Atrioventricular septal defect
- Brachial plexus repair
- Fallot's tetralogy (depends on age)
- Laryngectomy
- Mastectomy: radical
- Maxillectomy
- Myomectomy
- Nephrectomy or graft nephrectomy
- Ovarian carcinoma
- Patent ductus arteriosus
- Prostatectomy: suprapubic
- Pyelolithotomy: 1st operation
- Renal transplantation
- Spinal fusion
- Thoracotomy: pneumonectomy
  wedge resection
- Total or hemicolectomy or anterior resection of rectum

Group, screen and cross-match three units of blood
- Adrenalectomy
- Femoropopliteal bypass
- Gastrectomy: partial

Table 19.5 (Cont'd)

Hip: arthroplasty
Hysterectomy: Wertheim
Pulmonary valvulotomy
Group, screen and cross-match four units of blood
Aorto-iliac or aortofemoral bypass
Commando operation
Coronary vein graft
Gastrectomy: total
Hip prosthesis: change of
Mitral commissurotomy
Pancreatectomy: partial
Pyelolithotomy: repeat operations
Group, screen and cross-match six units of blood
Coronary vein grafts: repeat operations
Oesophagectomy
Pancreatectomy: total
Partial hepatectomy
Radical cystectomy
Valve replacement: single
Ventricular aneurysm
Group, screen and cross-match eight units of blood
Aortic aneurysm: abdominal
Aortic aneurysm: thoracic
Valve replacement: double
Vein graft and valve replacement

effected at the preoperative visit by establishment of rapport, explanation of events which occur in the perioperative period and reassurance regarding the patient's expressed anxieties and fears. There is good evidence that psychotherapy has a significant calming effect.

In some patients, reassurance and explanation may be insufficient to allay anxiety. Thus it is customary and traditional to prescribe anxiolytic medication; the benzodiazepine drugs are the most effective for this purpose.

Reduction in secretions

The older anaesthetic agents, ether and cyclopropane, stimulate the production of secretions from pharyngeal and bronchial glands. This effect occurs only to a minor degree with modern anaesthetic agents and so anticholinergic premedication is not essential. However, many anaesthetists continue to prescribe anticholinergic drugs to reduce the secretions produced by the presence of an airway or tracheal tube in the mouth and larynx.

Ketamine tends to promote secretions and an anticholinergic premedication should be prescribed before using this agent.

Sedation

Sedation is not synonymous with anxiolysis. Some drugs, e.g. the barbiturates and to a lesser extent the opioids, possess sedative but no anxiolytic properties. In general, it is unnecessary to use a sedative preoperatively unless the patient expresses a preference for this. An exception to this may be in paediatric practice.

Postoperative antiemesis

Nausea and vomiting are extremely common after anaesthesia. Opioid drugs administered during and after operation are often responsible. Occasionally, antiemetics may be given with the premedication, but they are more effective if administered intravenously during anaesthesia.

Amnesia

Under some circumstances it may be desirable for patients, especially children, to be amnesic for the immediate perioperative period in case unpleasant memories cause difficulties if subsequent operations are required. However, some anaesthetists believe that amnesia should not be induced in children, otherwise they may associate natural sleep with awakening to find a surgical incision.

Although claims have been made for retrograde amnesia, it is unlikely that this is ever achieved. However, anterograde amnesia (after administration of a drug) is produced commonly by the benzodiazepines; in this respect, lorazepam is two to five times more potent than diazepam. It is totally inappropriate to prescribe an amnesic drug with the object of reducing the risks of awareness during anaesthesia.

Reduction in gastric volume and elevation of gastric pH

In patients who are at risk of vomiting or regurgitation (e.g. emergency patients with a full stomach or elective patients with hiatus hernia or pharyngeal pouch), it may be desirable to promote gastric emptying and elevate the pH of residual gastric contents. Gastric emptying may be enhanced by the administration of metoclopramide, which also possesses some antiemetic properties, whilst elevation of the volume of gastric contents may be produced by administration of sodium citrate. This topic is described in greater detail in Chapter 14.

Reduction in vagal reflexes

Vagal bradycardia, which may be severe, may occur in several situations:

1. Traction on the eye muscles, particularly the rectus medialis during squint surgery, leads to bradycardia and/or arrhythmias (the oculocardiac reflex). Premedication with atropine protects against this, but it is not as effective as the i.v. administration of atropine at induction of anaesthesia or in anticipation of traction on the muscles.
2. Repeated administration of suxamethonium commonly gives rise to bradycardia, which may proceed to asystole. Administration of atropine should always precede the administration of a second dose of suxamethonium.
3. Induction of anaesthesia with halothane, particularly in children, may be associated with bradycardia.
4. Surgical stimulation during an opioid/relaxant technique employing one of the newer muscle relaxants (atracurium or vecuronium) may be associated with bradycardia.

Limitation of sympathoadrenal responses

Induction of anaesthesia and tracheal intubation may be associated with marked sympathoadrenal activity, manifest by tachycardia, hypertension and elevation of plasma catecholamine concentrations. These responses are undesirable in the healthy individual and may be harmful in patients with hypertension or ischaemic heart disease. β-Blockings drugs are sometimes given with the premedication in order to attenuate these responses.

Some of the objectives listed above may be achieved by administration of drugs at induction or during maintenance of anaesthesia. The only essential requirement of premedication in the period before anaesthesia is anxiolysis. The ability to achieve all objectives by administration of a variety of drugs either preoperatively or at induction is responsible for the wide variation in prescribing habits amongst anaesthetists. The commonest regimens used for premedication are shown in Table 19.6.

Drugs used for premedication

Benzodiazepines

The benzodiazepines possess several properties which are useful for premedication, including anxiolysis, sedation and amnesia. The extent of each of these effects differs among individual drugs. Lorazepam produces a greater degree of

Table 19.6 Common premedication regimens (doses are suitable only for healthy adult male)

Drug (combination)	Dose (mg)	Route of administration	Comments
Papaveretum Hyoscine	20 0.4	i.m. i.m.	Profound sedation. 'Omnopon & scopolamine' still very commonly used combination.
Diazepam	10–15	oral	Good anxiolysis but effect variable
Lorazepam	2–3	oral	Marked anterograde amnesia. Prolonged action
Diazepam Metoclopramide	10 10	oral oral	Metoclopramide increases the tone of the lower oesophageal sphincter and possesses antiemetic effect
Morphine Atropine	10 0.6	i.m. i.m.	Frequently used when less profound sedation is required than 'Omnopon & scopolamine'
Promethazine Atropine	50 0.6	i.m. i.m.	Frequently prescribed for asthmatic patients

amnesia than diazepam. In addition, diazepam and lorazepam may produce anxiolysis in doses that do not produce excessive sedation. The drugs are thought to increase brain receptor sensitivity to γ-aminobutyric acid (GABA).

Absorption of diazepam after i.m. administration is relatively poor; absorption from the gastrointestinal tract is more reliable. This accounts for the popularity of the oral route for administration of diazepam. In contrast, lorazepam is absorbed equally well after i.m. or oral administration. Standard preparations of diazepam should not be given by the i.v. route because of the high incidence of thrombophlebitis; the incidence is reduced substantially if diazepam is administered in a lipid emulsion (Diazemuls).

In patients who are particularly anxious, it is common practice to prescribe a benzodiazepine as a hypnotic on the night before operation and to employ the same drug for premedication the following morning.

Cimetidine delays the plasma clearance of diazepam but not lorazepam.

Unfortunately, there is a very wide variation in response to benzodiazepines and effects may be unpredictable. Although physostigmine has been used in the past to reverse excessive sedation produced by benzodiazepines, a specific antagonist (flumazenil) is now available.

Opioid analgesics

It is necessary to prescribe opioid analgesic drugs for premedication only when patients are in pain preoperatively. This is uncommon except in the emergency situation; nevertheless, opioid drugs are employed commonly for premedication.

The opioids cause sedation, but are not good anxiolytic agents. Although they produce euphoria in the presence of pain, they tend to cause dysphoria in its absence. Because of their long duration of action, they contribute to a smoother intraoperative course and provide some analgesia in the early postoperative period. Tachypnoea, which occurs during spontaneous breathing of volatile agents, is reduced, and a lower concentration of anaesthetic agent is required for maintenance of anaesthesia. However, it is more logical in many respects to administer opioids intravenously at or after induction of anaesthesia rather than intramuscularly for premedication.

There are several important side effects of the opioids:

1. Depression of ventilation and delayed resumption of spontaneous ventilation at the end of N_2O/O_2-relaxant techniques.
2. Nausea and vomiting produced by stimulation of the chemoreceptor trigger zone in the medulla are extremely common. Opioids should always be used in combination with an antiemetic agent, such as hyoscine, a phenothiazine or a butyrophenone.
3. Morphine causes spasm of the sphincter of Oddi and this may result in right upper quadrant pain, particularly in patients presenting for surgery on the biliary tract.
4. Morphine causes histamine release and is generally regarded as contraindicated in asthmatics.

Butyrophenones

Of the two butyrophenones, haloperidol and droperidol, only the latter enjoys current popularity in anaesthetic practice. This drug possesses neuroleptic effects (which may be manifest as withdrawal and seclusion), α-blocking actions and antiemetic effects. Occasionally, droperidol may produce dose-dependent dysphoric reactions and extrapyramidal side effects.

Butyrophenones possess a very long duration of action and this may delay recovery from anaesthesia, particularly in elderly patients. The commonest use for droperidol in anaesthetic practice is as an antiemetic agent, administered either with the premedication in a dose of 2.5 mg or intravenously during anaesthesia in a dose of 1.25 mg.

Phenothiazines

These are useful agents for premedication because they produce the following effects:

1. Central antiemetic action.
2. Sedation.
3. Anxiolysis.
4. H_2-receptor antagonism.
5. α-Adrenergic antagonism.

6. Anticholinergic properties.
7. Potentiation of opioid analgesia.

Disadvantages include extrapyramidal side effects, synergism with opioids which may delay postoperative recovery and potentiation of the hypotensive effects of anaesthetic agents. Postoperatively (particularly in children given trimeprazine) the patient may exhibit pallor with mild tachycardia and hypotension, mimicking the signs of hypovolaemia.

Anticholinergic agents

The three anticholinergic agents used commonly in anaesthesia are atropine, hyoscine and glycopyrronium. Atropine and hyoscine are tertiary amines that cross the blood–brain barrier; pyrronium is a quarternary amine, does not cross the blood–brain barrier and is not absorbed from the gastrointestinal tract. Although atropine is absorbed from the gastrointestinal tract, this occurs in an unpredictable manner and is dependent upon gastric content, pH and motility.

These three drugs differ with respect to their dose–response effects at various cholinergic receptors. In standard clinical doses, hyoscine 0.4 mg differs from atropine 0.6 mg in that there is greater antisialagogue effect and little action on cardiac vagal receptors. Hyoscine possesses sedative and amnesic actions and in contrast to atropine does not cause stimulation of higher centres. Hyoscine should be avoided in the elderly (over 60 years) as it produces dysphoria and restlessness. Glycopyrronium has no central effects, a much longer duration of action and in a standard clinical dose of 0.4 mg causes less change in heart rate than atropine 0.6 mg.

Anticholinergic drugs are used clinically to produce:

1. *Antisialagogue effects*. Glycopyrronium and hyoscine are more potent in this respect than atropine. These drugs block secretions when irritant anaesthetic gases are used and reduce excessive secretions and bradycardia associated with suxamethonium when it is given either repeatedly or as an infusion.
2. *Sedative and amnesic effects*. In combination with morphine, hyoscine produces powerful sedative and amnesic effects.
3. *Prevention of reflex bradycardia*. Anticholinergics are given for both prophylaxis and treatment of bradycardia. Atropine is used very commonly as premedication in ophthalmic surgery to block the oculocardiac reflex in patients undergoing squint surgery, and is used also in small children to reduce the bradycardia which may occur in association with halothane anaesthesia.

Side effects of anticholinergic drugs include:

1. *CNS toxicity*. The *central anticholinergic syndrome* is produced by stimulation of the CNS (usually by atropine). Symptoms include restlessness, agitation and somnolence and in extreme cases convulsions and coma. With hyoscine there is more commonly prolonged somnolence. Physostigmine 1–2 mg i.v. has been recommended to reverse the central anticholinergic syndrome and should be given in combination with glycopyrronium to prevent profound muscarinic effects produced by physostigmine.
2. *Reduction in lower oesophageal sphincter tone*. Theoretically, a reduction in tone may lead to increased risk of gastro-oesophageal reflux, although in clinical practice there is no suggestion that the use of anticholinergics for premedication is associated with an increased incidence of preoperative aspiration.
3. *Tachycardia*, which should be avoided in cardiac conditions, (e.g. obstructive cardiomyopathy, valvular stenosis and ischaemic heart disease) or when a hypotensive anaesthetic technique is planned.
4. *Mydriasis and cycloplegia*, which lead to visual impairment. This may be troublesome, but is not a serious side effect. Theoretically, mydriasis may be associated with reduced drainage of aqueous from the anterior chamber of the eye, thereby increasing intraocular pressure in patients with glaucoma. However, this effect is not important in practice, and atropine may be prescribed safely to patients with glaucoma provided that appropriate therapy is maintained.
5. *Pyrexia*. By suppressing secretion of sweat,

anticholinergics predispose to elevation in body temperature. These drugs should therefore be avoided in the presence of pyrexia, particularly in children.

6. *Excessive drying.* Although anticholinergics are given for the specific purpose of producing antisialagogue effects, this may be most unpleasant for the patient.

7. *Increased physiological deadspace.* Atropine and hyoscine increase physiological deadspace by 20–25% but this is compensated for by an increase in ventilation.

FURTHER READING

Buck N, Devlin H B, Lunn J N 1987 The report of a confidential enquiry into perioperative deaths (CEPOD). Nuffield Provincial Hospitals Trust, London

Derrington M C, Smith G 1987 A review of studies of anaesthetic risk, morbidity and mortality. British Journal of Anaesthesia 59: 815

Goldman L, Caldera D L, Southwick F S et al 1977 Multifactorial index of cardiac risk in non-cardiac surgical procedures. New England Journal of Medicine 297: 845

Vacanti C J, van Houten R J, Hill R C 1970 A statistical analysis of the relationship of physical status to postoperative mortality in 68 388 cases. Anesthesia and Analgesia 49: 564

20. The practical conduct of anaesthesia

Planning the conduct of anaesthesia starts normally after details concerning the surgical procedure and the medical condition of the patient have been ascertained at the preoperative visit. Preoperative assessment and selection of appropriate premedication are discussed in Chapter 19.

PREPARATION FOR ANAESTHESIA

Before embarking on the anaesthetic, consideration should be given to the induction and maintenance of anaesthesia, the position of the patient on the operating table, equipment necessary for monitoring, the use of intravenous fluids or blood for infusion, and the postoperative care and recovery facilities which will be required.

Table 20.1 Equipment required for tracheal intubation

Correct size of laryngoscope and spare (in case of light failure)
Tracheal tube of correct size + an alternative smaller size
Tracheal tube connector
Wire stilette
Gum elastic bougies
Magill forceps
Cuff-inflating syringe
Artery forceps
Securing tape or bandage
Catheter mount(s)
Local anaesthetic spray — 4% lignocaine
Cocaine spray/gel for nasal intubation
Tracheal tube lubricant
Throat packs
Anaesthetic breathing system and face masks — tested with O_2 to ensure no leaks present

The availability and function of all anaesthetic equipment should be checked before starting (see Table 20.1). After the patient's arrival in the anaesthetic room, the anaesthetist should be satisfied that the correct operation is being performed upon the correct patient, and that consent has been given. The patient must be on a tilting bed or trolley and the anaesthetist should have a competent assistant.

INDUCTION OF ANAESTHESIA

Anaesthesia is induced using one of the following techniques.

Inhalational induction

The most common indications for induction of anaesthesia by an inhalational technique are listed in Table 20.2.

The proposed procedure should be explained to the patient before starting. A 'no-mask' technique using a cupped hand around the fresh gas delivery tube may be preferred for young children; some anaesthetists favour allowing the child to play with the mask before connecting the anaesthetic tubing. The mask or hand is introduced *gradually* to the face from the side as the sight of a black

Table 20.2 Indications for inhalational induction

Young children
Upper airway obstruction, e.g. epiglottitis
Lower airway obstruction with foreign body
Bronchopleural fistula or empyema
No accessible veins

mask descending on to the face may be disturbing. While talking to the patient and encouraging him to breathe normally, the anaesthetist adjusts the mixture of the fresh gas flow and observes the patient's reactions. Initially, nitrous oxide 70% in oxygen is used and anaesthesia is deepened by the gradual introduction of increments of a volatile agent, e.g. halothane 1–3%, enflurane 1–3% or isoflurane 1–3%. Maintenance levels of halothane (1–2%), enflurane (1.5–2.5%) or isoflurane (1–2%) are used when anaesthesia has been established.

A single-breath technique of inhalational induction has been advocated for patients who are able to cooperate. One vital capacity breath from a prefilled 4-litre reservoir bag containing a high concentration of volatile agent (e.g. halothane 5%) in oxygen (or nitrous oxide 50% in oxygen) results in smooth induction of anaesthesia within 20–30 s.

Observation of the colour of the patient's skin and pattern of ventilation, palpation of the peripheral pulse, ECG monitoring and measurement of arterial pressure are important accompaniments to the technique of inhalational induction.

If spontaneous ventilation is to be maintained throughout the procedure, the mask is applied more firmly as consciousness is lost and the airway is supported manually. Insertion of an oropharyngeal airway or a tracheal tube may be considered when anaesthesia has been established.

Difficulties and complications

1. Slow induction of anaesthesia.
2. Problems particularly during stage 2 (vide infra).
3. Airway obstruction, bronchospasm.
4. Laryngeal spasm, hiccups.
5. Environmental pollution.

Intravenous induction

Induction of anaesthesia with an i.v. agent is suitable for most routine purposes and avoids many of the complications associated with the inhalational technique. It is the most appropriate method of rapid induction for the patient undergoing emergency surgery, in whom there is a risk of regurgitation of gastric contents during induction. All drugs which may be required at induction should be prepared and a cannula inserted into a suitable vein before starting.

If an existing i.v. cannula is to be used, its function must be checked. 'Butterfly' type needles or cannulae with a side injection port ('Venflon' type) are useful; large cannulae (e.g. 16G, 14G) are necessary for transfusion of fluids or blood. A vein in the forearm or back of the hand is preferable; veins in the antecubital fossa are best avoided because of the risks of intra-arterial injection. After selection of a suitable vein, skin preparation is performed using iodine or alcohol. Subcutaneous local anaesthetic may be used where a large cannula is to be employed. Intravenous entry is confirmed with blood aspiration and the device secured firmly with tape. 'Opsite' dressing may be used when long-term use is anticipated. Arterial pressure should be measured, and ECG monitoring may be attached to the patient at this stage. Preoxygenation is carried out, if appropriate, by administration of 100% oxygen by face mask.

Doses of the common i.v. agents are shown in Table 20.3. The induction dose varies with the patient's weight, age, state of nutrition, circulatory status, premedication and any concurrent medication. A small test dose is administered commonly and its effects are observed. Slow injection is recommended in the aged and in those with a slow circulation time (e.g. shock, hypovolaemia, cardiovascular disease) while the effects of the drug on the cardiovascular and respiratory systems are monitored.

A rapid-sequence induction technique is indicated for patients undergoing emergency surgery and for those in whom vomiting or regurgitation is a potential problem. After i.v. induction, a rapid transition to stage 3 anaesthesia (vide infra)

Table 20.3 Intravenous induction agents

Agent	Induction dose (mg/kg)
Thiopentone	3–5
Methohexitone	1–1.5
Etomidate	0.3
Propofol	1.5–2.5
Ketamine	2

is achieved; this is maintained by the introduction of an inhalational agent or by repeated bolus injections or a continuous infusion of an i.v. anaesthetic agent. Emergency anaesthesia is discussed fully in Chapter 32.

Complications and difficulties

1. *Regurgitation and vomiting.* If regurgitation occurs, the patient should be placed immediately into the Trendelenburg position and material aspirated with suction apparatus. Should inhalation of gastric contents occur, treatment with 100% oxygen, bronchodilators, tracheal suction and toilet, steroids, and antibiotics should be started immediately. Continued IPPV may be required if the resultant pneumonitis is severe.

2. *Intra-arterial injection of thiopentone.* This causes pain and blanching in hand and fingers as a result of crystal formation in the capillaries. The needle should be left in the artery and 5 ml 0.5% procaine and 40 mg papaverine injected. Further treatment includes stellate ganglion block, brachial plexus block or sympathetic block with i.v. guanethidine.

3. *Perivenous injection.* This causes blanching and pain and may result in a small degree of tissue necrosis. Methohexitone and propofol produce less tissue damage than thiopentone. Hyaluronidase may be used to speed dispersal of the drug.

4. *Cardiovascular depression.* This is likely to occur particularly in the elderly, the hypovolaemic or the untreated hypertensive patient. Caution should be exercised especially in the use of propofol or thiopentone in these patients. Infusion of i.v. fluid (e.g. 500 ml colloid or 1000 ml crystalloid solution) is usually successful in restoring arterial pressure.

5. *Respiratory depression.* Slow injection of an induction agent may reduce the extent of respiratory depression. Respiratory adequacy must be assessed carefully, and the anaesthetist should be ready to assist ventilation of the lungs if necessary.

6. *Histamine release.* Thiopentone or methohexitone may cause release of histamine with subsequent formation of typical weals. Severe reactions may occur to individual agents, and appropriate drugs and fluids should be available in the anaesthetic room for treatment.

7. *Porphyria.* An acute porphyric episode may be precipitated by barbiturates in susceptible individuals.

8. *Other complications.* Pain on injection (especially with methohexitone, etomidate or propofol), hiccup or muscular movements may occur.

POSITION OF PATIENT FOR SURGERY

After induction of anaesthesia, the patient is placed on the operating table in a position appropriate for the proposed surgery. When positioning the patient, the anaesthetist should take into account surgical access, patient safety, anaesthetic technique, monitoring and position of i.v. lines, etc.

Some commonly used positions are shown in Figure 20.1. Each may have adverse effects in terms of skeletal, neurological, ventilatory and circulatory effects.

1. The *lithotomy* position may result in nerve damage on the medial or lateral side of the leg from pressure exerted by the stirrups, which must be well padded. Care must be taken to elevate both legs simultaneously so that pelvic asymmetry and resultant backache are avoided. The sacrum should be supported on the operating table and not allowed to slip off the end.

2. The *lateral* position may result in asymmetrical lung ventilation (see Ch. 39). Care is required with arm positon and i.v. infusions. The pelvis must be supported to prevent the patient from rolling either backwards (with a risk of falling from the table) or forwards into the recovery position.

3. The *prone* position may cause abdominal compression which may result in ventilatory and circulatory embarrassment. To prevent this, support must be provided beneath the shoulders and iliac crests. Excessive extension of the shoulders should be avoided. The face, and particularly the eyes, must be protected from trauma. The tracheal tube must be secured firmly in place as it is almost impossible to reinsert it with the patient in this position.

4. The *Trendelenburg* position may produce upward pressure on the diaphragm because of the weight of the abdominal contents. Damage to the

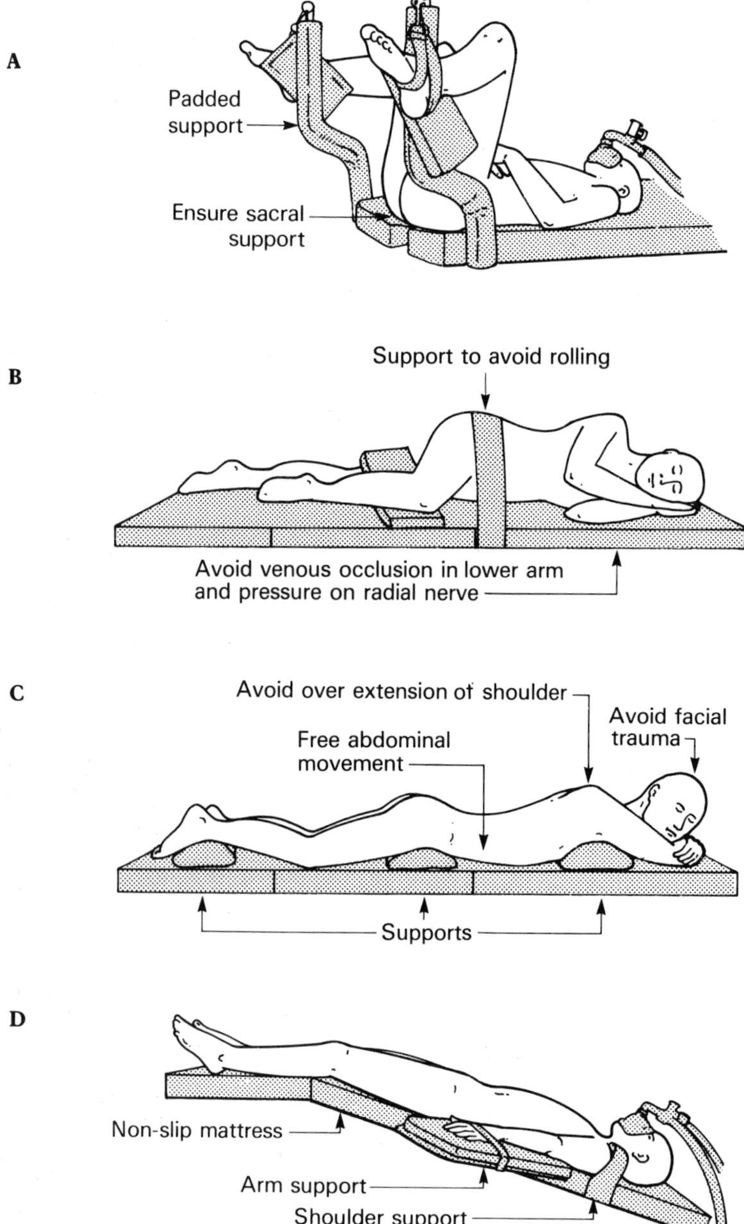

Fig. 20.1 Positions on the operating table: (a) lithotomy, (b) lateral, (c) prone, (d) Trendelenburg.

brachial plexus may occur as a result of pressure from shoulder supports, especially if the arms are abducted.

5. The *sitting* position requires careful support of the head. In addition, venous pooling and resultant cardiovascular instability may occur.

6. The *supine* position carries the risk of the supine hypotensive syndrome during pregnancy (see Ch. 33) or in patients with a large abdominal mass.

MAINTENANCE OF ANAESTHESIA

Anaesthesia may be continued using inhalational agents, i.v. anaesthetic agents, or i.v. opioids either alone or in combination. Tracheal intubation with or without muscle relaxants may be employed. Regional anaesthesia may be used to supplement any of these techniques.

Inhalational anaesthesia with spontaneous ventilation

This is an appropriate form of maintenance for superficial operations, minor procedures which produce little reflex or painful stimulation, and operations for which profound muscle relaxation is not required.

Conduct

After induction of anaesthesia, inhalational and/or volatile agents may be used in the spontaneously breathing patient. Depending on the nature of surgery, the provision of analgesia in the premedication and the patient's response (assessed by observation of ventilation, circulation and heart rate and rhythm), halothane 1–2% may be employed in a mixture with nitrous oxide 70% in oxygen; enflurane 1.5–2.5% or isoflurane 1–2% are alternatives to halothane. Trichloroethylene possesses a greater analgesic effect but is more soluble in blood; consequently, it is slower in onset and must be administered initially in a relatively high concentration (1–1.5%) relative to its MAC value (vide infra), although this concentration may be reduced subsequently to 0.4–0.6%.

Minimum alveolar concentration (MAC)

MAC is the minimum alveolar concentration of an inhaled anaesthetic agent which prevents reflex movement in response to surgical incision in 50% of subjects. MAC values of commonly used inhalational agents are shown in Appendix II (p. 723). MAC varies little with metabolic factors but is reduced by opioid premedication and in the presence of hypothermia. MAC is higher in neonates and is reduced in the elderly (see Ch. 9).

The effects of inhalational anaesthetics are additive; thus 1 MAC-equivalent could be achieved by producing an alveolar concentration of 70% nitrous oxide (0.67 MAC) and 0.25% halothane (0.33 MAC).

The rate at which MAC is attained may be increased by raising the inspired concentration and by avoidance of airway obstruction. Increasing ventilation at a constant inspired concentration produces more rapid equilibration between inspired and alveolar concentrations. The time taken for equilibration increases with the blood/gas solubility coefficient of the agent; those with a high blood/gas solubility coefficient do not reach equilibrium for several hours (see Ch. 9). It follows therefore that the inspired concentration must be considerably higher than MAC to produce an adequate alveolar concentration when such agents are used.

Control of depth of anaesthesia by varying the inspired concentration of volatile agent requires constant assessment of the patient's reaction to anaesthesia and surgery to produce adequate anaesthesia while avoiding overdosage and excessively 'deep' anaesthesia. This rapid control is one of the main advantages of inhalational anaesthesia. The signs of inadequate depth of anaesthesia include tachypnoea, tachycardia, hypertension and sweating.

Signs of anaesthesia (Fig. 20.2)

Guedel's classical signs of anaesthesia are those seen in patients premedicated with morphine and atropine, and breathing ether in air. The clinical signs associated with anaesthesia produced by other inhalational agents follow a similar course, but the divisions between the stages and planes are less precise.

Stage 1: the stage of analgesia. This is the stage attained when using nitrous oxide 50% in oxygen, as employed in the technique of relative analgesia (see Ch. 35).

Stage 2: stage of excitement. This is seen with inhalational induction, but rapidly passed during i.v. induction. Respiration is erratic, breath-holding may occur, laryngeal and pharyngeal reflexes are active and stimulation of pharynx or

STAGE	RESPIRATION	PUPILS	EYE REFLEXES	URT & RESPIRATORY REFLEXES
1 Analgesia	Regular Small volume	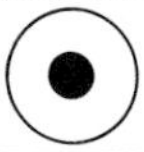		
2 Excitement	Irregular	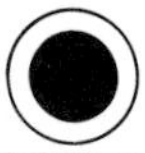	Eyelash absent	
3 Anaesthesia Plane I	Regular Large volume	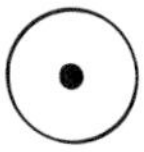	Eyelid absent Conjunctival depressed	Pharyngeal & vomiting depressed
Plane II	Regular Large volume	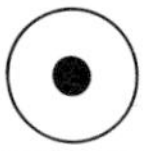	Corneal depressed	
Plane III	Regular Becoming diaphragmatic Small volume			Laryngeal depressed
Plane IV	Irregular Diaphragmatic Small volume	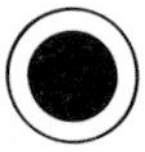		Carinal depressed
4 Overdose	Apnoea	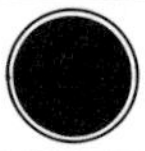		

Fig. 20.2 Stages of anaesthesia (modified from Guedel).

larynx can produce laryngeal spasm. The eyelash reflex (used as a sign of unconsciousness with i.v. induction) is abolished in stage 2, but the eyelid reflex (resistance to elevation of eyelid) remains present.

Stage 3: surgical anaesthesia. This deepens through 4 planes (in practice 3 — light, medium, deep) with increasing concentration of anaesthetic drug. Respiration assumes a rhythmic pattern and the thoracic component diminishes with depth of anaesthesia. Respiratory reflexes become suppressed but the carinal reflex is abolished only at plane IV (therefore a tracheal tube which is too long may produce carinal stimulation at an otherwise adequate depth). The pupils are central and gradually enlarge with depth of anaesthesia. Lacrimation is active in light planes but absent in planes III and IV — a useful sign in a patient not premedicated with an anticholinergic.

Stage 4: stage of impending respiratory and circulatory failure. Brainstem reflexes are depressed by the high anaesthetic concentration. Pupils are enlarged and unreactive. The patient should not be permitted to reach this stage. Withdrawal of the anaesthetic agents and administration of 100% oxygen lightens anaesthesia.

Observation of other reflexes provides a guide to depth of anaesthesia. Swallowing occurs in the light plane of stage 3. The gag reflex is abolished in upper stage 3. Stretching of the anal sphincter produces reflex laryngospasm even at plane III of stage 3.

Complications/difficulties during inhalational anaesthesia

Airway obstruction. Relieved by appropriate positioning and equipment (vide infra).

Laryngeal spasm. This may occur as a result of stimulation above light–medium stage 3. Treatment is to stop the stimulation and gently deepen anaesthesia. If spasm is severe, 100% oxygen is applied with the face mask held tightly, while the airway is maintained by hand and pressure is applied to the reservoir bag. Attempts to ventilate the patient's lungs usually result only in gastric inflation. However, as the larynx partially opens, 100% oxygen flows through under pressure. Further gentle deepening of anaesthesia may then take place. In severe laryngeal spasm, suxamethonium may be required and after the lungs have been inflated with oxygen it is advisable to intubate the trachea.

Bronchospasm. This may occur if volatile anaesthetic agents are introduced rapidly, particularly in smokers with excessive bronchial secretions. Humidification and warming of gases may minimise the problem. Bronchospasm may accompany laryngospasm. Administration of bronchodilators may be required. These respiratory reflexes are induced more readily in the presence of an upper respiratory tract infection.

Malignant hyperpyrexia. Volatile agents, suxamethonium or amide-type local anaesthetic agents may trigger this syndrome in susceptible individuals (see Ch. 23).

Raised intracranial pressure (ICP). All volatile agents may produce an increase in ICP, and this is accentuated by retention of CO_2 which accompanies the use of volatile agents in the spontaneously breathing patient. A spontaneous ventilation technique is therefore contraindicated in patients with an intracranial space-occupying lesion or cerebral oedema.

Atmospheric pollution. The use of the appropriate scavenging apparatus helps to reduce levels of theatre pollution by volatile and gaseous agents (see Ch. 17).

Airway maintenance during inhalational anaesthesia

Maintenance of the airway is one of the most important aspects of the anaesthetist's task. Inhalational anaesthesia usually involves the use of a face mask; these take many forms, and selection of the correct size is important to provide a gas-tight seal. For children, a mask with excessive dead space should be avoided. Nasal masks are required during dental anaesthesia. The patient's head position during mask anaesthesia is important; the mandible is held 'into' the mask by the anaesthetist, with his fingers holding the mandible itself rather than pressing into the soft tissues, which may result in airway obstruction (especially in children). The mandible is held forward, helping to prevent obstruction of the airway by posterior movement of the tongue.

The importance of observation of the airway during mask anaesthesia cannot be overemphasised. Soft tissue indrawing in the suprasternal and supraclavicular areas is evidence of obstruction of the upper airway. Noisy ventilation or inspiratory stridor provides further evidence that airway obstruction requires correction. Maintenance of the airway is assisted by the use of an oropharyngeal (Guedel) airway. The patient must be anaesthetised adequately before insertion of the airway as stimulation of the pharynx may produce coughing, breath-holding or laryngeal spasm. The use of local anaesthetic spray or jelly to coat the airway may permit its insertion at an earlier stage. A nasopharyngeal airway may be tolerated better.

When the airway has been established and the patient's ventilatory pattern is regular, the use of a Clausen harness to provide airway support frees the anaesthetist's hands. The straps should be applied carefully and symmetrically for success. Support for the mandible may be achieved with a well-padded tongue spatula or an oropharyngeal airway inserted between the straps. The use of a laryngeal mask (see p. 19) overcomes many of the problems of airway maintenance associated with conventional face masks and airways.

Tracheal intubation

Indications

1. Provision of a clear airway, e.g. anticipated difficulty in using mask anaesthesia in the edentulous patient.
2. An 'unusual' position, e.g. prone or sitting. A reinforced non-kinking tube may be necessary.
3. Operations on the head and neck, e.g. ENT, dental. A nasotracheal tube may be required.
4. Protection of the respiratory tract, e.g. from blood during upper respiratory tract or oral surgery and from inhalation of gastric contents in emergency surgery or patients with oesophageal obstruction. The use of a cuffed tube for adults is mandatory in these circumstances.
5. During anaesthesia using IPPV and muscle relaxants.

6. To facilitate suction of the respiratory tract.
7. During thoracic operations.

Contraindications

There are few contraindications. In emergency situations, hypoxaemia must be relieved if at all possible before insertion of a tracheal tube.

Preparation

Before starting, the anaesthetist must check the availability and function of the necessary equipment. He should have a 'dedicated' and experienced assistant. Laryngoscopes of the correct size are chosen and the function of bulb and batteries checked, the patency of the tracheal tube is checked and the integrity of the cuff ensured. Various aids to intubation must also be present (see Table 20.1).

Choice of equipment

Laryngoscopes. Laryngoscopes are manufactured in many shapes and sizes. There are two basic types of blade — straight or curved. Straight-blade laryngoscopes (e.g. Magill) are favoured for children, in whom the epiglottis is floppy, and are designed to pass posterior to the epiglottis and to lift it anteriorly, exposing the larynx. The curved blade (e.g. Macintosh) is designed so that the tip lies anterior to the epiglottis in the vallecula, pressing on the hyo-epiglottic ligament and moving it anteriorly to expose the larynx and vocal cords (Fig. 20.3).

Tracheal tubes. Most tracheal tubes are made of either rubber or plastic. The latter are disposable and less irritant to the tracheal mucosa. In some circumstances, e.g. head and neck or throat surgery, the tracheal tube may be subject to direct or indirect pressure, and standard tubes may kink or become compressed. It may be appropriate to use a tube which is reinforced with nylon or steel in such cases. Tracheal tubes are introduced usually through the mouth, although it may be preferable to pass the tube through the nose, particularly for oral surgery. The length of disposable tubes exceeds that required normally for oral intubation, and the tube should be cut to the appropriate length before use. During thoracic surgery, it may be necessary to ventilate the lungs independently, and a bronchial or double-lumen tube is required (see Ch. 39).

In order to seal the airway, most tracheal tubes are manufactured with an inflatable cuff at the distal end. The cuff may be of low or high volume; low-volume cuffs produce a seal over a smaller area of tracheal mucosa, and tend to exert a high pressure on the mucosal cells, reducing the capillary blood supply and rendering the cells potentially ischaemic. High-volume cuffs cover a wide area of mucosa; the pressure exerted varies

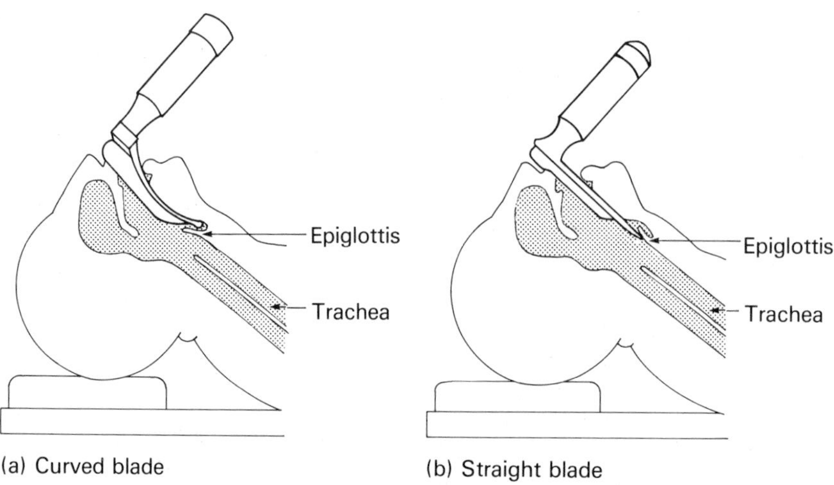

Fig. 20.3 Use of the laryngoscope.

during the respiratory cycle, but on average is lower than that produced by a low-volume cuff.

Tracheal tubes of different sizes are required. The size quoted usually is the internal diameter (ID). Adult males require normally a tube of 9–10 mm ID, and females 8–8.5 mm. For oral intubation, the tube should be 20–23 cm in length. The appropriate internal diameter of tube for paediatric use can be calculated from the formula (Age/4) + 4 mm. This is an approximation, and a tube 0.5 mm smaller and 0.5 mm larger should also be prepared. The length of tube required for oral intubation in children is approximately equal to (Age/2) + 12 cm. A tube of slightly smaller internal diameter may be required for nasal intubation, and its length may be calculated from the formula (Age/2) + 15 cm.

An appropriate connector is required between the tracheal tube and the anaesthetic breathing system, e.g. curved connector for nasal tube, lightweight plastic with low deadspace for children, or a connector with a suction port for thoracic surgery.

Anaesthesia for tracheal intubation

Tracheal intubation may be performed with the patient awake (e.g. neonates), under local anaesthesia (using topical spray, transtracheal spray and superior laryngeal nerve block) or under general anaesthesia (either i.v. or inhalational, with or without the use of muscle relaxation). The usual approach is to provide general anaesthesia and muscle relaxation, to perform laryngoscopy and direct vision intubation, and then to maintain anaesthesia via the tracheal tube with spontaneous or controlled ventilation. Adequate anaesthesia and muscle relaxation must be provided for laryngoscopy.

Inhalational technique for intubation. Adequate depth of anaesthesia is necessary to depress the laryngeal reflexes and provide a degree of relaxation of the laryngeal and pharyngeal muscles. Halothane in concentrations up to 4% may provide rapid attainment of the necessary depth, which can be judged from a pattern of respiration with predominance of diaphragmatic breathing (a useful sign in children is the 'dissociation' of the thoracic and abdominal excursion). The mask is removed and laryngoscopy and intubation performed. The anaesthetic circuit is then connected to the tracheal tube and anaesthesia maintained at a depth appropriate for surgery.

Relaxant anaesthesia for intubation. After i.v. or inhalational induction of anaesthesia, the short-acting depolarising muscle relaxant suxamethonium may be used to provide relaxation for tracheal intubation. After loss of consciousness, the patient breathes 100% oxygen or 50% nitrous oxide in oxygen and suxamethonium is administered in a dose of 1–1.5 mg/kg. Assisted ventilation is maintained via the face mask until muscle relaxation occurs (except in emergency patients and those likely to regurgitate) and laryngoscopy and intubation are performed. Inhalational anaesthesia may be continued with manual ventilation until the effects of the relaxant have ceased, whereupon spontaneous ventilation is resumed. Alternatively, non-depolarising neuromuscular blockade is instituted and ventilation controlled.

Conduct of laryngoscopy

The position of the patient's head and neck is important. The neck should be flexed and the head extended with support of a pillow; thus the oral, pharyngeal and tracheal axes are brought into alignment (Fig. 20.4). The laryngoscope is designed for left hand use and is introduced into the right side of the mouth while the right hand opens the mouth, parting the lips to avoid interposing them between laryngoscope and teeth. The teeth may be protected from blade trauma with the fingers or the use of a plastic 'guard'. The

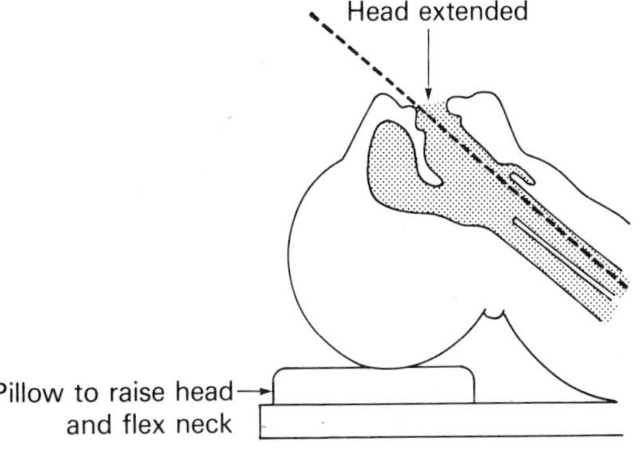

Fig. 20.4 Head position for laryngoscopy.

laryngoscope blade deflects the tongue to the left and the length of the blade is passed over the contour of the tongue. The laryngoscope is lifted upwards and forwards, avoiding a levering movement which can damage the upper teeth. Using a straight blade, the tip is passed posterior to the epiglottis, which is lifted anteriorly and the vocal cords visualised. With a curved blade, the tip is inserted into the vallecula and pressure on the hyo-epiglottic ligament moves the epiglottis to expose the vocal cords. External pressure on the thyroid cartilage by an assistant may aid laryngeal visualisation at this stage.

Conduct of intubation

After laryngeal visualisation, the supraglottic area and cords may be sprayed with local anaesthetic solution (lignocaine 4%). The tracheal tube is passed from the right side of the mouth (which may be held open by the assistant's finger if necessary, permitting a clear view of the midline) and between the vocal cords into the trachea until the cuff is below the vocal cords. A semirigid stilette may be used during intubation to provide the correct degree of curvature of the tracheal tube to facilitate intubation.

The tube cuff is inflated sufficiently to abolish audible gas leak on inflation of the lungs. The correct position of the tube must now be confirmed. If the tube has been seen clearly at laryngoscopy to pass through the vocal cords into the trachea, then equal movement of both sides of the chest during ventilation should be confirmed and auscultation in each axilla for breath sounds should be performed to ensure that the tip of the tracheal tube has not passed too far distally to enter, or occlude, one of the main bronchi (see p. 406); if there is unilateral air entry, the tube should be withdrawn slowly and carefully until air entry is equal in both lungs. If the tube has not been seen clearly to enter the trachea, or if there is *any* reason to suspect that its distal end is not in the trachea, then the steps outlined in Chapter 23 (p. 410) must be undertaken immediately to identify possible oesophageal intubation.

After its correct position has been determined, the tube is secured with either cotton tape or bandage, or sticking plaster strips. Correct fixation of the tube is important, particularly if the head is inaccessible during surgery, e.g. when the patient is in the prone position.

Nasal intubation

Nasal intubation may be employed for dental operations, ENT operations, etc., and may be preferred for long-term intubation by providing easier tube fixation, easier oral toilet and greater patient comfort.

A slightly smaller tube is used, and is introduced preferentially to the right nostril since the left-facing bevel of the tube favours this approach. The tube is passed along the floor of the nose and advanced *gently* into the pharynx, avoiding excessive force. Laryngoscopy takes place, and the tube is advanced into the trachea by manipulation of the proximal end or by grasping the tip with Magill's intubating forceps to pass it between the cords.

Packing of the throat may be employed after intubation especially for oropharyngeal operations. The moist gauze pack is introduced using the laryngoscope and Magill forceps. The pharynx should be packed on each side of the tracheal tube. The pack should be applied gently to avoid abrasion of the mucosa. A 'tail' of the pack is left protruding from the mouth and the anaesthetist must accept responsibility for removal of the pack before extubation. A latex 'foam' pack may be used as an alternative to cotton gauze.

Difficult intubation

Difficult intubation may be anticipated or unanticipated. Difficulty may be expected from evidence sought at the preoperative visit. The unexpected case should be acknowledged as such at the time of intubation and the anaesthetist should have contingency plans to overcome the situation. This subject is discussed in Chapter 23.

Complications of tracheal intubation

Complications may be mechanical, respiratory, or cardiovascular and may occur early or late.

Early complications. Trauma may occur to lips and teeth or dental crowns. Jaw dislocation and dislocation of arytenoids may be produced. Trauma during intubation may result in damage to larynx and vocal cords. Nasal intubation may produce epistaxis, trauma to the pharyngeal wall or dislodgement of adenoid tissue. Obstruction or kinking of the tube can occur and carinal stimulation or bronchial intubation may take place if the tube is too long. Laryngeal trauma may produce postoperative croup, bronchospasm or laryngospasm, especially in children. Mechanical complications may be avoided with a careful technique. Broken teeth must be retrieved and the event documented. Immediate postoperative respiratory complications may be minimised by humidification of inspired gases. Cardiovascular complications of intubation include arrhythmias and hypertension, especially in untreated hypertensive patients.

Late complications. These are more common after long-term intubation. Tracheal stenosis is rare, but damage to tracheal mucosa from a cuffed tube may be related to its design; high-volume low-pressure cuffs may be preferred for long-term intubation. Trauma to vocal cords may result in ulceration or granulomata which may require surgical removal. Cord trauma may be more common in the presence of an upper respiratory tract infection.

Relaxant anaesthesia

Indications for relaxant anaesthesia

As an alternative to deep anaesthesia with spontaneous ventilation and volatile agents leading to multisystem depression, the triad of sleep, suppression of reflexes and muscle relaxation may be provided separately with specific agents. Relaxation anaesthesia provides muscle relaxation, permitting lighter anaesthesia with less risk of cardiovascular depression. Thus the technique is appropriate for major abdominal, intraperitoneal, thoracic or intracranial operations, prolonged operations in which spontaneous ventilation would lead to respiratory depression and operations in a position in which ventilation is impaired mechanically.

Conduct of relaxant anaesthesia

Induction of anaesthesia is followed by tracheal intubation after administration of a depolarising muscle relaxant. When its action has subsided relaxation is provided by a longer-acting non-depolarising relaxant (Table 12.1). The choice of agent depends upon operative indications (e.g. tubocurarine has been employed traditionally during induced hypotension) or the patient's condition (e.g. vecuronium and atracurium produce little cardiovascular depression).

Controlled ventilation is instituted, first manually by compression of the reservoir bag, and then by a mechanical ventilator delivering the appropriate tidal and minute volume (see Appendix VII, p. 740). Anaesthesia and analgesia are provided usually by nitrous oxide/oxygen, together with a volatile agent and/or i.v. analgesic. Analgesia may be provided by opioid premedication. Volatile agents are used in an inspired concentration less than MAC when ventilation is controlled. Intravenous opioids, e.g. morphine, papaveretum, phenoperidine or fentanyl may be employed in small doses.

Assessment of relaxant anaesthesia

Light anaesthesia with preservation of reflexes permits the use of physical signs for the continued assessment of the adequacy of anaesthesia.

Adequacy of anaesthesia. Autonomic reflex activity with lacrimation, sweating, tachycardia, hypertension, or reflex movement in response to surgery, indicate 'light' anaesthesia and response to surgical stimulation and warn that the depth of anaesthesia should be increased or further increments of i.v. analgesic given.

Awareness during anaesthesia. The possibility of conscious or unconscious awareness exists in a patient who is under the influence of a neuromuscular blocking drug if nitrous oxide/oxygen anaesthesia is unsupplemented, or is supplemented by an opioid with little or no volatile agent. The anaesthetist should ensure that this possibility is avoided by constant observation of the patient for clinical signs of light anaesthesia and by judicious use of small concentrations of a volatile agent. Up to 1% of patients may recall intraoperative events spontaneously if a mixture of nitrous oxide 67% in oxygen is administered, even with an i.v. opioid, and a proportion of these patients experience pain. Awareness during anaesthesia is now a common source of litigation. An appropriate concentration of volatile anaesthetic agent should be used routinely during elective surgery.

Adequacy of muscle relaxation. Clinical signs of return of muscle tone include retraction of the wound edges during abdominal operations and abdominal muscle, diaphragmatic or facial movement. An increase in airway pressure (with a time- or volume-cycled ventilator) may indicate a return of muscle tone. Quantitative estimation of neuromuscular status may be obtained with a peripheral nerve stimulator (see Ch. 12). Small increments (e.g. 25–35% of the original dose of muscle relaxant) may be given to maintain relaxation; alternatively, an infusion of vecuronium or atracurium may be a more convenient method of administration, but the use of a peripheral nerve stimulator is mandatory with this technique.

Adequacy of ventilation. Clinical signs of inadequate ventilation and an increase in Pa_{CO_2} include venous dilatation, wound oozing, tachycardia, hypertension and attempts at spontaneous ventilation by the patient.

Measurements of arterial P_{CO_2}, end-expired P_{CO_2}, or minute volume provide more objective information to guide adjustment of mechanical ventilation.

Reversal of relaxation

At the end of operation, residual neuromuscular blockade is antagonised and spontaneous ventilation established before the tracheal tube is removed and the patient awakened. Residual neuromuscular block is antagonised with neostigmine 2.5–5 mg (0.05–0.08 mg/kg in children). Atropine 1.2 mg or glycopyrrolate 0.5 mg counteracts the muscarinic side effects of the anticholinesterase and may be given before, or with, neostigmine. Care should be exercised in the use of an anticholinergic agent in the presence of existing tachycardia, pyrexia, carbon dioxide retention or ischaemic heart disease.

Resumption of spontaneous ventilation is aided by adding 5% CO_2 to the inspired gas mixture to restore normocapnia if hyperventilation has been employed. Tracheobronchial suction (vide infra) has the beneficial side effect of stimulating respiration.

Extubation

This may take place with the patient supine if the anaesthetist is satisfied that airway patency can be maintained by the patient in this position and there is no risk of regurgitation. In patients at risk of regurgitation and potential aspiration, the lateral position is preferred. However, it is safer to employ the lateral recovery position after extubation (Fig. 20.5). Return of respiratory reflexes is signified by coughing and resistance to the presence of the tracheal tube.

Tracheobronchial suction via the tracheal tube is carried out using a soft sterile suction catheter with an external diameter less than half the internal diameter of the tube. Preoxygenation precedes suctioning as the oxygen stores may be depleted by tracheal suction. The catheter is occluded during insertion and suction applied during withdrawal.

Pharyngeal suction is performed best under direct vision, avoiding trauma to the pharyngeal mucosa, uvula or epiglottis.

Oxygen 100% replaces the anaesthetic gas mixture before extubation to avoid the potential effects of diffusion hypoxia (p. 429) and to provide a pulmonary reservoir of oxygen in case breath-holding or coughing occurs.

Extubation is performed preferably during an inspiration when the larynx dilates; the cuff is deflated and the tube withdrawn along its curved

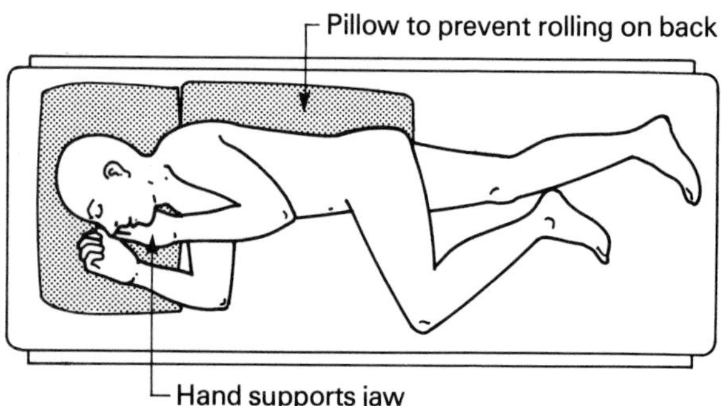

Fig. 20.5 Recovery position.

axis. Some anaesthetists generate a positive pressure in the trachea during this manoeuvre by 'squeezing the bag' in order to propel secretions into the pharynx.

After extubation, the patient's ability to maintain the airway is ensured, the ability to cough and clear secretions is assessed and an oropharyngeal airway employed if required. Administration of oxygen is continued by facemask. Preparations are made for recovery.

Precautions and complications associated with extubation

Laryngeal spasm. This may follow stimulation during extubation. Extubation during deep anaesthesia and subsequent maintenance with a mask may be used. Local anaesthetic spray to the larynx may block the reflex, and pharyngeal suction before extubation removes the secretions which cause stimulation.

Regurgitation/inhalation. Aspiration via the nasogastric tube (if present) should be performed before tracheal extubation to remove gastric liquid. In emergency patients, extubation should be performed with the patient awake so that airway control is continuous. Partial incompetence of laryngeal reflexes may occur in the immediate post-extubation period, especially if local anaesthetic spray has been employed. In this event, recovery should take place with the patient in the lateral head-down position, with facilities at hand for suction, oxygenation and reintubation.

EMERGENCE AND RECOVERY

After tracheal extubation or at the end of mask anaesthesia, anaesthetic agents are withdrawn and oxygen 100% is delivered via the face mask. The patient's airway is supported until respiratory reflexes are intact. The patient's muscle power and coordination are assessed by testing hand grip, tongue protrusion or lifting the head from the pillow in response to command. Return of adequate muscle power must be ensured before the patient leaves theatre (Ch. 12, Table 12.5).

The patient is then ready for transfer from the operating table to a bed or trolley and further recovery takes place in a recovery area of theatre or in the recovery ward (Ch. 24).

The lateral recovery position (Fig. 20.5) is adopted unless the anaesthetist is satisfied that this is unnecessary. The patient is turned on one side, upper leg flexed and lower extended; the head is on one side and the tongue falls forward under gravity, thus avoiding airway obstruction.

FURTHER READING

Adams A P, Henville J D 1979 Anaesthetic circuits and flexible pipelines for medical gases. In: Langton Hewer C, Atkinson R S (eds) Recent advances in anaesthesia and analgesia 13. Churchill Livingstone, Edinburgh

Birmingham P K, Cheney F W, Ward R J 1986 Esophageal intubation: a review of detection techniques. Anesthesia and Analgesia 65: 886

Brit B 1979 Malignant hyperthermia. International Anesthesiology Clinics 17. Little, Brown, Boston

Dundee J W, Wyant G M 1977 Intravenous anaesthesia. Churchill Livingstone, Edinburgh

Editorial 1987. New awakening in anesthesia — at a price. Lancet 1: 1469

Martin J T 1978 Positioning in anaesthesia and surgery. W B Saunders, Philadelphia

Stenquist O, Nilsson K 1982 Postoperative sore throat related to tracheal cuff design. Canadian Anaesthetists Society Journal 29: 384

Utting J E 1982 Awareness during surgical operations. In: Atkinson R S, Langton Hewer C (eds) Recent advances in anaesthesia and analgesia 14. Churchill Livingstone, Edinburgh

White D C 1985 Appraisal of inhalational anaesthetic agents. In: Kaufman L (ed) Anaesthesia review 3. Churchill Livingstone, Edinburgh

21. Monitoring during anaesthesia

The word 'monitor' is derived from the Latin verb *monere* — to warn. The purpose of a monitoring device is to measure a physiological variable and to indicate trends of change, thus enabling appropriate therapeutic action to be taken.

As the derivation suggests, a monitor can only warn. No mechanical or electrical device can replace conscientious observations of the patient by the anaesthetist. Information from monitoring equipment requires clinical interpretation.

It is essential to ensure that all monitoring equipment is maintained correctly and that it functions accurately, so that the information which it provides is reliable. The user should understand the basic principles on which monitoring equipment is based and be able to interpret the information provided.

The anaesthetic record

Varying levels of complexity of monitoring are appropriate during anaesthesia in different clinical situations; for instance, major cardiovascular surgery and dilatation and curettage represent opposite ends of the monitoring spectrum.

The importance of meticulous record-keeping for all patients undergoing anaesthesia cannot be stressed too highly. Detailed, accurate charts provide not only a valuable record of trends occurring during anaesthesia, but are useful also for reference purposes, if further administration of anaesthesia is necessary. In addition, they may be required for medicolegal purposes. Litigation may arise many years after the event and claims are almost impossible to defend in the absence of comprehensive records. A suitable chart is shown in Figure 21.1. The basic requirements of a chart are that it should provide space to record:

1. Details of preoperative assessment including drug history.
2. Cardiovascular variables, including heart rate, arterial pressure, CVP and urine output.
3. Respiratory variables, including ventilator settings, airway pressures and F_{IO_2}.
4. Details of apparatus employed.
5. Dosages of all drugs, including the concentrations of nitrous oxide and volatile agent employed.
6. Details of all i.v. fluids.
7. Volume of blood lost.
8. Any problems or difficulties encountered.
9. Postoperative instructions.

THE CARDIOVASCULAR SYSTEM

Electrocardiography

Valuable information concerning cardiac rhythm may be obtained by monitoring the ECG. Most ECG machines calculate ventricular rate. This should not distract the anaesthetist from monitoring peripheral pulse rate.

ECG monitors have become increasingly reliable and less subject to interference. As the technique is non-invasive, simple and accurate, it is now regarded as mandatory that the electrocardiogram should be monitored in all patients undergoing anaesthesia, no matter how minor the surgical procedure.

Standard lead II monitoring is used widely. However, the CM_5 lead configuration (Fig. 21.2) has been advocated for routine intraoperative

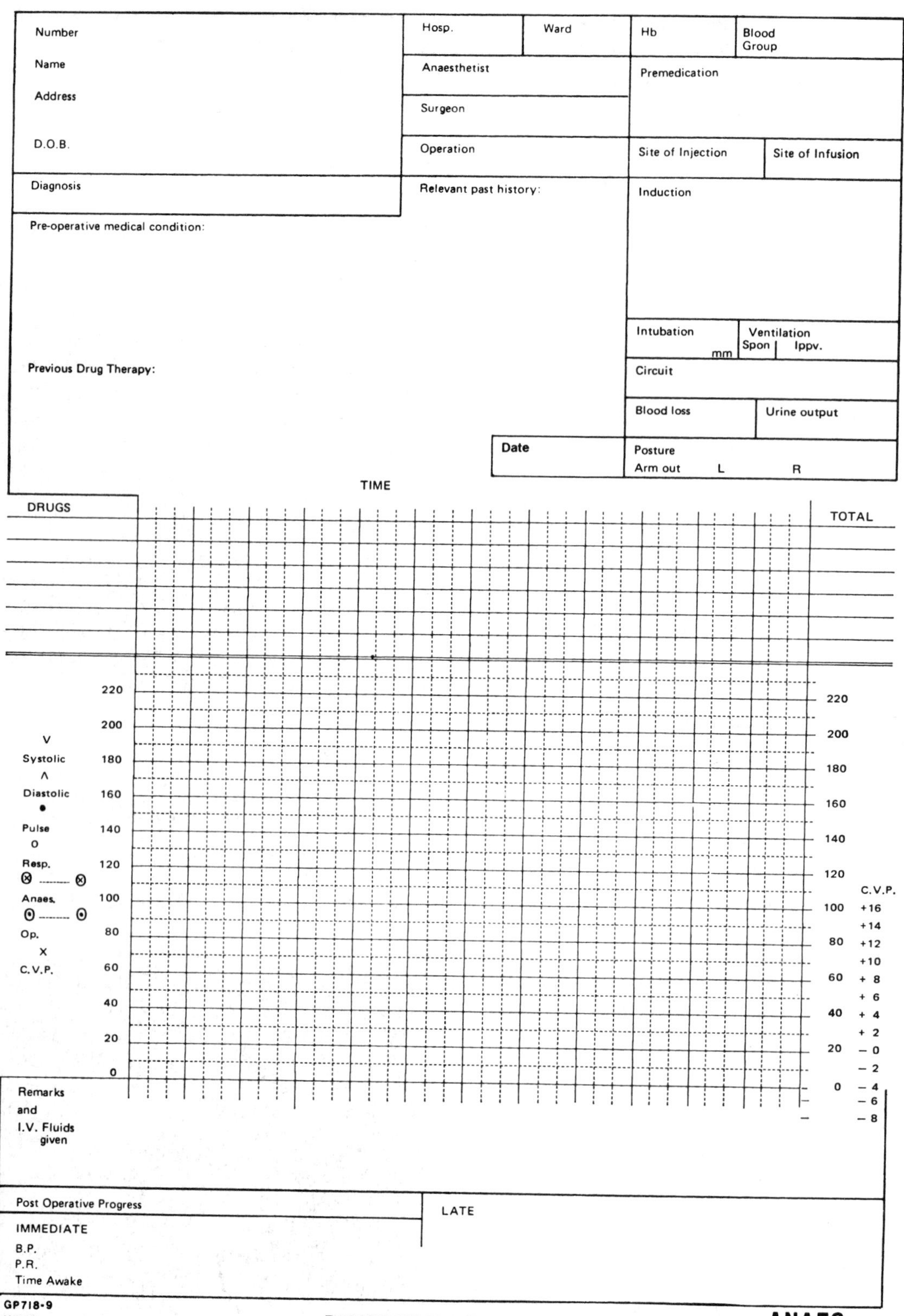
Number
Name
Address
D.O.B.
Hosp.
Ward
Hb
Blood Group
Anaesthetist
Premedication
Surgeon
Operation
Site of Injection
Site of Infusion
Diagnosis
Relevant past history:
Induction
Pre-operative medical condition:
Intubation mm
Ventilation Spon | Ippv.
Previous Drug Therapy:
Circuit
Blood loss
Urine output
Date
Posture
Arm out L R
TIME
DRUGS
TOTAL
220
200
V Systolic
180
Λ Diastolic
160
● Pulse
140
O Resp.
120
⊗ ------ ⊗ Anaes.
100
⊙ ------ ⊙ Op.
80
X C.V.P.
60
40
20
0
C.V.P.
+16
+14
+12
+10
+ 8
+ 6
+ 4
+ 2
− 0
− 2
− 4
− 6
− 8
ANAESTHETIC RECORD
Remarks and I.V. Fluids given
Post Operative Progress
IMMEDIATE
B.P.
P.R.
Time Awake
LATE
Sheet No. 46
GP718-9
W146
THIS COPY FOR CASE-NOTES (TOP)
ANAES

Fig. 21.1 Anaesthetic record.

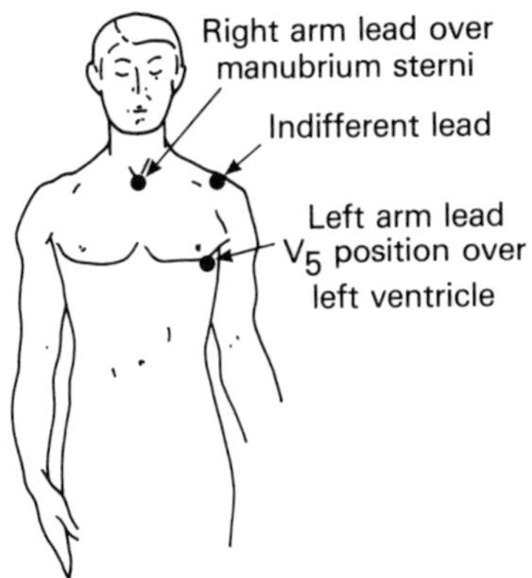

Fig. 21.2 CM_5 lead configuration for ECG monitoring.

monitoring because it reveals more readily ST segment changes produced by left ventricular ischaemia.

It is important to appreciate that the ECG is an index only of electrical activity. It is possible for a normal electrical waveform to exist in the presence of a negligible cardiac output. Consequently, information from the ECG should be used in conjunction with data acquired from monitoring of perfusion.

Monitoring the circulation

Maintenance of perfusion of vital organs is one of the principal tasks of the anaesthetist during surgery. Adequate perfusion is dependent on adequate venous return to the heart, cardiac performance and arterial pressure.

Direct measurements of cardiac output and blood volume are difficult during anaesthesia and require invasive procedures which are inappropriate in many situations. However, adequacy of cardiac output and circulating blood volume may be inferred indirectly from observation of the following variables:

1. Peripheral pulse.
2. Peripheral oxygen saturation.
3. Peripheral perfusion.
4. Urine production.
5. Arterial pressure.

The peripheral pulse

Regular palpation of the peripheral pulse is one of the simplest and most useful methods of monitoring during anaesthesia and is mandatory for even the most minor surgery. Information may be obtained by observation of the rate, volume and rhythm.

Pulse plethysmography

Automated devices are available for monitoring peripheral pulsation. They are based on the principle of photoplethysmography. The skin of a suitable digit, or of the pinna of the ear, is illuminated by a weak source of light. The intensity of light transmitted through, or reflected by, the digit waxes and wanes with each capillary pulsation, and this is detected by a photoelectric cell, the signal of which is transduced to display a waveform on an oscilloscope. When a finger is used, inflation of an arterial pressure recording cuff causes the waveform from the pulse meter to flatten. Oscillations reappear when the cuff is deflated below systolic arterial pressure.

The pulse monitor provides a guide to the pulse pressure. Thus an increased signal may be seen in peripheral vasodilatation or increased cardiac output, and a low pulse pressure is seen during vasoconstriction or low cardiac output states.

Pulse oximetry

Reliable pulse oximetry instruments are now available which measure the arterial oxygen saturation and the pulse rate non-invasively and accurately to within $\pm 2\%$. A simple probe is attached to a finger (Fig. 21.3) or ear lobe, flexed across the

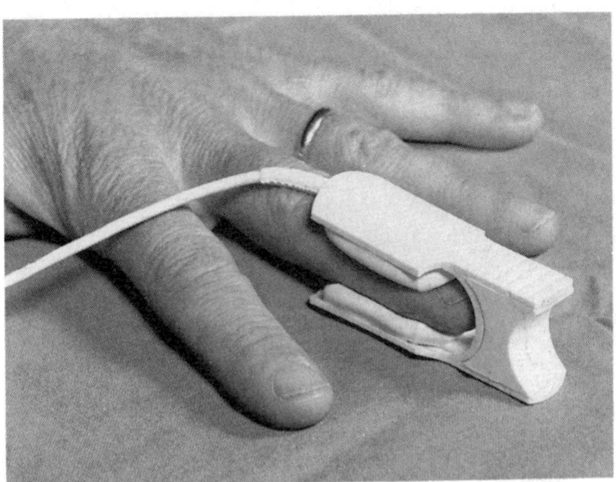

Fig. 21.3 Finger probe for pulse oximeter.

nasal bridge, or wrapped around a child's digit (Fig. 21.4) and connected to the oximeter (Fig. 21.5). The probe contains two light-emitting diodes, one for red and one for infrared light, and a single detector positioned on the opposite side of the digit or ear lobe.

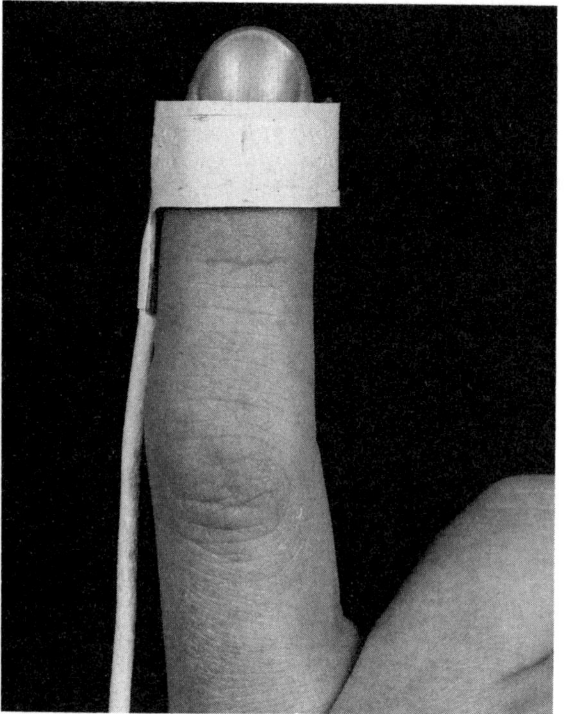

Fig. 21.4 Disposable finger probe for pulse oximeter.

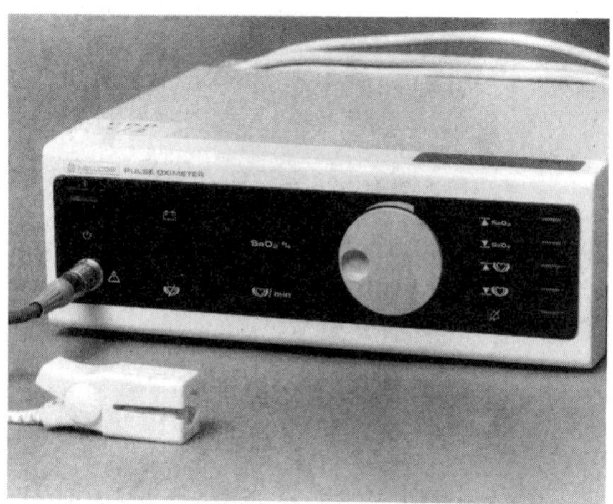

Fig. 21.5 Pulse oximeter control and display module.

The function of the instrument is based on the following principle. The proportion of light absorbed by blood depends on two factors; the wavelength of the light, and the ratio of oxyhaemoglobin to deoxyhaemoglobin (Fig. 21.6). At the isobestic point, absorption is identical; at other wavelengths, the absorption is different but the ratio of absorptions is known. As both forms of haemoglobin are present within a sample of blood the saturation of haemoglobin may be calculated by measuring the absorption at two different wavelengths. Developments in electronics have made it possible to separate the incident light absorbed by the tissues from that absorbed by the

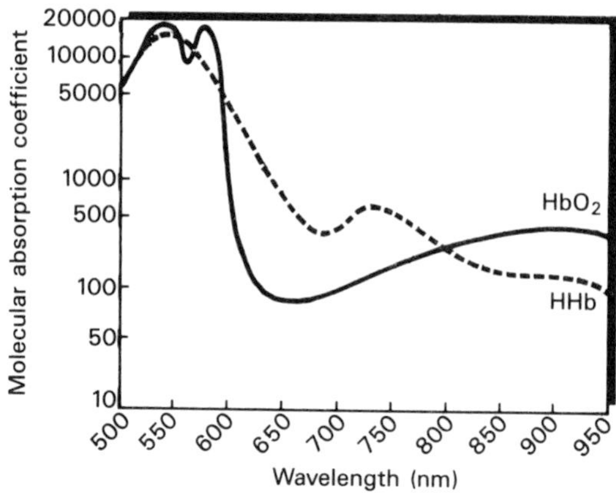

Fig. 21.6 Absorption spectra of reduced (HHb) and oxygenated (HbO_2) haemoglobin.

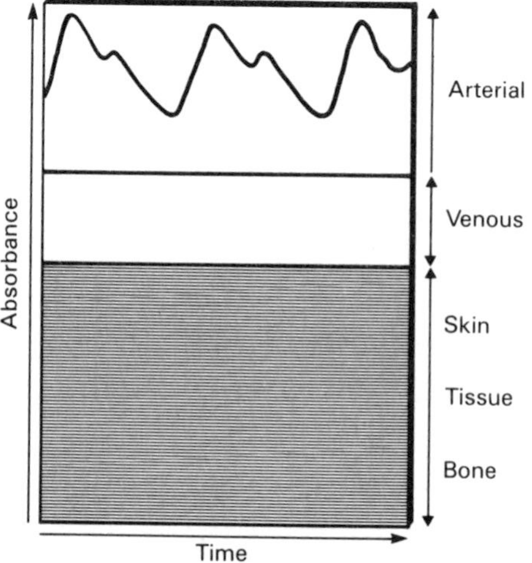

Fig. 21.7 Schematic representation of the contribution of various body components to absorbance of light.

pulsatile arterial component (Fig. 21.7). Thus, the pulse oximeter records only the saturation of arterial blood.

The software is designed to recognise the shape of the pulse waveform so that the saturation of arterial blood only is assessed and in order to minimise errors caused by movement artefact. Recently, a pulse oximeter linked to an ECG signal has been introduced in an attempt to increase the accuracy of pulse detection.

Advantages. Pulse oximeters are simple to use, non-invasive and require no warm-up time. They provide an overall assessment of the integrity of all the systems involved in delivering oxygen to the tissue:

1. Oxygen supply to the patient.
2. Oxygen uptake by the lungs.
3. Oxygen delivery to the tissues via the circulatory system.

Their function is unaffected by pigmented skin. This is a significant advantage in patients of African or Asian origin, in whom hypoxaemia is more difficult to detect clinically.

Disadvantages. Because of the sigmoid shape of the oxyhaemoglobin dissociation curve, there may be a substantial decrease in Pa_{O_2} before saturation begins to decrease; a large change in Pa_{O_2} above 10 kPa (75 mmHg) produces a small change in saturation, but if Pa_{O_2} is less than 10 kPa a small change produces a large change in saturation. A saturation of 94% corresponds to a Pa_{O_2} of 10 kPa. Therefore, the lower alarm limit should be set at this point.

Pulse oximeters read inaccurately in the presence of other forms of haemoglobin, e.g. carboxyhaemoglobin, methaemoglobin or other pigments, e.g. bilirubin. Some models are inaccurate in the presence of poor tissue perfusion or excessive vasoconstriction because of attenuation of the light signal, and also in the presence of excessive incident light.

Pulse oximeters are useful particularly in the following circumstances:

1. Anaesthesia in infants and children.
2. Situations in which rapid fluctuations in oxygen saturation may occur, e.g. during recovery from anaesthesia.
3. One-lung anaesthesia.
4. Conditions of reduced lighting, e.g. in the X-ray department or during ENT procedures.
5. During regional anaesthesia with accompanying sedation.
6. Endoscopic examination.
7. Transport of the critically ill patient.
8. Exacerbations of chronic respiratory disease.
9. Sleep studies.

Peripheral perfusion

Peripheral perfusion is assessed most usefully by observation of the patient's extremities. Warm, dry, pink skin indicates adequate peripheral perfusion; cold white peripheries imply the converse. This is true particularly in children, in whom cool peripheries usually indicate a degree of hypovolaemia. Other methods exist for estimating peripheral blood flow, including ultrasound and venous occlusion plethysmography, but these are not useful for routine monitoring.

The core–peripheral temperature gradient is a useful index of adequacy of peripheral perfusion. One temperature probe is placed centrally (e.g. in the nasopharynx) and the other peripherally (e.g. on the great toe). The temperature gradient increases with vasoconstriction and low cardiac output, and decreases gradually as vasodilatation occurs with increasing limb blood flow consequent upon increasing cardiac output.

Urine output

Adequacy of renal perfusion may be inferred from the volume of urine produced. The kidney is the only organ whose function may be monitored directly in this way. Adequate production of urine implies that perfusion of other vital organs is likely to be adequate. Accurate measurement of urine volumes with, for example, a urimeter, is indicated particularly in the following situations:

1. Major vascular surgery.
2. Massive fluid or blood loss.
3. Major trauma.
4. Critically ill/shocked patients.
5. Cardiac surgery.
6. Surgery in the jaundiced patient.

The aim is to achieve a urine production of 0.5–1 ml kg^{-1} h^{-1}.

Systemic arterial pressure

Measurement of arterial pressure may be classified into indirect or direct methods (Table 21.1).

Measurement of arterial pressure is mandatory during anaesthesia in all patients. It is an indirect method of estimating adequacy of cardiac output, because:

cardiac output = arterial pressure × peripheral resistance

In conjunction with estimation of peripheral perfusion, it is an invaluable measurement. Indirect, non-invasive methods of measurement are appropriate for most types of surgery.

Palpation. Palpation of the radial pulse as the sphygmomanometer cuff is deflated is simple, but inaccurate at low pressures or when vasoconstriction is present.

Auscultation. Auscultation of the Korotkoff sounds is too cumbersome for routine use during anaesthesia.

Oscillotonometry. Von Recklinghausen's oscillotonometer (Figs 21.8 and 21.9) is used widely

Table 21.1 Classification of methods of arterial pressure measurement

Indirect	Direct
Palpation	Intra-arterial manometry
Auscultation	
Oscillotonometry	
Oscillometry	
Doppler ultrasound	

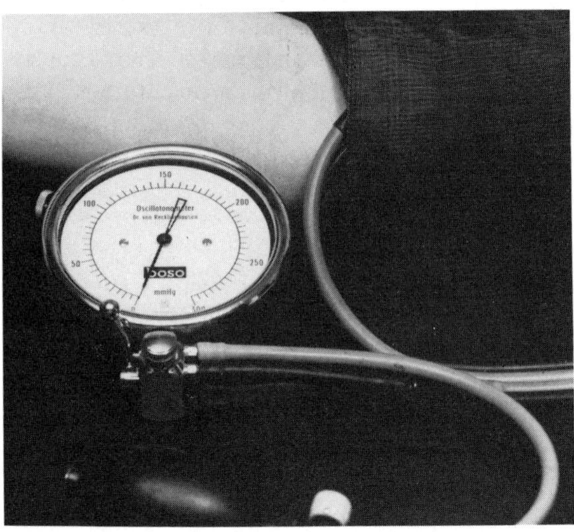

Fig. 21.8 Von Recklinghausen's oscillotonometer.

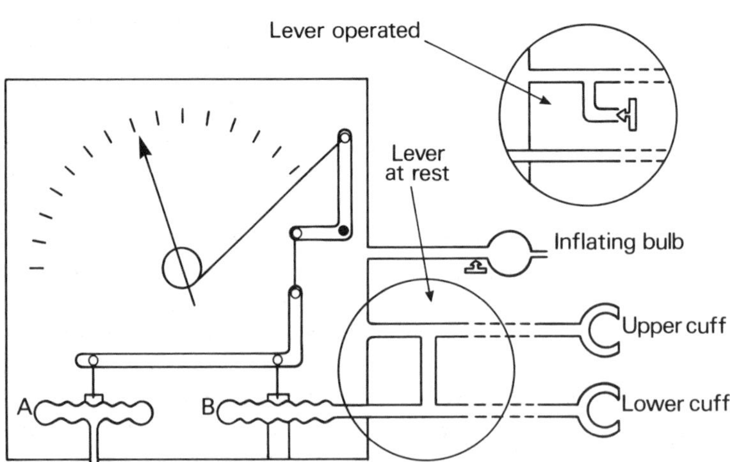

Fig. 21.9 Principle of oscillotonometer. With the control lever at rest, air is pumped into the cuffs and the airtight case of the instrument using the inflating bulb to a pressure exceeding systolic arterial pressure. By operating the lever, the lower cuff is isolated, and the pressure in the upper cuff and instrument case is allowed to decrease slowly through an adjustable leak. As systolic pressure is reached, pulsation of the artery under the lower cuff results in an increase of pressure within the cuff and anaeroid capsule B. The pressure changes are transmitted by a mechanical amplification system to the pointer, which swings with each pulsation. As the pressure in the upper cuff decreases below diastolic pressure, the pulsation ceases. Aneroid capsule A is connected to atmosphere, and changes in pressure inside the instrument case (and upper cuff) result in deflection of the pointer. Although systolic and diastolic pressures are detected when the lever is operated, the true pressure in the upper cuff is recorded with the lever at rest. The lever is therefore operated intermittently, and readings made on detection of pulsatile movement of the pointer.

in anaesthetic practice, and exemplifies the principles of oscillotonometry.

A double cuff, consisting of an upper small occluding cuff which overlaps a lower and longer sensing cuff, is connected to the oscillotonometer. The cuffs are inflated above the anticipated systolic pressure and a slow leak from both cuffs is obtained by unscrewing the case valve and depressing the lever. A complex mechanical amplification system enables the pressure waves arriving at the lower cuff to be displayed as oscillations of the needle. When the needle begins to oscillate, the lever is released and the pressure recorded on the gauge approximates to systolic pressure. The significance of the maximum oscillation point which occurs as the cuffs are deflated is uncertain, and the diastolic pressure cannot be measured accurately with this device.

The oscillotonometer is reliable at low arterial pressures and no stethoscope is necessary. However, it is prone to artefact, e.g. as a result of patient movement or pressure from a surgeon's arm. It is also delicate, and must be serviced regularly.

Oscillometry. The indirect measurement of arterial pressure using automated oscillometry has become popular, although the accuracy of the various machines now available is no better, and in some cases worse, than conventional methods. However, these devices may free the anaesthetist to perform other tasks.

An example of an automated oscillometer is shown in Figure 21.10. These devices incorporate a microprocessor which controls the inflation and deflation sequence. An air pump inflates the cuff; a bleed-valve then deflates it in discrete decrements of pressure. A pressure transducer records the pressure signals, which in turn are interpreted by the microprocessor.

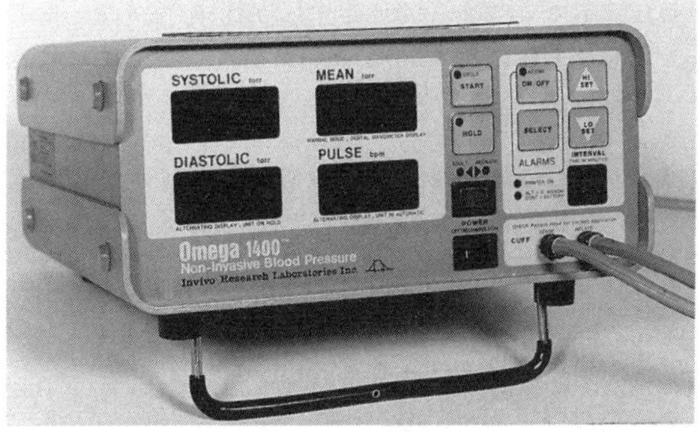

Fig. 21.10 An automated oscillometer.

The single-bladder cuff possesses two tubular connections. Inflation of the cuff occurs through one, and pressure fluctuations are sensed through the other, which is connected to the pressure transducer. An example of the signal generated is shown in Figure 21.11. Systolic, diastolic and mean pressures can be estimated, mean pressure being the minimum pressure at which maximal arterial wall expansion occurs. Heart rate is determined as the median rate calculated from an analysis of all the pressure pulses received during a single determination sequence. Measurements may be instituted at preset intervals ranging from 1/min to 1/h.

A recent review showed that all models tested were inaccurate at a systolic pressure of less than 60 mmHg. In addition, under-reading occurred at high systolic pressures. Invasive methods of measurement are preferable in the shocked patient. Determinations may be impossible during episodes of arrhythmia, and the oscillometer is unable to follow rapid swings in arterial pressure.

Frequent repeated cuff inflations have resulted in ulnar nerve palsy, and may cause petechial haemorrhages of the skin immediately beneath the cuff. Clearly, it is imprudent to apply the cuff to an arm with an intravenous infusion in progress.

Doppler ultrasound. The Doppler principle is utilised in the Arteriosonde. An ultrasound emitter and receiver are placed over the brachial artery and surrounded by an inflatable cuff. As the cuff deflates from just above systolic pressure, the vessel walls begin to move apart during systole. Each movement generates a signal detected by the machine. As the pressure in the cuff decreases further, the vessel walls remain open for longer during each pulsation, and when the cuff pressure equals diastolic pressure, they do not move. Two mercury columns display systolic and diastolic pressures. The main advantages of the method are that it is accurate at low pressures, and that it is suitable for use in children. Disadvantages include its expense and size.

Direct measurement of arterial pressures. This is achieved by attaching a transducer to an intra-arterial cannula inserted percutaneously into a peripheral artery. This is an invasive procedure

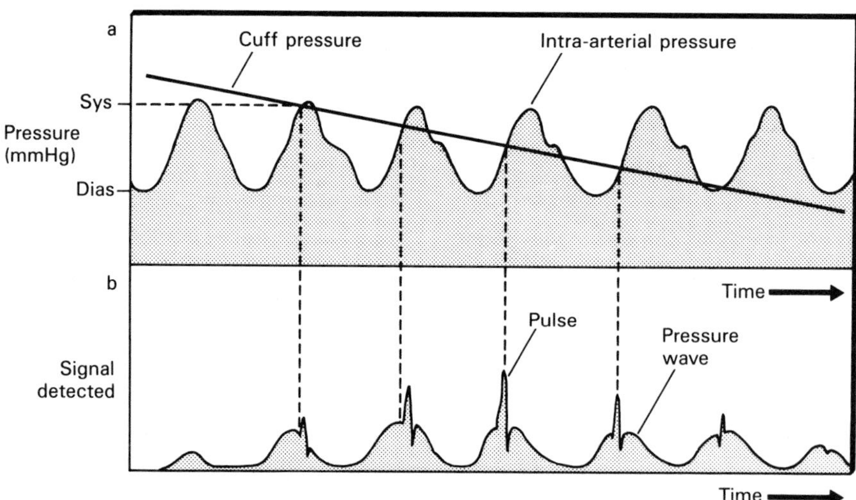

Fig. 21.11 Diagram showing: (a) relationship between cuff pressure and intra-arterial pressure as cuff pressure decreases during oscillometry; (b) the signal created by the relative pressure changes in (a). The sharp spikes of pressure in (b) are created by the walls of the artery opening and closing. These spikes are detected by a transducer first when the cuff pressure is just below systolic arterial pressure; their amplitude reaches a peak at mean arterial pressure and they cease when the cuff pressure is below diastolic arterial pressure.

Table 21.2 Common indications for arterial cannulation

Major vascular surgery
Cardiothoracic surgery
Induced hypotension
Critically ill and shocked patients
Surgery for phaeochromocytoma
Neurosurgery
Necessity for frequent blood gas analysis

Table 21.3 Morbidity associated with long-term arterial cannulation

Arterial wall damage and thrombosis
Embolisation
Disconnection and haemorrhage
Sepsis
Tissue necrosis

which carries potential morbidity. Thus, the method is justified only when rapid changes in arterial pressure are anticipated during anaesthesia. Some indications for arterial cannulation are shown in Table 21.2.

The radial or dorsalis pedis arteries are selected most frequently for cannulation. When using the radial artery, the non-dominant hand should be used if possible. Complications of short-term cannulation (up to 48 h) are relatively minor and infrequent. Long-term cannulation carries risks of morbidity (Table 21.3). Most of these may be minimised by meticulous attention to antisepsis, continuous slow flushing of the cannula with heparinised saline, the use of a Teflon, parallel-sided cannula of small diameter (20- or 22-gauge), and the use of Luer–Lok connections.

The availability of accurate, low volume-displacement miniature strain-gauge transducers has helped to simplify recording of arterial pressure. The transducer should be zeroed, i.e. placed at the same level as the left ventricle, and the system should be calibrated. The transducer is connected to the arterial cannulae via a short piece of stiff-walled, saline-filled manometer tubing. The pressure signal is displayed usually as a waveform on an oscilloscope screen (Fig. 21.12) and systolic, diastolic and mean arterial pressures displayed digitally.

Damping of the system should be adjusted carefully in order to reproduce pressures accurately.

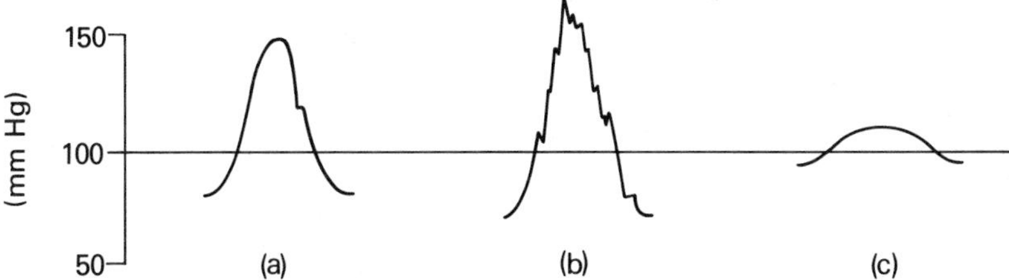

Fig. 21.12 Arterial pressure waveform. (a) Correct, optimally damped waveform. (b) Underdamped waveform, resulting in overestimation of systolic and underestimation of diastolic pressure. (c) Overdamped waveform, resulting in underestimation of systolic and overestimation of diastolic pressure.

The commonest causes of a 'damped' trace are:

1. Air bubbles/blood in the system.
2. Kinking of the cannula.
3. Arterial spasm.

Central venous pressure (CVP)

The placement of a central venous catheter with its tip in the lower superior vena cava or right atrium provides valuable information concerning the volume status of the circulation during anaesthesia. Measurement of CVP is useful in situations similar to those warranting direct measurement of arterial pressure.

Catheters are usually inserted percutaneously via one of the following routes:

1. *Peripheral arm vein*. This route is the least likely to provide correct placement of the catheter (approximately 40%). However, it avoids most of the serious complications of other routes of insertion. Thrombophlebitis and sepsis are common when a peripheral arm vein is used, particularly if the catheter is left in place for more than 48 h.

2. *Internal jugular vein* (Fig. 1.8). This route is associated with the highest incidence of correct catheter placement (approximately 90%). Numerous techniques have been described for insertion of a catheter into the internal jugular vein. Common complications are listed in Table 21.4. Secure fixation of an internal jugular catheter is difficult.

3. *Subclavian vein*. This approach is more hazardous than the internal jugular, and less likely to provide correct catheter placement. However, it is the most suitable route if long-term cannulation is contemplated, e.g. to facilitate parenteral feeding. The main complications of insertion at this site are shown in Table 21.5.

Table 21.4 Complications of internal jugular cannulation

Air embolism
Carotid artery puncture
Brachial plexus/phrenic nerve damage
Ectopic placement (numerous sites)
Sepsis
Pneumothorax

Table 21.5 Complications of subclavian vein cannulation

Pneumothorax
Subclavian artery puncture
Air embolism
Damage to thoracic duct (left side)

Whichever route is chosen, meticulous attention to antisepsis is necessary. Backflow of blood should always be confirmed before starting infusion of fluid. Numerous complications have been documented, associated particularly with routes of entry in the neck, and these approaches are unsuitable for the unskilled unless properly supervised.

The position of any central venous catheter should be confirmed by chest X-ray as soon as possible after insertion. Oscillations of pressure should be observed with ventilation. Large oscillations in time with heart rate may indicate insertion into the right ventricle, and the catheter should be withdrawn accordingly.

Measurement of CVP. The catheter is connected to a fluid-filled water manometer column via a three-way stopcock (Fig. 21.13). Alternatively, the catheter may be connected to a transducer, as with arterial pressure monitoring, and the waveform displayed on a screen. The surface markings of the right atrium, the true zero reference point, are shown in Figure 21.14. The normal range of values is 0–6 cmH_2O. It is sometimes simpler to use the manubriosternal junction as the reference point, in which case the value obtained for central venous pressure is 5–10 cm lower than the true right atrial measurement at the mid-axillary line.

Trends in measured observations are more valuable than absolute values. For example, in a patient undergoing major arterial surgery, a decrease in CVP from +5 to +1 cm H_2O indicates considerable fluid loss which warrants therapeutic intervention, even though the lower value is still within the 'normal' range.

Measurement of CVP is a valuable aid to blood and fluid replacement. If CVP increases above normal and remains high with no improvement in arterial pressure, it is likely that myocardial failure has occurred and inotropic support may be required.

Pulmonary artery pressure monitoring

In the normal individual, CVP measurement provides a reasonably accurate estimate of the filling pressures of both right and left atria. In some clinical situations, however, the central venous or right atrial pressure does not correlate with pressure in the left atrium, and infusion of fluids or inotropic agents titrated against CVP may not result in optimum cardiac function. Dissociation between left atrial and central venous (right atrial) pressures occurs in:

1. Left ventricular failure with pulmonary oedema.
2. Interstitial pulmonary oedema of any aetiology.
3. Chronic pulmonary disease.
4. Valvular heart disease.

If such patients are about to undergo major surgery, it may be desirable to monitor pressures in the pulmonary circulation and left side of the heart. This is achieved by the use of a balloon-tipped flow-directed pulmonary artery catheter (Figs 21.15 and 21.16).

The simplest form of catheter has two channels, one for inflation of the balloon and one for

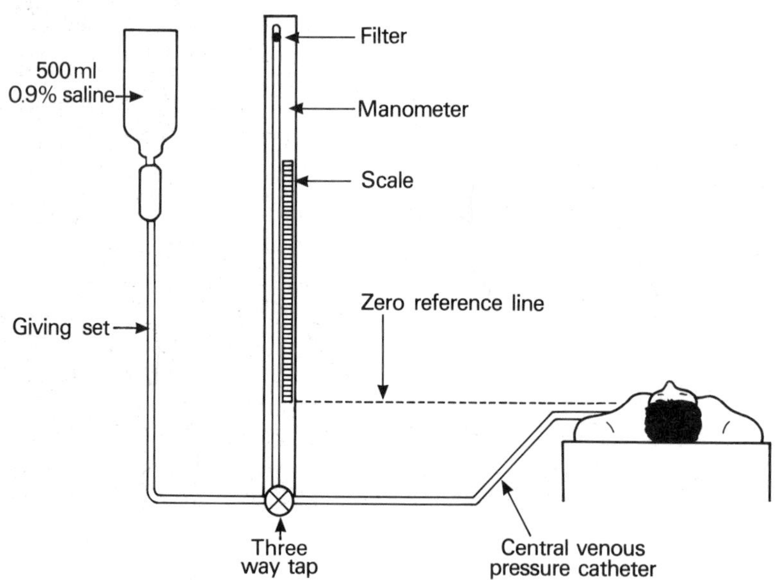

Fig. 21.13 Measurement of CVP using a manometer. The manometer tubing is filled from the infusion bag and the tap turned to connect the manometer to the central venous catheter. The fluid level in the manometer falls until the height of the fluid column above the zero reference point is equal to the central venous pressure.

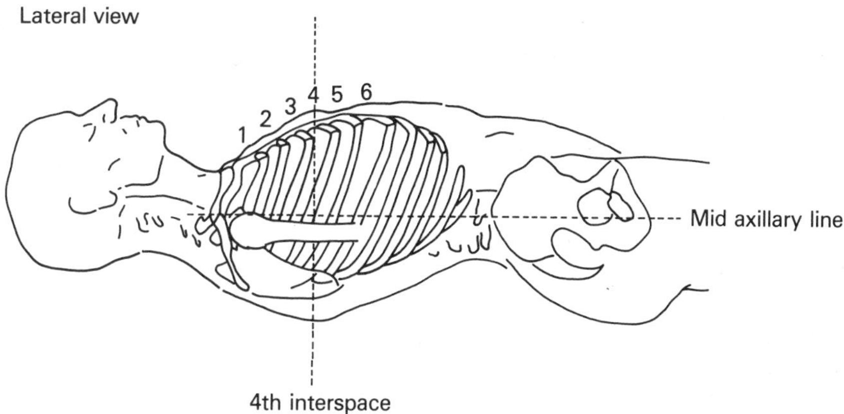

Fig. 21.14 Surface markings used to identify the position of the right atrium.

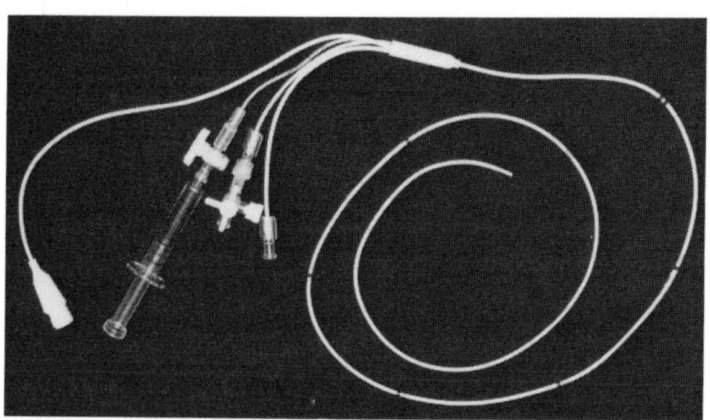

Fig. 21.15 Pulmonary artery catheter.

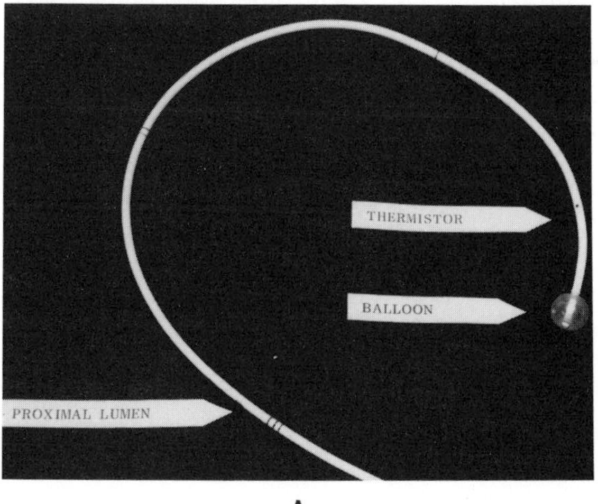

A

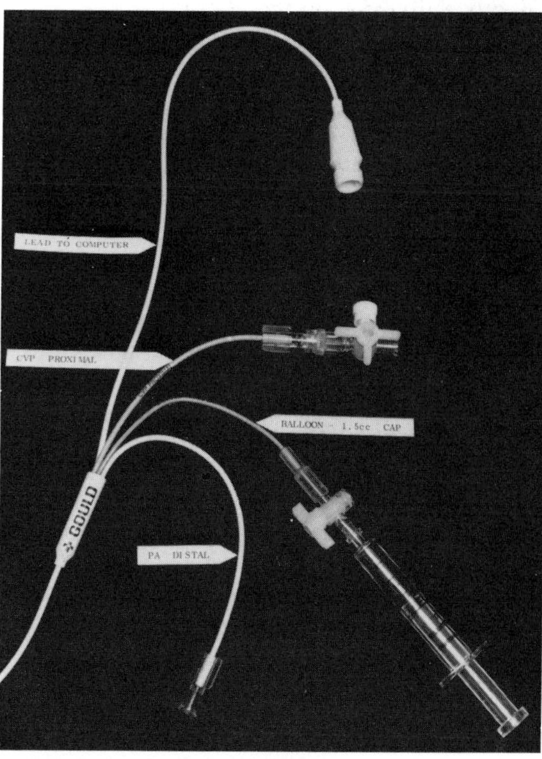

B

Fig. 21.16 (a) Distal end of pulmonary artery catheter, showing inflated balloon, thermistor and position of end of the proximal lumen. (b) Proximal end of pulmonary artery catheter. The proximal lumen may be used for measurement of CVP and the distal lumen for measurement of pulmonary artery pressure. The connection from the thermistor is used in conjunction with a cardiac output computer. The balloon capacity is normally 1–1.5 ml.

measurement of pressure at the tip. It is marked at 10 cm intervals in order to facilitate insertion. More sophisticated versions of this device have four lumina:

1. *The proximal lumen.* This is situated approximately 25 cm from the tip and should lie in the right atrium after final placement of the catheter. CVP may be measured using this lumen.
2. *The distal lumen.* Situated at the tip of the catheter, this lumen lies in a major branch of the pulmonary artery when the catheter is placed correctly and is used to measure pulmonary artery pressure by connecting it to a suitable transducer.
3. *The balloon lumen.* This lumen permits the introduction of approximately 1 ml of air into the balloon which surrounds the distal tip of the catheter.
4. *Thermistor lumen.* A bead thermistor is situated 4 cm from the tip of the catheter and measures the temperature of blood at this site. This is used in measurement of cardiac output (vide infra).

The pulmonary artery catheter is inserted via a central vein, usually the internal jugular or subclavian. A vein dilator is necessary to facilitate its introduction. The port of the distal lumen is connected to a pressure transducer and the pressure signal displayed on an oscilloscope screen. When the catheter reaches the right atrium (indicated by a venous pressure waveform on the screen; Fig. 21.17) the balloon is inflated and the catheter advanced slowly and gently. The balloon helps to 'float' the catheter through the right ventricle, where the typical ventricular waveform replaces that of the atrium. The catheter then passes into the pulmonary artery, when the waveform again alters. Further advancement of the catheter into a branch of the pulmonary artery should show typical 'wedging' of the waveform. At this stage, a continuous column of fluid connects the left atrium via the pulmonary veins and capillaries to the catheter. Thus, the pressure measured reflects left atrial pressure. As soon as this pressure is obtained, the balloon is deflated. Constant inflation may cause pulmonary infarction.

Occasionally, arrhythmias may be encountered during insertion, and suitable therapeutic agents should be available.

Uses of the pulmonary artery catheter include:

1. The assessment of the volume status of the patient in conditions where CVP is unreliable (vide supra).
2. Sampling of mixed venous blood in order to calculate shunt fraction (see Ch. 3).
3. Measurement of cardiac output using the thermodilution method.

Measurement of cardiac output. The thermistor lead is connected to a cardiac output computer. 10 ml of glucose 5% at room temperature are injected as quickly as possible through the proximal lumen. The temperature of the blood arriving at the thermistor near the tip of the catheter is measured. The computer calculates the degree of dilution of the relatively cold injectate,

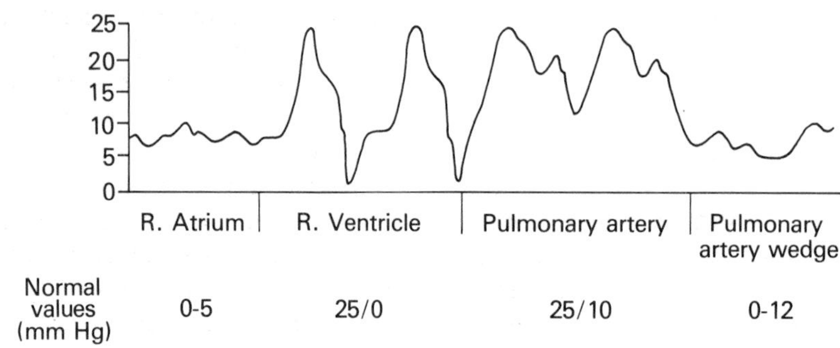

Fig. 21.17 Diagrammatic representation of pressure waveforms seen on an oscilloscope as the tip of a pulmonary artery catheter is advanced through the right atrium and right ventricle to lie in the pulmonary artery. The 'pulmonary artery wedge' waveform is seen when the balloon is inflated with the tip of the catheter in a branch of the pulmonary artery. Normal values shown represent pressures in a spontaneously breathing patient.

and from this extrapolates the cardiac output. This method has been shown to correlate well with the Fick method of measuring cardiac output.

Complications of pulmonary artery catheterisation are not negligible and include:

1. Arrhythmias on insertion.
2. Knotting of the catheter in the right ventricle .
3. Balloon rupture.
4. Pulmonary infarction.
5. Infection.

The device should be used for as short a period of time as necessary, and only in exceptional circumstances for longer than 48 h.

Non-invasive measurement of cardiac output

Thoracic impedance cardiography. If a high-frequency alternating current is applied across the chest, cyclical changes occur in transthoracic impedance during the cardiac cycle because of ejection of blood, which possesses a relatively high conductance, into the thoracic cavity. These changes are related to stroke volume. Two electrodes are used to apply the alternating current, and the voltage changes are detected by a second pair of electrodes. Impedance cardiography is less accurate than thermodilution in measuring absolute cardiac output, but provides a reliable indication of trends.

Doppler systems. Doppler ultrasound provides a non-invasive and virtually continuous method of measuring cardiac output. Two values must be determined; the blood velocity and the aortic diameter; the first may be measured, but the second must be calculated (albeit from known measurements), and this results in the major inaccuracy of the technique. The probe may be placed over the suprasternal notch, which may not be accessible easily during anaesthesia, or it may be mounted at the tip of an oesophageal stethoscope and placed behind the descending aorta. Information related to changes in cardiac output are useful, but absolute measurements are inaccurate, with the devices currently available.

Two-dimensional echocardiography. This technique may also be used to measure ventricular volumes, cardiac output, ejection fraction and regional myocardial muscle performance. The probe may be applied either over the relevant part of the precordium or mounted on an oesophageal stethoscope and placed in the oesophagus behind the ventricle. The usefulness of this device remains to be assessed fully in anaesthetic practice.

Measurement of blood loss

Losses of up to 10% of blood volume (i.e. approximately 7 ml/kg in the adult) are tolerated well and may be replaced by an appropriate volume of crystalloid solution. Blood loss in excess of 10% of blood volume during surgery should be replaced as whole blood.

It is prudent to weigh wet swabs when losses appear to be mounting and then subtract the weight of an equivalent number of dry swabs in order to obtain an estimate of blood loss. This is particularly important in children. However, the method is notoriously inaccurate; it ignores blood lost on drapes, gowns, etc., and unless weighing is carried out promptly, weight is lost because of evaporation of water. A more accurate method is that which employs colorimetry; swabs, gowns and drapes are washed with a known volume of fluid, and the haemoglobin content measured colorimetrically. Clearly, this can be performed only at the end of the procedure.

THE RESPIRATORY SYSTEM

Clinical monitoring of ventilation

Continuous observation should be made of the following: the patient's colour, respiratory rate, adequacy of chest movement and the movement of the reservoir bag or ventilator bellows. Auscultation of both lung fields should also be performed frequently in order to detect equality of air entry, intubation of a bronchus, presence of secretions or the occurrence of a pneumothorax. In addition, the anaesthetist must check regularly for signs of respiratory obstruction as evidenced by tracheal tug, paradoxical abdominal movement and absence of bag deflation. Some ventilators make a regular noise during part of the ventilating cycle and this is a valuable audible monitor.

Oesophageal stethoscope

This method of monitoring the cardiovascular and respiratory systems (Fig. 21.18) is in common use in the USA, but is not employed with sufficient frequency in the UK. It permits the anaesthetist to monitor heart and breath sounds continuously. A moulded earpiece renders the device more comfortable. Alterations in heart sounds, air entry to the tracheobronchial tree and the development of abnormal breath sounds, e.g. crepitations or rhonchi, may be detected readily. In procedures subject to the risk of air embolism, e.g. hip joint replacement and some neurosurgical operations, air is audible if it enters the great veins or cardiac chambers.

The oesophageal stethoscope is simple, cheap, safe, non-invasive and free from electrical interference. Its routine use is recommended in intraoperative monitoring.

Measurement of airway pressure

A simple manometer which measures the pressure of the gases delivered to the airway is incorporated into most mechanical ventilators. Observation of changes in this pressure is vital. Airway pressure may reflect changes in lung and chest wall compliance if the ventilator is of the volume-cycled, or time-cycled volume-preset, variety (see Ch. 17). Chest wall compliance may be influenced by the degree of muscle paralysis, surgical manipulation and the position of the patient, and lung compliance by accumulation of secretions, or the development of a pneumothorax. Increased resistance to airflow caused by bronchospasm or obstruction of the tracheal tube is reflected by an increased peak airway pressure.

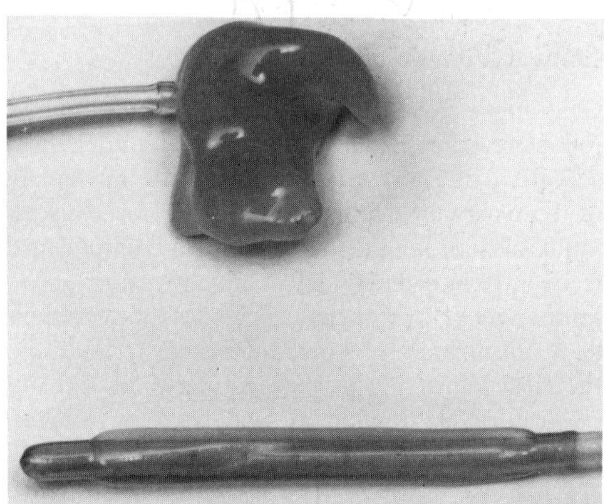

Fig. 21.18 An oesophageal stethoscope.

Causes of excessive elevation of airway pressure

1. Kinking of ventilator tubing or tracheal tube.
2. Overinflation of tracheal tube cuff with consequent obstruction of the lumen of the tube.
3. Increased secretions.
4. Pneumothorax.
5. Bronchospasm.
6. Inadequate muscle relaxation.

Disconnection alarm

When the lungs are ventilated mechanically, the continuity of the anaesthetic breathing system, and thus of gas delivery to the patient, should be monitored using a disconnection alarm. An example is shown in Figure 21.19. The alarm is activated if the airway pressure decreases below a preset minimum for a preset time interval. A large leak, or total disconnection, is indicated if the alarm is triggered. In addition, most of these devices sound an alarm if excessive airway pressures are generated. A disconnection alarm does not obviate the need for visual surveillance of the continuity of the breathing system.

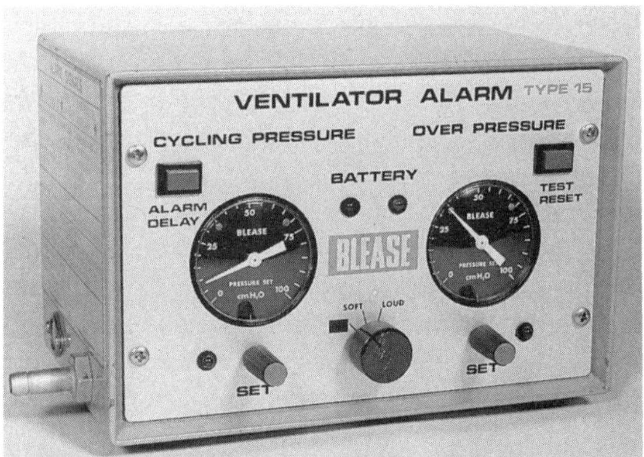

Fig. 21.19 A ventilator disconnection alarm.

Measurement of inspired and expired volumes

A device for measuring inspired and expired lung volumes should always be incorporated into the breathing system when a patient receives intermittent positive pressure ventilation (IPPV). A Wright respirometer (Fig. 21.20) is used commonly and is mounted usually in the expiratory limb of the breathing system, so that leaks which occur in the inspiratory limb are eliminated from the evaluation of expired minute volume. It should be sited as near to the tracheal tube as possible to minimise the effects of system compliance on its function.

A

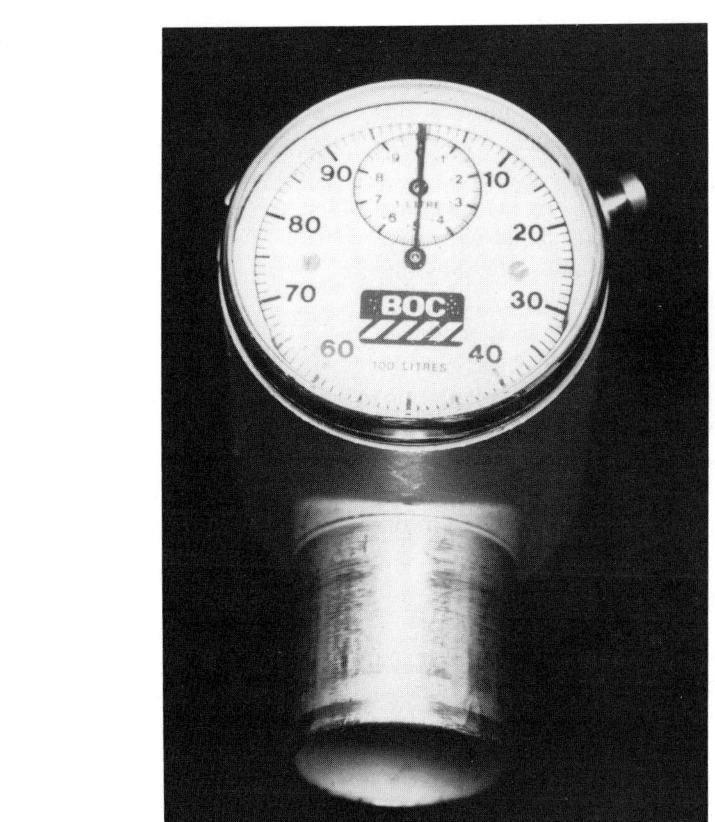

B

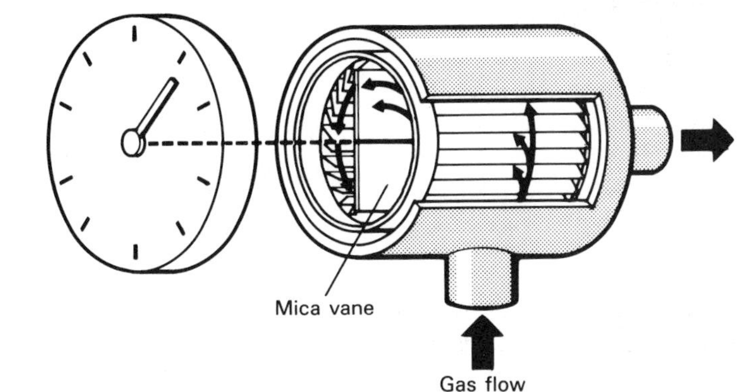

Fig. 21.20 (a) Wright respirometer. (b) Diagrammatic representation of mechanism (see text for details).

The Wright respirometer is a vane anemometer. The vane rotates within a small cylinder, the walls of which are perforated with a number of tangential slits, so that the air stream causes the vane to rotate. Rotation of the vane drives the pointer around the dial and gas volume is recorded. It tends to over-read at high tidal volumes and under-read at low volumes as a result of its inertia. Its function is affected by moisture, which causes the pointer to stick; thus, it should be switched off when not in use. In the electronic version, rotation of the vane is detected electronically; this reduces the inaccuracies caused by water condensation.

The pneumotachograph (Fig. 16.15) measures gas flow rate and integrates this signal with time to produce a calculated gas volume. The flow rate is derived from the pressure decrease across a resistance (see p. 276). Laminar flow is produced by using multiple small tubes. The head may be heated electrically to avoid water condensation, which increases resistance to flow. This instrument is expensive and requires expert calibration and maintenance. Consequently, it is not used routinely, although pneumotachographs are incorporated into some ventilators used in the intensive therapy unit.

MONITORING GAS DELIVERY AND EXCRETION

Oxygen delivery

1. To the patient

Before using an anaesthetic machine, the anaesthetist must assess whether it is functioning correctly, particularly with regard to delivery of oxygen (see Ch. 17). All anaesthetic machines should be fitted with an oxygen failure alarm which provides an audible and/or visual warning if the oxygen pressure decreases. A full spare cylinder of oxygen should always be available on the anaesthetic machine when piped gases are in use.

Inspired oxygen concentration

An oxygen analyser should be used in every anaesthetic breathing system to ensure that the required

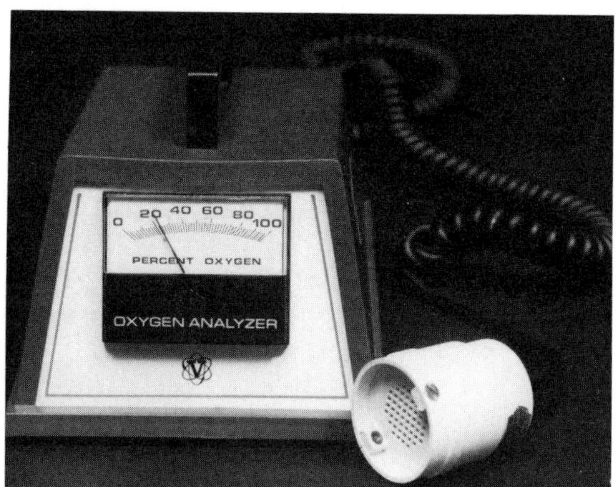

Fig. 21.21 A fuel cell oxygen analyser.

concentration of oxygen is delivered to the patient. A galvanic (fuel cell) oxygen analyser (Fig. 21.21) generates a current proportional to the partial pressure of oxygen; this is achieved by reduction of oxygen at a silver cathode connected through a thin film of electrolyte solution to a lead anode. These instruments may be placed in the inspiratory limb of the breathing system, and have a 90% response time of approximately 20 s. They are accurate to within ±3%, are calibrated simply using air, are not affected by humidity and are powered by battery.

It is important to appreciate that oxygen analysers measure partial pressure, although the display is calibrated in percentage of oxygen. If these devices are positioned between the gas outlet port of an anaesthetic machine and a gas-driven ventilator (e.g. Munley), the total gas pressure to which the detector is subjected increases by 25–30%. The partial pressure of oxygen increases by the same percentage, and the display indicates an erroneously high oxygen concentration. The analyser should be positioned in the inspiratory limb of the breathing system to overcome this problem.

2. To the tissues

Pulse oximetry

This has become the standard method of measuring oxygen delivery to the tissues. It is described fully on page 365.

Transcutaneous P_{O_2}(TcP_{O_2}) measurement

The instrument used to measure this parameter is a modified Clark electrode (Fig. 21.22) applied to the skin surface. However, to ensure that TcP_{O_2}approximates to Pa_{O_2}, the skin must be rendered hyperaemic by heating to 45°C. The transcutaneous P_{O_2} electrode provides a continuous, non-invasive estimate of arterial oxygen tension.

The instrument requires a warm-up period of 15 min, calibration and subsequently a 5-min equilibration period. There is good correlation, at least in infants, between $TcP_{O_2}$and Pa_{O_2}. The response time is 10–15 s when the skin is thin, and the device is reliable in following trends. However, the equipment is cumbersome and expensive. In adults with a thicker skin, correlation is less good and decreases with increasing age.

Carbon dioxide excretion

1. In expired gas

It is important to ensure adequate carbon dioxide elimination during anaesthesia because of the deleterious effects of raised arterial carbon dioxide tension (Pa_{CO_2}).

End-tidal CO_2 tension (Pe'_{CO_2})

Pe'_{CO_2} correlates well with Pa_{CO_2} in patients who have no significant pulmonary disease. The normal Pa_{CO_2}–Pe'_{CO_2} gradient is approximately 0.7 kPa (5 mmHg). End-tidal CO_2 concentration may be measured using the principle of infrared absorption spectrophotometry. Infrared rays are passed through two identical channels; one contains the sampled gas and the other acts as a reference. Carbon dioxide absorbs infrared light and the extent of absorption is measured as a reduction in heat generated at a detector. Infrared light is absorbed by many gases, including nitrous oxide and anaesthetic vapours, and appropriate measures are taken to minimise errors caused by their presence in the sample.

A number of machines are marketed which measure CO_2 concentration breath by breath. The example shown in Figure 21.23 determines also the concentrations of nitrous oxide and oxygen in the inspired gas, and computes the respiratory rate. The sampling probe is placed as near as poss-

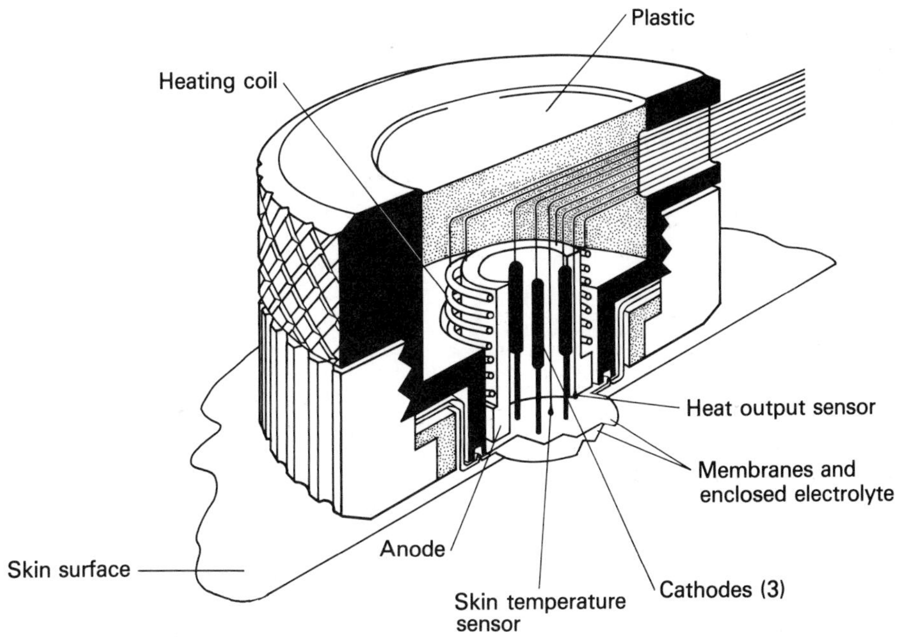

Fig. 21.22 Diagram of a transcutaneous P_{O_2} electrode.

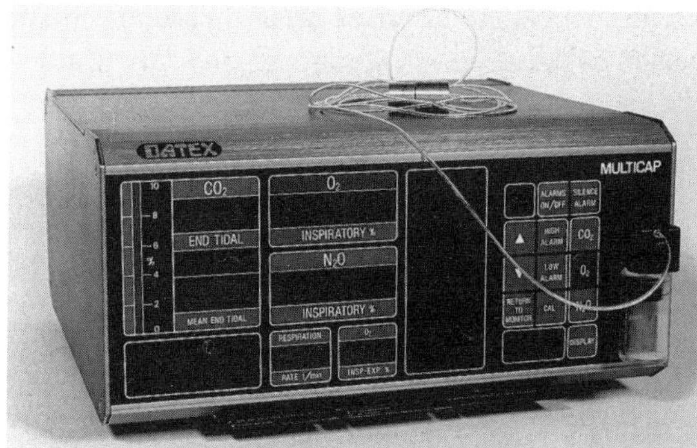

Fig. 21.23 A capnograph for measurement of CO_2 concentration in a gas mixture. This model also measures nitrous oxide and oxygen concentrations.

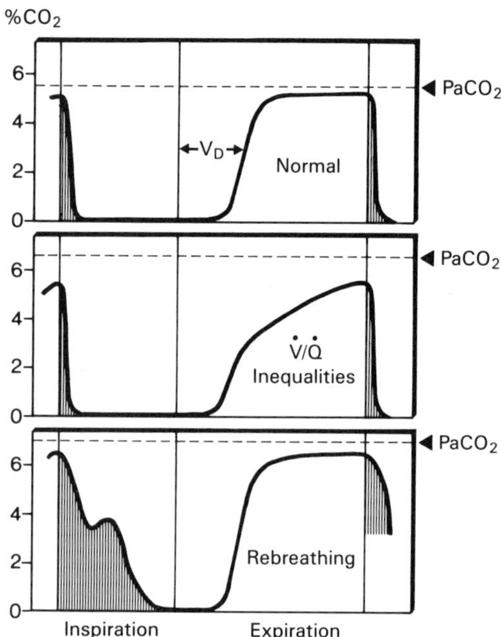

Fig. 21.24 CO_2 traces recorded from the proximal end of the tracheal tube to illustrate the altered pattern of alveolar plateau in a patient with ventilation/perfusion ($\dot{V}/\dot{Q}$) inequalities. The bottom trace shows the presence of CO_2 in inspired gas during spontaneous ventilation with a Bain breathing system supplied with an inadequate flow rate of fresh gas.

ible to the patient's mouth. Tracheal tubes are available which incorporate a pilot tube to sample gas near the tip; these ensure a more representative end-tidal sample. A digital or analogue signal of end-tidal CO_2 is displayed by the capnograph.

A printer may be used to provide a permanent record of expired CO_2 concentrations, permitting trended information to be obtained. Information regarding $\dot{V}/\dot{Q}$ inequalities and rebreathing may be gleaned from the printed capnogram (Fig. 21.24).

Capnography is useful particularly in the following circumstances:

1. To provide evidence of correct placement of the tracheal tube. Capnography is the only method available which provides rapid diagnosis of intubation of the oesophagus.
2. For routine monitoring of the adequacy of ventilation and the effects of IPPV.
3. To detect rebreathing.
4. To detect air, fat or pulmonary embolism; a sudden decrease in Pe'_{CO_2} occurs as a result of increased deadspace.
5. To detect malignant hyperpyrexia; a progressive increase in Pe'_{CO_2} is produced by increased muscle metabolism.
6. To ensure normocapnia in elderly patients in an attempt to maintain adequate cerebral perfusion.
7. To maintain normal Pe'_{CO_2} during carotid artery surgery in order to maintain cerebral perfusion.

The technique may provide inaccurate measurements in the presence of:

1. Respiratory frequency greater than 15 breaths/min (e.g. children).
2. Chronic respiratory disease ($\dot{V}/\dot{Q}$ abnormalities)
3. Hypotension and blood loss ($\dot{V}/\dot{Q}$ abnormalities)
4. High inspired oxygen concentrations.

2. In tissues

Transcutaneous P_{CO_2}(TcP_{CO_2}) monitoring

Devices for measurement of TcP_{CO_2} are at present undergoing clinical trials and have already proved useful in the management of acutely ill neonates. In adults, there are numerous technical problems.

Pa_{CO_2} changes much less rapidly than Pa_{O_2} after apnoea, making TcP_{CO_2} less useful as an emergency warning device. In addition, the instrument has a slow response time: 5 min to 90% response.

TcP_{CO_2} consistently reads higher than arterial P_{CO_2}, but there is a good correlation over a wide range of values up to 8 kPa. The skin must be heated to increase blood flow and reduce arterial-capillary P_{CO_2} gradient.

Anaesthetic vapour delivery

Inspired and expired concentrations of halothane, enflurane and isoflurane may be measured on a breath-by-breath basis. Devices may be classified into two categories, based on the physical principle employed.

Infrared analysers

An example of this type of machine is shown in Figure 21.25. Gas is sampled from the breathing system into a measuring chamber, where the concentration of vapour is measured using infrared absorption spectrophotometry (vide supra). Volatile vapours absorb infrared light to varying degrees depending on their concentration and composition. The resulting transmitted radiation is converted into an electrical signal. Sample flow is approximately 200 ml/min but this gas can be returned to the breathing system; thus, these instruments are suitable for use during closed-circuit anaesthesia. Readings are unaffected by the presence of nitrous oxide or carbon dioxide. Water vapour has a negligible effect. The response time of this instrument is inadequate to give accurate breath-by-breath monitoring if the respiratory frequency exceeds 15/min.

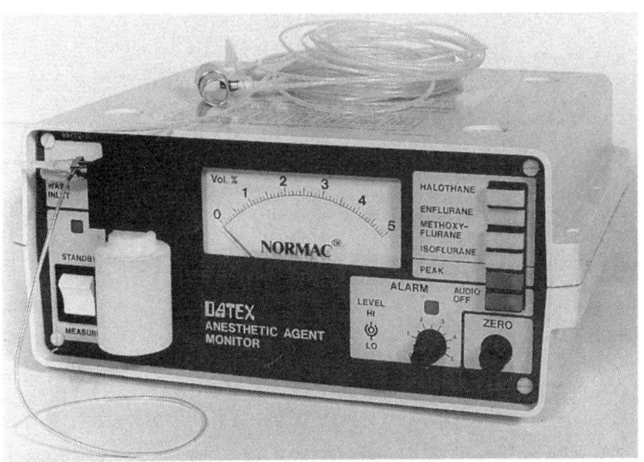

Fig. 21.25 An infrared monitor for measurement of concentrations of volatile anaesthetic agents.

Quartz crystal oscillators

The EMMA multigas analyser is an example of this type of machine. The resonant frequency of a highly stable quartz crystal oscillator changes as a result of interaction between the coating of the crystal and its surrounding gas. This oscillation produces an electrical signal proportional to the vapour concentration. The crystal is mounted in a compact measuring head which is positioned in the anaesthetic breathing system. Water vapour produces some artefact, and this, together with the weight of the measuring head, makes the device less suitable for use with the closed circuit.

Both types of instrument may be used to check the calibration of vaporisers.

Mass spectrometer

At present, this versatile but bulky and expensive instrument is used mainly as a research tool. It provides extremely rapid and accurate measurements of a number of gases simultaneously. Smaller, cheaper devices will be available in the near future for use in the operating theatre.

THE NERVOUS SYSTEM

Central nervous system

Monitoring of the central nervous system during anaesthesia is concerned primarily with estimation of depth of unconsciousness, in order to avoid awareness or vivid unpleasant dreams.

Clinical monitoring

Observations of the signs of sympathetic overactivity (lacrimation, sweating, increase in pupil size, increase in heart rate or arterial pressure) and reflex movements indicate that anaesthesia is too 'light'. However, numerous investigations have shown that these signs are unreliable indicators of inadequate narcosis.

A more sophisticated attempt to detect the occurrence of awareness comprises isolation of one arm from the remainder of the circulation by inflation of a tourniquet on the upper arm before injection of relaxant into the systemic circulation. It is suggested that in this way contact may be maintained with the patient, who indicates when he or she is aware by responding to the anaesthetist's questions with a squeeze of the isolated hand. However, many anaesthetists regard this technique as unsatisfactory.

Lower oesophageal contractility

It has been suggested that lower oesophageal contractility may act as an indicator of the depth of anaesthesia. The smooth muscle of the lower oesophagus is unaffected by muscle relaxants. Two types of activity occur during anaesthesia and these may be measured simply and non-invasively by passing a balloon-tipped catheter into the oesophagus. Tertiary activity (spontaneous, non-peristaltic contractions) occur with a frequency which is stress-related, and secondary, peristaltic waves may be provoked by inflation of a second, air-filled balloon in the oesophageal lumen. The frequency of tertiary contractions and the amplitude of secondary contractions decrease with increasing concentrations of i.v. or volatile anaesthetic agents, and increase in response to surgical stimulation. However, there is enormous interindividual variability in oesophageal contractions, and the method cannot be used reliably to indicate depth of anaesthesia.

Cerebral function monitor

The conventional electroencephalograph (EEG) is too cumbersome for routine theatre use. The cerebral function monitor (CFM) is a device which integrates the total electrical activity in the brain.

Two parietal needle electrodes record the electrical signal for display on an X-Y plotter. The height of the signal against the axis is proportional to the amplitude of cerebral electrical rhythms. Changes in the height and width of the trace correspond to changes in cerebral electrical function (Fig. 21.26). This device appears to be capable of detecting changes in depth of total i.v. anaesthesia, but is unreliable when volatile agents are used. It is employed principally in situations in which cerebral ischaemia may occur, e.g. carotid artery or cardiac surgery.

A more recent model, the cerebral function analysing monitor (CFAM), provides the facility to display both the amplitude and frequency of cerebral electrical activity separately, again indicating trends in cerebral activity. Separate electrodes enable the function of each hemisphere to be monitored. The data provided are amenable to statistical analysis by computer. This device is also capable of computing evoked potentials (see Ch. 5) and of measuring the spontaneous scalp electromyogram (EMG). Increasing amplitude of the EMG reflects an increase in patient activity. Facial and scalp muscles are less sensitive to muscle relaxants than peripheral muscles and this may be a promising way of detecting pain and awareness during relaxant anaesthesia.

The CFM may be useful in:

1. Cardiac surgery.
2. Carotid artery surgery.
3. Neurosurgery.
4. Total i.v. anaesthesia.
5. Status epilepticus — if neuromuscular blockers are used.
6. Hypotensive anaesthesia.
7. Drug overdose.

Cerebral blood flow (CBF)

The measurement of CBF using a gamma camera and radioactive isotope injection provides the most accurate measurement of cerebral perfusion. However, this method is too cumbersome and complicated for routine application.

MONITORING THE NEUROMUSCULAR JUNCTION

See Chapter 12.

MONITORING OF METABOLISM

Homeostasis of the main metabolic processes of the body must be assured during anaesthesia. Monitoring of the following functions should be considered for all but minor surgery.

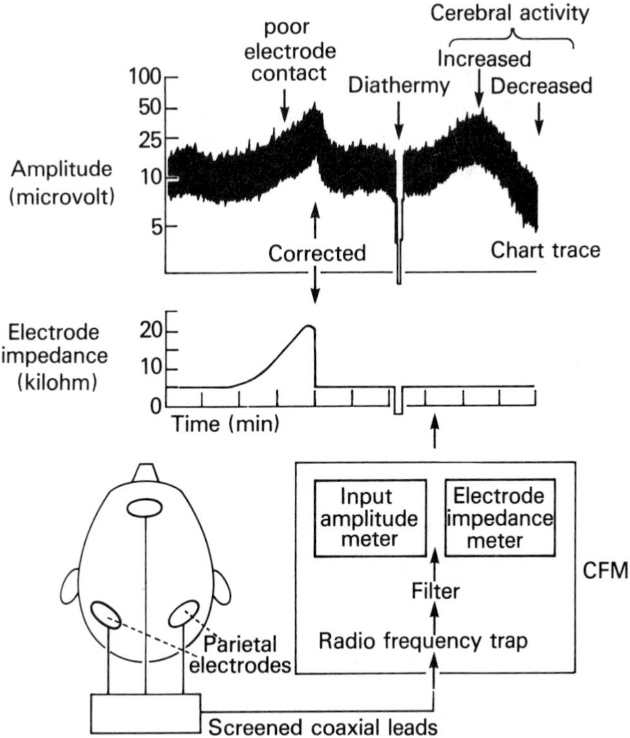

Fig. 21.26 The cerebral function monitor. Screened electrical signals displayed on the upper trace depict cerebral activity. Allowance must be made for alterations in electrode impedance and interference from extraneous electrical sources.

Temperature regulation

General anaesthesia inhibits the patient's ability to maintain body temperature by depressing the thermoregulatory centre in the hypothalamus. Heat loss during anaesthesia is potentiated by surgery of long duration and exposure of large surface areas of tissue, e.g. the abdominal contents during gastrointestinal operations. The use of wet packs and dry inspired gases compounds the problem. These sources of heat loss assume even more importance in children, especially small babies, whose surface area is much larger in proportion to body weight than in the adult.

During operations where these factors are important, core temperature must be monitored and efforts made to minimise heat loss. Measures to minimise heat loss include the following:

1. The operating room temperature should be as high as is comfortable for the theatre staff.
2. A warming mattress should be placed beneath the patient.
3. Exposed surfaces should be swaddled with warm gauze or foil, especially in neonates.
4. All i.v. infusion fluids should be warmed.
5. Inspired gases should be warmed and humidified.

The thermistor probe is the most commonly used type of temperature measuring device. It consists of a bead of a mixture of non-metal oxides which is thermally sensitive and the resistance of which varies non-linearly with temperature.

The probe may be placed in the following positions in order to measure core temperature:

1. The nasopharynx (approximates to brain temperature).
2. The oesophagus (approximates to cardiac temperature).
3. The tympanic membrane (best for core temperature, but the membrane is delicate and easily damaged).
4. The rectum.

It is useful also to measure the temperature of the inspired gases when an efficient humidifer is employed in order to avoid thermal burns to the respiratory tract.

If core temperature decreases during anaesthesia, this may result in intense shivering during recovery. This in turn results in increased oxygen consumption (5–10 times normal), disturbances of blood gas homeostasis, increased demands on the cardiovascular system, and discomfort to the patient.

Rarely, a rapid increase in temperature occurs during anaesthesia. This is associated usually with the rare inherited disorder of malignant hyperpyrexia. The rapid increases in muscle metabolism and temperature result in profound metabolic acidosis, hypercapnia and hyperkalaemia. Prompt therapeutic action is required to prevent a fatal outcome (see p. 417).

Fluid and electrolyte status

Blood and fluid losses may be considerable during surgery and empirical calculations of electrolyte losses may be erroneous. Estimation of fluid losses includes measurement of blood loss on swabs and drapes (vide supra), fluid collection in suction jars, and an allowance for evaporative loss. Fluid input and output must be measured as accurately as possible in babies and young children.

Measurement of serum sodium and potassium concentrations in the laboratory is relatively simple and this provides guidance on replacement with appropriate i.v. fluids. However, there may be some delay in obtaining laboratory results. Flame photometers and ion-specific electrodes are now available for measurement of serum and urine electrolytes in the operating theatre suite or ITU.

Blood gas and acid–base status

Monitoring of oxygen and carbon dioxide contents in blood is achieved most accurately by the measurement of arterial blood gases. This is facilitated by the presence of an arterial cannula and the availability of an automated blood gas analyser. Modern blood gas analysers use microelectrode systems and require very small quantities (approximately 0.2 ml) of heparinised blood. These machines provide results within 2–3 min and have helped to improve the management of patients undergoing major surgery.

Measurement of blood gases or acid–base status is indicated in:

1. Major vascular surgery, including cardiac surgery.
2. One-lung anaesthesia.
3. Hypotensive anaesthesia.
4. Critically ill patients.
5. Neurosurgical anaesthesia.

Monitoring of hormonal status

The metabolic response to anaesthesia and surgery consists of an elevation of the plasma concentrations of all the catabolic hormones (cortisol, catecholamines, growth hormone) and depression of the secretion of insulin. The magnitude of this response is proportional to the extent and duration of surgery.

The resulting elevation of blood sugar concentration may be detrimental, particularly to the diabetic patient and to patients who are critically ill and already in a catabolic phase. In such patients, blood sugar concentrations should be monitored at appropriate intervals and an insulin infusion administered as appropriate. Blood sugar concentration may be estimated rapidly and accurately if a sample of blood from a thumb prick is applied to a test strip, e.g. Dextrostix or BM Test.

Assessment of clotting status

Assessment of the adequacy of blood coagulation is of obvious importance during surgery. However, in specific situations, e.g. patients with inherent disorders of clotting, those given a massive blood transfusion, those receiving anticoagulant therapy, or those suspected of developing disseminated intravascular coagulation (DIC), it is mandatory to monitor clotting status.

Massive transfusion

Storage of blood induces the following changes:

1. Decrease in platelet count.
2. Decrease in labile clotting factors (mainly V and VIII).
3. Decrease in 2,3-DPG.

4. Increase in extracellular K^+.
5. Decrease in Ca^{2+}.
6. Decrease in pH (6.6–7.1).

When large quantities of stored blood are transfused, coagulation may be affected adversely. The following tests may be helpful in assessing the necessity for platelet transfusion, transfusion of fresh frozen plasma, or calcium therapy.

1. Platelet count (normal range 150–300 × 10^9/litre).
2. Prothrombin time (normal range 12–15 s) or INR (normal range 1.0–1.2) — tests extrinsic system.
3. PTT (normal range 35–45 s) — tests intrinsic system.

If PTT is prolonged by more than 10 s above the upper limit of normal, infusion of fresh frozen plasma is indicated. Spontaneous bleeding may not occur until the platelet count is less than 10 × 10^9/litre but platelet transfusion should be considered if the platelet count is less than 50 × 10^9/litre and the patient is bleeding actively. If DIC is suspected the fibrinogen level (normally 1.5 g/litre) and fibrin degradation product titre (normally <10 mg/litre) should also be measured.

Anticoagulant therapy

Patients receiving oral anticoagulants should not be considered for surgery until the international normalised ratio (INR) is less than twice normal. If emergency surgery is necessary, fresh frozen plasma should be available.

Peroperative heparin therapy may be monitored by measuring the activated clotting time. A commercially available kit (Haemochron) may be used in the operating theatre. It consists of a test tube which contains a magnet and some diatomaceous earth. The blood sample is injected into the test tube, which is placed in the machine. The test tube is rotated slowly and when a clot forms it enmeshes the magnet which then rotates along with the tube and activates a detector. The activated clotting time is kept at two to three times normal (normal range 80–135 s) for adequate heparin anticoagulation.

Table 21.6 Essential and desirable patient monitoring in addition to that incorporated in the breathing system and ventilator (see Table 21.7)

Operation category	Monitoring	
Minor	*Essential*	*Desirable*
Less than 30 min	Pulse	Pulse oximeter
Inhalational face mask GA	Palpation	
	Stethoscope { oesophageal / precordial	
	Finger plethysmograph	
	ECG	
	Indirect arterial pressure	
Standard		
Less than 3 h	As for minor	End-tidal CO_2
Relatively healthy patient	Expired volume (if IPPV employed)	Neuromuscular blockade
Endotracheal anaesthesia		Temperature
Blood loss <10% of blood volume		
Major		
Longer than 3 h	ECG	Neuromuscular blockade
Blood loss >10% of blood volume	Pulse oximeter	
Operations on:	Direct arterial pressure	
chest	Central venous pressure	
central nervous system	Blood loss measurement	
cardiovascular system	Urine output	
	Temperature	
	— patient	
	— blood warmer, mattress	
	— inspired gas	
	Blood gas analysis	
	Serum potassium concentration	
	Coagulation status	

ESSENTIAL MONITORING

The question of what constitutes generally applicable minimum standards for monitoring has generated much recent debate on both sides of the Atlantic. This debate has arisen because of an increasingly litiginous climate over the past few years, which has resulted in an escalation of awards for damages, and consequently of insurance premiums. Adequate monitoring appears to be one of the more critical factors in preventing injury to patients during anaesthesia in that analysis of anaesthetic mishaps often identifies events which might have been prevented by the use of an appropriate monitor.

Analysis of anaesthesia-related mishaps at the Harvard University Hospitals, Departments of Anaesthesia led to the establishment of standards for minimal monitoring during the conduct of any anaesthetic.

1. Continuous presence of the anaesthetist.
2. Arterial blood pressure monitoring.
3. Frequent heart rate monitoring (at least every minute).
4. Continuous ECG display.
5. Continuous monitoring of:

   (a) Ventilation — observation of reservoir bag or measurement of expired gas flow.
   (b) Circulation — palpation of the pulse or pulse plethysmography or arterial oxygen saturation measurement.

6. Breathing system disconnection monitoring (when using IPPV).
7. Inspired oxygen concentration monitoring.
8. Temperature monitoring should always be available.

End-tidal carbon dioxide monitoring was considered to be an emerging standard.

As yet, no such minimum standards have been defined in the UK. However, Sykes has suggested a categorisation of operative procedures, together with a list of essential and desirable monitoring techniques suitable for each category. His classification is shown in Table 21.6. In addition to this level of patient monitoring, it is suggested that the usual monitoring of both machine function and the breathing system should be used (Table 21.7).

Table 21.7 Recommended machine/breathing system/ventilator monitors

Monitor	System monitored
Machine	
O_2 supply pressure failure alarm	Fresh gas oxygen supply
Fresh gas O_2 concentration	Fresh gas oxygen concentration
Flowmeters	Fresh gas composition and flow
Fresh gas vapour analysis*	Fresh gas vapour concentration
Breathing system/ventilator	
Circle system $F\text{I}_{O_2}$	Fresh gas input; O_2/N_2O uptake, N_2 accumulation
Circle system inspired anaesthetic concentration	Fresh gas input; vapour delivery/uptake
Expired volume	Breathing system–patient leaks Tidal or minute ventilation
End-tidal CO_2	CO_2 transport to sampling site Alveolar ventilation/CO_2 production Rebreathing (IPPV)
Expired volume and end-tidal CO_2	Rebreathing (spontaneous ventilation)
Airway pressure	Expiratory valve function Ventilator function Lung/chest wall compliance and airway resistance

*Desirable but not essential.

Clearly, modification, and possibly extension, of these recommendations may be dictated by preoperative assessment of the patient's condition, and the physiological changes caused by specific operations.

The adoption of these standards demands enormous expenditure on the part of hospital authorities, and not all are likely to acquiesce to the requests of anaesthetists for purchase of new equipment. However, it is likely that if any mishap occurs during an anaesthetic in which monitoring does not meet the published standards, the anaesthetist may be judged to have been negligent.

FURTHER READING

Barash P G 1985 Update on noninvasive cardiac monitoring techniques. ASA Annual Refresher Course Lectures

Cheney F W 1987 Anaesthesia and the law: The North American experience. British Journal of Anaesthesia 59: 891

Eichhorn J H, Cooper J B, Cullen D J, Maier W R, Philip J H, Seeman R G 1986 Standards for patient monitoring during anesthesia at Harvard Medical School. Journal of the American Medical Association 256: 1017

Jawson C J H Kerr J H 1985 Automatic blood pressure monitors. Anaesthesia 40: 471

Saidman L J, Smith N T 1978 Monitoring in anesthesia. Wiley, New York

Sykes M K 1987 Essential monitoring. British Journal of Anaesthesia 59: 901

Taylor M D, Whitwam J G 1986 The current status of pulse oximetry. Anaesthesia 41: 943

22. Fluid, electrolyte and acid-base balance

The realisation that the enzyme systems and metabolic processes responsible for the maintenance of cellular function are dependent on an environment with stable electrolyte and hydrogen ion concentrations led Claude Bernard over 100 years ago to describe the 'milieu interieur'. Complex homeostatic mechanisms have evolved to maintain the constancy of this internal environment and thus prevent cellular dysfunction.

Basic definitions

Osmosis refers to the movement of *solvent* molecules across a membrane into a region in which there is a higher concentration of *solute*. This movement may be prevented by applying a pressure to the more concentrated solution — the effective osmotic pressure. This is a colligative property; the magnitude of effective osmotic pressure exerted by a solution depends on the *number* rather than the type of particles present.

The amounts of osmotically active particles present in solution are expressed in *osmoles*. One osmole of a substance is equal to its molecular weight in grams (one mole) divided by the number of freely moving particles which each molecule liberates in solution. Thus, 180 g of glucose in 1 litre of water represents a solution with a molar concentration of 1 mol/litre and an *osmolarity* of 1 osmol/litre. Sodium chloride ionises in solution and each ion represents an osmotically active particle. Assuming complete dissociation into Na^+ and Cl^-, 58.5 g of NaCl dissolved in 1 litre of water has a molar concentration of 1 mol/litre and an osmolarity of 2 osmol/litre. In body fluids, solute concentrations are much lower (mmol/litre) and dissociation is incomplete. Consequently, a solution of NaCl containing 1 mmol/litre contributes slightly less than 2 mosmol/litre.

The term *osmolality* refers to the number of osmoles per unit of total weight of solvent and, unlike osmolarity, is not affected by the volume of various solutes in solution. Confusion regarding the apparently interchangeable use of the terms osmolarity (measured in osmol/litre) and osmolality (measured in osmol/kg) is caused by their numerical equivalence in body fluids; plasma osmolarity is 280–310 mosmol/litre and plasma osmolality is 280–310 mosmol/kg. This equivalence is explained by the almost negligible solute volume contained in biological fluids and the fact that most osmotically active particles are dissolved in water, which has a density of one, i.e. osmol/litre = osmol/kg). As the number of osmoles in plasma is estimated by measurement of the magnitude of freezing point depression, the more accurate term in clinical practice is osmolality.

Cations (principally Na^+) and anions (Cl^- and HCO_3^-) are the major osmotically active particles in plasma. Glucose and urea make a smaller contribution. Plasma osmolality (P_{osm}) may be estimated from the formula:

$$P_{osm} = \underset{\text{(mmol/litre)}}{2\,[Na^+]} + \underset{\text{(mmol/litre)}}{\text{Blood glucose}} + \underset{\text{(mmol/litre)}}{\text{Blood urea}} = 290\ \text{mosmol/kg}$$

Osmolality is a chemical term and may be confused with the physiological term of *tonicity*. This term is used to describe the effective osmotic pressure of a solution relative to that of plasma. The critical difference between osmolality and tonicity is that *all* solutes contribute to osmolality but only solutes that do not cross the cell membrane contribute to tonicity. Thus, tonicity expresses the osmolal activity of solutes restricted to the extracellular compartment, i.e. those which exert an osmotic force affecting the distribution of water between ICF and ECF. As urea diffuses freely across cell membranes, it does not alter the distribution of water between these two body fluid compartments and does not contribute to tonicity. Other solutes that contribute to plasma osmolality but not tonicity include ethanol and methanol, both of which distribute rapidly throughout the total body water. In contrast, mannitol and sorbitol are restricted to the ECF and contribute to both osmolality and tonicity. The tonicity of plasma may be estimated from the formula:

$$\text{Plasma tonicity} = 2\,[Na^+]\ (\text{mmol/litre}) + \text{Blood glucose}\ (\text{mmol/litre}) = 285\ \text{mosmol/kg}$$

Compartmental distribution of total body water

The volume of total body water (TBW) may be measured using radioactive dilution techniques involving either deuterium or tritium, both of which cross all membranes freely and equilibrate rapidly with hydrogen atoms in body water. Such measurements show that approximately 60% of lean body mass (LBM) is water in the average 70-kg male adult. As fat contains little water, females have proportionately less TBW (55%) relative to LBM. TBW decreases with age, falling to 45–50% in later life.

The distribution of TBW between the main body compartments is illustrated in Table 22.1. One-third of TBW is contained in the extracellular fluid volume (ECFV) and two-thirds in the intracellular fluid volume (ICFV). The ECFV is subdivided further into the interstitial and intravascular compartments. In addition to the absolute volumes of each compartment, Table 22.1 shows the relative size of each compartment compared with body weight.

Solute composition of body fluid compartments

Extracellular fluid (ECF)

The capillary endothelium behaves as a freely permeable membrane to water, cations, anions and many soluble substances such as glucose and urea (but *not* protein). As a result, the solute compositions of interstitial fluid and plasma are similar. Each contains sodium as the principal cation and chloride as the principal anion. Protein behaves as a non-diffusible cation and is present in a higher concentration in plasma. The concentration of Cl^- is slightly higher in interstitial fluid in order to maintain electrical neutrality (Donnan equilibrium).

Table 22.1 Distribution of total body water related to body weight (BW).

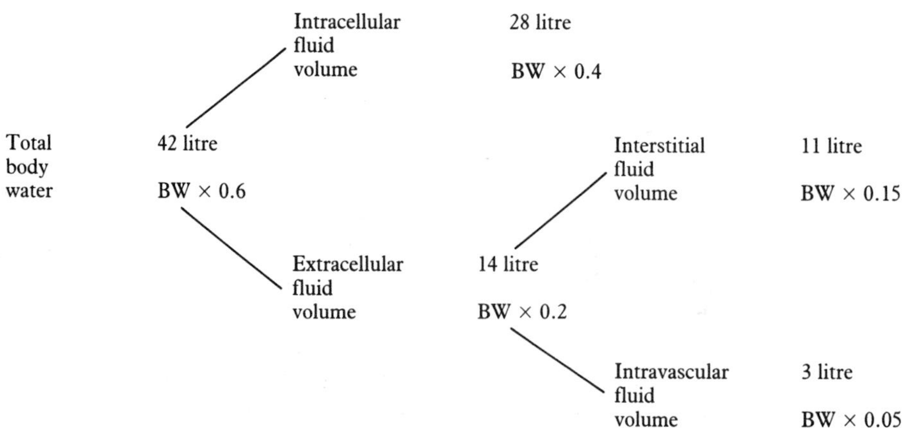

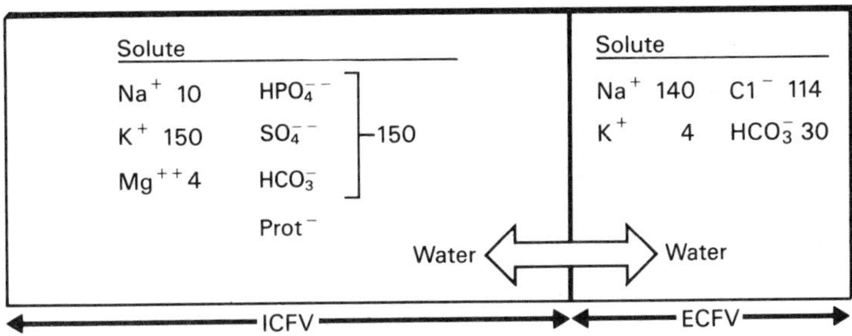

Fig. 22.1 Principal solute composition of body fluid compartments. All concentrations are expressed in mmol/litre.

Intracellular fluid (ICF)

This differs from ECF in that the principal cation is potassium and the principal anion is phosphate. In addition, there is a high protein content. In contrast to the capillary endothelium, the cell membrane is permeable *selectively* to different ions and freely permeable to water. Thus, equalisation of osmotic forces occurs continuously and is achieved by the movement of water across the cell membrane. The osmolalities of ICF and ECF at equilibrium must be equal. Water moves rapidly between ICF and ECF to eliminate any induced osmolal gradient. This principle is fundamental to an understanding of fluid and electrolyte physiology.

Figure 22.1 shows the solute composition of the main body fluid compartments. Although the total concentration of intracellular ions exceeds that of extracellular ions the numbers of osmotically active particles (and thus the osmolalities) are the same on each side of the cell membrane (290 mosmol/kg of solution).

Water homeostasis

Normal day-to-day fluctuations in TBW are small (<0.2%) because of a fine balance between input, controlled by the thirst mechanisms, and output, controlled mainly by the renal–ADH system.

The principal sources of body water are ingested fluid, water present in solid food and water produced as an end product of metabolism. Intravenous fluids are another common source in hospital patients. Actual and potential outlets for water are classified conventionally as sensible and insensible losses. Insensible losses emanate from the skin and lungs; sensible losses occur mainly from the kidneys and gastrointestinal tract. Figure 22.2 depicts the daily water balance in a 70-kg adult in whom input and output balance. It should be noted that sources of potential loss are not evident in this diagram. For example, over 5 litres of fluid are secreted daily into the gut in the form of saliva, bile, gastric juices and succus entericus, yet only 100 ml of fluid is present in faeces. This illustrates the potential that exists for significant fluid loss in the presence of disease.

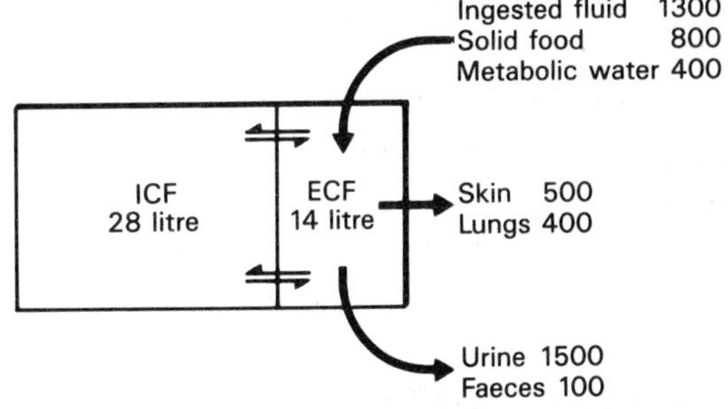

Fig. 22.2 Daily water balance. Input and output in ml.

PRACTICAL FLUID BALANCE

Calculation of the daily prescription of fluid is an arithmetic exercise to balance the input and output of water and electrolytes.

Table 22.2 shows the electrolyte contents of five intravenous solutions used commonly in the United Kingdom. These solutions are adequate for most clinical situations. Two self-evident but important generalisations may be made regarding solutions for intravenous infusion.

Table 22.2 Electrolyte contents of commonly used intravenous fluids

Solution	Electrolyte content (mmol/litre)	Osmolality (mosmol/kg)
Saline 0.9% ('normal saline')	Na^+ 154 Cl^- 154	308
Saline 0.45% ('half-normal saline')	Na^+ 77 Cl^- 77	154
Glucose 4%/saline 0.18% (glucose–saline)	Na^+ 31 Cl^- 31	284
Glucose 5%	nil	278
Compound sodium lactate (Hartmann's solution)	Na^+ 131 Cl^- 112 K^+ 5 HCO_3^- 29 Ca^{2+} 4 (as lactate)	281

Rule 1

All infused Na^+ remains in the ECF; Na^+ cannot gain access to the ICF because of the sodium pump. Thus, if saline 0.9% is infused, all Na^+ remains in the ECF. As this is an isotonic solution, there is no change in ECF osmolality and therefore no water exchange occurs across the cell membrane. Thus, saline 0.9% expands ECFV only. However, if saline 0.45% is given, ECF osmolality decreases; this causes a shift of water from ECF to ICF. If saline 1.8% is administered, all Na^+ remains in the ECF, its osmolality increases and water moves from ICF to ECF to maintain osmotic equality.

Rule 2

Water without sodium expands the TBW. After infusion of a solution of glucose 5%, the glucose enters cells and is metabolised. The infused water enters both ICF and ECF in proportion to their initial volumes.

Table 22.3 illustrates the results of infusion of 1 litre of saline 0.9%, saline 0.45% or glucose 5% in a 70-kg adult.

Assessment of daily fluid requirements may be allocated usefully into three processes:

1. Normal maintenance needs.
2. Abnormal losses resulting from the underlying pathology.
3. Correction of pre-existing deficits.

Table 22.3 Compartmental expansion resulting from infusion of 1 litre of saline 0.9%, saline 0.45% or glucose 5%

Intravenous infusion of 1000 ml	Change in volume (ml)		Remarks
	ECF	ICF	
Saline 0.9%	+1000	0	Na^+ remains in ECF
Glucose 5%	+333	+666	66% of TBW is ICF
Saline 0.45%	+666	+333	33% of TBW is ECF

Normal maintenance needs

Water

Regardless of the disease process, water and electrolyte losses occur in urine and as evaporative losses from skin and lungs. It is evident from Figure 22.2 that a normothermic 70-kg patient with a normal metabolic rate may lose 2500 ml of water per day. Allowing for a gain of 400 ml from water of metabolism, this hypothetical patient needs 2000 ml H_2O/day. As a rule of thumb, a volume of 30–35 ml H_2O kg^{-1} day^{-1} is a useful estimate for daily maintenance needs.

Sodium

The normal requirement is 1 mmol kg^{-1} day^{-1} (50–80 mmol/day) for adults.

Potassium

The normal requirement is 1 mmol kg^{-1} day^{-1} (50–80 mmol/day) for adults.

Thus, a 70-kg patient requires daily provision of 2000–2500 ml of water, and approximately 70 mmol each of Na^+ and K^+. This could be administered as:

1. 2000 ml of glucose 5% + 500 ml of saline 0.9%; or
2. 2500 ml of glucose 4%/saline 0.18%;

plus potassium as KCl, 1 g (13 mmol) added to each 500 ml of fluid.

Abnormal losses

These are common in surgical patients. They may be sensible or insensible and either overt or covert.

Losses from the gut are common, e.g. nasogastric suction, diarrhoea and vomiting or sequestration of fluid within the gut lumen (e.g. intestinal obstruction). Although the composition of gastrointestinal secretions is variable, replacement should be with saline 0.9% with 13–26 mmol/litre of potassium as KCl. If losses are considerable (>1000 ml/day), a sample of the appropriate fluid should be sent for biochemical analysis so that electrolyte replacement may be rationalised.

Increased insensible losses from the skin and lungs occur in the presence of fever or hyperventilation. The usual insensible loss of 0.5 ml kg^{-1} h^{-1} increases by 12% for each degree Celsius rise in temperature.

Sequestration of fluid at the site of operative trauma is a form of fluid loss which is common in surgical patients. Plasma-like fluid is sequestered in any area of tissue injury; its volume is proportional to the extent of trauma. This fluid is referred to frequently as 'third-space' loss because it ceases to take part in normal metabolic processes. However, it is not contained in an anatomically separate compartment; it represents an expansion of ECFV. Third-space losses are not measured easily. Sequestered fluid is reabsorbed after 48–72 h.

Existing deficits

These occur preoperatively and arise primarily from the gut. The difficulty in correcting these deficits relates to an inability to quantify their magnitude accurately. Fluid and electrolyte deficits occur directly from the ECF. If the fluid lost is isotonic, only ECFV is reduced; however, if water alone or hypotonic fluid is lost, redistribution of the remaining TBW occurs from ICF to ECF to equalise osmotic forces.

Dehydration with accompanying salt loss is a common disorder in the acute surgical patient.

Assessment of dehydration

This is a clinical assessment based upon:

1. *History*. How long has the patient had abnormal loss of fluid? How much has occurred, e.g. frequency of vomiting?
2. *Examination*. Specific features are thirst, dryness of mucous membranes, loss of skin turgor, orthostatic hypotension or tachycardia, reduced JVP or CVP and decreased urine output; in the presence of normal renal function, dehydration is associated usually with a urine output of less than 0.5 ml kg^{-1} h^{-1}. The severity of dehydration may be described clinically as mild, moderate or severe and each category is associated with the following water loss relative to body weight.

Mild. Loss of 4% body weight (approximately 3 litres in a 70-kg patient); reduced skin turgor, sunken eyes, dry mucous membranes.

Moderate. Loss of 5–8% body weight (approximately 4–6 litres in a 70-kg patient); oliguria, orthostatic hypotension and tachycardia in addition to the above.

Severe. Loss of 8–10% body weight (approximately 7 litres in a 70-kg patient); profound oliguria and compromised cardiovascular function.

Laboratory assessment.

The degree of haemoconcentration and increase in albumin concentration may be helpful in the absence of anaemia and hypoproteinaemia. Increased blood urea concentration and urine osmolality (>650 mosmol/kg) confirms the clinical diagnosis.

Perioperative fluid therapy

In addition to normal maintenance requirements of water and electrolytes, patients may require fluid in the perioperative period to restore TBW after a period of fasting and to replace small blood losses, loss of ECF into the 'third space' and losses of water from the skin, gut and lungs.

Blood losses in excess of 15% of blood volume in the adult are replaced usually by infusion of stored blood. Smaller blood losses may be replaced by a crystalloid electrolyte solution such as compound sodium lactate; however, because these solutions are distributed throughout ECF, blood volume is maintained only if at least three times the volume of blood loss is infused. Alternatively, a colloid solution (human albumin solution or a synthetic substitute) may be infused in a volume equal to that of the estimated loss.

'Third-space' losses are replaced usually as compound sodium lactate. In abdominal surgery (e.g. cholecystectomy), a volume of 5 ml kg^{-1} h^{-1} during operation, in addition to normal maintenance requirements (approximately 1.5 ml kg^{-1} h^{-1}) and blood loss replacement, is usually sufficient. Larger volumes may be required in more major procedures, but should be guided by measurement of CVP.

In the postoperative period, normal maintenance fluids should be administered (vide supra). Additional fluid (given as saline 0.9% or compound sodium lactate) may be required in the following circumstances:

1. If blood or serum is lost from drains (colloid solutions should be used if losses exceed 500 ml).
2. If gastrointestinal losses continue, e.g. from a nasogastric tube or a fistula.
3. After major surgery (e.g. total gastrectomy, repair of aortic aneurysm), when additional water and electrolytes may be required for 24–48 h to replace continuing 'third-space' losses.
4. During rewarming if the patient has become hypothermic during surgery.

Normally, potassium is not administered in the first 24 h after surgery as endogenous release of potassium from tissue trauma and catabolism warrants restriction. The postoperative patient differs from the 'normal' patient in that the stress reaction modifies homeostatic mechanisms; stress-induced release of ADH, aldosterone and cortisol causes retention of Na^+ and water and increased renal excretion of potassium. However, restriction of fluid and sodium in the postoperative period is inappropriate despite a low urine output because of increased losses by evaporation and into the 'third space'. The stress response lasts for 24–72 h and recovery is heralded usually by a diuresis.

After major surgery, assessment of fluid and electrolyte requirements is achieved best by measurement of CVP and serum electrolyte concentrations.

Fluid and electrolyte requirements in infants and small children differ from those in the adult (see Ch. 34).

Patients with renal failure require fluid replacement for abnormal losses, although the total volume of fluid infused should be reduced to a degree determined by the urine output.

SODIUM AND POTASSIUM

Sodium balance

Daily ingestion amounts to 50–300 mmol. Losses in sweat and faeces are minimal (approximately 10 mmol/day) and final adjustments are made by the kidney. Urine sodium excretion may be as little as 2 mmol/day during salt restriction or may exceed 700 mmol/day after salt loading. Sodium balance is related intimately to ECFV and water balance.

Disorders of sodium/water balance

Hypernatraemia

Hypernatraemia is defined as a plasma sodium concentration of more than 150 mmol/litre and may result from pure water loss, hypotonic fluid loss or salt gain. In the first two conditions, ECFV is reduced, whereas salt gain is associated with an expanded ECFV. For this reason, the clinical assessment of volaemic status is important in the diagnosis and management of hypernatraemic states. The common causes of hypernatraemia are summarised in Table 22.4. The abnormality common to all hypernatraemic states is intracellular dehydration secondary to ECF hyperosmolality. Primary water loss resulting in hypernatraemia may occur during prolonged fever, hyperventilation or during severe exercise in hot, dry climates.

Table 22.4 Causes of hypernatraemia

Pure water depletion	
Extrarenal loss	Failure of water intake (coma, elderly, postoperative) Mucocutaneous loss Fever, hyperventilation, thyrotoxicosis
Renal loss	Diabetes insipidus (cranial, nephrogenic) Chronic renal failure
Hypotonic fluid loss	
Extrarenal loss	Gastrointestinal (vomiting, diarrhoea) Skin (excessive sweating)
Renal loss	Osmotic diuresis (glucose, urea, mannitol)
Salt gain	
	Iatrogenic ($NaHCO_3$, hypertonic saline) Salt ingestion Steroid excess

However, a more common cause is the renal water loss that occurs when there is a defect in either the production or release of ADH (cranial diabetes insipidus) or an abnormality in response to ADH (nephrogenic diabetes insipidus).

The administration of osmotic diuretics results temporarily in plasma hyperosmolality. An osmotic diuresis may occur also in hyperglycaemia. During an osmotic diuresis, the solute causing the diuresis (e.g. glucose, mannitol) constitutes a significant fraction of urine solute and the sodium content of the urine becomes hypotonic relative to plasma sodium. Thus, osmotic diuretics cause hypotonic urine losses which may result in hypernatraemic dehydration.

Hypertonic dehydration may occur also in paediatric practice. Diarrhoea, vomiting and anorexia lead to loss of water in excess of solute (hypotonic loss). Concomitant fever, hyperventilation and the use of high-solute feeds may combine to exaggerate the problem. ECFV is maintained by movement of water from ICF to ECF to equalise osmolality, and clinical evidence of dehydration may not be apparent until 10–15% of body weight has been lost. Rehydration must be undertaken gradually to prevent the development of cerebral oedema.

Measurement of urine and plasma osmolalities and assessment of urine output help in the diagnosis of hypernatraemic, volume-depleted states. If urine output is low and urine osmolality exceeds 800 mosm/kg, then both ADH secretion and the renal response to ADH are present. The most likely causes are extrarenal water loss (e.g. diarrhoea, vomiting or evaporation) or insufficient intake. High urine output and high urine osmolality suggest an osmotic diuresis. If urine osmolality is less than plasma osmolality, reduced ADH secretion or impairment of the renal response to ADH should be suspected; in both cases, urine output is high.

Usually, hypernatraemia caused by salt gain is iatrogenic in origin. It occurs when excessive amounts of hypertonic sodium bicarbonate are administered during resuscitation or when isotonic fluids are given to patients who have only insensible losses. Treatment comprises induction of a diuresis with a loop diuretic if renal function is normal; urine output is replaced in part with glucose 5%. Dialysis or haemofiltration is necessary in patients with renal dysfunction.

Hyponatraemia

This is defined as a plasma sodium concentration of less than 135 mmol/litre. Hyponatraemia is a common finding in hospital patients. It may occur as a result of water retention, sodium loss or both; consequently, it may be associated with an expanded, normal or contracted ECFV. As in hypernatraemia, the state of ECFV is important in determining the cause of the electrolyte imbalance.

As plasma osmolality decreases, an osmolal gradient is created across the cell membrane and results in movement of water into the ICF. The resulting expansion of brain cells is responsible for the symptomatology of hyponatraemia or 'water intoxication': nausea, vomiting, lethargy, weakness and obtundation. In severe cases (plasma Na^+ < 115 mmol/litre), seizures and coma may result.

A scheme depicting the causes of hyponatraemia is shown in Table 22.5. True hyponatraemia must be distinguished from pseudohyponatraemia. Sodium ions are present only in plasma water, which constitutes 93% of normal plasma. In the laboratory the concentration of sodium in plasma is measured in an aliquot of whole plasma and the concentration is expressed in terms of plasma volume (mmol/litre of whole plasma). If the percentage of water present in plasma is decreased, as in hyperlipidaemia or hyperproteinaemia, the amount of Na^+ in each aliquot of plasma is decreased also, even if its concentration in plasma water is normal. A clue to this cause of hyponatraemia is the finding of a normal plasma osmolality.

True hyponatraemic states may be classified conveniently into *depletional* and *dilutional* types. Depletional hyponatraemia occurs when a deficit in TBW is associated with an even greater deficit of total body sodium. Assessment of volaemic status reveals hypovolaemia. Losses may be *renal* or *extrarenal*. Excessive renal loss of sodium occurs in Addison's disease, diuretic administration, renal tubular acidosis and salt-losing nephro-

Table 22.5 Causes of hyponatraemia.

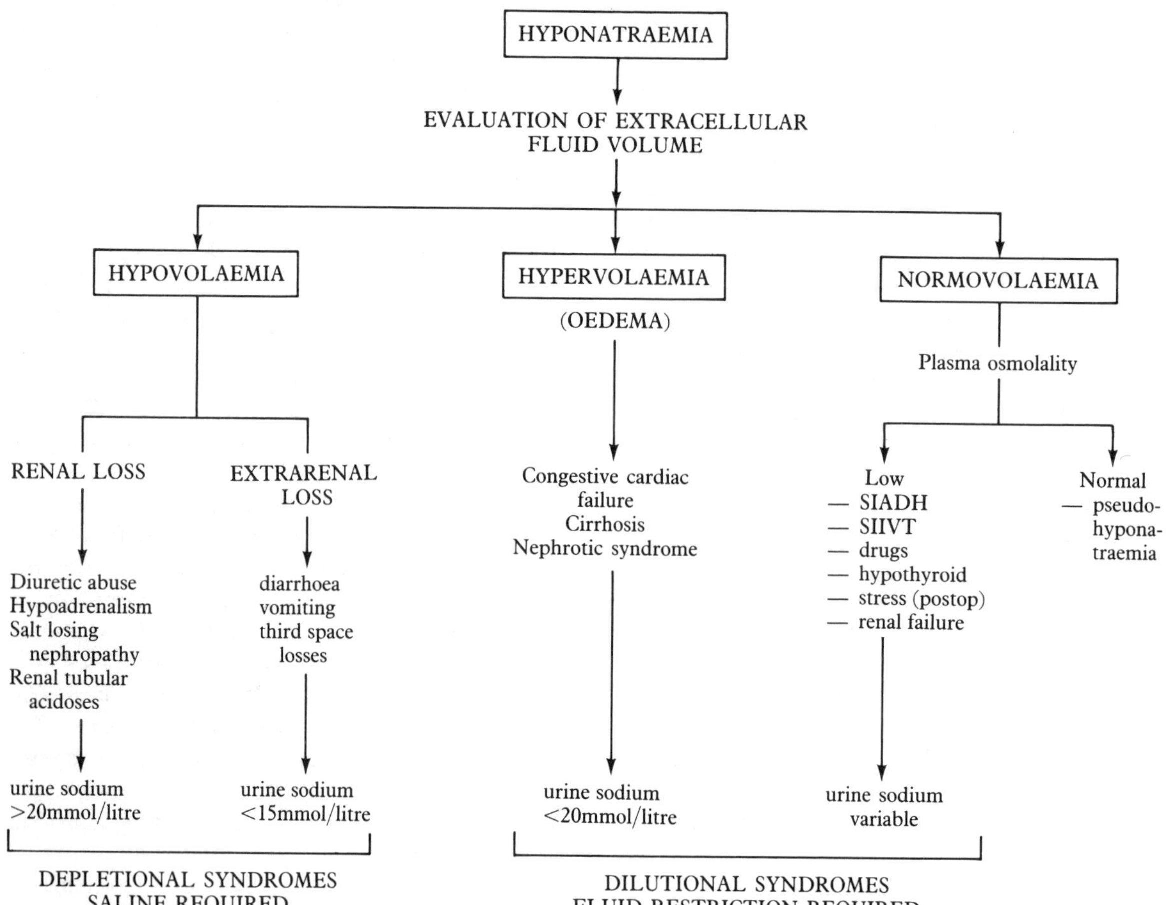

pathies; usually, urine sodium concentration exceeds 20 mmol/litre. Extrarenal losses occur usually from the gastrointestinal tract (e.g. diarrhoea, vomiting) or from sequestration into the 'third space' (e.g. peritonitis, surgery). Normal kidneys respond by conserving sodium and water to produce a urine that is hyperosmolal and low in sodium. In both situations, treatment should be directed at expanding the ECFV with saline 0.9%.

Dilutional hyponatraemic states may be associated with hypervolaemia and oedema, or with normovolaemia. Again, assessment of volaemic status is important. If oedema is present, there is an excess of total body sodium with a proportionately greater excess of TBW. This is seen in congestive heart failure, cirrhosis and the nephrotic syndrome and is caused by secondary hyperaldosteronism. Treatment comprises salt and water restriction and spironolactone.

In normovolaemic hyponatraemia there is a modest excess of TBW and a modest increase in ECFV associated with a normal total body sodium. Pseudohyponatraemia is excluded by finding high protein or lipid levels and a normal plasma osmolality. True normovolaemic hyponatraemia is commonly iatrogenic in origin. The syndrome of inappropriate intravenous therapy (SIIVT) is caused usually by administration of intravenous fluids with a low sodium content to patients with isotonic losses.

A more chronic water overload may occur in patients with hypothyroidism and in conditions associated with an inappropriately elevated level of ADH. The syndrome of inappropriate ADH secretion (SIADH) is characterised by hyponatraemia, low plasma osmolality and an inappropriate antidiuresis, i.e. a urine osmolality higher than anticipated for the degree of hyponatraemia. It occurs in the presence of malignant tumours which produce ADH-like substances (e.g. lung, prostate, pancreas), in neurological disorders (e.g. head injury, tumours, infections) and in some severe pneumonias. A number of drugs are associated with increased ADH secretion or potentiate the effects of ADH (Table 22.6). In patients with SIADH, the urine is concentrated in spite of hyponatraemia. Management comprises restriction of fluid intake to encourage a negative fluid balance. In severe or refractory cases, demeclocycline or lithium may result in improvement. Both drugs induce a state of functional diabetes insipidus and have been used effectively in SIADH if the primary disease cannot be treated.

Acute symptomatic hyponatraemia is a medical emergency and warrants the use of hypertonic saline (3%). Because of the danger of precipitating pulmonary oedema and cerebral haemorrhage, sufficient Na^+ should be given to return the plasma concentration to 125 mmol/litre only, and this should be administered over a period of no less than 12 h.

Potassium balance

The normal daily intake of potassium is 50–200 mmol. Minimal amounts are lost via the skin and faeces; the kidney is the primary regulator. However, the mechanisms for the retention of potassium are less efficient than those for sodium. In periods of K^+ depletion, daily urinary excretion cannot decrease to less than 5–10 mmol. A considerable deficit of total body potassium occurs if intake is not restored. Hypokalaemia is a more common abnormality than hyperkalaemia.

Table 22.6 Drugs associated with antidiuresis and hyponatraemia

Increased ADH secretion
- Hypnotics — barbiturates
- Analgesics — opioids
- Hypoglycaemics — chlorpropamide, tolbutamide
- Anticonvulsants — carbamazepine
- Miscellaneous — phenothiazines, tricyclics

Potentiation of ADH at distal tubule
- Paracetamol
- Indomethacin
- Chlorpropamide

Hypokalaemia

This is defined as a plasma potassium concentration of less than 3.5 mmol/litre. Non-specific symptoms of hypokalaemia include anorexia and nausea, effects on skeletal and smooth muscle (muscle weakness, paralytic ileus) and cardiac conduction (delayed repolarisation with ST segment depression, reduced height of the T wave, increased height of the U wave and a widened QRS complex).

The causes of hypokalaemia are summarised in Table 22.7. Management includes diagnosis and treatment of the underlying disorder in addition to repletion of total body potassium stores. As a general rule, a reduction in plasma K^+ concentration by 1 mmol/litre reflects a total body K^+ deficit of approximately 100 mmol. Potassium supplements may be given orally or i.v. The maximum infusion rate should not exceed 0.5 mmol kg^{-1} h^{-1} to allow equilibration with the intracellular compartment; much slower rates are employed usually.

The potassium salt used for replacement therapy is important. In most situations, and

Table 22.7 Causes of hypokalaemia

Cause	Comments
Reduced intake	Usually only contributory
Tissue redistribution	Insulin therapy, alkalaemia, β_2-adrenergic agonists, familial periodic paralysis, vitamin B_{12} therapy
Increased loss	
gastrointestinal (urine K^+ < 20 mmol/litre)	Diarrhoea, vomiting, fistulae, nasogastric suction, colonic villous adenoma
renal	Diuretic therapy, primary or secondary hyperaldosteronism, malignant hypertension, renal artery stenosis (high renin), renal tubular acidosis, hypomagnesaemia, renal failure (diuretic phase)

especially in the presence of alkalosis, potassium should be replaced as the chloride salt. Supplements are available also as the bicarbonate and phosphate salts.

Hyperkalaemia

This is defined as a plasma potassium concentration exceeding 5 mmol/litre. Vague muscle weakness progressing to flaccid paralysis may occur. However, the major clinical feature of an increasing plasma potassium concentration is the characteristic sequence of ECG abnormalities. The earliest change is the development of tall, peaked T waves and a shortened QT interval, reflecting more rapid repolarisation (6–7 mmol/litre). As plasma K^+ increases (8–10 mmol/litre), abnormalities in depolarisation become manifest as widened QRS complexes and widening, and eventually loss, of the P wave; the widened QRS complexes merge finally into the T waves (*sine wave pattern*). Plasma concentrations in excess of 10 mmol/litre are associated with ventricular fibrillation. The cardiac toxicity of K^+ is enhanced by hypocalcaemia, hyponatraemia or acidaemia. The causes of hyperkalaemia are summarised in Table 22.8.

Immediate treatment is necessary if the plasma potassium concentration exceeds 7 mmol/litre or if there are any serious ECG abnormalities. Specific treatment may be achieved by four mechanisms:

1. Chemical antagonism of the membrane effects.
2. Enhanced cellular uptake of K^+
3. Dilution of ECF.
4. Removal of K^+ from the body.

Methods by which the plasma potassium concentration may be reduced are summarised in Table 22.9.

Table 22.8 Causes of hyperkalaemia

Factitious (pseudohyperkalaemia)	– in vitro haemolysis – thrombocytosis – leucocytosis – tourniquet – exercise
Impaired excretion	– renal failure – acute or chronic hyperaldosteronism – Addison's disease – K^+-sparing diuretics – indomethacin
Tissue redistribution	– tissue damage (burns, trauma) – rhabdomyolysis – tumour necrosis – hyperkalaemic periodic paralysis – massive intravascular haemolysis – suxamethonium
Excessive intake	– blood transfusion – excessive i.v. administration

Table 22.9 Treatment of hyperkalaemia

Calcium gluconate 10% i.v. (0.5 ml/kg to maximum of 20 ml) given over 5 min. No change in plasma $[K^+]$. Effect immediate but transient
Glucose 50 g (0.5–1.0 g/kg) plus insulin 20 units (0.3 unit/kg) as single i.v. bolus dose. Then infusion of glucose 20%, plus insulin 6–20 units/h (depending on blood glucose)
Sodium bicarbonate 1.5–2.0 mmol/kg i.v. over 5–10 min
Calcium resonium 15 g p.o. or 30 g p.r. 8-hourly
Peritoneal or haemodialysis

ACID-BASE BALANCE

The concentration of hydrogen ions (H^+) in body fluids is extremely small and the pH notation was adopted for the sake of practicality. This system expresses H^+ concentration $[H^+]$ on a logarithmic scale:

$$pH = -\log_{10}[H^+]$$

A more logical arithmetic convention which expresses $[H^+]$ in nmol/litre is gaining popularity. Table 22.10 compares values of $[H^+]$ expressed as pH and nmol/litre and reveals a number of disadvantages of the pH notation. The most obvious disadvantage is that it moves in the opposite direction to $[H^+]$; a decrease in pH is associated with increased $[H^+]$ and vice versa. It is also apparent that the logarithmic scale distorts the quantitative estimate of change in $[H^+]$; for example, twice as many hydrogen ions are required to reduce pH from 7.1 to 7.0 as are needed to reduce it from 7.4 to 7.3. The pH scale gives the false impression that there is relatively little difference in the

Table 22.10 Comparison of logarithmic and arithmetic methods of expressing hydrogen ion concentration in the range of blood $[H^+]$ compatible with life

pH	$[H^+]$ (nmol/litre)	
7.8	16	
7.7	20	
7.6	25	*Alkalaemia*
7.5	32	
7.4	**40**	*Normal*
7.3	50	
7.2	63	
7.1	80	*Acidaemia*
7.0	100	
6.9	125	
6.8	160	

sensitivity of biological systems to an equivalent increase or decrease in $[H^+]$. However, when $[H^+]$ is expressed in nmol/litre, it becomes apparent that tolerance is limited to a reduction in $[H^+]$ of only 24 nmol/litre from normal, but to an increase of up to 120 nmol/litre. Nevertheless, the pH notation remains the most widely used system, and is employed in the remainder of this chapter.

Basic definitions

An *acid* is a substance that dissociates in water to produce H^+; a *base* is a substance that can accept H^+. Strong acids dissociate completely in aqueous solution, whereas weak acids (e.g. carbonic acid, H_2CO_3) dissociates only partially. The *conjugate base* of an acid is its dissociated anionic product. For example, bicarbonate ion (HCO_3^-) is the conjugate base of carbonic acid:

$$H_2CO_3 \rightleftharpoons H^+ + HCO_3^-$$

A *buffer* is a combination of a weak acid and its conjugate base (usually as a salt) which acts to minimise any change in $[H^+]$ that would occur if a strong acid or base was added to it. Buffers in body fluids represent an important defence against $[H^+]$ change. The carbonic acid/bicarbonate system is an important buffer in blood. The pH of a buffer system may be determined from the Henderson–Hasselbalch equation which, for the carbonic acid/bicarbonate system, relates pH, $[H_2CO_3]$ and $[HCO_3^-]$:

$$\text{pH} = \text{p}K + \log_{10} \frac{[HCO_3^-]}{[H_2CO_3]}$$

where K = dissociation constant and $\text{p}K = -\log_{10}K$.

This equation shows that $[H^+]$ in body fluids is a function of the *ratio* of base to acid. For the bicarbonate buffer system, pK is 6.1. As most of the carbonic acid pool exists as dissolved CO_2, the equation may be rewritten:

$$\text{pH} = 6.1 + \log_{10} \frac{[HCO_3^-]}{0.225 \times P\text{CO}_2}$$

The value 0.225 represents the solubility coefficient of CO_2 in blood (ml/kPa). Normally, $[HCO_3^-]$ is 24 mmol/litre and Pa_{CO_2} is 5.3 kPa. Thus:

$$\text{pH} = 6.1 + \log_{10} \frac{24}{0.225 \times 5.3} = 7.4$$

Most acid–base disorders may be formulated in terms of the Henderson–Hasselbalch equation. The pH of plasma is kept remarkably constant at 7.36–7.44, i.e. a hydrogen ion concentration of 40 ± 5 mmol/litre. This is achieved by:

1. Regulation of H^+ excretion and bicarbonate regeneration by the kidney.
2. Regulation of CO_2 by the alveolar ventilation of the lungs.

Cellular metabolism poses a constant threat to buffer systems by the production of 'volatile acid', i.e. CO_2, from cellular respiration and the formation of 'fixed' or 'non-volatile' acids by intermediary metabolism. Thus, the acid–base status of body fluids reflects the metabolism of both H^+ and CO_2.

Acid-base disorders

The normal pH of body fluids is 7.36–7.44. Conventional acid-base nomenclature involves the following definitions:

1. An *acidosis* is a process that causes acid to accumulate.

2. An *acidaemia* is present if pH < 7.36.
3. An *alkalosis* is a process that causes base to accumulate.
4. An *alkalaemia* is present if pH > 7.44.

Simple acid–base disorders are common in clinical practice and their successful management requires logical analysis of pH, $[HCO_3^-]$ and Pa_{CO_2}. The first step involves diagnosis of the primary disorder; this is followed by an assessment of the extent and appropriateness of any compensation.

Primary acid–base disorders are either *respiratory* or *metabolic*. The disorder is respiratory if the primary disturbance involves CO_2 and metabolic if it involves HCO_3^-. Thus, four potential primary disturbances exist (Table 22.11) and each may be identified by analysis of pH, $[HCO_3^-]$ and Pa_{CO_2}. Both pH and Pa_{CO_2} are measured directly by the blood gas machine. $[HCO_3^-]$ is measured directly on the electrolyte profile but is derived in most blood gas machines. Other derived parameters include *standard bicarbonate* and *base excess*. The standard bicarbonate is not the actual bicarbonate of the sample but an estimate of bicarbonate concentration after elimination of any abnormal respiratory contribution to $[HCO_3^-]$, i.e. an estimate of $[HCO_3^-]$ at a Pa_{CO_2} of 5.3 kPa. The base excess (in alkalosis) or base deficit (in acidosis) is the amount of acid or base (in mmol) required to return the pH of 1 litre of blood to normal at a Pa_{CO_2} of 5.3 kPa; it is a measure of the magnitude of the metabolic component of the acid–base disorder.

Table 22.11 Compensatory mechanisms in acid–base disturbances. ↓ ↓ or ↑ ↑ denotes the primary abnormality. The final pH depends on the degree of compensation. Respiratory compensation for metabolic disorders is rapid; renal compensation for respiratory disorders is slow

Primary disorder		pH	HCO_3^-	Pa_{CO_2}	Compensation
Metabolic	acidosis	↓	↓ ↓		Hyperventilation ↓ Pa_{CO_2}
	alkalosis	↑	↑ ↑		Hypoventilation ↑ Pa_{CO_2}
Respiratory	acidosis	↓		↑ ↑	Renal retention of HCO_3^-
	alkalosis	↑		↓ ↓	Renal elimination of HCO_3^-

After the primary disorder has been identified, it is necessary to consider if it is acute or chronic and if any compensation has occurred. The body defends itself against changes in pH by compensatory mechanisms which *tend* to return pH towards normal. Primary respiratory disorders are compensated by a metabolic mechanism, and vice versa. For example, a primary respiratory acidosis is compensated for by renal retention of HCO_3^-, whereas a primary metabolic acidosis is compensated by hyperventilation and a decrease in Pa_{CO_2}. Thus, in each case the *acidaemia* produced by the primary acidosis is reduced by a compensatory alkalosis. The response to a respiratory alkalosis is increased renal elimination of HCO_3^-, and a metabolic alkalosis results in hypoventilation and increased Pa_{CO_2}. pH is restored towards normal by the compensatory respiratory acidosis. In each case, the efficiency of compensatory mechanisms is limited; compensation is usually only partial and rarely complete. Overcompensation does not occur.

Metabolic acidosis

This is characterised by decreased $[HCO_3^-]$ and a variable degree of acidaemia. The extent of the acidaemia depends upon the nature, severity and duration of the initiating pathology in addition to the efficiency of compensatory mechanisms. An important clue to the nature of the abnormality is given by the measurement of the *anion gap* in plasma:

$$\text{anion gap} = ([Na^+] + [K^+]) - ([Cl^-] + [HCO_3^-])$$

In reality, the numbers of cations and anions in plasma are the same and an anion gap exists because negatively charged proteins, together with phosphate, lactate and organic anions (which maintain electrical neutrality) are not measured. The normal anion gap is 12–18 mmol/litre.

Clinically, it is useful to divide the metabolic acidoses into those associated with a normal anion gap and those with an increased anion gap. The former are caused by loss of HCO_3^- from the body and replacement with chloride. In acidoses associated with an increased anion gap, HCO_3^- has

Table 22.12 Types and causes of metabolic acidosis

High anion gap	
Overproduction of acid	– diabetic ketoacidosis – lactic acidosis type A (hypoxia, shock) or type B (biguanides) – starvation
Exogenous acid	– salicylates – methanol – ethylene glycol
Reduced excretion	– renal failure
Normal anion gap	
Bicarbonate loss	– *Extrarenal* diarrhoea biliary/pancreatic fistula ileostomy ureterosigmoidostomy
	– *Renal* renal tubular acidosis carbonic anhydrase inhibitors
Addition of acid (with chloride)	– HCl, NH_4Cl, arginine or lysine hydrochloride

been titrated by either endogenous, e.g. lactic, or exogenous acids, thus increasing the number of unmeasured plasma anions without altering the plasma chloride concentration (Table 22.12).

Clinical effects and treatment. Metabolic acidosis results in widespread physiological disturbances, including reduced cardiac output, pulmonary hypertension, arrhythmias, Kussmaul respiration and hyperkalaemia; the severity of the disturbances are related to the extent of the *acidaemia*. Treatment should be directed initially at identifying and reversing the cause. If acidaemia is considered to be life-threatening (pH < 7.2, $[HCO_3^-]$ < 10 mmol/litre), measures may be required to restore blood pH to normal. Over-zealous use of sodium bicarbonate may lead to rapid correction of blood pH, with the risks of tetany and convulsions in the short term, and volume overload and hypernatraemia in the longer term. The required quantity of bicarbonate should be calculated:

$$\text{bicarbonate requirement (mmol)} = \text{body weight (kg)} \times \text{base deficit (mmol/litre)} \times 0.3$$

Administration of sodium bicarbonate should be followed by repeated measurements of plasma $[HCO_3^-]$ and pH. Sodium bicarbonate is available as isotonic (1.4%; 163 mmol/litre) and hypertonic (8.4%; 1000 mmol/litre) solutions. Slow infusion of the hypertonic solution is advisable to minimise adverse effects.

Metabolic alkalosis

This is characterised by a primary increase in plasma $[HCO_3^-]$ and a variable degree of alkalaemia. The compensatory response of hypoventilation is limited and not very effective. For diagnostic and therapeutic reasons it is usual to subdivide metabolic alkalosis into the chloride-responsive and chloride-resistant varieties (Table 22.13). The differential diagnosis of metabolic alkalosis, and in particular the separation of patients on the basis of the urinary chloride concentration, is important because of the differences in treatment of the two groups. In chloride-responsive alkalosis, the administration of saline causes volume expansion and results in the excretion of excess bicarbonate; if potassium is required, it should be given as the chloride salt. In patients in whom volume administration is contraindicated, the use of acetazolamide results in renal loss of HCO_3^- and an improvement in pH. H_2-receptor antagonists may be helpful if nasogastric suction is contributing to hydrogen ion loss.

Table 22.13 Types and causes of metabolic alkalosis

Chloride-responsive (urine chloride < 20 mmol/litre)	
Loss of acid	– vomiting – nasogastric suction – gastrocolic fistula
Chloride depletion	– diarrhoea – diuretic abuse
Excessive alkali	– $NaHCO_3$ administration – antacid abuse
Chloride-resistant (urine chloride > 20 mmol/litre)	
Primary or secondary hyperaldosteronism	
Cushing's syndrome	
Severe hypokalaemia	
Carbenoxolone	

Severe alkalaemia with compensatory hypoventilation may result in seizures or CNS depression. In life-threatening metabolic alkalosis, rapid correction is necessary and may be achieved by administration of hydrogen ions in the form of dilute hydrochloric acid. Acid administration requires central vein cannulation as peripheral infusion causes sclerosis of veins. Acid is given as 0.1 normal HCl in glucose 5% at a rate no greater than 0.2 mmol kg^{-1} h^{-1}.

Respiratory acidosis

This abnormality is characterised by a primary increase in Pa_{CO_2} which results in acidaemia to an extent proportional to the degree of hypercapnia. Buffering processes are activated rapidly in acute hypercapnia and may remove enough H^+ from the extracellular fluid to result in a secondary increase in plasma HCO_3^-. The compensation is less efficient than in metabolic alkalosis and pH is seldom more than 7.35.

Usually, hypoxaemia and the manifestations of the underlying disease dominate the clinical picture but hypercapnia *per se* may result in coma, raised intracranial pressure, and a hyperdynamic cardiovascular system (tachycardia, vasodilatation, ventricular arrhythmias) resulting from release of catecholamines.

There are many causes of respiratory acidosis; the most important are classified in Table 22.14. Treatment consists of reversing the underlying pathology if possible and mechanical ventilatory support if required.

Respiratory alkalosis

This is characterised by a primary decrease in Pa_{CO_2} (alveolar ventilation in excess of metabolic needs) which increases pH above 7.44. Usually, hypocapnia indicates a disturbance of ventilatory control (in patients not receiving mechanical ventilation). As in respiratory acidosis, the manifestations of the underlying disease usually dominate the clinical picture. Acute hypocapnia results in cerebral vasoconstriction and reduced cerebral blood flow, and may cause lightheadedness, confusion and, in severe cases, seizures.

Table 22.14 Causes of respiratory acidosis

Central nervous system	
Drug overdose	
Trauma	
Tumour	
Degeneration or infection	
Cerebrovascular accident	
Cervical cord trauma	
Peripheral nervous system	
Polyneuropathy	
Myasthenia gravis	
Poliomyelitis	
Botulism	
Tetanus	
Organophosphorus poisoning	
Primary pulmonary disease	
Airway obstruction	– asthma
	– laryngospasm
	– chronic obstructive airways disease
Parenchymal disease	– ARDS
	– pneumonia
	– severe pulmonary oedema
	– chronic obstructive airways disease
Loss of mechanical integrity	– flail chest

Table 22.15 Causes of respiratory alkalosis

Supratentorial	
Voluntary/hysterical hyperventilation	
Pain, anxiety	
Specific conditions	
CNS disease	– meningitis/encephalitis
	– cerebrovascular accident
	– tumour
	– trauma
Respiratory disease	– pneumonia
	– pulmonary embolism
	– early pulmonary oedema or ARDS
	– high altitude
Shock	– cardiogenic
	– hypovolaemic
	– septic
Miscellaneous	– cirrhosis
	– Gram-negative septicaemia
	– pregnancy
	– IPPV
Drugs/hormones	– salicylates
	– aminophylline
	– progesterone

Circumoral paraesthesia, hyperreflexia and tetany are common. Cardiovascular manifestations include tachycardia and ventricular arrhythmias secondary to the alkalaemia.

The causes of respiratory alkalosis are summarised in Table 22.15. Treatment comprises correction of the underlying cause, and thus differential diagnosis is important.

FURTHER READING

Askanazi J, Starker P M, Weissman C (eds) 1986 Fluid and electrolyte balance in critical care. Butterworths, Boston

Walmsley R N, Guerin M D 1984 Disorders of fluid and electrolyte balance. Wright, Bristol

Willatts S M 1987 Lecture notes on fluid and electrolyte balance, 2nd edn. Blackwell, Oxford

23. Complications during anaesthesia

RESPIRATORY OBSTRUCTION

Respiratory obstruction is a very common and potentially hazardous complication in the anaesthetised patient. If allowed to persist it may lead to coughing, straining and regurgitation or vomiting, resulting in hypoxaemia. In addition, the depth of anaesthesia may be reduced. Airway obstruction should be suspected when there is snoring, inadequate movement of the reservoir bag associated with respiration, or an obstructed respiratory pattern (paradoxical chest and abdominal movements which result in little or no gas exchange). In the artificially ventilated patient, an excessive inflation pressure is required to deliver the preset tidal volume. It may be difficult to inflate the lungs manually and, in extreme cases, the duration of expiration may be prolonged.

Airway causes

The lips may close tightly together in the edentulous patient as the mandible is supported in order to maintain the airway.

The tongue

As consciousness is lost, the tongue falls back into the oropharynx. In the overweight, short-necked individual, it may be difficult to pull the tongue and floor of the mouth forward sufficiently to maintain a clear airway.

Supraglottic structures

Swelling, oedema, tumours of the supraglottic area, or strictures may render maintenance of the airway difficult. Irradiation may result in rigidity and irritability of the structures of the floor of the mouth, so that the airway cannot be maintained when consciousness is lost. In epiglottitis, airway obstruction may be so severe that it is difficult to deepen anaesthesia sufficiently to permit intubation of the trachea.

A tumour of the larynx may act as a flap valve in the anaesthetised patient and cause intermittent obstruction. Alternatively, the laryngeal narrowing may result in turbulent flow which decreases the rate of induction of anaesthesia. In laryngotracheobronchitis, inflammation and oedema narrow the airway at both glottic and subglottic levels.

A large goitre may cause tracheal compression or deviation, and malignant thyroid tumours may infiltrate the trachea.

Mechanical obstruction

This usually occurs when the trachea has been intubated. The catheter mount may twist and obstruct. The tracheal tube itself may kink. This is most likely to occur close to the connector, particularly when PVC tracheal tubes of small diameter are used. These become more pliable when they reach body temperature. Armoured latex tubes contain an unreinforced area at the proximal end; if the connector is not inserted fully to reach the nylon reinforcement spiral, the soft latex may kink.

A Boyle Davis gag or palatal gag used in plastic surgery may obstruct the tracheal tube near the lips.

Red rubber tubes and to a lesser extent PVC tubes may kink in the oropharynx. While the degree of narrowing of the airway is likely to be small, the resulting obstruction may be sufficient to increase Pa_{CO_2}.

Overinflation of the cuff may cause herniation of the cuff over the distal end of the tube with resulting obstruction; in nylon latex tubes, herniation may obstruct the internal diameter of the tube. On occasions, the distal orifice of the tube may lie against the wall of the trachea.

BRONCHIAL INTUBATION

Unintentional bronchial intubation leads to hypoxaemia, may precipitate bronchospasm, and increases the risk of postoperative pulmonary collapse and infection. At induction of anaesthesia with volatile agents, rate of induction may be slowed considerably in comparison with the anticipated rate.

When the tracheal tube has not been cut to the appropriate length, inadvertent bronchial intubation is more likely to occur. This seems to be most common when intubation has been performed as an emergency by non-anaesthetic personnel.

To avoid bronchial intubation, it is important to cut the tracheal tube to the appropriate length for each patient, and to listen to both lung fields with a stethoscope before securing the tube and after any change of posture. Usually, the tracheal tube passes into the right main bronchus.

BRONCHOSPASM

Bronchospasm during anaesthesia is an undesirable, sometimes severe complication. It may be so intense that oxygenation of the patient is impossible and death may ensue.

Preoperative assessment and adequate preparation of the asthmatic or wheezy bronchitic patient diminish intraoperative problems and allow an appropriate anaesthetic technique to be selected. Bronchodilator therapy should be continued until immediately before anaesthesia. Respiratory function tests may demonstrate a reversible element in the respiratory obstruction of a bronchitic which should be treated by bronchodilator agents. Physiotherapy is required when chest secretions are present.

Bronchospasm may be triggered by chemical, mechanical or neurogenic factors. Halothane and enflurane are relatively non-irritant to the bronchial tree compared with ether or trichloroethylene. Bronchial secretions tend to increase during anaesthesia and may trigger an already irritable bronchial tree. The presence of a tracheal tube near the carina often initiates bronchospasm. Surgical stimulation may act as a trigger, either when the incision is made in a patient who is too lightly anaesthetised or during upper abdominal operations. Pneumothorax may mimic bronchospasm and should always be excluded. Unsuspected aspiration of stomach contents on induction or during the course of anaesthesia may precipitate bronchospasm, as may drugs, either as a side effect or as part of an adverse reaction.

The presence of bronchospasm should be suspected if there is an audible wheeze and prolonged expiratory phase, or if an increased inflation pressure is required to deliver a preset tidal volume. However, bronchospasm is not a common cause of respiratory obstruction and the diagnosis should be made only after the position and patency of the tracheal tube have been checked, secretions aspirated and the possibility of a pneumothorax eliminated.

Intravenous aminophylline 250 mg (50 mg/min) or salbutamol 250 μg (50 μg/min) are the drugs of first choice and both may be continued in an infusion. Hydrocortisone 100 mg i.v. may be useful. Intractable bronchospasm sometimes responds to halothane, enflurane or ether.

It is important to achieve adequate oxygenation while treating bronchospasm.

Anaesthesia and the wheezy patient

A preoperative visit helps to allay anxiety, and premedication should be designed to aid bronchodilation. Most induction agents have been both recommended and deemed to be unsuitable for the patient with bronchospasm; the role of propofol remains to be assessed. It is accepted generally that an inhalational induction is more likely to increase anxiety and therefore to trigger bronchospasm. If surgery is essential in the presence of severe bronchospasm, etomidate or ketamine together with pancuronium is an appropriate combination. Alternatively, a regional technique with adequate sedation may be employed.

LARYNGEAL SPASM

Partial laryngeal spasm is manifest as a crowing inspiratory noise and may progress to complete spasm resulting in hypoxaemia. Laryngeal spasm occurs most commonly during induction. The stimulus may be premature insertion of an airway or laryngoscope, pharyngeal secretions or vomit irritating the larynx, or surgical incision when anaesthesia is too light. Although i.v. barbiturates are not primary stimulants, they enhance respiratory reflexes during light anaesthesia. In contrast, premature insertion of an airway is often tolerated after induction of anaesthesia with propofol.

Some surgical operations, particularly anal stretch, breast surgery or dilatation of the cervix, often produce a degree of laryngeal spasm in the apparently well-anaesthetised patient.

At the end of surgery, laryngeal spasm may be encountered after extubation. Rarely, trauma to the recurrent laryngeal nerves at the time of thyroid surgery produces adduction of the vocal cords and stridor.

Minor degrees of laryngeal spasm are treated with 100% oxygen with respiratory assistance. The operation should be stopped until control is regained if surgical stimulation is the cause. On rare occasions it may be necessary to administer suxamethonium to allow intubation of the larynx.

Doxapram has been shown to be effective in treating laryngeal spasm when it occurs after tracheal extubation.

HICCUPS

Hiccups result from uncoordinated diaphragmatic movements, often as a result of vagal stimulation. Their incidence is increased when muscle relaxants are used. Patients undergoing subarachnoid or extradural techniques may also suffer this complication. Hiccups occur less commonly when atropine or hyoscine are used for premedication. Methohexitone is more likely to produce hiccups than thiopentone or propofol.

Hiccup is most commonly encountered during upper abdominal surgery and has been ascribed to hypocapnia, unduly light anaesthesia and insufficient dosage of non-depolarising muscle relaxants. The suggested remedies reflect these views; hand ventilate, administer more muscle relaxant, or deepen anaesthesia. Stimulation of the postnasal space with a suction catheter may be successful when other methods have failed.

Hiccup may be remarkably difficult to treat during anaesthesia. The trainee should beware of the temptation to administer excessive quantities of muscle relaxant. If hiccup is not inconveniencing the surgeon, the best course of action may be to ignore this problem.

PNEUMOTHORAX

The presence of pneumothorax may cause serious problems during anaesthesia. As nitrous oxide diffuses into the pleural space, a pneumothorax enlarges, producing haemodynamic disturbances. Positive pressure ventilation augments the problem and a tension pneumothorax may result as additional gas enters the pleural space.

The common causes of pneumothorax during anaesthesia are listed in Table 23.1. Iatrogenic pneumothorax is the most common cause of problems during anaesthesia, especially when a subclavian catheter has been inserted. The anaesthetist should inspect the chest X-ray before inducing anaesthesia.

A chest drain should be inserted before induction of anaesthesia in the presence of a known pneumothorax or recent rib fractures, particularly if IPPV is to be employed. On rare occasions this rule may be ignored and ketamine or a continuous inhalational technique avoiding nitrous oxide may be used if spontaneous respiration is maintained.

Table 23.1 Common causes of pneumothorax during anaesthesia

Traumatic	Chest injury Rib fracture	
Iatrogenic	Sublavian cannulae Internal jugular cannulae Brachial plexus block Inadvertent barotrauma	Cervical surgery Thoracic surgery
Spontaneous	Localised disorder, e.g. congenital bullae Marfan's syndrome Generalised emphysema Spontaneous mediastinal emphysema Asthma Rapid decompression of divers	

Detection of pneumothorax

Pneumothorax may present during anaesthesia as unexplained tachycardia, hypotension, bronchospasm, altered pattern of breathing, cyanosis and surgical emphysema. Diagnosis is made by clinical examination of the chest, surgery being suspended if necessary to allow the anaesthetist adequate access. Pulse oximetry may demonstrate sudden desaturation.

Action

Nitrous oxide should be discontinued immediately, and oxygen 100% administered while the diagnosis is confirmed by percussion of the chest and by needle aspiration of the suspected side via the 2nd intercostal space in the midclavicular line. A tension pneumothorax may be relieved by inserting an i.v. cannula at this site temporarily while the underwater seal and intercostal drain are prepared.

Pneumomediastinum

Air in the mediastinum may result from trauma or barotrauma. In barotrauma, it usually precedes the development of a pneumothorax. Pneumomediastinum is common after tracheostomy.

DIFFICULT INTUBATION

Relative ease of tracheal intubation reflects the experience and skill of the individual anaesthetist. However, from time to time every anaesthetist encounters a patient in whom tracheal intubation is either extremely difficult or impossible.

There are two problems; firstly recognising the potentially difficult intubation and planning how to overcome the problem, and secondly ensuring the safety of the patient when planned intubation has failed. Approximately 1 in 65 patients is likely to present difficulties in tracheal intubation.

Common anatomical causes of difficulty in intubation should be detected during the preoperative visit. A physical examination should be carried out in the following stages to determine the shape and size of the oropharyngeal cavity and whether or not normal laryngoscopy will reveal the vocal cords:

1. Examine the patient's face from lateral and anterolateral aspects for maxillary or mandibular abnormalities.
2. Examine the neck for swelling, scarring or tracheal deviation. If the distance from the chin to the suprahyoid notch is < 6 cm, laryngoscopy will be difficult.
3. Examine the neck for full extension.
4. Examine the neck for full flexion.
5. Examine mouth opening, the condition of the teeth and the oral cavity. Laryngoscopy should be possible if the fauces can be seen with the patient seated upright and the tongue protruded.

Causes

Congenital

Pierre Robin syndrome
Cystic hygroma
Treacher Collins syndrome
Gargoylism
Achondroplasia
Marfan's syndrome

Anatomical

Eight anatomical features associated with difficult intubation have been identified, some of which may be seen only on X-ray:

1. A short muscular neck and full set of teeth.
2. Receding lower jaw with obtuse mandibular angles.
3. Protruding incisors, with relative overgrowth of the premaxilla.
4. Long high arched palate with a long narrow mouth.
5. Increased alveolar–mental distance requiring wide opening of the mandible for laryngoscopy.
6. Poor mobility of the mandible.
7. Increase in posterior depth of the mandible hindering displacement of the mandible.
8. Decreased distance between the occiput and the spinous process of Cl.

Recent work suggests that the last cause is the most important factor.

Acquired

Restricted jaw opening. Trismus is caused by spasm of the medial pterygoid and masseter muscles and is often secondary to an infective cause, e.g. dental abscess. Fibrosis may follow infection, and restrict temporomandibular joint (TMJ) movement. Rheumatoid or osteoarthritis affecting the TMJ also restricts mouth opening. Mandibular fractures may impede TMJ movement and also produce trismus.

Restricted neck movement. Osteoarthritis commonly affects the cervical spine, and undue neck movement during anaesthesia may worsen the patient's symptoms. Ankylosing spondylitis is less common, but may result in total rigidity of the cervical spine. This may be encountered also in patients who have undergone fusion of the cervical spine.

Neck instability. Intubation may be made difficult if neck movement (especially the flexion required for tracheal intubation) is prohibited because it may cause cord damage, e.g. in the presence of a cervical spine injury or severe rheumatoid arthritis.

Soft tissue swelling. Facial swelling occurs with dental infections, trauma and immediately after burns. There may be associated intra-oral swelling which distorts the upper airway and makes it difficult to see the larynx.

Bleeding after thyroidectomy or other neck operations produces both compression of neck structures and oedema of the oropharynx and larynx, making intubation hazardous.

Scarring. Skin and soft tissue contractures develop after burns, making the floor of the mouth rigid. Radiotherapy also produces a 'wooden' mouth floor which cannot be displaced easily to allow laryngoscopy.

Other causes. Laryngeal and tracheal causes are discussed above.

In the morbidly obese individual, direct laryngoscopy may be physically difficult to perform. Excessive weight gain in pregnancy may limit the range of movements necessary for easy laryngoscopy as the laryngoscope handle infringes on the anterior chest wall.

Management

There are three questions the trainee should ask himself on approaching a patient in whom intubation may prove difficult:

1. Is the patient likely to regurgitate as a result of a full stomach following recent ingestion of food or liquid, or because of pregnancy or gastrointestinal pathology, e.g. pharyngeal pouch, hiatus hernia, pyloric stenosis, paralytic ileus?
2. Is intubation likely to prove difficult because of respiratory tract obstruction?
3. Is intubation likely to be difficult because of difficulty in laryngoscopy, e.g. inability to open the mouth or extend the atlanto-occipital joint?

The trainee should never attempt to perform tracheal intubation using an i.v. induction agent and long-acting muscle relaxant in any of the above situations.

Tracheal intubation and a failed intubation drill in obstetric anaesthesia are described in detail in Chapter 33 (p. 551), whilst difficult intubation in emergency anaesthesia is described in Chapter 32 (p. 532).

The following manoeuvres are used in non-emergency anaesthesia. Items 1 to 5 represent progressive anticipated difficulty in laryngoscopy and/or tracheal intubation.

1. Where there is minimal difficulty anticipated in either laryngoscopy or intubation, the following may be attempted. After setting up an i.v. infusion and following preoxygenation for 3 min, a small dose of induction agent is administered i.v. and manual ventilation of the lungs via a face mask is attempted. If satisfactory ventilation of the lungs is achieved, suxamethonium may be given before laryngoscopy. If laryngoscopy is difficult, anaesthesia should be maintained with nitrous oxide, oxygen and halothane. In most instances a bougie may be passed into the trachea and a tracheal tube 'railroaded' over it. If this fails, blind nasal intubation should be considered with the patient breathing spontaneously a volatile

agent, e.g. halothane. Alternatively, if visualisation of the larynx is impossible, it may be possible to thread a tracheal tube over an extradural catheter passed through the cricothyroid membrane via an extradural needle and passed up through the oropharynx.

2. In the presence of respiratory tract obstruction severe enough to cause dyspnoea on exercise, i.v. agents should not be used and anaesthesia should be induced with a volatile agent with 50% nitrous oxide in oxygen. The reason for this is that minor degrees of respiratory tract obstruction may progress to complete obstruction when muscle tone decreases following loss of consciousness. The use of a gas induction is beneficial as muscle tone diminishes gradually with progressive loss of consciousness, and if ventilation ceases because of total respiratory tract obstruction the patient wakes up rapidly.

3. Following sedation with an i.v. benzodiazepine, local anaesthetic solution may be applied to the nose, pharynx and trachea to enable a tracheal tube to be passed blindly in the awake patient before anaesthesia is induced. This is an appropriate technique in patients when laryngoscopy is impossible, e.g. severe trismus.

4. A fibreoptic laryngoscope may be used under local anaesthesia and a tracheal tube threaded over the laryngoscope before insertion. However, the anaesthetist requires considerable practice with this instrument in order to be able to acquire familiarity with the normal anatomical landmarks.

5. Tracheostomy may be performed surgically under local anaesthesia and the airway maintained safely via the tracheostomy tube.

In respiratory tract obstruction which is severe enough to cause dyspnoea at rest, only manoeuvres 3–5 should be contemplated.

If it is anticipated that the level of difficulty in intubation warrants manoeuvres 2–5, surgery should be undertaken under local anaesthesia if appropriate.

Failed intubation drill

If intubation fails when neither experienced help nor alternative aids to intubation are available, it is essential to have a contingency plan. The failed intubation drill was devised for obstetric patients undergoing general anaesthesia, but deserves to be applied more widely. In emergency anaesthesia, cricoid pressure must be maintained from the moment of loss of consciousness, and the patient positioned head down on the left side. Manual ventilation is continued via the facemask and pharyngeal secretions aspirated if necessary. Surgical anaesthesia is established using nitrous oxide, oxygen and a volatile agent until spontaneous respiration returns, or if oxygenation is difficult the patient is allowed to wake up and the situation reassessed.

It is essential to record in the patient's notes that intubation has proved to be difficult.

Oesophageal intubation

The most reliable way of ensuring that the tracheal tube is in the trachea is to see directly that it has passed through the vocal cords. Oesophageal intubation may be misdiagnosed as bronchospasm, with tragic consequences. Clinical signs may be misleading; the chest may move and breath sounds may be heard in all four quadrants even if the oesophagus has been intubated. If the patient's lungs have been pre-oxygenated, cyanosis may not be detected for up to 5 min. The presence of expiratory condensation on the tracheal tube and refilling of the anaesthetic reservoir bag are unreliable signs of trachea intubation. A consistent rise and fall of end-tidal carbon dioxide concentration with a *normal capnograph waveform* is the most reliable sign that the tube is in the trachea. A recently described and simple test of correct tracheal placement uses a 50 ml syringe attached to a catheter mount; air may be aspirated easily from the trachea, but not from the oesophagus.

HYPOTENSION

Hypotension during anaesthesia may be defined as a decrease in systolic arterial pressure below 70 mmHg.

Causes (see Table 23.2)

Preoperative resuscitation of a patient for emergency anaesthesia may have been inadequate. This is most likely to occur when the magnitude of fluid loss has been underestimated, e.g. in the

Table 23.2 Common causes of hypotension during anaesthesia

Hypovolaemia	Preoperative hypovolaemia Surgical haemorrhage
Induction agents	Relative overdosage in very young, very old, very ill, or patients with cardiovascular disease Absolute overdosage
Volatile agents	Halothane, enflurane, isoflurane
Muscle relaxants	D-Tubocurarine
SAB and extradural	Hypotension proportional to height of block
Cardiovascular disease	Myocardial infarction Arrhythmias Pulmonary embolus
Respiratory disease	Pneumothorax
Hypersensitivity reactions	Induction agent Muscle relaxants Blood or colloid infusions

patient with intestinal obstruction, intra-abdominal haemorrhage or multiple fractures of long bones or pelvis. Induction of anaesthesia produces vasodilatation and abolishes compensatory vasoconstriction, resulting in hypotension.

When given in equipotent doses, all induction agents, with the exception of ketamine and possibly etomidate, produce similar cardiovascular effects, viz. an increase in heart rate and decreases in systolic and diastolic arterial pressures, central venous pressure and cardiac output.

Excessive dosage is likely to lead to a decrease in arterial pressure, particularly when propofol is used in the elderly. Those who have coexisting myocardial disease or inadequately treated hypertension often develop greater arteriolar dilatation and are much more susceptible to the hypotensive effects of induction agents.

Volatile anaesthetic agents, particularly halothane, enflurane and isoflurane, produce myocardial depression, and may result in hypotension. This is more likely to occur if large concentrations are used or IPPV is employed. The concurrent use of *d*-tubocurarine with its ganglion blocking properties may compound the hypotensive effect. IPPV may cause hypotension resulting from a decrease in cardiac output caused by increased intrathoracic pressure. This responds usually to infusion of i.v. fluids.

Subarachnoid or extradural anaesthesia produces vasodilatation because of sympathetic blockade. Hypotension and bradycardia may require correction with i.v. fluids and ephedrine. Hypotension during anaesthesia may be caused also by surgical manoeuvres (e.g. haemorrhage, pressure on great veins), anaphylactic reactions to drugs or blood transfusion, pneumothorax, myocardial infarction, or cardiac arrhythmias.

HYPERTENSION

Hypertension during anaesthesia is an undesirable complication because of the risk of myocardial ischaemia or infarction, or vascular damage. Some causes are listed in Table 23.3.

There is no doubt that poorly controlled hypertension intra- and postoperatively leads to an increased mortality and morbidity. However, moderate hypertension with a diastolic arterial pressure <110 mmHg does not increase risk provided that it is controlled during surgery and the early post-operative period.

In patients with a phaeochromocytoma, coarctation of the aorta or renal artery stenosis, particular attention should be paid to preoperative

Table 23.3 Common causes of hypertension during anaesthesia

Light anaesthesia	Inadequate analgesia Inadequate hypnosis Coughing, straining on tracheal tube
Coexisting hypertension	Untreated Treated Undiagnosed phaeochromocytoma
Aortic cross-clamping	
Hypercapina	
Drugs adrenaline ergometrine ketamine	
Pre-eclampsia	

treatment if intraoperative fluctuations are to be avoided.

A hypertensive response to laryngoscopy occurs commonly. β-Blockers given at induction may partly attenuate this. Coughing and straining on the tracheal tube may be diminished by topical analgesia of the larynx with lignocaine provided that sufficient time elapses for surface analgesia to become effective.

Surgical stimulation results in hypertension if the depth of anaesthesia is inadequate.

Ketamine should be avoided in patients with ischaemic heart disease or hypertension. Ergometrine is contraindicated in the obstetric patient with pre-eclampsia.

Cross-clamping the aorta (e.g. during repair of aortic aneurysm) greatly increases peripheral resistance and afterload. Increased myocardial work may result in hypertension and subendocardial ischaemia. A volatile anaesthetic agent or sodium nitroprusside may be used to control arterial pressure at a level that is normal for that patient.

Hypercapnia may lead to hypertension, tachycardia or ventricular arrhythmias. In the absence of end-tidal CO_2 monitoring, it is essential to ensure that the carbon dioxide cylinder on the anaesthetic machine is not accidentally in operation and that fresh gas flows are appropriate for the anaesthetic breathing system in use.

CARDIAC ARRHYTHMIAS (see also Ch. 41, p. 650)

As perioperative disturbances of cardiac rhythm are common, all anaesthetised patients warrant continuous ECG monitoring in conjunction with the other standard aspects of monitoring including capillary refill, arterial pressure and pulse. Electrocardiographic evidence of sinus rhythm implies normal cardiac impulse generation and conduction, and is not indicative of adequate cardiac output or tissue perfusion.

The ECG allows early and accurate detection and analysis of abnormal rhythms, some of which may go unnoticed clinically. For example, ventricular bigeminy may exist in the presence of a normal radial pulse.

Aetiology

There are many potential causes of arrhythmias during anaesthesia (Table 23.4). Most can be avoided by adequate preoperative assessment and skilful intraoperative management. However, there are some arrhythmias that occur despite good anaesthesia.

Table 23.4 Common causes of arrhythmia during anaesthesia

Surgical	Ophthalmic, Nasal, Dental } Surgery Mesenteric traction Anal stretch
Metabolic	Hyperthyroidism Hypercapnia Hypokalaemia
Disease	Ischaemic heart disease Rheumatic heart disease Congenital heart disease
Drugs	Atropine Adrenaline Halothane

Ischaemic heart disease is by far the commonest cardiac disorder encountered in the surgical population. In its presence, any change in circulatory status that adversely affects the myocardial oxygen supply:demand ratio (e.g. hypertension, hypotension, bradycardia, tachycardia) may precipitate ventricular arrhythmias. Pharmacological suppression of an ectopic focus should be accompanied by attempts to improve myocardial metabolism.

Patients with inadequately treated hypertension are also prone to perioperative arrhythmias, as are patients with chronic rheumatic heart disease associated with valvular stenosis or regurgitation. The pre-excitation syndromes, e.g. the Wolff–Parkinson–White syndrome, which are not as uncommon as once supposed, may present with a supraventricular tachycardia during anaesthesia. Similarly, sino-atrial dysfunction is being increasingly recognised and may result in sinus bradycardia and sinus arrest which predispose to junctional escape rhythms. Paroxysmal tachycardia followed by a prolonged period of sinus arrest may also be a prominent feature of this syndrome.

Patients with undiagnosed hyperthyroidism may develop atrial fibrillation in the perioperative period, whereas unheralded hypertensive crises together with malignant ventricular arrhythmias are the hallmarks of an unsuspected phaeochromocytoma.

Apart from pre-existing cardiac or endocrine disease, the two commonest causes of perioperative rhythm disturbances are arterial hypoxaemia and hypercapnia. Hypercapnia provokes the release of endogenous catecholamines which may trigger ventricular arrhythmias especially in the presence of halothane in a spontaneously breathing patient. This interaction between adrenaline and halothane is also important in the context of exogenous adrenaline injected to reduce blood loss. In the presence of halothane the maximum dose of adrenaline for infiltration should not exceed 100 μg (i.e. 10 ml of 1:100 000) during any 10-min period. Isoflurane and enflurane are much safer in this respect and problems are unlikely if oxygenation and ventilation are guaranteed.

Halothane, and to a lesser extent enflurane, cause a dose-dependent depression of sinus node automaticity. This suppression of the dominant pacemaker may encourage the emergence of a secondary pacemaker in AV junctional tissue. The resulting junctional escape rhythm is a common occurrence in patients anaesthetised with these agents. Treatment is necessary only if the junctional focus is very slow (less than 50 beats/min), or if the concomitant loss of 'atrial kick' causes hypotension. Small doses of atropine (0.3 mg) usually restore sinus rhythm.

Hyperventilation and hypocapnia are associated with transcellular potassium shifts resulting in relative extracellular hypokalaemia. Serum potassium concentrations may decrease by 0.5 mmol/litre for every 1.3 kPa decrease in P_{CO_2} and the resulting hypokalaemia increases the resting membrane potential of excitable tissues, causing hyperpolarisation of cell membranes. The overall effect is an irritable, excitable myocardium that is more prone to arrhythmias. This situation exists in hypokalaemia of any aetiology including that commonly seen in the surgical population.

Hyperkalaemia decreases the resting membrane potential and the resulting membrane hypopolarisation predisposes to arrhythmias. An increased serum potassium concentration is seen typically in renal insufficiency when excretion of potassium is limited, but can also occur with ionic redistribution. In patients with burns, extensive denervation of skeletal muscle (paraplegia), or some neuromuscular or myopathic diseases, large amounts of potassium are released from muscle in response to suxamethonium. This may result in acute hyperkalaemia and cardiac arrest.

Many non-anaesthetic drugs predispose to arrhythmias — digoxin, tricyclic antidepressants, aminophylline and some sympathomimetic inotropes. In each instance, toxicity should be excluded prior to anaesthesia.

If anaesthesia is too light, surgical stimulation may result in extreme reflex sympathetic and parasympathetic activity, and this may be associated with arrhythmias. However, more extreme rhythm abnormalities occur in the form of traction reflexes presenting during specific surgical manipulations. Traction on hollow viscera during laparotomy, or on the external ocular muscles during squint surgery, may produce extreme bradycardia which, although usually transient, can result in asystole. Atropine may be used both to prevent and to treat these disturbances. In neuroanaesthetic practice, severe rhythm abnormalities are seen when the brain stem and/or cranial nerves are encroached upon in posterior fossa explorations. More importantly to general anaesthetists, stimulation and traction on the pharynx and larynx are associated commonly with transient ventricular arrhythmias. These are seen during tracheal intubation and are reflected in the high incidence of arrhythmias during ENT, oral and dental surgery.

Treatment

Whilst arrhythmias which compromise cardiac function, e.g. ventricular tachycardia, always require immediate treatment, some arrhythmias do not. Treatment is required in the following situations:

1. When they interfere significantly with cardiac output and tissue perfusion, i.e. in the presence of hypotension.
2. When they predispose to ventricular fibril-

lation or asystole (which are associated with circulatory standstill and may be difficult to treat).

3. When they are associated with significant myocardial ischaemia.

Supraventricular tachyarrhythmias, e.g. atrial fibrillation, flutter or supraventricular tachycardia may result in heart rates sufficiently fast to embarrass cardiac function and these should probably not be allowed to persist untreated. It should be remembered that antiarrhythmic drugs are potent depressants of cardiac conduction and contractility and should not be used unless there is a good indication. In this context any underlying factors which may precipitate or perpetuate arrhythmias (hypoxaemia, hypercapnia, electrolyte disturbances, light anaesthesia) should be corrected before resorting to drug therapy. (See Appendix IV (c) for doses of drugs.)

Perioperative arrhythmias are rarely primary cardiac events and often may be attributed to extracardiac factors. Sinus tachycardia may result from hypovolaemia, sepsis, pain or light anaesthesia and treatment should be directed at the underlying cause. Atrial premature contractions do not usually warrant specific treatment but on occasion herald atrial fibrillation which may be associated with haemodynamic deterioration.

Ventricular fibrillation should be treated immediately with DC shock as should ventricular tachycardia if cardiac function is compromised. Premature ventricular contractions and ventricular tachycardia with a well-preserved cardiac output should be treated with lignocaine.

EMBOLISM

Venous

Venous embolism during anaesthesia is uncommon. However, prophylactic measures should be used to decrease the incidence of postoperative venous thrombosis and embolism. Preoperatively, subcutaneous heparin is used most frequently. Intraoperatively, the venous return may be improved by squeezing the calves mechanically or stimulating the calf muscles electrically.

The choice of anaesthetic technique influences the incidence of DVT. DVT may be more common when IPPV and a muscle relaxant are used than when a regional or spontaneously breathing technique is employed.

Arterial

The most common source of arterial emboli during anaesthesia is an indwelling cannula, and is often associated with excessive flushing of an arterial line with either a 2 ml syringe or an automatic flushing device. Rapid injection of a volume of more than 1 ml may flush clots retrogradely from the radial artery into the more proximal arterial tree.

Air

The possibility of an air embolism exists in many types of surgical operation (Table 23.5), whenever atmospheric pressure is greater than intravascular pressure. In many situations, careful positioning of the patient so that the heart is higher than, or at the same level as, the operation site prevents this complication.

Pathophysiology

Symptoms of venous air embolism are produced if air enters a vessel at a rate of 0.5 ml kg^{-1} min^{-1} or greater. A hissing sound may be heard in the wound. As the air enters the right side of the heart, mechanical distension is produced, cardiac

Table 23.5 Surgical and other causes of air embolism

Neurosurgery	Posterior fossa operations in sitting position
Abdominal surgery	Laparoscopy Hysterectomy D & C and insufflation
Orthopaedic surgery	Arthrography Hip surgery
Chest	Open heart surgery Breast operations
Miscellaneous	Middle ear surgery Neck surgery Blood transfusion CVP lines Hyperbaric situations Arterial monitoring Extradural injection

output and arterial pressure decrease, heart rate increases and a 'millwheel' murmur is heard. The air passes into the pulmonary vein producing coughing, gasping and cyanosis. End-tidal CO_2 decreases, and pulmonary artery and central venous pressures increase. Asphyxia results from obstruction to the pulmonary circulation. Paradoxical air embolism may occur via a 'probe patent' foramen ovale, or air may cross the pulmonary capillary bed, to enter the coronary or cerebral circulations causing myocardial ischaemia or convulsions.

Detection

Precordial or oesophageal stethoscope; end-tidal CO_2 monitoring; Doppler studies — chest wall, oesophageal; echocardiography.

Treatment

Haemostasis is achieved by compression, or the operative field may be flooded by the surgeon. The patient is tipped head down on the left side so that air may be aspirated from the right atrium via a central venous line. In extreme situations, a cannula may be inserted percutaneously into the right ventricle for aspiration of air. Neurosurgical air embolism may be obviated almost completely if the patient is placed prone and not in the sitting position.

HYPOVOLAEMIA

Prior to anaesthesia, it is essential to assess the extent of fluid deficit and to correct hypovolaemia. Thirst, apathy, a dry tongue, inelastic tissue and a decreased urine output indicate fluid depletion which may be confirmed biochemically and haematologically. Poor peripheral perfusion, decreased urine production (<0.5 ml kg^{-1} h^{-1}) in the presence of a raised heart rate, hypotension and low central venous pressure confirm the diagnosis. β-Blocking drugs may prevent a compensatory tachycardia and obscure the diagnosis.

Induction of anaesthesia in a hypovolaemic patient may result in cardiovascular collapse as peripheral vasodilatation occurs and as the adrenergic vasoconstrictor response is depressed by barbiturates. Therefore, fluid losses should be replaced preoperatively; CVP measurement is essential if large volumes are required.

Table 23.6 indicates some common causes of fluid loss in the perioperative period.

Haemorrhage

In children a blood loss greater than 10% of circulating blood volume (wt in kg × 80 ml) should be replaced with blood. In adults, blood losses up to 1 litre may be replaced by crystalloid or plasma substitutes, but larger losses should be replaced with warmed blood.

Allowance must be made for additional fluid loss by sequestration as interstitial fluid when increased vascular permeability in damaged areas is likely to occur, e.g. crush injuries, intestinal obstruction. 5 ml kg^{-1} min^{-1} of a balanced electrolyte solution is usually sufficient to cover these losses.

Evaporation

Insensible loss from skin and lungs forms part of normal body fluid losses and 0.5–2 litres of water per day may be lost. Electrolyte loss is increased significantly by sweating. Evaporative losses are

Table 23.6 Causes of fluid loss

Pre-existing deficit	
Haemorrhage	Trauma Gastrointestinal Obstetric Major vessel rupture
Gastrointestinal	Vomiting Obstruction Fistula Diarrhoea
Other causes	Diuretics
Continuing physiological loss	
Evaporation	
Sequestration of fluids	
Continuing current abnormal losses	
Haemorrhage	
Drainage of ascites	
Decompression of obstructed bowel	
Burns	

increased during anaesthesia and surgery. The patient loses fluid and latent heat of vaporisation in humidifying dry inspired gas and from exposed abdominal contents. Humidification of inspired gas decreases respiratory heat and water loss and helps to maintain body temperature. Condenser humidifiers are suitable, but they achieve only 70% relative humidity and an airway temperature of 32°C. They may also increase airway resistance on becoming blocked, and represent an additional site of potential disconnection.

HYPERVOLAEMIA (Table 23.7)

Fluid should be administered according to the requirements of the individual patient. Over-enthusiastic administration of crystalloid may lead to pulmonary oedema if the interstitial fluid volume is expanded by more than 30%. Special care should be taken when crystalloid is used to correct hypotension produced by anaesthetic drugs. Myocardial failure may occur, particularly in the elderly patient with ischaemic heart disease.

During anaesthesia, hypervolaemia may be suspected if an elevated CVP, tachycardia and low arterial pressure are present after rapid fluid infusion. Distended neck veins, a third heart sound, pulmonary crepitations and raised inflation pressure confirm the diagnosis. During longer procedures, facial oedema may develop.

Inotropic support should be provided with dopamine and digoxin, and loop diuretics used to excrete the excess fluid. If CVP monitoring is misleading and does not reflect left heart function, pulmonary capillary wedge pressure measurement should be considered.

Table 23.7 Factors resulting in hypervolaemia

Myocardial failure
Overenthusiastic replacement in response to:
drug-induced hypotension
caval compression
Inability to excrete a fluid load
Misleading monitoring, CVP not indicating left ventricular function
Pregnancy — circulatory changes at delivery
Hypoproteinaemia
Water intoxication following transurethral resection of prostate

HYPOTHERMIA

Induced hypothermia is used to reduce metabolic rate and oxygen consumption to increase the ability of the brain to withstand hypoxia without producing irreversible damage, e.g. in cardiac surgery, neurosurgery and intensive therapy. Surface cooling is used in small children before induction of profound hypothermia (15–20°C) and circulatory arrest to allow repair of congenital heart defects. Non-depolarising muscle relaxants are used to prevent shivering, and carbon dioxide added to inspired gases to shift the oxygen dissociation curve to the right, thereby allowing greater oxygen release in the tissues.

Inadvertent hypothermia

During surgery a patient loses heat to the cooler theatre environment. This heat loss may be increased by evaporative loss from exposed viscera, the use of dry anaesthetic gases, and replacement of fluid loss with cold i.v. solutions.

The temperature may decrease to 33–34°C during prolonged surgery. Drugs are metabolised more slowly and their duration of action is prolonged. At the end of surgery, a cold patient has to expend energy to regain body temperature, and may shiver. Shivering increases oxygen consumption significantly and may compromise myocardial oxygen supply because cardiac output is depressed by the residual effects of anaesthesia. Measures which may be employed to reduce heat loss during anaesthesia and surgery are shown in Table 23.8.

Table 23.8 Prevention of heat loss

Swaddling of small children
Warming mattress
Space blanket
Humidification
Swedish nose
heated water bath
Enclose exposed viscera in plastic bags
Warm surgical preparation fluids
Warm irrigation fluids
Warm i.v. solutions
Increase ambient temperature and humidity

MALIGNANT HYPERPYREXIA

This is a potentially fatal condition in which, as a result of an inherited abnormality in skeletal muscle cells, exposure to some anaesthetic agents may precipitate a rapid increase in body temperature of at least 2°C/h.

Aetiology

Susceptible individuals inherit a defect in calcium binding in the sarcoplasmic reticulum of skeletal and possibly cardiac muscle cells. In the presence of specific trigger agents, calcium is released into the cytoplasm, producing myofibrillar contraction, depletion of the high-energy phosphate reserves in muscle, accelerated lactic acid and carbon dioxide production, increased oxygen consumption, a profound metabolic acidosis, and the production of heat. Membrane stability is lost, and potassium leaks from the cells into the extracellular fluid causing hyperkalaemia.

The pattern of inheritance varies from recessive to dominant. Susceptible individuals may have muscular disorders or myopathies, or frequently are normal on clinical examination.

Trigger agents

Most drugs used in anaesthesia have been incriminated in the precipitation of malignant hyperpyrexia. Halothane and suxamethonium are the two agents most likely to produce the condition, although all volatile anaesthetic agents should be avoided in an individual who is known to be susceptible. Lignocaine is probably unsafe.

Clinical signs

There may be increased muscle tone and a precipitous increase in end-tidal carbon dioxide concentration after the injection of suxamethonium, particularly in young patients. Less than 10% progress to the full syndrome. In other patients, hyperpyrexia with or without rigidity appear later during the anaesthetic, or in the early postoperative period, and are accompanied by tachycardia, hyperpnoea, cyanosis, hypoxaemia, metabolic acidosis, hyperkalaemia, hypocalcaemia, tetany, myoglobinuria, acute renal failure, and cardiac failure. Arrhythmias may occur at any time. With the prompt use of dantrolene, the mortality may be reduced from 64% to zero.

Treatment

Volatile agents should be discontinued. 100% oxygen should be administered, if necessary by IPPV. Attempts should be made to reduce body temperature using ice or ice-packs, and sodium bicarbonate should be infused to treat the metabolic acidosis. Insulin may be required to treat hyperkalaemia.

Dantrolene is the only drug available for the specific treatment of malignant hyperpyrexia. As soon as the diagnosis is made, it should be administered i.v. in a dose of 1 mg/kg and repeated every 5 min up to a maximum dose of 10 mg/kg or until control of the condition has been obtained.

Investigation of susceptible individuals

Although measurement of serum creatine kinase has been recommended as a screening test for susceptible individuals, the results are unreliable. Susceptible individuals, and members of their family, require muscle biopsy for histological evidence of the condition and for in vitro exposure to trigger agents. These investigations are highly specialised, and the patient and his family should be referred to a malignant hyperpyrexia investigation centre.

Anaesthesia in the susceptible individual

In a patient known to be susceptible to the condition, or a relative of such a patient, all attempts should be made to prevent triggering of malignant hyperpyrexia. Diazepam is a suitable premedication, but anticholinergic agents should not be administered. Induction with a barbiturate, muscle relaxation using pancuronium, and maintenance of anaesthesia with nitrous oxide supplemented by an opioid agent, appears to be the safest technique available. Although regional anaesthesia may have advantages, malignant hyperpyrexia has been reported in patients undergoing spinal nerve block. Throughout the course of the anaesthetic, temperature should be monitored using needle probes inserted into muscle, and an oesophageal or nasopharyngeal temperature probe. Dantrolene and all necessary resuscitation equipment should be immediately available.

HYPERSENSITIVITY

Hypersensitivity reactions refer to uncommon, unpredictable drug toxicity, in most cases involving the release of histamine, and not exaggerated normal pharmacological actions resulting from relative or absolute overdosage. Reactions occur most commonly to induction agents and muscle relaxant drugs.

Anaphylactic or type I hypersensitivity

Type I hypersensitivity to a drug, e.g. thiopentone, involves production of specific IgE antibodies as a result of previous exposure. Occasionally a primary IgG-mediated response is seen.

Anaphylactoid

This is a descriptive term used for responses which are clinically similar to a type I response but which involve pharmacological as opposed to immunological release of histamine.

Recognition

There is an equal sex incidence but reactors are generally from a younger age group. Allergies (particularly to cosmetics), atopy and asthma are more common in barbiturate reactors than in the general population. Most reactions present within the first 5 min of anaesthesia, but in 10% the onset is delayed. The first apparent feature is variable, but flushing over the upper half of the body, absent peripheral pulses, bronchospasm or transient difficulty in lung inflation are the most common (Table 23.9).

Treatment

This is designed to prevent hypoxaemia and restore the circulation. In many reactions, spontaneous recovery occurs but a severe reaction comprising hypotension and bronchospasm may be fatal. When a severe reaction occurs, the following steps should be followed:

Table 23.9 Manifestations of hypersensitivity

Cutaneous	Flushing Large urticarial weals Rash
Oedema	Early (within minutes) affecting head, eyelids, upper airway, with significant loss of fluid Late (slow to resolve); generalised
Cardiovascular collapse	Vasodilatation — absent peripheral pulses ECG — tachycardia asystole VF
Bronchospasm	Mild — transient difficulty in ventilation Severe — likely to be asthmatic
Gastrointestinal symptoms	Cramping abdominal pain Nausea, vomiting Diarrhoea
Haematological abnormalities	Present in 10–15% ? Should surgery proceed

1. Administer 100% oxygen.
2. Intermittent positive pressure ventilation and external cardiac massage if necessary.
3. 500–1500 ml human albumin solution i.v. — crystalloid escapes via leaky capillaries.
4. Consider administering adrenaline 0.3–0.5 ml 1:1000 i.v. or i.m. to counter vasodilatation.
5. Steroids, Aminophylline, Sympathomimetic drugs } may be required for bronchospasm.
6. Surgery should not commence after treatment of a severe reaction because there is increased risk of abnormal coagulation. In one series, the average length of treatment was 143 min.

Investigation

The mechanism of the reaction may be elucidated by detecting complement conversion or formation of IgE antibodies in sequential blood samples taken into EDTA bottles at time 0, 3 h, 6 h and 24 h after the reaction.

Some anaesthetists advocate intradermal testing on the basis that it is safe, highly sensitive, and a ready source of antigen is provided. Others query the safety and particularly the reliability for drugs which have the capacity to release histamine. Intradermal testing is performed one month after the reaction when all drugs which might modify the result have been discontinued.

Prevention

The patient should be advised to wear a warning bracelet describing sensitivity to drugs. Prophylaxis with antihistamines and steroids is not usually successful. The evidence for the efficacy of H_2-receptor antagonists is ill-defined. It has been suggested that disodium cromoglycate may have a role.

Blood transfusion reactions

Most transfusion reactions are febrile or urticarial in nature and are induced by leucocyte or platelet antigens. Microfiltration of blood recovers 90% of the granulocytes and decreases the incidence of reactions. Pretreatment with chlorpheniramine or other antihistamines may be indicated in a patient who has had a previous reaction.

Anaesthesia masks the signs of incompatible transfusion but tachycardia, hypotension, cyanosis or unexplained oozing from the wound shortly after a transfusion has started may be indicative of mismatched blood. At times of stress, the wrong blood may be given to a patient and surveys have shown that this is most likely to occur in the operating theatre or ITU.

Plasma substitutes

Haemaccel (mol. wt 35 000) and Dextran 70 (av. mol. wt 70 000) are most likely to produce hypersensitivity, urticaria, tachycardia and hypotension when they are infused rapidly. The incidence of these reactions varies according to different surveys but the most commonly quoted figures are:

0.26% for Dextrans
0.068% for Haemaccel
0.003% for plasma protein solutions.

FURTHER READING

Clarke R S J 1988 Hypersensitivity to intravenous anaesthetics. In: Dundee J W, Wyant G M (eds) Intravenous anaesthesia. Churchill Livingstone, Edinburgh

Gray T C 1985 Thoughts on some serious anaesthetic errors. Journal of the Medical Defence Union, 10

Hirsham C A 1983 Airway reactivity in humans. Anesthetic implications. Anesthesiology 58: 170

Kerr J H 1987 Is the tube in the trachea? British Medical Journal 285: 400

McIntyre J W R 1987 The difficult tracheal intubation. Canadian Journal of Anaesthesia 34: 204

Plasma substitutes: the choice during surgery and intensive care. Drug and Therapeutics Bulletin 1987 25: 37

Symposium on malignant hyperthermia. British Journal of Anaesthesia 1988 60: 253–319

Taylor T H, Major E (eds) 1987 Hazards and complications of anaesthesia. Churchill Livingstone, Edinburgh

Tunstall M E 1976 Failed intubation drill. Anaesthesia 31: 850

Willatts S M 1982 Lecture notes on fluid and electrolyte balance. Blackwell, Oxford

24. Postoperative care

In modern anaesthetic practice, the patient is monitored and supervised closely and continuously during induction and throughout the operative procedure. However, many problems associated with anaesthesia and surgery may occur in the immediate postoperative period, and it is essential that supervision by adequately trained and experienced personnel is continued during the recovery period. In addition, some major and minor complications of anaesthesia and surgery may occur at any time in the first few days after operation.

THE EARLY RECOVERY PERIOD

Many hospitals have a recovery ward in close proximity to the operating theatre suite (see Ch. 18). A large number of recovery areas are closed at night and at weekends; at these times, and in hospitals with no recovery ward, the patient is supervised usually in a corridor close to the operating theatre and often by inadequately trained staff. This section describes common problems which occur in the immediate postoperative period and refers specifically to their management in a recovery ward; however, the same principles are applicable to recovery in other locations.

The recovery period starts as soon as the patient leaves the operating table and the direct supervision of the anaesthetist. All the complications listed below may occur at any time, including the period of transfer from operating theatre to recovery ward; in some operating theatre suites, the transfer to the recovery ward may last for several minutes, and it is essential that the standard of observation does not diminish during the journey. The patient must be supervised and monitored closely *at all times*.

Systems affected

Central nervous system

Consciousness may not return for several minutes after the end of general anaesthesia, and may be impaired for a longer period of time. During this period, a patent airway must be maintained. There is a risk of aspiration into the lungs of any material, e.g. gastric content or blood, which is present in the pharynx. Consciousness may be depressed also in patients who have received sedation to facilitate endoscopy or regional anaesthesia.

Excitement and confusion may occur during recovery and may result in injury. Pain may be severe if long-acting analgesics have not been given during surgery.

Cardiovascular system

Peripheral resistance and cardiac output may be reduced because of residual effects of anaesthetic drugs in the absence of surgical stimulation. Hypovolaemia may be present because of inadequate fluid replacement during surgery, continued bleeding postoperatively or expansion of capacitance of the vascular system as a result of rewarming. Cardiac output may be reduced also as a result of arrhythmias or pre-existing disease. Hypertension may occur as a result of increased sympathoadrenal activity after restoration of consciousness, especially if analgesia is inadequate.

Respiratory system

Hypoventilation occurs commonly, usually as a result of residual effects of anaesthetic drugs or incomplete antagonism of neuromuscular blocking drugs. Hypoxaemia may result from hypoventilation, ventilation/perfusion imbalance or increased oxygen consumption produced by restlessness or shivering.

Gastrointestinal

Nausea and vomiting are common in the immediate postoperative period.

Staff, equipment and monitoring

The recovery ward should be staffed by trained and experienced nurses; one nurse must remain with each patient at all times. The responsibility for the patient's welfare remains with the anaesthetist. In many hospitals, an anaesthetist is designated to be available immediately to treat complications detected by the nursing staff.

The patient is nursed in a bed if a prolonged stay is anticipated, but more commonly on a trolley (Fig. 24.1). All beds and trolleys must have the facility to be tipped head-down. Suction apparatus, including catheters, an oxygen supply with appropriate facemask, a self-inflating resuscitation bag and anaesthetic mask, and a sphygmomanometer must be available for each patient. In addition, there should be a complete range of resuscitation equipment within the recovery area; this includes an anaesthetic machine, a range of laryngoscopes, tracheal tubes, bougies, i.v. cannulae, fluids, emergency drugs, ECG monitor and defibrillator. Facilities for cricothyroid cannulation, e.g. minitracheotomy set, or for formal tracheostomy should be available also.

A wide range of drugs should be stored in the recovery area for the treatment of common complications and also emergency events (Table 24.1).

All patients should be monitored by measurement of heart rate, arterial pressure and respiratory rate and by assessment of level of consciousness, peripheral circulation and adequacy of ventilation; in some circumstances, minute volume may be measured using a respirometer (e.g. Wright's). Depending on the nature of work undertaken in the theatre suite, a proportion of bed stations should have the facility for monitoring ECG, systemic and pulmonary arterial pressures and CVP continuously; this may be required in high-risk patients or those who have

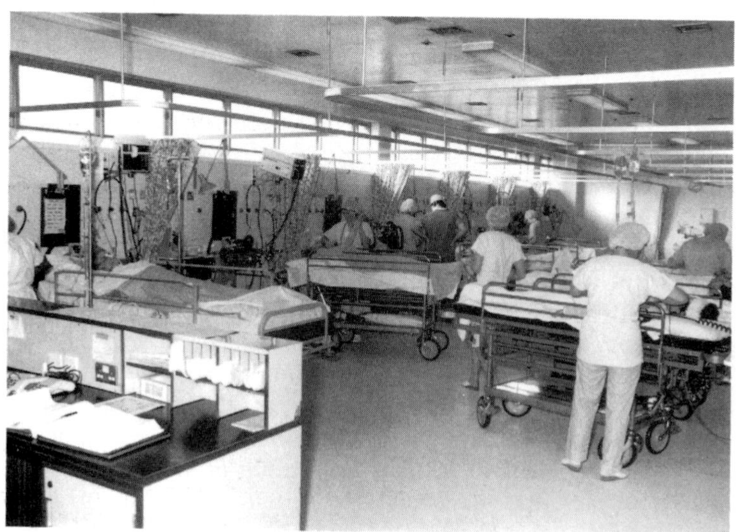

Fig. 24.1 A recovery ward. Most patients are nursed on a trolley, but a bed is used for those who require to stay for several hours.

Table 24.1 Drugs which should be available in the recovery room

Adrenaline	Hydrocortisone
Aminophylline	Insulin
Atenolol	Isoprenaline
Atracurium	Lignocaine
Atropine	Mannitol
Bupivacaine	Metoprolol
Calcium	Midazolam
Chlorpromazine	Morphine
Diazemuls	Naloxone
Digoxin	Neostigmine
Dobutamine	Papaveretum
Dopamine	Pethidine
Doxapram	
Ephedrine	Saline 0.9%
Frusemide	Sodium bicarbonate
Glucose 50%	Sodium nitroprusside
Glyceryl trinitrate	Suxamethonium
	Vecuronium

undergone major surgery. At least one mechanical ventilator should be available. Pulse oximetry is valuable, particularly in children, the elderly, patients with pulmonary disease and those with cardiovascular instability. Urine output should be measured routinely in patients who have undergone major surgery.

Wounds and surgical drains should be inspected regularly for signs of bleeding.

The patient should not be discharged to the surgical ward until:

1. Consciousness has returned fully, and a patent airway can be maintained.
2. Ventilation is adequate and stable.
3. The cardiovascular system is stable.
4. Excessive surgical blood loss has stopped.

High-risk patients, or those who have undergone major surgery, should stay in the recovery ward for up to 24 h. If this is not feasible, or if instability persists for longer than 24 h, the patient should be transferred to a high-dependency or intensive therapy unit.

The remainder of this chapter is devoted to the diagnosis and management of common problems which occur in the postoperative period. Some of these occur most frequently in the immediate recovery period, while others may occur at any time during the patient's convalescence from surgery. Some surgical procedures are associated also with specific complications.

CENTRAL NERVOUS SYSTEM

Conscious level

Many patients are unconscious on arrival in the recovery ward because of residual effects of anaesthetic drugs. The duration of impaired consciousness depends on:

1. *The drugs used.* Recovery of consciousness may be delayed if the following agents have been used:

   (a) Volatile anaesthetics with high blood/gas solubility coefficient.
   (b) Barbiturates, particularly if large total doses have been given.
   (c) Benzodiazepines.
   (d) Opioids with a long duration of action, including large doses of fentanyl.

2. *The timing of drug use.* Delayed recovery may occur if a long-acting i.v. anaesthetic or analgesic drug has been given towards the end of the procedure, or if volatile agents have been continued until the end of surgery.
3. *Pain.* The presence of pain speeds recovery of consciousness. Recovery may be delayed after minor procedures or if potent analgesia has been provided by administration of opioids or by regional anaesthesia.

Undue prolongation of consciousness should not be attributed to these factors alone. Other causes should be considered, as their early recognition may prevent serious sequelae.

Hypoglycaemia

This occurs most commonly in diabetic patients treated with oral hypoglycaemic agents or insulin, and an inadequate intake of glucose. The perioperative management of the diabetic patient is discussed in Chapter 41.

Hyperglycaemia

Hyperglycaemia in known diabetics may occur as a result of inadequate provision of insulin or injudicious infusion of glucose. However, coma is unusual in acute hyperglycaemia. Undiagnosed diabetics with hyperglycaemia and ketosis may present for surgery because of abdominal pain, and prolonged postoperative coma may occur unless the metabolic defect is diagnosed and treated.

Cerebral pathology

Consciousness may be impaired by functional or structural cerebral damage. Possible causes include:

1. Episodes of cerebral ischaemia (e.g. carotid artery surgery, profound hypotension) or hypoxia during anaesthesia.
2. Intracranial haemorrhage, thrombosis or infarction. These may occur fortuitously, or may have been associated with intraoperative hypertension, hypotension or arrhythmias.
3. Pre-existing cerebral lesions, e.g. tumour, trauma. Anaesthetic techniques which increase ICP are likely to impair cerebral function.
4. Epilepsy. Convulsions may have been masked by anaesthesia or neuromuscular blocking drugs.
5. Air embolism.
6. Intracranial spread of local anaesthetic solution after subarachnoid injection. Introduction into the subarachnoid space may be accidental, e.g. during extradural block or rarely interscalene brachial plexus block. Unconsciousness is accompanied almost always by apnoea.

Other causes

1. *Hypoxaemia*. In the presence of an adequate circulation, coma occurs only if profound hypoxaemia is present.
2. *Hypercapnia*. Unconsciousness may occur if Pa_{CO_2} exceeds 9–10 kPa.
3. *Hypotension*.
4. *Hypothermia*.
5. *Hypo-osmolar or 'TURP' syndrome*. This results most commonly from absorption of water from the bladder during transurethral resection of the prostate (TURP). The investigation and management of this condition are described on p. 489.
6. *Hypothyroidism*.
7. *Hepatic or renal failure*.

Confusion and agitation

These occur occasionally during emergence from an otherwise uncomplicated anaesthetic. They are more common in elderly patients, particularly if hyoscine has been given as a premedicant. Atropine also crosses the blood–brain barrier and may result in the 'central anticholinergic syndrome', characterised by restlessness and confusion together with obvious antimuscarinic effects. Glycopyrronium does not cross the blood–brain barrier, and is preferable to atropine for antagonism of the muscarinic effects of neostigmine in elderly patients; in addition to its lack of central effects, it produces less tachycardia and antagonises the effects of neostigmine for a longer period.

All the factors listed above as causes of prolonged coma may result also in confusion and agitation. Pain may also contribute, although it is seldom responsible alone. Emergence delirium is associated particularly with the use of ketamine, and may occur after the administration of etomidate. Septicaemia may result in confusion, as may distension of the stomach or bladder.

A lightly sedated, conscious patient with inadequate antagonism of neuromuscular blocking drugs may appear to the inexperienced observer to be agitated and confused. Movements are uncoordinated. The condition is distressing to the patient and is an indication of a poor anaesthetic technique. It should never be allowed to develop.

Pain

This subject is discussed fully in Chapter 25. The effects of pain should be differentiated from those of hypercapnia and hypovolaemia (Table 24.2).

RESPIRATORY SYSTEM

Hypoventilation

Common causes of hypoventilation in the immediate postoperative period are listed in Table 24.3. Hypoventilation results in an increase in

Table 24.2 Common problems in the recovery room: symptoms and signs

	Pain	Hypercapnia	Hypovolaemia
Conscious level	May be restless May be quiescent if severe pain	Comatose	Restless or quiescent depending on extent of analgesia and residual anaesthesia
Periphery	Vasoconstriction, pallor ± sweating	Warm, flushed with bounding pulse (if normovolaemic)	Vasoconstriction, pallor ± sweating
Heart rate	Tachycardia	Tachycardia	Tachycardia
Arterial pressure	Systolic ↑ Diastolic ↑ Pulse pressure normal	Systolic ↑ Diastolic ↑ ↓ Pulse pressure ↑	Systolic and diastolic may be normal until marked reduction in stroke volume then ↓ Pulse pressure ↓

Table 24.3 Causes of postoperative hypoventilation

Factors affecting airway	Factors affecting ventilatory drive	Peripheral factors
Upper airway obstruction: tongue laryngospasm oedema foreign body tumour Bronchospasm	Respiratory depressant drugs Preoperative CNS pathology Intra- or postoperative cerebrovascular accident Hypothermia Recent hyperventilation (Pa_{CO_2} low)	Muscle weakness: residual neuromuscular block preoperative neuromuscular disease electrolyte abnormalities Pain Abdominal distension Obesity Tight dressings Pneumo/haemothorax

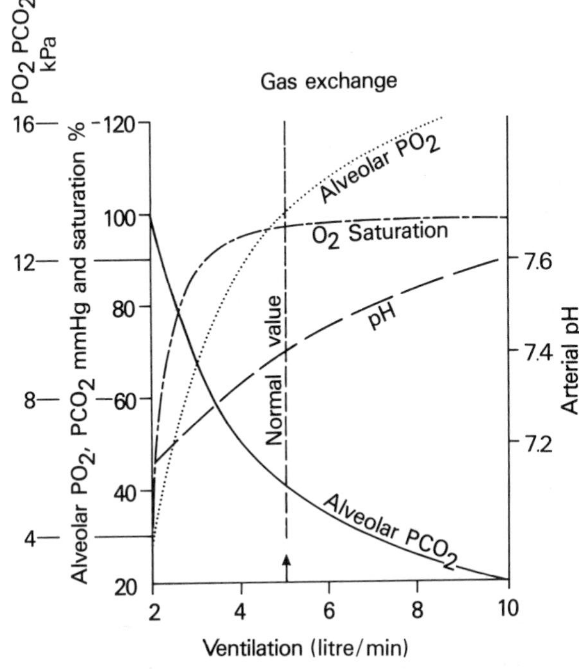

Fig. 24.2 Gas exchange during hypoventilation. Note the relatively rapid increase in alveolar P_{CO_2} compared with the slow decrease in arterial oxygen saturation.

Pa_{CO_2} (Fig. 24.2), and a decrease in PA_{O_2}, and thus hypoxaemia, which may be corrected by increasing the inspired concentration of oxygen.

Airway obstruction

Airway obstruction caused by the tongue, by indrawing of the pharyngeal muscles or by blood or secretions in the pharynx, is ameliorated by placing the patient in the lateral or recovery position (Fig. 20.5). This position should be used for all unconscious patients who have undergone oral or ENT surgery, and for patients at risk of gastric aspiration.

Partial obstruction of the airway is characterised by noisy ventilation. As the obstruction increases, tracheal tug and indrawing of the supraclavicular area occur during inspiration. Total obstruction is signalled by absent sounds of breathing and paradoxical movement of the chest wall and abdomen.

In many patients, a clear airway is maintained only by displacing the mandible anteriorly and extending the head. In some, it is necessary also to insert an oropharyngeal airway, although this may stimulate coughing, gagging and laryngospasm during recovery of consciousness. A nasopharyngeal airway is often tolerated better, but there is a risk of causing haemorrhage from the nasopharyngeal mucosa. Very occasionally, tracheal intubation is necessary to maintain the airway until consciousness has returned fully.

Blood, oral secretions or regurgitated gastric fluid which have accumulated in the pharynx should be aspirated and the patient placed in the recovery position to allow any further fluid to drain anteriorly.

Foreign bodies, such as dentures (particularly partial dentures) or throat packs may cause airway obstruction. It may be difficult to maintain a patent airway in unconscious patients with an oral, pharyngeal or laryngeal tumour.

Obstruction of the upper airway occurs intermittently after recovery from anaesthesia. Obstructive sleep apnoea is common in the postoperative period, and may result in decreases of Sa_{O_2} to less than 75%. Episodes occur with the greatest frequency in the first 4 h after anaesthesia, and are more common and severe in patients who receive opioids for postoperative analgesia than those in whom analgesia is provided by a regional technique.

Airway obstruction may result from haemorrhage after surgery to the neck, including thyroid surgery; the wound should be opened urgently, and the haematoma drained. Occasionally, tracheal collapse occurs after thyroidectomy in patients who have developed chondromalacia of the cartilaginous rings of the trachea caused by pressure from a large goitre. Inspiratory stridor may be present or there may be total obstruction during inspiration; the trachea must be re-intubated immediately.

Laryngeal spasm

This complication is relatively common after general anaesthesia. It may be partial or complete, and is caused usually by direct stimulation of the cords by secretions or blood, or of the epiglottis by an oropharyngeal airway. It may follow extubation of the trachea in the semiconscious patient. It may be difficult to differentiate this condition from airway obstruction caused by the tongue; if airway obstruction persists despite implementation of the measures described above, laryngoscopy should be undertaken.

Any obvious foreign material causing laryngospasm should be removed by aspiration, and oxygen 100% administered. If obstruction is complete, positive pressure ventilation by mask may force some oxygen through the cords to maintain arterial oxygenation until the spasm has subsided; there is a significant risk of inflating the stomach with oxygen during this procedure. If attempts to oxygenate the lungs fail, suxamethonium should be administered, and the lungs ventilated with oxygen. When oxygenation has been achieved, it may be advisable to intubate the trachea to reduce the risk of regurgitation of gastric contents, as the stomach may have been inflated with oxygen, and to administer 60–65% nitrous oxide in oxygen to minimise the risk of awareness if the patient regains consciousness before muscle power returns. When the effects of suxamethonium have terminated, oxygen 100% is administered, and the trachea extubated when the patient regains consciousness.

Rarely, laryngeal obstruction occurs after thyroid surgery if both recurrent laryngeal nerves have been traumatised.

Laryngeal oedema

This occurs occasionally after tracheal intubation and may result in severe obstruction, particularly in a child. Treatment depends on the severity of the obstruction; immediate re-intubation may be required if obstruction is complete, but partial obstruction may subside if the patient is treated with heated humidified gases. Dexamethasone may hasten resolution of the oedema.

Bronchospasm

This may result from stimulation of the airway by inhaled material. It is commoner in asthmatic or bronchitic patients, and in smokers. It may result directly from intrinsic asthma, or may be part of an anaphylactic reaction. Several drugs used in anaesthetic practice may precipitate bronchospasm either by a direct effect on bronchial muscle or by releasing histamine; these include barbiturates, *d*-tubocurarine, morphine and atracurium. Treatment comprises the removal of any predisposing factor and the administration of oxygen and bronchodilators.

Ventilatory drive

There are several possible causes of reduced ventilatory drive during recovery from anaesthesia (Table 24.3). The presence of intracranial pathology, e.g. tumour, trauma or haemorrhage, may affect ventilatory drive in the postoperative period. Ventilation is reduced in the presence of hypothermia, although it is usually appropriate for the metabolic needs of the body. Hypoventilation occurs in the hypocapnic patient, e.g. after a period of hyperventilation, until Pa_{CO_2} is restored to normal, and in the presence of primary metabolic alkalosis.

The most important cause of reduced ventilatory drive during recovery is the effect of drugs administered by the anaesthetist in the perioperative period. All the volatile and i.v. anaesthetic agents, with the exception of ketamine, depress the respiratory centre; significant concentrations of these drugs remain in the brain stem during the early postoperative period.

All opioid analgesics depress ventilation. With most opioids the effect is dose-dependent, although the agonist–antagonist agents are claimed to have a 'ceiling' effect. In the majority of patients opioids do not produce apnoea, but result in decreased ventilatory drive and an increase in Pa_{CO_2} which plateaus at an elevated value. The elderly are particularly sensitive to drug-induced ventilatory depression.

Spinal opioids, particularly lipid-insoluble agents such as morphine, may produce ventilatory depression some hours after administration. Patients who have received subarachnoid or extradural opioids should remain in the recovery ward or high-dependency unit for at least 12 h after administration of the last dose.

Reduced ventilatory drive is easy to diagnose if the ventilatory rate or tidal volume are clearly reduced. However, lesser degrees of hypoventilation may be difficult to detect, and the signs of moderate hypercapnia, e.g. hypertension and tachycardia, may be masked by the residual effects of anaesthetic agents, or misdiagnosed as pain-induced (Table 24.2).

Mild hypoventilation is acceptable provided that oxygenation remains adequate; this can be achieved easily by a modest increase in FI_{O_2} (see below). If ventilatory drive is reduced excessively by opioids, with an increasing Pa_{CO_2} or delayed recovery of consciousness, naloxone in increments of 1.5–3 μg/kg should be administered every 2–3 min until improvement occurs. Administration of excessive doses of naloxone reverses the analgesia induced by systemic, but not spinal, opioids; large doses may cause severe hypertension and have been associated with cardiac arrest on rare occasions. The effects of i.v. naloxone last only for 20–30 min; in order to prevent the recurrence of reduced ventilation after long-acting opioids, an additional dose (50% of the effective i.v. dose) may be administered i.m., or an i.v. infusion instituted.

Peripheral factors

The commonest peripheral factor associated with hypoventilation is residual neuromuscular blockade. This may be exaggerated by disease of the neuromuscular junction, e.g. myasthenia gravis, or by electrolyte disturbances. Inadequate reversal of neuromuscular blockade is associated usually with uncoordinated, jerky movements, although these may occur occasionally during recovery of consciousness in patients with normal neuromuscular function. Measurement of tidal volume is not a reliable guide to adequacy of reversal of neuromuscular blockade; a normal tidal volume may be achieved with only 20% return of diaphragmatic power, but the ability to cough remains severely impaired. If the patient is able to lift his head from the trolley for 5 s or can maintain a good hand-grip, it is likely that there is sufficient return of neuromuscular function for adequate ventilation and maintenance of the airway. Some more objective means of assessment are listed in Table 24.4, but these require

Table 24.4 Assessment of the adequacy of antagonism of neuromuscular block

Grip strength Adequate cough	subjective
Ability to sustain head lift for at least 5 s	
Ability to produce vital capacity of at least 10 ml/kg body weight	

the cooperation of the patient. In the unconscious or uncooperative patient, nerve stimulation (Ch. 12) provides the best means of assessing neuromuscular function, although there are differences among the non-depolarising relaxants in the relationship between their actions in the forearm and diaphragm.

If residual non-depolarising blockade is confirmed, further doses of neostigmine may be administered (with atropine or glycopyrronium) up to a total of 5 mg. If the block persists, artificial ventilation must be maintained while the cause is sought.

Factors responsible most commonly for difficulty in antagonism of neuromuscular block include overdosage with muscle relaxant, too short an interval between administration of the drug and the antagonist, hypokalaemia, respiratory or metabolic acidosis, administration of aminoglycoside antibiotics, local anaesthetic agents, diseases affecting neuromuscular transmission and muscle disease.

Delayed elimination of all non-depolarising muscle relaxants (except atracurium) has been reported, and causes prolonged neuromuscular block. Delayed elimination occurs most frequently in the presence of renal or hepatic insufficiency, or in dehydrated patients with low urine output. Muscle paralysis may recur 30–60 min after administration of neostigmine if elimination of the relaxant is inadequate, even if antagonism appears to be satisfactory initially. A similar phenomenon may occur if acidosis develops, or when patients who have been hypothermic are rewarmed.

Prolonged neuromuscular block after suxamethonium occurs in the presence of atypical plasma cholinesterase, or a low concentration of normal plasma cholinesterase. Paralysis may persist for up to 8 h, although in most instances recovery occurs within 2 h. Neostigmine should not be administered.

Artificial ventilation of the lungs must be maintained or resumed in any patient who has inadequate neuromuscular function. Anaesthesia should be provided to prevent awareness; this is achieved most easily with nitrous oxide and a low concentration of volatile anaesthetic agent.

Hypoventilation may be caused also by restriction of diaphragmatic movement resulting from abdominal distension, obesity, tight dressings or abdominal binders. Pain, particularly from thoracic or upper abdominal wounds, may cause reduced ventilation.

The presence of air or fluid in the pleural cavity may result in hypoventilation. Pneumothorax may occur during IPPV. It is an occasional complication in healthy patients, but is a particular risk in those with chronic obstructive airways disease, especially if bullae are present, and after chest trauma. It may complicate brachial plexus nerve block, central venous cannulation or surgery of the kidney or neck. Haemothorax may result from chest trauma or central venous cannulation. Hydrothorax may be caused by pleural effusions or inadvertent infusion of fluids through a misplaced central venous catheter. These rapidly remediable causes of hypoventilation are often overlooked.

Treatment

This consists primarily of treatment of the cause. Mild or moderate hypoventilation resulting from residual effects of anaesthetic drugs may respond to a bolus dose or infusion of doxapram. Artificial ventilation should be reinstituted if severe hypercapnia is present or Pa_{CO_2} continues to rise, or if the clinical condition of the patient is deteriorating.

Hypoxaemia

A functional classification of causes of hypoxaemia in the early recovery period is shown in Table 24.5. An inspired oxygen concentration of less than 21% should never occur, although PA_{O_2} is decreased when air is breathed at high altitudes.

Table 24.5 Functional classification of the causes of hypoxaemia in the postoperative period

Reduced inspired oxygen concentration
Ventilation–perfusion abnormalities
Shunting
Hypoventilation
Diffusion deficits
Diffusion hypoxia after nitrous oxide anaesthesia

Ventilation–perfusion abnormalities

These are the commonest cause of hypoxaemia in the recovery room. Cardiac output and pulmonary arterial pressure may be reduced after general or regional anaesthesia, causing impaired perfusion of some areas of the lungs. FRC is reduced during and immediately after anaesthesia, and closing capacity (see p. 28) may encroach on the tidal breathing range, resulting in reduced ventilation of some lung units, particularly those in dependent alveoli. Thus the scatter of ventilation/perfusion ($\dot{V}/\dot{Q}$) ratios is increased. Areas of lung with increased $\dot{V}/\dot{Q}$ ratios constitute physiological deadspace; unless there is central depression of ventilation, an increase in deadspace is followed usually by an increase in minute volume. Areas of lung with low $\dot{V}/\dot{Q}$ ratios increase venous admixture, which results in hypoxaemia.

Shunt

Physiological shunt may be increased in the immediate postoperative period if small airways closure has been extreme. Shunting may be present also in patients with pulmonary oedema of any aetiology, or if there is consolidation in the lung. More commonly, shunt is increased in the later postoperative period secondary to retention of secretions and underventilation of the lung bases because of pain; these changes lead to alveolar consolidation and collapse.

Hypoventilation

This has been discussed in detail above. Moderate hypoventilation, with some elevation of Pa_{CO_2}, leads to a modest reduction in Pa_{O_2} (Fig. 24.2). Obstructive sleep apnoea may produce profound transient but repeated decreases in arterial oxygenation. Sa_{O_2} may decrease to less than 75%, corresponding to a Pa_{O_2} of less than 5 kPa (40 mmHg). These repeated episodes of hypoxaemia cause temporary, and possibly permanent, defects in cognitive function in elderly patients, and may contribute to perioperative myocardial infarction.

Diffusion defects

Interstitial oedema produced by overtransfusion of fluids or by left ventricular dysfunction may cause hypoxaemia by impairment of oxygen transfer across the alveolar–capillary membrane.

Diffusion hypoxia

Nitrous oxide is 40 times more soluble in blood than nitrogen. When administration of nitrous oxide is discontinued at the end of anaesthesia, nitrous oxide diffuses out of blood into the alveoli in larger volumes than nitrogen diffuses in the opposite direction. Consequently, the alveolar concentrations of other gases are diluted. PA_{O_2} is reduced and arterial oxygenation impaired if the patient breathes air; PA_{CO_2} is reduced also, causing hypoventilation. Sa_{O_2} is reduced below baseline to values as low as 90% for several minutes in normal individuals after breathing 50% nitrous oxide in oxygen. Arterial desaturation is greater in elderly patients, if higher concentrations of nitrous oxide have been used, or if Pa_{CO_2} is low initially because of hyperventilation.

Diffusion hypoxia is avoided by the administration of oxygen for 10 min after discontinuation of nitrous oxide anaesthesia.

Reduced venous oxygen content

Assuming that oxygen consumption remains unchanged, anaemia and reduced cardiac output result in increased oxygen extraction from circulating arterial blood, and consequently a reduction in mixed venous oxygen content. In the presence of increased ventilation/perfusion scatter or intrapulmonary shunt, this causes a variable degree of arterial hypoxaemia. Similarly, if cardiac output remains constant, increased oxygen utilisation by the tissues (as may occur during shivering, restlessness or malignant hyperpyrexia) causes a reduction in mixed venous oxygen content and a worsening of arterial hypoxaemia if any shunt is present.

Tissue hypoxia

Oxygenation of the tissues is a function of arterial oxygenation, oxygen carriage in blood, delivery of blood to the tissues and transfer of oxygen from the blood. It may be impaired by respiratory or cardiovascular dysfunction, by severe anaemia or by a leftward shift of the oxyhaemoglobin dissociation curve (reduced P_{50}).

Pulmonary changes after abdominal surgery

Patients with previously normal lungs suffer impairment of oxygenation for at least 48 h after abdominal surgery. The extent of this impairment is related to the site of operation. It is less marked after lower abdominal surgery and worst after thoraco-abdominal procedures, or midline or paramedian incisions in the upper abdomen. In these circumstances, the differences between pre- and postoperative Pa_{O_2} may be as much as 4 kPa.

Impairment of oxygenation in the postoperative period is related to a reduction in functional residual capacity (FRC). After induction of anaesthesia there is an abrupt decrease in FRC. The exact cause is not known, but the magnitude of the decrease is similar for anaesthetic techniques in which the patient breathes spontaneously and those in which IPPV is employed. Postoperatively, this decrease is maintained by wound pain, which causes spasm of the expiratory muscles, and abdominal distension leading to diaphragmatic splinting. This is influenced also by the site of surgical incision; the greatest reduction follows thoracic or upper abdominal surgery. The supine position also reduces FRC.

The reduction in FRC may lead to closing capacity impinging upon the tidal breathing range. This results in small airways closure during normal tidal ventilation. Gas trapping occurs in the affected airways and subsequent absorption of air may lead to the development of small, discrete areas of atelectasis which are not visible radiologically. This occurs mainly in the dependent parts of the lung. The end result is an increase in the number of areas of low $\dot{V}/\dot{Q}$ ratio within the lungs. The relationship between changes in FRC and Pa_{O_2} postoperatively is shown in Figure 24.3.

In most patients, these abnormalities return towards normal by the fifth or sixth postoperative day. However, if the changes have been marked, the areas of low $\dot{V}/\dot{Q}$ ratio may become a focus for infection, particularly in the presence of retained secretions. Factors which contribute to the retention of secretions after surgery are:

1. *Inability to cough*. This results mostly from wound pain. However, excessive sedation may contribute also. Postoperative electrolyte imbalance, especially hypokalaemia and hypophosphataemia, may compound the situation by interfering with muscle function.
2. *Suppression of bronchial mucosal ciliary activity*. This results primarily from the use of unhumidified anaesthetic gases.
3. *Antisialagogue drugs*. When antisialagogue premedicants have been used the secretions become more viscid. The dry mucosa itself is more prone to inflammatory reaction. If this occurs, the exudate produced increases the problem still further.
4. *Infection*. If pulmonary infection supervenes, impairment of oxygenation may contribute to a lack of co-operation in clearing secretions.

A combination of these factors may result in retention of secretions, leading to areas of radiologically visible pulmonary collapse, and an increase in the work of breathing. Ultimately, oxygenation of the blood may become inadequate despite oxygen therapy, or carbon dioxide retention may occur. The sequence of events that culminate in ventilatory failure is shown in Figure 24.4.

Predisposing factors

1. *Site of surgery*. Pulmonary complications occur more commonly after upper abdominal surgery than after lower abdominal operations.

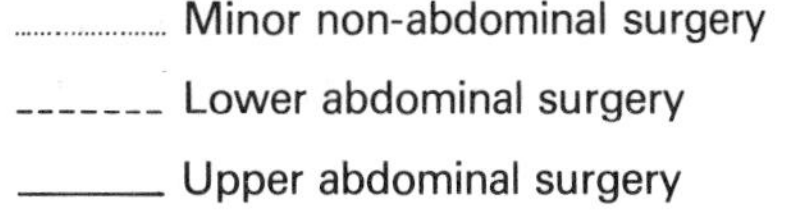

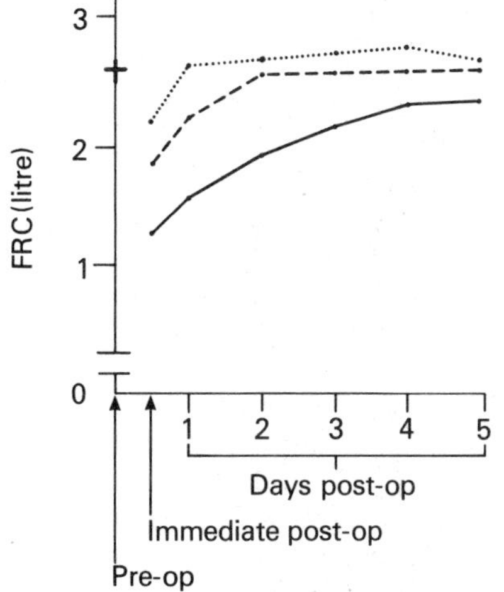

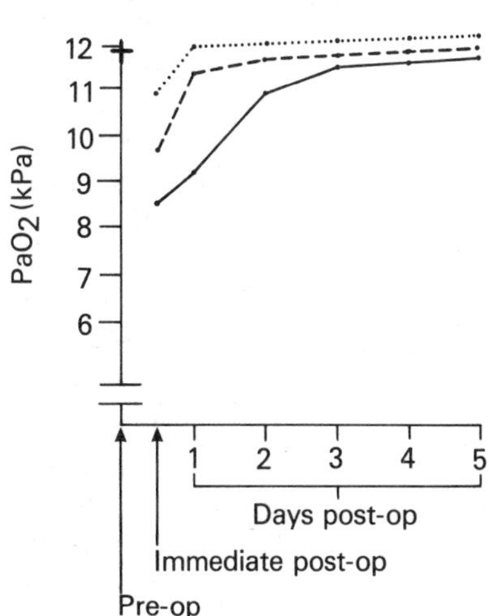

Fig. 24.3 Changes in FRC and Pa_{O_2} postoperatively.

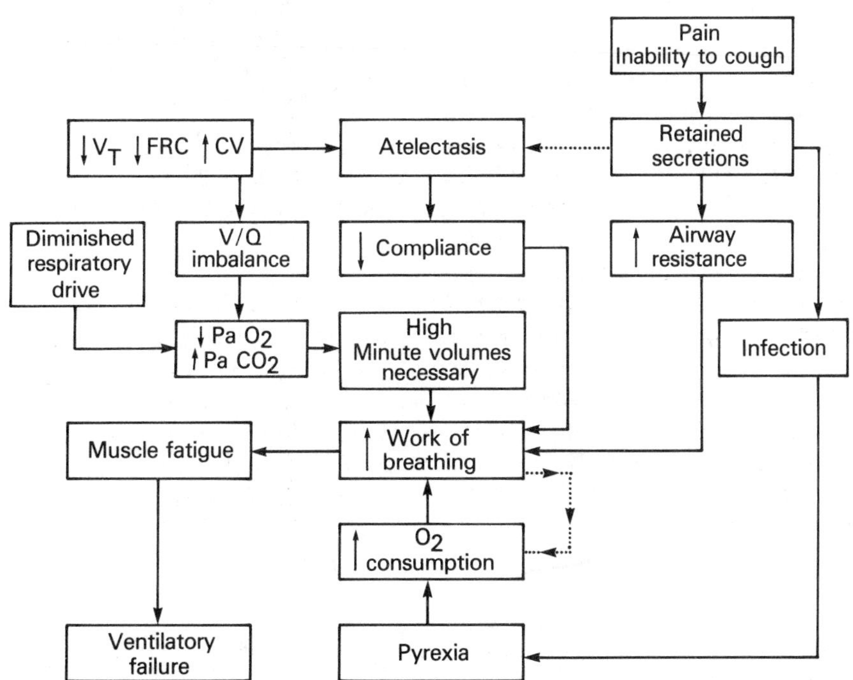

Fig. 24.4 Diagrammatic representation of events that result in postoperative ventilatory failure.

2. *Pre-existing respiratory disease* increases the complication rate. This is so particularly in the presence of concurrent infection or excessive secretions.

3. *Smokers* have an increased incidence of pulmonary complications compared with non-smokers.

4. *Obesity* is associated with a high incidence of pulmonary complications. Obese patients have a low FRC and increased work of breathing postoperatively.

The anaesthetic technique has little effect on the incidence of postoperative pulmonary complications.

Clinical findings

Collapse of lung units. In patients who develop clinical symptoms, the first signs of atelectasis are seen usually within 24 h of operation. The triad of pyrexia, tachycardia and tachypnoea is often present. Temperature is usually in the range of 38–39°C. There is often a productive cough. If atelectasis is extensive, the patient is cyanosed. On physical examination, localising signs are uncommon unless the area of involvement is large. Chest X-ray reveals patchy areas of atelectasis.

Pneumonia. Lobar pneumonia is rarely seen postoperatively. Bronchopneumonia is more common, especially in the elderly. The onset of symptoms is not as rapid as in atelectasis. There is usually fever and associated tachycardia with an increase in the ventilatory rate. Physical examination usually reveals areas of consolidation, predominantly at the lung bases, which are evident radiologically.

Treatment

If a pulmonary complication is suspected, a sputum sample should be sent to the laboratory for bacteriological analysis. Appropriate antibiotic therapy may then be started. Intensive physiotherapy should be prescribed in an attempt to remove secretions and re-expand atelectatic areas of the lung.

Patients with pulmonary collapse are usually hypoxaemic, but Pa_{CO_2} remains normal or may be low as a result of tachypnoea, at least in the early stages. Usually, oxygen in moderate concentrations (30–40%) is sufficient to correct hypoxaemia, but this should be confirmed by blood gas analysis. If the patient fails to respond to these measures, signs of respiratory distress develop. The patient becomes drowsy and ventilation is laboured, with rapid shallow breathing involving the accessory muscles. Pa_{CO_2} increases and arterial oxygenation deteriorates despite oxygen therapy. The presence of continued deterioration in blood gases is an indication for ventilatory support.

Reducing pulmonary complications

Preoperative

Measures to reduce pulmonary complications should begin preoperatively. Upper and lower respiratory tract infections should be treated before surgery. Dental sepsis and sinus infections should be eradicated. Pre-existing chronic respiratory disorders should be treated so that the patient is in optimal condition before surgery. Spirometry is useful to monitor such treatment, but arterial blood gas analysis is the only assessment which has been demonstrated to correlate well with the need for postoperative ventilatory support. Smoking should be discouraged and weight loss encouraged where indicated. In patients with increased risk factors, heavy premedication should be avoided to ensure minimal ventilatory depression at the end of the procedure.

Intraoperative

At induction, care should be taken not to introduce infection by contaminated equipment. During prolonged procedures, the anaesthetic gases should be humidified. If neuromuscular blocking agents are used, particular care should be taken to ensure that antagonism is adequate.

Postoperative

Analgesia should be optimal to ensure adequate coughing and cooperation during physiotherapy, which should be started as soon as possible after operation.

Oxygen therapy

Hypoxaemia may occur to some degree in *any* patient during the early recovery period as a result of one or more of the mechanisms described above. Consequently, *all* patients should receive additional oxygen for the first 10 min after general anaesthesia has been discontinued. Oxygen therapy should be continued for a longer period in the presence of any of the conditions listed in Table 24.6.

Oxygen therapy is beneficial particularly in treating hypoxaemia caused by hypoventilation; $P\text{A}_{O_2}$ is increased substantially by a modest increase in $F\text{I}_{O_2}$. In contrast, higher concentrations are required in the presence of a shunt fraction in excess of 0.1–0.15 (Fig. 24.5). Known concentrations of oxygen may be administered by a tightly fitting mask supplied with metered flows of air and oxygen via either an anaesthetic breathing system or a CPAP system (see Ch. 42). In small children, an oxygen tent or headbox may be used. However, oxygen is administered usually by less cumbersome disposable equipment.

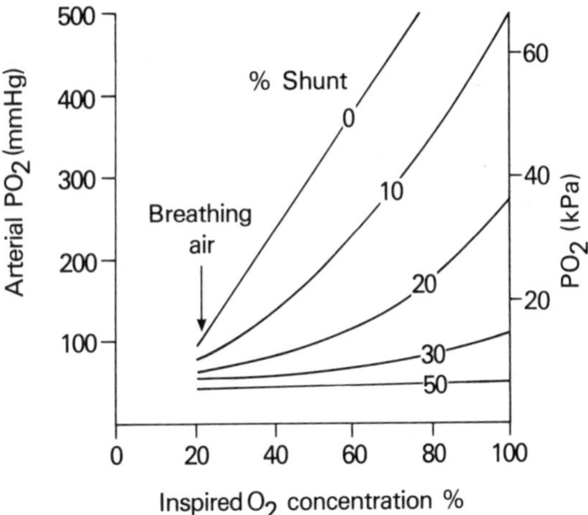

Fig. 24.5 Response of Pa_{O_2} to increased inspired oxygen concentrations in the presence of various degrees of shunt. Note that Pa_{O_2} remains well below the normal value when 100% oxygen is breathed. Nevertheless, useful increases in arterial oxygenation occur with a shunt of up to 30%.

Oxygen therapy devices

The characteristics of oxygen facemasks depend predominantly on their volume, the flow rate of gas supplied and the presence of holes in the side of the mask. If no gas is supplied, facemasks act as increased deadspace and result in hypercapnia unless minute volume is increased; the increase in deadspace is proportional to the volume of the mask. If the mask contains holes, air is entrained readily during inspiration.

Table 24.6 Conditions in which prolonged oxygen therapy is required after operation

Hypotension
Ischaemic heart disease
Reduced cardiac output
Anaemia
Obesity
Shivering
Hypothermia
Hyperthermia
Pulmonary oedema
Airway obstruction
After major surgery

When oxygen is supplied, the inspired oxygen concentration increases, but to an extent which depends upon the relationship between the oxygen flow rate and the ventilatory pattern. If there is a pause between expiration and inspiration, the mask fills with oxygen and a high concentration is available at the start of inspiration; during inspiration, the inspired oxygen is diluted by air drawn in through the holes when the inspiratory flow rate exceeds the flow rate of oxygen. During normal tidal ventilation, the peak inspiratory flow rate (PIFR) is 20–30 litres/min, but is considerably higher during deep inspiration or in the hyperventilating patient. If there is no expiratory pause, alveolar gas may be rebreathed from the mask at the start of inspiration; this occurs especially when the oxygen flow rate is low, or no holes are present in the mask. A predictable and constant inspired oxygen concentration may be achieved only if the total gas flow to the mask exceeds the patient's PIFR.

Fixed-performance devices. These masks, termed also 'high air flow oxygen enrichment' (HAFOE) devices, provide a constant and

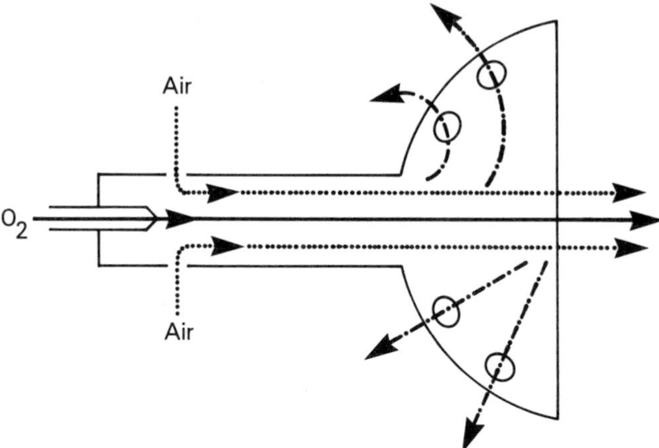

Fig. 24.6 Diagram of HAFOE mask. See text for details.

predictable inspired oxygen concentration irrespective of the patient's ventilatory pattern. This is achieved by supplying the mask with oxygen and air at a high total flow rate. Oxygen is passed through a jet which entrains air (Fig. 24.6). The mask is designed in such a way that the total flow rate of gas to the mask exceeds the expected PIFR of the majority of patients who require oxygen therapy. For example, if a jet designed to supply 28% oxygen is supplied with an oxygen flow rate of 4 litres/min, approximately 41 litres/min of air are entrained and a total flow of 45 litres/min passes to the patient's face.

Various types of HAFOE device are available; some examples are shown in Figure 24.7. Ventimasks are the most accurate, but a different mask is required for each of the range of oxygen concentrations available. Some manufacturers produce masks in which the jet device can be changed by the user, so that the oxygen concentration may be adjusted as appropriate.

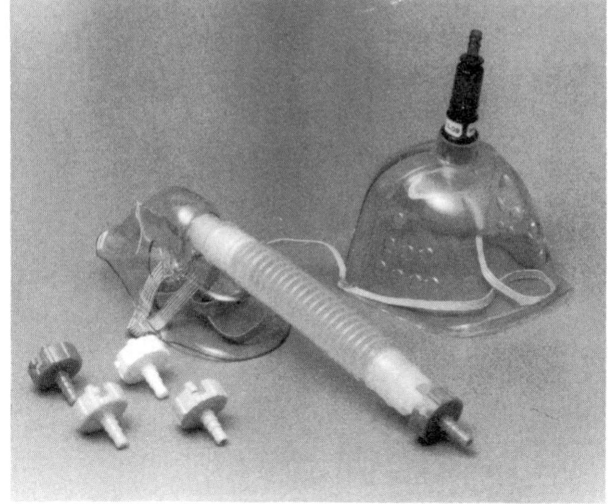

Fig. 24.7 HAFOE masks.

The air-entraining jets of HAFOE devices provide a relatively constant oxygen concentration irrespective of the flow rate of oxygen. The recommended oxygen flow rates are large when jets providing a high concentration are used (e.g. 8 litres/min for 40%, 15 litres/min for 60%) so that the total flow rate supplied to the mask remains adequate despite the smaller proportion of air entrained. The total flow rates through masks which deliver more than 28% oxygen are between 20 and 30 litres/min when the recommended oxygen flow rates are provided; higher flow rates of oxygen may be used in patients who are thought to have an increased PIFR.

Because of the high fresh gas flow rate, expired gas is flushed rapidly from the mask. Thus, rebreathing does not occur, i.e. fixed performance devices do not act as an additional deadspace.

Variable-performance devices. All other disposable oxygen masks, and nasal cannulae, provide an oxygen concentration which varies with the oxygen flow rate and the patient's ventilatory pattern. Although there is no increase in deadspace when nasal cannulae are used, all variable-performance disposable facemasks add deadspace,

Table 24.7 Oxygen masks, flow rates and approximate O_2 concentrations delivered

Type of mask	Oxygen flow (litres/min)	Oxygen concentration (%)
Edinburgh	1	24–29
	2	29–36
	4	33–39
Nasal cannulae	1	25–29
	2	29–35
	4	32–39
Hudson	2	24–38
	4	35–45
	6	51–61
	8	57–67
	10	61–73
M.C.	2	28–50
	4	41–70
	6	53–74
	8	60–77
	10	67–81

the magnitude of which depends on the patient's pattern of ventilation. Table 24.7 gives an indication of the range of oxygen concentrations achieved with a number of commonly used variable-performance devices; some examples are shown in Figure 24.8.

Oxygen therapy in the recovery ward

The large majority of patients recovering after anaesthesia require only a modest increase in $F\text{I}_{O_2}$ to overcome the combined effects of mild hypoventilation, diffusion hypoxia and some degree of increased $\dot{V}/\dot{Q}$ scatter. Usually, an inspired concentration of 30% is adequate and this may be achieved in most instances by supplying an oxygen flow rate of 4 litres/min to any of the variable-performance devices (Table 24.7). However, in a small proportion of patients, it is necessary to control the $F\text{I}_{O_2}$ more strictly.

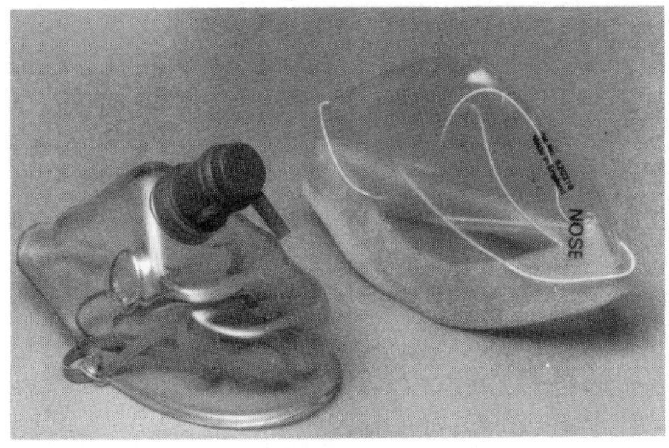

Fig. 24.8 Variable-performance masks.

Controlled oxygen therapy. This is required in two categories of patient:

1. Some patients with chronic bronchitis develop chronic hypercapnia, and ventilatory drive is produced largely by hypoxaemia. If Pa_{O_2} increases above the level which stimulates respiration, ventilatory depression may occur. However, these patients may become dangerously hypoxaemic after anaesthesia, and oxygen therapy is required so that adequate oxygenation of the tissues is maintained. The aim of oxygen therapy in these circumstances is to increase arterial oxygen content without an excessive increase in Pa_{O_2}. This is achieved by a modest increase in $F\text{I}_{O_2}$. In the hypoxaemic patient, the relationship between arterial oxygen tension and saturation (and therefore oxygen content) is represented by the steep portion of the oxyhaemoglobin dissociation curve, and a small increase in oxygen tension results in a significant increase in saturation and oxygen content (Fig. 24.9).

The use of a variable-performance device in these patients is unsatisfactory, as an unacceptably high $F\text{I}_{O_2}$ may be delivered. A fixed-performance device delivering 24% oxygen should be used initially, and the response assessed. If the patient remains clinically well, and the Pa_{CO_2} does not increase by more than 1–1.5 kPa, 28% oxygen, and subsequently higher concentrations, may be administered if further increases in Pa_{O_2} are desirable.

Most patients with chronic bronchitis do not depend on hypoxaemia for respiratory drive, and should not be denied adequate concentrations of oxygen. Patients at risk may usually be detected preoperatively by the presence of central cyanosis; hypoxaemia and hypercapnia are confirmed by blood gas analysis.

2. Patients with increased shunt, e.g. those with ARDS, pulmonary oedema or pulmonary consolidation, may require a high inspired oxygen concentration (Fig. 24.5), which cannot be guaranteed if a variable-performance device is used. In addition, serial blood gas analysis is used normally to assess improvement or deterioration in their

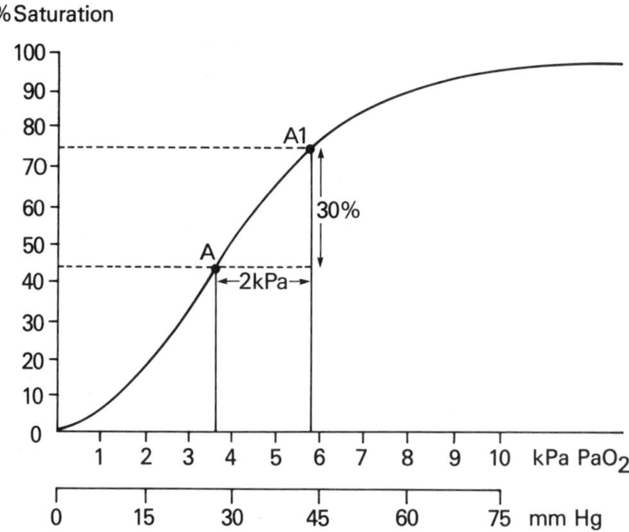

Fig. 24.9 Effect of controlled oxygen therapy on oxygen saturation in a hypoxaemic chronic bronchitic patient. A small increase in inspired oxygen concentration produces a modest increase in Pa_{O_2} but a substantial increase in arterial oxygen saturation.

condition. Changes in Pa_{O_2} and the degree of shunt may be interpreted accurately only if the FI_{O_2} is known. Thus, controlled oxygen therapy should be employed, using a fixed-performance device which delivers 40% oxygen or more.

CARDIOVASCULAR SYSTEM

Hypotension

Residual effects of anaesthetic drugs

Hypotension may result from the residual vasodilator effect of i.v. or inhalational anaesthetic drugs, particularly in patients who are experiencing little pain. Subarachnoid or extradural nerve block may also cause hypotension which persists into the postoperative period. Heart rate is seldom elevated, and the peripheries are warm if anaesthetic drugs or regional anaesthesia are the cause of the hypotension. A systolic arterial pressure of 80–90 mmHg is tolerated well except by the elderly or patients with myocardial disease. No treatment is required in most patients. Elevation of the legs often increases arterial pressure by increasing venous return. Intravenous infusion of 7–10 ml/kg of colloid solution is usually effective in restoring normotension if there is concern; infusion should be undertaken cautiously in elderly patients and in those with cardiovascular disease.

Other causes of hypotension in the recovery period are more sinister, and must be excluded before it may be assumed that residual anaesthesia is responsible.

Hypovolaemia

This may result from inadequate or inappropriate replacement of preoperative or intraoperative fluid and blood losses, or from postoperative haemorrhage. Surgical bleeding may be obvious from inspection of wounds and drains, but may be concealed, particularly in the abdomen, retroperitoneal space or thorax even when drains are present.

Inadequate surgical haemostasis is the usual cause of postoperative bleeding but coagulation disorders may be present in the following circumstances:

1. After massive blood transfusion, which results in decreased concentrations of clotting factors and reduced platelet numbers.
2. Pre-existing bleeding tendency, e.g. haemophilia.

3. Disseminated intravascular coagulation produced by sepsis, amniotic fluid embolism, etc.

4. If anticoagulant drugs have been administered.

A coagulation disorder is associated frequently with prolonged bleeding after venepuncture, oozing from the wound and the development of petechiae or bruises. The investigation and management of coagulation disorders are discussed in Chapter 7.

Hypotension caused by hypovolaemia is accompanied by signs of poor peripheral perfusion, e.g. cold, clammy extremities and pallor. Tachycardia may be present but is masked not infrequently by the effects of drugs (e.g. anticholinesterases, β-blockers). CVP may be low or normal. Urine output is reduced (<30 ml/h). The effects of hypovolaemia on arterial pressure are more pronounced in the presence of vasodilatation or reduced myocardial contractility resulting from the effects of residual anaesthetic drugs, or antihypertensive, calcium channel or β-blocker therapy. In patients who have undergone prolonged surgery, and particularly if the core temperature is below normal, vasoconstriction may be profound and hypovolaemia may be unmasked at a relatively late stage, as normal vasomotor tone returns with rewarming.

Treatment comprises elevation of the legs and administration of appropriate crystalloid or colloid solutions; in elderly or high-risk patients, or if hypovolaemia is profound, administration of fluids should be monitored by measurement of CVP. Clotting factors or platelets should be administered if appropriate, and surgical bleeding treated by re-operation if necessary.

Arrhythmias

These are discussed below.

Ventricular failure

Left or right ventricular failure may cause hypotension. The latter is uncommon, and is secondary usually to acute pulmonary disease, e.g. ARDS.

Left ventricular failure in the postoperative period is associated most commonly with perioperative myocardial infarction or overtransfusion. The peripheral circulation is poor. Usually, tachycardia is present, and there is clinical and radiological evidence of pulmonary oedema. Jugular venous pulse and CVP are elevated usually, but they may remain normal despite a substantial increase in left atrial pressure, particularly if right ventricular hypertrophy is present. Thus, left ventricular failure may be misdiagnosed as hypovolaemia in some patients, and in some instances the two conditions coexist. If there is doubt about the diagnosis, a small fluid load may be administered (no more than 200 ml), and the response of arterial and central venous pressures monitored; if the diagnosis remains uncertain, a pulmonary artery catheter should be inserted to measure pulmonary artery and left atrial pressures.

Treatment comprises administration of oxygen, fluid restriction, diuretics and if necessary inotropic support or vasodilator therapy. ECG, arterial pressure and CVP should be monitored. The possibility of myocardial infarction should be investigated.

Septic shock

In this condition, hypotension is accompanied by raised cardiac output and peripheral vasodilatation in the early stages, followed by vasoconstriction and reduced cardiac output caused partly by loss of fluid from the circulation. Central venous pressure monitoring is essential and a pulmonary artery catheter desirable. Treatment includes infusion of appropriate volumes of colloid, inotropic support, antibiotic therapy and if necessary surgical treatment of the source.

Hypertension

Arterial hypertension is a common complication in the early postoperative period. The causes include:

1. Pain.
2. Pre-existing hypertension, particularly if controlled inadequately.
3. Hypoxaemia.
4. Hypercapnia.
5. Administration of vasopressor drugs.
6. After aortic surgery, as a result partly of increased plasma concentrations of renin.

A combination of these causes may be present. Hypertension results in increased cardiac work and myocardial oxygen consumption, and may result in myocardial ischaemia or infarction, left ventricular failure or cerebral haemorrhage. The cause should be elicited rapidly and treated if possible. Oxygen should be administered. If no remediable cause is found, vasodilatation with hydralazine, sodium nitroprusside or glyceryl trinitrate should be started. Alternatively, labetalol may be used, particularly if there is a degree of tachycardia. Such treatment may unmask hypovolaemia (vide supra) and additional i.v. fluids may be required.

Arrhythmias (see also p. 650)

These are common during and immediately after anaesthesia. The majority are benign and require no treatment. However, the cause should be sought and their effect on the circulation assessed. Common causes include:

1. Residual anaesthetic agents, especially halothane.
2. Hypercapnia.
3. Hypoxaemia.
4. Electrolyte or acid–base disturbance.
5. Vagal stimulation, e.g. by tracheal tube or suction catheters.
6. Myocardial ischaemia or infarction.
7. Pain.

Sinus tachycardia is common, and may be a reflex response to hypovolaemia or hypotension. It occurs also in the presence of hypercapnia, anaemia or hypoxaemia, and if the metabolic rate is elevated by fever, shivering, restlessness or malignant hyperpyrexia. The commonest cause is pain. Tachycardia increases myocardial oxygen consumption, and decreases coronary artery perfusion by reducing diastolic time. The combination of arterial hypertension and tachycardia is dangerous in the presence of ischaemic heart disease and should *not* be allowed to persist as it may result in myocardial infarction. Sinus tachycardia should be treated specifically only if it persists after therapy for specific causes has been given; a small i.v. dose of a cardioselective β-blocker (e.g. metoprolol 1–2 mg) should be administered slowly. The ECG must be monitored.

Sinus bradycardia may result from inadequate antagonism by atropine of vagal stimulation by neostigmine, pharyngeal stimulation during suction or the residual effects of volatile anaesthetic agents. Other causes include hypoxaemia (especially in neonates and infants), raised intracranial pressure, myocardial infarction and some cardiac drugs, e.g. β-blockers, digoxin. Oxygen should be administered. Intravenous atropine is effective usually, and should be given in a dose of 0.4–0.6 mg in adults if heart rate is less than 45 beats/min, or if there is associated hypotension.

Bradycardia may occur also as a result of complete heart block.

Supraventricular arrhythmias, including atrial fibrillation, flutter or supraventricular tachycardia, are treated as in other circumstances. Rapid arrhythmias are treated best by cardioversion, but may require pharmacological therapy to prevent recurrence. Nodal rhythm with a normal heart rate is common in the perioperative period, particularly when volatile anaesthetic agents have been used. Supraventricular arrhythmias may cause moderate hypotension because of the loss of synchronisation between atrial and ventricular contractions.

Ventricular arrhythmias. Premature ventricular contractions (PVCs) may require treatment with i.v. lignocaine 1–1.5 mg/kg if they are frequent (>5/minute), multifocal or occur close to the preceding T-wave; however, most cardiologists regard PVCs as benign if cardiac output is adequate. Ventricular tachycardia requires immediate treatment with lignocaine or cardioversion. The management of ventricular fibrillation and asystole are discussed in Chapter 44.

Conduction defects

In the perioperative period these occur usually in patients with pre-existing heart disease (see p. 651). Heart rate and cardiac output in complete heart block may increase in response to isoprenaline, but a transvenous pacemaker should be inserted as soon as possible. Patients who develop second-degree heart block during anaesthesia or in the recovery ward should be transferred to a coronary care or intensive therapy unit for an appropriate period of observation.

Myocardial ischaemia

This occurs most commonly in patients with pre-existing coronary artery disease, and most often in the presence of hypoxaemia, hypotension, hypertension or tachycardia. The ECG should be monitored throughout the recovery period in patients known to be at risk, and precipitating factors should be avoided. Angina occurring during the recovery period should be treated by elimination of any predisposing factor and administration of glyceryl trinitrate sublingually or intravenously.

Myocardial infarction

The incidence of myocardial infarction (MI) is 0.7% in patients over 50 years of age without a history of ischaemic heart disease. Pre-existing coronary artery disease, and in particular, evidence of a previous MI, result in a significantly higher risk. Mortality in patients who suffer a perioperative MI may be as high as 60%. Perioperative MI occurs most commonly on the third postoperative day, but may happen at any time during or after surgery.

A number of factors which may be detected during preoperative assessment are known to increase the likelihood of perioperative MI. The most important of these is the time interval between surgery and a previous MI (Table 24.8). One extensive study of risk factors which might predict major cardiac complications (including, but not exclusively, MI) showed that preoperative evidence of cardiac failure, arrhythmias (of any type) or aortic stenosis, and age were associated also with a high risk. In addition, there is evidence that pre-existing uncontrolled hypertension is associated with increased risk, and that in elderly patients haemodynamic abnormalities detected only by pulmonary artery catheterisation (e.g. elevated left atrial pressure) may affect the incidence of MI in the perioperative period. These problems are discussed more fully in Chapter 19.

Table 24.8 Incidence of perioperative reinfarction in relation to time after previous infarction

Time after previous infarct (months)	Incidence of reinfarction (%)
0–3	27
4–6	11
7–12	6
>12	4

The incidence of perioperative MI is related also to intraoperative and postoperative factors. The magnitude of surgery is an important determinant; in patients with a history of previous MI, the incidence of perioperative reinfarction associated with major vascular surgery is 16%, but only 4% when surgery is performed outside the thorax and abdomen. In patients with ischaemic heart disease, postoperative MI is more likely if there is evidence of ischaemic changes on ECG during operation. Such changes are associated most commonly with episodes of intraoperative hypotension, hypertension or tachycardia; the last two occur most frequently in response to noxious stimuli, e.g. tracheal intubation, surgical incision. The drugs used, and the manner in which they are employed by the anaesthetist, influence the incidences of both intraoperative ischaemia and perioperative MI. Regional anaesthesia is not associated with a reduction in risk.

Reduction of risk

The incidence of perioperative MI may be reduced by:

1. *Identification of patients at risk*. Elective surgery should be postponed if possible until at least 6 months after a previous MI.
2. *Treatment of risk factors*. Cardiac failure, hypertension and arrhythmias should be controlled before surgery. If necessary, the operation should be postponed until control is achieved. Coronary artery bypass grafting or aortic valve replacement may be required in patients with severe coronary artery disease or aortic stenosis respectively, before other major abdominal or thoracic surgery is undertaken.
3. *Avoidance of ischaemia*. The anaesthetic technique and postoperative management should ensure adequate oxygenation of the myocardium and should minimise myocardial oxygen demand (see Ch. 41).
4. *Monitoring*. ECG must be monitored throughout anaesthesia, including induction, in all patients at risk; the CM_5 electrode configuration

(Fig. 21.2) is suitable for detection of ischaemic changes. Arterial pressure should be monitored regularly, and continuously in patients undergoing major surgery. Monitoring of right and left atrial pressures by central venous and pulmonary artery catheterisation, and prompt treatment of abnormalities which occur during operation and in the first 72 h postoperatively, reduce substantially the incidence of perioperative MI.

Diagnosis

Perioperative MI may be difficult to diagnose. It occurs most commonly on the third postoperative day. The classical distribution of pain is present in only 25% of patients.

The diagnosis should be considered in any patient at risk who develops an arrhythmia or becomes hypotensive in the postoperative period. Premature ventricular contractions occur in 90% of patients who experience an MI; sinus bradycardia and the development of any degree of atrioventricular conduction defect are also common. There is often a pyrexia of up to 39°C. The diagnosis is confirmed by changes in serial ECG recordings and/or cardiac enzymes.

OTHER MAJOR POSTOPERATIVE COMPLICATIONS

Deep venous thrombosis (DVT)

The main factors postulated by Virchow as contributing to the formation of venous thrombi are:

1. Changes in the composition of blood.
2. Damage to walls of blood vessel.
3. Decreased blood flow.

However, the exact 'trigger' mechanism which initiates thrombosis remains unknown.

Risk factors

A higher incidence of DVT has been reported in patients with:

1. Extensive trauma.
2. Infection.
3. Heart failure.
4. Blood dyscrasias.
5. Malignancy.
6. Metabolic disorders.

DVT is commoner after hip, pelvic and abdominal surgery than other types of surgery. There is a well-established association between spontaneous DVT and oestrogen, and DVT may occur in women who take the oral contraceptive pill. The number of women who develop this complication is small. However, the incidence increases if surgery is performed while the patient is currently taking the drug. The risk is reduced but not abolished if a low-oestrogen (50 μg or less) preparation is used.

Diagnosis

Approximately 70% of patients with a DVT have neither symptoms nor signs. Fifty per cent of patients with calf pain and tenderness on dorsiflexion of the foot do not have a DVT. Often there is mild pyrexia.

Investigations

Venography. This is an effective method for demonstrating most thrombi of clinical importance.

Radioactive fibrinogen uptake. Iodine-labelled fibrinogen is taken up preferentially by a growing thrombus. The investigation is quick to perform and may detect small thrombi in the calf vessels. Its main disadvantage is that it cannot be used to detect iliac and pelvic vein thrombi, although most thrombi in surgical patients occur in the calf. It does not correlate well with either venography or the development of pulmonary embolism and is associated with a high incidence of false-positive results.

Ultrasonography. This is non-invasive and simple to perform. However, it is insensitive and is useful only for confirming the diagnosis of a major thrombus.

Prophylaxis

Elimination of stasis. The efficacy of early ambulation after operation in reducing the incidence of DVT is not clear. Attempts directed at preventing stasis, including physiotherapy, elastic stockings and elevation of the feet may reduce the incidence of DVT but have not been shown to influence the incidence of pulmonary embolism.

Two methods are used currently for increasing venous return from the lower limbs during surgery:

1. *Electrical stimulation of the calf muscles.* A low-voltage current is applied across the calf to contract the muscles every 2–4 s.
2. *Pneumatic compression of the calves.* The legs are encased in an envelope of plastic material, which is inflated and deflated rhythmically, thus squeezing the calves intermittently. This technique may be continued postoperatively.

Although the incidence of DVT is reduced substantially by these techniques, there is no reduction in the incidence of, or mortality from, pulmonary embolism.

Alteration of blood coagulability

Platelet aggregation. Various drugs which interfere with different aspects of platelet function have been investigated. These include dextran 70, dipyridamole, aspirin and chloroquine. There is no evidence to suggest that dipyridamole or aspirin prevents DVT. Infusion of dextran during and after surgery may reduce the incidence of fatal postoperative pulmonary embolism but its role in the prevention of peripheral venous thrombosis is undetermined.

The coagulation mechanism. Oral anticoagulant therapy instituted before operation is the only well-substantiated method of reducing venous thrombosis. However, there is a risk of increased surgical haemorrhage. Low-dose heparin, 5000 units s.c. 2 h before operation and subsequently at 8- or 12-h intervals until the patient is mobile, is the most promising regimen for prevention of DVT and carries little risk of major haemorrhage. If DVT does occur, it is more likely to be confined to the calf if heparin has been given. Subcutaneous heparin reduces the incidence of fatal pulmonary embolism. It is possible that low molecular weight heparin is a more effective antithrombotic than standard heparin but may carry less risk of haemorrhage.

Pulmonary embolism (PE)

This term covers a range of events from sudden circulatory collapse and death, through minor episodes of pleurisy and haemoptysis, to the long-standing disability of patients with chronic thromboembolic pulmonary hypertension. The acute forms of PE are encountered after anaesthesia and surgery. In the elderly, multiple small pulmonary emboli may be misdiagnosed as bronchopneumonia.

The common sites of origin for thrombi which result in pulmonary embolus are the veins of the pelvis and lower extremities. The most common time for presentation of a postoperative PE is during the second week. In some patients, predisposing factors may have existed preoperatively for some time, and the whole time-scale of events may be shifted; the embolus may occur at the time of, or shortly after, surgery.

Diagnosis

Presenting features. The principal features are circulatory collapse and sudden dyspnoea, associated often with chest pain. If the embolus is large, the pulmonary artery outflow is blocked and sudden death results. If the embolus involves more than 50% of the main pulmonary arteries it is termed 'massive'.

Physical signs. A low cardiac output state develops. Tachypnoea and central cyanosis are usual. There is arterial hypotension, sinus tachycardia and constricted peripheral circulation. The jugular venous pressure is elevated. A fourth heart sound is present usually on auscultation.

Investigations

ECG (Fig. 24.10). This reflects acute right ventricular strain, with features that often include right axis deviation, T wave inversion in leads V_1–V_4 and sometimes right bundle branch block. The classical S_1–Q_3–T_3 pattern is less common.

Chest X-ray. This is often unremarkable but may show areas of oligaemia reflecting pulmonary vascular obstruction.

Arterial blood gases. There is usually hypoxaemia because of ventilation–perfusion imbalance, and hypocapnia resulting from hyperventilation.

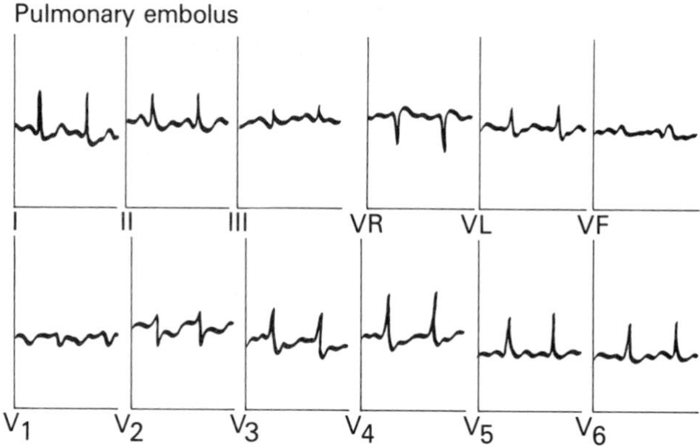

Fig. 24.10 Typical ECG changes in pulmonary embolism.

Perfusion and ventilation lung scans. The perfusion scan shows uneven circulation, with perfusion defects delineating the emboli. A simultaneous ventilation scan is usually normal.

Pulmonary angiography. This provides a definitive diagnosis of major obstruction in the pulmonary circulation. This investigation is useful particularly if the patient is critically ill and the diagnosis is in doubt, and is essential if pulmonary embolectomy is planned. However, it is invasive and normally requires transfer of the patient to the X-ray department.

Treatment

DVT. The mainstay of therapy is anticoagulation. Initially, i.v. heparin is infused in a dose of 40 000 units per day. At the same time, oral anticoagulant therapy is started. Warfarin is used most commonly. Heparin may be discontinued after 48 h. Oral anticoagulants are continued for at least 3 months.

Pulmonary embolism. Immediate treatment consists of administration of oxygen in a high concentration and i.v. heparin. Digoxin is often useful. Sometimes it is necessary to use additional inotropic support for the circulation. Heparin is continued for 5–6 days. Oral anticoagulant therapy is started as soon as possible and is continued for at least 6 months.

Massive pulmonary embolus which does not respond to the above measures may warrant the use of thrombolytic agents, e.g. streptokinase. The risk of haemorrhage with these agents is considerably higher than with heparin. If the cardiovascular effects of the embolism are life-threatening, open pulmonary embolectomy under cardiopulmonary bypass may be considered.

Postoperative renal dysfunction

The kidney is vulnerable to a wide range of drugs and chemicals. It is susceptible particularly to toxic substances for the following reasons:

1. Large blood flow per unit mass.
2. High oxygen consumption.
3. Non-resorbable substances concentrated by tubules.
4. Permeability of tubular cells.

All anaesthetic techniques depress renal blood flow and, secondary to this, interfere with renal function. Provided that prolonged hypotension is avoided, the effects are temporary. However, some anaesthetic agents may produce permanent renal damage.

Methoxyflurane

The administration of this volatile anaesthetic agent is associated with a relatively high incidence of renal dysfunction. Clinically, the defect is characterised by failure of the concentrating ability of the kidney. In certain instances this may progress to high-output renal failure. The nephrotoxicity of methoxyflurane is dose-dependent, and is caused by inorganic fluoride ions which are produced during its metabolism. Administration of methoxyflurane in combination with other nephrotoxic drugs, e.g. aminoglycosides, is particularly hazardous.

Fluoride ions are produced also during metabolism of enflurane. However, only approximately 2% of enflurane undergoes metabolism, compared with up to 45% of methoxyflurane. At present, there is little evidence to suggest that enflurane causes permanent renal dysfunction.

Postoperative hepatic dysfunction

There are many causes of postoperative hepatic dysfunction (Table 24.9). Most patients show no evidence of hepatic damage after anaesthesia and surgery. If it occurs, it is attributable usually to one of the causes shown in Table 24.9. However, if other causes are excluded, consideration should be given to the possibility of hepatotoxicity from anaesthetic drugs.

Chloroform was the first anaesthetic agent to be suspected of causing hepatic damage. In large doses, chloroform is a direct hepatotoxin, and after anaesthesia a hepatitis-like syndrome, with histological evidence of centrilobular hepatic necrosis, occurred occasionally. Methoxyflurane was associated also with hepatic damage, causing a syndrome similar clinically to viral hepatitis. Two of the volatile agents in current use have been implicated in cases of postoperative hepatic dysfunction.

Halothane

Attention was focused first on halothane-associated hepatitis in the early 1960s. Numerous case reports prompted institution in 1969 of the largest retrospective anaesthetic study ever undertaken (United States National Halothane Study). The incidence and causes of fatal hepatic necrosis occurring within six days of anaesthesia were reviewed. The overall incidence was 1 in 10 000; that associated with halothane was 1 in 35 000, and was no greater than the incidence associated with other anaesthetic agents. However, it is believed at present that there is a small number of patients who develop postanaesthetic jaundice in which halothane is the aetiological agent.

The histological picture of halothane-associated hepatitis is similar to that seen in type-A viral hepatitis. Clinically, there is hepatocellular jaundice, with elevation of the aminotransferase enzymes. The exact mechanism of liver damage is not known. At present, there are two main hypotheses:

1. Metabolites of reductive halothane metabolism bind covalently to hepatocyte macromolecules, causing hepatocellular damage.
2. Halothane or its metabolites react with hepatocyte proteins to form antigenic compounds, against which the body mounts an immune response that results in hepatocellular damage.

Antibodies to halothane have been demonstrated recently in patients who have suffered hepatic damage after administration of the drug. At present, this is the most promising method for evaluating the aetiology of a condition which has been a source of great controversy in recent years.

The following groups of patients are believed to be at the greatest risk of developing hepatic dysfunction after halothane anaesthesia:

1. Patients subjected to repeated halothane anaesthetics, especially within a 3-month period.

Table 24.9 Causes of postoperative hepatic dysfunction

Increased bilirubin load	Hepatocellular damage	Extrahepatic biliary obstruction
Blood transfusion	Pre-existing liver disease	Gallstones
Haemolysis and haemolytic disease	Viral hepatitis	Ascending cholangitis
Abnormalities of bilirubin metabolism	Sepsis	Pancreatitis
	Hypotension/hypoxia	Surgical misadventure
	Drug-induced hepatitis	
	Congestive heart failure	

2. Patients who have developed unexplained pyrexia or jaundice after a previous halothane anaesthetic.

3. Obese patients, particularly women.

Enflurane

A number of cases of unexplained jaundice have been reported after the use of enflurane.

OTHER COMPLICATIONS (Table 24.10)

Local vascular complications

Haematoma formation is probably the commonest complication of i.v. injection. This results usually from inadequate pressure at the injection site after removal of the needle. Phlebitis, thrombosis or thrombophlebitis may occur after the use of some i.v. induction agents. Etomidate, propanidid and methohexitone are probably the most troublesome, although some studies have shown little difference between the various induction agents. Intravenous diazepam is a potent cause of phlebitis, although the formulation of diazepam in a fat emulsion (Diazemuls) has overcome this problem.

Table 24.10 Minor morbidity resulting from anaesthesia

Nausea and vomiting related to operation site females > males
Sore throat up to 70% of patients
Hoarseness
Laryngeal granulomata
Headache up to 60% of patients
Backache
Discomfort from catheters, drains, nasogastric tubes
Anxiety
Muscle pains up to 100% of those who receive suxamethonium
Shivering
Drowsiness
Anorexia
Disorientation
Thrombophlebitis at injection site
Bruised or cut lip
Chipped teeth
Corneal abrasions

Intravenous infusions commonly cause thrombophlebitis. The incidence is related to the duration of infusion, and this is more important than the type of cannula used. Thrombophlebitis is rare if the infusion site is changed every 12 h. If it is changed every 72 h, the incidence of thrombophlebitis is 70%. Cannulae constructed from polytetrafluorethylene (Teflon) appear to be the least thrombogenic of those available.

Arterial cannulation is performed commonly to permit continuous monitoring of systemic arterial pressure during major surgery. Unfortunately, it is not without adverse sequelae. Intimal damage may lead to thrombosis and occasionally aneurysm formation. Recannulation of the vessel generally occurs, even when the vessel has been occluded completely. Nevertheless, gangrene of the extremities is an occasional complication, particularly if the brachial artery is used rather than the radial. Ischaemia of the hand or fingers may occur after radial artery cannulation if there is inadequate collateral circulation.

It has been suggested that a modified Allen's test should be performed to assess the adequacy of the collateral circulation through the ulnar artery before radial artery cannulation. The patient is asked to clench his fist, and radial and ulnar arteries are compressed by the examiner. The patient is instructed subsequently to unclench his fist; the examiner releases the ulnar artery and observes the palm of the hand. If there is adequate collateral flow, prompt return of colour to the palm is seen; if there is little or no return of colour within 15 seconds, the collateral flow is poor. However, there is some doubt about the relationship between the results of Allen's test and the incidence of ischaemic episodes after radial artery cannulation.

The incidence of thrombosis after arterial cannulation is reduced by the use of a cannula made of Teflon and of a diameter that is small relative to the size of the artery. A 20-gauge cannula is appropriate in the adult, and a 22- or 24-gauge in children. Arterial damage is reduced also by avoiding multiple punctures of the artery during cannulation. The incidence of radial artery thrombosis is highest in the presence of sepsis, low cardiac output states and when the duration of cannulation is prolonged beyond 24 h.

Nausea and vomiting

Although regarded often by medical and nursing staff as only a minor complication of anaesthesia and surgery, nausea and vomiting are frequently the cause of great distress to patients. In severe cases, fluid and electrolyte imbalance may result. In some circumstances, e.g. after intraocular surgery, vomiting may prejudice the result of the operation.

Many studies have been undertaken to investigate nausea and vomiting after anaesthesia and surgery. The incidence varies from 14 to 82%, the wide range resulting partly from differences in design of studies. Several factors contribute to the aetiology of postoperative nausea and vomiting.

1. *The patient.* Some individuals are particularly susceptible to sickness after the most minor events. Those who are prone to motion sickness are more likely to vomit postoperatively. Women are more likely to vomit than men, and children more so than adults.
2. *Perioperative drugs.* All the opioids possess marked emetic properties. The use of an anticholinergic, especially hyoscine, for premedication reduces the incidence of post-operative vomiting caused by opioids.
3. *Anaesthetic agents.* Ether, cyclopropane and trichloroethylene were associated with high incidences of postoperative vomiting. However, there is little difference in this respect between the volatile anaesthetics used currently, or between techniques in which the patient breathes spontaneously compared with those in which a relaxant and IPPV are used.
4. *Site of operation.* Vomiting is more likely after abdominal procedures than those in most other areas. Middle-ear surgery is associated with a high incidence of vomiting, presumably because of the proximity of the vestibular apparatus. Surgery for correction of strabismus is associated with more vomiting than other ocular procedures. Dilatation of the cervix may also cause postoperative emesis.
5. *Other factors.* The duration of surgery is related to the incidence of postoperative vomiting. Gastric dilatation, e.g. caused by inflation of the stomach with anaesthetic gases, may result in emesis in the postoperative period. Intraoperative or postoperative hypoxaemia may cause vomiting. Hypotension during regional anaesthesia induces vomiting, as does the administration of ergometrine, e.g. during Caesarean section. Premature resumption of oral fluids may make emesis worse.

Prevention and treatment

The incidence of postoperative vomiting may be reduced by careful selection of drugs in the perioperative period, and the prophylactic use of antiemetic agents. The most effective drugs in the prevention and treatment of postoperative vomiting are the phenothiazines and butyrophenones; these are described in Chapter 14.

Headache

The reported incidence of severe headache after anaesthesia and surgery ranges from 12 to 35%, but up to 60% of patients complain of some headache. Individuals who are susceptible to headaches caused by stress, etc. are more likely to complain of postoperative headache. Most investigations have failed to identify any single agent as being responsible for postoperative headache.

Sore throat

Up to 80% of patients complain of sore throat after anaesthesia and surgery. Some of the common causes include:

1. *Trauma during tracheal intubation.* Damage to the pharynx and tonsillar fauces may be caused by the laryngoscope blade.
2. *Trauma to the larynx.* This is more likely if a red rubber tracheal tube is used rather than a plastic disposable tube. A poorly stabilised tube causes more frictional damage to the larynx than one which is stabilised securely.
3. *Trauma to the pharynx.* This may occur during passage of a nasogastric tube or insertion of an oropharyngeal airway, and is common particularly when a throat pack has been used.

Sore throat is likely if a nasogastric tube remains *in situ* during the postoperative period.

4. *Other factors*. The mucous membranes of the mouth, pharynx and upper airway are sensitive to the effects of unhumidified gases; the drying effect of anaesthetic gases may cause postoperative sore throat. The antisialagogue effect of anticholinergic drugs may also contribute to this symptom.

The use of topical local anaesthetics does not reduce the incidence of sore throat. Lubrication of the tracheal tube is effective in reducing the incidence, although there is no difference in this respect between plain or local anaesthetic jellies. However, there is little difference in the incidence of sore throat between an anaesthetic technique in which tracheal intubation is employed and one in which only an oropharyngeal airway is used.

In the absence of a nasogastric tube, postoperative sore throat is usually of short duration; most patients are symptom-free within 48 h.

Hoarseness

This should not be confused with sore throat. It is almost always associated with tracheal intubation, and is caused predominantly by prolonged abduction of, and pressure on, the vocal cords.

Laryngeal granulomata

These may occur after tracheal intubation, and arise from areas of ulceration, usually on the posterior aspect of the vocal cords. The ulcers are caused by pressure and consequent ischaemia. Granulomata are reported most frequently after thyroidectomy.

If hoarseness persists for longer than one week, indirect laryngoscopy should be performed. If ulceration is present, complete voice rest is indicated. Any granulomata present should be excised; untreated granulomata may grow to such a size as to obstruct the airway.

Dental trauma

This is the commonest cause of litigation against anaesthetists. Damage occurs usually during laryngoscopy, especially if tracheal intubation is difficult. Loose teeth, crowns, caps and bridges are particularly susceptible to damage. Preoperative enquiry and examination should alert the anaesthetist to the possibility of damage.

Ocular complications

Carelessness is the commonest cause of damage to the eyes; corneal abrasion is the most frequent lesion. The eyes are often allowed to remain open during anaesthesia. The cornea is thus exposed and vulnerable to the irritant effects of skin preparations, dust and surgical drapes. This type of damage is prevented easily by securing the eyelids in a closed position with adhesive tape.

Retinal infarction has occurred on rare occasions as a result of pressure on the eyeball from a facemask.

Muscles

Problems associated with inadequate reversal of neuromuscular blocking drugs have been discussed above. The detection and treatment of malignant hyperpyrexia are described in Chapter 23; it is important to appreciate that this condition may present during recovery.

Shivering

This is a common complication in the recovery room. It may occur in patients who are hypothermic as a result of prolonged surgery and during injection of local anaesthetic solution into the extradural space. It may also complicate recovery after anaesthesia with volatile anaesthetic agents, particularly halothane. It is essential to administer oxygen throughout the period of shivering.

Shivering increases oxygen consumption and carbon dioxide production, and may result in hypoxaemia and hypercapnia if the response of the respiratory centre to carbon dioxide is impaired by drugs. Oxygen should be administered.

Suxamethonium pains

Muscle pains after suxamethonium are very common, occurring in at least 50% of patients who receive the drug. The muscles involved most frequently are those of the shoulder girdle, neck and thorax. The pain is similar in nature to that caused by viral-related myositis. The incidence is influenced by the following factors:

1. *Age*. Suxamethonium pains are unusual in young children and the elderly.
2. *Gender*. Women are more susceptible than men. The incidence is reduced during pregnancy.
3. *Type of surgery*. There is an increased incidence after minor procedures, when early ambulation is likely.
4. *Physical fitness*. The incidence is higher in individuals who are physically fit.
5. *Repeated doses*. The incidence is increased if repeated doses of suxamethonium are administered.

The exact cause of muscle pains after suxamethonium is unknown, although it is thought that fasciculations produced by depolarisation of the motor nerve end-plate are involved in the pathogenesis. However, the visible extent of fasciculations does not correlate with the severity of subsequent pain. Myoglobinuria occurs after administration of suxamethonium, demonstrating that muscle cell injury does occur.

After minor surgery, the patient may be disturbed by the muscle pains to a greater extent than the discomfort caused by the operative procedure.

It is possible to reduce, but not to eliminate, the incidence of suxamethonium pains by pretreatment with one of the following agents:

1. A small dose of non-depolarising muscle relaxant (usually 10% of the normal dose) 2–3 min before induction of anaesthesia.
2. A small dose of suxamethonium (0.1 mg/kg).
3. Lignocaine 1 mg/kg.
4. Diazepam 0.15 mg/kg i.v. before induction of anaesthesia.
5. Dantrolene 2 h pre-operatively.

Surgical considerations

During the recovery period, a number of surgical complications may occur. These include haemorrhage, blockage of drains or catheters and soiling of dressings. Prosthetic arterial grafts may block, resulting in ischaemia of the limbs. Recovery ward nurses and anaesthetists must be aware of potential surgical complications, as rapid surgical intervention may be required.

The recovery period may be used also to institute orthopaedic traction before the patient returns to the ward.

FURTHER READING

Drain C B, Christoph S S 1987 The recovery room, 2nd edn. W B Saunders, Philadelphia

Hedges A R, Kakkar V V 1988 Prophylaxis of pulmonary embolus and deep vein thrombosis. Hospital Update 14: 1159

Hindmarch I, Jones J G, Moss E (eds) 1987 Aspects of recovery from anaesthesia. Wiley, Chichester

Nimmo W S, Smith G (eds) 1989 Anaesthesia. Blackwell Scientific Publications, Oxford

Nunn J F 1987 Applied respiratory physiology, 3rd edn. Butterworths, London

25. Postoperative pain

Pain is an extraordinarily complex sensation which is difficult to define and equally difficult to measure in an accurate objective manner. It has been defined as the sensory appreciation of afferent nociceptive stimulation which elicits an affective (or autonomic) component; both are subjected to rational interpretation by the patient. It may be represented as a Venn diagram (Fig. 25.1), the shaded area of which represents the quantum of suffering experienced by the patient. The advantage of describing pain by means of the Venn diagram is that it may be seen instantly that the sensation of pain differs among individual patients; the emotional component may vary according to the patient's psychological composition, and the rational component varies with the patient's previous experience, insight and motivation.

Postoperative pain differs from other types of pain in that it is usually transitory, with progressive improvement over a relatively short time-course. Typically, the affective component tends towards an anxiety state associated with diagnosis of the condition, and fear of delay in provision of analgesic therapy by attendants. In contrast, chronic pain is persistent, frequently with fluctuating intensity, and the affective component contains a greater depressive element. Thus, acute pain is more easily amenable to therapy than chronic pain.

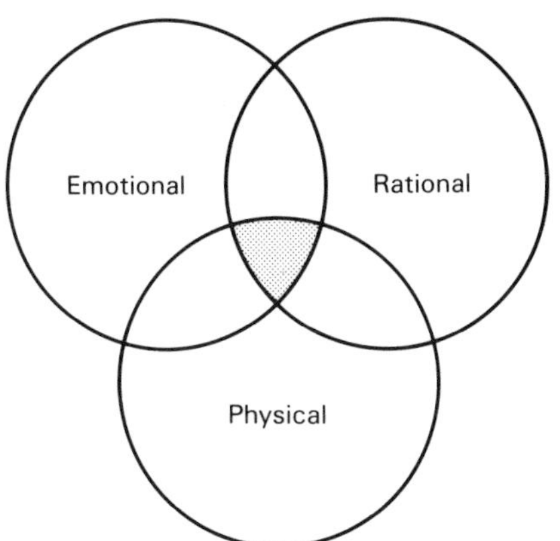

Fig. 25.1 The interrelationship between emotional, rational and physical components of pain. Perceived pain is represented by the area of intersection of all three components.

The traditional management of postoperative pain comprises the prescription of a standard dose of an opioid, to be given i.m. on demand by a nurse when the patient's pain threshold has been exceeded. This leads to poor control of postoperative pain for the following reasons:

1. Responsibility for management of pain is delegated to the nursing staff who err on the side of caution in the administration of opioids. They tend to give too small a dose of drug too infrequently because of fears of producing ventilatory depression or addiction.
2. Because the administration of drugs is left entirely to the discretion of the nursing staff, the degree of empathy between nurse and patient affects analgesic administration. This explains the common observation that the mean dosage of morphine given for a standard operation varies among hospitals and even among wards in the same hospital.
3. Because the measurement of pain is difficult, it is seldom possible to adjust the dosage of drug to match the extent of pain.
4. There are enormous variations in the extent of analgesic requirements depending upon the type of surgery, pharmacokinetic variability, pharmacodynamic variability, etc.

Causes of variation in analgesic requirements

Using patient-controlled analgesic apparatus (vide infra), it has been shown that there is marked interindividual variation in analgesic requirements. Thus after cholecystectomy some patients may require no morphine within the first 24 h, whereas others may require as much as 120 mg. Unfortunately, there is no way of predicting in advance the extent of opioid requirements of an individual patient. In clinical practice, requirements are assessed on a trial-and-error basis; anaesthetists are therefore in an ideal position to be involved in prescribing postoperative analgesia, as they obtain a 'feel' for dose requirements during management of anaesthesia.

Site and type of surgery

In general, upper abdominal surgery produces greater pain than lower abdominal surgery, which in turn is associated with greater pain than peripheral surgery. This generalisation is not entirely accurate; operations on the richly innervated digits may be associated with quite severe pain.

The type of pain may differ with different types of surgery. Operations on joints are associated with sharp pain; in contrast, abdominal surgery is associated with two types of pain: a continuous dull nauseating ache (which responds well to morphine) and sharper pain induced by coughing and movement (which responds poorly to morphine). Pain associated with surgery on the digits may respond relatively poorly to opioids but well to non-steroidal anti-inflammatory drugs.

Table 25.1 Duration and severity of postoperative pain

Site of operation	Duration of opioid use (h)	Severity of pain (0–4)
Abdominal:		
upper	48–72	3
lower	up to 48	2
inguinal	up to 36	1
Thoracotomy	72–96	4
Limbs	24–36	2
Faciomaxillary	up to 48	2
Body wall	up to 24	1
Perineal	24–48	2
Hip surgery	up to 48	2

Table 25.1 provides an approximate guide to the duration and severity of postoperative pain.

Age, gender and body weight

The analgesic requirements of males and females are identical for similar types of surgery. However, there is a reduction in analgesic requirements with advancing age. Consequently, it is essential that the anaesthetist reduces the dosage of opioid drugs in elderly patients.

The established anaesthetic practice of prescribing the potent opioid drugs on a mg or μg per body weight basis lacks scientific validity. There is no evidence to suggest that variations in body weight in the adult population affect opioid requirements.

Psychological factors (Table 25.2)

The patient's personality affects pain perception and response to analgesic drugs. Thus, patients with a low anxiety and low neuroticism score on a personality scale exhibit less postoperative pain and require smaller doses of opioid than patients who rate highly on these scales. Patients with high scores may exhibit a higher incidence of postoperative chest complications.

The extent of a patient's anxiety also affects pain perception; increased anxiety results in a greater degree of perceived postoperative pain and increased opioid requirements.

These psychological factors help to explain the efficacy of preoperative psychotherapy. Anxiety and postoperative analgesic requirements are reduced if the preoperative visit by the anaesthetist includes an explanation of forthcoming perioperative events and details regarding the provision of pain relief.

Table 25.2 Psychological factors which influence postoperative analgesic requirements

Personality
— more pain if high neuroticism/extroversion
Social background
Culture
Motivation
Preoperative psychotherapy

Pharmacokinetic variability

After the intramuscular injection of an opioid, there is a three- to seven-fold difference between patients in the rate at which peak plasma concentrations of the drug occur and a two-to five-fold difference in the peak plasma concentration achieved. This is illustrated in Figure 25.2, which shows the mean change in plasma concentration after the first and second, and seventh and eighth injections. The variability in the plasma concentration is reflected by the large standard deviation of the mean. In addition, average concentrations increase after each of the first few injections; oscillation around a steady mean concentration does not occur until after approximately the fourth injection.

This pharmacokinetic variability helps to explain the relatively poor response to a single intramuscular injection given in the postoperative period.

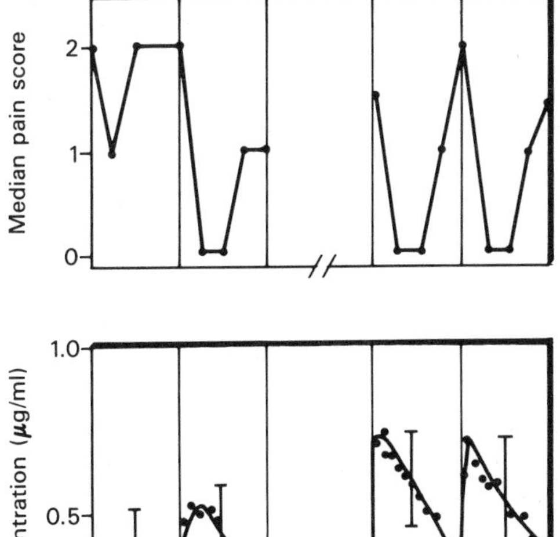

Fig. 25.2 Blood concentrations of pethidine and pain score after surgery; a pain score of 0 indicates no pain. Doses of pethidine 100 mg have been given 4-hourly. Mean blood concentration of pethidine continues to rise for 24 h before a plateau is reached. Little pain relief is provided by the first dose. Even after 24 h, significant pain is present 3 and 4 h after each injection, as blood concentrations decline.

Pharmacodynamic variability

Although there are widespread pharmacokinetic variations between patients in response to administration of opioids, the major reason for variation in opioid sensitivity is pharmacodynamic, i.e. a difference in the inherent sensitivity of opioid receptors.

Using continuous infusions of opioids to achieve equilibrium between receptor drug concentration and plasma concentration, it is possible to define a steady-state plasma concentration of opioid at which analgesia is produced. This is termed the minimum effective analgesic concentration (MEAC); values of MEAC for the commonly available opioids are shown in Table 25.3. MEAC levels vary four-to five-fold between individual patients, and are affected by age and differences in psychological profile.

Table 25.3 Minimum effective analgesic concentration (MEAC) in blood for a number of analgesic drugs. Note the wide range of values for each agent

Drug	MEAC (ng/ml)
Fentanyl	1–3
Alfentanil	100–300
Pethidine	300–650
Morphine	12–24
Methadone	30–70

METHODS OF TREATING POSTOPERATIVE PAIN (Table 25.4)

Conventional administration of opioids

Intramuscular administration of opioids on a *pro re nata* (p.r.n.; as required) basis is the method used most commonly for prescribing postoperative analgesia. However, for the reasons noted above, this leads frequently to inadequate pain relief. Almost 60% of patients report dissatisfaction with the quality of postoperative analgesia administered in this way.

Intramuscular injection results in variable absorption, particularly in patients with hypothermia, hypovolaemia or hypotension. In addition, there is inevitably a considerable delay between request for analgesia and subsequent administration while controlled drugs are checked and

Table 25.4 Methods of treating postoperative pain

1. 'Conventional administration of opioid'
   i.m. on-demand bolus
2. Newer opioid agonist/antagonist drugs
3. Newer parenteral routes of administration of opioid:
   (a) Bolus i.v. administration
   (b) Continuous i.v. infusion
   (c) PCA:
      bolus } i.v./i.m./s.c.
      bolus + infusion }
4. Non-parenteral administration of opioid:
   buccal/sublingual
   oral
   rectal
   transdermal
5. Local anaesthetic techniques
6. Subarachnoid/extradural opioids
7. Respiratory route of administration of volatile/gaseous agents
8. Non-pharmacological methods:
   cryotherapy
   TCNS
   acupuncture
   psychological methods

drawn into a syringe. Although it is customary to prescribe opioids on a 4-hourly p.r.n. basis, there are frequently much longer periods between injections and this may lead to considerable 'breakthrough' pain.

The commonest cause of postoperative nausea and vomiting is the administration of opioids either intraoperatively or in the postoperative period. It should therefore be standard practice to prescribe antiemetic drugs regularly for administration with opioids.

Regular administration of i.m. opioids provides improved analgesia, although care must be taken to avoid overdosage in debilitated patients and those at the extremes of age.

The advantages and disadvantages of repeated p.r.n. administration of opioids are listed in Table 25.5. Drugs used commonly for postoperative pain and antiemesis are listed in Table 25.6; their pharmacological properties are discussed fully in Chapters 11 and 14.

Properties of morphine and morphine-like drugs

1. Analgesia. Morphine produces analgesia by binding with opioid receptors which are present in high concentrations in the periaqueductal area and limbic system of the brain and in the region of the substantia gelatinosa of the spinal cord.

Table 25.5 Advantages and disadvantages of intramuscular p.r.n. administration of opioids

Advantages	Disadvantages
Familiar practice	Fixed dose not related to pharmacovariability
Gradual onset of side effects	I.m. administration causes profound pharmacovariability
Nursing assessment before administration	Painful injections
Inexpensive	Fluctuating plasma concentrations Delayed onset of analgesia

Table 25.6 Drugs used systemically for postoperative pain relief and antiemesis

Drug	Dose i.m. (healthy adult)
Opioids	
Morphine	10 mg 4-hourly
Papaveretum	20 mg 4-hourly
Pethidine	100 mg 3-hourly
Buprenorphine (sublingual)	0.4 mg 6-hourly
Moderate analgesics	
Pentazocine	60 mg 4-hourly
Dihydrocodeine	50 mg 4-hourly
Antiemetics	
Prochlorperazine	12.5 mg 6-hourly
Perphenazine	5 mg 6-hourly
Cyclizine	50 mg 6-hourly
Metoclopramide	10 mg 6-hourly

2. Ventilatory depression.
3. Sedation.
4. Cough suppression.
5. Vasodilatation.
6. Release of histamine.
7. Constipation.
8. Nausea and vomiting.
9. Pupillary constriction.
10. Biliary spasm.
11. Urine retention.
12. Tolerance.
13. Physical dependence.

The most important side effects of morphine are ventilatory depression and nausea and vomiting. Morphine should not be administered to patients with biliary or renal colic (occasionally it may precipitate pain in patients with gall-bladder disease when administered as premedication) and should be avoided in patients with head injury and perhaps in asthmatics.

Alternative drugs are described in Chapter 11. Despite manufacturers' claims to the contrary, there is no evidence that any of the newer opioid agonist/antagonist drugs produce analgesia equivalent to that of morphine with lesser degrees of ventilatory depression. Some of the newer drugs produce a higher incidence of side effects such as nausea, vomiting and sedation than equianalgesic doses of morphine.

Buprenorphine is a particularly interesting drug. By virtue of its very high lipid solubility it is absorbed readily across membranes and can be administered by the sublingual route. However, it undergoes a high degree of first-pass metabolism in the gut wall and liver; thus the drug is largely inactivated if the tablet is swallowed. Buprenorphine is a partial agonist with a much higher affinity for μ receptors than morphine. In low doses it displaces morphine from the receptors, thereby apparently 'antagonising' the morphine. In slightly higher doses it produces excellent analgesia in its own right. Sublingual buprenorphine 0.4 mg 6-hourly provides reasonable analgesia after abdominal surgery. A major disadvantage of buprenorphine is the greater degree of sedation compared with that produced by morphine, and this accounts for its relative unpopularity for patients who are mobilised rapidly after surgery (e.g. herniorrhaphy). Because of its high receptor affinity it is recommended that the use of buprenorphine should not be combined with that of morphine.

Newer parenteral routes of opioid administration

Bolus i.v. administration

It is possible to improve the quality of analgesia in the postoperative period by giving small incremental doses of opioid i.v. when required. However, this carries the risk of rapid induction of ventilatory depression and in the majority of hospitals cannot be undertaken by nursing staff. In general, this technique is employed only by anaesthetists in the immediate recovery period.

Continuous i.v. infusion (Table 25.7)

This technique is employed to provide analgesia in patients receiving artificial ventilation in ITU. An infusion rate designed to exceed MEAC in all patients is clearly safe, and ventilatory depression is an advantage in this situation.

Continuous infusions have been used in general surgical wards for the provision of postoperative analgesia in spontaneously breathing patients. The dosage rate is determined by the medical attendant on a trial-and-error basis, and a fixed infusion rate prescribed. However, this carries great risks of producing ventilatory depression and cannot be recommended in spontaneously breathing patients outside a high-dependency or intensive therapy unit.

Patient-controlled analgesia (PCA)

The main problem with continuous i.v. infusion is that there is no way of predicting an individual patient's MEAC. With PCA, the patient determines the rate of i.v. administration of the drug, thereby providing feedback control.

PCA equipment comprises an accurate source of infusion, coupled to an i.v. cannula and controlled by a patient–machine interface device. Safety features are incorporated to limit the preset dose, the number of doses which may be administered and the 'lock-out' period between doses. Accidental triggering of the patient control is prevented usually by a requirement for the patient to make two successive presses on a hand control within 1 s.

The Cardiff palliator was the first commercially available device and has been used principally with pethidine, delivering boluses of approximately

Table 25.7 Advantages and disadvantages of continuous i.v. infusions

Advantages	Disadvantages
Rapid onset of analgesia	Fixed dose not related to pharmacodynamic variability
Steady-state plasma concentrations	Errors may be fatal
Painless	Expensive fail-safe equipment required May result in less frequent assessment by nursing staff

Table 25.8 Advantages and disadvantages of patient-controlled analgesia (PCA)

Advantages	Disadvantages
Dose matches patient's requirements and therefore compensates for pharmacodynamic variability	Technical errors may be fatal
Doses given are small and therefore fluctuations in plasma concentrations are reduced	Expensive equipment
Reduces nurses' workload	Requires ability to cooperate and understand
Painless	
Placebo effect from patient autonomy	

10–20 mg (for a healthy adult patient) with a lock-out period of 10 min.

The major disadvantage of this type of PCA equipment is that the patient stops demanding the drug when asleep; the plasma concentration then declines below the analgesic threshold, and the patient wakes up with pain. Newer PCA machines provide the facility for a continuous low-dose background infusion, on which the patient superimposes patient-activated boluses. Advantages and disadvantages of PCA are listed in Table 25.8.

Non-parenteral opioid administration

Sublingual opioids

Sublingual administration requires cooperation. With buprenorphine, good analgesia can be provided without the necessity for painful injections, making this route popular with patients and convenient for nursing staff.

This route is confined largely to buprenorphine. Combination with morphine may result in dysphoria and withdrawal phenomena. If this route is chosen, it is preferable to use buprenorphine as the sole opioid in the perioperative period.

Oral route

In the immediate postoperative period there is invariably a reduction in the rate of gastric emptying (caused mainly by the intraoperative or preoperative use of opioids). For this reason, opioids should not be used orally for pain relief in the immediate postoperative period because:

1. Absorption is delayed, with poor analgesia.
2. If opioids have been given orally on a regular basis, there is a danger of a large dose being dumped into the upper gastrointestinal tract when gastric motility returns to normal, resulting in overdosage and ventilatory depression.

Oral administration of opioids may be used in the late postoperative period. However, it is more customary to use less potent drugs such as dihydrocodeine or paracetamol because the severity of the pain is generally declining by this time.

All the opioids undergo extensive metabolism in the gut wall and liver (first-pass metabolism) and therefore the bioavailability is relatively low (e.g. 20–30% for morphine).

The rectal route

The rectal route may be used as a means of delivering morphine but there is marked variability in the plasma concentrations achieved. Venous blood from the lower part of the rectum drains directly into the systemic circulation, but the upper part drains into the portal circulation. Thus, bioavailability varies according to the site of a suppository within the rectum. However, this route avoids the problems of reduced gastrointestinal motility. Probably the best indication for the rectal route is the treatment of chronic intractable pain particularly where there is dysphagia.

Transdermal

Because of the high lipid solubility and high potency of fentanyl, this drug may be absorbed across the skin in sufficient quantities to produce effective plasma concentrations. Several centres are currently investigating transdermal administration of fentanyl using a rate-controlled delivery system.

Local anaesthetic techniques

Many local anaesthetic techniques, administered for the purpose of operative surgery or during the course of general anaesthesia, may provide excellent analgesia in the early postoperative period. However, it is usually necessary for the anaesthetist to administer an opioid to the patient before the block regresses to reduce the likelihood of severe pain when the block wears off.

Many local anaesthetic techniques may be used for the primary purpose of providing analgesia in the early postoperative period. However, a major disadvantage is that the duration of blockade with a 'single-shot' technique is relatively short. Bupivacaine (0.25% or 0.5%) is the drug of choice and may produce peripheral nerve blockade lasting for 8–12 h, and occasionally for as long as 18 h. The duration of action for extradural nerve block is 4–6 h.

Adrenaline may be added to a local anaesthetic solution to prolong the block, although this produces relatively little effect on the duration of analgesia produced by bupivacaine. The most effective means of prolonging the block is by the use of a catheter to permit either repeated bolus doses or a continuous infusion of local anaesthetic to be administered.

Local anaesthetic blocks in common use are described in Chapter 26. The following blocks represent those which are employed most usefully for postoperative analgesia.

Spinal nerve block

Subarachnoid analgesia rarely lasts more than 3–4 h with the drugs currently available, and is therefore of limited use for postoperative analgesia. Although the insertion of a catheter into the subarachnoid space is employed in the United States, this is not a popular manoeuvre in the United Kingdom because of the risk of infection.

Extradural block

Extradural block is popular for postoperative analgesia because of familiarity with the technique, and ease of insertion of a catheter. Repeated injections may be made through the catheter, or a dilute solution of local anaesthetic infused continuously. Initially, bupivacaine produces analgesia lasting up to 4 h, but by 24–48 h some tolerance develops and single-bolus administrations may last for only 2 h.

Bupivacaine 0.25% injected at L2/3 provides good analgesia after lower abdominal or perineal surgery, e.g. hysterectomy or transurethral resection of prostate. Upper abdominal procedures require a higher block; 15 ml of bupivacaine 0.5% produces analgesia up to T7.

For thoracic surgery, an extradural catheter may be inserted in the thoracic region between T6 and T8 and volumes of bupivacaine of 6–12 ml may provide excellent postoperative analgesia.

It is recommended that extradural catheter techniques should be employed only when the patient is nursed in an intensive therapy or high-dependency unit, because of the risks of hypotension after extradural injections and total spinal block if the catheter migrates into the subarachnoid space.

Caudal block

Caudal administration of local anaesthetic drugs is useful for child day-case surgery, e.g. circumcision, or in patients undergoing anal or perineal surgery. It is customary to administer only a single dose of local anaesthetic; catheter techniques are unpopular in the United Kingdom because of the risk of infection. Suitable dosage of local anaesthetic solution for use by the caudal route are shown in Table 25.9.

Table 25.9 Doses of bupivacaine (0.25% plain) for caudal analgesia

Adult	Child
0.3–0.4 ml/kg	0.5–0.7 ml/kg (or 0.1 ml/year for each segment to be blocked)

N.B. Dosage of bupivacaine should *never* exceed 2 mg/kg.

Other regional blocks used for postoperative analgesia

1. *Intercostal nerve blockade*. Blocks from T4 to T8 or 9 provide satisfactory analgesia for pain relief after subcostal incision for cholecystectomy. Intercostal blocks may be repeated at regular intervals; the use of catheters for repeated administration has been employed. Bilateral blockade should not be carried out because of the risk of pneumothorax.

2. *Paravertebral block.* This may be used to provide analgesia after thoracic or abdominal surgery. Local anaesthetic solution is injected into the region of the paravertebral space to block the dorsal sensory nerve roots as they emerge from the vertebral foramina. This technique may be performed using single or repeated injections, or with an indwelling catheter.

3. *Femoral nerve block* may be performed during anaesthesia for analgesia after arthroscopy of the knee but is not very effective.

Spinal and extradural opioids (see also p. 200).

In recent years there has been great interest in the use of opioids by the subarachnoid or extradural routes. After injection of opioid into the CSF drug is taken up in the region of the substantia gelatinosa within the dorsal horn. It is thought that opioids act predominantly on the presynaptic enkephalin receptors, although opioid is absorbed from the CSF into the circulation. After extradural administration of opioids, the drug diffuses through the dura into CSF and produces analgesia by the same mechanism as that associated with subarachnoid injection. However, there is more rapid uptake of opioid into the circulation via the rich network of blood vessels in the extradural space. Consequently, there is a rapid increase in both CSF and blood concentrations of the drug after extradural administration.

Uptake into the dorsal horn, and rate of passage through the dura, are dependent upon lipid solubility. Thus the more highly lipid-soluble drugs (e.g. fentanyl) have a more rapid onset and a shorter duration of action. The less lipid-soluble drugs (e.g. morphine) have a slower rate of onset of action; in addition there is a greater dispersion within the CSF because of reduced uptake into spinal cord and the drug may reach the medulla to cause delayed ventilatory depression.

Subarachnoid opioids

This route is less popular than the extradural route of administration for opioids because of the production of spinal headache. However, smaller doses are required than when the extradural route is used and therefore systemic concentrations are lower. The quality of analgesia is not as good as that achieved with subarachnoid local anaesthetic drugs.

Extradural opioids

The administration of extradural opioids is more popular because spinal headache is avoided and a catheter technique may be employed. It is possible to achieve analgesia without the motor or autonomic block produced by local anaesthetic injected into the extradural space. Thus, postural hypotension and changes in heart rate do not occur. Early ventilatory depression may occur as a result of systemic absorption (e.g. within the first 1–2 h) but late ventilatory depression (8–20 h) is a result of rostral spread of opioid within the CSF to the medulla. Prolonged duration of action of analgesia is produced by a single injection (up to 24 h).

Side effects of extradural opioids

1. Early ventilatory depression — occurs more commonly with lipid-soluble agents.
2. Late ventilatory depression — occurs more commonly with agents of lower lipophilicity.
3. Coma — occurs relatively late, usually in association with late ventilatory depression, and can be reversed by naloxone.
4. Urinary retention.
5. Itching — this is reversed only partially by naloxone.
6. Nausea and vomiting.

Inhalation of volatile or gaseous anaesthetics

This technique was very popular in the past to provide analgesia during childbirth. Vaporisers were designed for the administration of methoxyflurane (Cardiff inhaler) or trichloroethylene (Tecota), and apparatus was designed also for the administration of nitrous oxide with oxygen.

For non-obstetric pain relief, the only gaseous technique used currently comprises 50% O_2/50% N_2O (Entonox). This is used in the field situation, (e.g. by ambulance personnel to provide analgesia at the site of an accident), or for changing burns dressings in hospital practice. The use of this technique in the intensive care unit was discontinued many years ago because continuous or frequent intermittent use of nitrous oxide may cause neutropenia as a result of the toxic effect of nitrous oxide on vitamin B_{12} metabolism.

Non-pharmacological methods

Cryotherapy

This may be applied to intercostal nerves exposed during a thoracotomy. The nerve is surrounded by an iceball produced by intense sub-zero temperatures at the end of a probe. The neuronal disruption produced by this method is temporary, and sensation returns after some months, although it may be accompanied by unpleasant paraesthesiae and occasionally by persistent neuralgia.

Transcutaneous electrical stimulation

A small alternating current is passed between two surface electrodes at low voltage and at a frequency between 0.2 and 200 Hz. It is thought that the technique acts by increasing CNS concentrations of endorphins. Acupuncture may work in a similar manner. The technique produces only moderate analgesia.

FURTHER READING

Cousins M J, Phillips G D (eds) 1986 Acute pain management. Churchill Livingstone, New York

Harmer M, Rosen M, Vickers M D (eds) 1985 Patient-controlled analgesia. Blackwell Scientific Publications, Oxford

Smith G 1989 The management of postoperative pain. In: Nimmo W S, Smith G (eds) Anaesthesia. Blackwell Scientific Publications, Oxford

Smith G, Covino B G (eds) 1985 Acute pain. Butterworths, London

26. Local anaesthetic techniques

The efficacy of local anaesthetic techniques has increased greatly within the past two decades as a result of advances in drugs, equipment and the anatomical approaches to nerve blocks. This chapter outlines the basic principles of patient management and the methods employed in the performance of a variety of blocks which are undertaken commonly by the trainee anaesthetist.

Regional techniques for obstetrics and dental surgery are described in other chapters.

FEATURES OF LOCAL ANAESTHESIA

In some circumstances, regional anaesthesia may have distinct advantages over general anaesthesia, as for example in the use of axillary block for hand surgery in a respiratory cripple. However, rather than view a local anaesthetic technique as a 'rival' to general anaesthesia, it is more useful to consider it as part of an individually selected technique which may include the use of sedative or centrally acting anaesthetic drugs. Although the trainee may consider local anaesthesia as having 'advantages and disadvantages', it becomes apparent with experience that an advantage in one situation may be a disadvantage in another.

Preservation of consciousness is considered often to be an advantage of regional anaesthesia. For example, the patient undergoing Caesarean section is able to protect her own airway and experience the birth of the child. However, patients who require other forms of surgery may be unhappy at the prospect of being awake; in this situation the combination of a regional block and light general anaesthesia may be valuable.

One benefit of a regional block is the quality of early postoperative analgesia, but this may carry disadvantages. Some patients are distressed by the accompanying numbness, although correct preoperative explanation should minimise this concern; in addition, it is important that nursing staff are aware of the risk of trauma to the blocked segments.

Other features of regional anaesthesia include simplicity of administration, sympathetic blockade, attenuation of the stress response and minimal depression of ventilation. Some studies have suggested that the net effect of these features may be a reduction in the incidence of major postoperative complications, but this is controversial.

COMPLICATIONS OF LOCAL ANAESTHESIA

The incidence of complications may be minimised by ensuring adequate supervision and training in local anaesthetic techniques, and by exercising care in the performance of each block. Sufficient expertise and equipment must always be available to deal with potential complications. Complications common to many techniques are discussed in this section; more specific problems are considered later.

Local anaesthetic toxicity

This results usually from accidental intravascular injection, an excessive dose of local anaesthetic or faulty technique, particularly during performance of Bier's block at the injection site.

Features and treatment

These are described in Chapter 15.

Prevention

Correct technique, careful and repeated aspiration, and the use of a test dose are important, but the main safety measure is *slow injection* of the local anaesthetic. This prevents rapid production of very high plasma concentrations even if the injection is intravascular. By this means, toxicity may be diagnosed early, the injection discontinued and a major reaction avoided. Rapid injection of local anaesthetic is not necessary for the performance of any block.

Test dose

This may be used before administration of the main dose of local anaesthetic drug. It is indicated particularly for extradural block, where it should be capable of demonstrating inadvertent i.v. or subarachnoid injection. A test dose of 4 ml of 2% plain lignocaine is sufficient to cause mild symptoms in most patients after accidental i.v. injection; during performance of extradural block this test dose should provide evidence of significant blockade (impairment of straight-leg raising) within 5 min if inadvertent subarachnoid injection has occurred. No test dose is infallible; slow administration of the main dose is the most important factor in avoiding local anaesthetic toxicity.

Hypotension

There are several possible mechanisms by which a local anaesthetic technique may cause hypotension. The anaesthetist must always remember that surgical factors may be responsible.

Sympathetic blockade

A limited sympathetic block may be produced by peripheral nerve anaesthesia, but only central blocks are likely to produce hypotension by this mechanism.

Total spinal blockade

This is discussed on page 475. It occurs occasionally during subarachnoid block if excessive spread of local anaesthetic solution occurs, and is a recognised complication of extradural block if the dura has been penetrated. Apnoea may occur if local anaesthetic solution reaches the CSF during interscalene brachial plexus block, or the ventricular system during retrobulbar nerve block.

Vasovagal attack

This is particularly likely to occur in an anxious patient with a rapidly ascending spinal block. Pallor, nausea and bradycardia are associated with the hypotension. The supine position is no guarantee against this complication. Rapid resolution results from placing the patient head-down and the administration of i.v. ephedrine 5–6 mg with cautious i.v. sedation (e.g. midazolam 1–2 mg).

Anaphylactoid reaction

This is very rare with amide local anaesthetics. Treatment is discussed in Chapter 23.

Local anaesthetic toxicity

This is considered above and in Chapter 15.

Motor blockade

To avoid unnecessary distress, patients must be warned of the possibility of lower limb weakness or paralysis which may persist for some time after operation.

Pneumothorax

This is a potential hazard of supraclavicular brachial plexus, intercostal and paravertebral blocks. The possibility of its occurrence is an absolute contraindication to the use of these techniques in outpatients and also to the performance of these blocks bilaterally.

Urinary retention

This may follow the use of central blocks. It is important to avoid overhydration, as bladder distension may require catheterisation.

Neurological complications

Carefully performed blocks result rarely in neurological complications.

Neuritis with persisting sensory changes and/or weakness may result from trauma to the nerve, intraneural injection, or bacterial, chemical or particulate contamination of the injected solution. Injection of the incorrect solution has caused some of the most severe neurological complications. To avoid this serious error, all drugs must be checked personally by the anaesthetist immediately before injection.

Anterior spinal artery syndrome may follow an episode of prolonged, severe hypotension and results in painless permanent paraplegia. *Adhesive arachnoiditis* has been described after subarachnoid and extradural blockade and may lead to permanent pain, weakness, and bladder or bowel dysfunction. It is suspected that this complication results from injection of the incorrect solution. *Haematoma* or *abscess* formation in the spinal canal after subarachnoid or extradural anaesthesia results in weakness and sensory loss below the level of spinal cord compression. It is associated with intense back pain and is a neurosurgical emergency which demands immediate decompression to avoid permanent disability.

Equipment problems

Needles are most likely to break at the junction with the hub and therefore should never be inserted fully. Catheters may also break, but exploratory surgery to find small pieces of catheter is inappropriate, as complications are very unlikely.

GENERAL MANAGEMENT

Patient assessment and selection

Careful preoperative evaluation is as important before a local anaesthetic as it is before general anaesthesia, and the same principles of preoperative management apply. Therapy to improve the patient's condition before surgery should be instituted if appropriate. It is inappropriate to proceed with surgery under local anaesthesia for the sake of convenience in the poorly prepared patient. A decision on the need for immediate surgical intervention should be made before the anaesthetic technique is chosen.

The preoperative visit should be used to establish rapport with the patient. A clear description of the proposed anaesthetic should be given in simple terms, but there is rarely a need for excessive detail. Occasionally patients require some explanation of the reasons for selecting a regional technique before accepting it, but there should be no attempt at coercion.

Potential problems related to the intended block should be sought. Anatomical deformities may render some blocks impractical. A history of allergy to amide local anaesthetics is rare, but is an absolute contraindication, as is infection at the site of needle insertion. For most blocks, anticoagulant therapy and bleeding diatheses are also absolute contraindications, and the use of major blocks in patients with distant infection or receiving low-dose s.c. heparin requires careful consideration. Sympathetic blockade with consequent vasodilatation may lead to profound hypotension in patients with aortic or mitral stenosis because of the relatively constant cardiac output. Hypovolaemia must be corrected before contemplating subarachnoid or extradural anaesthesia.

There is no evidence that neuromuscular disorders or multiple sclerosis are affected adversely by local anaesthetic techniques, but most anaesthetists use regional anaesthesia in such patients only if there are obvious benefits to be gained; any perioperative deterioration in the neurological condition is often associated by the patient with the local anaesthetic procedure. Raised intracranial pressure is a contraindication to central blockade.

Selection of technique

Local anaesthetic drugs may be administered by:

1. Single dose.
2. Intermittent bolus:

(a) repeated injections.
(b) indwelling catheter for repeat administration.

3. Continuous infusion (with optional bolus doses) via a catheter.

If regional anaesthesia has been selected primarily to provide analgesia during and after surgery under general anaesthesia, a distal technique is appropriate and is associated with least complications.

Because a local anaesthetic technique renders only part of the body insensible it is essential that the method employed is tailored to, and sufficient for, the planned surgery. Account must be taken of the duration of surgery, its site (which may be multiple, e.g. the need to obtain bone grafting material from the iliac crest), and the likelihood of a change of procedure in mid-operation. The problem of multiple sites of surgery may be met by one block which covers both sites, or by more than one regional procedure. The duration of anaesthesia may be tailored to the anticipated duration of surgery by selection of an appropriate local anaesthetic agent, or may require the use of a technique which allows further administration of drug.

Premedication

Manipulation of fractures and other short emergency procedures are often carried out using a local anaesthetic technique in the unpremedicated patient, as rapid recovery is desirable. However, premedication is helpful before inpatient elective or emergency surgery. An oral benzodiazepine allays anxiety, but an opioid (e.g. morphine) alleviates the discomfort of prolonged immobility which may be required during a long procedure. Opioids are indicated also in the emergency situation to relieve pain before surgery, and are best administered intravenously. Patients should be fasted for all but the most minor peripheral nerve blocks.

Timing

It is essential that sufficient time is allowed to perform the block without undue haste on the part of the anaesthetist. This is largely a matter of organisation, and the experienced practitioner seldom causes delay to an operating list. Any preoperative delay is compensated for by the ability to return the patient to bed immediately after completion of surgery.

Resuscitation equipment

A full range of resuscitative equipment must be in working order and available immediately. This includes:

1. An anaesthetic breathing system through which oxygen may be administered under pressure via a face mask or tracheal tube.
2. A laryngoscope with two sizes of blade, a range of tracheal tubes and an introducer.
3. A table which can be tilted head-down rapidly.
4. Suction apparatus.
5. Intravenous cannulae and fluids.
6. Thiopentone to control convulsions.
7. Drugs to treat hypotension, especially atropine, ephedrine and methoxamine.

A cannula must be inserted intravenously before *any* local anaesthetic block is performed in case emergency therapy is required.

Regional block equipment

Regional anaesthesia may be employed with basic equipment, but some special items increase the success rate and reduce the risk of complications.

Needles

Very fine spinal needles (26G) have reduced significantly the incidence of post-spinal headache. Disposable prepacked spinal and extradural needles ease preparation and ensure sterility. Short-bevelled needles (Fig. 26.1) reduce the likelihood of nerve damage and are recommended for plexus and peripheral nerve blockade. Sheathed needles are valuable for use with nerve stimulators.

Immobile needle technique

For plexus and major nerve blocks, local anaesthetic drug is drawn into labelled syringes and connected to the block needle by a short length

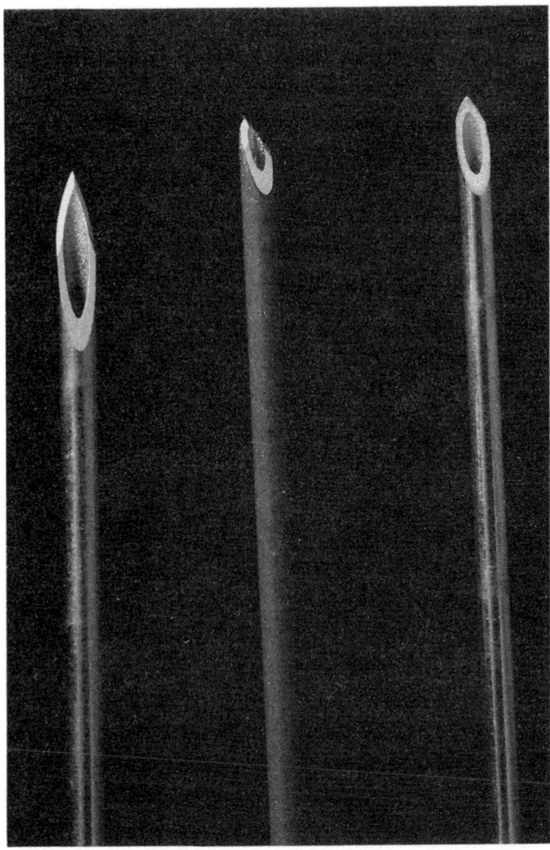

Fig. 26.1 Left to right: standard-bevelled, and sheathed and unsheathed short-bevelled, needles.

of tubing (see Fig. 26.14). This allows the anaesthetist to hold the needle steady while aspiration tests are performed and syringes changed. The system must be primed to avoid air embolism.

Catheters

Continuous administration of local anaesthetic drugs has been made possible by the development of high-quality catheters, which are introduced through a needle and left in position for many hours.

Nerve stimulators

Many anaesthetists prefer to elicit paraesthesiae when performing a major nerve block. However, a nerve stimulator (Fig. 26.2) is a useful aid,

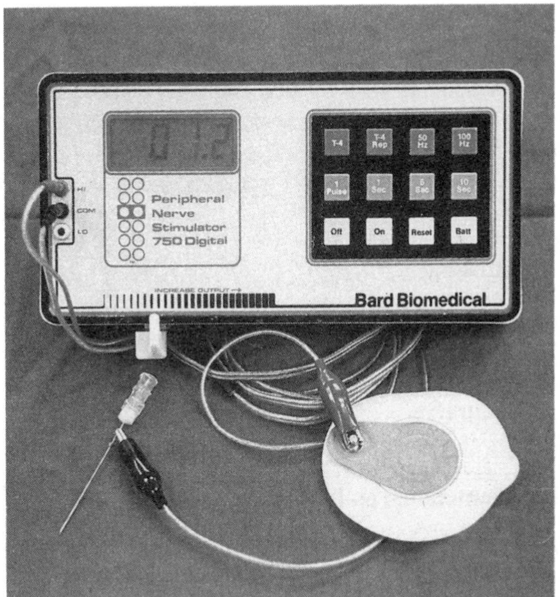

Fig. 26.2 Nerve stimulator and stimulating needle.

especially for the beginner. It is important to explain to the patient the sensation elicited by stimulation.

Stimulators that deliver a constant current and give a digital display of the current used are readily available. One lead is attached to an ECG electrode on the patient's skin, and the other to the shaft of the needle. After skin puncture, the stimulator is set to a frequency of 1 Hz and an initial current of 3 mA. As the nerve is approached, motor fibre stimulation causes muscle movement. This procedure is not painful unless the nerve is touched, when paraesthesiae result.

The current is reduced gradually until movement is still present at a current of, optimally, less than 1 mA. At this point, an aspiration test is performed and 2 ml of local anaesthetic solution injected. Movement should cease immediately. If it does not, and an unsheathed needle is being used, the tip may be beyond the nerve; the needle should be withdrawn slightly and the procedure repeated. Severe pain on injection suggests intraneural injection and the needle should be repositioned. When the correct position has been found, the remainder of the anaesthetic solution should be injected slowly with repeated aspiration tests.

Asepsis

A 'no-touch' technique is essential. Drapes should be used for all major blocks and gloves and gown worn by the beginner. Gown and gloves are advisable for all central blocks, even with a 'no-touch' technique, especially when a catheter is inserted.

Monitoring

It is essential that the anaesthetist remains with the patient. Monitoring equipment should be appropriate to the anaesthetic and surgical procedure.

Supplementary techniques

A local anaesthetic may be the only drug administered to the patient, or it may form part of a balanced anaesthetic technique. During surgery, patients may be awake, or sedated by i.v. or inhalational means. Midazolam, chlormethiazole and low concentrations of nitrous oxide are employed commonly. General anaesthesia may be used as a planned part of the procedure. Experienced anaesthetists use a combination of regional and general anaesthesia to obtain advantages from both.

When a surgical tourniquet is used, the chosen block must extend to the tourniquet site unless the procedure is brief. Discomfort from prolonged immobility on a hard table is relieved by the administration of an opioid either as a premedicant or intravenously during surgery; this type of discomfort is not relieved by sedative drugs, which often result in the patient becoming confused and uncooperative.

Aftercare

Clear instructions should be given to the nurses caring for the patient.

After day-case surgery, the patient must be in a safe condition at the time of discharge. Plexus blockade with a long-acting agent is inappropriate because of the risk of the patient injuring the anaesthetised limb, but is suitable for postoperative pain relief in supervised inpatients. Patients who have received central blockade should have routine nursing observations at least until the block has worn off.

Continuous infusion techniques are suitable for use only by experienced anaesthetists. When used correctly, administration by infusion is safer than repeated bolus injection of drug, but regular observations are essential and the nursing staff must have an adequate level of knowledge to appreciate possible complications. An anaesthetist must be available within the hospital at all times.

INTRAVENOUS REGIONAL ANAESTHESIA (IVRA)

Ideally, IVRA (Bier's block) should be the first local anaesthetic technique learnt by a trainee, because its technical simplicity allows him to concentrate on acquiring the skills of patient management. Bier's block is simple, safe and effective when performed correctly using an appropriate drug in correct dosage. Deaths from IVRA have resulted from incorrect selection of drug and dosage, incorrect technique and the performance of the block by personnel unable to treat toxic reactions. The drug involved in these deaths, bupivacaine, was not the most suitable agent and is no longer recommended. The lessons to be learned from these deaths are applicable to all local anaesthetic techniques, and emphasise that expert guidance is essential even when learning the most basic blocks.

Indications

IVRA is suitable for short procedures when postoperative pain is not marked, e.g. manipulation of Colles' fracture or carpal tunnel decompression. Recovery is rapid, and the technique is appropriate for outpatient surgery. Premedication is generally undesirable as it delays discharge.

Method (Fig. 26.3)

IVRA involves isolating an exsanguinated limb from the general circulation by means of an arterial tourniquet and then injecting local anaesthetic solution intravenously. Analgesia and weakness occur rapidly and result predominantly

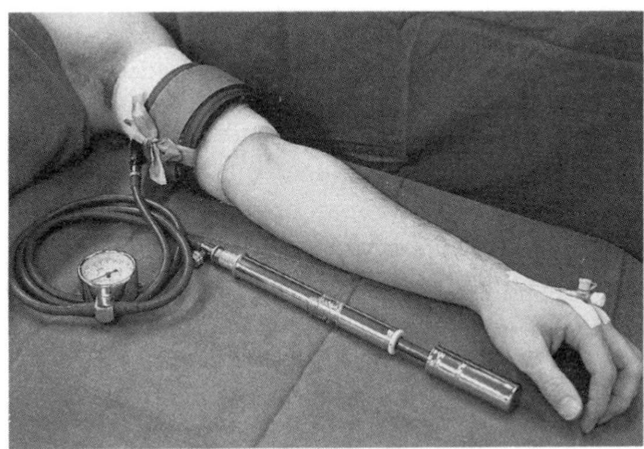

Fig. 26.3 Tourniquet and i.v. cannula for Bier's block.

from local anaesthetic action on peripheral nerve endings.

An orthopaedic tourniquet of the correct size is applied over padding on the upper arm. All connections must lock, and the pressure gauge should be calibrated regularly. A cannula is inserted intravenously in the contralateral arm in case administration of emergency drugs is required. An indwelling cannula is inserted into a vein of the limb to be anaesthetised; scalp vein needles (e.g. Butterfly) are best avoided as they are liable to penetrate the vein during exsanguination. A vein on the dorsum of the hand is preferred; injection into proximal veins reduces the quality of the block and increases the risk of toxicity. Exsanguination by means of an Esmarch bandage improves the quality of the block and increases the safety of the technique by reducing the venous pressure developed during injection. In patients with a painful lesion (e.g. Colles' fracture), elevation combined with brachial artery compression is adequate. The tourniquet should be inflated to a pressure 100 mmHg above systolic arterial pressure.

In an adult, 40 ml of prilocaine 0.5% are injected over 2 min with careful observation that the tourniquet remains inflated. Analgesia is complete within 10 min, but it is important to inform the patient that the feeling of touch is often retained at this time. The anaesthetist must be ready to deal with toxicity or tourniquet pain throughout the surgical procedure. The tourniquet should not be released until at least 20 min after injection, even if surgery is completed. This delay allows for diffusion of drug into the tissues so that plasma concentrations do not reach toxic levels after release of the tourniquet. The technique of repeated reinflation and deflation of the cuff during release has little effect on plasma concentrations, and is not necessary.

Reinstitution of the block within 30 min of tourniquet release is possible using 50% of the initial dose, because some drug is retained within the limb. Bilateral blocks may be performed without exceeding the maximum recommended doses, but it is preferable to do this consecutively rather than concurrently.

Tourniquet pain

This may be troublesome if the cuff remains inflated for longer than 30–40 min. It is alleviated sometimes by inflating a separate tourniquet below the first on an area already rendered analgesic by the block; the first cuff is then deflated. Failing this, light general anaesthesia is preferable to administration of large and often ineffective doses of opioids and sedatives.

Choice of drug

The agent of choice for this procedure is prilocaine 0.5% plain. It has an impressive safety record with no major reactions reported after its use, although minor side effects such as transient lightheadedness after release of the tourniquet are not uncommon. The drug has distinct pharmacokinetic advantages in IVRA (see Ch. 15). Methaemoglobinaemia does not result from the doses employed for IVRA.

Lower limb

IVRA of the foot can be produced using the same dose of prilocaine and a calf tourniquet positioned carefully to avoid compression of the common peroneal nerve on the neck of the fibula.

CENTRAL NERVE BLOCKS

Spinal anaesthesia is a term that may be used to denote all forms of central blockade, although it refers usually to intrathecal administration of local anaesthetic. Thus, the term subarachnoid block (SAB) is preferred. The technique itself is basically that of lumbar puncture, but a knowledge of factors which affect the extent and duration of anaesthesia, and experience in patient management, are essential. Extradural (also termed epidural) nerve block may be performed in the sacral (caudal block), lumbar, thoracic or cervical regions, although lumbar block is employed most commonly. Local anaesthetic solution is injected through a needle after the tip has been introduced into the extradural space. The anatomy of the spinal canal is described in Chapter 1.

Physiological effects of SAB

Differential nerve blockade

As spinal anaesthetic solutions spread away from the site of injection the concentration of the solution declines as mixing occurs with cerebro spinal fluid (CSF). A differential blockade of fibres occurs because small fibres are blocked by weaker concentrations of local anaesthetic solution. Sympathetic fibres are blocked to a level two segments higher than the upper segmental level of sensory blockade. Motor blockade tends to extend to within two segments caudal to the upper level of sensory block. Thus sensory levels of spinal anaesthesia to T3 are associated with total blockade of the T1–L2 sympathetic flow.

Respiratory system

Low spinal block has no effect on the respiratory system and thus the technique is used frequently for patients with chest disease.

Blocks extending as high as the roots of the phrenic nerve (C 3,4,5) cause total apnoea.

Blocks which reach the thoracic level cause loss of intercostal muscle activity. This has little effect on tidal volume (because of diaphragmatic compensation) but there is a marked decrease in vital capacity resulting from a significant decrease in expiratory reserve volume. A thoracic block leads also to reduction in cardiac output and pulmonary artery pressure, and increased ventilation/perfusion imbalance results in a decrease in Pa_{O_2}. Thus awake patients with a high spinal block should always be given oxygen-enriched air to breathe.

Cardiovascular system

The cardiovascular effects are proportional to the height of the block and result from denervation of the sympathetic outflow tracts (T1 to L2). This produces dilatation of resistance and capacitance vessels and results in hypotension. In awake patients, compensatory vasoconstriction above the height of the block may compensate almost completely for these changes, thereby maintaining arterial pressure, but loss of consciousness produced by the smallest dose of anaesthetic drug may abolish this compensation with consequent profound hypotension.

Hypotension is augmented by:

1. The use of head-up posture.
2. Any degree of hypovolaemia — pre-existing or induced by surgery.

Prevention of hypotension

Both the incidence and the degree of hypotension are reduced by limiting the height of the block and, in particular, by keeping it below the sympathetic supply to the heart (T1–5). Many authorities advise that all patients who receive subarachnoid or extradural block should be placed in a slight head-down position (5–10°) throughout the procedure. This small degree of tilt has little effect on distribution of block, but has a significant effect on venous return.

It is common practice to attempt to minimise hypotension during SAB or extradural anaesthesia by 'preloading' the patient with 500–1000 ml of crystalloid solution i.v. before or during the institution of the block. This may compensate in part for the 'relative' hypovolaemia induced by increased capacitance of the circulation.

Bradycardia may occur because of:

1. Neurogenic factors in awake patients, i.e. vasovagal syndrome.
2. Block of the cardiac sympathetic fibres (T1–T4).

SAB has no direct effect on the liver or kidneys,

but reductions in hepatic and renal blood flow occur in the presence of hypotension associated with high spinal blocks.

Gastrointestinal system

The vagus nerve supplies parasympathetic fibres to the whole of the gut as far as the transverse colon. A spinal or extradural causes sympathetic denervation (proportional to height of block) and unopposed parasympathetic action leads to a constricted gut with increased peristaltic activity. This is regarded by some as advantageous for surgery.

Nausea, retching or vomiting may occur in the awake patient and is often the first symptom of impending or established hypotension.

If nausea or retching occurs, the anaesthetist must measure arterial pressure and heart rate immediately and take appropriate measures.

Physiological effects of extradural block

The physiological effects of extradural blockade are similar to those following SAB. However, there may be important differences resulting from the much larger volumes of anaesthetic solutions used, as there is appreciable systemic absorption leading to myocardial depression. These effects are complicated by the use of adrenaline-containing solutions.

In summary, the cardiovascular effects comprise:

1. A reduction in cardiac output with plain solutions but an increase with adrenaline-containing solutions.
2. A reduction in heart rate with plain solutions but maintenance of heart rate or tachycardia with adrenaline-containing solutions.
3. A greater decrease in mean and diastolic arterial pressures with adrenaline than with plain solutions (although systolic arterial pressure may be greater with adrenaline-containing solutions).
4. Severe myocardial depression with plain solutions in the presence of haemorrhagic hypovolaemia; this is less marked with adrenaline-containing solutions.

Indications for SAB

Blockade is produced more consistently and with a lower dose of drug by the subarachnoid route than by extradural injection. However, it is not customary in the UK to use a catheter in the subarachnoid space and therefore prolonged analgesia (>2–3 h) cannot be produced. SAB is most suited to surgery below the umbilicus and in this situation the patient may remain awake. Surgery above the umbilicus in the presence of SAB generally necessitates a general anaesthetic in addition, in order to abolish unpleasant sensations from visceral manipulation resulting from afferent impulses transmitted by the vagus nerves.

Types of surgery

Urology. SAB is well suited to urological procedures such as transurethral prostatectomy, but it should be remembered that a block to T10 is required for surgery involving bladder distension. Perineal and penile operations may be carried out more conveniently under peripheral blockade or caudal anaesthesia.

Gynaecology. Minor procedures such as dilatation and curettage may be performed reliably with a block to T10. For major intra-abdominal gynaecological procedures and for diagnostic laparoscopy, light general anaesthesia is usually necessary in addition.

Obstetrics. The rapid onset of SAB may be advantageous in some circumstances, but this should be weighed against the high incidence of post-lumbar puncture headache in this group of patients.

Any surgical procedure on the lower limbs or perineum.

For patients with medical problems, low SAB may be the anaesthetic technique of choice, e.g.:

1. *Metabolic disease.* Diabetes mellitus, thyrotoxicosis.
2. *Respiratory disease.* Low SAB has no effect on ventilation and obviates the requirement for anaesthetic drugs with depressant properties.
3. *Cardiovascular disease.* Low SAB may be valuable in patients with ischaemic heart disease or congestive cardiac failure, in whom a small reduction in preload and afterload may be beneficial. SAB is effective in preventing cardiovascular responses to surgery (e.g. hypertension,

tachycardia) which are undesirable, particularly in patients with ischaemic heart disease.

Indications for extradural blockade

The indications for extradural anaesthesia are widespread because it is an extremely versatile technique which can be tailored to suit a variety of situations. The duration of analgesia may be prolonged as necessary by means of an indwelling catheter and the use of intermittent 'top-ups' or a continuous infusion. Bupivacaine is the drug of choice when one of these continuous techniques is employed. The pharmacokinetic properties of bupivacaine are such that with the doses necessary to maintain adequate blockade, systemic accumulation of the drug is slow and the risk of toxicity is small. Either local anaesthetic drugs or opioids may be used extradurally, but the latter are most suited to provision of postoperative analgesia and are inadequate for surgery in most circumstances. Almost all opioids have been tried by the extradural route with success.

Contraindications to SAB and extradural anaesthesia

Most contraindications are relative, but are best regarded as absolute by the trainee.

1. Bleeding diathesis.
2. Hypovolaemia.
3. Sepsis close to site of lumbar puncture.
4. Severe stenotic valvular heart disease. The patient may be unable to compensate for vasodilatation because of a fixed cardiac output.
5. Pre-eclamptic toxaemia. Extradural block has been used with great benefit in this condition, but a platelet count of less than 100×10^9/litre usually precludes extradural or subarachnoid anaesthesia.

Performance of SAB

Intravenous access

An intravenous infusion must be instituted before lumbar puncture is performed.

Positioning the patient

Lumbar puncture for SAB may be performed with the patient sitting or in the lateral decubitus position (Fig. 26.4). If it is anticipated that lumbar puncture may be difficult, the midline is usually more discernible with the patient in the sitting position. The technique of lumbar puncture for the patient in the lateral position is described in the next section.

Technique of lumbar puncture

For the right-handed anaesthetist, the patient is positioned on the operating table in the left lateral position. The patient's back should lie along the edge of the table and must be vertical (Fig. 26.5a). A curled position opens the spaces between the lumbar spinous processes. An assistant stands in front of the patient to assist with positioning and to reassure the patient. The anaesthetist must inform the patient before performing each part of the procedure.

A line between the iliac crests lies on the 4th lumbar spinous process or interspace; lumbar

Table 26.1 Techniques of subarachnoid block (SAB)

Type of block	Upper level of analgesia	Position during lumbar puncture	Volume of solution
Saddle block	SI	Sitting 5 min	1 ml hyperbaric solution
Low thoracic	T10–12	Sitting/lateral decubitus	3–4 ml*
High thoracic	T4–6	Lateral decubitus Sitting (immediately supine)	2–3 ml hyperbaric solution
Unilateral	Not possible with hyperbaric solutions which eventually affect both sides after the patient is placed supine. Hypobaric solutions, e.g. amethocaine in water, may be used when the patient can remain with the operative side uppermost throughout, e.g. hip replacement surgery.		

*Plain bupivacaine is slightly hypobaric at body temperature and the eventual block height is difficult to predict. Plain amethocaine, available in some countries, is truly isobaric, gives a more predictable height of block and is often used in volumes of 2 ml to achieve low thoracic blockade.

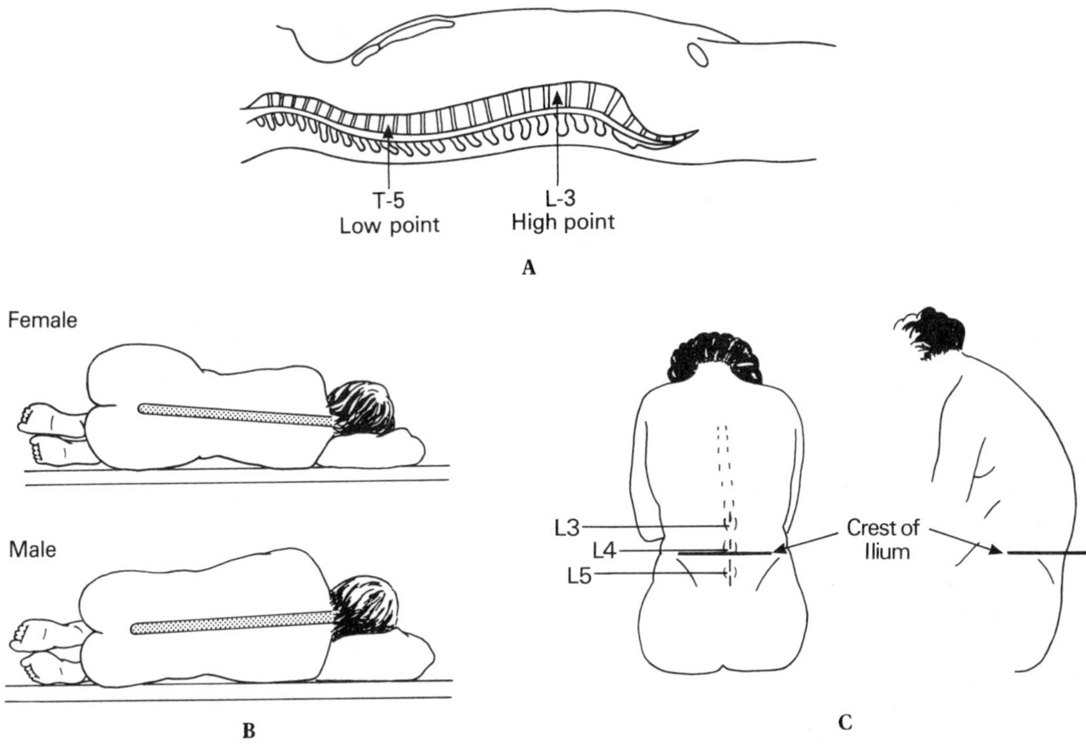

Fig. 26.4 Spinal curvature in: A — supine; B — lateral; C — sitting positions.

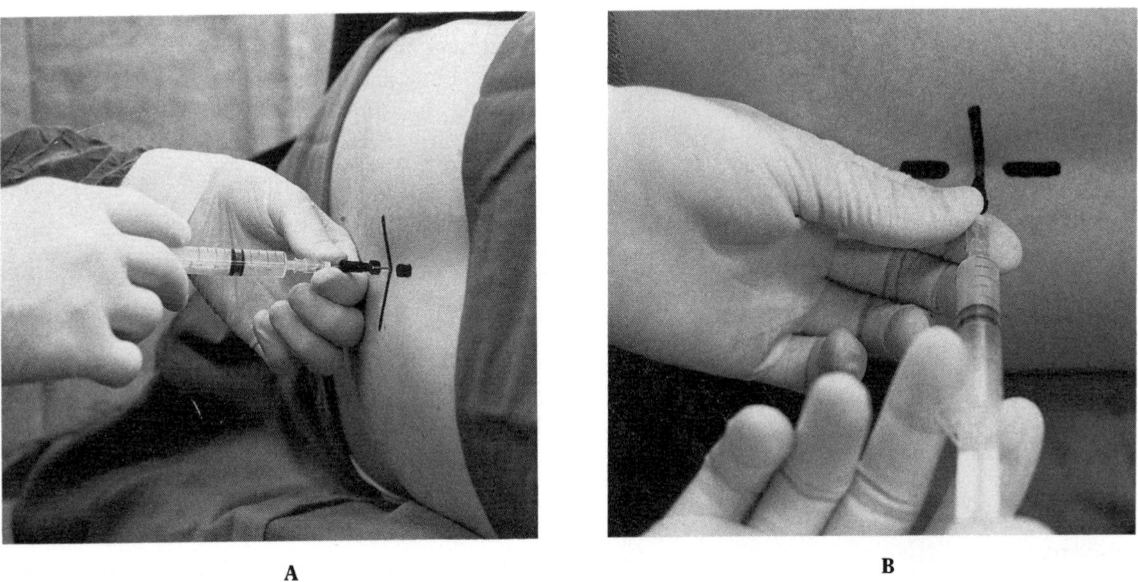

Fig. 26.5 Injection of local anaesthetic solution into the subarachnoid space. Note that the needle is horizontal. The third lumbar interspace is marked.

puncture should be performed at the 3rd or 4th space. A full sterile technique (with gown, gloves and surgical drapes) is adopted. All drugs should be drawn into syringes directly from sterile ampoules which are double wrapped and autoclaved only once. A selection of spinal needles (22-gauge to 26-gauge) should be available.

The skin and subcutaneous tissues are infiltrated with local anaesthetic using a small needle. The spinal needle is inserted in the midline, midway between two spinous processes. In the well-positioned patient, the needle is directed at right angles to the skin. Passage through the interspinous ligament and ligamentum flavum into the spinal canal is appreciated easily with a 22-gauge needle. With some practice these structures are discernible usually with a 26-gauge needle, which all anaesthetists should aspire to use. The use of an introducer (19-gauge needle) is advisable to brace the 26-gauge needle, which is very flexible. The spinal needle should be inserted with the bevel facing laterally to minimise the risk of post-spinal headache. When the needle tip has entered the spinal canal, the stilette is withdrawn from the needle and the hub is observed for flow of CSF; a needle with a transparent hub makes this easier. A gentle aspiration test should be performed if a free flow of CSF is not observed.

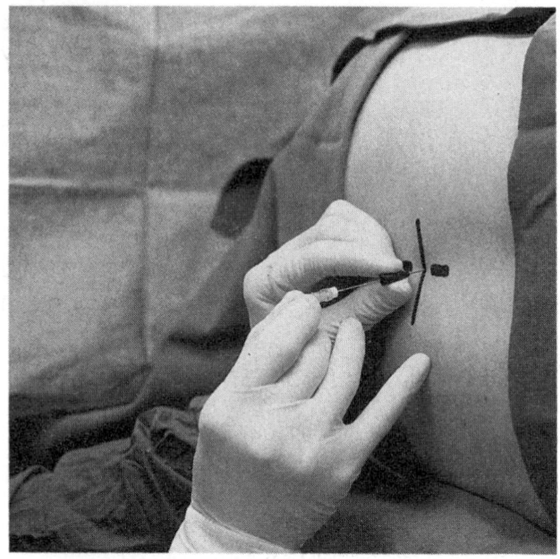

Fig. 26.6 Incorrect needle angulation during lumbar puncture for subarachnoid block.

The three most common reasons for difficulty are poor patient position, failure to insert the needle in the midline, and directing the needle laterally. This last fault is seen most easily from one side (Fig. 26.6), and is apparent usually to onlookers, but not to the anaesthetist, who looks only along the line of the needle.

When CSF is obtained, the syringe containing the local anaesthetic solution should be attached firmly to the needle. Gentle aspiration confirms the needle position and the solution is injected at a rate of 1 ml every 5 s. Aspiration after injection confirms that the needle tip has remained in the correct place. Needle and introducer are withdrawn and the patient placed supine.

Factors affecting spread (Table 26.2)

The most important factor which affects the height of block in SAB is the baricity of the solution, which may be made hyperbaric (i.e. denser than CSF) by the addition of glucose. The specific gravity (SG) of CSF is 1.004. The addition of glucose 5% or 6% to a local anaesthetic produces a solution with SG of 1.024 or greater. A patient who assumes the sitting position for 5 min after injection of 1 ml of hyperbaric solution develops a 'saddle block' which affects the perineum only. Conversely, a patient placed supine immediately after injection develops a block to the mid-thoracic region. Slightly larger volumes are advisable to ensure spread above the lumbar curvature (Fig. 26.4).

Within the range normally used for SAB (2–4 ml), the volume of solution has only a minor effect on spread. Obesity, pregnancy and a high site of injection are minor factors which increase the height of the block; lower volumes may be desirable in these situations. Barbotage and rapid injection may produce high blocks, but increase the unpredictability of spread.

Factors affecting duration

The duration of anaesthesia depends on the drug used and the dose of drug employed. Vasoconstrictors added to the local anaesthetic solution increase significantly the duration of action of

Table 26.2 Factors influencing spread of hyperbaric spinal solutions

Factor	Effect
Position of patient	Sitting position produces perineal block only, provided that low volumes are used
Spinal curvature	With standard volumes (2–3 ml) the block often spreads to T4. With low volumes (1 ml) the block may affect only the perineum even when the patient is placed supine immediately
Dose of drug	Within the range of volumes usually employed (2–4 ml) increasing the dose of drug increases the duration of anaesthesia rather than the height of the block
Interspace	Minor factor affecting height of block
Obesity	Minor factor affecting height of block. Obese patients tend to develop higher blocks
Speed of injection	Rapid injection makes the height of block more variable
Barbotage	No longer employed. Makes the height of block more variable

amethocaine (tetracaine), which is used widely in the USA, but this is not so for other agents.

Agents

Only three agents are readily available for SAB in the UK. Plain bupivacaine 0.5% is slightly hypobaric at body temperature and this leads to unpredictable spread and a higher incidence of inadequate blocks. It is used in volumes of 3–4 ml and lasts 2–3 h. Hyperbaric bupivacaine 0.5% is much more predictable and consistently produces a block to the umbilicus (and usually to T5) in supine patients. As with all hyperbaric solutions, hypotension is encountered more frequently because of higher levels of sympathetic blockade. Volumes of 2–3 ml are used and a duration of 2–3 h is usually assured. Plain lignocaine 2% usually provides analgesia of the lower limbs and perineum. Volumes of 3–4 ml are used and duration is approximately 1 h.

Complications

Acute

1. *Hypotension*. Significant hypotension should be anticipated with SAB. Changes in position, e.g. turning the patient from the supine to the prone position, may result in a sudden increase in the height of block, with consequent extension of sympathetic blockade. This may occur even after 15–20 min. Treatment (Table 26.3) may not be necessary; moderate hypotension may help to reduce operative blood loss and is tolerated well by most patients. Severe or unwanted hypotension may be treated by i.v. fluids or drugs. The use of large volumes of crystalloid or colloid in this situation is not recommended as urinary retention may occur postoperatively or circulatory overload may result when the block wears off. However, it is essential that operative blood losses are replaced promptly, and when blood losses are expected (e.g. Caesarean section) it is wise to administer fluid in advance of the loss. Hypotension is associated commonly with bradycardia and ephedrine 5–6 mg i.v. is the most appropriate treatment. Atropine may be useful, but sympathomimetic drugs are usually more effective than vagolytics.

2. *Oversedation*. This may occur when sedative drugs have been administered before performance of SAB. When the block is established the previously satisfactory level of sedation may become excessive, with the attendant risks of respiratory obstruction or aspiration. Reports of cardiac arrest associated with SAB may be related to hypoxaemia produced in this manner.

Postoperative

1. *Headache*. This is more common in young adults and particularly in obstetric patients. It may occur up to 2–7 days after lumbar puncture, and may persist for up to 6 weeks. Charac-

Table 26.3 Management of hypotension

1. 5° head down tilt
2. Maintain blood volume
3. Heart rate

<60	Atropine 0.3 mg
60–80	Ephedrine 3 mg
>80	Methoxamine 2 mg

teristically, it is worse on sitting, occipital in distribution and very disabling. The incidence is reduced by using small-gauge needles and ensuring that the bevel of the needle penetrates the dura in a sagittal plane. Simple analgesics may be the only treatment required, but occasionally an extradural blood patch is necessary. The incidence of post-spinal headache is not reduced by keeping the patient supine for 24 h; the patient should remain supine only until the anaesthetic has worn off and the risk of postural hypotension is minimal. If headache is severe and persistent, an extradural blood patch may be performed by removing 20 ml of the patient's own blood under aseptic conditions and injecting it extradurally at the same interspace as SAB was performed. Injection should be stopped if discomfort is experienced. This is an effective cure for lumbar puncture headache and appears to be remarkably free from adverse effects.

2. *Urinary retention.* This may be associated with the surgical procedure. Large volumes of i.v. fluids may increase the frequency of this complication.

3. *Labyrinthine disturbances.*

4. *Cranial nerve palsy.* Sixth nerve palsy may occur and is usually temporary. This complication is more common with larger needles.

5. *Meningitis and meningism.*

6. *Transverse myelitis* and *cauda equina syndrome* resulting from adhesive arachnoiditis. Fortunately these conditions, giving rise to permanent neurological damage or paraplegia, are extremely rare.

Extradural block

By virtue of its great versatility, extradural analgesia is probably the most widely used regional technique in the UK. It may be used for procedures from the neck downwards and the duration of analgesia can be tailored to meet the needs of surgery and postoperative pain relief by using a catheter system.

The major differences between SAB and extradural block are summarised in Table 26.4. Further expansion of the technique has taken place with the advent of extradural administration of opioids (see Ch. 11).

Table 26.4 Differences between subarachnoid and extradural block

	SAB	Extradural
Dose of drug employed	Small. Minimal risk of systemic toxicity	Large. Possibility of systemic toxicity after intravascular injection or total spinal blockade after subarachnoid injection
Rate of onset	Fast. 2–5 min for initial effect. 20 min for maximum effect	Slow. 5–15 min for initial effect. 30–45 min for maximum effect
Intensity of block	Usually complete anaesthesia	Often not complete anaesthesia for all segments
Pattern of block	May be dermatomal for first few minutes, but rapidly develops appearance of cord transection	Dermatomal
Addition of vasoconstrictor	Reliably prolongs block with amethocaine, but not with other drugs	Reliably prolongs block with lignocaine. May prolong block with bupivacaine, but not in all patients

Equipment

Extradural anaesthesia is performed usually using a Tuohy needle (Fig. 26.7). The needle is marked at 1-cm intervals and has a Huber point which allows a catheter to be directed along the long axis of the extradural space. Disposable catheters are available with a single end hole or with a sealed tip and three side holes distally.

Technique

Extradural block may be performed at any level of the spinal cord to provide segmental analgesia over an area that can be predetermined with reasonable success. Initial experience should be gained in the lumbar region before progressing to

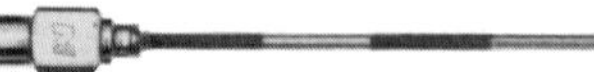

Fig. 26.7 16-Gauge Tuohy extradural needle.

sites above the termination of the spinal cord.

The pressure in the extradural space is usually subatmospheric, particularly in the thoracic region, because of communications by valveless veins between the extradural and intrathoracic spaces. Some older methods of identifying the extradural space (e.g. Odom's indicator, Macintosh's balloon) relied on detection of the subatmospheric pressure in the extradural space. However, methods which depend on loss of resistance to injection of air or saline as the tip of the needle penetrates the ligamentum flavum and enters the extradural space have become more popular. A midline approach is described here, using loss of resistance to saline to detect the extradural space.

The patient is positioned as for SAB and the vertebral level is identified from the iliac crests. The skin and subcutaneous tissues of the third lumbar interspace are infiltrated with local anaesthetic solution in the midline. A sharp needle is used to puncture the skin and the Tuohy, round-ended extradural needle is introduced through the skin puncture, subcutaneous tissue and supraspinous ligament. The common reasons for difficulty are the same as those for SAB. When inserted into the interspinous ligament, the unsupported needle remains steady. The stilette is withdrawn and a 20-ml plastic syringe filled with saline is attached and advanced using firm, but gentle pressure on the plunger. The needle must be gripped tightly at all times (Fig. 26.8) to prevent sudden forward movement. When the needle penetrates the ligamentum flavum there is a sudden loss of resistance to pressure on the plunger, but the needle must not be allowed to advance further. The needle must not be rotated after its tip has entered the extradural space, as this increases the risk of penetration of the dura.

Single-dose technique

The syringe containing local anaesthetic is connected to the extradural needle, and after aspiration a test dose is administered to detect intravascular or subarachnoid placement. After an appropriate pause, the remainder of the solution is injected at a rate not exceeding 10 ml/min while verbal contact is maintained with the patient.

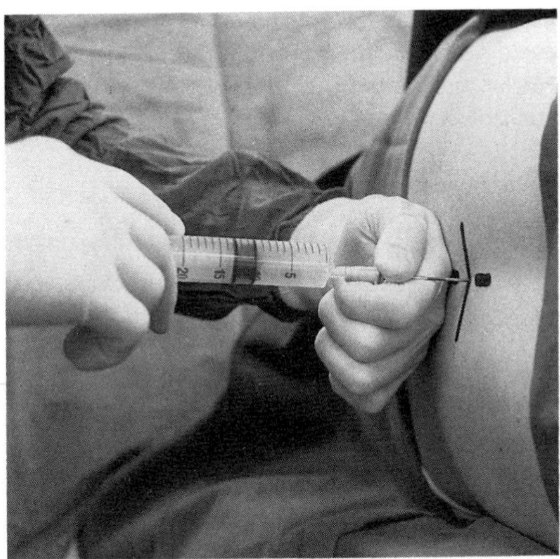

Fig. 26.8 Loss-of-resistance technique to identify the extradural space. See text for details.

Catheter insertion

An extradural catheter should pass freely through the needle into the extradural space. If the catheter does not thread easily, the needle should be repositioned, as forcing the catheter into the extradural space makes intravascular placement more likely. When a sufficient length of catheter (2–3 cm) is in the space, the needle is withdrawn carefully over the catheter. After ensuring that there is no flow of blood or CSF down the catheter, the hub is attached, and an aspiration test performed; if blood or CSF is obtained, the catheter should be reinserted in an adjacent space. A filter is connected and a test dose given. If this is satisfactory, the catheter is fixed to the patient's back with adhesive strapping and the main dose is administered. Application of Nobecutaine spray before strapping the catheter in position helps to prevent dislodgement.

Factors affecting spread

Extradural spread is variable and the initial dose depends on the clinical situation. The volume of solution has a relatively minor effect on spread, and increasing the dose of local anaesthetic is more likely to prolong duration of the block than to increase spread. Posture has a minimal effect on spread, but patients who are pregnant or aged over 60 years may have an increased likelihood of a high block with a given dose of local anaesthetic.

Factors affecting onset

Onset time is reduced by increasing the concentration of the local anaesthetic and by the addition of adrenaline 1:200 000.

Factors affecting duration

The choice of local anaesthetic agent has a major effect on the duration of anaesthesia. The concentration of the drug also has an effect; the higher concentrations of bupivacaine produce a more prolonged block. To some extent this is a reflection of increased dose, which is known to increase the duration of anaesthesia. The addition of adrenaline 1:200 000 to lignocaine also increases duration.

Agents

Lignocaine. This drug is used in concentrations of 1.5–2% with or without adrenaline 1:200 000. Without adrenaline, the duration of action is approximately 1 h; a duration of approximately 2–2.5 h may be expected when solutions containing adrenaline are used.

Bupivacaine. This agent is available in concentrations of 0.25%, 0.5% and 0.75%. The 0.75% concentration is no longer recommended for obstetric use. Increasing the concentration results in a faster onset, a denser block, more profound motor block (and therefore muscle relaxation) and increased duration of anaesthesia. A block lasting more than 4 h may be achieved with 0.75% solution. The addition of adrenaline 1:200 000 prolongs analgesia with 0.75% bupivacaine; the block may last for 6–8 h.

Complications

Intraoperative

1. Dural tap. The incidence should be less than 0.5% in experienced hands. It occurs usually with the needle rather than the catheter and is obvious immediately because of the free flow of CSF. Puncture of the dura with a large extradural needle leads to a high incidence of headache. If this occurs, extradural block should be instituted at an adjacent space, and 0.9% saline 40 ml/h should be infused extradurally for 36 h after surgery or labour to reduce the likelihood of headache. Simple analgesics may suffice if headache occurs; if not, an extradural blood patch should be performed. Accidental total spinal anaesthesia (vide infra) is rare because the dural tap is usually obvious.

2. Total spinal anaesthesia. This may occur if the large volume of solution used for extradural anaesthesia is injected into the subarachnoid space. The consequences may be

a. Profound hypotension.

b. Apnoea, unconsciousness and dilated pupils secondary to local anaesthetic action on the brain stem.

Paralysis of the legs should alert the physician to the possibility of subarachnoid injection. When using a test dose, motor function should be tested by asking the patient to raise the whole leg and not merely to wiggle the toes; movement of the toes may not be abolished for 20 min after SAB, if at all. It should be noted that relatively large volumes of local anaesthetic solution, e.g. 10 ml of bupivacaine 0.25%, may be injected into the subarachnoid space without total spinal anaesthesia occurring in all patients.

Provided that skilled resuscitation is undertaken rapidly, a total spinal should be followed by complete recovery. Appropriate personnel and equipment should be present before extradural analgesia is instituted and whenever top-up injections are administered.

3. Massive extradural block and subdural block. A very high block may occur in the absence of subarachnoid injection. This may be associated with Horner's syndrome.

4. Intravenous toxicity (see Ch. 15).

5. Hypotension.

6. Shivering.

7. Nausea/vomiting. This may result from hypotension or visceral manipulation in the awake patient.

Postoperative

1. Headache following dural tap.

2. Extradural haematoma. The spinal canal acts as a rigid box and an expanding haematoma within the canal compresses the spinal cord, resulting in loss of neurological function unless the compression is relieved surgically at a very early stage. Decompression within 6 h is completely effective in virtually all patients, but after 12 h is almost totally ineffective.

3. Neurological complications.

Anticoagulants and SAB or extradural anaesthesia

1. *Oral anticoagulants*. The half-life of coumarin-type drugs is 1–4 days and 2–3 weeks for diphenadione. Anticoagulation should be stopped at an appropriate time before surgery if SAB or extradural anaesthesia is planned.

2. *Platelets*. The platelet count should probably be in excess of 150×10^9/litre.

3. *Heparin*. The half-life of heparin given i.v. is 58–160 min, depending on dose. When given s.c. blood concentrations vary widely; in some patients plasma concentrations are in the anticoagulant range. At present it is regarded as imprudent to use SAB or extradural analgesia with 'minihep' regimens.

4. *Intraoperative heparinisation*. Extradural analgesia and SAB offer advantages for major vascular surgery but the routine use of heparin introduces the theoretical risk of haemorrhage if an extradural catheter is in place. The precise risk is unknown as prospective trials would require in excess of 10 000 cases. Some large series (3000 patients) have been conducted under extradural analgesia without haematoma formation.

Caudal anaesthesia

Caudal block involves injection of local anaesthetic into the extradural space through the sacral hiatus to obtain anaesthesia of sacral and coccygeal nerve roots. Injection of very large volumes to obtain anaesthesia of lumbar and thoracic roots is practised seldom in adults because there is a high incidence of side effects and failure to achieve a sufficiently high block. With appropriate volumes, caudal blockade affects the lower limbs infrequently, does not cause sympathetic blockade and has a low risk of dural puncture. The anatomy (Ch. 1) is variable and difficulty is experienced in approximately 5% of subjects.

Indications

Caudal anaesthesia is suitable for perineal operations, e.g. haemorrhoidectomy. Regional anaesthesia for circumcision is achieved better with a penile block.

Method

Caudal blockade may be performed with the patient in the prone position, but the left lateral position is usually more acceptable to the patient. Palpation down the sacral spine leads to the depression of the sacral hiatus at S5, flanked by the sacral cornua, through which the needle is inserted. A 21-gauge hypodermic needle is introduced through skin and sacrococcygeal ligament in a cephalad direction at 45° to the skin (Fig. 26.9). When the membrane is penetrated, the needle hub is depressed toward the natal cleft, and the needle inserted 2–3 mm along the sacral canal; it must be remembered that the dura may extend to S3. Lignocaine 2% with or without adrenaline, or bupivacaine 0.5%, are suitable agents. In an

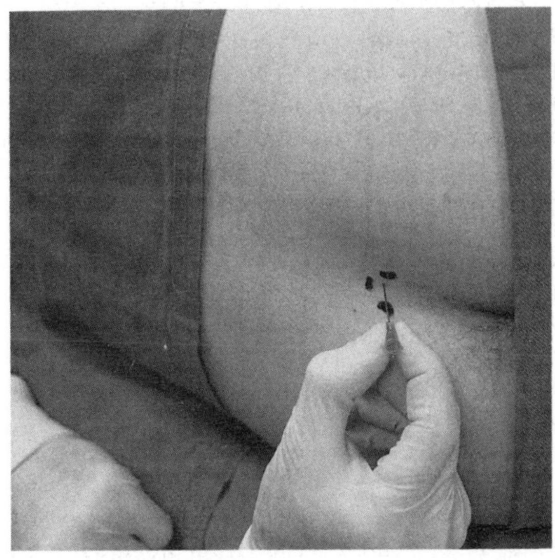

Fig. 26.9 Initial needle position for caudal anaesthesia. The sacral hiatus is marked.

adult, 10 ml of solution blocks anal sensation consistently.

In conjunction with light general anaesthesia, caudal anaesthesia provides smooth operating conditions and good postoperative analgesia. With this combined technique it is preferable to perform caudal block before induction of general anaesthesia because:

1. The patient does not need to be lifted while anaesthetised.
2. Subperiosteal injection is reported by the patient.
3. Accidental i.v. injection is detected before the full dose is given.

Avoidance of complications

Misplaced needle. Injection into subcutaneous tissue causes a swelling with fluid, or surgical emphysema with 2–3 ml of air. Intraosseous and subperiosteal injection results in marked resistance to injection. Penetration of rectum and fetal head (in obstetric practice) have been reported but should not occur if the technique is performed carefully.

Dural tap. This is rare, but the procedure should be abandoned if CSF is aspirated.

PERIPHERAL BLOCKS

Head and neck blocks

These are mostly specialised blocks which are used in ophthalmic and plastic surgery. Only the technique of local anaesthesia for awake intubation is described here.

Awake intubation

This may be the safest option in a patient with upper airway obstruction or a history which suggests difficulty with intubation. Sedation with midazolam or a combination of fentanyl and droperidol is desirable if this is not likely to exacerbate airway obstruction. A fibreoptic or rigid technique of laryngoscopy may be employed, but considerable experience is necessary with the former.

The patient sucks a benzocaine lozenge, or the mouth and pharynx are sprayed with lignocaine 1%. The laryngoscope blade and tube are smeared with 4% lignocaine gel. This may suffice in sick patients, but in robust subjects a cricothyroid injection is necessary. A 25-gauge needle is advanced through the cricothyroid membrane (Fig. 26.10) and air is aspirated to confirm position. Two millilitres of lignocaine 2% are injected and the needle is withdrawn immediately. A vigorous cough results and spreads the solution. The total dose of lignocaine must be kept as low as possible because absorption from mucous membranes is rapid.

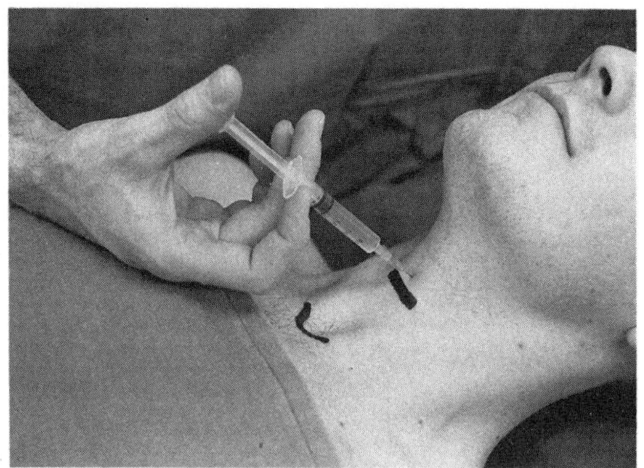

Fig. 26.10 Cricothyroid injection. The sternal notch and cricoid cartilage are marked.

Upper limb blocks

The upper limb is well suited to local anaesthetic techniques, as it is possible to block almost the whole arm with a single injection. Percutaneous approaches to the brachial plexus were described first in 1911, but approaches based on the concept of a sheath surrounding the brachial plexus are more effective.

Anatomy of the brachial plexus

The nerve supply of the upper limb is derived mainly from the brachial plexus, which is formed from the anterior primary rami of the 5th to 8th cervical and lst thoracic nerve roots. The roots of the plexus divide repeatedly and recombine to form trunks, divisions, cords and terminal nerves (Fig. 26.11). The roots emerge from the intervertebral foramina and combine into three trunks above the first rib. Each trunk separates above the

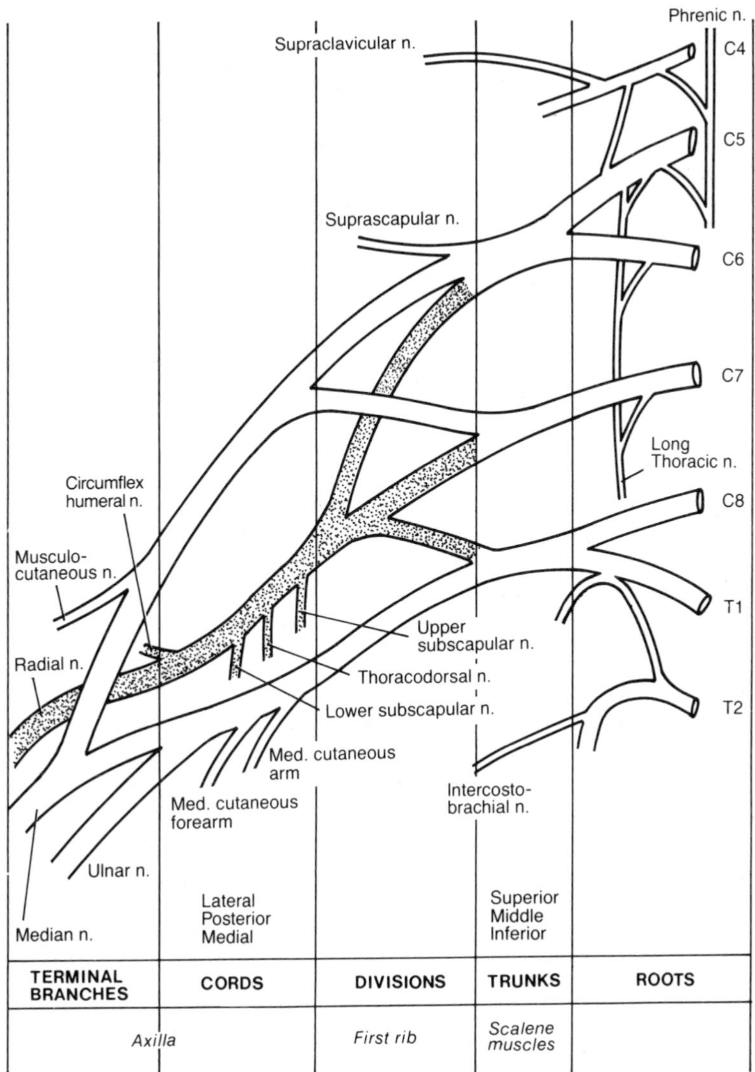

Fig. 26.11 Formation of the brachial plexus.

clavicle into anterior and posterior divisions; anterior divisions supply the flexor structures of the arm and posterior divisions the extensor structures. The divisions recombine into three cords, which surround the second part of the axillary artery behind the pectoralis minor and then form the terminal nerves (Fig. 26.12).

The roots lie between the anterior and middle scalene muscles and are invested in a sheath, derived from the prevertebral fascia, which splits to enclose the scalenes. This fascial covering extends into the axilla and causes solution injected anywhere within the sheath to spread along the line of the plexus. The cutaneous and deep nerve supplies of the upper limb are depicted in Figure 26.13.

Part of the cutaneous nerve supply of the upper limb is not derived from the brachial plexus; the upper medial part of the arm is supplied by the intercostobrachial nerve (T2) and has to be blocked separately if a tourniquet is to be used for a prolonged period. The reader is referred to standard texts for a more detailed anatomical description.

Acromio-
thoracic trunk
Trapezius
1st and
2nd rib
Deltoid
Musculocutaneous n.
Sublavian a.and v.
Cephalic v.
Lat. and med. pectoral ns.
Pectoralis minor
Pectoralis major
Pectoralis major cut
and turned back
Lateral thoracic a.
Med. cut.n.of
forearm
N. to serratus antr.
Median nerve
N. to latissimus dorsi
Lower subscapular n.
Brachial artery
and vein
Median cut. n. of arm
Ulnar nerve

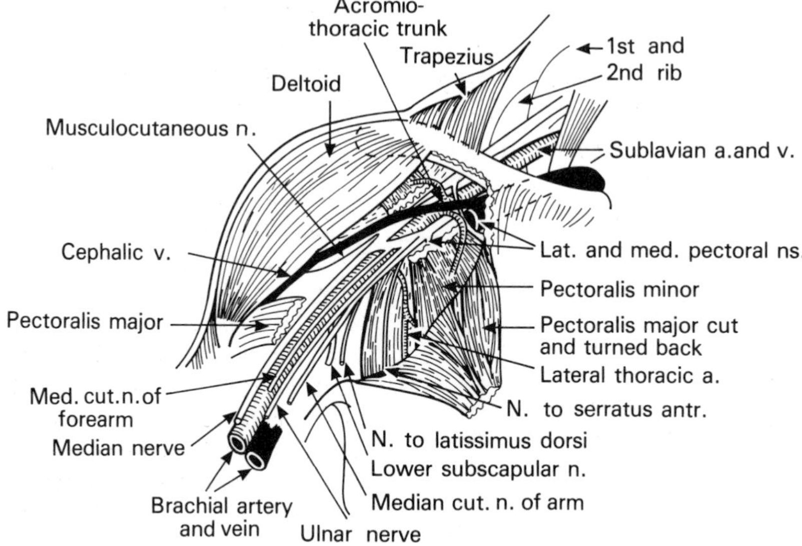

Fig. 26.12 Relationship of the brachial plexus to adjacent structures.

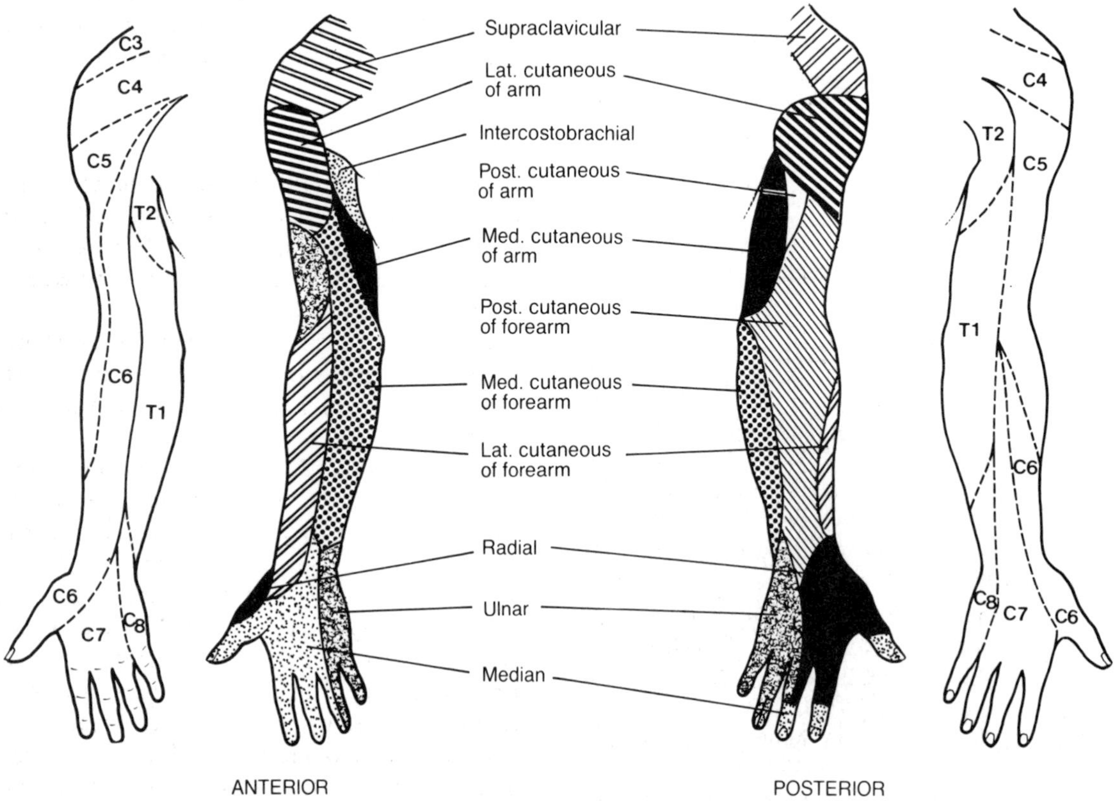

C3
C4
C5
T2
C6
T1
C6
C7
C8
Supraclavicular
Lat. cutaneous
of arm
Intercostobrachial
Post. cutaneous
of arm
Med. cutaneous
of arm
Post. cutaneous
of forearm
Med. cutaneous
of forearm
Lat. cutaneous
of forearm
Radial
Ulnar
Median
C4
T2
C5
T1
C6
C8
C7
C6
ANTERIOR
POSTERIOR

Fig. 26.13 Dermatomal innervation of the upper limb. Outer: innervation of the skin. Inner: innervation of deep structures.

Axillary block

Positioning. The patient lies supine with the arm to be blocked abducted to no more than 90° and the elbow bent to 90° (Fig. 26.14). Further abduction with the hand placed behind the head is convenient but the axillary vessels become stretched and distorted, and performance of the block is more difficult.

Method. The axillary artery is palpated and followed as far medially as possible. A skin weal is raised with local anaesthetic at this point just above the palpating finger. A short-bevelled block needle is introduced through this weal after puncturing the skin with a standard 19-gauge needle. A nerve stimulator is attached and the needle is directed towards the apex of the axilla at an angle which places it alongside, but does not penetrate, the axillary artery. A click may be felt as the needle enters the sheath. Stimulation causes flexion or extension at the wrist or elbow. When this is produced by a suitably low current, the local anaesthetic is injected.

Thirty-five to 40 ml of solution are required in an adult to achieve consistent blockade of the musculocutaneous and axillary nerves which leave the sheath at the level of the coracoid process. Digital pressure should be applied just distal to the needle during and immediately after injection to promote proximal flow of solution; a venous tourniquet is ineffective for this purpose. After completion of injection, the arm should be returned to the patient's side and digital pressure maintained. This manoeuvre may allow further spread of local anaesthetic beyond the humeral head.

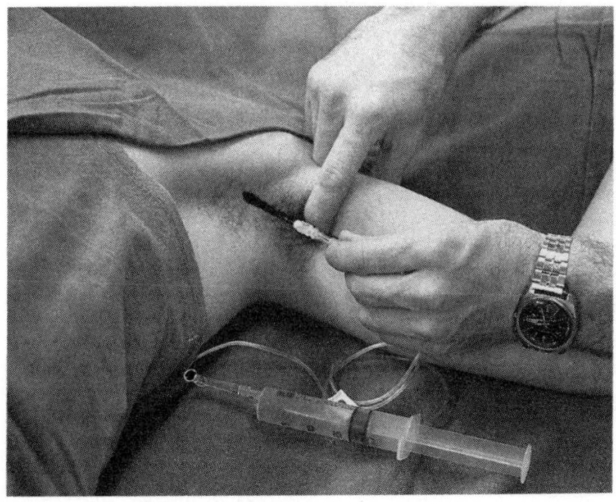

Fig. 26.14 Correct position and approach for axillary block. The axillary artery is marked.

The intercostobrachial nerve is blocked using 5 ml of solution. This can be performed without further skin puncture by redirecting the needle in the subcutaneous tissues around the medial side of the arm.

Disadvantages and complications. The onset time may be as long as 30–40 min. If the musculocutaneous nerve is not blocked, there is no analgesia on the lateral border of the arm. Puncture of the axillary artery is rarely a problem, but may lead to haematoma formation or inadvertent intravascular injection. The block should not be abandoned if the axillary artery is punctured; local anaesthetic solution is injected after penetrating the posterior wall of the artery and performing a careful aspiration test. Nerve damage occurs rarely, and results usually from malposition of the anaesthetised limb or failure to recognise a compression syndrome postoperatively.

Supraclavicular block

Supraclavicular approaches to the brachial plexus are favoured by many anaesthetists and the relatively recent description by Winnie of the subclavian perivascular approach has increased the safety of this technique.

Advantages. Onset time may be as short as 10–15 min, analgesia of the whole arm is more likely and 25–30 ml of solution is sufficient in an adult.

Disadvantages. The risk of pneumothorax is always present, but is very small in experienced hands. Phrenic nerve paralysis is probably common, but is usually asymptomatic. However, axillary block is the method of choice if there is diminished respiratory reserve. If bilateral blocks are intended, one should be performed by the axillary route. Recurrent laryngeal nerve block may result in hoarseness. Sympathetic block is relatively common, and results in Horner's syndrome. Subarachnoid or extradural spread of local anaesthetic solution is possible, but rare.

Interscalene block

This is the highest approach to the brachial plexus and may be the most suitable block for proximal procedures on the arm. Block of the C8 and T1 roots may prove difficult, and this approach is therefore less suitable for hand surgery. Complications are similar to those for supraclavicular blocks. Vertebral artery puncture and direct intraspinal injection are also possibilities.

Agents

Lignocaine or prilocaine 1.5–2% with or without adrenaline 1:200 000, or bupivacaine 0.375–0.5%, are suitable. The more dilute solutions are necessary when larger volumes are required.

Blocks in the trunk

Intercostal and paravertebral blocks have potentially important roles in abdominal and thoracic surgery, but there is a significant risk of pneumothorax when they are performed by unskilled personnel. Paravertebral block is a relatively difficult procedure. These methods are suitable only for the more experienced anaesthetist and are not considered further.

Field block for inguinal hernia repair

The main nerves which supply the groin are the subcostal (T12), iliohypogastric (L1) and ilioinguinal (L1). Their blockade produces good postoperative analgesia, but supplementary infiltration, especially around the internal ring and hernial sac, is usually necessary during surgery if this is the only anaesthetic employed.

A needle is inserted 3 cm medial and inferior to the anterior superior iliac spine (Fig. 26.15) and 15 ml of local anaesthetic are injected in a fan shape down to the inner surface of the ilium between the abdominal muscle layers. Further injections superficial and deep to the external oblique aponeurosis are made medially from this point and laterally from a point above the medial end of the inguinal ligament. Fan-shaped injections are made using a further 20 ml of solution. Bupivacaine 0.25% is a suitable agent for postoperative analgesia.

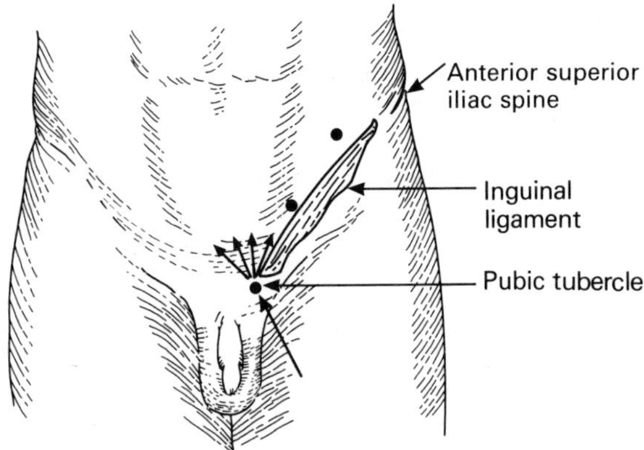

Fig. 26.15 Landmarks for field block for inguinal hernia repair.

Local infiltration is employed routinely as the sole anaesthetic in some centres and may be the method of choice in the unfit patient or in the day-case unit.

Penile block

The dorsal nerves to the penis are derived from the pudendal nerves and are blocked with 5–10 ml of local anaesthetic solution injected inferior to the symphysis pubis in the midline at a depth of 3–4 cm. Care must be taken to avoid intravascular injection in this area and vasoconstrictors *must not* be used. Plain bupivacaine 0.5% is suitable. The base of the penis is innervated by the genital branch of the genitofemoral nerve, which may be blocked if necessary by subcutaneous infiltration around the penis.

Penile block is quick and simple, produces a limited effect and is the block of choice for circumcision or other minor penile surgery such as meatotomy. It is used commonly in combination with light general anaesthesia and provides good postoperative pain relief. However, a simpler technique is to smear lignocaine jelly over the wound on a regular 4–6-hourly basis in the postoperative period.

Lower limb blocks

Lower limb blocks are practised less frequently than upper limb blocks for three reasons.

1. It is not possible to block the whole of the lower limb with one injection.
2. Subarachnoid or extradural anaesthesia may prove simpler.
3. There is an impression among anaesthetists that lower limb blocks are difficult and unreliable.

However, new approaches to the peripheral nerves of the lower limb have simplified the subject and the blocks considered below are appropriate for the junior anaesthetist.

Sciatic nerve block

Anatomy. The sciatic nerve (L4, 5, S1, 2, 3) arises from the sacral plexus, passes through the great sciatic foramen and descends in the posterior thigh to the popliteal fossa, where it divides into the tibial and common peroneal nerves. In the thigh it supplies muscles and the hip joint. The posterior cutaneous nerve of the thigh (S1,2,3) may run with the sciatic nerve or separate from it proximally; this nerve supplies the skin of the posterior thigh and upper calf. The tibial and common peroneal nerves, together with the saphenous nerve, supply all structures below the knee.

Method. There are four approaches to the sciatic nerve; the supine approach described by Raj is the most straightforward. After leaving the pelvis the sciatic nerve lies in a groove between the greater trochanter and the ischial tuberosity covered only by skin, subcutaneous tissue and gluteus maximus. The patient lies supine with both the hip and knee of the leg flexed to 90°. This manoeuvre stretches the nerve and holds it firmly in the groove while making the gluteus maximus thinner. After infiltration of the skin, a short-bevelled 3-inch needle is inserted midway between the greater trochanter and the ischial tuberosity, at right angles to the skin (Fig. 26.16). A nerve stimulator simplifies this technique; stimulation should cause plantar or dorsiflexion of the foot.

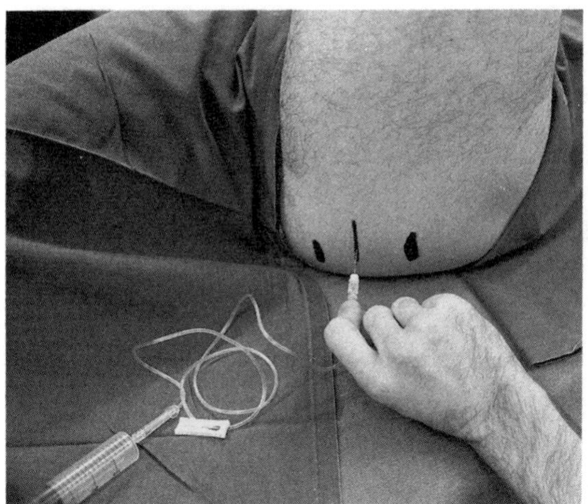

Fig. 26.16 Position and approach for Raj's supine sciatic nerve block. The ischial tuberosity and medial border of greater trochanter are marked.

This block has a high success rate with few complications. In combination with femoral nerve block it is suitable for operations below the knee. The posterior cutaneous nerve is not blocked if it does not run with the sciatic.

Lignocaine 1.5–2% with or without adrenaline 1:200 000, prilocaine 1.5–2% or bupivacaine 0.375–0.5% are suitable agents. Fifteen to 20 ml of solution are necessary. The more dilute solutions are required when other blocks are performed concurrently.

Femoral nerve block

Anatomy. The femoral nerve (L2,3,4) arises from the lumbar plexus and runs between psoas and iliacus to enter the thigh beneath the inguinal ligament, 2–3 cm lateral to the femoral artery, and at a slightly greater depth. Branches of the anterior division include the intermediate and medial cutaneous nerves of the thigh and the supply to the sartorius. The posterior division supplies the quadriceps, the hip and knee joints and terminates as the saphenous nerve, which supplies the skin of the medial side of the calf as far as the medial malleolus and sometimes the medial side of the dorsum of the foot.

Method. The patient lies supine and the inguinal ligament and femoral artery are ident-

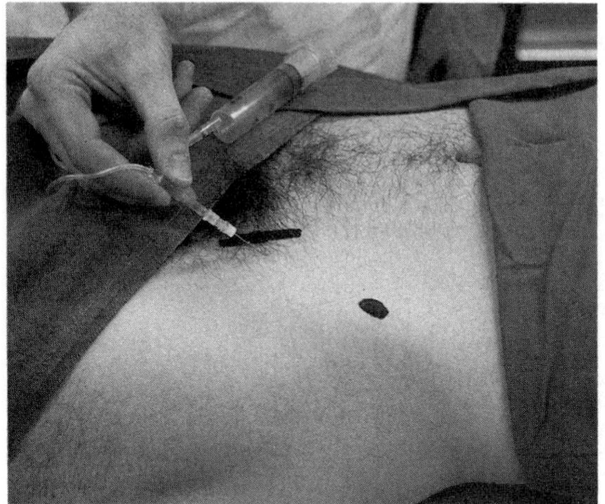

Fig. 26.17 Position and approach for femoral nerve block. The anterior superior iliac spine and femoral artery are marked.

ified. The skin is anaesthetised just lateral to the femoral artery, 1 cm below the inguinal ligament. A short-bevelled needle is inserted parallel to the artery in a slightly cephalad direction (Fig. 26.17). Patellar twitching is observed when the femoral nerve is stimulated. Care should be taken not to confuse this movement with the movement obtained by direct stimulation of the sartorius. Ten to 15 ml of solution are required.

Femoral nerve block is combined usually with sciatic block for operative procedures. Analgesia after femoral fracture or knee surgery may be satisfactory with femoral nerve block alone.

The inguinal perivascular technique of lumbar plexus anaesthesia (3-in-1 block) provides anaesthesia in the distribution of the femoral, lateral cutaneous and obturator nerves from a single injection and is an extension of the femoral nerve block technique. Twenty to 30 ml of solution are necessary and digital pressure is applied below the needle to encourage cephalad spread of the solution between iliacus and psoas.

Suitable local anaesthetic agents for femoral or 3-in-1 block are the same as for sciatic nerve block.

Mid-tarsal block

In comparison with the traditional ankle block, mid-tarsal block has the advantages of clear landmarks, a supine position and reliability. If performed after induction of light general anaesthesia, it provides good postoperative analgesia and is ideal for operations such as removal of metatarsal heads.

Anatomy. Five nerves supply the forefoot. The medial and lateral plantar nerves are the terminal branches of the tibial nerve and enter the foot posterior to the medial malleolus; they supply deep structures within the foot and all of the sole. The common peroneal nerve divides into deep and superficial branches; the deep peroneal nerve supplies the web space between 1st and 2nd toes, and the superficial branch supplies the dorsum of the foot. The saphenous nerve may supply a variable area of skin on the medial side of the dorsum of the foot. The sural nerve is a branch of the tibial nerve; it runs posterior to the lateral malleolus and supplies skin over the lateral side of the foot and 5th toe.

Method. The posterior tibial artery is palpated as far distally as possible. Injection of 3 ml of local anaesthetic to each side of it, below deep fascia, blocks medial and lateral plantar nerves. Injection of 2 ml of local anaesthetic to each side of the dorsalis pedis artery, below deep fascia, blocks the deep peroneal nerve. The saphenous, superficial peroneal and sural nerves are blocked by subcutaneous infiltration at the level of the ankle joint in a line extending from a point anterior to the medial malleolus to a point posterior to the lateral malleolus as for a classical ankle block (Fig. 26.18). A complete block of the foot requires 15 ml of solution; bupivacaine 0.375–0.5% is most suitable for postoperative analgesia. It is probably advisable to avoid this block when the circulation to the foot is impaired.

Special situations

Paediatric techniques

Most blocks employed in adult practice are suitable for use in children, but because of the nature of most paediatric surgery and the understandable difficulties that may be experienced with patient cooperation, only a limited number of techniques are used commonly. Many of these are used for postoperative analgesia and are performed after

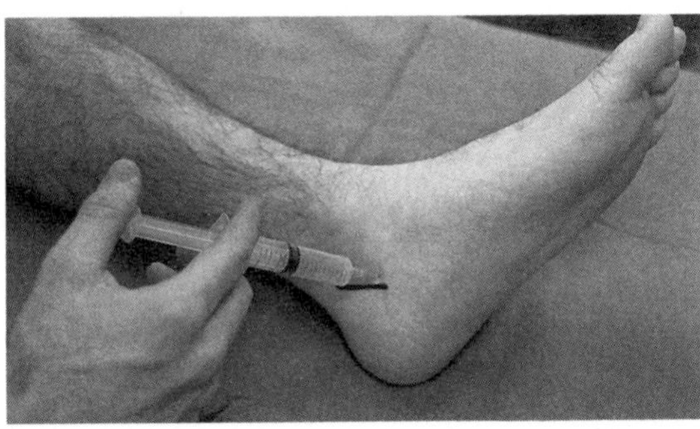

A

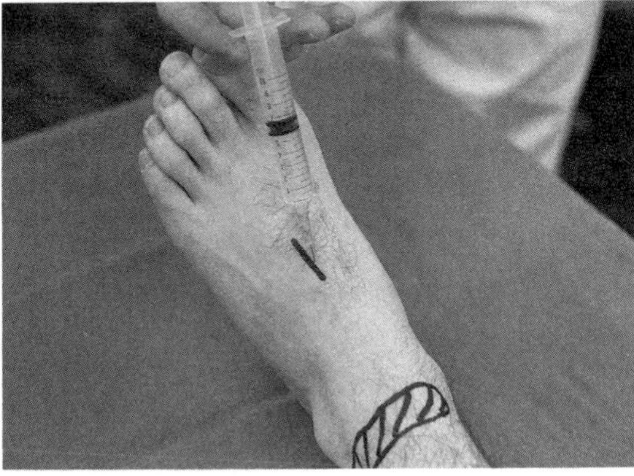

B

Fig. 26.18 Mid-tarsal block. The posterior tibial and dorsalis pedis arteries are marked. The area of subcutaneous infiltration is outlined.

induction of light general anaesthesia; they should be performed only by experienced anaesthetists.

The disposition of local anaesthetic agents in children differs from that in adults. Recent work suggests that in children of less than 1 year of age, and particularly in the neonate, very high plasma concentrations of local anaesthetic may ensue after standard doses based on weight. In children over 1 year of age, plasma concentrations are consistently lower than would be expected from adult data.

Agents and doses for paediatric blocks are shown in Table 26.5.

Table 26.5 Agents and doses of local anaesthetics used in paediatric practice

Caudal anaesthesia	
0.25% bupivacaine	
0.5 ml/kg	Sacral block
1.0 ml/kg	Low thoracic block
0.19% bupivacaine (3 parts bupivacaine 0.25% :1 part saline)	
1.25 ml/kg	Mid-thoracic block
Penile block	
0.5% bupivacaine *plain*	
Body weight	Dose
2.5 kg	0.5 ml
10 kg	1.0 ml
20 kg	2.0 ml
40 kg	4.0 ml
Axillary block	
0.25% bupivacaine	
Body weight	Dose
10 kg	6 ml
20 kg	12 ml
30 kg	18 ml
40 kg	24 ml

Topical anaesthesia

The introduction of EMLA (eutectic mixture of local anaesthetics) cream allows anaesthesia of intact skin. The cream must remain in contact with the skin for at least 1 h and is held in place with an occlusive dressing. This technique is particularly useful before venepuncture in children.

FURTHER READING

Arthur D S, McNicol L R 1986 Local anaesthetic techniques in paediatric surgery. British Journal of Anaesthesia 58 :760

Cousins M J, Bridenbaugh P O 1980 Neural blockade in clinical anesthesia and management of pain. Lippincott, Philadelphia

Ellis H, Feldman S 1983 Anatomy for anaesthetists, 4th edn. Blackwell Scientific Publications, Oxford

Eriksson E 1979 Illustrated handbook in local anaesthesia. Lloyd-Luke, London

Sharrock N E, Waller J F, Fierro L E 1986 Midtarsal block for surgery of the forefoot. British Journal of Anaesthesia 58: 37

Wildsmith J A W, Armitage E N 1987 Principles and practice of regional anaesthesia. Churchill Livingstone, Edinburgh

Winnie A P 1984 Plexus anesthesia Vol I. Perivascular techniques of brachial plexus block. Churchill Livingstone, New York

27. Anaesthesia for gynaecological, genitourinary and orthopaedic surgery

These three specialties provide a large proportion of the anaesthetist's workload. The types of operation performed vary widely from short minor procedures to lengthy major operations. Most of the procedures are well defined and many are performed in otherwise healthy patients. The majority of all day-case surgery comes from these three specialties. In gynaecology and urology, emergency surgery plays only a small role, and the anaesthetic management of gynaecological and urological patients is similar in many respects. The anaesthetic management of patients who require orthopaedic surgery is discussed separately.

Table 27.1 Specific complicating factors related to anaesthesia for gynaecological and urological surgery

Gynaecology	Urology
Anaemia	Anaemia (renal disease)
Pregnancy Contraceptive pill	Cardiovascular disease, especially hypertension
Nausea and vomiting	Renal dysfunction
Intra-abdominal pressure (laparoscopy)	Old age (prostatic disease, bladder tumour)
Massive haemorrhage (ectopic pregnancy)	Absorption of irrigating fluid (transurethral procedures)
Day-case surgery (D & C, cautery of cervix)	Day-case surgery (cystoscopy, urethral dilatation)
Position for operation	Position for operation

GYNAECOLOGICAL AND GENITOURINARY SURGERY

Preoperative assessment

As with all patients undergoing anaesthesia and surgery, it is mandatory to assess general medical fitness with particular attention to cardiopulmonary function, concurrent illness, past medical history and drug history. Investigations may be required also.

When assessing any patient who presents for surgery, it is important to consider specific factors which may give rise to anaesthetic complications. Some of the problems associated particularly with gynaecology and urology are shown in Table 27.1.

Anaemia

Anaemia has a wide variety of aetiologies and may be found in any preoperative patient; however, anaemia secondary to menorrhagia is relatively common in gynaecological patients. In an elective case, a haemoglobin concentration below 10 g/dl should be corrected either by oral iron or by blood transfusion at least 48 h before surgery. Anaemia is common also in old age.

Pregnancy

Young women present commonly for gynaecological surgery and it is important to establish if they are either pregnant or taking the contraceptive pill. Pregnancy is a relative contraindication to elective surgery but it is sometimes necessary to give an anaesthetic to a pregnant patient during the first or second trimester. Because of the possible teratogenic effect of anaesthetic drugs, anaesthesia should be avoided during the first 12 weeks of pregnancy; for this reason, a menstrual history should be taken from all female patients in their fertile years. Spontaneous abortion has been associated with surgery, but not with the use of any specific anaesthetic agent. It has been suggested that halothane, which relaxes the pregnant uterus, may reduce the risk of spontaneous abortion associated with surgery.

Oral contraceptive

Both the contraceptive pill and surgery increase the risk of thromboembolism and their effects should be considered additive. The risk is reduced if preparations containing 50 μg or less of oestrogen are used. The manufacturers recommend that oral contraceptive therapy should be discontinued at least 6 weeks before elective surgery.

Renal dysfunction

This is often the end result of diseases that require urological surgery for either palliation or treatment. Chronic renal failure may be found coincidentally in other surgical patients. Many of the effects of renal failure have an important influence on anaesthesia. The potassium-releasing effect of suxamethonium is dangerous in the presence of pre-existing hyperkalaemia; acidosis changes both the pharmacokinetics and dynamics of many drugs; reduced drug clearance requires reduced drug dosage; and anaemia and hypertension occur frequently in renal failure. Preoperative evaluation of these patients must therefore include assessment of the cardiovascular system and drug therapy, a full biochemical profile, and measurement of the acid–base status and haemoglobin concentration.

Important factors in the preoperative assessment of the patient with renal disease are discussed in detail in Chapter 41.

Premedication

Premedication is influenced by the type of operation, the psychological and physical state of the patient and the intended length of stay in hospital. In elective surgery, analgesic premedication is usually unnecessary. Often anxiolysis is important in younger patients undergoing gynaecological procedures; an antiemetic should be considered also. Oral premedication is preferred by most patients, especially those undergoing minor surgery. A benzodiazepine (e.g. temazepam 10–20 mg) together with droperidol 2.5–5 mg or metoclopramide 10 mg is often appropriate. Elderly patients and those with renal failure are more sensitive to the effects of sedative drugs and either light premedication or none is indicated. Anxiolysis with a short-acting benzodiazepine may be desirable in some day-case patients, but usually it is best to avoid premedication in order to achieve full and rapid recovery.

Day-case surgery

A number of minor gynaecological and genitourinary procedures are suitable for day-case surgery (Table 27.1). Laparoscopy for diagnosis or for female sterilisation has been performed on a day-case basis, but postoperative pain may be distressing, and in most cases necessitates analgesia and an overnight stay in hospital. There is a risk of haemorrhage or uterine rupture after vaginal termination of pregnancy, but in some centres patients return home on the same day.

The anaesthetic technique for day-case surgery demands a short recovery. The first requirement for this is a short duration of surgery. Any i.v. induction agent may be used. Maintenance of anaesthesia may be achieved by continued administration of a rapidly metabolised induction agent such as propofol or by the use of volatile agents with nitrous oxide. Tracheal intubation is not contraindicated in day-case surgery but is usually unnecessary. If appropriate, local anaesthesia is useful. Antiemetics may be required, particularly after short gynaecological procedures. Oxytocics administered during termination of pregnancy have an emetic effect as do prostaglandins, which are given commonly to soften the pregnant cervix before dilatation. Ergometrine is the most emetic of the oxytocic drugs and syntocinon (in a dose of 10 units i.v.) is to be preferred.

Gynaecological surgery

Either the lithotomy or Trendelenburg position is necessary for most gynaecological procedures, and these positions may have adverse respiratory and cardiovascular effects. In both positions, respiratory excursions are limited by restriction of diaphragmatic movement, a disadvantage exaggerated in the obese, and a potential cause of hypercapnia. Any concomitant reduction in functional residual capacity induced by these positions may result in dependent airways collapse and hypoxaemia, thus reducing further the efficiency of respiratory gas exchange. On completion of surgery, removal of the patient's legs from the lithotomy stirrups, or resumption of the supine position from Trendelenburg, results in pooling of blood in the extremities, thus reducing venous return. The resultant decrease in cardiac output and hypotension may occasionally be clinically significant. It should be apparent that all changes in body position should be accomplished gradually and gently if these untoward effects are to be avoided.

Minor procedures

Dilatation and curettage (D and C), vaginal termination of pregnancy and evacuation of retained products of conception (ERCP) are common minor procedures for which patients require anaesthesia. All involve dilatation of the cervix, a painful stimulus associated with reflex changes including laryngospasm and bradycardia if a relatively deep plane of anaesthesia has not been achieved.

During D and C, blood loss is not a problem and uterine relaxation is permissible. Mask anaesthesia with N_2O and O_2 supplemented with halothane or isoflurane 1–2% or enflurane 1.5–3% is satisfactory. Fentanyl 50–75 μg given on induction results in a smoother anaesthetic.

During termination of pregnancy, haemorrhage is the major complication. As vigorous uterine contraction is necessary after expulsion of the conceptus, high inspired concentrations of volatile agents, which cause profound uterine relaxation, are contraindicated. A commonly employed technique involves fentanyl 1 μg/kg followed by a sleep dose of propofol (2–2.5 mg/kg), and inhalation of N_2O and O_2. Anaesthesia is maintained with N_2O and O_2 and increments of propofol 20–30 mg. Syntocinon 5–10 units is administered i.v. to produce uterine contraction when the uterus has been cleared; ergometrine is not recommended as it results in a high incidence of nausea and vomiting in the postoperative period. Inadvertent perforation of the uterus by the surgeon may cause profound shock.

Similar anaesthetic considerations apply to evacuation of retained products of conception, which is often necessary after spontaneous abortion. However, preoperative blood loss may be significant in these patients and, as the procedure is performed as an emergency, there may be considerable gastric residue. Although the i.v. technique described above is often suitable, hypovolaemia and the likelihood of aspiration may render a technique employing tracheal intubation and light anaesthesia with muscle relaxation more appropriate. If intermittent suxamethonium is used, administration of atropine i.v. is mandatory before the second dose of suxamethonium.

Laparoscopy

This procedure permits inspection of the abdominal cavity via a telescope passed through a small incision in the abdominal wall. It is undertaken commonly for sterilisation, for investigation of infertility and in patients suspected of having a tubal pregnancy (vide infra). Blind insertion of the laparoscope may injure intraperitoneal structures and the aorta or other large blood vessels. The bladder must be emptied before insertion of the cannula.

To minimise the risk of intra-abdominal damage and to obtain clear visualisation of the pelvic organs, a pneumoperitoneum is induced by insufflating CO_2 (or N_2O) into the peritoneal cavity through a Verres' needle. The gas is introduced at a rate not exceeding 4 litres/min and adequate abdominal distension is obtained with a total of 3–5 litres. Diathermy may be used during laparoscopy (e.g. for sterilisation), and CO_2 is usually preferred as the insufflating gas because it does not support combustion.

The anaesthetic problems associated with this procedure are related predominantly to the CO_2 pneumoperitoneum. These include:

1. Reduced thoracic compliance from diaphragmatic splinting.

2. Inferior vena caval compression from increased intraperitoneal pressure (especially if intraperitoneal pressure is greater than 50 cmH_2O).

3. Hypercapnia from accumulation of CO_2. The peak Pa_{CO_2} concentration may not occur until after the end of the procedure.

In addition, pulmonary function is impaired by the use of the Trendelenburg position.

Most of these adverse effects are overcome by an anaesthetic technique employing tracheal intubation and mild hyperventilation. Gastric dilatation caused by overenthusiastic manual mask ventilation may increase the likelihood of gastric perforation by the laparoscope or trocar. Careful monitoring of the circulation is essential. Intraperitoneal pressure is monitored also, and should not be allowed to exceed 30 cmH_2O. Immediate deflation of the pneumoperitoneum is warranted if hypotension occurs as a result of compression of the inferior vena cava. Hypotension is more likely to occur in the hypovolaemic patient (e.g. suspected ruptured ectopic pregnancy).

The procedure is often of short duration and there may be difficulty in antagonising the residual effects of muscle relaxant drugs. Intermittent suxamethonium may be used but it is more common to employ a small dose of a non-depolarising agent, e.g. vecuronium 75 $\mu g/kg$.

Other rare complications of laparoscopy include gas embolism (a more serious problem if N_2O is used as the insufflating gas), haemorrhage, mediastinal emphysema, pneumothorax and perforation of an abdominal viscus. The peritoneal cavity should be evacuated as much as possible at the end of the procedure as residual intraperitoneal gas causes shoulder-tip pain referred from the diaphragm.

Major procedures

Abdominal hysterectomy

Total abdominal hysterectomy (with or without salpingoophorectomy is a standard abdominal procedure, and a balanced technique involving muscle paralysis and controlled ventilation is suitable. Some anaesthetists employ lumbar extradural block in combination with light general anaesthesia and spontaneous ventilation. During hysterectomy, blood loss may be considerable and blood should be cross-matched. Some patients may be anaemic because of preoperative uterine blood loss.

Major vaginal procedures

Pelvic floor repair and vaginal hysterectomy may result in considerable bleeding also, and lumbar extradural or caudal block together with light general anaesthesia or sedation may improve surgical conditions. Alternatively, a balanced technique with controlled ventilation may be employed. Some gynaecologists insist on infiltrating adrenaline locally, and in these cases the use of halothane should be avoided. These procedures are undertaken in the lithotomy position, and particular care must be taken when the legs are lowered at the end of the procedure because of the risk of hypotension if hypovolaemia is present.

Ectopic pregnancy

Emergency laparoscopy or laparotomy is often necessary for suspected rupture of a tubal pregnancy. Patients with a suspected tubal pregnancy should be anaesthetised with the utmost caution as catastrophic haemorrhage may occur. Some patients may complain only of trivial lower abdominal pain, but others are in a state of near exsanguination. Even if volaemic status is judged to be normal, a large-gauge i.v. cannula should be inserted before induction of anaesthesia and the status of the circulation monitored closely.

A rapid-sequence induction technique (see p. 531) with controlled ventilation is appropriate in most instances but those with profound cardiovascular collapse represent a major anaesthetic challenge. These patients may exsanguinate very quickly and resuscitation may be impossible until bleeding has been stemmed surgically (clamping of the internal iliac artery may be required). Consequently, it may be necessary to induce anaesthesia in a hypovolaemic patient, and to delay definitive resuscitation until after surgical haemostasis has been secured. Two large-gauge cannulae are inserted i.v. and colloid given as necessary. As sudden reduction in abdominal muscle tone may result in even more profound hypotension, anaesthesia should be induced in the operating theatre, with the patient towelled and the surgeons gowned. Appropriate monitoring is instituted. After a period of preoxygenation, ketamine 0.5–2.0 mg/kg is given i.v. and suxamethonium administered to facilitate tracheal intubation. Anaesthetic agents may be introduced gradually as the patient's circulatory status allows. These otherwise healthy patients respond quickly to transfusion after the bleeding vessel has been clamped.

Urological procedures

Cystoscopy and transurethral resections

Operations performed through a cystoscope require continuous bladder irrigation, sometimes with large quantities of fluid. It is usual for sterile water to be used during cystoscopy. However, a solution of glycine 1.5% is used during resection of a bladder tumour or hypertrophic prostate because of its greater osmolality, although it is hypotonic. Absorption of water may cause complications during and after operation; the extent of these depends on the duration of the procedure, the hydrostatic pressure of the fluid and the number and size of venous sinuses opened during the operation.

Intravascular absorption of large volumes of water from the bladder may result in haemolysis or water intoxication. The latter causes hyponatraemia and cerebral oedema and is referred to sometimes as the 'TURP (transurethral resection of prostate) syndrome'; a serum sodium concentration of less than 120 mmol/litre is diagnostic. Intraoperative haemolysis is difficult to detect under general anaesthesia and may lead to acute tubular necrosis later. The greater osmolality of glycine helps to reduce the incidence of these problems but does not prevent them. Intravascular absorption of water or glycine solution also increases intravascular volume, and may result in cardiac failure. If neurological signs or signs of circulatory overload develop, prompt treatment is required with diuretics and cautious administration of hypertonic saline.

Irrigation of the bladder with large volumes of fluid may result in hypothermia. In addition, it is very difficult to assess blood loss during transurethral resections, and hypovolaemia may occur; this may be masked initially by the increased circulating volume caused by absorption of irrigation fluid. Postoperative haemorrhage may be considerable also.

The anaesthetic technique for cystoscopy is similar to that employed for D and C (vide supra). However, many patients who present for cystoscopy are elderly and drug doses should be reduced accordingly.

The anaesthetic management of patients who undergo transurethral resection is determined by the condition of the patient and the anticipated duration of surgery. In otherwise healthy individuals, a technique may be selected in which the patient breathes spontaneously; however, it may be preferable in patients with other diseases to use muscle relaxants and to employ IPPV. Subarachnoid or extradural block is suitable also for this procedure.

Renal surgery

Open surgery of the kidney is performed usually with the patient in the lateral position and a bridge placed under the operative site so as to open up the renal bed. The upper arm is suspended above the patient. This position may be associated with cardiovascular instability because of obstruction of the inferior vena cava. Careful monitoring is necessary during positioning of the patient and adjustments should be made slowly to ensure that venous obstruction does not occur. A number of nerve injuries may occur in this position. The brachial plexus may be damaged when an arm is suspended on a frame above the patient if there is excessive abduction of the shoulder. Padding must be used over all promontories of the upper and lower limbs, especially around the course of the major nerves.

The anaesthetic technique employed is similar to that for any intra-abdominal procedure. If renal function is impaired, selection and dosage of anaesthetic, analgesic and neuromuscular blocking drugs should be adjusted accordingly (see p. 660).

Pneumothorax is caused occasionally by damage to the pleura during the surgical approach to the kidney and this may require postoperative drainage.

ORTHOPAEDIC SURGERY

Preoperative assessment

Patients who present for orthopaedic surgery may have associated conditions which are of importance to the anaesthetist.

Arthritic diseases

Apart from general difficulties encountered in ensuring the safe positioning of a patient with stiff and painful joints, the arthritic diseases have an influence on anaesthesia in three major areas:

1. Intubation and the airway.
2. Pulmonary dysfunction.
3. Association with systemic disease.

The airway may be complicated by arthritic disease in several ways. There may be ankylosis of the cervical vertebrae, resulting in limited or absent extension; this may render tracheal intubation difficult. The arthritic process may cause destruction and instability of the cervical vertebral joints (particularly the atlanto-axial joint) and this may make extension of the neck inherently dangerous. Involvement of the joints of the larynx and upper airway may make laryngoscopy difficult. Arthritis at the temporomandibular joint affects particularly the forward gliding motion of the condylar head on the articular cartilage and restricts mouth opening, which may render laryngoscopy difficult or even impossible.

Restrictive lung disease may occur in arthritic diseases as a result of either deformity of the chest wall or reduced joint movements. Long-established extrapulmonary restrictive diseases may lead to intrapulmonary fibrosis. Restrictive lung disease is associated also with arthritic diseases such as rheumatoid arthritis and ankylosing spondylitis.

Ankylosing spondylitis may be encountered in patients who present for corrective surgery of the hips or knees. There is restricted movement of the costovertebral joints, which reduces vital capacity and results eventually in total dependence on the diaphragm for ventilation. Usually, pulmonary function is well maintained, although intrapulmonary fibrosis may occur. The risk of postoperative respiratory complications is increased. Ankylosis of the cervical vertebrae is often complete; although tracheal intubation is made very difficult, it is usual for the airway to be maintained well in the patient without a tracheal tube.

Rheumatoid arthritis is a disease predominantly of peripheral joints; the vertebral joints are often spared. However, the cervical spine is an exception, and instability and subluxation of the atlanto-axial joint occurs frequently in advanced disease. There may be involvement also of the temporomandibular joint and the cricoarytenoid joints. Rheumatoid arthritis does not cause pulmonary dysfunction usually, but as an immune disease it is associated with dysfunction in a number of organ systems and renal and myocardial function may be impaired. Patients with rheumatoid arthritis may be receiving steroid therapy.

Other pre-existing conditions

Kyphoscoliosis has many causes, including congenital deformity, neuromuscular disease, rheumatoid arthritis and neurofibromatosis. The progressive deformity may result in severe extrapulmonary restrictive lung disease.

Paget's disease of bone is found commonly in patients presenting for total hip replacement or surgery for long bone fractures. Because of the hyperaemic bone, arteriovenous anastomoses may develop; these cause low peripheral resistance and eventually high-output cardiac failure.

Haemophilia is a rare disease which may necessitate surgery to correct the deformities caused by multiple haemarthroses. At present, approximately 50% of haemophiliac patients in the UK are HIV-positive.

Malignant hyperpyrexia is also a rare disease and is caused by an inherited myopathy. A surprisingly large percentage of cases (approximately 30%) present for the first time during orthopaedic surgery, although this may reflect only the fact that orthopaedics is often the first exposure of a patient to surgery and anaesthesia. The detection and management of this condition are discussed in Chapter 23.

Special considerations during orthopaedic surgery

Tourniquets

Tourniquets are an indispensable aid to orthopaedic surgery of the limbs. They must be applied carefully in order to avoid tissue damage. The correct position is the midpoint of the thigh or upper arm, where muscle bulk is greatest. In thin patients, extra protection underneath the tourniquet is essential. Exsanguination of the limb may be achieved with an Esmarch bandage, but lower limb exsanguination increases the central venous pressure, especially if performed bilaterally. Care should be taken in patients with cardiac insufficiency. Simple elevation of the limb may suffice if an Esmarch bandage is contraindicated.

The tourniquet is inflated to a pressure of 50 mmHg above systolic arterial pressure for the upper limb and 100 mmHg above systolic pressure for the lower limb. Pressures recommended on most tourniquet machines are higher than necessary. It is usual to use a pneumatic cuff; the modern types which maintain a preset pressure are preferable to the older manual varieties, which need constant vigilance. The maximum length of time for tourniquet inflation is 2 h but it is usual to try to limit the time to 1.5 h.

Incorrect application or prolonged inflation may lead to soft tissue damage. Severe bruising may occur, and arteries and nerves may be damaged. Pressure and ischaemia caused by the tourniquet result in considerable pain; consequently, the patient must receive general anaesthesia or the area of the tourniquet must be blocked by local anaesthesia. There is a reactive hyperaemia after release of the tourniquet and this may result in haemorrhage if haemostasis during surgery has been inadequate. Release of the tourniquet is accompanied by the release of acids, produced by anaerobic metabolism, into the circulation. This seldom causes clinical problems unless bilateral lower limb tourniquets have been used.

Severe peripheral vascular disease with incipient limb ischaemia is a contraindication to the use of a tourniquet. Usually, sickle cell disease is considered to be a contraindication, although there have been several reports of the uneventful use of a tourniquet in patients with this condition.

Bone cement

Prosthetic joints are cemented to the bone usually with methylmethacrylate cement. The application of the cement has been associated with severe cardiovascular disturbances, including profound hypotension and sometimes cardiac arrest. These disturbances occur usually during total hip replacement or Thompson prosthetic replacement, most commonly when the femoral component is cemented into the femur. The cause is probably multifactorial. The liquid monomer component causes vasodilatation, hypotension and tachycardia if absorbed into the circulation. The reaction of the monomer with the methylmethacrylate polymer is exothermic and the heat produced in the confines of the femoral shaft may cause air embolism. In addition, methylmethacrylate is a fat solvent which may cause the absorption of fat from the marrow, resulting possibly in fat embolism.

These problems are minimised if the surgical technique includes venting of the femoral shaft and if the cement mix is sufficiently stiff. Arterial pressure must be monitored continuously and hypovolaemia should be avoided. Some anaesthetists advocate the withdrawal of nitrous oxide before insertion of cement to avoid an increase in the size of any air embolus. A precordial or oesophageal stethoscope is useful in detecting the presence of air embolism.

Spinal surgery

These procedures present some very demanding problems for the anaesthetist. The procedures undertaken most commonly are:

1. Application of traction.
2. Reduction of fractures — open or closed.
3. Spinal fusion at any level.
4. Decompressive laminectomy at any level.
5. Correction of scoliosis.

Access to the airway is restricted during spinal surgery because of the position of the patient;

tracheal intubation is essential and the tube must be fixed firmly in place. Fixed deformities of the cervical spine may result in difficulties in intubating the trachea. If the cervical spine is unstable, intubation becomes hazardous and difficult, and the utmost care, gentleness and vigilance are required to avoid producing quadriplegia.

The unstable vertebral column is jeopardised further by the use of muscle relaxants; all passive movements of the patient should be performed with the advice of the orthopaedic surgeon. Patients who are already quadriplegic may develop autonomic hyperreflexia and maintenance of cardiovascular stability may be difficult. A rapid and dangerous increase in serum potassium concentration may occur in paraplegic patients when suxamethonium is used between 24 h and 6 months after the injury. During surgery for correction of scoliosis, it may be necessary to wake the patient in order to assess spinal cord function. Clearly, this requires careful psychological preparation of the patient and a suitable anaesthetic technique.

Posture

Variations from the supine are required for many orthopaedic operations and there is an increased risk of damaging the patient accidentally. Injury to superficial nerves, eyes, pressure areas, hair and genitalia may occur in any anaesthetised patient. Those with backache may suffer severe pain after short periods in a relaxed supine posture. Positioning of limbs or turning the patient may increase the risk of joint dislocation, stretching nerve plexuses or overstressing the spine. The effects of abnormal postures on intra-abdominal pressure and the diaphragm influence the choice of anaesthetic technique. Spontaneous ventilation may be unsuitable in obese patients with a flexed spine because of the resultant reduction in vital capacity. In the lateral position, increased ventilation/perfusion inequalities may occur, especially during IPPV (see p. 620).

It may be necessary to induce anaesthesia while the patient is in bed and surrounded by traction devices. Not all hospital beds may be tilted into the Trendelenburg position. Subsequent movement on to the operating table may be hazardous.

Anaesthetic techniques

Local anaesthetic techniques

In the absence of infection, i.v. regional anaesthesia and specific peripheral nerve blocks are suitable for surgery of the upper limb. Extradural or subarachnoid blocks are useful for surgery of the hip and lower limb, although careful maintenance of haemodynamic balance is essential, particularly in the elderly patient. Local anaesthetic techniques are discussed in detail in Chapter 26. The advantages and disadvantages of local and regional techniques in the orthopaedic patient are listed in Table 27.2.

General anaesthetic techniques

1. *Intravenous agents for short procedures*. Manipulation of stiff joints and reduction of dislocations may be performed after a single dose of i.v. induction agent. It may be necessary to use a small dose of suxamethonium to provide a brief period of muscle relaxation. If this is required, the trachea should be intubated, and the lungs ventilated with an oxygen/nitrous oxide mixture, supplemented by a volatile anaesthetic agent, until adequate spontaneous ventilation has resumed.

2. *Spontaneous ventilation with inhalational agents*. This technique is suitable for short procedures including meniscectomy, open reduction of fractures under tourniquet or surgery of soft tissues.

Table 27.2 Advantages and disadvantages of local anaesthetic techniques (excluding subarachnoid and extradural blocks) in orthopaedic surgery

Advantages
Avoids CVS depression from general anaesthesia
Minimises respiratory changes:
no reduction in FRC
hypoxic pulmonary vasoconstriction maintained
ciliary function maintained
Reduces risk of inhalation of gastric contents
Improves postoperative analgesia
Disadvantages
Block may be incomplete
Time-consuming
Nerve damage may occur
Patient unacceptability
Sedation/light general anaesthesia may be necessary

3. *Relaxant/IPPV*. For long or complex procedures, e.g. joint replacement, spinal operation or major bone graft, it is preferable to employ muscle relaxants and IPPV with nitrous oxide in oxygen, supplemented by a volatile anaesthetic agent and an opioid analgesic.

A local block combined with a general anaesthetic may result in excellent operating conditions and profound analgesia in the immediate post-operative period.

Application of dressings or plaster of Paris casts and institution of traction are often required immediately after surgery, and anaesthesia should not be terminated until these have been completed.

Emergency orthopaedic surgery

The majority of patients who require surgery for trauma have orthopaedic injuries. The urgency of initial surgery depends on the nature of the injury. Surgery should be performed with the minimum of delay if there is vascular damage which may cause haemorrhage or ischaemia or if there is a compound fracture with the risk of infection. However, most emergency orthopaedic surgery can be performed on a semi-urgent basis. The decision to operate is reached jointly between surgeon and anaesthetist, consideration being given to the surgical problems and the possibility of improvement in the patient's condition before surgery.

Many anaesthetic considerations associated with emergency orthopaedic surgery are similar to those of any emergency surgery (see Ch. 32). Factors of particular relevance to anaesthesia for trauma surgery include:

1. Preoperative assessment of:

(a) Cardiovascular system, particularly volaemic status.
(b) Respiratory system.
(c) Neurological status, bearing in mind the possibility of a head injury.
(d) Past medical and drug history, if available.

2. Management of major blood loss.
3. Prevention of aspiration of gastric contents. The stomach may not empty for many hours, even after minor trauma.
4. The possibility of hidden but major internal injuries.

Many of the problems posed by these factors may be overcome by delaying surgery until the condition of the patient is optimal.

Some emergency orthopaedic operations are associated with specific anaesthetic problems.

Fractured neck of femur

This is one of the most common operations performed in a trauma surgery unit. It occurs almost invariably in the elderly patient, who may have other medical problems. There may be limited physiological reserves, restricting the patient's ability to cope with major blood loss and general trauma of a long bone fracture. Usually, it is possible for surgery to be delayed so that a stable cardiovascular state may be achieved. Surgical fixation or hip replacement for this condition permits early mobilisation. Many of these patients would not survive if they were confined to bed for a prolonged period.

The choice of anaesthetic technique is determined by the proposed surgical technique (internal fixation or joint replacement), the anticipated duration of surgery and the condition of the patient. There is no evidence that regional anaesthesia improves long-term survival after surgery for fractured neck of femur.

Spinal fractures

The possibility of fractured vertebrae must be considered in any patient who has suffered major trauma. An unstable fracture is more liable to dislocation, resulting in spinal cord damage. Although this applies to the whole vertebral column, the cervical region is particularly vulnerable to anaesthetic manoeuvres. Any patient with a serious head injury must be assumed to have a cervical fracture until radiological studies prove otherwise. Both flexion and extension movements must be avoided, preferably by application of some form of fixation. This may render tracheal intubation difficult.

Anaesthesia in the accident and emergency department

The services of an anaesthetist may be requested in the accident and emergency department for patients who require closed manipulation and setting of fractures, relocation of dislocated joints, or other procedures which orthopaedic surgeons consider as minor. However, these patients pose a number of potential problems to the anaesthetist:

1. The stomach may not be empty even after the requisite period of starvation because pain and trauma cause gastric stasis.
2. Preoperative assessment in the outpatient is, of necessity, brief, but must be thorough to ensure that any medical condition of anaesthetic importance is detected.
3. The patient in pain may be difficult to anaesthetise without the use of large quantities of anaesthetic and analgesic drugs that delay recovery. This is undesirable, as the patient will be discharged after completion of surgery.
4. The manifestations of another injury, particularly a head injury, may be masked by the effects of a general anaesthetic.

Most of these difficulties may be averted by the use of local anaesthesia, although this is time-consuming in an area of the hospital which is often very busy. In addition, local anaesthesia is unacceptable to some patients, and is unsuitable for small children. Consequently, general anaesthesia is often necessary. The general principles of day-case anaesthesia (see Ch. 31) should be followed. However, if there is concern regarding the possibility of a full stomach, a rapid-sequence induction technique should be employed and the trachea intubated.

FURTHER READING

Loach A 1983 Anaesthesia for orthopaedic patients. Arnold, London

Hatch D P 1987 Surgical and anaesthetic considerations in transurethral resection of the prostate. Anaesthesia and Intensive Care 15: 203

Nimmo W S, Smith G (eds) 1989 Anaesthesia. Blackwell Scientific Publications, Oxford

28. Anaesthesia for ENT surgery

Two hundred and seventy thousand ear, nose and throat operations are performed in the United Kingdom each year, accounting for approximately 5% of the workload of an anaesthetic department. Patients are usually young and healthy and the average hospital stay is short (less than three days). Many operations are performed as day cases, thereby reducing the need for inpatient admission.

Children and young adults are frequently apprehensive and require reassurance. Some may have an atopic history which influences the choice of premedication and anaesthetic technique. Older patients may have hypertension or ischaemic heart disease and require careful preoperative assessment.

Smooth anaesthesia and a clear airway are essential as coughing and straining result in venous congestion which may persist during surgery and cause increased bleeding. Partial obstruction of the airway may lead to hypoxaemia, hypercapnia and unduly light anaesthesia.

THE SHARED AIRWAY

Special problems are caused when the airway is shared by both anaesthetist and surgeon. If bleeding is anticipated, the airway *must* be protected by the use of a tracheal tube and the oropharynx packed to obviate contamination of the larynx with blood, pus and other debris. Techniques which rely on insufflation of anaesthetic vapours to an unintubated, unprotected trachea are no longer in common use and are not described here.

Sometimes, a Boyle Davis gag may compress the tracheal tube and cause partial airway obstruction. During IPPV this is detected by a decrease in compliance and increased inflation pressure and in the spontaneously breathing patient by decreased movement of the reservoir bag.

At the end of the procedure the pack must be removed and the pharynx cleared of blood and debris before the trachea is extubated with the patient in a head-down lateral position.

TONSILLECTOMY

Each year 80 000 adenotonsillectomies are performed in the UK with a rate of 8 per 1000 children under the age of 15. This frequency is 40% of that 15 years ago. In 1968 there were 6 deaths, a mortality rate of 1 in 28 000 but this has now been reduced to less than 1 in 100 000.

It is customary to prescribe a premedication prior to tonsillectomy. This is administered most conveniently to the younger child as a syrup (trimeprazine 3 mg/kg or diazepam 0.3 mg/kg are effective). Most anaesthetists combine this with atropine 0.1–0.3 mg orally (except in hot weather) to decrease salivation during operation. Induction of anaesthesia may be either by inhalation or by the intravenous route, whichever is appropriate for the individual child; the application of an EMLA patch (p. 266) is advisable if i.v. induction is planned. Oral tracheal intubation is advisable, performed either under deep volatile anaesthesia or facilitated by suxamethonium; on occasions it may be difficult to maintain a patent airway because of respiratory obstruction produced by enlarged tonsils.

Relaxation provided by suxamethonium may assist the surgeon who guillotines (as opposed to dissects) tonsils before achieving haemostasis.

Analgesia should be given at the end of surgery, if none has been given previously, so that the child awakens in a pain-free state. Tracheal extubation is performed with the patient slightly head-down in a lateral position after suction has ensured that the pharynx is free from blood. Postoperative vomiting occurs frequently.

Blood loss during tonsillectomy is not usually measured but may be deceptively large. Particular care should be exercised in the 3–4 year-old child, weighing 13–15 kg. In this age range, blood transfusion is required after the loss of only 100 ml of blood.

The postoperative bleeding tonsil

Diagnosis is made usually on the basis of clinical signs of hypovolaemia — tachycardia, pallor and sweating. Swallowing is not uncommon, followed by vomiting of a large quantity of blood. Anaesthesia for such a child is difficult and the assistance of an experienced anaesthetist must be sought.

An i.v. infusion is essential and blood transfusion is required. After resuscitation, the patient is placed head-down in a lateral position and suction apparatus is positioned within grasp. After preoxygenation, a small dose of thiopentone (2–3 mg/kg) is given followed by suxamethonium 1 mg/kg and cricoid pressure applied, although this may make laryngoscopy difficult. Alternatively, a gaseous induction with halothane in oxygen may be used and pharyngeal suction and tracheal intubation undertaken under deep halothane anaesthesia. When bleeding has been controlled surgically the stomach is emptied with a nasogastric tube. At the end of the procedure the trachea is extubated with the child in a lateral position.

It should be emphasised that induction of anaesthesia with thiopentone must *never* be attempted before adequate resuscitation has been undertaken and the intravascular volume restored.

ADENOIDECTOMY

Adenoidectomy is often combined either with tonsillectomy or examination of the ears under anaesthesia. Premedication is similar to that for tonsillectomy and anaesthesia is induced either by inhalation or by the i.v. route. Oral tracheal intubation is advisable either under deep anaesthesia or facilitated by suxamethonium, and a small throat pack is inserted by the surgeon. The adenoids are curetted and the postnasal space is packed to achieve haemostasis. After 3 min, this pack is removed, and after removal of the throat pack, the patient is turned into the lateral position and the trachea extubated.

MICROLARYNGOSCOPY

The operating microscope revolutionised the treatment of laryngeal disorders. The Kleinsasser laryngoscope is supported on the chest by rests and the operating microscope allows detailed examination and assessment of the larynx.

Premedication with pethidine and promethazine has been suggested if there is no evidence of airway obstruction. The most popular technique uses a Coplan's tube (5 mm i.d., 31 cm long, constructed from soft plastic, with a 10-ml cuff volume). Anaesthesia is induced with thiopentone followed by a non-depolarising muscle relaxant; the vocal cords are sprayed with 3 ml lignocaine 4% to assist smooth anaesthesia and to minimise the possibility of postextubation laryngospasm. The Coplan's tube is passed nasally. The lungs are ventilated artificially with 66% N_2O in O_2 supplemented either with a volatile agent or analgesic drug. The small-diameter tube does not impede the surgeon's view and allows good access to the larynx. The cuff prevents contamination of the trachea with blood or debris.

At the end of the procedure, the pharynx is cleared with suction under direct vision, muscle relaxants are antagonised and tracheal extubation performed in a lateral position. Oxygen is administered to minimise the risk of hypoxaemia if laryngeal stridor occurs.

Other techniques used for microlaryngoscopy include:

1. Topical analgesia to the larynx with insufflation of N_2O/O_2 and halothane via a fine catheter.
2. Neuroleptanalgesia combined with topical analgesia.
3. Venturi ventilation with O_2 using a catheter and a Sanders injector. Hypnosis is maintained

with increments of a rapidly metabolised induction agent.

4. A conventional or Pollard's tracheal tube and controlled ventilation.

The lumen of the Pollard's tube differs in size at the proximal and distal ends. It is constructed of latex reinforced with a nylon spiral. The proximal internal diameter is 10 mm, narrowing to 5, 6 or 7 mm for the distal laryngeal portion.

In children, microlaryngoscopy is performed using spontaneous ventilation via an oral tracheal tube one size smaller than would be used normally. The larynx should be sprayed with a measured quantity of lignocaine in an attempt to prevent postoperative laryngospasm. Occasionally the surgeon requests that he observe the larynx without a tracheal tube in situ; in these circumstances the tube is removed during deep anaesthesia, allowing examination to take place during emergence or during Venturi ventilation via the operating microscope.

LARYNGECTOMY

The incidence of carcinoma of the larynx is 3–4 per 100 000 population. Many tumours may be treated with radiotherapy and therefore surgery is relatively uncommon for this condition. Airway obstruction by tumour is the major anaesthetic problem; alcohol and smoking are aetiological factors which may influence anaesthesia.

Respiratory function should be assessed preoperatively although this is difficult to measure accurately if there is airway obstruction. Chest physiotherapy should always be prescribed since it aids clearance of secretions pre- and postoperatively.

When respiratory obstruction is present, opioid or sedative premedication should always be avoided. If awake intubation is contemplated, successful topical anaesthesia of the mouth and pharynx requires an anticholinergic agent in addition. There is a risk of mechanical obstruction on induction of anaesthesia; consequently, if an i.v. agent is used, it should be given slowly in minimal dosage until consciousness is lost. If subsequently the patient's lungs can be inflated using a face mask, suxamethonium may be given to facilitate tracheal intubation; if not, anaesthesia is deepened slowly with nitrous oxide and halothane in oxygen until laryngoscopy is possible. If there is any doubt regarding the patient's ability to maintain a patent airway after loss of consciousness, the anaesthetist must *not* use an i.v. induction even with the smallest dose of thiopentone. Instead, an inhalational technique should be used; if there is progression to severe respiratory tract obstruction, awake intubation should be employed. A selection of non-cuffed tracheal tubes should be available as the lumen of the trachea may be narrowed at the level of the cords or subglottically. Tracheal intubation may be more difficult if preoperative radiotherapy has reduced the mobility of the floor of the mouth.

Monitoring of ECG and arterial pressure should be instituted in the anaesthetic room before induction of anaesthesia, which is maintained using controlled ventilation with nitrous oxide in oxygen supplemented by a volatile agent or opioid analgesic. Induced hypotension is often used to facilitate dissection of the neck (see Ch. 37). When the larynx has been dissected free, it is important to check that a sterile tracheal tube and compatible connections are available before the trachea is divided. The patient's lungs are ventilated with 100% oxygen for 2 min, the tracheal tube is withdrawn into the larynx, the trachea is divided and a second tracheal tube is placed rapidly in the trachea and secured firmly. This tube should be positioned carefully within the shortened trachea to prevent inadvertent one-lung anaesthesia.

At the end of surgery, residual neuromuscular blockade is antagonised and the tracheal tube changed for a laryngectomy or tracheostomy tube. Adequate humidification is essential postoperatively. Enteral nutrition is provided via a nasogastric tube.

PHARYNGOLARYNGECTOMY

Pharyngolaryngectomy is performed for tumours of the postcricoid region. The pharynx and larynx are removed and the stomach mobilised and anastomosed in the neck behind the tracheostomy. There are two surgical approaches: in one, after initial laparotomy, the stomach is passed through a mediastinal tract which is formed by blunt dissection; in the other more common procedure the stomach is mobilised via a thoraco-abdominal incision to be anastomosed in the neck. Thus several problems may arise:

1. Difficulty in intubation.
2. Temperature loss resulting from a large surgical incision, a prolonged operative procedure and extensive blood loss.
3. Pneumothorax if the pleura is damaged during dissection.
4. Rupture of the trachea causing difficulty in ventilation and mediastinal emphysema.

LASER SURGERY

The laser is used to strip polyps or tumours from the vocal cords accurately and with immediate control of bleeding. There are two anaesthetic problems:

1. *Damage to the tracheal tube*. It has been found that in the presence of oxygen PVC microlaryngoscopy tubes may be ignited by the intensity of the laser beam. Wrapping the tracheal tube in aluminium foil or using an aluminised PVC tube does not remove this threat completely. The introduction of an uncuffed flexible stainless steel tube (Hunton) for oral or nasal use has solved the problem.
2. *Retinal damage*. The DHSS recommends that all personnel should wear protective spectacles to prevent retinal damage.

NASAL OPERATIONS

Preparation of the nose with local anaesthetic

In 1942 Moffatt described a method of topical anaesthesia of the nose using cocaine as an alternative to spraying or packing the nose. There were three advantages of his method: minimal patient discomfort during preparation, a low risk of cocaine toxicity and a bloodless surgical field. In 1952 Curtiss simplified Moffatt's method as follows:

The patient lies supine with his head extended fully over the end of a trolley and supported by an assistant. A round-ended angulated needle is inserted with its tip directed along the floor of the nose. When the angle of the needle is reached, the tip is directed towards the roof of the nose and 2 ml of solution deposited when the tip has made contact. The procedure is repeated in the second nostril. The patient remains in this position for 10 min and is advised not to swallow any solution which may have trickled into the pharynx. Then he sits upright and spits out any residual solution.

Analgesia is produced by accumulation of cocaine in the region of the sphenopalatine ganglion, thereby blocking most of the sensory supply to the nose, including the anterior ethmoidal nerve. The columella is not affected, and requires a separate injection. Arterial blood supply to the nose accompanies the nerve supply, and is therefore constricted by the cocaine, producing good haemostasis.

Preparation of the nose in this manner enables any operation to be performed and dispenses with the need to use hypotensive techniques to control surgical bleeding.

Anaesthetic technique for nasal operations

Adequate premedication is essential and may be given either orally or i.m. A smooth induction is desirable to avoid coughing and straining. Suxamethonium or a non-depolarising muscle relaxant may be used to facilitate tracheal intubation. The larynx is not sprayed with local anaesthetic before intubation so that full laryngeal reflexes return as soon as possible after surgery.

Anaesthesia may be maintained using either spontaneous or controlled ventilation, depending on the duration of surgery. It is important to use a non-kinking tracheal tube and to pack the pharynx with 2-inch ribbon gauze so that blood, pus or debris does not contaminate the larynx. The presence of the pack should be marked in writing on the strapping which secures the tube to remind the anaesthetist to remove it at the end of the operation.

The patient is positioned 10° head-up and all breathing system connections are checked before surgery begins. An ECG should be used to detect the presence of arrhythmias which occur commonly during operations on the face. When surgery has been completed, the pack is removed, the pharynx cleared and the patient is turned into a lateral position for tracheal extubation.

Preparation of the nose is omitted frequently for nasal polypectomy and diathermy of the turbinates because the nasal mucosa can be shrunk to such a degree that surgery becomes difficult.

For submucosal resection of the nasal septum, or rhinoplasty (altering the external shape of the nose), the use of a preformed oral tube removes the connection from the operative field; careful nasal preparation minimises bleeding and improves operating conditions.

Epistaxis

Surgical intervention may be necessary to control bleeding from the nose and may involve packing the nose or postnasal space, or ligation of the maxillary artery.

The patient is often elderly, may be hypertensive and may have been sedated heavily with either barbiturates or benzodiazepines which render further premedication unnecessary. It is essential that the blood volume is restored before induction of anaesthesia. The problems inherent in haemorrhage from the upper airway and a stomach containing swallowed blood are similar to those of the bleeding tonsil, and the anaesthetic technique used is similar.

The sinuses

Bacterial infection of the paranasal sinuses occurs when the self-cleansing mechanism becomes impaired and mucus accumulates and stagnates. Antral washouts and intranasal antrostomies are performed to aid restoration of normal mucosal activity. In a Caldwell Luc operation a radical antrostomy is performed via a buccal incision above the canine tooth.

In all these procedures, the airway is protected by means of an oral tracheal tube and pharyngeal pack. Ethmoidectomy may require hypotensive anaesthesia.

Maxillectomy

Excision of the maxilla for tumour is a major procedure and hypotensive anaesthesia is used to reduce bleeding; ECG monitoring using a CM_5 lead is advisable. Accurate measurement of arterial pressure requires radial artery cannulation. A pack or obturator is inserted into the maxillectomy cavity at the end of surgery; first a mould is fashioned from a rapidly setting plastic compound in situ and additional debris may be deposited in the pharynx as a result. Usually, the patient is anaesthetised on a second occasion one week later to insert the permanent prosthesis.

EARS

Myringotomy

Examination of the ears together with myringotomy and insertion of grommets is carried out commonly in children who have secretory otitis media. This operation may be performed as an outpatient. Premedication with trimeprazine or diazepam often settles the fretful child. Either inhalational or i.v. induction may be used and anaesthesia is maintained with spontaneous ventilation via a face mask for myringotomy alone; if adenoidectomy is performed also, oral tracheal intubation is essential. The use of nitrous oxide increases middle ear pressure significantly, especially when combined with IPPV, and this may alter the appearance of the tympanic membrane.

Middle ear surgery

Smooth anaesthesia is essential for operations on the middle ear. Coughing, straining or bucking increase venous pressure and produce oozing which may persist for some time. Premedication may be given orally or i.m., omitting atropine for hypotensive anaesthesia. After induction of anaesthesia with thiopentone, suxamethonium is used to facilitate intubation with a non-kinking oral tracheal tube; the trachea and larynx are sprayed with lignocaine to aid tolerance of the tube. Often, sufficient reduction in arterial pressure is obtained using nitrous oxide in oxygen with halothane, enflurane or isoflurane in combination with *d*-tubocurarine and IPPV. Small doses of a β-blocker to reduce heart rate are often effective adjuvants. A 10° head-up tilt aids venous drainage. When induced hypotension is used, ECG and accurate arterial pressure monitoring are essential.

The middle ear is a closed cavity and nitrous oxide diffuses rapidly into the middle ear causing an increase in pressure. The maximum pressure is reached approximately 40 min after induction. There is concern that this may cause grafts to become dislodged. Such complications have led some authors to suggest that O_2/N_2 should be used in place of O_2/N_2O gas mixtures.

Bandaging the ear at the end of surgery involves movement of the head. This should be anticipated and supervised by the anaesthetist to prevent undue movement which may lead to gagging on the tracheal tube. If labyrinthine function has been disturbed, an antiemetic may be necessary to control postoperative vertigo and vomiting.

FURTHER READING

Atkinson R S 1976 Anaesthesia for endoscopy. In: Atkinson R S, Langton Hewer C (eds) Recent advances in anaesthesia and analgesia, 12. Churchill Livingstone, Edinburgh

Davis I, Moore J R M 1979 Nitrous oxide and the middle ear. Anaesthesia 34: 147

Flood L M, Astley B 1982 Anaesthetic management of acute laryngeal trauma. British Journal of Anaesthesia 54: 1339

Hospital Inpatient Inquiry Series MB4, 27. DHSS Office of Population Censuses and Surveys, Welsh Office, ENT Microfiches 24, 25

Hunton J, Oswal V H 1985 Metal tube for ear nose and throat carbon dioxide laser surgery. Anaesthesia 40: 1210

Morrison J D, Mirakhur R K, Craig H J L 1985 Anaesthesia for eye, ear, nose and throat surgery, 2nd edn. Churchill Livingstone, Edinburgh

Puttick N, Van der Walt J H 1987 The effect of premedication on the incidence of postoperative vomiting in children after ENT surgery. Anaesthesia and Intensive Care 15: 158

Van der Spek A L, Spargs P M, Norton M L 1988. The physics of lasers and implications for their use during airway surgery. British Journal of Anaesthesia 60: 709

29. Anaesthesia for ophthalmic surgery

The anaesthetist plays a crucial role in the production of suitable operating conditions for ophthalmic surgery. Careful attention to details of technique is therefore essential, particularly for intraocular procedures; e.g. cataract extraction, intraocular lens implantation, corneal grafting.

Many patients requiring surgery of the eye are at the extremes of age, and this presents associated problems for the anaesthetist. Ophthalmic surgical procedures may be categorised into intraocular and extraocular.

INTRAOCULAR SURGERY

Surgical requirements

When the globe is opened, intraocular pressure (IOP) becomes equal to atmospheric pressure. In the presence of a raised IOP, the sudden reduction in pressure on incision of the globe may lead to expression of ocular contents, including iris and vitreous, through the wound. On rare occasions, the sudden release of pressure may also cause disastrous expulsive haemorrhage from the short ciliary blood vessels in the posterior aspect of the eye.

Thus, control of IOP is essential, and moderate reduction is desirable for most procedures involving opening of the globe. Retinal detachment surgery is facilitated also by some reduction in IOP to allow the positioning of plombs, straps, etc. However, in corneal graft surgery, excessive reduction in IOP may cause difficulty in suturing. Complete immobility of the eye is essential for the microsurgical techniques which are now undertaken commonly for the majority of intraocular procedures.

Meticulous attention to control of intraoperative IOP is essential for patients who are at particular risk of ocular complications, including: those who have high myopia or diabetes; those who are aphakic; those with only one functioning eye, and adults of less than approximately 60 years of age. Particular care is necessary also in lens implant surgery as bulging of the vitreous, or loss of vitreous, may render the implant procedure impossible.

The factors controlling IOP are similar to those controlling intracranial pressure, as both involve manipulation of the volume of contents contained in a semirigid container. When the eye is opened, IOP is equal to atmospheric pressure and the *volume* of contents (particularly intravascular volume) assumes prime importance.

Control of intraocular pressure

The main factors involved in the regulation of IOP include: external pressure, the volume of arterial and venous vasculature (choroidal volume), and the volumes of aqueous and vitreous.

External pressure

Accidental pressure on the eye, e.g. from anaesthetic masks or retractors, should be avoided. Relaxation of the extraocular muscles with non-depolarising muscle relaxants may help to reduce IOP; this effect may be caused by a reduction in arterial pressure. However, suxamethonium causes a transient increase in IOP (see below).

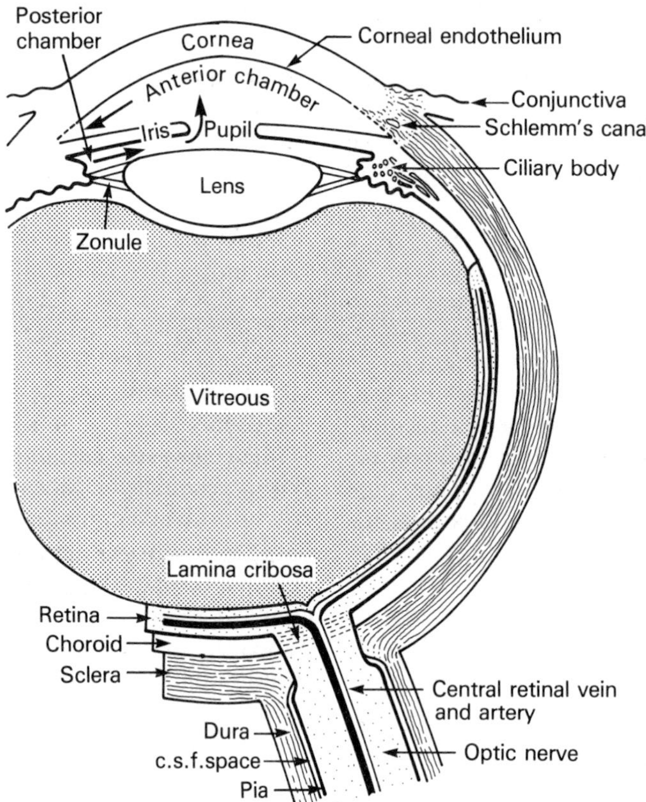

Fig. 29.1 Cross-section of the eye. Heavy arrows indicate flow of aqueous.

Vascular (or choroidal) volume

Variation in volume may result from vasoconstriction, dilatation of the choroid or changes in central venous pressure transmitted to the eye via its valveless venous drainage.

Venous pressure. Changes in venous pressure are transmitted to the ocular vasculature and are accompanied by immediate changes in ocular pressure and vascular volume. Raised venous pressure also impedes aqueous drainage by increased back pressure on the veins which drain the canal of Schlemm (Fig. 29.1), causing a further secondary gradual increase in IOP. During anaesthesia, venous pressure is influenced mainly by posture and transmitted intrathoracic pressure. A 15° head-up (anti-Trendelenburg) tilt causes a significant decrease in IOP.

Situations mimicking a Valsalva manoeuvre (e.g. airway obstruction, coughing or retching) cause immediate increases in venous and arterial pressures, and are reflected by immediate elevations in ocular pressure and vascular volume. These conditions must therefore be avoided.

Intermittent positive pressure ventilation (IPPV) produces a small increase in venous pressure secondary to the elevation in mean intrathoracic pressure, but this may be compensated for by regulation of arterial $P\text{CO}_2$.

Arterial blood gases. Arterial $P\text{CO}_2$ is a major influence in the control of choroidal vascular volume and IOP. A reduction in Pa_{CO_2} constricts the choroidal vessels and prevents forward displacement of the vitreous. This results in a reduction in IOP, if the eye is intact, and reduces the likelihood of prolapse of vitreous or other contents if it is open. Elevation of Pa_{CO_2} results in a proportional and linear increase in IOP. Increased Pa_{CO_2} may result also in raised central venous pressure.

Hypoxia produces intraocular vasodilatation and an increase in IOP.

Arterial pressure. Stable values of arterial pressure within the physiological range have little effect on IOP. However, when systolic arterial pressure decreases below 85–90 mmHg, IOP diminishes progressively and profoundly towards atmospheric pressure, which is reached at a systolic arterial pressure of 50–60 mmHg. Sudden increases or decreases in arterial pressure produce small, rapid, parallel but transient fluctuations in IOP and are therefore undesirable. The arterial pressure oscillations are buffered by expression of venous blood from the eye and, more slowly, by changes in aqueous volume. It should be noted that the effects of changes in venous pressure on IOP cannot be buffered by compression of the arterial vasculature of the eye.

Aqueous and vitreous volumes

Control of aqueous volume is important in the treatment of glaucoma, but is of less importance during surgery because the rate of change is relatively slow.

Reduction of vitreous volume by osmotic dehydrating agents (mannitol or sucrose) may be useful for controlling IOP during surgery. Mannitol (20–60 g) should be started 45 min before surgery. The diuresis produced necessitates catheterisation of the bladder. The usual precautions should be taken in administration of mannitol to patients with cardiovascular disease. Sucrose 50% (1 g/kg) i.v. produces a fairly rapid decrease in IOP (within 5 min) without a diuresis.

Reduction in IOP using acetazolamide, which reduces aqueous production and facilitates drainage, is of questionable benefit during surgery as it leads to increased intrachoroidal vascular volume. Thus, when the eye is open, a tendency to prolapse of contents may still exist.

Effects of anaesthetic drugs on IOP

Premedication. Drugs used for premedication have little effect on IOP, with the exception of those which alter Pa_{CO_2}. The use of opioid analgesics is unnecessary and their inherent properties of producing vomiting, retching and ventilatory depression are undesirable. Anticholinergic agents (in the doses used in premedication) have no effect on the glaucomatous eye provided that existing topical treatment is maintained. The commonly used anxiolytic and antiemetic drugs have little effect on IOP.

Induction agents. Thiopentone causes a moderate but transient decrease in IOP. Etomidate produces an immediate and prolonged decrease in IOP of approximately 40% from baseline values with little effect on cardiovascular stability, and the decrease in IOP persists for at least 20 min. The IOP does not seem to be affected by the myoclonic movements which may occur with this agent. Propofol also decreases IOP.

Ketamine may produce an increase in IOP and is therefore contraindicated if intraocular surgery is undertaken.

Muscle relaxants. Suxamethonium produces an increase in IOP which is maximal 2 min after injection, but the pressure returns to baseline by 5 min. This effect is thought to be caused by increased tone of the extraocular muscles and intraocular vasodilatation. Pretreatment with a small dose of non-depolarising muscle relaxant to prevent muscle fasciculation does not obtund this elevation of IOP reliably. Suxamethonium may be used safely if the eye is intact as IOP returns to normal before the incision is made. The problems involved in using suxamethonium in the presence of a penetrating eye injury are discussed below.

Non-depolarising muscle relaxants have no direct effects on IOP, but may produce alterations secondary to cardiovascular changes. Thus, tubocurarine causes a marked decrease in IOP but no change occurs with other non-depolarising relaxants.

Volatile agents. Both halothane and enflurane cause a decrease in IOP, this effect being more marked with enflurane. Ether and isoflurane also decrease IOP. The mechanism of these changes is unknown. Nitrous oxide has no effect in the absence of air or sulphur hexafluoride in the globe.

Opioids. Opioids cause a moderate reduction in IOP in the absence of significant ventilatory depression.

Suggested techniques for elective intraocular surgery

Table 29.1 summarises a suitable technique for adults. Premedication by the oral route (e.g. diazepam) is satisfactory except in babies. Usually sedative premedication is not given to babies or patients undergoing 'day-case' surgery. Anticholinergic agents are not essential in adults but are desirable in young children.

Induction of anaesthesia may be preceded by fentanyl (1–2 μg/kg). This reduces the doses required of induction and maintenance agents and helps to obtund the cardiovascular response to tracheal intubation. It may also reduce the likelihood of coughing after extubation of the trachea.

The benefits of induction with etomidate (reduction of IOP, cardiovascular stability and rapid recovery) are offset by the high frequency of pain on injection. The addition of 1–2 ml (20–40 mg) of lignocaine 2% to a 20 mg ampoule of etomidate helps to reduce this problem. The use of a large vein is also helpful. The advantages of etomidate are noticeable particularly in the elderly, unfit patient. It is unwise to use etomidate in children because of pain on injection, and thiopentone is a satisfactory alternative in both adults and children.

Suxamethonium provides ideal conditions for tracheal intubation with minimal risk of coughing or straining, and usually the transient increase in IOP has passed when the surgical procedure starts.

Topical anaesthesia of the larynx and trachea should be undertaken with a lignocaine spray before the trachea is intubated as this may help to reduce postoperative coughing. Patients should not eat or drink for 3 h subsequently because of the danger of aspiration. Topical local anaesthetic is unnecessary in children and indeed may cause increased coughing after tracheal extubation.

ECG monitoring is essential, and an audible 'beep' facilitates early detection of the oculocardiac reflex.

Table 29.1 Suggested technique for anaesthesia in elective intraocular surgery in adults

Premedication (oral)	Diazepam 0.1–0.2 mg/kg
Induction	Fentanyl 1–2 μg/kg Etomidate 0.3 mg/kg Suxamethonium 100 mg
Spray larynx and trachea	Lignocaine 4% (3–4 ml)
IPPV (moderate hyperventilation)	N_2O/O_2 + halothane 0.5%, enflurane 1% or isoflurane 0.8% Vecuronium 0.1 mg/kg
Antiemetic	Prochlorperazine 6.25–12.5 mg i.m. (20 min before completion of surgery)
Reversal	Atropine 1.2 mg or glycopyrronium 0.5 mg Neostigmine 2.5 mg

Ventilation — spontaneous or controlled?

The choice of spontaneous or controlled ventilation is controversial. There is no doubt that for the 'high-risk' eye, the combination of moderate hyperventilation and a 15° head-up tilt provides excellent conditions. IPPV with muscle relaxation virtually guarantees that no coughing or straining occurs whilst the eye is open, and reduction in Pa_{CO_2} can be achieved. In addition, smaller doses of anaesthetic agents are required with consequently improved cardiovascular stability and more rapid recovery from anaesthesia.

Spontaneous ventilation requires deeper levels of anaesthesia to ensure that coughing or straining on the tracheal tube do not take place when the eye is open. Carbon dioxide retention, hypotension and slow recovery from anaesthesia are often associated with this technique. If a head-up tilt and a non-rebreathing circuit are used, operating conditions may be adequate for many procedures, but the technique is unpredictable and may be unsatisfactory for the 'high-risk' eye.

Thus, IPPV is the method of choice to ensure good operating conditions for every patient. It has few disadvantages except for occasional delay in resumption of spontaneous ventilation after hyperventilation. Administration of the non-depolarising relaxant before the action of suxamethonium has ceased ensures that no coughing or straining takes place. The use of a peripheral nerve stimulator is recommended. No technique is completely reliable in preventing coughing after antagonism of residual neuromuscular blockade and tracheal extubation. Continuation of the volatile agent until reversal is helpful; i.v. lignocaine may also be useful. It is the surgeon's responsibility to ensure watertight closure of the wound.

An antiemetic should be administered i.m. approximately 20 min before the end of the procedure and further doses should be given during the postoperative period if necessary.

Prochlorperazine is an effective antiemetic for adults and also produces a useful degree of sedation. A small dose of cyclizine may be substituted for children.

Opioid analgesia is not usually required, but, if necessary, a small dose of papaveretum (with an antiemetic) is satisfactory.

Penetrating eye injury

The anaesthetic management of the patient with a penetrating injury causes potentially great problems to the anaesthetist, and experienced help should always be sought. If an increase in IOP is produced during induction of anaesthesia, loss of ocular contents may occur. As repair is carried out as an emergency procedure, the patient may have a full stomach. However, suxamethonium is contraindicated theoretically, as it produces an increase in IOP. Thus, the choice of muscle relaxant for tracheal intubation must balance the risks to the eye(s) against those of pulmonary aspiration. If it is anticipated that tracheal intubation will be uneventful, a large dose of non-depolarising agent can be substituted for suxamethonium in the usual 'crash induction' technique. Care should be taken not to exert pressure on the injured eye with the mask during preoxygenation. Vecuronium or atracurium are suitable choices of non-depolarising relaxant. However, if difficulties with tracheal intubation are anticipated, suxamethonium should be used despite the theoretical risk to the eye. If intubation is difficult and ventilation with a face mask is not efficient, the resulting hypoxaemia and hypercapnia produce far more risk to the eye than a single dose of suxamethonium. Recent evidence suggests that suxamethonium has not been proven to affect surgical outcome adversely.

Spraying of the larynx with local anaesthetic is undesirable in the emergency patient as airway protective reflexes are obtunded. Management is otherwise as for an intraocular procedure, but extubation of the trachea should be performed with the patient on his side and almost awake.

EXTRAOCULAR SURGERY

The most common procedures are squint surgery, examination under anaesthesia (EUA) and dacrocystorhinostomy (DCR).

Squint surgery

Any technique of anaesthesia with tracheal intubation is satisfactory. Traction on the extraocular muscles or pressure on the globe may provoke bradycardia via the oculocardiac reflex, which is mediated by the vagus. Prevention of the reflex by premedication with atropine is only partially effective, and careful intraoperative monitoring of heart rate is essential. Treatment of the bradycardia consists of cessation of traction and/or i.v. atropine, although the atropine may itself cause arrhythmias. Patients with squint may have an increased risk of developing malignant hyperpyrexia (see p. 417) and have a high incidence of postoperative vomiting.

EUA

EUA is undertaken mainly in children as day cases, and repeated anaesthetics at fairly short intervals may be required. Inhalational anaesthesia by mask is often satisfactory, but may limit surgical access. Tracheal intubation provides ideal access but it is seldom required. The view expressed in the past that this might induce laryngeal oedema and postextubation stridor is now disputed. Ketamine is a very appropriate agent for small children as intervention to maintain the airway is seldom required, but premedication with atropine is mandatory to reduce the risk of secretions provoking laryngeal spasm. IOP under ketamine anaesthesia is normal or slightly raised, and this is useful if repeated pressure measurements are required (as in buphthalmos) as falsely low pressure readings are avoided.

DCR

The main complication during DCR is haemorrhage which obscures the surgical field. Preparation of the nose with cocaine paste or other vasoconstrictor is helpful, and a throat pack is mandatory, as blood trickles into the nasopharynx. Hypotensive anaesthesia has been used to improve operating conditions in this procedure, but seems unjustified. The surgeon may infiltrate the operation site with adrenaline and the precautions indicated below should be noted.

DRUG INTERACTIONS

Patients with eye disease, especially glaucoma, are often receiving medication which may pose potential problems to the anaesthetist.

1. Acetazolamide, a carbonic anhydrase inhibitor, is used both acutely and chronically in the treatment of glaucoma. It is a diuretic and may produce dehydration and, less commonly, electrolyte imbalance.
2. Adrenaline is used topically in the long-term treatment of glaucoma, or intraoperatively by the surgeon to reduce bleeding. Systemic absorption may be significant and caution is necessary in the use of volatile agents, particularly halothane. Hypercapnia should be avoided.
3. Ecothiopate iodine (phospholine iodide) is a potent anticholinesterase used in the treatment of glaucoma. It depletes pseudocholinesterase and thus prolongs the action of suxamethonium.
4. Timolol maleate (Timoptol), a topical β-blocker, is used in some patients with raised IOP. Systemic absorption may be significant and precautions should be taken as for patients on oral β-blockers.

FURTHER READING

Adams A K, Jones R M 1980 Anaesthesia for eye surgery: general considerations. British Journal of Anaesthesia 52: 663

Arthur D S, Dewar K M S 1980 Anaesthesia for eye surgery in children. British Journal of Anaesthesia 52: 681

Barry Smith G 1983 Ophthalmic Anaesthesia. Edward Arnold, London

Foulds W S 1980 The changing pattern of eye surgery. British Journal of Anaesthesia 52: 643

Holloway K B 1980 Control of the eye during general anaesthesia for intraocular surgery. British Journal of Anaesthesia 42: 671

Jay J L 1980 Functional organization of the human eye. British Journal of Anaesthesia 52: 649

Libonatti M M, Leahy J J, Ellison N 1985 The use of succinylcholine in open eye surgery. Anesthesiology 62: 637

30. Anaesthesia for radiology, radiotherapy and psychiatry

General considerations

Many problems encountered in the radiology department, radiotherapy suite and psychiatric hospital are similar:

1. In most hospitals, radiology, radiotherapy and ECT suites have not been designed with anaesthetic requirements in mind. Anaesthetic apparatus often competes for space with bulky equipment, and in general, conditions are less than optimal.
2. Monitoring equipment may not be available readily, and is often the oldest in the hospital. Clinical observation may be limited by poor lighting.
3. Preparation of the patient may be inadequate because the patient comes from a ward in which staff are unfamiliar with preoperative protocols. Mentally disturbed patients may fail to comply with fasting instructions. Consequently, the patient may have a full stomach and may not be premedicated.
4. Anaesthetic assistance and maintenance of anaesthetic equipment may be less than ideal. Consequently, the anaesthetist must be particularly vigilant in checking the anaesthetic machine, changing empty gas cylinders (only the most modern suites have piped gases) and ensuring the presence of spare laryngoscope blades and batteries if required.
5. Communication between radiologist, radiotherapist or psychiatrist and the anaesthetist may be poor, with failure to recognise the other's requirements.
6. Often, recovery facilities are inadequate and the anaesthetist may have to recover his own patients. Consequently, he must be familiar with the siting of suction apparatus and supplementary oxygen supply within the recovery area.

ANAESTHESIA FOR RADIOLOGICAL PROCEDURES

The traditional role of the radiology department has changed in recent years. Conventional use of X-rays has been augmented by the introduction of new non-invasive diagnostic imaging techniques. Magnetic resonance imaging (MRI) (previously called nuclear magnetic resonance) and computerised tomography (CT) scanning have reduced the use of angiography and pneumoencephalography in neurodiagnosis. Whilst the main focus of clinical interest in these techniques has been centred on the brain, application has extended into delineation of thoracic and abdominal lesions. The major requirement of all these imaging techniques is that the patient remains almost motionless. Thus, anaesthesia may be necessary when these investigations are performed on children, the critically ill or the uncooperative patient.

Computerised tomography (CT scan)

General principles

Computerised tomography has become the most widely used neuroradiological procedure. A CT scan provides a series of tomographic axial 'slices' of the head and/or body. Each image is produced by computer integration of the differences in the radiation absorption coefficients between different normal tissues and between normal and abnormal tissues. The image of the structure under investigation is generated by a cathode ray tube, the brightness of each area being proportional to the absorption value.

One rotation of the gantry produces an axial slice or 'cut'. A series of cuts is made usually at intervals of 7 mm but may be larger or smaller, depending on the diagnostic information sought. The first-generation scanners took 4.5 min per cut, but the newest scanners take only 2–4 s.

Anaesthetic management

Neither sedation nor anaesthesia is required for most adult patients. However, young children and confused, demented or restless patients may need general anaesthesia to prevent movement, which degrades the image. Anaesthetists may be asked to assist also in the supervision of critically ill patients from the ITU in the CT scan room.

General anaesthesia is preferable to sedation when there are potential airway problems or when control of intracranial pressure (ICP) is critical. As the patient's head is inaccessible during the CT scan, it is mandatory to intubate the trachea. The scan itself requires only that the patient remains motionless and tolerates the tracheal tube. If ICP is high, controlled ventilation is essential to induce hypocapnia and decrease cerebral blood flow.

A thiopentone, nitrous oxide, oxygen and relaxant technique with orotracheal intubation and mild hyperventilation is acceptable. Anaesthetic complications include kinking of the tracheal tube (especially during extreme degrees of head flexion required for examination of the posterior fossa), hypothermia in paediatric patients and acute brain stem compression if the head is flexed excessively in the presence of an infratentorial tumour.

Computerised tomography involves exposure to ionising radiation, and access to the patient is limited. Consequently, a breathing system disconnection alarm, ECG display and automatic arterial pressure monitoring are essential. Pulse oximetry is recommended.

Magnetic resonance imaging

General principles

Magnetic resonance imaging (MRI) is a new imaging modality that does not use ionising radiation, but depends on magnetic fields and radiofrequency pulses for the production of its images.

An MRI imaging system requires a large-bore magnet in the form of a tube which is capable of accepting the entire length of the human body (Fig. 30.1). A radiofrequency transmitter coil is incorporated in the tube which surrounds the patient; the coil acts also as a receiver to detect the energy waves from which the image is constructed. In the presence of the magnetic field, protons in the body align with the magnetic field in the longitudinal axis of the patient. Additional perpendicular magnetic pulses are applied by the radiofrequency coil; these cause the protons to rotate into the transverse plane. When the pulse is discontinued, the nuclei relax back to their original orientation, and emit energy waves which are detected by the coil. The magnet is over 2 m in length, and weighs approximately 500 kg.

MRI can differentiate clearly between white and grey matter in the brain, thus making possible the in vivo diagnosis of demyelination. It can display images in the sagittal, coronal or transverse planes (Fig. 30.2) and, unlike the CT scanner, is capable of detecting disease in the posterior fossa.

Anaesthetic management

The indications for general anaesthesia during MRI are similar to those for computerised tomography. However, unique problems are presented by MRI. These include relative inaccessibility of the patient and the magnetic properties of the equipment. The body cylinder of the scanner surrounds the patient totally; manual control of the airway is impossible and tracheal intubation is essential, preferably with a Rae pattern oral tube. The patient may be observed from both ends of the tunnel and may be extracted quickly if necessary. As there is no hazard from ionising radiation, the anaesthetist may approach the patient in safety.

The magnetic effects of MRI impose some restrictions on the selection of anaesthetic equipment. Any ferromagnetic object distorts the magnetic field sufficiently to degrade the image. It is also likely to be propelled towards the scanner and held tightly against it. Of relevance to anaes-

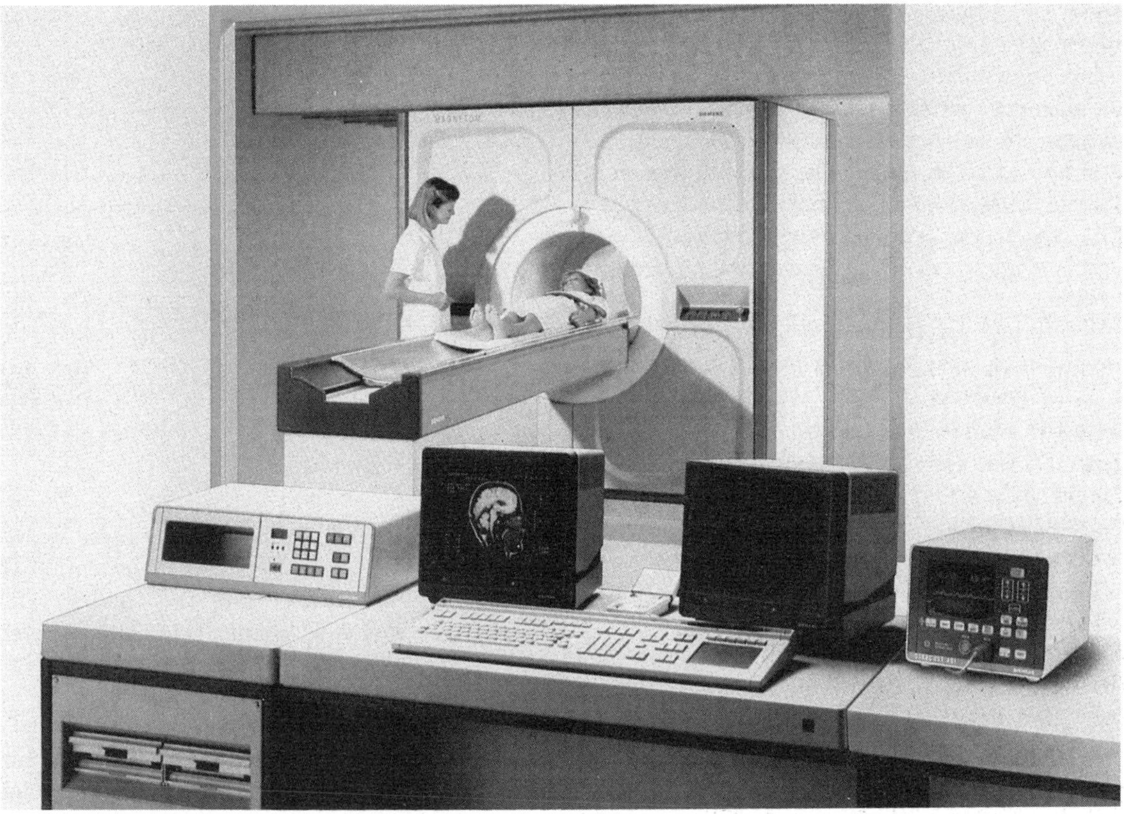

Fig. 30.1 MRI scan room.

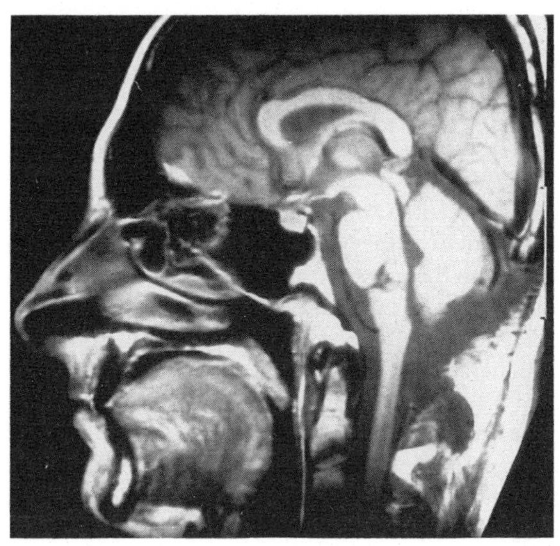

A

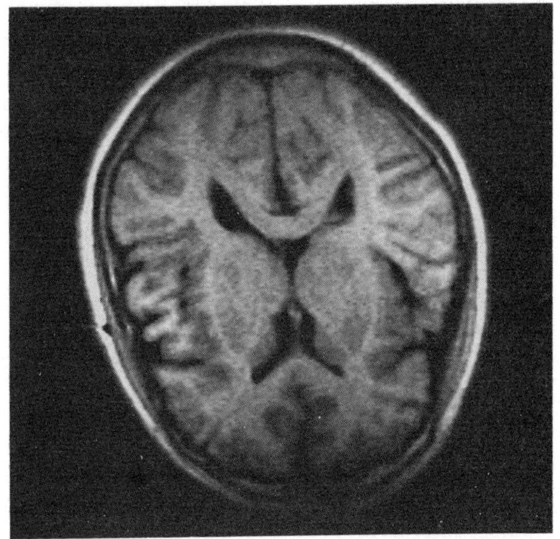

B

Fig. 30.2 Sections of the brain in the (a) sagittal and (b) coronal imaging planes.

thetists are such items as intravenous fluid stands, oxygen and nitrous oxide cylinders and monitoring equipment. Although laryngoscopes are non-magnetic, batteries are strongly magnetic, and laryngoscopy and intubation are difficult in close proximity to the scanner. The safest approach is to avoid all metallic equipment, e.g. use pipeline gases rather than cylinders, and to substitute apparatus of plastic or nylon manufacture whenever possible.

Monitoring may be difficult. Conventional ECG monitoring is not possible. A pulse oximeter may be used provided that the sensor lead is long enough to prevent the oximeter from affecting the magnetic field, and thus the image. Heart rate and ventilatory rate may be monitored with an oesophageal stethoscope, although the sounds may be obscured by the noise of the equipment. If the patient is allowed to breathe spontaneously, movement of the reservoir bag may be used as an index of ventilation. A non-invasive automated arterial pressure monitor, in which metallic tubing connectors are replaced by nylon connectors, is useful.

Hazards

The static magnetic field may prove dangerous in patients with implanted ferromagnetic devices. Patients fitted with a demand cardiac pacemaker should not be exposed to MRI because induced electrical currents may be mistaken for natural electrical activity of the heart and may inhibit pacemaker output. Metallic implants, e.g. intracranial vascular clips, may be dislodged from blood vessels.

Angiography

General principles

Computerised tomography has reduced the need for angiography in neurodiagnosis. However, angiography is indicated for the investigation of a suspected cerebral aneurysm, arteriovenous malformation or vascular tumour. Vertebral angiography is used if a posterior fossa lesion is suspected and carotid angiography is required for detection of supratentorial lesions (Fig. 30.3).

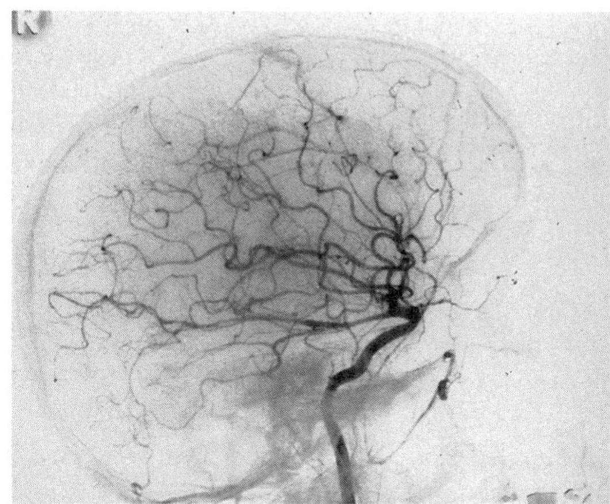

Fig. 30.3 Carotid angiogram.

Direct puncture of the common carotid or vertebral arteries has been replaced almost entirely by insertion of a catheter into the femoral artery using a Seldinger technique. This allows several vessels to be investigated through a single puncture site.

Most contrast media are exceedingly hypertonic (osmolarity 2000 mosmol/litre) and consequently produce expansion of the circulating blood volume. Injection of contrast medium causes burning pain in the face and eye, and vasodilatation produces headache and flushing. Newer agents, such as metrizamide, are less hypertonic and therefore preferable.

Anaesthetic management

Angiography is regarded generally as an unpleasant procedure and most patients prefer general anaesthesia. Sedation to augment local anaesthesia must be avoided in the presence of intracranial hypertension as the increased Pa_{CO_2} leads to vasodilatation and a further increase in ICP; in addition, vasodilatation results in poor-quality angiography.

General anaesthesia for angiography is more comfortable for the patient and ensures complete immobility during X-ray exposures. A relaxant/IPPV technique with moderate hyperventilation to induce hypocapnia (Pa_{CO_2} 4.0–4.5 kPa) is used. A moderate reduction in Pa_{CO_2} causes vasoconstriction of normal vessels, slows cerebral circulation and contrast medium transit time, and improves delineation of small vascular lesions. The failure of autoregulation within tumours increases blood flow relative to that in other areas because of an intracerebral steal phenomenon, and allows better visualisation of their vascularity.

Complications

Local. Haematoma and haemorrhage, vessel wall dissection, thrombosis, embolism of air or atheroma and the development of Horner's syndrome are all recognised complications.

General. The hypertonicity of contrast medium may exacerbate cerebral oedema. Circulatory responses occur occasionally during angiography and result either from manipulation or puncture of the artery, or the injection of contrast medium. Transient hypotension is common and cardiac arrhythmias including bradycardia, ventricular extrasystoles and asystole have been reported also.

Contrast encephalography

General principles

Encephalography is performed rarely in centres which possess a CT scanner. However, it is used occasionally to delineate small mass lesions in the suprasellar region and cerebellopontine angles.

These diagnostic studies are accomplished by injecting a contrast agent either into the lumbar subarachnoid space or directly into the ventricles via a burr hole, and employ gravity to manoeuvre the agent so that the ventricular system is outlined. Most commonly, air or oxygen is employed as the contrast agent, although iodinated compounds are used occasionally.

Lumbar air encephalography is performed by the injection of air into the lumbar subarachnoid space with the patient in the sitting position. The air rises, and by appropriate positioning of the head, it enters the cisterna magna and the ventricular system of the brain, outlining its size, shape and symmetry. The technique is contraindicated in patients with raised ICP because medullary 'coning' may be precipitated.

Ventriculography is performed usually on patients with obstructive hydrocephalus or those with raised ICP, in whom lumbar encephalography is considered too dangerous. There is a high risk of convulsions if iothalamate (Conray) is used as contrast medium.

Anaesthetic management

Encephalography is a very uncomfortable and unpopular procedure. Although performed occasionally under local anaesthesia and sedation, encephalography is distressing to most patients because of the protracted nature of the investigations (1–1.5 h), frequent changes of position and invariable headache and vomiting caused by the injection of air. Consequently, general anaesthesia is preferable, although there are difficulties. Nitrous oxide diffuses into any air-filled body cavity much more rapidly than nitrogen diffuses out, because of the difference between their blood/gas solubility coefficients. Nitrous oxide anaesthesia is contraindicated if air is used as the contrast medium, as distension of the ventricular system occurs and ICP increases.

If nitrous oxide is used as the contrast agent, there is no contraindication to its use as an anaesthetic gas. This modification reduces morbidity, as the rapid absorption of nitrous oxide from the ventricles after the procedure shortens the duration of headache. If air has been used as the contrast medium, any subsequent anaesthetic administered within one week of the study should not include nitrous oxide.

Miscellaneous procedures

Translumbar aortography (TLA)

TLA is a common investigation in the assessment of patients with peripheral vascular disease. Although it may be carried out under local anaesthesia with sedation, general anaesthesia is desirable. The patient is placed prone and therefore tracheal intubation and controlled ventilation are essential. The patient and operating table move rapidly by up to 2 m during radiological exposure so that additional lengths of ventilator tubing and an intravenous drip extension are necessary. Serious complications are infrequent but include pneumothorax, perforation of the bowel and renal puncture. Often, patients who require TLA have generalised vascular disease and most are heavy smokers with associated pulmonary pathology; consequently, anaesthesia may be hazardous.

Bronchography

Bronchography is used mainly for the diagnosis and evaluation of bronchiectasis and its use is declining. Most bronchograms are carried out using local anaesthesia, but children and anxious adult patients require general anaesthesia.

Commonly, respiratory function in these patients is compromised and additional hypoxaemia is inevitable after inhalation of the oil-based contrast medium.

Intravenous or inhalational induction is followed by tracheal intubation without any local anaesthetic spray, so that the cough reflex returns rapidly at the end of the procedure. Spontaneous ventilation is preferred, as it allows contrast medium to be drawn gradually into the bronchi to provide even distribution; controlled ventilation tends to disperse the dye too rapidly and delineates the bronchial tree poorly. Contrast medium is instilled through a catheter passed down the lumen of the tracheal tube. The posture of the patient is altered sequentially to fill the various lobes of the lung.

As much contrast material as possible is removed at the end of the procedure by suction and physiotherapy. The tracheal tube remains in situ until there is an active cough reflex. Humidified oxygen should be given during the recovery period and the patient should be nursed in a head-down position with the healthier lung uppermost.

Intussusception

This condition occurs usually between the ages of 6 and 18 months. Commonly, the ileum invaginates into the caecum because of small bowel lymphadenopathy. General anaesthesia may be necessary in the radiology department during attempted reduction of the intussusception by instillation of rectal barium.

The major problems are those of anaesthetising any young child in an unfamiliar environment. Precautions should be taken to minimise the decrease in body temperature. Fluid losses are always greater than expected and plasma (or substitute) may be needed to restore circulating blood volume.

ANAESTHESIA FOR RADIOTHERAPY

Adults may require general anaesthesia for insertion of radioactive sources locally to treat some types of tumour. The commonest tumours to be treated in this way are carcinoma of the cervix, breast or tongue. These procedures are undertaken in the operating theatre, and the anaesthetic management is similar to that for any type of surgery in these anatomical sites. However, the patients may have undergone anaesthesia recently for a diagnostic procedure and may require more than one anaesthetic for radiotherapy treatment; consequently, halothane should be avoided. In addition, the anaesthetist may be exposed to radiation and appropriate precautions should be taken.

Radiotherapy is used increasingly in the management of a variety of malignant diseases which occur in childhood. These include the acute leukaemias, Wilms' tumour, retinoblastoma and central nervous system tumours. High-dose X-rays are administered by a linear accelerator, but all staff must remain outside the room to be protected from radiation.

Anaesthesia in paediatric radiotherapy presents several problems:

1. Treatment is administered daily over a 4–6-week period and necessitates repeated doses of sedation or general anaesthesia.
2. The patient must remain alone and motionless for short periods during treatment, but immediate access to the patient is required in an emergency.
3. Monitoring is difficult as the child can be observed only on a closed-circuit television screen during treatment.
4. Recovery from anaesthesia must be rapid, as treatment is organised usually on an outpatient basis and disruption of normal activities should be minimised.

Before treatment begins, the fields to be irradiated are plotted and marked so that the X-rays can be focused on the tumour without damaging surrounding structures. This procedure requires the child to remain still for 20–40 min and takes place in semi-darkness. Radiotherapy treatment is of much shorter duration; two or three fields are irradiated for 30–90 s each, but a considerably longer period of anaesthesia is required so that the child can be positioned correctly and the radiation source focused precisely. A typical treatment session lasts 20–30 min.

Anaesthetic management

A wide range of techniques has been employed for this purpose.

Intravenous or intramuscular administration of ketamine is distressing for children. Ketamine produces excessive salivation, even if an antisialagogue is prescribed, and there is a risk of airway obstruction or laryngospasm. Tachyphylaxis occurs with repeated use, and sudden purposeless movements are not infrequent. The use of ketamine as a sole anaesthetic agent is unsatisfactory.

Often, children who require repeated daily anaesthesia have a Hickman line in situ to ensure reliable i.v. access for induction of anaesthesia. If establishment of i.v. access is required daily, venepuncture becomes not only technically difficult, but also increasingly distressing for the patient, parent and anaesthetist. Inhalational induction with the child sitting on the parent's knee is an alternative technique.

When anaesthesia has been induced, the child is placed on a trolley and anaesthesia maintained with nitrous oxide, oxygen and volatile agent delivered by facemask. Halothane remains the most suitable inhalational agent for repeated anaesthesia in children as the risk of hepatic damage is very low and airway complications are much less frequent than with enflurane or isoflurane. No analgesia is required and tracheal intubation is not necessary. During the period when the patient is unattended anaesthesia is continued by insufflating a low dose of anaesthetic in oxygen via a nasopharyngeal catheter.

Monitoring during radiotherapy under general anaesthesia is not easy. Closed-circuit television cameras provide visual monitoring of the patient's respiratory movements. Continuous ECG and automatic arterial pressure monitoring are essential. The pulse oximeter is a useful non-invasive monitor, especially if the trachea is not intubated. Ideally a microphone transmits the audible ECG signal and the saturation-dictated pitch of the oximeter signal.

ANAESTHESIA AND PSYCHIATRIC DISEASE

Patients who require anaesthesia and surgery usually experience some degree of anxiety and apprehension. Often a professional attitude, together with a friendly and humane approach by the anaesthetist, alleviates much of this anxiety.

The management of the patient with pre-existing psychological illness requires specific anaesthetic considerations. Patients with disorders of affect may require a course of treatment with electroconvulsive therapy (ECT), and thus repeated anaesthesia. The safe management of these patients demands an understanding of potential drug interactions between anaesthetic agents and psychotropic drugs such as tricyclic antidepressants, monoamine oxidase inhibitors and lithium. The prevalence of alcoholism is increasing, and the close association between alcohol consumption and acute trauma results commonly in the presentation of alcoholic patients for emergency surgery. Many patients with Down's syndrome and mentally subnormal individuals survive into late adulthood and may require anaesthesia for correction of associated medical conditions or dental care. Finally, the management of the narcotic addict is an area of increasing personal concern for the anaesthetist in view of the blood-borne transmission of hepatitis B and HIV.

Drug Interactions

The concomitant administration of psychotropic drugs is frequent in psychiatric patients scheduled for anaesthesia. The drugs encountered most commonly are tricyclic antidepressants, monoamine oxidase inhibitors, phenothiazines and lithium.

Tricyclic antidepressants

Tricyclic antidepressants inhibit the reuptake of noradrenaline into the presynaptic nerve terminals. Most of these drugs have anticholinergic effects also.

Tricyclic antidepressants may produce tachycardia and arrhythmias even in therapeutic doses, and the hypertensive response to directly acting sympathomimetic amines is increased dramatically. Although it has been recommended that tricyclic antidepressants are discontinued 2 weeks before anaesthesia, this may not be possible in many psychiatric patients.

Side effects of tricyclic therapy include sedation and anticholinergic symptoms (dry mouth, blurred vision, constipation, urinary retention). Centrally acting anticholinergic drugs (atropine, hyoscine) should be avoided in premedication because the additive effect may precipitate confusion, especially in the elderly.

Monoamine oxidase inhibitors (MAOIs)

Monoamine oxidase is responsible for the intraneuronal metabolism of sympathomimetic amines. Inhibition of this enzyme by drugs such as phenelzine and tranylcypromine is responsible for their antidepressant action. Usually, these agents are used when the response to tricyclic antidepressants has been unsatisfactory.

Tyramine, a precursor of noradrenaline, is known to precipitate hypertensive crises in the presence of MAOIs. Similarly, indirectly acting sympathomimetic amines e.g. ephedrine, result in unpredictable changes in arterial pressure. These hypertensive responses may be eliminated by withdrawal of MAOIs 2 weeks before anaesthesia, but, as with tricyclic drugs, this may not always be practical in the psychiatric patient.

The interaction between MAOIs and pethidine is important also, although uncommon. Agitation, restlessness, hypertension, rigidity, convulsions and hyperpyrexia may result. Morphine appears to be safe.

Phenothiazines

Phenothiazines possess antipsychotic, antiemetic, antihistamine and sedative properties. Interactions with anaesthetic drugs are common. The central depressant actions of opioids are potentiated, and opioid requirements are decreased. Central anticholinergic effects are additive with those of atropine and hyoscine, so that glycopyrrolate is the preferred antisialagogue. Moderate α-adrenoceptor blockade aggravates the hypotensive effect of anaesthetic agents.

Lithium

Lithium carbonate is used predominantly in the long-term treatment of mania. Its mode of action is inhibition of the release, and increased reuptake, of noradrenaline.

As lithium tends to act as an imperfect sodium ion, potentiation of both depolarising and non-depolarising muscle relaxants occurs, and close monitoring of neuromuscular function is necessary.

Lithium is excreted by the kidneys. Toxicity may ensue in hyponatraemic states, when there is intense renal conservation of sodium, and consequently lithium. The risk may be minimised by establishing a saline infusion during the perioperative period.

Electroconvulsive therapy (ECT)

ECT is used widely in psychiatric practice, primarily for the treatment of endogenous depression when drug therapy has failed. The aim of ECT is to produce a grand mal seizure; it is the seizure rather than the electrical stimulus which is responsible for the therapeutic effect.

Originally, seizures were induced chemically and electrical stimulation was not introduced until the late 1930s. Further advances involved the use of muscle relaxants (initially curare and later suxamethonium) to modify the convulsion. By the 1960s, the technique of using a short-acting i.v. barbiturate and a depolarising muscle relaxant became accepted as a simple, safe regimen for modified ECT.

Administration of ECT

The electrical stimulus produced by all ECT devices comprises short pulses of current interrupted by longer periods of electrical inactivity.

The electrical transmission lasts for only a fraction of the total stimulus duration, and this results in a decrease in the amount of electrical energy required to provoke a generalised seizure. Typical settings are a pulse of 60 Hz of 0.75 ms duration, with a total stimulus time of 1.25 s.

The electrical stimulus is applied to the patient's head by hand-held electrodes of low impedance. Traditionally, electrodes are placed in the bifrontotemporal region for bilateral ECT, whereas both electrodes are placed over the non-dominant hemisphere to produce unilateral ECT.

Physiological effects of ECT (Table 30.1)

Cardiovascular system. Activation of the autonomic nervous system is responsible for the profound cardiovascular changes during ECT. The autonomic disturbance consists of a parasympathetic–sympathetic sequence; this results in an initial bradycardia followed by tachycardia and hypertension secondary to intense sympathetic stimulation. This, together with the increased muscle activity of the convulsion, increases myocardial oxygen demand and may result in myocardial ischaemia in susceptible individuals unless hypoxaemia is avoided by administration of supplementary oxygen during the convulsion.

Cerebrovascular system. Cerebral blood flow increases dramatically to 1.5–7 times the basal level. This increased flow represents mainly a response to the increase in cerebral oxygen consumption that accompanies the seizure. There is an associated increase in ICP which may prove hazardous in patients with a space-occupying lesion.

Table 30.1 Physiological effects of electroconvulsive therapy

Cardiovascular effects	
Immediate	
Parasympathetic stimulation	Bradycardia Hypotension
Late (after 1 min)	
Sympathetic stimulation	Tachycardia Hypertension Arrhythmias Myocardial oxygen consumption increases
Cerebral effects	
Cerebral oxygen consumption	
Cerebral blood flow	
Intracranial pressure	
Intraocular pressure	
Intragastric pressure	

Anaesthetic considerations

In an effort to avoid or minimise the physiological sequelae and attendant complications of ECT, a technique of modified ECT has evolved gradually in which drugs are employed to reduce the detrimental effects of ECT without the abolition of the essential beneficial effects.

Preanaesthetic assessment. All patients should receive a visit and evaluation by the anaesthetist before treatment. Special attention should be paid to cardiorespiratory function, symptoms of oesophageal reflux, allergies and previous anaesthetic experiences. The presence of loose or missing teeth should also be noted.

The patient must be fasted for a period of at least 6 h before anaesthesia. This may seem simple, but many of these patients are extremely unreliable and occasionally uncooperative, so that careful supervision is required to ensure that fasting does occur.

Premedication with sedatives or opioids is not required and may serve only to prolong the anaesthetic recovery time. The routine administration of atropine is no longer considered to be necessary.

Anaesthetic management. Anaesthetic requirements include smooth induction, autonomic stability, safety with repeated administration and rapid recovery.

Methohexitone is the induction agent used most commonly. It is a barbiturate with a rapid onset and short duration of action that decreases the duration of, and raises the threshold to, electrically induced seizures. Thiopentone offers no advantages over methohexitone, and prolongs the recovery time. Propofol appears to be unsuitable as it shortens the duration of the seizure and may limit the therapeutic benefits.

The use of muscle relaxants in ECT has virtually eliminated the risk of fractures. Suxamethonium is used most commonly; the usual dose is 0.5 mg/kg, but a record should be kept of the dose and degree of modification of the seizure so that subsequent adjustments may be made if necessary.

When neuromuscular blockers are used it may be difficult to ascertain if a convulsion has occurred. The most effective way to record a seizure is by monitoring EEG activity; this is possible with modern ECT machines. Alternatively, an isolated forearm technique may be used.

After induction of anaesthesia and administration of suxamethonium, the lungs are ventilated with 100% oxygen using facemask and anaesthetic breathing system. When the limbs are flaccid, a rubber 'bite block' is inserted between the teeth before electrical stimulation is applied. During the seizure, artificial ventilation with oxygen is continued to avoid arterial desaturation, and continued until adequate spontaneous ventilation has returned.

Patients should be recovered in the lateral position by trained nursing staff with equipment available immediately for treatment of any emergency.

Contraindications

There is no general agreement regarding conditions which constitute relative or absolute contraindications to ECT (Table 30.2). However, the consensus is that patients with an intracranial mass lesion, or those who have suffered a myocardial infarction or cerebrovascular accident within the last 3 months, should not undergo ECT. The decision to proceed with ECT is determined after balancing the risks of treatment and the risks associated with progression of the psychiatric disease and long-term therapy with antidepressants.

Table 30.2 Contraindications to electroconvulsive therapy

Absolute
Recent myocardial infarction (<3/12)
Recent cerebrovascular accident (<3/12)
Intracranial mass lesion
Relative
Angina pectoris
Congestive cardiac failure
Severe pulmonary disease
Severe osteoporosis
Major bone fractures
Glaucoma
Retinal detachment
Pregnancy

Morbidity after ECT

Modified ECT in association with skilled anaesthetic management is safe and effective. Patients may complain of headache, muscle aches and confusion for 1–2 h after treatment, but memory disturbances may persist for several weeks. The latter are minimised by unilateral ECT over the non-dominant cerebral hemisphere.

Other mental disorders

Mental subnormality

Mentally subnormal patients should be assessed in the presence of parents or a guardian. Relevant medical history can be obtained, consent for surgery given (if the patient is unable to give this himself), and rapport with the patient established.

Pharmacological premedication is usually unnecessary. The interval between arrival in the anaesthetic room and induction of anaesthesia should be minimised, and the presence of a reassuring parent may be invaluable. A flexible approach by the anaesthetist is required during induction of anaesthesia, which may have to be performed with the patient in the sitting position or even lying on the floor! Adequate help must be available to lift or restrain the patient if necessary. Induction of anaesthesia should be as smooth and rapid as possible; either an inhalational or i.v. technique may be employed. Occasionally, i.m. ketamine is required.

Poor dental hygiene and difficulty with tracheal intubation should be anticipated.

Patients must be allowed to recover undisturbed, and the presence of parents in the recovery area is to be encouraged.

Down's syndrome

Down's syndrome is associated with a variety of medical abnormalities including congenital heart disease, and duodenal or choanal atresia. Patients with this condition have a large tongue, small mandible and increased incidence of subglottic stenosis; consequently, airway management and tracheal intubation may prove difficult. Antibiotics are necessary in the prophylaxis of endocarditis. No abnormal responses to anaesthetic agents have been substantiated.

Alcohol withdrawal

Denial of alcohol intake in the perioperative period may result in disturbances associated with acute withdrawal. Delirium tremens is characterised by extreme disorientation, increased psychomotor activity, hallucinations, marked autonomic activity and hyperpyrexia. Usually, the syndrome lasts for 7–10 days.

Delirium tremens should be treated by correction of fluid and electrolyte imbalance and administration of vitamins, particularly thiamine. Control is achieved most readily by i.v. sedation with 0.8% chlormethiazole; barbiturates should be avoided.

A nitrous oxide, oxygen and relaxant technique with analgesic supplementation is suitable if anaesthesia is required for a surgical procedure, although maintenance of anaesthesia may require the administration of larger doses of anaesthetic agents than normal.

FURTHER READING

Bydder G M 1983 Clinical nuclear magnetic resonance imaging. British Journal of Hospital Medicine 29: 348

Casey W F, Price V, Smith H S 1986 Anaesthesia and monitoring for paediatric radiotherapy. Journal of the Royal Society of Medicine 79: 454

Edwards R, Mosher V B 1980 Alcohol abuse, anaesthesia, and intensive care. Anaesthesia 35: 474

Freeman C P L 1979 Electroconvulsive therapy: its current clinical use. British Journal of Hospital Medicine 21: 281

Gaines Y G, Rees D I 1986 Electroconvulsive therapy and anaesthetic considerations. Anesthesia and Analgesia 65: 1345

Hutton P, Cooper G 1985 Psychiatry. In: Guidelines in clinical anaesthesia. Blackwell Scientific Publications, Oxford

Marks R J 1984 Electroconvulsive therapy: physiological and anaesthetic considerations. Canadian Anaesthetists' Society Journal 31: 541

Nixon C, Hirsch N P, Ormerod E C, Johnson G 1986 Nuclear magnetic resonance: its implications for the anaesthetist. Anaesthesia 41: 131

Weston G, Strunin L, Amundson G M 1985 Imaging for anaesthetists: a review of the methods and anaesthetic implications of diagnostic imaging techniques. Canadian Anaesthetists' Society Journal 32: 552

Willatts S M, Walters F J M 1986 Anaesthesia for neuroradiology. In: Anaesthesia and intensive care for the neurosurgical patient. Blackwell Scientific Publications, Oxford

31. Day-case anaesthesia

Day-stay surgery comprises the admission of a patient, surgical treatment, recovery and discharge within the same day. This concept has become popular since 1960 for the reasons noted in Table 31.1.

Although there are few disadvantages with this system, it is essential that the patient reports any complications to a doctor. Some relatives feel insecure if left alone at home with the patient. The fear of increased medicolegal risk has not proved to be justified.

In addition to surgical indications, anaesthesia for day-stay patients may be required for haematological, radiological and other investigations.

TYPES OF UNIT

There are three common types:

1. A unit within a hospital complex, but with separate wards and operating theatre. This is functionally the most flexible type as it may be adapted to the varying requirements of day-patients.
2. A unit with a separate ward, but using the hospital's main operating theatre complex.
3. Outside the United Kingdom, it is common for a separate centre to have its own operating theatres and wards remote from a conventional hospital.

Table 31.1 Advantages of day-stay surgery

Party	Advantage
Patient	Shorter waiting time for operation than as inpatient. Recovery in own home
Child	Avoids psychological trauma of prolonged separation from parents and home
Surgeon	Shortens inpateint operation waiting lists. Lower infection rate
Health economist	No 'hotel' costs and lower nursing costs, therefore economical
Nurses	No night or weekend duty
Relatives	No repeated hospital visiting

In some units, most patients are discharged after only a half-day stay. In many hospitals which lack a special unit, day-stay patients are admitted to the ordinary wards.

Whatever the system employed, the staff and facilities for surgery, anaesthesia and recovery should be of the same standard as for inpatients and complete facilities for resuscitation must be provided.

Standing arrangements should exist for admitting a day-patient immediately to a standard hospital bed if he is not fit to be discharged at the end of the day.

PATIENT SELECTION

Selection of patients for day surgery is dependent on both the surgical procedure and also the physical state of the patient. Practically any surgical procedure expected to last less than 1 h may be undertaken provided that undue haemorrhage and severe postoperative pain are not anticipated. Patients should be of a fitness rating of ASA grade I or II, although very short examinations under anaesthesia may be performed on grade III patients (see Table 19.1). It is essential that the home background is adequate and that relations or friends are available to provide postoperative monitoring and care.

Initial selection is made by the surgeon who advises operation. In some centres, the patient may then be assessed immediately at an outpatient anaesthetic clinic. If selection is delegated to the surgeon, he must instigate appropriate investigations. However, cancellation of surgery after a patient's admission to a day-care unit rarely results from incorrect selection, but more often is occasioned by recent ingestion of food, an upper respiratory tract infection or the disappearance of the lesion requiring surgery.

The letter calling the patient for surgery should contain an outline of what he (or she) should expect (see Table 31.2). It should also stress that the patient must:

1. Refrain from eating and drinking for 6 h before operation (modified for infants, where 3–4 h abstention is preferable to avoid hypoglycaemia).
2. Bring current medication to hospital so that it may be identified.
3. Be accompanied home.
4. Have company in the house on the night of operation.
5. Abstain from alcohol for 24 h after operation.
6. Not drive a car or work machinery for 24 h after operation.

Although minor behavioural changes have been noted for up to 48 h after anaesthesia, most anaesthetists consider a 24-h abstention from driving as reasonable.

Abstention from food is very important and although early studies suggested that patients may ignore this instruction, this has not been confirmed recently.

Fear of the risks involved has prompted some

Table 31.2 An explanatory letter sent to the parents of children undergoing day-stay surgery at Leicester Royal Infirmary

DAY CASE SURGERY FOR CHILDREN

Dear Parent,

Your child requires a minor operation which can probably be done in a single day in hospital, thus reducing the unpleasantness of a long hospital stay.

In order to make the visit to hospital as happy as possible, your help would be appreciated in making things run as smoothly as they can. The following notes are provided to give you some idea of what to do in preparation for the visit.

Please do explain to your child, if old enough, that he is going into hospital, but do not enter into elaborate details which will only confuse and frighten him, and may well be wrong. Try to present the hospital admission as an interesting experience. Try to control your own natural anxiety. If you are obviously worried, then your child will think that something awful is about to happen.

On the day of the operation you will be asked to arrive in good time to enable the necessary preparations to be made.

Most of the operations will be done under general anaesthesia. It is essential that your child should have nothing at all to eat or drink for some hours before the operation. The exact arrangements depend on the child's age. Please follow the instructions below.

On arrival in the ward, there will be some essential paperwork to complete.

Your child will then be seen by a member of the surgical team and an anaesthetist. Normally there will be NO injections or medicines to take on the ward before the operation.

Children are taken to the operating theatre in their beds or cots. You may, if you wish, accompany them as far as the theatre entrance. However, the design of our theatres is such that parents cannot come into the anaesthetic rooms.

Anaesthesia and surgery will take a variable time, depending on the operation, but all children are kept in the recovery area of the theatre suite, under careful supervision, until they are safely awake again.

If the operation is likely to cause any pain afterwards a pain-killer will be given while the child is still asleep. This may result in your child being quite sleepy after the operation.

Before discharge from hospital children are again visited by an anaesthetist and surgeon, at which time instructions for postoperative care will be given.

EATING AND DRINKING BEFORE OPERATION — MORNING CASES

1. *Children over 4 years of age*
   Nothing to eat or drink after midnight on the day before operation.
2. *Children between 2 and 4 years of age*
   Wake when you go to bed and give a milk drink and biscuits. After this — nothing to eat or drink.
3. *Children less than 2 years of age*
   Wake very early on the morning of operation and give a milk drink (up to $\frac{1}{2}$ pint of milk). This must be completed by 6.00 a.m.

REMEMBER

1. The aim is to make the admission as pleasant as possible.
2. If you do not understand anything, please ask for more details.
3. If you have any helpful suggestions for improving the service, please let us know.

anaesthetists to insist that the patient signs a special consent form indicating agreement to these limitations.

In some centres, patients are asked to complete a questionnaire (Table 31.3) providing details of medical history and medication. This is brought with the patient on admission, and speeds clerking. Such a form is particularly valuable for children if the person accompanying the child is not a parent.

Table 31.3 Example of form for completion by the parents, used by the Toronto Hospital for Sick Children (Reproduced by permission)

HOSPITAL FOR SICK CHILDREN

Ambulatory Services
Outpatient surgery

Instructions:
— Check one answer to each question
— Please complete this side only
— Please bring this form with you on the day of surgery

	Yes	No	Don't Know
1. Has your child ever been in hospital?	☐	☐	☐
2. Has he been in this hospital before?	☐	☐	☐
3. Has your child ever had an anaesthetic?	☐	☐	☐
4. Did your child have any problems with the anaesthetic?	☐	☐	☐
5. Does your child have any allergies?	☐	☐	☐
6. Was the allergy due to:			
a) A drug or medicine?	☐	☐	☐
b) Any type of food?	☐	☐	☐
c) Other things?	☐	☐	☐
7. If he had an allergy, did he have:			
a) A skin rash or hives?	☐	☐	☐
b) Wheezing or trouble breathing?	☐	☐	☐
c) Hay fever or a runny nose?	☐	☐	☐
d) A high fever?	☐	☐	☐
8. Has this child had a head cold or cough within the past week?	☐	☐	☐
9. Does your child wear a dental plate or bridge?	☐	☐	☐
10. Has your child had a cortisone type drug within the past two years?	☐	☐	☐
11. Is your child receiving any medicine just now?	☐	☐	☐
12. Is there anyone in the family with a bleeding problem?	☐	☐	☐
13. Has the patient had any minor injuries, operations, or tooth extraction followed by an unusual amount of bleeding?	☐	☐	☐
14. Does the child bruise easily on body areas other than the legs?	☐	☐	☐
15. Has your child been exposed to any infectious disease within the past month?	☐	☐	☐
16. Has your child ever had:			
Diabetes	☐	☐	☐
Asthma	☐	☐	☐
Cystic fibrosis	☐	☐	☐
Tuberculosis	☐	☐	☐
Rheumatic fever	☐	☐	☐
Rheumatism	☐	☐	☐
Heart disease	☐	☐	☐
Liver disease	☐	☐	☐
Anemia	☐	☐	☐
Convulsions or fits	☐	☐	☐
Glaucoma	☐	☐	☐
Jaundice	☐	☐	☐
17. Is there any problem about your child not mentioned so far?	☐	☐	☐
18. Has anyone in your family ever had a problem with an anaesthetic?	☐	☐	☐

IF ANY QUESTIONS ABOVE RECEIVED A 'YES' ANSWER GIVE DETAILS BELOW:

____
____
____
____
____

DATE COMPLETED: __________
SIGNATURE OF PARENT: __________

Proposed Procedure: __________

History of Present Illness: __________

Physical Examination:

Under 6 years —	Over 6 years —
length ______ cm	height ______ cm
Weight: ______	Blood Pressure: ______
Temperature: ______	Hemoglobin: ______ gm%
Pulse: ______	Sickle Cell Test: ______
Respirations: ______	Urinalysis: ______

Nose and Throat: __________

Heart: __________

Lungs: __________

Other Physical Findings: __________

Diagnosis: ______ Date: Physician Signature ______

ADMISSION

Patients should be admitted to the day ward in adequate time for history-taking and examination. The results of any investigation requested as an outpatient should be noted. The patient should receive an identity bracelet and their name should be entered in the nursing record. The operation site should be marked.

Premedication

There is some controversy regarding premedication, both sedative and antisialagogue. Sedative premedicant drugs produce a 'hangover' effect which delays recovery and therefore departure from a day ward and often prevents discharge from a half-day ward. Preoperative explanation and psychotherapy usually render the use of sedatives unnecessary, but they may be required for the very anxious or retarded adult patient; intramuscular midazolam 0.1 mg/kg or oral temazepam 20 mg may be given, as they are least likely to delay discharge.

Children over 5 years are usually co-operative and do not require sedation. In children under 5 years, the greatest cause of distress is usually separation from the mother and if the theatre design allows it, the mother's presence in the anaesthetic room obviates this problem. If this is not possible, an oral premedication may be given 1–2 h before surgery. Some authors have prescribed diazepam 0.5 mg/kg for young children, given by the mother at home. Children under 1 year seldom require sedation.

Premedication with anticholinergic drugs is usually avoided in adults. In paediatric practice, their use is controversial and the same considerations discussed in Chapter 34 apply to outpatient as to inpatient paediatric practice.

Induction of anaesthesia

Induction of anaesthesia with an i.v. agent in unpremedicated patients requires slightly larger doses than normal. The incidence of excitatory phenomena (coughing, movement, or breath-holding) is much greater than in premedicated patients and care must be exercised to avoid moving any part of the patient, attempting to insert an oral airway too early, or increasing the dose of volatile agents too rapidly. Unpremedicated patients are more likely to experience cutaneous pain on i.v. injection of methohexitone, etomidate or propofol.

All the common i.v. induction agents have been used in day-case patients. The factors affecting their suitability are shown in Table 31.4.

None of the drugs currently available is the ideal induction agent, but sleep doses of propofol (2–2.5 mg/kg), methohexitone (1.5 mg/kg) or thiopentone (5 mg/kg) are popular. Although propofol most nearly meets the requirements for the ideal induction agent for day-stay surgery, the respiratory and cardiovascular depression which it causes preclude its use in some patients. Delayed recovery has been reported in day-stay patients. The use of ketamine for outpatients is controversial. As premedication is usually avoided, emergence phenomena are particularly likely to occur, so it is rarely used in adults. It is said that emergence effects are rare in children, although many paediatric nurses would disagree. The i.m. route (8–10 mg/kg) is convenient in the uncooperative small child without visible veins.

Children may be allowed to choose the method of induction, but the i.v. route is preferable if veins are prominent. If the child has chosen an inhalational induction, 66% N_2O in O_2 with the gradual introduction of 1–2.5% halothane is acceptable.

Rectal methohexitone (10% methohexitone in

Table 31.4 Side effects of the induction agents

Agent	Awakening	Hangover effect	Pain on injection	Smoothness of induction
Thiopentone	Fairly rapid	++		++
Methohexitone	Rapid	+	++	
Etomidate	Rapid		+++	
Propofol	Rapid		++	++

water = 100 mg/ml) in a dose of 25 mg/kg administered through a lubricated 14 G cannula has been recommended for the preschool child. Close monitoring of the patient is required during the slow induction, which may take up to 11 min and occasionally longer. The anaesthetist must be available immediately with ventilatory support if required. After 30 min, the rate of recovery is the same as that for children given i.v. methohexitone.

Tracheal intubation

Tracheal intubation does not produce subsequent airway problems at home, even in children, provided that an unduly large tube is not used. However, as patients are young, healthy and mobilise quickly, suxamethonium is particularly prone to produce pain. Prior administration of a small dose of a non-depolarising neuromuscular blocking agent (e.g. gallamine 20 mg) reduces the incidence, but a larger dose of suxamethonium (up to 2 mg/kg) is required for equivalent relaxation. When artificial ventilation is intended, a medium-duration competitive agent (e.g. vecuronium or atracurium) may be used from the outset, provided that the anaesthetist is experienced and that difficulty in intubation is not anticipated.

Maintenance of anaesthesia

The technique used for maintenance is less important than the choice of anaesthetic agents. Maintenance by inhalation with spontaneous respiration, a total i.v. technique, and a nitrous oxide/oxygen/muscle relaxant technique supplemented by short-acting opioids or volatile agents have all been used successfully. The principle employed is that every sedative agent used should be either excreted rapidly or metabolised rapidly to inactive metabolites. When analgesia is required, a short-acting analgesic, e.g. fentanyl or alfentanil, should be used.

Of the volatile agents, enflurane and isoflurane are theoretically preferable to halothane as they have lower blood/gas solubility coefficients and recovery of consciousness is slightly quicker. However, halothane provides a smoother induction, which is often more rapid because the maximum vaporiser setting is a greater multiple of MAC than is the case for the other agents. There are no differences between these agents in respect of recovery to 'street fitness'.

Local analgesia

Local analgesic techniques are particularly valuable in day surgery. These include local infiltration, Bier's block (i.v. regional analgesia for the forearm and hand), blocks of nerve trunks (e.g. axillary brachial plexus block) or spinal nerve blockade, e.g. caudal block. Subarachnoid anaesthesia has been performed in day-stay patients, although this is rare in the United Kingdom.

Local anaesthesia may be employed in many patients without the use of sedatives. However, the use of a local anaesthetic technique in combination with general anaesthesia enables a lighter depth of unconsciousness to be maintained and provides prolonged analgesia postoperatively, reducing the requirement for systemic analgesics. A common and successful example is the use of penile dorsal nerve block or caudal block with light inhalational analgesia for circumcision.

Monitoring during anaesthesia

There is no reason to accept a lower standard of monitoring than that employed for inpatient surgery. The patient's colour, respiration and pulse, and the functioning of the anaesthetic machine should be observed. Arterial pressure should be monitored regularly and ECG monitoring should be routine.

Recovery

Recovery of unconscious patients should be undertaken by trained nursing staff. There should be one nurse to each unconscious patient. Standard resuscitation equipment (oxygen masks, suction equipment, defibrillator) and standard resuscitation drugs must be available. The patient must recline on a bed or trolley capable of tilting to a Trendelenburg position. The anaesthetist must be available to deal with complications.

Patients should not leave the recovery area until they are awake with restoration of all protective reflexes. Babies should be awake before leaving the operating theatre.

Analgesia

Provided that recovery of consciousness is rapid, the patient is soon able to take simple oral analgesics (aspirin or paracetamol). These drugs usually provide adequate analgesia, and the patient is advised to continue to take them at home. When a nerve block has been used, simple analgesics should be ingested before the block is expected to wear off (e.g. 4 h for caudal bupivacaine).

There remains a small number of patients for whom systemic analgesia (e.g. pethidine 1 mg/kg) is required, with the disadvantage that the consequent sedation may delay discharge. Occasionally it is necessary for community nurses to administer strong analgesics to the patient at home under the supervision of the general practitioner.

Complications

Although modern, well-organised day-stay surgery is well tolerated by patients (only 9% of patients in one study wished to stay longer, and only 1.4% in another study would refuse further surgery as a day-case), there is a relatively high incidence of minor complications (Table 31.5).

Table 31.5 Complications of day-case surgery. Percentage of patients reporting symptoms in three studies

Symptom %	Ogg (1972)	Study Routh (1979)	Dawson (1980)
Headache	27	38	
Drowsiness	26	39	
Muscle stiffness	15	24	
Nausea	22	17	30
Vomiting	8	6	20
Dizziness	11	15	
Sore throat	6	15	
Injection site pain	17	3	

Nausea is a common minor complication of anaesthesia particularly when opioids have been employed. It is especially common in patients susceptible to travel sickness. Some anaesthetists employ antiemetic drugs routinely.

Migraine sufferers are particularly likely to develop headache. Deep anaesthesia and the use of volatile agents may be predisposing factors.

Nonetheless, the commonest complaint is of pain at the operation site.

Discharge

Every patient should be seen by the anaesthetist before discharge. Although day-stay patients are generally healthy, and surgery is relatively minor and of short duration (less than 1 h), a decision is required for every patient regarding discharge.

Elaborate tests have been devised to compare the hangover effects of different agents. These are research tools and are not necessarily relevant to the fitness of a patient for discharge. The patient who is ready to go home is obviously conscious, communicating well, and steady on his feet. Enquiry should be made for pain, headache or nausea and treatment prescribed if necessary.

After circumcision, with or without a caudal block, micturition is often delayed. As the child is more likely to pass urine in familiar surroundings, he is allowed to go home, with instructions to the parents to contact their general practitioner should the child become distressed (which rarely occurs).

To reinforce previous written instructions, patients must be warned against driving, operating machinery or ingesting alcohol for 24 h. They must be accompanied home and if a child is being taken home by car, a second adult is required to prevent distraction of the driver.

FURTHER READING

Burn J M 1979 A blue print for day surgery. Anaesthesia 34: 790

Dawson B, Reed W A 1980 Anaesthesia for adult surgery outpatients. Anaesthesia for day-care surgery; a symposium in 4 parts. Canadian Anaesthetists' Society Journal 27: 409

Edelist G, Urbach G 1980 Organisation of the outpatient surgical facility. Anaesthesia for day-care surgery; a symposium in 4 parts. Canadian Anaesthetists' Society Journal 27: 406
Korttila K 1981 Recovery and driving after brief anaesthesia. Der Anaesthesist 30: 377
Ogg T W 1972 An assessment of postoperative outpatient cases. British Medical Journal 4: 573
Routh G S 1979 Day care surgery under general anaesthesia in a purpose-built unit. Anaesthesia 34: 809
Shah C P 1980 Day care surgery in Canada. Anaesthesia for day-care surgery; a symposium in 4 parts. Canadian Anaesthetists' Society Journal 27: 399
Steward D J 1980 Anaesthesia for paediatric outpatients. Anaesthesia for day-care surgery; a symposium in 4 parts. Canadian Anaesthetists' Society Journal 27: 412

32. Emergency anaesthesia

Patients scheduled for elective surgery are usually in optimal physical and mental condition, with a definitive surgical diagnosis and with concomitant medical illness well controlled. In contrast, the patient with a surgical emergency may have an uncertain diagnosis and uncontrolled concomitant medical illness, with consequent cardiovascular and metabolic derangements.

Thus a major principle governing the practice of emergency anaesthesia is to be prepared for all potential complications, including vomiting and regurgitation, hypovolaemia and haemorrhage and abnormal reactions to drugs in the presence of electrolyte disturbances and renal impairment.

PREOPERATIVE ASSESSMENT

The objective of emergency anaesthesia is to permit correction of the surgical pathology with the minimum of risk to the patient. This requires adequate and accurate preoperative evaluation of the patient's general condition, with particular attention to specific problems which may influence anaesthetic management.

It is essential to ascertain the likely surgical diagnosis, the magnitude of the proposed surgery, and how urgently surgery is required, as these dictate both the extent of preoperative preparation and the method of anaesthesia.

A pertinent past medical and drug history is elicited. In particular, enquiry is made into the presence and severity of specific symptoms relevant to cardiopulmonary reserve: angina, productive cough, dyspnoea of effort, orthopnoea or nocturnal coughing bouts. The presence of such symptoms should provoke detailed enquiry into the cardiovascular and respiratory systems (see Ch. 19 on preoperative assessment).

Depending upon the urgency of surgery, physical examination may be selective to identify significant cardiopulmonary dysfunction or any abnormalities which might lead to technical difficulties during anaesthesia. Basal crepitations, triple rhythm and raised jugular venous pulse signify impaired ventricular function and limited cardiac reserve, which increase significantly the risk of anaesthesia. It is also important to exclude arrhythmias and heart sounds indicative of valvular disease, as these influence the patient's response to physiological change and thus the anaesthetic management. Assessment of respiratory function is particularly difficult as the patient in pain (with or without peritoneal irritation) may be unable to be cooperative in pulmonary function testing.

It is important to cultivate the habit of airway evaluation if a rapid-sequence induction (see p. 531) is contemplated, since contingency plans are required for management of the patient in the event of failure to intubate the trachea.

Finally, a review of any laboratory investigations is made and urgent requests are made for further tests which may influence patient management.

Assessment of volaemic status

Assessment of intravascular volume is essential as underestimated or unrecognised hypovolaemia may lead to circulatory collapse during induction of anaesthesia, which causes reduction in the sympathetically mediated increases in arteriolar and venous constriction. In any patient in whom fluid is sequestered or lost (e.g. peritonitis, bowel obstruction), or in whom haemorrhage has occurred (e.g. trauma), efforts should be made to quantify the blood volume or extracellular fluid volume and to correct any deficit.

Intravascular volume deficit

Assessment of blood loss may be made from the history and any measured losses, but more commonly the anaesthetist has to rely on clinical evaluation. Useful indices include heart rate, arterial pressure (especially pulse pressure), the state of the peripheral circulation, central venous pressure and urine output. Table 32.1 describes approximate correlations between these clinical indices and the extent of haemorrhage, but it should be stressed that these refer to the 'ideal' patient. In young, healthy adults, heart rate and arterial pressure may be unreliable guides to volume status, and in elderly patients with widespread arterial disease, limited cardiac reserve and a rigid vascular tree (fixed total peripheral resistance), signs of severe hypovolaemia may become evident when blood volume has been reduced by as little as 15–20%.

In general, hypovolaemia does not become apparent clinically until blood volume has been reduced by at least 1000 ml (20% of blood volume). A reduction by more than 30% of blood volume occurs before the classical 'shock syndrome' is produced, with hypotension, tachycardia, oliguria and cold, clammy extremities. Haemorrhage in excess of 40% of blood volume may be associated with loss of the compensatory mechanisms that maintain cerebral and coronary blood flow and the patient becomes restless and agitated, and eventually comatose.

In patients with major trauma, it is valuable to compare the clinical assessment of the extent of haemorrhage with the measured or assumed loss. A marked disparity between these two estimates leads not infrequently to a diagnosis of a further concealed source of haemorrhage.

Extracellular volume deficit

Assessment of extracellular fluid volume deficit is difficult, as considerable losses must occur before clinical signs are apparent. Clinical acumen and a high index of suspicion are necessary to detect the subtle signs of lesser deficits.

Guidance is obtained from the nature of the surgical condition, the duration of impaired fluid intake, and the presence and severity of symptoms associated with abnormal losses (e.g. vomiting). At the time of the earliest radiological evidence of intestinal obstruction, there may be 1500 ml of fluid sequestered in the lumen of the bowel. If the obstruction is well established and vomiting has occurred, the deficit may exceed 3000 ml. At this stage, clinical signs are minimal but evident to the skilled observer.

Table 32.1 Clinical indices of extent of blood loss

Grade of hypovolaemia	1 minimal	2 mild	3 moderate	4 severe
Percentage blood volume lost	10	20	30	over 40
Volume lost (ml)	500	1000	1500	over 2000
Heart rate (beats/min)	normal	100–120	120–140	over 140
Arterial pressure (mmHg)	normal	orthostatic hypotension	systolic below 100	systolic below 80
Urinary output (ml/h)	normal ($1\ ml\ kg^{-1}\ h^{-1}$)	20–30	10–20	nil
Sensorium	normal	normal	restless	impaired consciousness
State of peripheral circulation	normal	cool and pale	cold and pale, slow capillary refill	cold and clammy peripheral cyanosis
CVP (cmH_2O)	normal	−3	−5	−8

For convenience, extracellular fluid volume loss may be graded into four degrees of severity; in each instance, loss is expressed as the percentage of the body weight lost as fluid. It may be seen from Table 32.2 that in minor degrees of extracellular fluid volume loss diagnosis is dependent on two highly subjective signs: diminished skin elasticity and reduced intraocular pressure. Loss of skin turgor is demonstrated best by pinching a fold of skin over a clavicle or tibia, areas where, under normal circumstances, there is little subcutaneous fat or redundant skin. Soft eyeballs resulting from lower intraocular pressure are assessed by asking the patient to close his eyes and look downwards; the examiner presses lightly on the eyeballs (above the tarsal plate), with the index finger of each hand.

It should be noted that the presence of orthostatic hypotension indicates considerable deficit which, if not corrected, may lead to severe hypotension on induction of anaesthesia. Orthostatic hypotension should be elicited with caution.

Laboratory investigations may help to confirm the extent of extracellular fluid volume deficit. Haemoconcentration results in an increased haemoglobin concentration and an increased packed cell volume. As dehydration becomes more marked, renal blood flow diminishes, reducing renal clearance of urea, and consequently increasing the concentration of blood urea. Under maximal stimulation from ADH and aldosterone, conservation of sodium and water by the kidneys results in excretion of urine of low sodium content (0–15 mmol/litre) and high osmolality (800–1400 mosmol/kg).

After estimation of the extent of blood volume or extracellular fluid volume deficit, correction is accomplished with the appropriate fluid. Hartmann's solution (compound sodium lactate) and 0.9% saline are isotonic, remaining predominantly in the extracellular space, and are suitable for replacement of extracellular fluid losses. Haemorrhage is treated preferably by blood transfusion, but alternative fluids may be used (see Ch. 7).

The optimal time for surgical intervention is when all fluid deficits have been corrected, but if there are urgent indications for surgery (e.g. presence of gangrenous bowel), compromise is necessary. As a general rule, the demonstration of orthostatic hypotension indicates that further fluid replacement is required.

Table 32.2 Indices of extent of loss of extracellular fluid

Percentage body weight lost as water	ml of fluid lost per 70 kg	Signs and symptoms
Over 4% (mild)	Over 2500	Thirst, reduced skin elasticity, decreased intraocular pressure, dry tongue, reduced sweating
Over 6% (mild)	Over 4200	As above, plus orthostatic hypotension, reduced filling of peripheral veins, oliguria, nausea, dry axillae and groins, low CVP, apathy, haemoconcentration
Over 8% (moderate)	Over 5500	As above, plus hypotension, thready pulse with cool peripheries
10–15% (severe)	7000–10 500	Coma, shock followed by death

THE FULL STOMACH

Of all the hazards of emergency anaesthesia, vomiting or regurgitation of gastric contents, followed by aspiration into the tracheobronchial tree whilst protective laryngeal reflexes are obtunded, is one of the commonest and most devastating.

Vomiting is an active process that occurs in the lighter planes of anaesthesia. Consequently, it is a potential problem during induction of, or emergence from, anaesthesia, but should not occur during maintenance if anaesthesia is sufficiently deep. In light planes of anaesthesia, the presence of vomited material above the vocal cords stimulates spasm of the cords, which prevents material from entering the larynx. Apnoea may persist until severe hypoxaemia occurs, at which point the vocal cords open and ventilation resumes. Thus the presence of laryngeal reflexes provides a margin of safety provided that the anaesthetist clears the oropharynx of all debris before ventilation resumes.

In contrast, regurgitation is a passive process that may occur at any time, is often 'silent' (i.e.

not apparent to the anaesthetist), and if aspiration occurs, may have clinical consequences ranging from minor pulmonary sequelae to fulminating aspiration pneumonitis. Because regurgitation occurs usually in the presence of deep anaesthesia or at the onset of action of muscle relaxant drugs, laryngeal reflexes are absent and the risk of aspiration is high.

In elective surgery, patients are usually starved of food and drink overnight, or at least for 4–6 h. However, in emergency surgery, it may be necessary to induce anaesthesia urgently before an adequate period of starvation occurs. In addition, the patient's surgical condition is often accompanied by delayed gastric emptying.

The most important factors determining the extent of gastric regurgitation are the function of the lower oesophageal sphincter and the rate of gastric emptying.

The lower oesophageal sphincter

The lower oesophageal sphincter (LOS) is an area (2–5 cm in length) of higher resting intraluminal pressure situated in the region of the cardia. The sphincter relaxes during oesophageal peristalsis to allow food into the stomach, but remains contracted at other times. The structure cannot be defined anatomically but may be detected using intraluminal pressure manometry.

The LOS is the main barrier preventing reflux of gastric contents into the oesophagus, and its resting tone is affected by many drugs used in anaesthetic practice. Reflux is related not to the LOS tone per se, but to the difference between gastric and LOS pressures; this is termed the barrier pressure. Drugs which increase barrier pressure decrease the risk of reflux. Prochlorperazine, cyclizine, anticholinesterases, α-adrenergic agonists and suxamethonium increase barrier pressure. For many years it was thought that the increase in intragastric pressure during suxamethonium-induced fasciculations predisposed to reflux. However, there is an even greater increase in LOS pressure with a consequent increase in barrier pressure.

Anticholinergic drugs, ethanol, ganglion blocking drugs, tricyclic antidepressants, opioids and thiopentone reduce LOS pressure and it is reasonable to assume that these drugs increase the tendency to gastro-oesophageal reflux.

Gastric emptying

Under normal circumstances, peristaltic waves sweep from cardia to pylorus at a rate of approximately 3/min, although temporary inhibition of gastric motility follows recent ingestion of a meal. The rate of gastric emptying is proportional to the volume of the stomach contents, with approximately 1–3% of total gastric content reaching the duodenum per minute. Thus, emptying occurs at an exponential rate. The presence of fat, acid or hypertonic solutions in the duodenum delays significantly the rate of emptying (the inhibitory enterogastric reflex), but both the nervous and humoral elements of this regulating mechanism are still poorly understood. Many pathological conditions are associated with a reduced rate of gastric emptying (Table 32.3). In the absence of any of these factors, it is reasonably safe to assume that the stomach is empty provided that solids have not been ingested within the preceding 6 h, or fluids consumed in the preceding 4 h, and provided normal peristalsis is occurring.

Table 32.3 Situations in which vomiting or regurgitation may occur

Cause	Mechanism
Full stomach	
1. Peritonitis of any cause	Absent or abnormal peristalsis
2. Postoperative ileus	Absent or abnormal peristalsis
3. Metabolic ileus: hypokalaemia, uraemia, diabetic ketoacidosis	Absent or abnormal peristalsis
4. Drug-induced ileus: anticholinergics, those with anticholinergic side effects	Absent or abnormal peristalsis
5. Small or large bowel obstruction	Obstructed peristalsis
6. Gastric carcinoma	Obstructed peristalsis
7. Pyloric stenosis	Delayed gastric emptying
8. Shock of any cause	Delayed gastric emptying
9. Fear, pain or anxiety	Delayed gastric emptying
10. Late pregnancy	Delayed gastric emptying
11. Deep sedation (opioids)	Delayed gastric emptying
12. Recent solid or fluid intake	Delayed gastric emptying
Other causes	
1. Hiatus hernia	
2. Oesophageal strictures — benign or malignant	
3. Pharyngeal pouch	

Vomiting and regurgitation during induction of anaesthesia are encountered most frequently in patients with an acute abdomen or trauma. All patients with minor trauma (fractures or dislocations) must be assumed to have a full stomach; gastric emptying virtually ceases at the time of significant trauma as a result of the combined effects of fear, pain, shock and treatment with opioid analgesics. In all trauma patients, the time interval between ingestion of food and the accident is a more reliable index of the degree of gastric emptying than the period of fasting. It is not uncommon to encounter vomiting up to 24 h after ingestion of food when trauma has occurred very shortly after the meal. Thus the 4–6 h rule is quite unreliable.

TECHNIQUES OF ANAESTHESIA

It is important to recognise any patient who may have significant gastric residue and is in danger of aspiration. The anaesthetic management of such a patient may be described in five phases: preparation, induction, maintenance, emergence and postoperative management.

Phase I — preparation

Whilst postponement of surgery in the emergency patient may be indicated in order to obtain investigations and institute resuscitation with i.v. fluids, there is usually no benefit to be gained in terms of reducing the risks associated with aspiration of gastric contents. However, two manoeuvres are available:

1. Insertion of a nasogastric tube and aspiration of the stomach contents. This is useful when gastric contents are liquid, as in bowel obstruction, but is less effective when contents are solid.
2. Neutralisation of the pH of gastric contents (e.g. with sodium citrate) or decreasing gastric acid secretion with an H_2-receptor antagonist to reduce the chance of acid aspiration syndrome occurring in the event of inhalation. Although this is standard practice in obstetric anaesthesia, few anaesthetists employ these measures for emergency general surgery. The regimens which may be used are described in Chapters 14 and 33.

Phase II — induction

Rapid-sequence induction

This is the technique employed most frequently for the patient with a full stomach, although it contravenes one of the fundamental rules of anaesthesia, namely that muscle relaxants are not given until control of the airway is assured. The decision to employ the rapid-sequence induction technique balances the risk of losing control of the airway against the risk of aspiration. It is therefore imperative to assess carefully whether or not difficulty is likely to be encountered in performing tracheal intubation. The anaesthetist must have prepared a contingency plan for management of the patient should intubation fail. If preoperative evaluation indicates a particularly difficult airway, the anaesthetist should consider alternative methods of proceeding, e.g. local anaesthetic techniques or 'awake intubation' under local anaesthesia.

For rapid-sequence induction to be consistently safe and successful it should be performed with meticulous attention to detail. The patient *must* be on a tipping trolley or table, preferably with an adjustable head piece so that the degree of neck extension/flexion may be altered quickly. Ideally, the patient's head should be in the classical 'sniffing position' with the neck flexed on the shoulders and the head extended on the neck. Failure to appreciate this point increases the likelihood of difficult intubation.

The anaesthetist *must* be aided by at least one skilled assistant to perform cricoid pressure, assist in turning the patient, obtain smaller tracheal tubes, supply stilettes for tubes, etc. Suction apparatus *must* be functional and the suction catheter within reach of the anaesthetist's hand.

As with any anaesthetic, the machine should have been checked before starting, the ventilator adjusted to appropriate settings and all drugs drawn up into labelled syringes before induction. The patient should breathe 100% O_2 for 3–5 min while appropriate monitoring devices are attached and an i.v. infusion started (if not already in place). The optimal inclination of the operating table is debatable as some authorities recommend the reverse Trendelenburg (head-up) position (to prevent regurgitation), and some the classical

Trendelenburg position (to prevent aspiration of any regurgitated or vomited material). In general, the optimum position is that in which the junior anaesthetist has gained greatest experience in performing intubation.

Preinduction measurement of heart rate, arterial pressure (and when appropriate central venous pressure), and inspection of the ECG are made and a skilled assistant is positioned on the patient's right side to perform Sellick's manoeuvre (cricoid pressure). It is important that the assistant can identify the cricoid cartilage, as compression of the thyroid cartilage distorts laryngeal anatomy and may render tracheal intubation very difficult. To perform Sellick's manoeuvre correctly, the thumb and forefinger of the right hand press the cricoid cartilage firmly in a posterior direction, thus compressing the oesophagus between the cricoid cartilage and the vertebral column. Because the cricoid cartilage forms a complete ring, the tracheal lumen is not distorted (Fig. 32.1).

Opinions differ with regard to the time at which cricoid pressure should be applied. Some prefer to inform the patient and apply it just before administration of the i.v. induction agent; others apply it as soon as consciousness is lost.

With the assistant in position, a predetermined sleep dose of i.v. induction agent is given (usually thiopentone, 2–4 mg/kg or less in the presence of hypovolaemia). Without waiting to assess the effect of the induction agent, a paralysing dose of suxamethonium (1.5 mg/kg) is administered immediately. As soon as the jaw begins to relax, laryngoscopy is performed and the trachea intubated with the aid of a stilette. Cricoid pressure *is maintained* until the cuff of the tracheal tube is inflated and correct placement of the tube ascertained by auscultation of both lungs. The lungs are *gently* ventilated manually as excessive increases in intrathoracic pressure may have harmful effects on circulatory dynamics. One of the main disadvantages of the rapid-sequence induction technique is the haemodynamic instability which may result if the dose of induction agent is excessive (hypotension, circulatory collapse) or inadequate (hypertension, tachycardia, arrhythmia). Unfortunately, selection of the correct dose is difficult and is dependent largely upon the experience of the anaesthetist. For thiopentone, a dose of 4 mg/kg may suffice for healthy, young patients, 2 mg/kg for the elderly, and less for the very frail. Alternatives are etomidate 0.1–0.3 mg/kg (which is less cardiodepressant than thiopentone) and methohexitone 1–1.5 mg/kg.

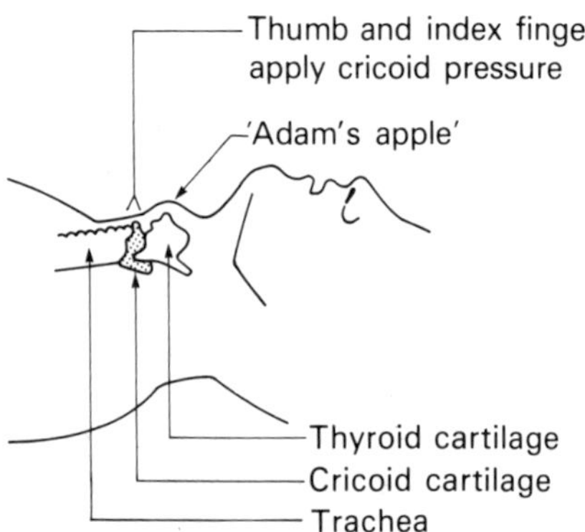

Fig. 32.1 Sellick's manoeuvre. The cricoid cartilage is palpated immediately below the thyroid cartilage.

Inhalational induction

If there is reasonable doubt about the ability to perform intubation or to maintain a patent airway in a patient with a full stomach (e.g. the patient with faciomaxillary trauma or the child with epiglottitis), an inhalational induction may be used with oxygen and halothane, followed by an attempt at tracheal intubation during spontaneous ventilation. Normally, the patient should be placed in the left lateral, head-down position, but if circumstances do not allow the lateral position then the supine posture with cricoid pressure may have to be accepted.

Awake intubation

Blind nasal intubation is a valuable skill which should be acquired by all anaesthetists. It is most useful in patients who are likely to develop unrelievable airway obstruction when loss of consciousness occurs (e.g. trismus from dental abscess or angioneurotic oedema) although it may be performed also on unconscious patients. Before embarking on blind nasal intubation in the awake subject it is necessary to render the upper airway insensitive so that introduction of a tracheal tube may be tolerated. This is accomplished in three stages:

1. The nasal mucosa is anaesthetised with cocaine solution 4% (maximum 2.5 ml/70 kg) which is sprayed into the more patent nasal passage. In addition to providing surface anaesthesia, this shrinks the nasal mucosa and greatly reduces the chance of bleeding.

2. The superior laryngeal branch of the vagus nerve is blocked as it sweeps around the hyoid bone. A 23 G needle is 'walked' off the inferior border of the greater cornu of the hyoid near its tip and approximately 3 ml of 1% lignocaine is deposited deep to the thyrohyoid membrane. A slight loss of resistance is felt as this membrane is penetrated by the needle. Successful bilateral block of the superior laryngeal nerve produces anaesthesia of the inferior surface of the epiglottis and the laryngeal inlet as far down as the vocal cords.

3. Anaesthesia of the tracheal mucosa below the vocal cords is accomplished best by transtracheal injection of local anaesthetic. A 21 G needle is introduced in the midline through the cricothyroid membrane. Entry into the trachea is confirmed by aspiration of air and a bolus of 3–5 ml of lignocaine 1% is injected rapidly. Invariably this results in a bout of coughing which aids spread of the local anaesthetic over the inferior surface of the vocal cords.

A simpler method to establish satisfactory anaesthesia of the upper airway is to nebulise 3–4 ml of lignocaine 4% through an oxygen face-mask. This process takes 10–20 min but is tolerated well by patients and requires less expertise.

Whichever technique is employed, anaesthesia of the upper airway increases the risk of pulmonary aspiration if vomiting or regurgitation occurs. Thus, these techniques should be employed in the emergency situation only after a full consideration of the potential benefits has been weighed against the risks of aspiration. For patients in whom there is a high risk of aspiration, it is possible with experience to perform awake blind nasal intubation after performing only step 1 above. However, this involves considerable discomfort for the patient and is not practised widely in the UK.

If a standard curved tracheal tube is advanced through the nose it enters the trachea in approximately 50% of patients without special manipulation. In the other 50% of patients, a sequence of manoeuvres increases the probability of success.

With the patient's head in the 'sniffing the morning air' position, a well-lubricated tube is inserted gently into the anaesthetised nostril and advanced towards the nasopharynx. The tube should be rotated slowly between thumb and forefinger (pill-rolling movement) and a distinct 'give' is felt on entry into the nasopharynx. As maximal vocal cord abduction occurs during inspiration, the tube is now advanced slowly in small steps coordinated with inspiration. Even with good upper airway anaesthesia, entry into the larynx results frequently in a violent cough but even if this occurs the position of the tube must be confirmed before general anaesthesia is induced.

If the tracheal tube does not enter the trachea it must be situated in the oesophagus or one or other pyriform fossa, or caught on the anterior commissure of the larynx. If it is in the oesophagus, no breath sounds emanate from the end of the tube after complete insertion. The tube should be withdrawn into the pharynx and re-advanced whilst the patient's head is extended slightly.

If the tip of the tube is lying in the pyriform fossa, a slight bulge is apparent in the neck just above the larynx, to the left or right of the midline. In this situation, successful intubation is achieved by withdrawal of the tube a few centimetres, rotation towards the midline and reinsertion.

If the tube cannot be inserted completely and sustained pressure does not produce a bulge on either side of the larynx, it is almost certainly caught on the anterior commissure. It should be withdrawn a few centimetres and reinserted after slight flexion of the patient's head.

In a small number of patients (e.g. those with severe neck deformity) blind nasal intubation is impossible. In this situation, use of the fibreoptic endoscope is valuable. However, considerable practice is needed in the operation of this instrument to ensure a successful outcome.

Regional anaesthesia

Anaesthetic expertise in the use of regional anaesthesia is lacking in many United Kingdom hospitals. This is unfortunate as local blocks are eminently suitable for emergency procedures on the extremities (e.g. to reduce fractures or dislocations).

Brachial plexus block by the axillary, supraclavicular or interscalene approach is satisfactory for orthopaedic manipulations or surgical procedures involving the upper extremity. It satisfies surgical requirements for analgesia, muscle relaxation and immobility. There is minimal effect on the cardiovascular system and there is a prolonged period of analgesia postoperatively. Similarly, i.v. regional anaesthesia (Bier's block, p. 464) is useful for orthopaedic reductions; prilocaine 0.5% plain is the drug of choice.

For regional anaesthesia of the lower extremity, techniques available include subarachnoid and extradural anaesthesia. These techniques are contraindicated if there is doubt about adequacy of ECF or vascular volumes, as large decreases in arterial pressure may result from the associated pharmacological sympathectomy.

It is a common surgical misconception that subarachnoid or extradural anaesthetic techniques are safer than general anaesthesia for patients in poor physical condition. It must be emphasised that for the *inexperienced* anaesthetist, these techniques are *invariably more dangerous* than general anaesthesia for the patient with moderate/major trauma or any intra-abdominal emergency condition.

Phase III — maintenance of anaesthesia

In emergency anaesthesia, there are strong arguments in favour of a balanced technique of anaesthesia combining:

1. Anaesthesia: loss of awareness.
2. Analgesia to attenuate autonomic reflexes in response to the painful stimulus.
3. Muscle relaxation.

If a rapid-sequence induction has been performed, the patient's lungs are gently ventilated manually whilst heart rate and arterial pressure measurements are repeated to assess the cardiovascular effects of the drugs used and of the insult of tracheal intubation. Nitrous oxide 50–66% (dependent upon the patient's condition) in oxygen contributes to loss of patient awareness but does not ensure it, and some anaesthetists advocate the use of either 0.5% halothane, 0.5–1% isoflurane or 0.5–1% enflurane in addition.

When there is evidence of return of neuromuscular transmission (by clinical signs or use of a nerve stimulator) as suxamethonium is degraded, a non-depolarising myoneural blocking agent is administered. The choice is dependent upon the patient's condition and the effect of the induction of anaesthesia on the patient's cardiovascular status. Vecuronium is an appropriate drug for routine use in a dose of 80–100 μg/kg. Pancuronium (dose 50–100 μg/kg) is useful in patients with hypovolaemia, as it tends to increase arterial pressure and heart rate. (The tachycardia it produces is undesirable in patients with ischaemic heart disease or valvular disease). Alcuronium (250–300 μg/kg) is an alternative drug, but it may produce hypotension which is not usually desirable in emergency anaesthesia. Atracurium has virtually no cardiovascular effects in clinical doses and is useful if renal impairment is present.

When the muscle relaxant has been administered, the tracheal tube is connected to a mechanical ventilator and minute volume adjusted to produce normo- or slight hypocapnia. There are few accurate means of estimating ventilatory requirement, but a minute volume of 100 ml kg^{-1} min^{-1} at a tidal volume of 8–12 ml/kg should be employed initially. The inspiratory flow rate should be adjusted to minimise peak airway pressure.

Before the initial surgical incision is made, analgesia may be supplemented by small incremental doses of morphine 1–5 mg, papaveretum 2–10 mg, or fentanyl 25–100 μg.

The use of supplemental doses of analgesic and muscle relaxant drugs are described in Chapters 11 and 12. The trainee should be aware that during emergency anaesthesia, particularly for intra-abdominal or trauma surgery, much smaller doses of drugs are usually required. As a general rule, it is safe practice to administer half the dose which might be considered appropriate for an elective patient, and to determine further doses by assessment of the subsequent response. If there are poor or inadequate recovery room facilities, it is also a good general rule to err on the side of caution in the use of i.v. drugs and consider supplementing anaesthesia with a volatile agent.

Fluid management

During emergency intra-abdominal surgery there may be large blood and fluid losses which exceed the patient's maintenance fluid replacement. These include evaporative losses from exposed gut and mesentery, blood loss on to swabs and into suction bottles, and the poorly defined 'third space losses' caused by sequestration of fluid in inflamed and traumatised tissue. Intraoperatively, maintenance requirements are supplied with Hartmann's solution (compound sodium lactate) at 2 ml kg^{-1} h^{-1}. An appropriate volume of replacement for third space loss and evaporative gut loss is given in addition. This volume depends on the degree of surgical trauma but is normally in the range 2–7 ml kg^{-1} h^{-1}.

Haemorrhage in excess of 15% blood volume in adults or 10% in children is usually an indication for blood transfusion.

Phase IV — reversal and emergence

Any volatile agent is discontinued 5–10 min before surgery finishes. On insertion of the last skin suture, direct pharyngoscopy is performed and secretions/debris removed from the pharynx; if a nasogastric tube is in situ, it is aspirated and left unspigoted. Atropine and neostigmine are given in one bolus of 20 μg/kg and 50 μg/kg respectively, and ventilation is undertaken manually (with an $F\text{I}_{O_2}$ of 1.0) so that spontaneous ventilatory activity may be detected. Because the risk of aspiration of gastric contents is as great on recovery as at induction, extubation of the trachea should not be performed until protective airway reflexes are intact. To demonstrate adequacy of reflexes, both level of consciousness and neuromuscular transmission should be assessed.

Level of consciousness. The patient should be awake and respond appropriately to verbal commands, e.g. eye opening.

Neuromuscular function. The adequacy of reversal of paralysis may be determined by observing the patient's ability to sustain a head lift for 5 s and ability to sustain a firm grip without fade (see Table 12.5). Preferably, a nerve stimulator is used to define reversal of neuromuscular transmission (see Ch. 12).

Immediately before tracheal extubation, the patient is turned to the lateral position (if possible) and asked to take a deep inspiration while gentle positive pressure is applied to the airway. At the peak of inspiration, the cuff is deflated and the tracheal tube removed as the patient exhales, thus assisting removal of any secretions which may have accumulated above the cuff. Oxygen 100% is administered until a regular ventilatory rhythm is re-established and the patient has demonstrated an ability to cough and maintain a patent airway. Breathing 40% O_2 he is transported in the lateral position to the recovery room and remains there until all vital signs are stable, postoperative shivering has ceased, core temperature is normal, and there is good perfusion as judged by warm extremities and good urine output.

If there is any doubt about the adequacy of ventilation after reversal of neuromuscular blockade, the patient is taken to the recovery room with the tracheal tube in situ and this is removed from the trachea only when ventilation and gas exchange are adequate.

Phase V — postoperative management

Postoperatively the patient requires analgesics, e.g. morphine 0.2 mg/kg i.m. 4-hourly, or papaveretum 0.3 mg/kg 4-hourly. If there is continued concern about the metabolic or volaemic state of the patient, these dosages should be reduced considerably.

Fluid balance should take into account maintenance needs plus compensation for abnormal fluid loss (e.g. gastric aspirate, loss from intestinal fistulae, or from surgical drains). This subject is discussed in Chapter 22.

The need for further blood replacement is assessed by regular observation of vital signs and drainage measurements, and postoperative Hb or haematocrit measurements.

Prophylactic postoperative IPPV

Continuation of IPPV should be considered electively in a number of ill-defined circumstances, some of which are listed in Table 32.4.

THE ANAESTHETIST AND MAJOR TRAUMA

The management of the patient with major trauma requires a multidisciplinary team effort. Successful treatment is often dependent on the efficacy of the initial resuscitation and rapid formulation of the correct priorities.

Immediate care

As soon as the patient arrives in the Accident and Emergency Department, resuscitation, diagnosis and specific treatment are required simultaneously.

The first priority for the anaesthetist is to establish the patency of the patient's airway. If upper airway obstruction is present, the pharynx is cleared of any debris, the jaw displaced forward (jaw thrust), and the neck extended gently. This manoeuvre must be performed very carefully in any patient with a potential cervical spine injury.

Once the airway is clear, attention is directed to the adequacy of ventilation and the need for tracheal intubation. If the patient is apnoeic, ventilation by mask with 100% oxygen is started immediately, as good oxygenation and correction of hypercapnia should be ensured before tracheal intubation is undertaken.

Patients with severe faciomaxillary trauma who are cooperative and awake despite their injuries may not require immediate tracheal intubation, but do need frequent and regular upper airway evaluation to assess the rate of progress of pharyngeal or laryngeal oedema which may proceed to complete airway obstruction with alarming rapidity.

Once the airway is under control, ventilation is deemed adequate, and any obvious external bleeding has been arrested, the next priority is evaluation of the cardiovascular system; this may be divided into assessment of blood volume status and pump function.

Table 32.4 Indications for continuation of ventilatory assistance postoperatively

1. Prolonged shock/hypoperfusion state of any cause
2. Massive sepsis (faecal peritonitis, cholangitis, septicaemia)
3. Severe ischaemic heart disease
4. Extreme obesity
5. Overt gastric acid aspiration
6. Previously severe pulmonary disease

Volume status

This has been described earlier in this chapter. Patients with major trauma often require urgent restoration of circulating blood volume. At least two large-bore (14-gauge) i.v. cannulae are inserted percutaneously into veins in one or two limbs, and at least one is attached to a blood warming coil. As soon as possible, a reliable CVP line is inserted. The right internal jugular vein is the preferred site for this purpose. Fluid is infused through the peripheral i.v. cannulae to produce a CVP of approximately 0–3 cmH_2O (manubrium being the zero reference).

Whilst whole blood is the ideal fluid for restoration of blood volume in haemorrhagic shock, substitute fluid should be given immediately while cross-matching is undertaken. If total exsanguination is imminent, type-specific blood may be given, as the chance of a reaction is less than 1% in males, but over 2% in parous females. If the patient has 20–30% blood volume depletion, 2 litres of Hartmann's solution may be infused rapidly whilst cross-matching is in progress. If this does not increase perfusion and arterial pressure significantly, and blood is still not available, either plasma or a plasma substitute should be considered. Human albumin solution is very expensive and probably has little advantage over gelatin solutions (p. 136). Their half-life in the circulation is approximately 4 h in the normal patient, but is shorter in the presence of shock. As 85% is excreted by the kidneys, gelatin solutions promote an osmotic diuresis and may therefore preserve urine output and renal function. Up to 1500 ml may be given initially; in most circumstances this is adequate to restore circulating blood volume until cross-matched blood is available. Warmed, stored blood is administered subsequently to maintain urine output, arterial pressure and CVP.

Pump function

The commonest cause of pump failure in major trauma is the presence of a tension pneumothorax, but other possibilities include severe myocardial contusion and traumatic pericardial tamponade.

Tension pneumothorax causes compression of the mediastinum (heart and great vessels) and presents with extreme respiratory distress, shock, unilateral air entry, a shift of the trachea towards the normal side and distension of the veins in the neck, although the last sign may not be seen in hypovolaemic shock. It may be relieved immediately by insertion of a 14-gauge cannula through the 2nd intercostal space in the midclavicular line but this should be followed by standard chest drainage. If there is any suspicion of tension pneumothorax, IPPV should not be instituted until decompression has been achieved, otherwise mediastinal compression is increased. Patients with blunt chest trauma and fractured ribs may develop a tension pneumothorax rapidly when positive pressure ventilation is instituted and consideration should be given to the prophylactic insertion of chest drains in such patients.

Definitive care

Whenever possible, hypovolaemia should be corrected before anaesthesia is induced, but if the rate of haemorrhage is likely to exceed the rate of transfusion, and continued transfusion results only in further bleeding (e.g. ruptured aorta), it may be necessary to induce anaesthesia in a hypovolaemic patient.

On arrival in theatre, the patient is placed on the operating table, which is covered by a warming blanket at 37°C. One hundred per cent oxygen is given whilst at least two large-gauge cannulae are inserted (one connected to a blood warming coil), if this has not already been accomplished. In patients with major trauma, anaesthesia should be induced in theatre so that surgery can start as soon as possible. Figure 32.2 illustrates standard monitoring which is necessary for the management of major trauma.

In the unconscious patient, the trachea may be intubated after administration of a paralysing dose of suxamethonium. If the patient is conscious, despite being severely hypovolaemic, a controlled rapid-sequence induction employing ketamine as the i.v. induction agent is preferred. The dose of ketamine is critical and often very small doses (0.3–0.7 mg/kg) suffice. If the dose is misjudged, cardiovascular decompensation similar to that seen with other i.v. induction agents may occur. The depressant effects of i.v. induction agents are exaggerated because the *proportion* of the cardiac output going to the heart and brain is increased. In addition, the rate of redistribution and/or metabolism is decreased as a result of reduced blood flow to muscle, liver and kidneys, and thus blood concentrations remain elevated for longer periods in comparison with healthy patients. Ketamine should not be used in patients with significant head injury. Etomidate (0.1–0.3 mg/kg) is an alternative for normovolaemic or marginally hypovolaemic patients with head injury, but is more likely to attenuate compensatory mechanisms. Even a single bolus dose of etomidate may interfere with adrenal function and recommendations concerning the use of this drug must be guarded.

After tracheal intubation, the lungs are ventilated at the lowest peak airway pressure consistent with an acceptable tidal volume. Pancuronium is given in small incremental doses of 1 mg to maintain relaxation. When the haemodynamic situation has stabilised and systolic arterial pressure exceeds 90 mmHg, consideration may be given to deepening anaesthesia. This should be undertaken cautiously and, in principle, agents which are rapidly reversible or rapidly excreted should be employed.

In the shock state, there is very rapid uptake of inhalational agents. As a result of chemoreceptor stimulation, the patient hyperventilates, thus accelerating the rate of increase of alveolar concentration of anaesthetic gas. Similarly, reduced cardiac output and pulmonary blood flow decrease the rate of removal of anaesthetic agent from the alveoli, producing a rapid increase in alveolar concentration. Thus the MAC value is

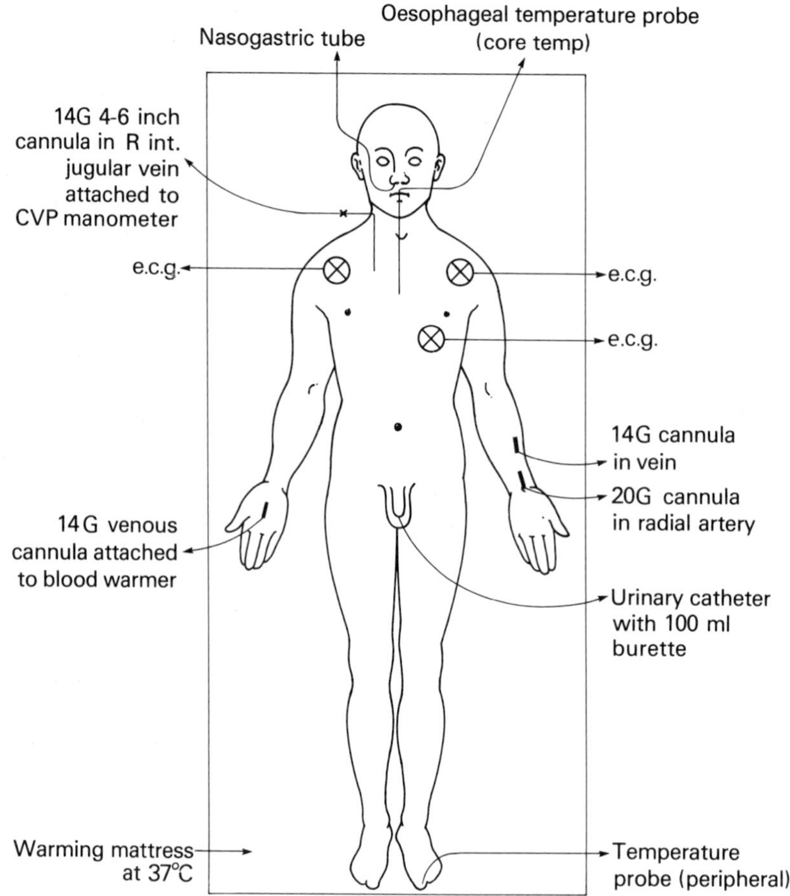

Fig. 32.2 Commonly used monitoring and resuscitation attachments in management of a patient with multiple injuries.

approached more rapidly than in normovolaemic patients.

Monitoring should be comprehensive in these patients (Fig. 32.2) and should be instituted before induction of anaesthesia when feasible. Blood may be sampled from the arterial line to monitor changes in blood gases, acid–base state, haemoglobin concentration, PCV and electrolyte concentrations. Requirements for further colloid replacement may be assessed from CVP measurement and urine output.

When surgical bleeding has been controlled, the patient's cardiovascular status should improve, but if hypotension persists despite apparently adequate fluid administration, other causes of haemorrhage should be sought (Table 32.5). It is important that the anaesthetist assesses the patient regularly during prolonged anaesthesia to exclude these latent complications of major trauma.

Table 32.5 Causes of persistent hypotension

Cause	
1. Continued overt bleeding	Surgical or medical (check platelets and clotting screen)
2. Continued concealed bleeding — chest, abdomen, retroperitoneal space, pelvis, soft tissues of each thigh	
3. Pump failure — haemothorax, pneumothorax, tamponade, myocardial contusion	
4. Metabolic problem — acidaemia (only correct pH less than 7.1) hypothermia (largely preventable) hypocalcaemia	

Massive transfusion

One definition states that if an amount greater than 50% of the patient's blood volume is replaced rapidly, the transfusion is deemed massive, e.g. 5 units of blood in 1 h in a 70-kg adult.

Stored blood is an unphysiological solution with a pH of 7.2–6.6, serum potassium concentration of 5–25 mmol/litre and a temperature of 4–6°C. It contains citrate as an anticoagulant. When stored for more than five days, it contains insignificant amounts of 2,3-DPG; consequently, the oxy-haemoglobin dissociation curve is shifted to the left. Blood stored for longer than 24 h has no functional platelets; concentrations of factors V and VIII are approximately 10% of normal and factor IX 20% of normal. Effete cells and platelets clump together forming debris which is potentially harmful when infused in sufficient quantity.

Many of these disadvantages of stored blood are not clinical problems; for example, citrate is removed by metabolic conversion in the liver (forming mostly bicarbonate), the transfused cells act as a 'potassium sink' and mop up excess potassium quickly and the post-transfusion alkalosis (resulting from citrate metabolism) may contribute to hypokalaemia in the post-transfusion period.

If the transfused blood is warmed near to body temperature before infusion and a 20 μm filter is used to remove unwanted cellular debris, the commonest problem is that of haemostatic failure.

Transfusion of bank blood in quantities approaching the patient's blood volume causes a dilutional thrombocytopenia and some measure of clotting factor deficiency, both of which affect haemostasis adversely. These abnormalities may be detected by a platelet count, prothrombin time and partial thromboplastin time, reflecting disorders of extrinsic and intrinsic systems as a result of dilutional loss of factors V and VIII. Treatment should be directed at correcting the dilutional coagulation change and consists of fresh frozen plasma (1 unit for every 4 units of blood) and, occasionally, platelet concentrate for severe thrombocytopenia (platelet count below 30×10^9/litre). Requests for these expensive blood components should be made early as there is often delay in obtaining them, and it is better, if possible, to prevent the development of coagulation failure.

FURTHER READING

Adams A P, Hewitt P B, Rogers M C (eds) 1986 Emergency anaesthesia. Arnold, London

Campbell D 1979 The anaesthetist and trauma. In: Atkinson R S, Langton-Hewer C (eds) Recent advances in anaesthesia and analgesia, 13. Churchill Livingstone, Edinburgh

Campbell D 1977 Immediate hospital care of the injured. British Journal of Anaesthesia 49: 673

Cotton B R, Smith G 1982 The lower oesophageal sphincter. In: Kaufman L (ed) Anaesthesia review. 1. Churchill Livingstone, Edinburgh

Giesecke A H 1986 Perioperative fluid therapy — crystalloids. In: Miller R D (ed) Anaesthesia, 2nd edn. vol 2. Churchill Livingstone, Edinburgh

Horsey P J 1982 Blood transfusion. In: Atkinson R S, Langton Hewer C (eds) Recent advances in anaesthesia and analgesia, 14. Churchill Livingstone, Edinburgh

Magill I W 1975 Lest we forget — blind nasal intubation. Anaesthesia 30: 476

Pavlin E 1989 Emergency anaesthesia in trauma. In: Nimmo W S, Smith G (eds) Anaesthesia. Blackwell Scientific Publications, Oxford

Sellick B A 1961 Cricothyroid pressure to control regurgitation of stomach contents during induction of anaesthesia. Lancet 2: 404

Sutcliffe A J 1983 Handbook of emergency anaesthesia. Butterworths, London

Thornton J A 1980 Blood loss, colloid infusion and blood transfusion. In: Gray T C, Nunn J F, Utting J E (eds) General anaesthesia, 4th edn. Butterworths, London

Walters F J M, Nott M R 1977 The hazards of anaesthesia in the injured patient. British Journal of Anaesthesia 49: 707

33. Obstetric anaesthesia and analgesia

The profound physiological effects of pregnancy have an important role in altering the maternal response to systemically administered analgesics, anaesthetic drugs and vertebral blocks. These changes are described in detail in Chapter 6.

History

Labour is painful for the majority of mothers, and extremely painful for some. Indeed, progress in labour in former years was related frequently to the degree of pain experienced by the mother. The successful outcome, the delivery of a healthy baby and survival of a healthy mother, reduced the subjective importance of the pain experienced by the mother during labour. However, not all mothers have a successful outcome. Before 1846, little could be done to relieve the distress and suffering undergone by those mothers. In that year, Simpson administered ether to a labouring mother and delivered her of a dead child. The significance of the benefits of general anaesthesia were apparent immediately and were welcomed in other fields of surgical practice, but considerable resistance to its adoption in obstetrics was manifest by the conservative clergy, and it says much for Simpson's strength of character and eloquence that he overcame the clergy's criticisms successfully.

Although ether was the first anaesthetic agent, chloroform was adopted quickly as the drug of choice. The importance and acceptance of general anaesthesia and analgesia by inhalational methods may be judged by the fact that chloroform was administered to Queen Victoria by Dr John Snow at the birth of her eighth child in 1853. The administration of chloroform was probably unnecessary but it was a powerful advertisement for its safety and propriety, and resistance crumbled subsequently.

Spinal anaesthesia, introduced by Bier in 1899, was popularised by Tuffier and gained widespread acceptance rapidly. By 1907, it had been used widely in almost all branches of surgery, including obstetrics. Complications such as ventilatory failure, hypotension and the high incidence of headaches were recognised but were outweighed by the benefits. Systemic analgesics were introduced in obstetrics in 1901; morphine was employed initially but the combination of papaveretum and hyoscine (twilight sleep) became the most popular technique. The value and safety of nitrous oxide/oxygen or air mixtures were known but the early apparatus was cumbersome and it was not until 1933, when Minnitt introduced a portable nitrous oxide/air machine, that inhalational analgesia became widespread. Unfortunately, the mixture of nitrous oxide and air was hypoxic. Nevertheless, the Minnitt apparatus was used widely in the UK. Extradural analgesia was not introduced to obstetric practice until 1941 and in the UK a continuous extradural analgesia service did not become available until 1964.

Innervation of the uterus and birth canal

This is depicted in Figure 33.1. Afferent nerves from the body of the uterus and the cervix are somatic sensory fibres, although they travel with sympathetic nerves. They emerge bilaterally from the uterus on each side of the cervix and pass laterally in the paracervical tissues to traverse the cervical plexus. The fibres continue in the base of the broad ligament, pass through the inferior, middle and superior hypogastric plexuses and

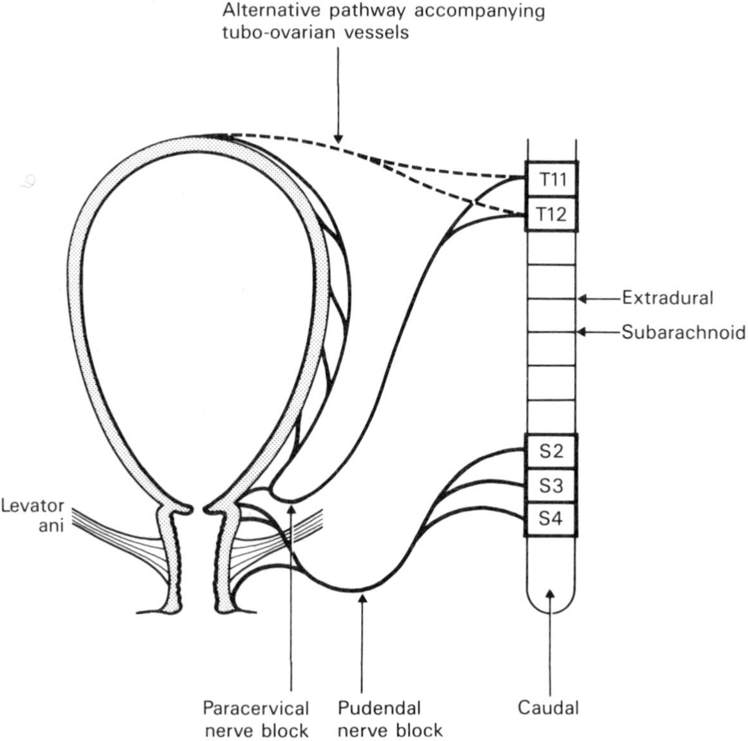

Fig. 33.1 Nerve supply of uterus and birth canal, and regional anaesthetic techniques which may be used to produce pain relief during labour and vaginal delivery.

enter the sympathetic chain in the lumbar and lower thoracic regions. The central connection from the sympathetic chain is via the white rami communicantes of the 11th and 12th thoracic nerves; in some women, a proportion of nerve fibres pass through the first lumbar nerve. There may be an additional afferent pathway from the cervix to S2–4 through the pelvic splanchnic nerves.

The haemorrhoidal and perineal nerves, and the dorsal nerve of clitoris, carry impulses from the vagina, vulva and perineum through the pudendal nerve bilaterally to S2–4; the pudendal nerves also provide the motor supply to levator ani. Some areas of perineal and vulval skin are innervated by the ileo-inguinal, genitofemoral and posterior femoral cutaneous nerves, and by cutaneous branches of S2–4.

Sympathetic (T5–L2) and parasympathetic fibres (S2–4) carry efferent impulses to the uterus and affect its motor function. However, uterine contractility during labour is largely independent of these impulses.

PAIN RELIEF IN LABOUR

Pain during the first stage of labour results both from uterine contractions and dilatation of the cervix. In the second stage, pain is caused by stretching, distension and tearing of fascia, skin and subcutaneous tissues, and by pressure on the skeletal muscle of the perineum.

This brief account of analgesia and anaesthesia in obstetrics does not deal in depth with the subject of preparation of the mother for labour. This should not deny or diminish the importance of adequate, skilled preparation. The aspirations and expectations of each mother differ and should be taken into account in the assessment of analgesic requirements. Preparation for labour must include adequate discussion of the methods available during labour and delivery, and the advantages and disadvantages of each method. It is clear from studies of pain relief in labour that the pain experienced by many mothers is extremely severe, but that the most effective method of pain relief, extradural analgesia, does not necessarily provide the greatest maternal satisfaction. Pethidine and Entonox have been shown to be relatively ineffective in relieving pain, but the proportion of satisfied mothers is similar among those who receive extradural analgesia and those given pethidine and Entonox for pain relief during labour. Clearly, pain is only one element of the distress of labour; however, it may be treated effectively and therapy must not be withheld. Psychological preparation and sympathetic support are essential during labour.

It is impossible to predict when emergency intervention may be required in obstetrics, and oral fluids are usually restricted in the interests of safety. Dehydration and thirst may be distressing. An i.v. infusion is mandatory if extradural analgesia is considered, and should be administered to any mother who is dehydrated. Ketosis is a normal accompaniment of labour and is not necessarily related to the degree of dehydration. The use of i.v. solutions that contain glucose to relieve ketosis is unnecessary and should be avoided; either saline 0.9% or compound sodium lactate solution should be used. Frequently, labour is augmented by i.v. syntocinon, which is best prepared in a concentrated form and administered by a syringe pump to limit the volume infused.

Systemic analgesics

The ideal analgesic drug should relieve pain without other effects on the mother and baby. Unfortunately, none of the available drugs is without side effects and all opioid analgesics share similar advantages and disadvantages. The disadvantages of opioid analgesic drugs include:

1. Transfer across the placental barrier.
2. Sedation of the baby.
3. Ventilatory depression of the mother.
4. Delay in maternal gastric emptying.

Pethidine is the most popular sedative analgesic used in British obstetric practice. It is administered most frequently by i.m. injection in a dose of 100–150 mg. It is most effective when given relatively early in labour, before patient distress is too severe. There is a rapid increase in the maternal serum pethidine concentration after i.m. injection, followed by a similar and parallel increase in fetal serum pethidine concentration as the drug crosses the placenta freely. Paediatric staff should be informed if pethidine has been administered within 3 h of delivery, as it may induce ventilatory depression in the neonate. Neonatal ventilatory depression resulting from opioid drugs administered to the mother may be reversed easily by naloxone (20 μg injected into the umbilical cord vein). Neurobehavioural assessment studies of neonates whose mothers have been given pethidine have shown that the influence of the analgesic may be detected for up to 48 h after delivery. The long-term significance of these effects (if any) is not known.

Pethidine may be administered intravenously, either as a single bolus injection or by patient-controlled analgesia (see p. 453). The volume and maximum frequency of administration are flexible, and preset on the machine by medical or nursing staff. Excessive demands by the mother are prevented, thus limiting the total dose to the preset maximum.

Extradural/subarachnoid opioids

The introduction of extradural or subarachnoid injection of opioid drugs was welcomed initially, but subsequent assessment has been disappointing. The non-selective blockade provided by local analgesic drugs injected into the extradural or subarachnoid space results in loss of sympathetic control and the development of motor block; these are undesirable. The extradural administration of a drug which would relieve only pain is most attractive but unfortunately the agents that are available currently have proved to be far from ideal. The drugs of low lipid solubility (pethidine and morphine) have undesirable side effects such as itching (which may be severe), nausea and the risk of delayed ventilatory depression. In addition, analgesia is not very effective during labour, and consequently their use has been limited.

Lipophilic drugs (fentanyl and methadone) have the theoretical advantage that they remain at the site of injection, being absorbed locally in the extradural fat and released slowly over a period of time; however, they have not been used extensively in pregnancy. Fentanyl is effective in providing pain relief after Caesarean section, but has proved to be of little benefit for pain relief in labour. Recent investigations have shown that extradural fentanyl combined with local anaesthetic solution is effective if administered at the onset of the second stage of labour.

Inhalational analgesia

Entonox, a mixture of nitrous oxide 50% in oxygen, is the most widely used inhalational analgesic agent in the UK. It has the advantages of providing a high inspired oxygen concentration and rapid onset of analgesia, and is self-administered. The rapid onset is attributable to the relatively insoluble nature of nitrous oxide in blood, and is mirrored by an equally rapid elimination; consequently, it is non-cumulative. The apparatus designed for its use is simple and safe, provided that the cylinders are kept at a temperature above 7°C (see p. 272). Nitrous oxide is not inert, but there are no physiological or biochemical consequences of note in the concentrations and durations used in obstetric practice. Entonox is used usually in conjunction with pethidine, and the majority of labours in the UK are conducted with pethidine and Entonox analgesia.

Formerly, low concentrations of trichloroethylene or methoxyflurane were administered by calibrated drawover vaporisers, but their use has been discontinued.

Local anaesthetic techniques

Many different local blocks have been described for use in obstetrics, but have been replaced to a large extent by extradural block.

Pudendal block

Pudendal block may be used to produce analgesia for low-cavity instrumental delivery. The block is performed usually by the obstetrician. Using the vaginal approach, the pudendal nerves are blocked as they pass under and slightly posterior to the ischial tuberosity. The major disadvantage is that the block is frequently unilateral. In addition, there is a distinct risk of exceeding the maximum dose of local anaesthetic agent if the perineum is infiltrated. For this reason, prilocaine 0.5% should be used to minimise the risk of toxic reactions. Otherwise the block is safe and is not associated with fetal risks. Anaesthesia is confined to the vagina; the block is suitable only for outlet or low forceps delivery. The pain of mid-cavity, rotational or Ventouse deliveries is not relieved.

Caudal block

Caudal block has not gained widespread popularity in the UK. It is most useful for providing rapid relief of pain when mothers are approaching, or in, the second stage of labour and require vaginal analgesia. It provides excellent analgesia for instrumental delivery.

The sacral hiatus lies caudal to the 4th sacral tubercle, between the two sacral cornua. The anaesthetist must be familiar with and able to identify the anatomical landmarks of the sacral hiatus before undertaking the block. If the patient is particularly obese, or if the landmarks cannot be identified, the anaesthetist should not proceed with the block. Under sterile conditions, the sacral hiatus is identified, the overlying skin infiltrated with local anaesthetic and a needle (e.g. 21-gauge) is inserted at an angle of 45° to the patient's back until the sacrococcygeal ligament is pierced. The direction of the needle is changed to 30° when loss of resistance is felt as the needle passes through the ligament into the extradural space. In other respects, the injection is identical to lumbar extradural analgesia and the same precautions are taken. After ensuring that neither CSF nor blood is aspirated, 10–15 ml of bupivacaine 0.25% are injected slowly. If continuous caudal block is required, the needle should be replaced with a 16- or 18-gauge i.v. cannula, through which an extradural catheter is inserted. Precautions, complications and their management are similar to those of continuous lumbar extradural analgesia.

Paracervical block

Paracervical block is simple to perform and is effective rapidly. It is performed by injecting 5 ml of bupivacaine 0.25% solution, superficially, on each side of the cervix, close to the uterine artery and venous plexus. However, absorption and transport of the local anaesthetic agent are rapid, and the block is associated frequently with profound fetal bradycardia. For this reason, paracervical block is used rarely in the UK.

Extradural analgesia

The advent of continuous lumbar extradural analgesia has given mothers the opportunity to benefit from a technique which can virtually eliminate the pain of labour. Studies of the effectiveness of the blocks vary slightly, but 70–80% of mothers experience complete relief of pain in labour when bupivacaine 0.5% plain is used; no other technique approaches this level of success. Bupivacaine plain solution is the local anaesthetic agent of choice, but the optimum concentration is a matter of debate. The use of low concentrations (0.25% or less) produces less motor block and a lower incidence of instrumental delivery, but provides less effective analgesia than 0.5% solution. The use of reduced concentrations has the added benefit of reducing the total mass of drug used during labour. Unless the mother wishes complete analgesia it is probably preferable to start with bupivacaine 0.25%; the volume of injection may be increased if analgesia is inadequate, and the higher concentration may be used if analgesia continues to be unsatisfactory. If an extradural block is ineffective, the anaesthetist should establish if any degree of block exists by mapping sensory and motor deficits; a frequent cause of failure is that the catheter does not lie within the extradural space.

Indications

Pain is the principal indication for extradural analgesia in normal labour. If pregnancy is complicated by hypertension or pre-eclampsia the use of extradural analgesia is almost mandatory, as the resulting sympathetic block reduces arterial pressure and eliminates that element of hypertension which is a consequence of pain and distress.

Contraindications

1. Mother opposed to extradural analgesia.
2. Presence of coagulopathy.
3. Anticoagulant therapy.
4. Sepsis in lumbar area.
5. Pre-existing neurological deficit. Not all patients with a neurological deficit need be denied the benefits of extradural analgesia. Patients with chronic, limited neurological deficits, e.g. resulting from poliomyelitis, may receive an extradural block. However, if the deficit is a consequence of active neurological disease, extradural analgesia should probably be avoided. Extradural block may have no effect on active disease, but it may be impossible to prove this if deterioration follows its administration.

Technique

The insertion of a Tuohy needle into the extradural space is a tactile technique. Optimum conditions for access are essential, and thus time and patience in obtaining complete patient co-operation are not wasted. A large-gauge i.v. cannula must be inserted and secured before the block is established.

The patient may be prepared either in the sitting or lateral position; the sitting position provides better access. The back is cleaned and draped and the L2/3 interspace identified. After local infiltration, a skin puncture is made, through which the Tuohy needle is passed, and advanced into the supraspinous ligament. It is essential to identify the supraspinous ligament and to be certain that the needle is placed correctly. A syringe in which the plunger moves freely is filled with sterile saline and attached to the extradural needle. The assembly is held in the right hand, and constant pressure applied to the barrel of the syringe with the thumb (Fig. 33.2). The left hand, which is braced against the back, is used to advance the needle. While the point of the needle is in the ligament, injection of saline is impossible.

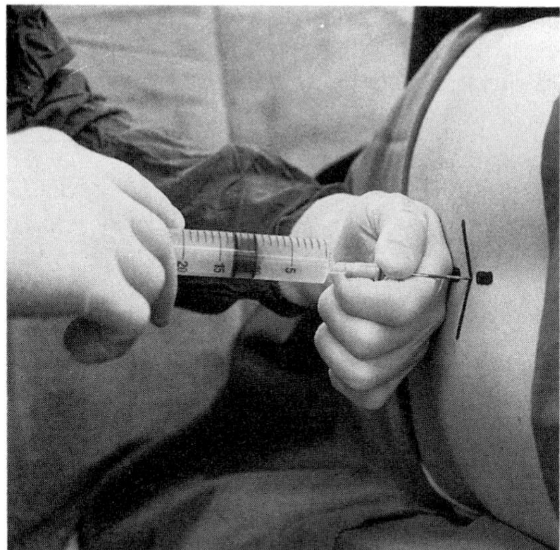

Fig. 33.2 Insertion of Tuohy needle into the extradural space using the loss-of-resistance method. See text for details.

If the point of the needle moves out of the ligament, intramuscular injection is possible, but there is resistance to injection. If in doubt, the needle should be withdrawn into the supraspinous ligament, repositioned slightly, and advanced again. Ligamentum flavum is felt as increased resistance to advancement of the needle; when this is detected, the left hand should be repositioned, and the needle advanced slowly.

Identification of the extradural space is characterised by a palpable click, felt with the left hand, and a simultaneous and unmistakable total loss of resistance to pressure on the barrel of the syringe. The volume injected should be minimal, and the syringe disconnected immediately from the needle to ensure that accidental dural puncture has not occurred. Any fluid leaking from the hub of the needle should be allowed to drop on to the back of the gloved hand; if cold, it is likely to be saline, and final identification may be made, if necessary, by using a Dextrostix (saline and local anaesthetic solutions do not contain glucose).

The initial dose of 5–7 ml of bupivacaine 0.25% plain should be injected slowly. The catheter is then passed through the needle and the needle withdrawn.

If bleeding occurs during insertion of the needle or the catheter, it is essential to ensure that it has ceased before local anaesthetic solution is injected, and that the catheter has not passed into a vein. Persistent bleeding is uncommon, but may be substantial; the block should be abandoned if it occurs. If there is a small quantity of blood in the catheter, this must be cleared by injecting sufficient saline, then repositioning the catheter by slight withdrawal until blood cannot be aspirated.

Intravenous injection of local anaesthetic resulting in a toxic reaction has been described in the USA but toxic reactions attributable to this cause have not been reported in the UK. An argument exists for using adrenaline-containing solutions of local anaesthetic for the initial dose, as inadvertent i.v. injection results in maternal tachycardia; however, this effect is rapid in onset and transitory, and is unlikely to be detected unless the maternal ECG is being monitored.

A sufficient length of catheter should be left in the extradural space to allow for movement of the tip, which occurs during labour. It is recommended that 4–5 cm should be inserted; this length is sufficient to permit repositioning if a unilateral block develops.

Caval occlusion must be avoided at all times, and the mother *must* be nursed in either a lateral position or in the modified supine position using a Crawford wedge.

Management of extradural analgesia

Careful monitoring of the mother is essential after the initial injection and also after the first dose injected through the catheter. Occasionally, extensive sensory, motor and sympathetic blocks follow extradural injection, even when there is no apparent dural puncture. In addition, the position of the catheter tip is unknown, and dural puncture may occur without detection. Some of the bizarre blocks which have been described in association with extradural analgesia may be the result of the catheter being inserted partially into the subarachnoid space; the block which develops then depends on the number of holes (if a typical three-hole catheter is used) which lie in the extradural or subarachnoid spaces, and through which the majority of the dose of local anaesthetic escaped.

Monitoring

1. Caval occlusion *must* be avoided.
2. Check arterial pressure at 5-min intervals if satisfactory, and more frequently if hypotension develops.
3. Check that the i.v. infusion is running satisfactorily.
4. The fetal heart should be monitored continuously.
5. The mother *must not* be left unattended.
6. The anaesthetist must be readily available.

Complications

1. *Hypotension*. The limited extradural block which follows the modest doses described above is accompanied by slight hypotension in approximately 5% of normal mothers. If the reduction in arterial pressure is more than 20 mmHg, or if the systolic pressure is less than 90 mmHg, active measures should be taken to limit any further reduction. Caval occlusion must be eliminated as a cause by turning the mother to the left lateral position. The rate of the i.v. infusion should be increased. The anaesthetist must be called if the arterial pressure continues to decrease. On arrival, the anaesthetist should ascertain the extent of the block immediately, as it is vital to differentiate between an unusual response to extradural injection and a subarachnoid injection. If the mother can move both legs and arms, subarachnoid injection is unlikely. If no arm weakness exists, ventilation will not be impaired. Subarachnoid injection is extremely rare, but early recognition is essential. The injection of an extradural dose of local anaesthetic solution into the subarachnoid space is likely to produce a total spinal block. Early recognition demands trained nursing and medical staff; prompt and skilled management obviates any morbidity or mortality.

2. *Total spinal block*. Total spinal blockade occurs when a dose of local anaesthetic intended for the extradural space is injected inadvertently into the subarachnoid space. Cardiovascular support should be provided immediately with i.v. fluids and i.v. ephedrine (5–10 mg) and the systolic arterial pressure maintained above 90 mmHg if possible. The development of arm weakness and advancing sensory loss often precedes ventilatory impairment. Before respiratory distress is marked, a standard general anaesthetic should be administered and controlled ventilation continued until recovery, which occurs usually within 45–60 min. Continual explanation to, and reassurance of, the mother are mandatory. Delivery is undertaken usually by Caesarean section. Subsequent recovery may be complicated by a spinal headache, which may require an extradural blood patch (vide infra) if it remains severe.

3. *Dural puncture*. This complicates 1–2% of extradural blocks. The frequency of the spinal headache that follows dural puncture is related to the diameter of the needle used. Extradural needles are large (16- or 18-gauge) and 75% of dural punctures caused by a needle of this diameter are followed by severe headache. This 'low-pressure' spinal headache is usually occipital initially. It is throbbing in nature, and is characterised by being most severe when standing or sitting, and relieved by lying down. If dural puncture occurs it is best to perform an extradural block in an adjacent interspace; the dermatomal spread of the block should be monitored carefully after top-up injections, as extensive blocks have been reported in patients with a dural puncture. Isotonic saline 500 ml over 24 h should be infused through the extradural catheter after delivery, and the patient should remain in bed.

If the headache is disabling, treatment by extradural blood patch should be considered. The injection of 15 ml of autologous blood into the extradural space under sterile conditions is thought to produce a fibrinous plug which prevents further escape of CSF. The headache is relieved in 95% of patients within 4–5 h.

4. *Unilateral block and unblocked segment*. An unblocked segment exists when there is evidence of a block above and below the segmental nerve root; a block is described as unilateral if it is more effective on one side. In the latter case, the dependent side usually has the most effective and

profound block. Unilateral block may be eliminated by the administration of a further top-up injection after positioning the mother on her other side. Unblocked segments are relatively rare, and the cause is not always clear. A further top-up injection or withdrawal of the catheter by 1–2 cm usually effects a cure. However, if adequate pain relief is not experienced, the catheter should be resited in an adjacent interspace. If an extradural block is totally ineffective, the anaesthetist should examine the patient and map sensory and motor deficits, as the catheter may not lie in the extradural space.

Analgesia may be maintained either by intermittent top-up injections when pain recurs or by continuous infusion of local anaesthetic agent. The advantages of top-up injections are that the injection may be given when required and the volume increased or decreased as necessary. The disadvantage is that close supervision of each top-up injection is required. Top-up injections should be given in divided doses; 3 ml should be injected initially, and the remainder administered 5–10 min later when assessment has been undertaken to ensure that injection into the subarachnoid space has not occurred.

Continuous injection by infusion pump appears to be an attractive solution, as top-up injections are not required and the pain experienced while waiting for a top-up injection is eliminated. However, the individual requirement of each mother for analgesia makes it difficult to identify correctly the optimum concentration and infusion rate of local anaesthetic which unfailingly relieves the pain without producing too extensive a block. The objective is to relieve the pain without further intervention by either medical or nursing staff. An effective technique is to establish an excellent block initially by injecting a bolus dose of bupivacaine 0.5% plain solution followed by an infusion of 10–14 ml/h of bupivacaine 0.125%. Monitoring of the mother is relatively simple and consists of checking the arterial pressure every 30 min. T8 should be marked, and sensory levels checked when the arterial pressure is being taken; if the block extends above the mark, or if motor block is severe, the infusion should be stopped and the anaesthetist informed.

Subarachnoid block

Subarachnoid block is not a suitable technique for pain relief in labour but is useful for high forceps delivery, Caesarean section (vide infra) or manual removal of placenta.

CAESAREAN SECTION

Risks of anaesthesia for Caesarean section

For the last 30 years the triennial Report on Confidential Enquiries into Maternal Deaths in England and Wales has provided a unique and valuable service to obstetrics. It contains an objective and detailed analysis of the causes of all maternal deaths and has played a seminal role in the development of obstetric services.

The percentage of maternal deaths attributable to general anaesthesia has increased (Table 33.1); anaesthesia is now the third most common cause of maternal death. Deaths associated with anaesthesia are related most frequently to difficulties with tracheal intubation or pneumonitis resulting from aspiration of gastric contents. Most of these deaths follow anaesthesia for Caesarean section. The increased use of extradural or subarachnoid anaesthesia obviates the risks of inadvertent oesophageal intubation and hypoxaemia produced by loss of an adequate airway when tracheal intubation is impossible. It is assumed, although not proven, that these techniques reduce the risk of aspiration of gastric contents. However, regional anaesthesia is not suitable for all patients, and general anaesthesia will always have an important role in obstetric practice. In addition, there is a small risk of loss of airway reflexes in patients who receive a high extradural or subarachnoid block for Caesarean section. Consequently, precautions must be taken to control the volume and pH of gastric contents in all patients who may require Caesarean section.

Control of gastric contents

The physiological changes of pregnancy cause a small reduction in gastric emptying, but the administration of opioids for pain relief in labour delays the rate of gastric emptying significantly, with an inevitable increase in the volume of acidic

Table 33.1 Maternal mortality figures obtained from the Confidential Enquiries into Maternal Deaths in England and Wales

Years	Maternal mortality per 1000 total births	Number of deaths from anaesthesia	Percentage true maternal deaths from anaesthesia	Percentage with avoidable factors
1952–54	0.53	49	4.5	—
1955–57	0.43	31	3.6	77
1958–60	0.33	30	4.0	80
1961–63	0.26	28	4.0	50
1964–66	0.20	50	8.7	48
1967–69	0.16	50	10.9	68
1970–72	0.13	37	10.4	76
1973–75	0.11	31	13.2	90
1976–78	0.11	30	13.2	93
1979–81	0.11	22	12.2	100

gastric fluid. It is thought that if gastric fluid has a pH of less than 2.5 and a volume of more than 0.4 ml/kg, aspiration may lead to potentially fatal pulmonary damage. The risks may be minimised by adoption of the following precautions:

1. *Dietary restriction.* The mother is allowed to suck ice during labour, but no food or drink is permitted. If fluids are required, these are administered intravenously. The precautions for elective surgery are similar to those in general surgery; breakfast is withheld.

2. *Elevation of pH of gastric contents.* This is achieved by the use of antacids and H_2-receptor antagonists. For many years magnesium trisilicate was the antacid of choice and was administered throughout labour at 2-hourly intervals, with an additional dose immediately before surgery. Clearly, the regular administration of magnesium trisilicate increases the volume of gastric contents if gastric emptying is delayed. In addition, experimental studies have shown that aspiration of particulate antacids causes a pneumonitis, and the use of magnesium trisilicate has failed to reduce mortality from aspiration of gastric contents. These observations have led to a reassessment of antacid therapy. The introduction of H_2-receptor antagonists has provided a method of controlling both gastric volume and pH. These drugs do not affect the volume and pH of the fluid already present in the stomach. However, 6-hourly administration of ranitidine 150 mg during labour reduces the volume of subsequent gastric secretions, and increases the pH by almost eliminating production of acid. Alternatively, treatment may be given selectively only to those mothers who require delivery by Caesarean section or those who need general anaesthesia. When the decision is made to deliver the mother by Caesarean section, cimetidine 200 mg is administered i.m. and 30 ml of 0.3 M sodium citrate is given orally 5 min before induction of anaesthesia. If surgery is being undertaken with extradural or subarachnoid anaesthesia, the citrate should be administered a few minutes before surgery is started.

3. *Cricoid pressure.* The correct application of cricoid pressure (see p. 532) reduces substantially the risk of regurgitation of gastric contents. Cricoid pressure must be applied to all obstetric patients who require general anaesthesia until the airway is secured by a cuffed tracheal tube, or whilst the patient is unconscious in the event that intubation proves to be impossible.

4. *Gastric emptying.* The stomach may be emptied using either a wide-bore gastric tube or the administration of apomorphine. However, these techniques are not required if the precautions listed above are taken.

Extradural analgesia

Successful extradural blockade for Caesarean section is a rewarding experience for the mother and the anaesthetist but is a most demanding technique.

Elective Caesarean section

The use of extradural analgesia for elective Caesarean section has increased in recent years, as it reduces the need for general anaesthesia and permits the mother to participate in the delivery of her child. The technique is similar to that described above, but the sensory, motor and sympathetic blocks are more extensive and thus the incidence and severity of complications are increased. Meticulous care and attention to detail are essential. Preparations for surgery begin on the previous day. The H_2-receptor antagonist ranitidine 150 mg should be administered on the evening before, and on the morning of surgery. In the 15 min preceding the insertion of the block, 1.5 litres of saline 0.9% or compound sodium lactate solution are infused. The block is inserted as described above using bupivacaine 0.5% plain solution. An initial injection of 10–12 ml is made through the needle, and a catheter is inserted for administration of subsequent doses. Following institution of the block, the mother is positioned on her side (as caval occlusion *must* be avoided) and the onset of the block is monitored at 5-min intervals.

Top-up injections of 7 ml are given when the level of the block can be determined by the anaesthetist, but the precautions described for the first top-up through the catheter must be followed. The onset of action of bupivacaine is relatively slow; on average, it is 45 min before the block is established. The block must extend from T6 to S5 to be effective. The dose required to achieve this degree of block is variable, but a total of 100 mg bupivacaine (20 ml of 0.5% solution) may be necessary.

Hypotension is common, the reported incidence ranging from 7 to 30%. Management is by judicious use of i.v. fluids and ephedrine 5–10 mg i.v., as described previously. Movement of the patient should be avoided when the block is effective to minimise the hypotensive effects of the extensive sympathetic block. During surgery, judicious use of sedatives and analgesics after delivery of the baby may make the procedure more pleasant for the mother, who should always be asked if she wishes sedation. Ergometrine should be avoided as its use is associated with a 50% incidence of vomiting, and syntocinon should be used as an alternative.

Emergency Caesarean section

If the mother is receiving continuous extradural analgesia for pain relief in labour, the local anaesthetic solution should be changed to bupivacaine 0.5% and top-up doses administered as described above to achieve a block extending from T6 to S5. Management should be identical.

In the absence of continuous extradural analgesia, the time required to produce a block as described above may be a limiting factor if Caesarean section is required for fetal distress. Lignocaine 2% with 1 in 200 000 adrenaline is equally effective and more rapid in onset than bupivacaine, and is a suitable alternative if surgery is urgent. It should be administered in similar volumes to bupivacaine 0.5%.

Subarachnoid block

The introduction of bupivacaine for subarachnoid block has served to stimulate interest in the UK, but the role of this block in obstetric practice has not yet been established. Subarachnoid anaesthesia offers a number of advantages over extradural anaesthesia for Caesarean section:

1. Onset of action is much faster (10 min cf. 45 min).
2. Less bupivacaine is required (15 mg).
3. It is arguably a simpler technique with a positive end-point.
4. Patient discomfort is less during performance of the block.

The disadvantages are:

1. Hypotension is common (up to 40%) and may be severe and rapid in onset.
2. Top-up doses are not possible.
3. The incidence of post-lumbar puncture headache is approximately 20%.

These disadvantages may be minimised but not eliminated. The frequency and severity of the hypotension may be modified by careful preloading with at least 1.5 litres of crystalloid in the 15 min preceding the block; an infusion of ephedrine is effective also in maintaining maternal arterial pressure. Post-spinal headache may be minimised by using a fine-gauge spinal needle (25-gauge or smaller), inserted with the bevel in the same plane as the ligaments, i.e. with the needle bevel parallel with the longitudinal axis of the spine, and by avoiding multiple punctures. Enforced 24 h bed rest is not necessary after subarachnoid anaesthesia.

General anaesthesia

The general anaesthetic technique used for Caesarean section comprises light general anaesthesia with a muscle relaxant, and is very similar to that used for most types of emergency surgery. Before anaesthesia is induced, the mother must be placed in the modified supine position with left lateral tilt to avoid caval occlusion. A secure i.v. route must be established, and grouped and cross-matched blood should be available. Appropriate antacid therapy must be administered. Adequate (5 min) preoxygenation is essential. Rapid-sequence induction of anaesthesia is achieved by i.v. injection of thiopentone 4–5 mg/kg and tracheal intubation with an 8-mm cuffed tracheal tube facilitated by suxamethonium 1.5 mg/kg. Cricoid pressure must be applied by a skilled assistant as soon as consciousness is lost, and must not be removed until the tracheal tube is in place and the cuff inflated. Positive pressure ventilation of the lungs is started immediately, using a 50% oxygen/nitrous oxide mixture and the addition of halothane 0.5% or an equipotent concentration of another volatile agent. The minute volume should ensure the maintenance of an end-tidal carbon dioxide concentration of 4%.

After delivery of the baby, the inspired oxygen concentration should be reduced to 30% and an opioid drug administered i.v. Muscular relaxation is maintained by small doses of either vecuronium or pancuronium. An appropriate concentration of volatile agent should be continued to minimise the risk of awareness.

Failed intubation

This occurs in approximately 1 in 300 general anaesthetics in obstetrics. The anaesthetist must acknowledge failure at an appropriate time and institute a failed-intubation drill. Skilled help should always be available, and Consultant assistance sought. All the equipment required must be available immediately:

1. A second laryngoscope.
2. A range of tracheal tubes of differing sizes.
3. Introducers.
4. Gum elastic bougies.
5. Minitracheotomy set.
6. Oesophageal obturator.
7. Magill forceps.
8. Range of oral airways.
9. Nasal airways.

A decision should be taken early that intubation is not possible; endless striving is dangerous. A failed intubation drill should be instituted immediately. The following measures are suggested:

1. Maintain cricoid pressure.
2. Place the patient head-down in the left lateral position.
3. Maintain oxygenation with 100% oxygen; manual ventilation of the lungs may be necessary until the effects of suxamethonium have ceased.
4. Allow the patient to waken, and summon help.
5. When senior help arrives, it may be appropriate to induce anaesthesia again, and to attempt to intubate the trachea using additional equipment, e.g. longer-bladed laryngoscope, bougies, etc. Alternatively, regional anaesthesia may be employed.

These measures are not suitable if it is essential that surgery proceeds rapidly, e.g. fetal distress or maternal haemorrhage. In these circumstances, anaesthesia is probably maintained best as follows:

1. Maintain cricoid pressure.
2. Place the patient in a head-down position.
3. Maintain anaesthesia using 40% oxygen in nitrous oxide and a volatile agent; the inexperienced anaesthetist is recommended to use the agent with which he/she is most familiar. Allow the patient to breathe spontaneously when the effects of suxamethonium have ceased.

If regurgitation and/or aspiration occurs, a sample of the aspirate should be obtained for measurement of pH, the operation concluded and the patient treated symptomatically. IPPV should be administered early if respiratory failure develops and the patient should be transferred to an ITU.

Awareness

In an effort to limit the transfer of anaesthetic agents to the baby, reduced doses of anaesthetic agents are administered compared with anaesthesia for other procedures and no premedication (other than H_2-receptor antagonists) is given. Consequently, the risk of awareness during obstetric general anaesthesia is high. Without volatile supplementation, an incidence of 17% has been reported, and as a consequence understandably aggrieved mothers have sued anaesthetists successfully. In normal circumstances the use of an appropriate concentration of volatile agent is essential. The incidence of awareness may be reduced significantly, but perhaps not entirely, by a meticulous anaesthetic technique.

General or regional anaesthesia for Caesarean section?

A local block should be used for elective Caesarean section if no contraindication to subarachnoid or extradural anaesthesia exists and the mother is willing to remain conscious during surgery. The mother should be informed of the advantages and disadvantages of local techniques and be permitted to participate in the decision-making process. General anaesthesia should be used only if the mother expressly wishes it or if there is some contraindication to a local technique. In the case of emergency Caesarean section, the critical factor is the time available to perform the block, or to extend the block if one is in place already. The anaesthetist should be aware of, and take part in, the activity of the labour suite and so should have a knowledge of any developing problems. Early warning should add a margin of time which allows the administration of a local block. If fetal distress is severe, the incidence and severity of hypotension following a subarachnoid block should be considered, although the rapid onset makes it an attractive technique if time is short.

COMMON OBSTETRIC PROBLEMS

Failure of pregnancy

Early failure of pregnancy at 8–14 weeks' gestation is relatively common and evacuation of the uterus under general anaesthesia is undertaken. The technique is simple and generally undemanding. An i.v. induction and mask anaesthesia with a spontaneously breathing patient is the most frequently used technique. Tracheal intubation is rarely necessary, as it is unusual for such patients to require urgent surgery, and the patient can be prepared adequately for theatre.

Termination of pregnancy for fetal abnormality is becoming more common as diagnostic precision in early pregnancy improves. If the diagnosis is made sufficiently early, the technique described above will suffice. In later pregnancy (greater than 20 weeks' gestation) termination of pregnancy is undertaken usually by the use of extra-amniotic prostaglandins. The anaesthetist is not involved often in these cases, but a prostaglandin-induced labour may be both extremely painful and slow; the patient may be very distressed and extradural analgesia offers some relief. Extradural analgesia should not be withheld, and sedative drugs should be administered freely.

Pregnancy-induced hypertension

Hypertension, arbitrarily defined as a diastolic arterial pressure exceeding 90 mmHg, complicates 5–8% of pregnancies; 1% of patients develop proteinuric hypertension. Fetal outcome is related to the severity of the hypertension and the gestational age of onset. The majority of mothers develop benign hypertension, manifested frequently as an increase in arterial pressure during labour. Extradural analgesia is almost mandatory for such patients, as it reduces arterial pressure and removes that element attributable to pain and distress.

Eclampsia and severe hypertension are associated frequently with a coagulopathy and, occasionally, impaired renal function. Careful monitoring of these patients is essential. The definitive treatment is delivery, but attempts may be made to prolong the pregnancy if the baby is not mature. Delivery may be required urgently under general anaesthesia. Difficulties may be experienced as a result of oedema and the hypertensive response to tracheal intubation.

Haemorrhage

Haemorrhage is defined in relation to the stage of pregnancy, as it may develop before, during or after labour and delivery.

Antepartum haemorrhage

Before delivery, haemorrhage is complicated by the presence of the baby. Clearly, the management of the haemorrhage is the same; resuscitation of the mother if necessary, and assessment of the cause and the condition of the baby.

Placenta praevia is diagnosed most frequently at an early ultrasound scan and the mother managed conservatively for as long as possible. The risk of bleeding is related to the position of the placenta and the extent to which it overlies the internal os of the uterus. Delivery is undertaken if bleeding becomes frequent or prolonged, or if pregnancy is near term and bleeding occurs. Fetal welfare is likely to be in jeopardy only if bleeding is severe.

Placental abruption occurs when part of the placenta separates from the wall of the uterus. It is associated with severe abdominal pain. External bleeding is not always obvious, but the degree of shock and hypotension is unrelated to the extent of external blood loss. Fetal well-being is severely jeopardised, and Caesarean section is undertaken as soon as possible. Maternal resuscitation should be vigorous. General anaesthesia should be administered rather than a regional technique, as a coagulopathy is associated frequently with this complication of pregnancy. Laboratory assistance is essential.

Postpartum haemorrhage

By definition, postpartum haemorrhage is said to have occurred if blood loss at delivery is greater than 500 ml. Severe blood loss is unusual, but vigorous management should be implemented at an early stage. This complication is associated most frequently with either a retained placenta or incomplete emptying of the uterus. If the placenta is not delivered and haemorrhage is slight, exploration and manual removal of the placenta may be undertaken under subarachnoid anaesthesia. If bleeding has occurred, the uterus should be explored under general anaesthesia when the patient's condition is satisfactory. Even in the presence of an extradural block, ergometrine should not be withheld if bleeding continues.

FURTHER READING

Bromage P R 1978 Epidural analgesia. W B Saunders, Philadelphia

Crawford J S 1978 Principles and practice of obstetric anaesthesia, 4th edn. Blackwell Scientific Publications, Oxford

Moir D D, Thorburn J 1986 Obstetric anaesthesia and analgesia, 3rd edn. Baillière Tindall, London

34. Paediatric anaesthesia and intensive care

Major differences in anatomy and physiology in the small infant have important consequences on many aspects of anaesthesia. These differences also cause different patterns of disease in small infants and children seen in the intensive therapy unit, in comparison with adult patients.

The physical disparity between the adult and child diminishes at 10–12 years of age although major psychological differences continue through adolescence.

PHYSIOLOGY IN THE NEONATE

Respiration

At birth the alveoli are thick-walled and number only approximately 10% of the adult total. Lung growth continues by alveolar multiplication until the age of 6–8 years. The airways remain relatively narrow up to this age, resulting in high airway resistance, and leading to a high incidence of airway disease in the young.

Ventilation is almost entirely diaphragmatic with soft horizontal ribs contributing little to gas movement in comparison with the bucket-handle movement in the adult.

Table 34.1 Lung mechanics of the neonate compared with the adult

	Neonate	Adult
Compliance (ml/cmH_2O)	5	100
Resistance (cmH_2O $litre^{-1}$ s^{-1})	30	2
Time constant (s)	0.5	1.3
Respiratory rate (breaths/min)	32	15

The high airway resistance and low compliance result in a short time constant (see p. 27). As a result, the ventilatory rate is rapid. The metabolic cost of respiration is higher in the infant and may reach 15% of total oxygen consumption.

The metabolic rate in infants is almost twice that of the adult and consequently alveolar minute ventilation is also greater, whilst FRC is a similar fraction of lung volume as that in the adult. Consequently, inhalational induction of anaesthesia and awakening at the termination of anaesthesia are more rapid than in the adult. Similarly, hypoxaemia occurs much more rapidly in a child.

The poor elastic qualities of the infant lung cause the closing volume (CV) to be greater than FRC until the age of 6–8 years; thus airways closure occurs during tidal ventilation, leading to an increase in the alveolar–arterial oxygen tension difference (A–a) P_{O_2} and a normal Pa_{O_2} in the newborn of approximately 9–9.5 kPa (70 mmHg).

Physiological deadspace is approximately 30% of tidal volume ($V_D/V_T = 0.3$) as in the adult but the absolute volume is small, so that any increase caused by apparatus deadspace has a disproportionately greater effect on a small child (Table 34.2). During anaesthesia, deadspace should be kept to a minimum and the resistance of breathing apparatus should be kept low. Secretions resulting

Table 34.2 Respiratory variables in the neonate

Tidal volume (V_T)	7 ml/kg
Deadspace (V_D)	$V_T \times 0.3$ ml
Respiratory rate	Neonate 32 breaths/min Age 1–13 (24 — age/2) breaths/min

either from cholinergic activity or upper respiratory infection may cause respiratory difficulty.

Cardiovascular system

Following the dramatic change from fetal to adult circulation at birth, the child establishes a high cardiac output (commensurate with the high metabolic rate) of approximately 200 ml kg^{-1} min^{-1}, which is 2–3 times the adult value. The small ventricles result in poor ventricular compliance; thus increased cardiac output is produced by an increase in heart rate. Babies tolerate heart rates of up to 200 beats/min without evidence of cardiac failure (Table 34.3).

Bradycardia may occur readily in the presence of hypoxaemia or vagal stimulation, and rapid treatment with oxygen or atropine is required. Arrhythmias are uncommon in the absence of cardiac disease, and cardiac arrest occurs usually in asystole rather than ventricular fibrillation.

Systemic arterial pressure is low at birth (approximately 80/50 mmHg) because of the low systemic vascular resistance resulting from the large proportion of vessel-rich tissues in the child. The pressure increases within the first month to approximately 90/60 mmHg and reaches adult levels of 120/70 mmHg at approximately 16 years of age.

Monitoring of the cardiovascular system

The cardiovascular system must always be monitored carefully in babies. Arterial pressure may be measured with a sphygmomanometer cuff or alternatively by an ultrasonic detector or an automatic oscillotonometer. Intra-arterial monitoring of arterial pressure is feasible in the neonate by percutaneous arterial catheterisation with a 22-gauge cannula. This invasive technique should be used only when regular blood gas estimations are required as the complication rate of arterial cannulation is significantly higher in children than in adults. Intermittent flushing has been shown to cause retrograde flow from the radial artery to the carotid artery with the risk of cerebral embolisation. Consequently, slow continuous flushing should be used and the volume of fluid administered measured carefully. Central venous pressure (CVP) monitoring is valuable in the treatment of fluid imbalance and haemorrhage; the internal jugular or subclavian veins are suitable for the introduction of CVP catheters.

Table 34.3 Variation of heart rate (beats/min) with age

Age	Mean value	Normal range
Neonate	140	100–180
1 year	120	80–150
2 years	110	80–130
6 years	100	70–120
12 years	80	60–100

Blood volume

Variations of up to ± 20% of blood volume occur at birth depending on the stage at which the cord is clamped. The average blood volume at birth is 90 ml/kg. This decreases in the infant and young child to 80 ml/kg and attains the adult level of 75 ml/kg at the age of 6–8 years. Blood losses of greater than 10% of blood volume should be replaced with blood.

Haemoglobin

At birth, 75–80% of haemoglobin is fetal haemoglobin (HbF). A decrease in blood volume and HbF occurs before adult haemoglobin (HbA) haemopoiesis is established fully at 6 months. HbF has a greater affinity for oxygen than HbA because of a lower content of 2,3-diphosphoglycerate (2,3-DPG) and the dissociation curve is shifted to the left (Fig. 34.1). The greater affinity of HbF for oxygen is overcome in the tissues of the fetus because of low tissue P_{O_2} and a metabolic acidosis. The acidosis, which persists into infancy (and the high CO_2 output as a result of the high metabolic rate) aid oxygen delivery to the tissues by shifting the dissociation curve to the right. Respiratory alkalosis caused by hyperventilation reduces oxygen availability and should be avoided both in the operating theatre and intensive care unit.

Blood for transfusion should be warmed and filtered. If required in small volumes, it may be

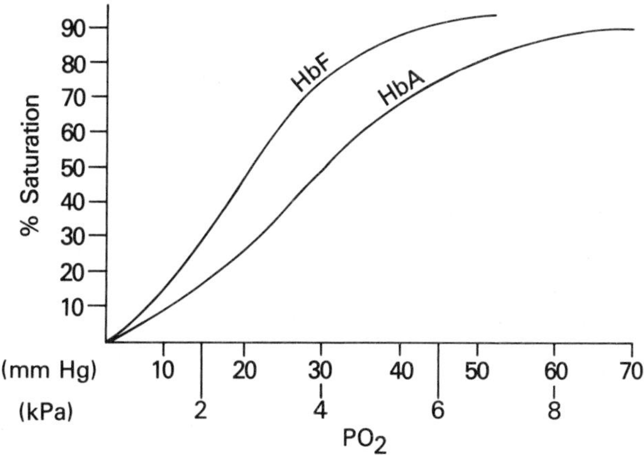

Fig. 34.1 Effects of HbF on oxygen dissociation curve.

given by syringe through a tap in the i.v. line. This system also allows rapid transfusion. In other cases, a burette type of infusion set should be used to minimise the risk of accidental overtransfusion and to permit careful monitoring of the volumes of blood administered.

As a result of the small blood volume of the neonate, haemorrhage should be monitored carefully. Swabs should be weighed, and all suction losses collected in a graduated container. Blood loss may be measured also by washing swabs and drapes in a fixed volume of fluid and measuring the haemoglobin content of the fluid.

Renal function and fluid balance

Body fluids constitute a greater proportion of body weight in the infant, particularly the premature infant, than the adult (Table 34.4).

The proportion of total body water present as extracellular fluid (ECF) exceeds that of intracellular fluid (ICF). This ratio reverses gradually with increasing age. Plasma volume remains constant, at approximately 5% body weight, throughout life.

Table 34.4 Distribution of water as percentage of body weight

Compartment	Premature	Neonate	Infant	Adult
ECF	50	35	30	20
ICF	30	40	40	40
Plasma	5	5	5	5
Total	85	80	75	65

The turnover of fluid is much greater in infants (15% total body water per day) than in adults. Thus, interruption of fluid intake in the infant results rapidly in dehydration.

The kidneys are immature at birth, both glomerular filtration and tubular reabsorption being reduced until the age of 6–8 months; as a result, there is inability to handle excessive water loads, and over transfusion may lead to oedema and cardiac failure. There is also diminished ability to handle sodium loads, which may occur with administration of excess sodium (e.g. sodium bicarbonate solutions.)

Immature renal function may lead to cumulation and toxicity of drugs excreted by the kidneys (e.g. digoxin and penicillin). Reduced doses or increased dosage intervals may be required in the neonate.

Fluid therapy

Normal maintenance requirements of fluid increase over the first few days of life (Tables 34.5 and 34.6) and thereafter reduce more slowly.

Suitable solutions are $\frac{1}{4}$ strength saline for the neonate and infant up to 1 year, and $\frac{1}{2}$ strength saline or $\frac{1}{2}$ strength Ringer lactate thereafter. Because of the high metabolic rate, all fluids should contain at least 5% glucose to avoid hypoglycaemia.

Table 34.5 Fluid requirements in the first week of life

Day	Rate
1	0
2, 3	50 ml kg^{-1} day^{-1}
4, 5	75 ml kg^{-1} day^{-1}
6	100 ml kg^{-1} day^{-1}
7	120 ml kg^{-1} day^{-1}

Table 34.6 Maintenance fluid requirements

Weight	Rate
Up to 10 kg	100 ml kg^{-1} day^{-1}
10 to 20 kg	1000 ml + 50 × [wt (kg) − 10] ml kg^{-1} day^{-1}
20 to 30 kg	1500 ml + 25 × [wt (kg) − 20] ml kg^{-1} day^{-1}

Clinical examination of skin turgor, tension of fontanelles, arterial pressure and venous filling may aid the estimation of hydration, but electrolyte and haemoglobin concentrations and haematocrit, urine volumes and plasma and urine osmolalities should be monitored if problems of fluid balance exist (Table 34.7).

During surgery, fluid administration should be increased by 10–20%; intake should be increased by 10% also in babies nursed under radiant heaters because of increased insensible loss, and in babies with pyrexia. Plasma proteins may require replacement (either as plasma or human albumin solution) in severe dehydration.

Calculation of replacement fluids, as opposed to maintenance fluids, should allow also for additional losses of water, protein and electrolytes which may occur with vomiting or diarrhoea. An i.v. infusion should be established for all but the briefest of procedures, to permit correction of preoperative dehydration and hypoglycaemia, to cover fluid requirements in the immediate postoperative period, and for administration of drugs.

Small doses of drugs should be given using either a 1 or 2 ml syringe or by dilution; overdilution should be avoided as excessive fluid administration may result. The drug and dilution should be labelled clearly on all syringes.

Intravenous fluids should be administered using a burette type of infusion set which (in the small infant) should deliver 60 drops per ml (Fig. 34.2), thus allowing the rate to be controlled down to very small volumes. Drip controllers of either mechanical or electrical type assist in the administration of small volumes (Fig. 34.3).

Temperature regulation and maintenance

The neonate has a surface area to volume ratio 2.5 times greater than the adult, and thus a greater area for heat loss. Heat is lost by conduction, by convection, and by evaporation from the skin and the respiratory tract. However, 70% of heat loss occurs by radiation to nearby surfaces e.g. the walls of an incubator.

In a thermoneutral environment, heat loss and energy expenditure are minimal. The temperature of such an environment is 34°C for the premature, 32°C for the neonate and 28°C for the adult. It is important therefore to raise the environmental temperature to reduce heat loss in the very young. Infants less than three months old do not shiver to generate heat if exposed to cold, but depend on non-shivering thermogenesis. This is achieved by increasing metabolism of brown fat which is

Table 34.7 Effects of dehydration in the young infant

	Mild	Moderate	Severe
Percentage loss of body weight	5%	10%	15%
Clinical signs	Dry skin and mucous membranes	Mottled cold periphery Loss of skin elasticity Depressed eyeballs and fontanelles Oliguria ++	Shocked Moribund Unresponsive to pain
Replacement	50 ml/kg	100 ml/kg	150 ml/kg

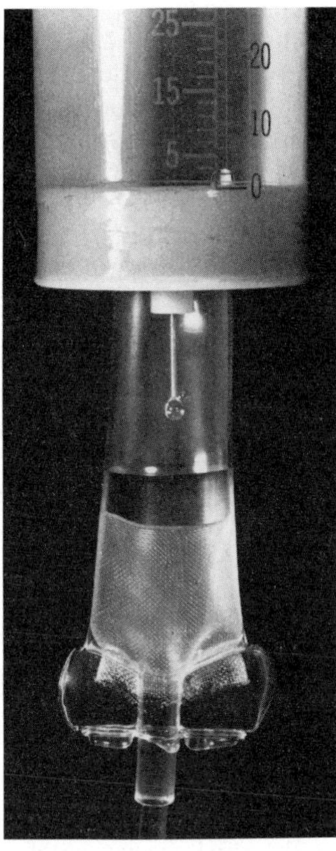

Fig. 34.2 Microburette for controlling i.v. infusion.

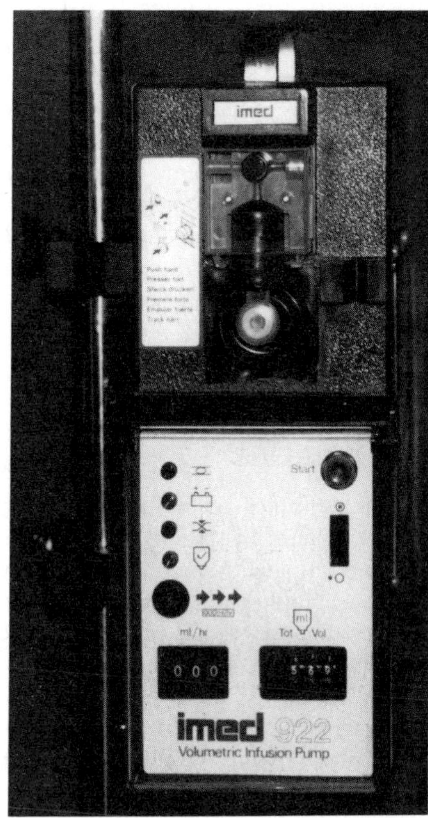

Fig. 34.3 Mechanical infusion pump.

present in the neck and upper thoracic area, and surrounds the great vessels. This metabolism is controlled by the sympathetic nervous system. As with the muscular activity of shivering, the increase in metabolism causes an increase in oxygen consumption which may stress the immature respiratory system and may even induce respiratory failure. The control of brown fat metabolism is compromised by general anaesthesia, and so it is important to maintain body temperature by other means during surgery. A decrease in temperature may lead to respiratory depression, reduced cardiac output, prolongation of the action of drugs (especially the muscle relaxants) and increased risks of hypoventilation, regurgitation and aspiration in the postoperative period.

At birth, subcutaneous fat is minimal (almost absent in the premature) and so natural insulation is poor. Heat loss may be reduced during surgery by wrapping the limbs in orthopaedic wool or padding, or by using a space blanket or silver swaddler. The child should be placed on a heating blanket; water or heated air is preferable to an electric blanket to avoid the danger of electric shock, hot spots and interference with monitoring equipment. Overhead radiant heaters may be used (as in modern intensive care incubators) before surgery, but are inconvenient for the surgeon during surgery. Humidification and warming of inspired gases reduce heat losses from evaporation.

Malignant hyperpyrexia is extremely rare under 3 years of age, although it has been reported in a child of 5 months.

Monitoring

Temperature should be monitored, even during the shortest procedure. An axillary probe is normally adequate. For longer surgery and in the intensive care area, core temperature should be monitored using a rectal, nasopharyngeal or oesophageal probe. The external auditory meatus should not be used in children because of the danger of damage to the tympanic membrane. If heating apparatus is in use, the temperature of the skin adjacent to the heating apparatus should be monitored closely and gradients of more than 10°C must be avoided at all temperatures to prevent burning. The core-skin temperature gradient is a useful monitor of cardiac output in the intensive care area. Decreases in cardiac output increase the gradient above the normal 3–4°C.

PHARMACOLOGY IN THE NEONATE

Central nervous sysem

At birth, the neurones are developed, but myelination is incomplete. In spite of this, the majority of body fat is contained within the central nervous system. Thus lipid-soluble drugs (e.g. anaesthetics) reach high levels in the central nervous system more rapidly than in the adult. The blood–brain barrier is more permeable in the newborn period, allowing the passage of drugs (including opioids) which should be given therefore with caution and in small doses. Antibiotics cross more readily, which is advantageous in the treatment of meningitis, but bilirubin also crosses the blood–brain barrier, leading to brain damage (kernicterus). The immaturity of the central nervous system (associated with the high metabolic rate) may be responsible for the increase in the minimum alveolar concentration (MAC) of the inhalational anaesthetic agents in young children (Table 34.8).

Liver

The liver is partly immature at birth but rapidly becomes the centre of protein production and drug detoxification. In the neonate, there is a quantitative and qualitative difference in the plasma proteins with a reduction in plasma albumin. There is therefore less protein binding in the neonate, allowing more drug to remain active. Some drugs (e.g. diazepam and vitamin K) may displace bilirubin from protein and increase the likelihood of kernicterus in the neonate.

The enzymes responsible for glucuronidation are immature; as a consequence the opioids (and chloramphenicol) are metabolised slowly, with consequent increase in toxicity.

The immaturity of the liver microsomal enzymes may be responsible for the extreme rarity of halothane-related hepatic damage in patients under 10 years of age. By the age of 1–2 years, the liver is twice the volume relative to body weight as in the adult. This may result in local anaesthetic agents being safer in youth than in later years.

Table 34.8 Minimum alveolar concentration of anaesthetic agents

Age	Halothane	Enflurane	Isoflurane
0–3 years	1.08	2.0	1.35
3–10 years	0.9	1.9	1.3
Adult	0.76	1.7	1.15

Specific drugs in relationship to paediatric anaesthesia

Inhalational agents

The greater alveolar ventilation in relation to FRC, and the preponderance of vessel-rich tissues, lead to more rapid increases in alveolar and brain concentrations of inhalational anaesthetics than in the adult. Induction is therefore more rapid, as is excretion of the agent at the termination of anaesthesia. The rapid increase in levels of depressant agents (e.g. halothane or enflurane) may lead to dramatic decreases in arterial pressure and cardiac output, particularly during controlled ventilation.

The minimum alveolar concentrations of inhalational anaesthetics are increased in the young (Table 34.8). This results in a more restricted therapeutic range between surgical anaesthesia and cardiovascular and respiratory depression. Great care should therefore be exercised in their use and the patient must be monitored closely.

Nitrous oxide. Nitrous oxide is used as a carrier gas and supplement for most inhalational anaesthetics. Because of the low solubility of nitrogen, an increase in the volume of air-containing spaces occurs during induction with N_2O/O_2. In the neonate this is important in lesions of the lung, especially pneumothorax and congenital lobar emphysema. Expansion of the bowel in diaphragmatic hernia, exomphalos or gastroschisis may increase diaphragmatic splinting after surgical correction. In necrotising enterocolitis, the gas within the bowel wall may expand and worsen the condition.

Halothane. Halothane is the most commonly used agent in paediatric anaesthesia. It produces a smooth, rapid induction of anaesthesia. The cardiovascular depressant properties are not normally marked in clinical anaesthesia, but are severe in the presence of cardiac failure. There is an increased tendency for laryngeal spasm to occur during tracheal intubation or extubation at light levels of anaesthesia; tracheal intubation should be undertaken at the level of surgical anaesthesia and the patient should be awake before extubation. However, extubation under deep anaesthesia is preferable in some circumstances, e.g. after intraocular surgery. Hepatic dysfunction after repeated halothane anaesthesia has been reported in children; however, the incidence is extremely small compared with that in adults. Halothane remains the drug of choice for emergency inhalational induction of anaesthesia in conditions such as acute epiglottitis or post-tonsillectomy haemorrhage.

Enflurane. This does not produce as smooth an induction as halothane and may induce breath-holding, coughing and laryngospasm. The high MAC value of enflurane in children, and particularly in infants, renders the drug of less value as a sole anaesthetic agent. Ventilatory and cardiovascular depression may occur. Central nervous system excitation occurs on EEG recordings and epileptiform seizures have been reported some hours after enflurane anaesthesia; thus the drug should not be used in children with a history of epilepsy.

Isoflurane. Isoflurane possesses cardiovascular and respiratory depressant properties similar to those of halothane. Recovery occurs more rapidly because of its lower blood/gas solubility coefficient. Unfortunately, isoflurane is irritant and thus inhalational induction is slow; breath-holding, coughing and laryngeal spasm may occur, particularly in the unpremedicated child. Laryngospasm occurs less commonly on extubation than after halothane.

Cyclopropane. This is still used occasionally for rapid induction of anaesthesia but it is explosive and may cause laryngospasm on induction and tracheal extubation.

Intravenous agents

Thiopentone is still the most frequently used i.v. induction agent for children. Very young infants are extremely sensitive to barbiturates, but older children are less sensitive, and a dose of 5–6 mg/kg is required.

Methohexitone 1 mg/kg may cause pain on injection; this can be abolished by adding lignocaine (1 mg/ml) to the solution before injection. Methohexitone may also cause central nervous system excitation which results in muscular twitching, and the drug should be avoided in patients with epilepsy.

Barbiturates may be given rectally in increased dosage, e.g. thiopentone 30 mg/kg, methohexitone 25 mg/kg, as 10% solutions. Onset of sleep is pleasant but slow, taking 5–10 min, during which time the child must be observed closely for signs of respiratory obstruction or depression.

Propofol 2 mg/kg may be used for induction of anaesthesia in older children; recovery is rapid. Unfortunately, pain on injection reduces the usefulness of the drug in children.

Etomidate has a rapid action and causes little cardiovascular or respiratory depression but does cause pain on injection. Involuntary movements and coughing are common. Because of its rapid metabolism, it has been advocated as an infusion agent for total i.v. anaesthesia. This technique is not used frequently in children because of rapid fluctuations in depth of anaesthesia and the volume of infusion required.

Ketamine may be used i.v. in a dose of 2 mg/kg, or i.m. 10 mg/kg. In the very young, increased doses are required as a consequence of poor cortical development. Following i.v. induction, respiratory depression may occur, and breath-holding is not uncommon. There is a risk of aspiration at this time. The presence of secretions or an airway in the mouth may cause laryngospasm because of increased airway reflex activity.

The psychic phenomena associated with emergence from ketamine anaesthesia in adults are less common in children and may be reduced further by premedication with diazepam and provision of a quiet, undisturbed recovery period. The analgesia and catatonia provided by ketamine are useful for skin grafting of burns and allow exposed skin grafts to become adherent while the child remains immobile after surgery. Ketamine tends to maintain or slightly increase intra-ocular pressure and can be used for examination of the eye under anaesthesia if the intra-ocular pressure is to be measured. Intracranial pressure is increased by ketamine and its use should be avoided if there is any possibility of pre-existing elevation of intracranial pressure.

Relaxants (see Appendix IX(a), p. 746)

Although it has been stated that the neonate is particularly sensitive to non-depolarising neuromuscular blockers, this is probably related to the more marked effect of small doses of relaxant on respiration because of poor respiratory reserve and dependence on the diaphragm, rather than a myasthenic response of neonatal neuromuscular function. Recent work shows a greater variation amongst neonates in their response to non-depolarising relaxants than occurs in the older child and adult, but the conclusion is that for surgical relaxation a 'scaled-down' adult dose should be used initially. Subsequent 'top-up' doses should be restricted to one-tenth of the initial dose. Residual paralysis or difficulty in reversal at the end of surgery are likely to be associated either with acid–base abnormalities or hypothermia, correction of which restores muscle activity to normal.

Curare (0.5 mg/kg) causes much less hypotension in the child than the adult. Histamine release does occur; thus there is a relative contraindication to the use of curare in the asthmatic child.

Pancuronium (0.1 mg/kg) is similar in action to curare but has the advantage of causing less histamine release. The tachycardia caused by pancuronium is a disadvantage in children, who normally have a rapid heart rate.

Atracurium (0.5 mg/kg) causes rapid onset of relaxation. The duration of action (approximately 30 min) is particularly appropriate for many paediatric surgical procedures. Release of histamine occurs, and anaphylactic reactions have been reported in children.

Vecuronium (0.1 mg/kg) has a similar onset and duration of action to those of atracurium. The incidence of histamine release is less. Vecuronium may be the muscle relaxant of choice for procedures that last 20–30 min. When given by infusion, vecuronium may be used for longer surgical procedures or in the ITU.

The neonate is said to be resistant to the depolarising relaxant suxamethonium. The dose required is normally approximately twice that used in adults on a body weight basis, i.e. 2 mg/kg. This is related to the distribution of the drug in the relatively larger extracellular fluid space. Bradycardia occurring after administration of suxamethonium may be avoided by prior administration of atropine.

ANAESTHETIC MANAGEMENT

Preoperative preparation

Every patient should be visited by the anaesthetist prior to surgery. The procedures involved in anaesthesia should be explained to the patient, in the presence of a parent if possible, and in suitable language if the child is old enough to understand. Older children may express a preference for the type of induction and this should be used if possible.

The patient should be assessed for fitness for anaesthesia. Upper respiratory infections are common, as are other viral infections, e.g. measles, mumps or chickenpox. These are a contraindication to anaesthesia for non-essential operations, but not for a more urgent procedure. The presence of pyrexia may indicate infection and is a contraindication to non-urgent surgery. The patient's weight should be noted as this is the

Table 34.9 Estimates of children's weights

Age	Body weight (kg) (approximate average values)
Neonate	3
4 months	6
1–8 years	2 × age + 9
9–13 years	3 × age

most reliable and simple guide to drug dosage (Table 34.9). Veins should be examined with regard to i.v. induction and the establishment of i.v. infusions.

Premedication

Premedication should be prescribed according to the needs of the patient. Many children do not require sedation or analgesia preoperatively, particularly the very young and outpatients. Secretions may contribute to respiratory obstruction in small airways and premedication with an antisialagogue may be required. Hyoscine (15 μg/kg) is an effective drying agent with sedative and antiemetic properties. Atropine (20 μg/kg) is a most effective drug for prevention of arrhythmias from cardiovagal stimulation resulting from the oculocardiac reflex or tracheal intubation, but is more useful for this purpose when given i.v. at the induction of anaesthesia. Atropine should not be given i.m. to patients with pyrexia, but may be used i.v. at induction. Glycopyrronium bromide is a suitable alternative in children; in a dose of 10 μg/kg i.v., it causes less tachycardia than atropine 20 μg/kg.

If analgesia is required preoperatively, an opioid premedication (morphine 0.2 mg/kg, or papaveretum 0.3 mg/kg) may be prescribed. The resultant respiratory depression may impede inhalational induction of anaesthesia.

The majority of older children require only sedation. The drugs used most frequently are trimeprazine 3 mg/kg, diazepam 0.2–0.4 mg/kg or droperidol 0.2–0.4 mg/kg administered orally.

Induction

Parents should be allowed to be present during induction of anaesthesia if they so wish.

Anaesthesia may be induced either by inhalation, i.v., i.m., or rectal administration of drugs. Intravenous induction is associated with decreased Sa_{O_2} in a significant proportion of children. Inhalational induction may be accomplished rapidly with halothane or cyclopropane; these may be administered directly by mask or by placing the T-piece in the anaesthetist's hands. The latter technique reduces anxiety in the patient, but causes greater pollution of the atmosphere.

There is no place for the use of gas mixtures containing less than 30% O_2 to increase the rapidity of induction. If laryngeal spasm occurs, the small reserves of oxygen are depleted further by such mixtures and very severe hypoxaemia may result.

The child should be monitored throughout an inhalational induction using a precordial stethoscope.

Intravenous induction may be virtually painless if a 25 or 27 needle is used. EMLA cream (see p. 266) applied at least 1 h preoperatively reduces the incidence of discomfort from venepuncture or insertion of an i.v. cannula. Intravenous injections in children may be difficult between the ages of 6 months and 2 years because of increased subcutaneous fat. The veins are very mobile in children and the skin should be stretched tightly to stabilise the veins. An assistant is essential to hold and squeeze the arm and to distract and immobilise the patient.

Rectal induction is slow, taking up to 15 min, and requires supervision for a prolonged period, during which the patient is at risk of developing respiratory depression and obstruction.

Airway management

The physiological deadspace of the young infant is small but the V_D/V_T ratio is the same throughout life (0.3). Any increase in deadspace from anaesthetic apparatus is more significant in the infant, and therefore must be kept to a minimum.

The Rendell–Baker–Soucek mask is designed specifically to minimise deadspace in infants. When holding the mask, it is important not to press upward on the tongue below the mandible (Fig. 34.4) as this may occlude the airway totally by pushing the tongue against the posterior pharyngeal wall. The chin should be supported by pressure on the mandible alone (Fig. 34.5).

The use of the Ayres' T-piece apparatus reduces deadspace to a minimum and also has the advantage of a low resistance to expiration because of the absence of valves. The T-piece may be used for anaesthesia using spontaneous ventilation, but

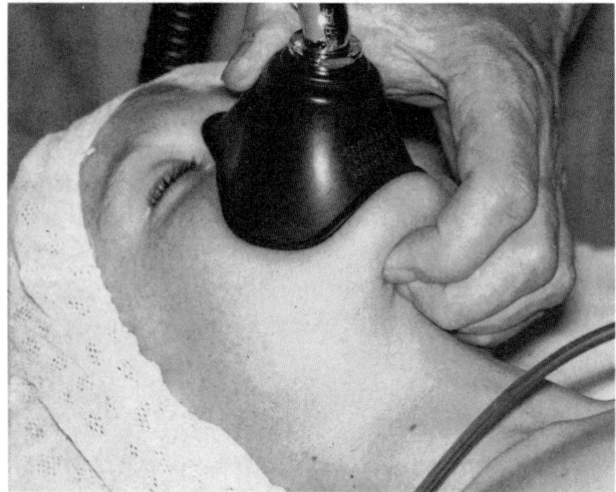

Fig. 34.4 Incorrect way of holding paediatric facemask.

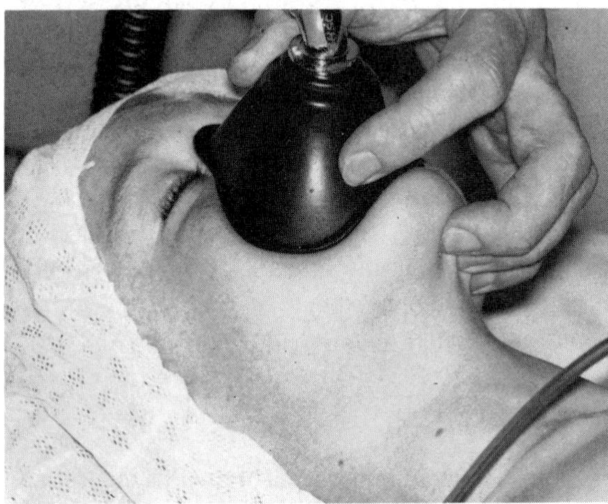

Fig. 34.5 Correct way of holding paediatric facemask.

only for short periods in the very young as even the small increase in deadspace causes an unacceptable level of rebreathing. The fresh gas flow should be calculated as 2.5 times the predicted minute volume.

Jackson Rees modified the T-piece by the addition of an open-ended reservoir bag, and this allows the apparatus to be used for controlled ventilation. Alternatively, a ventilator may be attached to the expiratory limb for controlled ventilation. In this mode, a fresh gas flow rate of 1000 ml + 100 ml/kg body weight per min results in an arterial P_{CO_2} of 4.8–5.3 kPa (35–40 mmHg). A minimum gas flow of 3 litres/min is required to operate the system satisfactorily.

The size of the small baby causes difficulty in maintenance of the airway during surgery with a mask. Most infants require tracheal intubation. The reduction in cross-sectional area of the airway caused by a 3.5- or 4.0-mm tube in a small infant causes an increase in resistance of approximately 16 times, compared with a threefold increase in an adult with a 9.5-mm tracheal tube. Thus controlled ventilation should always be undertaken in an infant subjected to tracheal intubation.

The very young are obligate nose-breathers and secretions caused by upper respiratory infection may lead to respiratory difficulty, particularly in the postoperative period. Enlarged tonsils and adenoids may cause difficulty with airway maintenance, especially in the older child. This may be overcome by the use of an oropharyngeal airway.

Tracheal intubation

The anatomy of the infant may cause difficulties in tracheal intubation. Infants have a relatively large head, short neck and large tongue. The mandible may be underdeveloped.

The larynx is higher in the neck (C3–4) than in the adult (C5–6) and is placed more anteriorly. The epiglottis is large, floppy and U-shaped and is not easily elevated using the conventional Macintosh laryngoscope in the valeculla (Fig. 34.6). Intubation in the very young is easier if the epiglottis is elevated using a laryngoscope with a straight blade.

The internal diameter of a tracheal tube for a child may be calculated from the formula:

$$\frac{\text{Age}}{4} + 4 \text{ mm}$$

INFANT LARYNX
U shaped epiglottis
Large arytenoids

ADULT LARYNX
Flat epiglottis

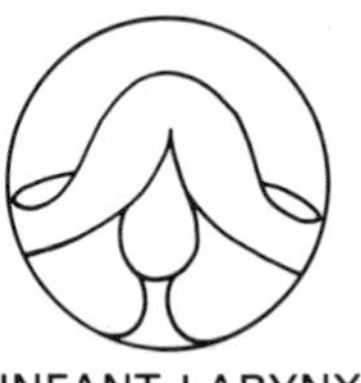

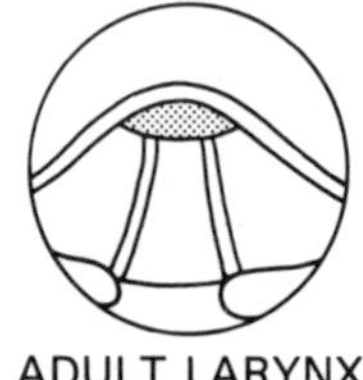

Fig. 34.6 The infant and adult larynx.

The tube should be small enough to allow a leak during the application of positive pressure, otherwise pressure on the tissues of the glottis or cricoid may lead to oedema following extubation. This may cause stridor up to 8 h later and require reintubation. For this reason, intubation, although not entirely contraindicated, should be avoided in outpatients or day cases. Tracheal tubes with shoulders (e.g. the Cole) may cause glottic oedema from pressure of the shoulder on the lax tissues of the glottis.

The tracheal tube should be secured firmly to avoid accidental extubation or bronchial intubation during anaesthesia. If adhesive tape is used, the tube should be secured to the maxilla and not the mandible, which is extremely mobile in small children (except where this is not feasible, e.g. cleft lip and palate surgery).

The trachea of the infant is short (4 cm) at birth. Both lung fields must be auscultated to confirm correct positioning of the tracheal tube. Although the angles between main bronchi and trachea are more nearly equal than in the adult, a tracheal tube still tends to enter the right main bronchus. Preformed tracheal tubes (e.g. the Oxford) have the disadvantage of a fixed length, which may result in bronchial intubation.

The narrowest part of the airway of the child is the cricoid ring. Because this is circular (unlike the diamond-shaped glottic opening which is the narrowest part of the adult airway) a cuff on the tracheal tube is unnecessary if the correct size has been selected. Thus, in children up to 5–6 years of age, a tube of the same diameter may be used for either nasotracheal or orotracheal intubation.

Monitoring

Direct observation of the patient is the most important single method of monitoring. The anaesthetist may see changes in the patient's colour (cyanosis or pallor). Movement or lacrimation may be detected if anaesthesia is too light, or a change in respiratory pattern if respiratory obstruction occurs. A clear plastic drape permits observation of the patient during head and neck surgery when normal drapes totally obscure the small patient (Fig. 34.7).

The stethoscope, precordial or oesophageal, is the single most valuable monitoring device available to the anaesthetist and should always be attached before induction. It allows continuous monitoring of heart sounds for rate, rhythm and intensity. In the infant, the intensity of sound varies with the stroke volume, and acts as a quali-

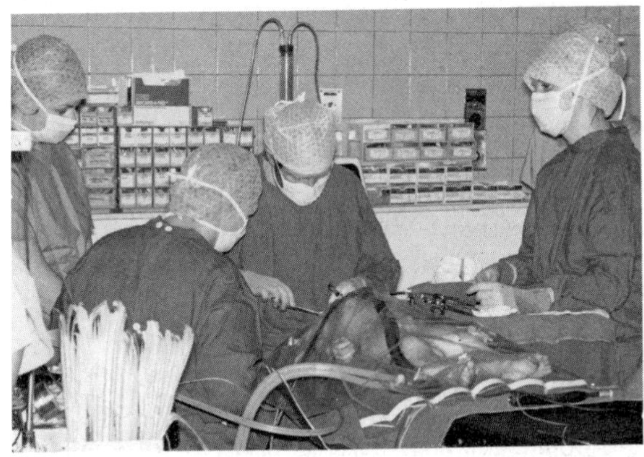

Fig. 34.7 Use of plastic surgical drapes to permit observation of child.

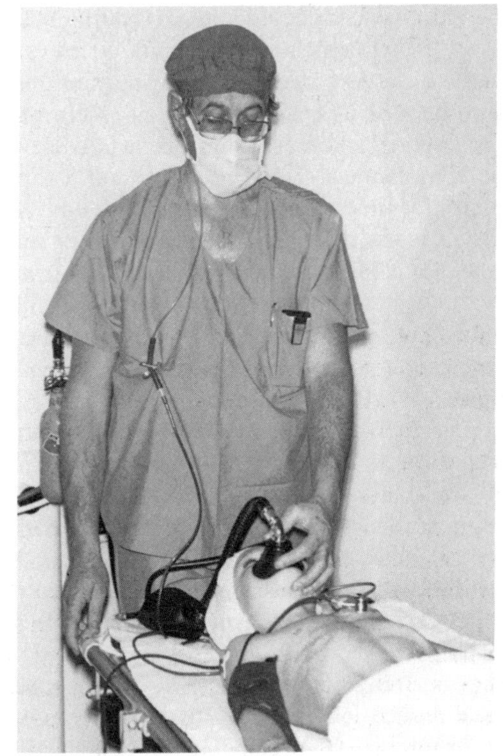

Fig. 34.8 Continuous use of precordial stethoscope.

tative monitor of cardiac output. The stethoscope should always be used to check both lungs following intubation to confirm that bronchial intubation has not taken place and it continues to give an indication of changes in ventilation during anaesthesia (Fig. 34.8).

The ECG provides less information than the stethoscope but may demonstrate arrhythmias. An arterial pressure cuff and temperature probe should always be attached before induction. Pulse oximetry is recommended strongly.

It is important to have an i.v. infusion established, all monitoring apparatus attached and the patient positioned correctly before draping, as access to the patient may be extremely limited during surgery.

NEONATAL ANAESTHESIA

Additional problems are associated with anaesthetising the neonate because of size and immaturity. Temperature maintenance mechanisms are immature, and the patient must be kept warm during transport, induction and anaesthesia. The temperature should be monitored continuously, and the environmental temperature elevated throughout surgery. Venous access may be more difficult because of small mobile veins; scalp veins can be used in addition to limb veins. A flexible 24 or 22 G cannula should be used with a three-way tap for injection of drugs or blood. Any extension to the i.v. line should have a very small volume. Care must be taken to avoid overtransfusion. Burette infusion sets should be filled initially only to a volume of 10 ml/kg. Sedative premedication is not required for the neonate. Atropine 15–20 μg/kg i.m. may be given to reduce secretions and prevent vagal stimulation during tracheal intubation and surgery. Vitamin K_1 1 mg should be given to reduce the neonatal bleeding tendency resulting from lack of vitamin K-dependent factors.

Ventilation by face mask should be carried out with extreme care to avoid inflation of the stomach.

The anatomy of the neonate may render tracheal intubation difficult. In the very small, weak or premature neonate, it is customary to perform intubation before induction of anaesthesia. This reduces the likelihood of aspiration of gastric contents and the need to ventilate by mask, with subsequent gastric distension. In addition, the baby is able to breathe if attempts to intubate fail. The disadvantages of awake intubation are that it is often traumatic and it may be more difficult to see the larynx than in the anaesthetised child.

A normal neonate requires a 3.5-mm tube, and a premature child a 3.0-mm or rarely a 2.5-mm tube.

Drugs should be prepared before anaesthesia and given from 1-ml or 2-ml syringes to avoid excessive administration of fluid. Cardiovascular monitoring must be continuous. Non-depolarising relaxants may be given in scaled adult doses initially (atracurium 0.5 mg/kg, vecuronium 0.1 mg/kg) but subsequent doses should be only one-tenth of the initial dose.

The neonate should not be allowed to breathe spontaneously under anaesthesia for any length of time; the inefficient respiratory system is depressed easily and the presence of a small tracheal tube greatly increases resistance. Controlled ventilation is carried out preferably by hand so that changes in compliance or resistance may be detected early.

Many neonatal surgical procedures affect pulmonary function. The major airways may be obstructed totally in repair of tracheo-oesophageal fistula, or compliance reduced greatly following the treatment of exomphalos or diaphragmatic hernia.

Bradycardia is usually a sign of hypoxaemia and should be treated by ventilation with 100% oxygen. Supplements of inhalational agents (halothane, enflurane or isoflurane) should be used in small doses to avoid hypotension, and should be discontinued several minutes before the end of anaesthesia to avoid residual depression.

Relaxants should be antagonised by neostigmine and atropine. If there is any doubt with regard to the quality of reversal, the temperature should be checked carefully and any abnormality in acid–base status treated appropriately. Any child whose respiration may be compromised after surgery should receive pulmonary ventilation electively. Opioid analgesics should be avoided postoperatively as they cause severe depression of respiration. Local anaesthetic techniques may provide excellent analgesia after many procedures in the neonate.

SPECIFIC OPERATIONS IN THE NEONATE

Pyloric stenosis

This occurs usually in babies of 3–8 weeks of age. In mild cases, the child may be well nourished and hydrated, but if severe, extreme dehydration and electrolyte imbalance are present, with hypokalaemia and severe metabolic alkalosis. Surgical treatment by pyloromyotomy is not an emergency and fluid and electrolyte imbalance should be corrected before anaesthesia. The child may have had a barium swallow, and a nasogastric tube should always be passed and aspirated before induction; the patient should nevertheless be treated as though he has a full stomach. If an i.v. infusion is in progress, i.v. induction should be used, the trachea intubated after suxamethonium (1.5–2 mg/kg) and paralysis maintained with a non-depolarising muscle relaxant or intermittent suxamethonium. Hyperventilation should be avoided to prevent worsening of the pre-existing alkalosis which may lead to slow onset of respiration at the termination of anaesthesia. The nasogastric tube should be aspirated before tracheal extubation.

Tracheo-oesophageal fistula and oesophageal atresia

The commonest form of this disorder is oesophageal atresia with a fistula between the trachea and the lower part of the oesophagus. The diagnosis may be made if the child aspirates secretions continually or chokes on his feed. The presence of a fistula may be detected by persistent pulmonary problems as a result of aspiration from the stomach. A large tube should be placed in the upper oesophageal pouch to aspirate secretions. Anaesthesia is similar to that for other neonates but particular problems are associated with intubation of the fistula and inflation of the stomach. The position of the tube must be checked by auscultation.

During surgery, large airways may be kinked or clamped accidentally and surgical retraction may cause dramatic decreases in cardiac output by compression of the left and right atria or vagus nerve. Respiratory and cardiovascular systems should be monitored closely. The respiratory problems resulting from aspiration through the fistula do not resolve until after surgery but tracheobronchial toilet should be performed both before and after surgery, and postoperative elective ventilation may be required.

Diaphragmatic hernia

The usual presentation is that of severe acute respiratory distress and cyanosis, with a flat or scaphoid abdomen. Chest X-ray is usually diagnostic. Resuscitation should be initially by tracheal intubation and controlled ventilation. Positive pressure ventilation must not be carried out using bag and mask, as expansion of the viscera in the hernia further compresses the contralateral lung and heart. Nitrous oxide should be avoided to prevent gas distension. Arterial or capillary blood gases should be monitored.

If the lungs expand well, the trachea may be extubated postoperatively when blood gases are normal. Some infants have a hypoplastic lung on the side of the hernia, usually the left. If the hernia occurred early in fetal life there may be some hypoplasia of the contralateral lung also; thus there may be insufficient pulmonary tissue to maintain life. Some children may survive after treatment in the ITU with controlled ventilation and a pulmonary arterial vasodilator, e.g. tolazoline. Bilateral chest drains should be inserted, as there is a danger of pneumothorax if high ventilatory pressures are required.

Exomphalos and gastroschisis

In these conditions there is herniation of the abdominal contents through the anterior abdominal wall. In exomphalos, the sac of the hernia is within the umbilical cord. In gastroschisis the hernia is lateral to the umbilicus and the bowel usually lacks any covering. If the defect is large, there is a likelihood of dramatic loss of heat and fluid from exposed bowel. It may not be possible to return the bowel to the small abdominal cavity; the bowel may be protected initially in a silastic pouch and replaced gradually into the abdomen over a few days.

Bowel obstruction

Obstruction may be the result of an atresia at any point from duodenum to anal canal. Malrotation, volvulus and reduplication of bowel may cause obstructive symptoms. Meconium ileus, a premonitory sign of cystic fibrosis, may cause neonatal obstruction, although the associated respiratory problems are not usually of significance in the neonate. The major anaesthetic problems are those of fluid and electrolyte imbalance and danger of regurgitation and aspiration.

Myelomeningocoele

This is a defect resulting from the failure of the neural tube to close in the fetus. If the defect is large, there may be severe problems of heat and fluid loss during surgery, and blood loss may be difficult to estimate because of mixture with CSF.

Hydrocephalus

Hydrocephalus may result from the closure of a myelomeningocoele or the associated Arnold–Chiari syndrome. A shunt procedure to drain CSF into the right atrium or peritoneal cavity may be required. Problems may be encountered in relation to raised intracranial pressure (ICP). In the very young with open fontanelles, tapping of the lateral ventricle may help reduce acute increases in pressure. Ketamine and volatile agents must be avoided. Hypertension resulting from raised ICP may disappear rapidly when ICP is reduced. Hypercapnia should be avoided at all stages. Blood loss is not usually a problem during shunt surgery.

Cleft lip and palate

This may cause airway problems which lead to difficult intubation, especially in association with Pierre Robin syndrome. Some surgeons treat these conditions during the neonatal period but it is more common to repair the cleft lip at 2–3 months and the palate at 18 months to 2 years.

Atropine 20 μg/kg should be given, as secretions may be a problem. The airway should be monitored closely, as the tracheal tube may be kinked or compressed by the gag used during cleft palate repair. A throat pack is inserted before surgery; its insertion and removal should be recorded. In some cases of Pierre Robin syndrome or mild micrognathia, closure of the soft palate may cause airway difficulty postoperatively, requiring tracheal intubation for a day or two. Blood may be required for cleft lip or palate surgery but losses do not usually exceed 15% of blood volume. Congenital heart disease is a commonly associated disorder in patients with cleft lip or palate.

The airway may be compromised after cleft palate closure and analgesic drugs must be given in reduced doses. The child should be admitted to the ITU or a 24-h recovery area overnight.

POSTOPERATIVE CARE

When adequate ventilation has been re-established after recovery from anaesthesia, the child should be nursed in the lateral position and the airway, cardiovascular system and temperature monitored closely in an adequately equipped postoperative recovery area (see Ch. 24). Oxygen should be administered during transfer from the operating theatre, and until the child awakens in the recovery area. The patient should be awake before return to the ward. Recovery from ketamine anaesthesia should take place in a quiet undisturbed manner. Diazepam 0.2 mg/kg may be required if there is evidence of psychological upset.

Laryngeal spasm

Laryngeal spasm is a relatively frequent complication of paediatric anaesthesia particularly after volatile agents have been used. Treatment comprises ventilation with 100% oxygen under positive pressure by bag and mask. If bradycardia occurs, the trachea should be reintubated rapidly and the lungs inflated with 100% oxygen. Laryngeal spasm may be avoided by extubating the trachea either when the patient is totally awake or when surgically anaesthetised. Extubation should not be carried out when the patient is only lightly anaesthetised or just beginning to cough. The pharynx should be cleared of all secretions under direct vision as these may precipitate this particularly dangerous hazard.

Postoperative pain

Pain is frequent although not usually as protracted or severe a problem in children as in adult patients. Analgesics should be prescribed as a routine, except for neonates and small infants. For severe pain, i.m. opioids are required while for less severe pain, milder drugs, e.g. paracetamol elixir orally, are preferable. Dihydrocodeine may be given also as an elixir.

Local anaesthesia

Blocks which are suitable include extradurals (thoracic or lumbar) with or without a catheter, and caudal, intercostal, ilioinguinal and penile blocks. For the upper limb, axillary block, and for the lower limb femoral, lateral cutaneous nerve of thigh, or sciatic nerve block may be useful. A local block can be used as the sole technique of anaesthesia in the severely ill child, or in circumstances in which it may be desirable to avoid the metabolic upset associated with general anaesthesia, e.g. the severely dehydrated child with pyloric stenosis. Caudal anaesthesia has been shown to be useful in the neonate with a low imperforate anus. Local techniques should be performed on the young child only by experienced anaesthetists.

INTENSIVE THERAPY

The total reliance of the newborn on the diaphragm for adequate ventilation may result in a requirement for prolonged controlled ventilation if the diaphragm is paralysed or splinted by high intra-abdominal pressure. This may occur after surgery for gastroschisis or exomphalos, where abdominal growth is not adequate to contain the entire bowel. Severe splinting may also occur with distension of the bowel as a result of necrotising enterocolitis, bowel obstruction or gastro-enteritis.

Controlled ventilation may be required for babies with cardiac or respiratory failure. Institution of controlled ventilation may be necessary irrespective of blood gas values because of a clinical diagnosis of exhaustion.

The newborn tolerates relatively high ventilatory and intrathoracic pressures without a decrease in cardiac output because of his large right ventricle, which regresses slowly following the change from fetal to adult type of circulation. However, there is a danger of lung rupture leading to pneumothorax.

The immature respiratory system with small, easily obstructed airways, is the factor responsible for the majority of admissions to the ITU. The child has little respiratory reserve and any increase in airway resistance or decrease in compliance may require respiratory support or assistance.

The method of choice for maintenance of the airway is nasotracheal intubation in preference to tracheostomy except when very prolonged airway control is required or a severe anatomical disorder of the upper airway or trachea is present. Narrow nasal tubes require meticulous care and attention to detail including fixation to prevent kinking or dislodgement of the tube and ulceration of the nares as a result of pressure. Humidification is of paramount importance if obstruction by secretions (requiring reintubation under emergency conditions) is to be avoided. If necessary the patient should be sedated to assist toleration of the tracheal tube. Aspiration of secretions should be carried out regularly using soft atraumatic catheters no larger than half the diameter of the tracheal tube. The duration of suction should be limited to a few seconds to prevent hypoxaemia. As with patients undergoing anaesthesia, a child should not be allowed to breathe through a small tracheal tube for prolonged periods without support either by positive pressure ventilation or continuous positive airways pressure (CPAP). Particular attention should be paid to adequate hydration of the patient in addition to humidification of inspired gas. The environmental temperature should be kept close to the neutral thermal environment to minimise oxygen requirements.

Respiratory distress syndrome (hyaline membrane disease)

This occurs particularly in the premature as a result of absence of pulmonary surfactant. This defect allows the alveoli to collapse, causing a decrease in compliance, and tachypnoea. Respiration is grunting in nature as the child breathes out against a closed glottis in an attempt to maintain alveolar patency. Mild cases may recover if the hypoxaemia is treated with humidified oxygen, and the acidosis is corrected. The arterial P_{O_2} should be maintained at a minimum of 9.5 kPa (70 mmHg). More severe cases require mechanical assistance to keep the alveoli patent either with spontaneous respiration using nasal catheters or tracheal intubation to induce CPAP. The most severe cases require IPPV with PEEP.

Acute epiglottitis

This condition results from bacterial infection, usually by *Haemophilus influenzae*. The child usually presents between the ages of 2 and 7 years. There is a rapid onset of severe respiratory obstruction and dysphagia resulting from glottic swelling. The patient cannot swallow saliva and has to sit to avoid choking. Toxaemia is usually present. Treatment is by tracheal intubation under general anaesthesia, and antibiotic therapy. An i.v. infusion should be started and atropine 20 μg/kg given i.v. to avoid the effects of vagal stimulation when the inflamed epiglottis is stimulated during intubation. Anaesthesia is induced by inhalation of 100% oxygen with halothane, with the child in the sitting position. Induction may be difficult and protracted in the presence of respiratory obstruction. Intubation may be extremely difficult because of the swollen epiglottis. An ENT surgeon should be standing by to perform emergency tracheostomy if total respiratory obstruction occurs. An oral tube should be used initially but this may be changed subsequently for a nasal tube when a clear airway has been established. Extubation is normally possible after antibiotic therapy for 24–48 h.

Laryngotracheobronchitis

This may be bacterial or, more commonly, viral in origin and is the most frequent cause of croup in children. It is a disorder of the larger airways. In mild conditions it may be treated with well-humidified oxygen but if severe the trachea should be intubated. If hypoxaemia is present, IPPV may be necessary. Stridor and an increase in the work of breathing leading to physical exhaustion may necessitate tracheal intubation and ventilation on purely clinical grounds before the establishment of biochemical evidence of hypoxia. Profuse viscid secretions are a major problem. Humidification is of the utmost importance, and additional quantities of water should be instilled into the airways before the aspiration of secretions to maintain patency of the tube. If the cause is viral, the course of the disease runs for 10 to 14 days during which time airway support may be required.

Bronchiolitis

This is a viral disorder of the smaller airways causing expiratory wheeze. Hypoxaemia tends to occur early and secretions are a problem. Tracheal intubation and ventilation are required frequently in this condition.

Cardiac arrest and resuscitation in children

The commonest causes of cardiac arrest in children are:

1. Hypoxaemia.
2. Hypovolaemia.
3. Electrolyte imbalance.
4. Overdose of drugs.

Prevention of cardiac arrest and its sequelae may be achieved to a great extent by ensuring that all seriously ill children are well oxygenated, the circulating volume is maintained and electrolyte imbalances are monitored continuously and treated when appropriate. Meticulous care should be taken with the doses of all drugs.

Cardiac arrest in children is associated more commonly with asystole than ventricular fibrillation. Thus treatment with adrenaline (1 in 10 000) should be used early, as acidosis reduces the effectiveness of catecholamines.

FURTHER READING

Arthur D S, McNicol L R 1986 Local anaesthetic techniques in paediatric surgery. British Journal of Anaesthesia 58: 760

Brown T C K, Fisk G C 1979 Anaesthesia for children. Blackwell Scientific Publications, Oxford

Hatch D, Sumner E 1986 Neonatal anaesthesia and perioperative care. Edward Arnold, London

Jackson Rees G, Gray T C 1981 Paediatric anaesthesia. Trends in current practice. Butterworths, London

Pang L M, Mellins R B 1975 Neonatal cardiorespiratory physiology. Anesthesiology 43: 171

Rackow H, Salanitre E 1969 Modern concepts in pediatric anesthesiology. Anesthesiology 30: 208

Rylance G 1981 Clinical pharmacology. Drugs in children. British Medical Journal 282: 50

Smith R M 1980 Anesthesia for infants and children. C V Mosby, St Louis

Steward D J 1984 Manual of paediatric anaesthesia. Churchill Livingstone, Edinburgh

Steward D J (ed) 1981 Some aspects of paediatric anaesthesia. Biochemical Press, Amsterdam

Vivori E, Bush G H 1977 Modern aspects of the management of the newborn undergoing surgery. British Journal of Anaesthesia 49: 51

Winter R W 1973 The body fluids in pediatrics. Little, Brown, Boston

35. Dental anaesthesia

The term 'dental anaesthesia' encompasses the administration of a general anaesthetic, local anaesthetic or sedation technique to an outpatient in a dental hospital or dentist's surgery. Extensive dental surgery is carried out normally by oral surgeons upon hospital inpatients, and the anaesthetic considerations for this treatment are similar to those of general anaesthesia for ENT surgery. This chapter describes only the techniques appropriate to the former categories.

In 1976, 1.2 million dental anaesthetics were administered in England and Wales for extractions, and a further 129 000 for conservation work. This workload could not be accommodated in hospital practice and, for the foreseeable future, a substantial and major proportion of dental anaesthetics will be given to outpatients. Much of this work could be avoided if patients attended for regular dental treatment, but the attitude to conservation is complex and relates to the influence of education, custom and previous experiences of the patient.

Local anaesthetic blocks are safer than general anaesthetic techniques and patients should be encouraged to have dental work performed under local anaesthesia. It has been estimated that more than 60 million local anaesthetics are given annually in the UK. However, local techniques are contraindicated in some conditions, notably infection, but this is present only in a small proportion of patients presenting for surgery.

The estimated mortality rate of dental anaesthesia is 1/260 000, which compares favourably with the extrapolated mortality rate for general anaesthetics of 1/10 000. Much of this difference results from the fact that dental anaesthesia is of very short duration and the patients are usually young and healthy.

Most patients experience marked anxiety whilst undergoing dental treatment. In an attempt to reduce this, many combinations of drugs and techniques (including acupuncture and hypnotism) have been employed to produce mental relaxation without loss of consciousness. Currently, the two most popular techniques comprise sedation either with nitrous oxide/oxygen or with a drug administered i.v.

GENERAL ANAESTHETIC TECHNIQUES

Anaesthetic equipment

Historically, dental anaesthetists have used intermittent flow anaesthetic machines, but these are less accurate than continuous flow machines and are less familiar to most hospital anaesthetists. Continuous flow machines have the advantages of economy, simplicity, reliability, familiarity to junior anaesthetists, accuracy and flexibility.

The anaesthetic equipment and facilities which should be available in a dental outpatient surgery have been detailed in the Wylie report and include a basic anaesthetic machine (Fig. 35.1) with an oxygen failsafe device and inability to provide less than 20% oxygen, a vaporiser, a suitable range of masks, valves, laryngoscopes, tracheal tubes and suction apparatus. All persons working in the anaesthetic area must be familiar with the emergency drug tray, the contents of which should be complete and unexpired. Lighting should be bright and enable the anaesthetist to see the patient and the anaesthetic machine clearly. The

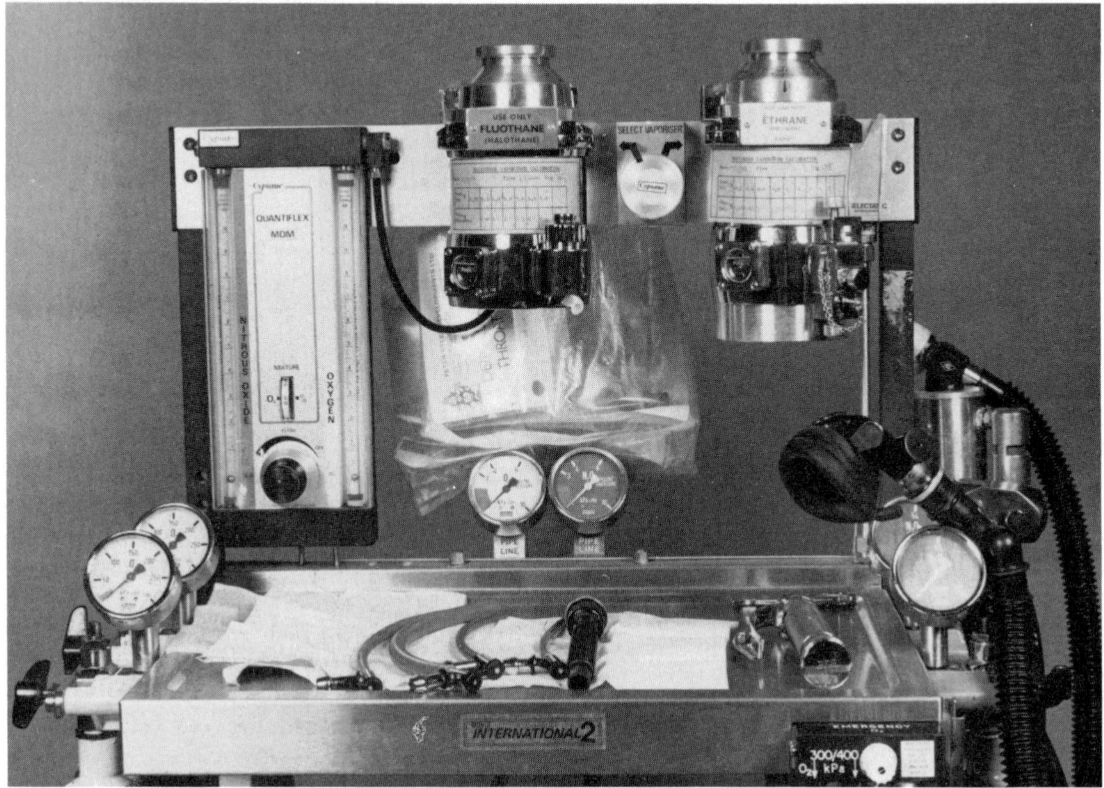

Fig. 35.1 Boyle international anaesthetic machine fitted with a Quantiflex rotameter head, with single dials to control both flow and mixture. This machine is ideal for both anaesthesia and relative analgesia. Note the reversed position of oxygen and nitrous oxide. This machine is fitted also with detachable vaporisers.

premises should be provided with easy access for emergency services.

It has been recommended that some provision be made for scavenging anaesthetic gases, particularly if volatile agents are used. Scavenging requires a collecting device round the anaesthetic breathing system valve (Fig. 35.2), and this may render the nasal mask rather cumbersome and awkward in use. The valve may be positioned at a different part of the breathing system, but the efficiency of the system is impaired. For these reasons many anaesthetists rely solely upon good ventilation of the surgery.

Outpatient anaesthesia

Outpatient dental anaesthesia is undertaken for the same reason as other forms of outpatient surgery, i.e. speed, economy, convenience and because there are insufficient facilities to enable the surgery to be undertaken on inpatients. Only predominantly healthy patients should be considered for outpatient dental anaesthesia. Most hospitals have inpatient facilities for dental emergencies and patients with recognised risk factors should be admitted for treatment.

Selection of patients

The majority of patients requiring outpatient anaesthesia are children. There are two distinct groups:

1. Those too young to cooperate for local anaesthesia, or with oral infection which renders a local technique inadvisable.
2. Uncooperative children, many of whom are handicapped, who require conservation dentistry.

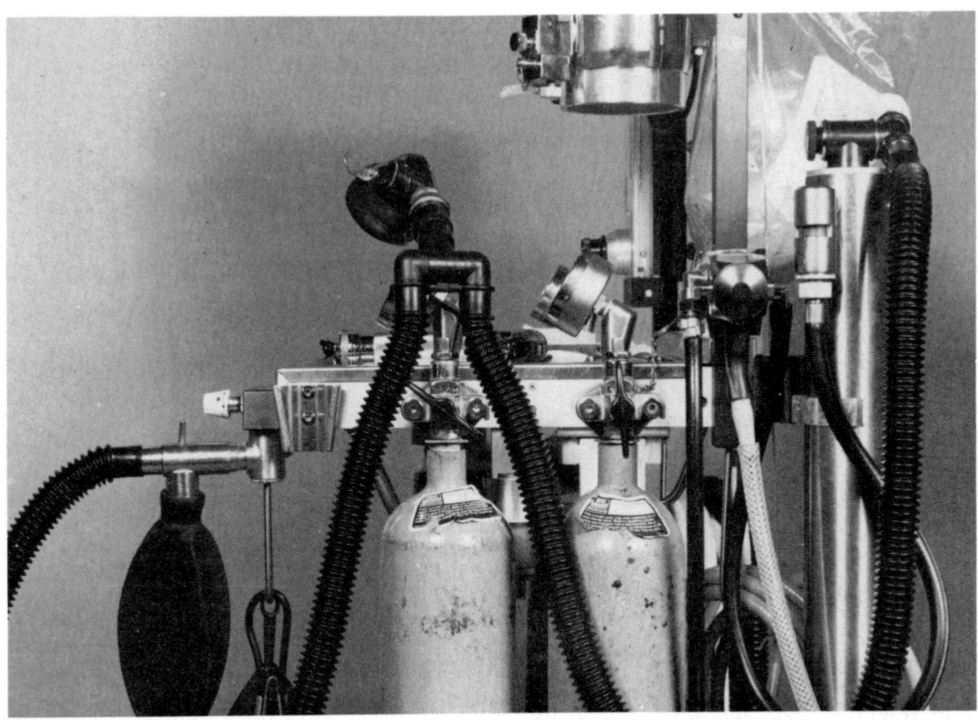

Fig. 35.2 View of anaesthetic machine showing the fitting of the active scavenging unit and the adapted breathing system.

These patients often require extensive work which should be undertaken only after tracheal intubation.

Adults are less likely to require general anaesthesia for emergency dental work but it may be necessary in the presence of infection.

Written consent should be obtained before undertaking treatment under general anaesthesia. This may be difficult to obtain from children, but a guardian's or parental consent is essential unless the condition is so serious that the child's life is in danger; this is virtually unknown in dental work. It should be remembered that most children presenting for either emergency or elective dental work have not been examined by a medical practitioner and the contact with the anaesthetist is the first meeting with a physician. It is common practice to ask the parent or guardian to complete a form with a series of questions about the health of the child, with particular emphasis on the respiratory and cardiovascular systems and the presence of known allergies (see Ch. 41). It is essential also to ensure that parents and adult patients are given both written and verbal instructions regarding the preparation and precautions which should be taken before and after surgery. It has been demonstrated that many outpatients presenting for surgery ignore instructions and one study noted that 9% of patients drove home, despite instructions to the contrary.

The anaesthetist should know the extent and likely duration of the proposed surgery. An attempt to assess the patency of the nasal airway should be made as tracheal intubation may be required if the nose is blocked. The dentist should have noted and brought to the attention of the anaesthetist the existence of loose teeth. However, it is sound practice to assume that some of the primary dentition of young children is likely to be loose, and great care should be taken in inserting gags and mouth props.

Induction of anaesthesia

The majority of anaesthetists use inhalational anaesthesia for induction in children, but some prefer to use an i.v. agent, e.g. methohexitone.

Some children find the insertion of an i.v. needle painful, and object strongly. Conversely, others dislike the anaesthetic mask and struggle to avoid inhalational anaesthesia. Usually, a combination of tact, persuasion and firmness suffices to induce acceptance of a mask.

Induction of anaesthesia with hypoxic mixtures of N_2O/O_2 (the so-called 'black gas') is now of historical interest only. The inspired concentration of oxygen should never be allowed to decrease below 30% at any time during anaesthesia. Halothane should be introduced early during induction in low concentrations and increased as rapidly as possible without provoking coughing. When the muscle tone of the lower jaw is diminished, the mouth prop or gag (Fig. 35.3) is inserted carefully.

The introduction of a throat pack (Figs 35.4, 35.5) may be undertaken by either the anaesthetist or the dentist, although the latter is usually positioned in front of the patient and has a better view of the oral cavity. The anaesthetist must observe the reservoir bag and ensure that the airway is not compromised during placement of the pack. Correct placement is essential; the pack should not push the tongue back against the posterior pharyngeal wall and should prevent any debris passing into the lower pharynx or larynx. It should prevent oral breathing. A tail from the pack must always protrude out of the mouth to alert staff of its presence. At the end of the procedure, the pack is removed, and the patient is transferred to the recovery room in the hori-

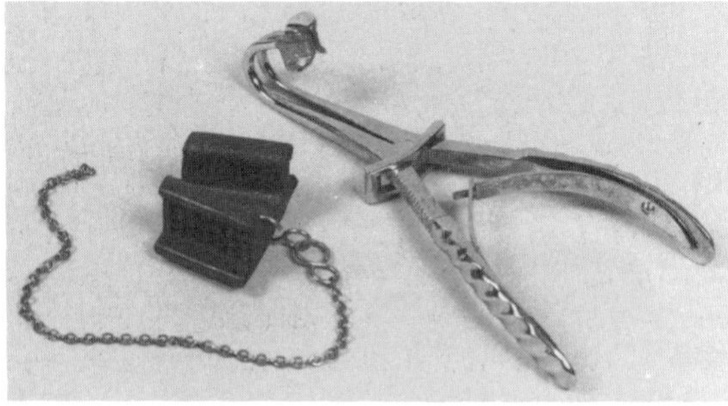

Fig. 35.3 The rubber mouth prop is usually placed in position before inducing i.v. anaesthesia. The Ferguson gag illustrated requires single-handed ambidextrous manipulation to achieve maximum benefit. This requires practice.

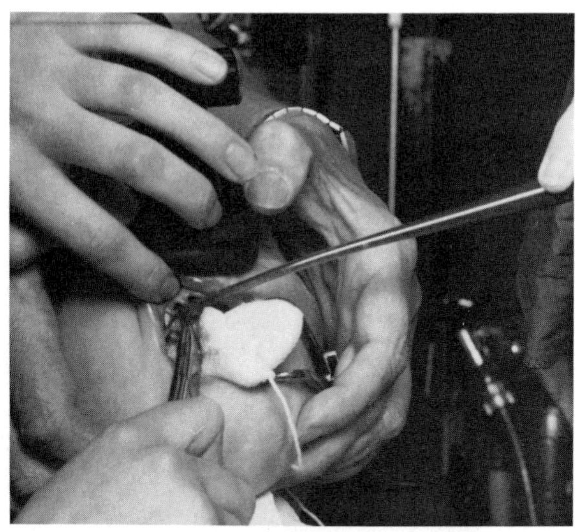

Fig. 35.4 This illustrates the position of the gag and throat pack. The suction is also in use. The nasal mask is positioned to avoid obstructing the external nares, but allowing access to the upper front teeth. Figures 35.4 and 35.5 demonstrate the advantages of the pack being placed by the dentist, who has a better view than the anaesthetist.

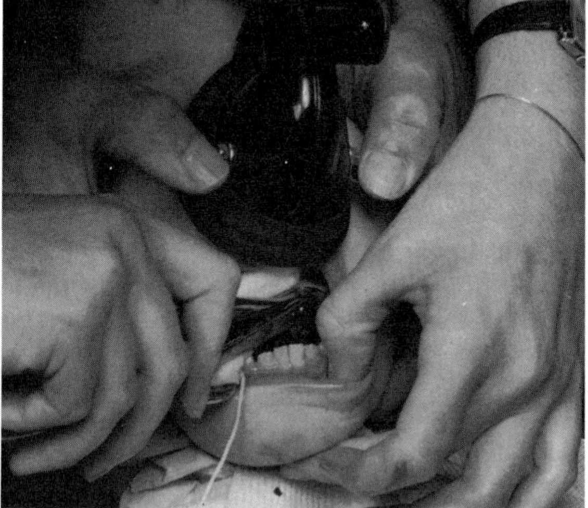

Fig. 35.5 The mouth can become crowded! The anaesthetist's hands support the head and pull the lower jaw forward to maintain the airway. The mouth gag is concealed by the dentist's right hand. The dentist supports the lower jaw. Note the position of the throat pack, with the tail hanging from the mouth. In placing the throat pack, the tongue is not forced back, and the pack is positioned to prevent material from falling posteriorly and also to prevent oral breathing.

zontal position on a trolley. Complete recovery must occur before the patient is discharged.

Monitoring

Careful monitoring is essential during dental anaesthesia. In addition to the normal hazards of anaesthesia, there are risks of airway obstruction resulting from interference with the oral airway, hypotension caused by posture and the effects of anaesthetic drugs, and arrhythmias induced by tooth extraction. Clinical monitoring of the patient's colour, pulse and ventilatory pattern should be routine. It may be awkward to institute instrumental monitoring in the fully clothed dental outpatient, but ECG monitoring is now regarded as essential. Facilities for measurement of arterial pressure should be available. Pulse oximetry is recommended strongly. In addition, the anaesthetic machine should be equipped with an oxygen monitor to ensure that an adequate inspired oxygen concentration is administered.

Problems

The most common difficulty is a problem with the airway, in the form of partial respiratory obstruction. Correct positioning of the jaw obviates much of the problem. It takes considerable practice to position the hands correctly. Initially, the anaesthetist finds great difficulty in simultaneously holding the jaw, operating the gag, applying the mask and adjusting the flows of anaesthetic gases. The ideal position is to hold the jaw well forward with the middle and ring fingers of both hands, whilst both thumbs apply the mask. Once the patient is anaesthetised, the position may be maintained with one hand, thereby allowing the other to insert the gag and open it, while still maintaining an airway. If a clear airway is not possible despite altering the position of the jaw, tracheal intubation should be undertaken.

Some children will have been crying and excessive salivation is not uncommon; this often results in some laryngospasm. Difficulty may then occur, as the spasm causes hypoventilation, diminished uptake of anaesthetic agents and reduction in depth of anaesthesia. Suction may be of some value, but care should be taken not to increase the extent of posterior pharyngeal stimulation.

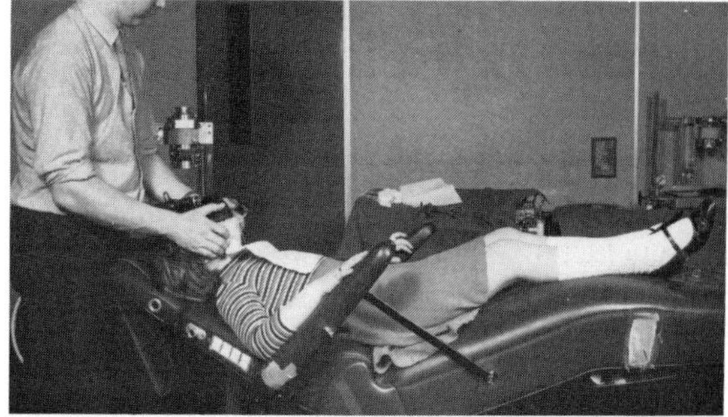

Fig. 35.6 The semisupine position. Note the position of the anaesthetist's fingers holding the jaw forward with both thumbs securing the nasal mask. The anaesthetic machine, suction and dental equipment are to the left. This leaves the right side clear and gives the dentist sufficient room to gain access to all quadrants of the mouth.

Position — horizontal/sitting. There has been considerable controversy regarding the most appropriate position for patients during dental anaesthesia. There is a danger of fainting and resultant cerebral hypoxia in the patient sitting in an upright dental chair. In the horizontal or semisupine position (Fig. 35.6), material is more likely to fall posteriorly down the throat and it has been demonstrated that the nasal airway is less well maintained in this position, as the soft palate acts as a 'curtain' obstruction. This may result in hypoxaemia. On balance it would seem that the position should be the one with which the anaesthetist and dentist are most happy and familiar.

Arrhythmias. Arrhythmias have been reported in approximately 30% of patients undergoing general anaesthesia in the dental chair. Most of these abnormalities are benign, and are usually focal extrasystoles. Neither atropine premedication nor differing anaesthetic techniques have been shown to alter significantly the frequency of arrhythmia. It has been suggested that the patients most at risk are those with increased sympathetic activity, often manifest as tachycardia and a pale frightened appearance.

In the extremely rare event of cardiovascular collapse with no evidence of peripheral perfusion, cardiopulmonary resuscitation should be instituted immediately. Defibrillation should be undertaken as soon as possible, as ventricular fibrillation is more likely to be encountered than asystole.

Induction agents

The choice of i.v. induction agent is limited to those with a rapid rate of induction and short duration of recovery. Many agents are available, but methohexitone is used most commonly. It is administered as a 1% solution in an approximate dose of 1 mg/kg. Its disadvantages are pain on injection and occasional movements of the patient. Methohexitone is probably the most popular drug for children as it produces a predictable response and few sensitivity reactions. Thiopentone causes delayed recovery, and propofol more cardiovascular instability, in comparison with methohexitone.

It is preferable to induce i.v. anaesthesia in the semi-reclining position.

Anaesthesia for adults

The majority of adults presenting for dental procedures under general anaesthesia are suffering from oral infections which contraindicate the use of local anaesthesia. Thus the majority of patients present as emergencies, but there is a small number of adults who are unable or unwilling to submit to local techniques. In addition, some adult mentally handicapped patients are unable to cooperate with the dentist. This last group presents usually for a mixture of conservation and dental surgical work (often extensive) generally requiring tracheal intubation.

Inhalational anaesthesia is not suitable for use in adults as it is not uncommon for some struggling to occur, and an i.v. induction is preferable. The most common reason for general anaesthesia is infection, often of one tooth, and this suggests that periodontal disease is present, which renders the tooth easily extractable. Thus a single tooth can usually be removed readily while the induction agent is effective. However, it is not always possible to extract the tooth easily and i.v. induction should always be followed by inhalation anaesthesia until surgery is complete. It is usual to insert a mouth prop before induction.

If infection is severe and trismus present, anaesthesia may not always relieve masseter spasm. It may be preferable in this case to assess adequacy of the airway by use of an inhalational induction. If access is too limited to allow extraction, antibiotics should be administered and the infection allowed to subside before surgery is undertaken.

Tracheal intubation

Formal tracheal intubation is undertaken much more commonly during dental anaesthesia now than in the past. Mental handicap, extended surgery, obstruction of nasal airways or difficulty in maintaining an airway are indications for tracheal intubation. A formal decision to intubate may be made if surgery is scheduled to extend beyond 15–20 min.

Tracheal intubation may be achieved during inhalational anaesthesia or by the use of an i.v. induction agent followed by a short-acting muscle relaxant. Conditions for intubation are arguably less ideal if inhalational methods are used, but suxamethonium pains are avoided. The tube may be passed either orally or nasally; the latter route allows access to both sides of the mouth without movement of the tube, and packing the throat is more secure. The pack may be placed more posteriorly than when no tracheal tube is used; thus it is mandatory to ensure that some evidence of packing is obvious, e.g. by leaving a tail of the pack hanging from the corner of the mouth. Prior to extubation, the nasopharynx should be sucked out carefully under direct vision and the pack removed.

All children should be examined before discharge, particularly if a nasal tube has been used, as bleeding from disrupted adenoids may sometimes be troublesome. Advice regarding analgesia and postoperative care must also be given before discharge.

SEDATION TECHNIQUES

The anxiety experienced by the majority of patients undergoing dental treatment has encouraged a search for effective methods of sedation. Nitrous oxide has become popular in the USA for this purpose. In the UK the Society for the Advancement of Anaesthesia in Dentistry was founded to establish satisfactory training facilities for dentists and dental anaesthetists using intermittent injections of i.v. methohexitone for sedation. Intravenous sedation has become more popular with the introduction of the benzodiazepines.

Relative analgesia

Relative analgesia is a misleading title. If painful operative dental surgery is undertaken, complete and not relative analgesia is necessary. However, the name was taken from the classical Guedel stages of inhalational anaesthesia, relative analgesia being the name given to the first phase before the onset of anaesthesia. Relative analgesia is essentially a technique of inhalational sedation, using low concentrations of nitrous oxide (20–35%) in oxygen. The use of such low concentrations results in sedation without anaesthesia; there is no loss of consciousness, and integrity of protective reflexes is maintained. It should be understood that this is not an anaesthetic technique. Both the dental work and the relative analgesia should be undertaken by the dentist, as he knows when discomfort is to be expected and can maintain the necessary rapport with the patient.

Whilst almost any anaesthetic machine may be used for this technique, few are really suitable. Intermittent-flow machines are probably too inaccurate for the low concentrations desired, and are wasteful of gases. Continuous-flow machines do not have the safety features which specifically designed machines possess. Purpose-built machines may also be used as anaesthetic machines by the addition of a vaporiser.

Specific apparatus operates as a continuous-flow machine and does not function if the O_2 supply fails (or if the cylinder empties); the valve at the position of the anaesthetic reservoir bag is designed to admit room air if the machine switches off (as a result of failure of the O_2 supply). If the fresh gas flow is inadequate and the reservoir bag empties, air is admitted to the circuit; the valve does not allow rebreathing. From the foregoing it can be seen that the valve is not one which is familiar to anaesthetists.

The technique of relative analgesia consists initially of acclimatising the patient to the lightweight nasal mask, while inhaling oxygen. After a short period, nitrous oxide is introduced, initially in concentrations of less than 10% for a few breaths. The nitrous oxide concentration is increased slowly whilst a steady stream of conversation is directed at the patient, indicating the sensations likely to be experienced (usually little until 10% N_2O is inhaled, although there are wide individual variations). The initial feelings comprise mild sedation, but part of this may result from suggestion by the dentist. The concentration is increased until the patient experiences a sense of floating, or paraesthesiae around the lips or fingers. At this point, the concentration of N_2O is decreased slightly.

The advantages of this technique are that no preparation of the patient is required and the rapid uptake and elimination of N_2O ensures that no hangover effect is experienced. There are two disadvantages. Equipment is expensive to install and to operate and it has also been suggested that in the absence of scavenging, the abortion rate is higher in female dental assistants in practices in which relative analgesia is used than in those in which it is not used.

There are few contraindications to the use of relative analgesia, although expense prohibits universal use. The mask may be distressing to some patients, but this is overcome usually by gentle persuasion. The technique cannot be used in the presence of nasal obstruction. It has also been suggested that it should be avoided in patients with a serious psychiatric history or severe obstructive airways disease.

Intravenous sedation

With this technique, the patient is given a small dose of a benzodiazepine, e.g. diazepam i.v. It is generally accepted that not more than 20 mg diazepam should be given to outpatients and sufficient time should be available to allow the drug to act before starting surgery. When teaching this technique to dentists, it is important to stress that a maximum dose should be selected which will not induce anaesthesia, as there is great patient variation in response to benzodiazepines. The use of diazepam is associated with pain on injection (>30%) and a substantial frequency of venous thrombosis. The introduction of an emulsion of diazepam ('Diazemuls') reduced the frequency of both these complications. It is inadvisable to drive or to operate machinery within 24 h of administration, as the metabolites of diazepam are active pharmacologically.

Midazolam is now preferred as its duration of action is shorter. However, it is more potent than diazepam and excessive doses cause cardiovascular and ventilatory depression, particularly in the elderly.

Patients must receive written guidance regarding the duration of action of the benzodiazepines; nonetheless it has been shown that approximately 10% of outpatients ignore this advice.

The relative merits and disadvantages of i.v. sedation and relative analgesia are summarised in Table 35.1.

Table 35.1 A comparison of inhalational sedation and i.v. benzodiazepines

	Relative analgesia	I.v. sedation
Advantages		
	No preparation	Simple equipment
	Rapid onset	Inexpensive
	Ease of control	Simplicity of use
	No escort required	
Disadvantages		
	Very expensive equipment	Venous access required
	Expensive to run	Injection may be painful
	Use of mask initially complicated	Slow onset
	Pollution	Prolonged action

CONCLUSION

It is appropriate to consider briefly the changes in dental anaesthetic practice which are likely to follow the relatively recent publication of reports on dental anaesthetic training. For some time it has been considered that it is not possible to train dental students to give safe anaesthesia without undertaking a considerably altered training programme as an undergraduate, and further training as a postgraduate.

In 1965 a Joint Subcommittee on Dental Anaesthesia was convened to consider the problem, and a report emerged in 1967. This led to the establishment with anaesthetists and dentists of a joint working party whose recommendations were published in 1969. No action was taken to implement the recommendations of these Committees.

In 1978, the Wylie report was published. The remit of this Committee was to consider the safety of patients under dental anaesthesia (all aspects including sedation techniques), to define the required training for a 'core anaesthetist', and to define the facilities required in any dental surgery where general anaesthesia is undertaken. It was the intention to institute the recommendations as a national policy, training programmes being subject to the joint approval of the Faculties of Dental Surgery and of Anaesthetists.

To implement the Wylie report, an interfaculty working party was formed under the chairmanship of Professor Seward, which reported in 1981. In Scotland similar steps were taken and published as the Spence report.

Unlike the earlier reports, there is firm resolve to implement their recommendations, although it is recognised that some time will be required, perhaps as long as 10 years. The result is a profound change in the training of dental undergraduates and the provision of postgraduate training courses for dentists interested in dental anaesthesia. In general terms a substantial upgrading will be required of equipment and premises in which dental anaesthesia is undertaken. This will, in time, alter the demand for skilled dental anaesthetic services, although it is too early to predict the final result. It is interesting to note that the Wylie report acknowledges that no evidence exists to indicate that implementation of the proposals would result in improved safety.

FURTHER READING

Danziger A M 1980 Intubation and/or the supine position for dental outpatients. Anaesthesia 35: 70

Dinsdale R C W, Dixon R A 1978 Anaesthetic services to dental patients in England and Wales. British Dental Journal 144: 271

Editorial 1981 General anaesthesia for dentistry. British Dental Journal 151: 357

Langa H 1976 Relative analgesia in dental practice, inhalational analgesia sedation with nitrous oxide, 2nd edn. W B Saunders, Philadelphia

Muir V M J, Leonard M, Haddaway E 1976 Morbidity following dental extraction: a comparative survey of local and general anaesthesia. Anaesthesia 31: 171

Seward report 1981 Report of the Interfaculty Working Party formed to consider the implementation of the Wylie report. British Dental Journal 151: 389

Spence report 1981 Report of the Joint Working Party on Anaesthesia in General Dental Practice. British Dental Journal 151: 392

Sykes P (ed) 1979 Drummond-Jackson's dental sedation and anaesthesia, 6th edn. Society for Advancement of Anaesthesia in Dentistry, London

Tomlin P J 1974 Deaths in outpatient anaesthetic practice. Anaesthesia 29: 551

Wylie report 1981 Report of the Working Party on Training in Dental Anaesthesia. British Dental Journal 151: 385

36. Anaesthesia for plastic, endocrine and vascular surgery

PLASTIC SURGERY

The term 'plastic surgery' is used to describe procedures which involve reconstitution of damaged or deformed tissues, removal of cutaneous tumours or cosmetic alteration of body features. Tissue may be deformed as a result of trauma, burns, infection or congenital abnormality. Division or removal of the abnormality often results in skin cover defects. Major plastic surgery includes the formation and repositioning of free and pedicle grafts and the movement of skin flaps.

General considerations

There are several important features common to many of these operations. The patient may be deformed grossly as a result of previous trauma or serious disease, and attention should be directed to the patient's psychological state, which is influenced by long periods of confinement and rehabilitation, concern over disfigurement or loss of limb function and occasionally chronic pain. Preoperative drug therapy should be controlled carefully and attention paid to removal of local or generalised infection, state of nutrition and haematocrit, which are important factors in the outcome of this form of surgery. Cosmetic surgery of the face, tattoo removal, breast augmentation and removal of unwanted adipose tissue are performed usually on healthy patients.

Haemorrhage is a common occurrence during plastic surgery and all but the most minor operations may necessitate blood transfusion. Operations (especially vascular reconstruction) may last many hours, and care must be taken to position the patient in such a way that ligament strain and pressure on skin over bony prominences are avoided. The use of lumbar support and soft padding minimises these risks. When surgery has been completed, wound dressing and bandaging may be lengthy procedures. It is common for bandages to be applied round the trunk, and the patient must be lifted carefully to avoid injury. Finally, there may be severe postoperative pain, especially from donor skin graft sites.

Head and neck

Tracheal intubation is mandatory for surgery in this area and a reinforced tube should be used. It is important to protect the eyes from pressure, the ears from blood and other fluids, and the teeth and anaesthetic tubing from dislodgement. It may be difficult to monitor chest movement, and access to the arms may be impossible. An i.v. infusion with extension tubing is essential; there should be access to a three-way tap for injection of drugs. A foot should be exposed to allow the anaesthetist to monitor colour, capillary filling and arterial pulse. Venous drainage is improved in surgery on the head or neck if the patient is positioned in a 10–15° head-up tilt, and this reduces surgical bleeding.

The anaesthetist should anticipate difficulties in tracheal intubation and a complete range of equipment should be available. Tumours or scarring of the neck, deformity of facial bones and cleft palate make tracheal intubation particularly difficult. Use of muscle relaxants in such patients may be unwise before intubation; the anaesthetist should consider the use of local anaesthesia for awake intubation or an inhalational technique. The method of maintenance should be determined by the condition of the patient, the type and duration of surgery and the experience and preference of the anaesthetist. Hypotensive techniques are employed frequently (see Ch. 37).

Trunk

Problems encountered in surgery on the trunk include the adoption of unusual postures and their attendant risks, haemorrhage, prolonged operation and restrictive dressings applied after surgery.

Limbs

Local anaesthesia may be an advantage for surgery on upper or lower limbs. However, Bier's block is of limited value as the surgeon often requires cuff deflation to identify bleeding points. The duration of some plastic operations may preclude local anaesthetic techniques, although prolonged neural blockade may be achieved by repeated injection (e.g. through an extradural catheter) or by employing an agent with a prolonged duration of action (e.g. bupivacaine). Sedative drugs or light general anaesthesia may be required to help the patient to remain motionless on the operating table. Specific nerve blocks may be useful, e.g. blockade of the femoral and lateral cutaneous nerve of thigh provides analgesia for skin graft donor sites during and after operation.

Surgical techniques of reimplantation and microsurgical repair of the limbs are well established and make specific demands upon the anaesthetist. These include maintenance of general anaesthesia for up to 24 h, control of vascular spasm and provision of optimum conditions for postoperative recovery.

Anaesthesia should be administered using humidified gases in a warmed theatre environment. Nitrous oxide may produce marrow depression with prolonged exposure and should be avoided. If a volatile agent is required, isoflurane is regarded by some as the agent of choice as it undergoes little biotransformation (0.2%), is eliminated rapidly and in normovolaemic patients produces vasodilatation which may be beneficial to the outcome of the operation. Fluid balance should be maintained scrupulously. Pressure areas should be protected by a ripple mattress. An arterial cannula should be inserted for measurement of arterial pressure and sampling of blood as a check that normocapnia is maintained. Measures should be taken to prevent DVT formation.

Vascular spasm in an isolated limb may be prevented by preoperative i.v. sympathetic blockade using guanethidine 15–20 mg. Normocapnia, normotension, adequate analgesia and maintenance of body temperature are important. Local anaesthetic block of the brachial plexus provides vasodilatation, but if surgery is prolonged a catheter technique may be required.

Burns

Hypoxaemia is the principal cause of rapid death in victims of fire. This may result either from a reduction in inspired oxygen concentration in a smoke-filled atmosphere or poisoning by products of combustion. Carbon monoxide has an affinity over 200 times greater than that of oxygen for haemoglobin and high concentrations cause reduced oxygen carriage in the blood. In addition, there may be direct thermal injury to the airway resulting in ciliary damage, mucosal oedema, loss of surfactant and epithelial destruction. These may result in mucosal sloughing and alveolar oedema.

It is not sufficient simply to replace fluid loss in the emergency management of the patient with burns. Account must be taken of disturbances in both ventilation and perfusion and a knowledge of $\dot{V}/\dot{Q}$ mismatch is essential when preparing these patients for emergency surgery. The aim of immediate treatment is to secure the airway and administer 100% oxygen; this may require tracheal intubation and IPPV until Pa_{O_2} is adequate. Such patients require humidification of inspired gas, physiotherapy, and bronchial suction. Bronchodilators and PEEP may be necessary.

Burning of flesh produces rapid fluid shifts and formation of tissue oedema, particularly during the first 36 h. The resulting depletion of intravascular volume is greatest in the first few hours and it is essential that a fluid replacement regimen is started as early as possible in order to avoid acute renal failure. An example of a suitable regimen is shown in Table 36.1.

Table 36.1 Fluid regimen for burned patients

1. Estimate/measure weight
2. Estimate percentage area of burns using 'rule of nines' for adults and 'rule of tens' for children
3. Transfuse if >15% burns (adults) or >10% burns (children)
   Measure:
   - haematocrit
   - haemoglobin
   - electrolytes
   - heart rate and arterial pressure
4. Give fluid replacement (at least 50% as human albumin solution) — weight in kg × % burns (ml) in each of the following six periods from time of burning:
   1. 0–4 h
   2. 4–8 h
   3. 8–12 h
   4. 12–18 h
   5. 18–24 h
   6. 24–36 h
5. If extensive full-thickness burns are present, some of the above fluid must be given as whole blood.

Initially, transfusion of whole blood increases the haematocrit and blood viscosity because increased capillary permeability is present, and this may result in reduced oxygen supply to the tissues.

The hormonal response to burning results in a hypercatabolic state with tachycardia, hyperpnoea and hyperpyrexia.

After the eschar has formed, there is loss of pure water from the body surface with a resultant increase in plasma concentration of aldosterone. The patient is at risk from water depletion and relative sodium overload. In addition, there is a rapid increase in serum potassium and urea concentrations (caused by cellular disruption in damaged tissue) and haemolysis, and these are accentuated by acidosis caused by infection. In the natural course of recovery, kalliuresis and anaemia result from continuing haemolysis of red cells.

The anaesthetist may be involved with the burns victim at an early stage when hypoxaemia is life-threatening and basic resuscitation is required. Thereafter, general anaesthesia may be required for:

1. Early excision of damaged tissue from 72 h after the burn.
2. Excision of granulation tissue and grafting.
3. Changes of dressing.
4. Reparative plastic procedures to relieve contractions, permit limb function or remove unsightly deformity.

Recovery from burns trauma may be protracted. The anaesthetist must be aware of the probable requirement for multiple administrations of general anaesthesia, frequent use of opioid analgesics in the early stages and the importance of psychological support throughout the patient's hospitalisation.

Anaesthetic problems

1. *Airway*. Thermal damage to the head and neck of a patient may provide the anaesthetist with a severe test of his ability. In the initial stages, raw, painful tissues may prohibit application of a facemask, while a rapid-sequence induction using a depolarising muscle relaxant drug may be inadvisable (vide infra). Later, as soft tissues fibrose and distort, the range of movement in the neck and temporomandibular joints may become grossly restricted, and render laryngoscopic intubation impossible (Fig. 36.1). Tracheostomy is regarded generally as undesirable because of the risk that infection may spread to damaged skin. Awake intubation may be necessary.

It may be difficult to secure the tracheal tube in place. Several ingenious methods have been devised, such as suspension of the anaesthetic breathing system from the ceiling, the use of umbilical tape to tie the tube in place and wiring the tube to the upper teeth.

In the early stages of the patient's treatment, and after prolonged surgery, it is wise to examine the pharynx closely before tracheal extubation. Oedema may form in the soft tissues around the base of the tongue and cause respiratory obstruction when the tracheal tube is removed.

2. *Ventilation*. Mechanical ventilation should be employed in the severely burned patient and careful monitoring of ventilation is required. Metabolic rate may be doubled in a patient with 40% burns; this results in large increases in oxgyen consumption and carbon dioxide production; i.v. alimentation increases the latter. Inhalational injury causes increased scatter of $\dot{V}/\dot{Q}$ ratios. A sophisticated ventilator, capable of

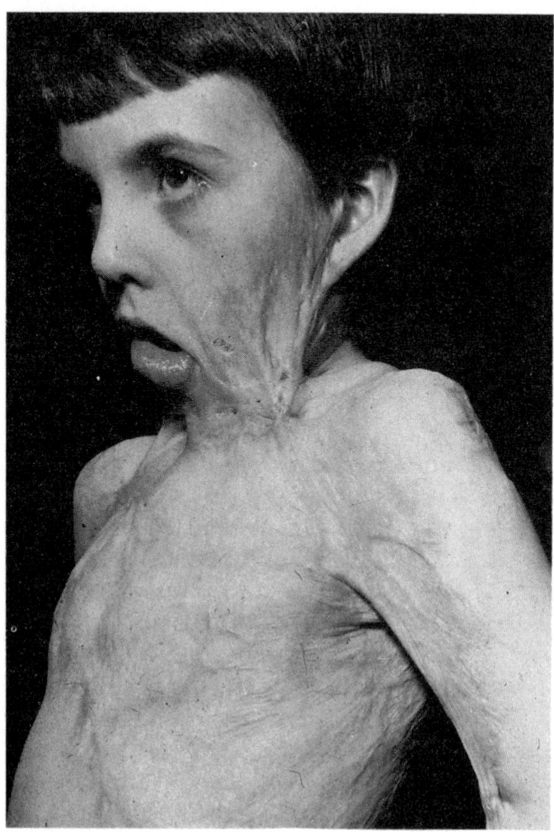

Fig. 36.1 Severe scar formation and contractions caused by burns to the thorax and neck.

providing PEEP and minute volumes up to 30 litres/min, is required. There should be continuous monitoring using a pulse oximeter and capnograph, with regular blood gas analysis.

3. *Fluid balance*. In addition to the fluid balance problems mentioned above, the modern practice of early tissue excision is accompanied by extensive and rapid blood loss. Cross-matched blood must be available before the operation is started, and it is wise to have two large-bore venous cannulae in situ and facilities for warming infused fluids.

4. *Temperature loss*. Heat loss is increased from a burned area by evaporation and inability of cutaneous vessels to constrict and prevent radiation. This loss is offset partly by the increased heat production which results from the raised metabolic rate, but the anaesthetist should minimise heat loss during anaesthesia and surgery by use of a warming blanket, foil blanket, blood warmer, gas humidifier and an ambient theatre temperature and humidity of 27°C and 50% respectively.

5. *Choice of anaesthetic agent*. This is governed by personal preference and the knowledge that repeated administration of some volatile agents may result in hepatic damage. Ketamine is useful; it may be used also as an infusion for analgesia during burns dressings. However, it is not safe to assume that the airway is preserved during ketamine anaesthesia and it is wise to premedicate the patient with an antisialagogue. Diazepam may control the emergence hallucinations suffered by some patients who receive ketamine.

Suxamethonium should be avoided in burned patients. In the presence of muscle damage its administration may cause release of potassium into the circulation in concentrations sufficient to cause cardiac arrest. It is thought that the most dangerous period in this respect is between 4 days and 10 weeks after thermal injury.

SURGERY OF TUMOURS OF THE ENDOCRINE SYSTEM

APUD (amine precursor uptake and decarboxylation) cells are thought to originate from neuroectoderm and are distributed widely throughout the body. Neoplastic change within these cells produces the group of tumours termed apudomas. These may be orthoendocrine or paraendocrine; the former produce amines and polypeptides associated normally with the constituent cells, while the latter secrete substances produced usually by other organs. There are two orthoendocrine apudomas which may produce significant difficulty for the anaesthetist.

Carcinoid tumour

Carcinoid tumours arise in the enterochromaffin cells of the intestinal tract, are commonly benign and are found most often in the appendix (Table 36.2). However, they may occur at any site in the gut and, rarely, in the gall-bladder or bronchus. Malignant change occurs in 4%, and may give rise to hepatic secondaries which are potentially resectable.

Table 36.2 Distribution of carcinoid tumours

Midgut	73% (appendix 45%; ileum 28%)
Rectum	16%
Bronchus	10%

Table 36.3 Symptoms and signs of carcinoid syndrome

Symptoms
Diarrhoea
Cutaneous flushing (especially in patients with hepatic metastases)
Venous telangiectasia (50% of patients have 'butterfly' distribution over the nose)

Clinical Signs
Endocardial lesions (50% of patients have fibrous deposits that interfere with valve function)
Bronchoconstriction
Pellagra
Hepatomegaly
Hyperactive borborygmi

Carcinoid tumours secrete over 20 substances with a variety of effects on vascular, bronchial and gastrointestinal smooth muscle activity. These include:

1. *Serotonin* (5-hydroxytryptamine, 5-HT) is responsible for abnormal gut motility and diarrhoea, and possibly for endocardial fibrosis which may result in pulmonary and tricuspid stenosis. Left-sided valvular lesions of the heart may be caused by the secretions of a bronchial carcinoid tumour. Serotonin also produces alteration in arterial pressure, and hyperglycaemia.
2. *Kallikrein* is an enzyme which acts on circulating plasma kininogen to produce bradykinin. This is a vasodilator which causes flushing and may contribute to bronchospasm, hypotension and oedema.
3. *Prostaglandins* produce diarrhoea and facial flushing.
4. *Histamine* may produce profound hypotension.
5. *Substance P* causes increased gastrointestinal motility and vasodilatation.

These compounds are metabolised normally in the liver. It is only when they escape the portal circulation (hepatic metastases, bronchial primary) that the clinical picture of carcinoid syndrome (Table 36.3) is seen.

Diagnosis is confirmed by high urinary excretion of 5-hydroxyindoleacetic acid (5-HIAA), a metabolite of 5-HT (a total of more than 27 mg/day is diagnostic). Liver scan may show filling defects caused by secondary tumours.

Treatment

The definitive treatment of carcinoid tumours is surgical removal. Specific problems for the anaesthetist occur only in patients presenting with the carcinoid syndrome. These patients may be receiving drug treatment (Table 36.4) to alleviate symptoms.

Many active compounds are produced by carcinoid tumours but their exact relationship to the production of symptoms is unclear. The mechanism of action of the drugs used to control the symptoms is also ill-defined and may result in serious unwanted side effects. Thus, the use of drugs which inhibit release of active substances, rather than those which block end-organ effects, is gaining popularity. Somatostatin is such a compound and is given by continuous i.v. infusion because its half-life is only 1–3 min. Octreotide, a somatostatin analogue, has a half-life of 45 min after i.v. injection; it may be given also by the s.c. route. This compound may be used peroperatively to control a carcinoid crisis.

Table 36.4 Drugs used in the treatment carcinoid syndrome

Drug	Symptom	Mode of action
Methysergide	Diarrhoea	5-HT antagonist
Cyproheptadine	Diarrhoea	5-HT antagonist and antihistamine
Parachlorophenylalanine	Diarrhoea	Tryptophan hydroxylase inhibitor (high incidence of allergic reaction)
5-Fluorotryptophan	Diarrhoea	5-HT analogue
Ketanserin	Diarrhoea Flushing	Adrenergic blockade
Phenothiazines (thorazine)	Flushing	
Glucocorticoids (for bronchial carcinoid)		
Methyldopa (for hypertension)		
Aprotinin — there is debate about the suitability of this drug in the treatment of carcinoid syndrome		

Conduct of anaesthesia

Acute attacks of carcinoid syndrome may be precipitated by fear, hypotension and handling of the tumour. The anaesthetist should be aware of the following factors:

1. Hypovolaemia and electrolyte imbalance may occur in patients with diarrhoea.
2. Adequate preoperative sedation with minimal cardiovascular disturbance is essential. A sedative with antihistamine properties, e.g. promethazine, is suitable.
3. Techniques which may cause hypotension, including extradural and subarachnoid block, should be avoided.
4. Sudden bronchospasm, arrhythmias and extreme fluctuations in arterial pressure may occur. Continuous monitoring of ECG and arterial pressure are mandatory. Bronchospasm may be particularly resistant to treatment.
5. Drugs which release histamine (e.g. curare or morphine) should be avoided. Volatile anaesthetics may prolong recovery time and their use may be hazardous in the presence of valvular lesions.

Promethazine, diazepam or droperidol are appropriate premedicants. Anaesthesia is induced most safely by an opioid agent such as fentanyl, and muscle relaxation may be achieved with vecuronium. After tracheal intubation, nitrous oxide and oxygen should be administered, and additional fentanyl given as required. IPPV should be delivered by a ventilator of the flow-generator type (see p. 311), which is capable of delivering the inspired gases at high pressure if bronchospasm develops. Monitoring should include ECG, direct arterial and central venous pressure measurement, pulse oximetry and capnography. IPPV may be required after operation, but in any event the patient should be observed in a high-dependency or intensive therapy unit.

Phaeochromocytoma

Ninety-four per cent of these rare tumours arise in the phaeochromocytes of the adrenal medulla; the remainder are associated with the paravertebral sympathetic ganglia. They produce adrenaline and noradrenaline, the hormones which cause the symptoms and signs of phaeochromocytoma (Table 36.5).

Table 36.5 Clinical symptoms and signs associated with phaeochromocytoma

Symptoms	Signs
Headache	Hypertension, paroxysmal or sustained
Palpitations	Increased basal metabolic rate
Excessive sweating	Haemoconcentration
Weight loss	Renal pathology
Pallor	Increased blood glucose, lactic acid and FFA concentrations
Visual disturbance	Cardiomyopathy

The presentation of the disease and its subsequent management depend on the total output of catecholamines and the relative proportions of adrenaline and noradrenaline.

Tachycardia, tachyarrhythmias and high-output cardiac failure are characteristic findings when the tumour secretes adrenaline predominantly; those which secrete predominantly noradrenaline result in a reduced circulating blood volume.

Diagnosis is confirmed by measurement of high plasma concentrations of catecholamines and high urinary excretion rates of catecholamines and their metabolite 3-methoxy-4-hydroxymandelic acid. It may be more practical to measure excretion of the intermediary metanephrines; increased concentrations in combination with the clinical findings and demonstration of raised circulating concentrations of catecholamines are diagnostic. Localisation of a tumour may be undertaken by selective venous catheterisation with sampling for raised catecholamine concentrations. Computerised tomography may be used to identify tumours greater than 1 cm in diameter. Uptake of $[^{131}I]$*meta*-iodylbenzylguanidine (MIBG), monitored by gamma camera, has been developed recently as a diagnostic aid.

Treatment

The aim is to control the effects of the tumour with drugs and then to remove it surgically. Pharmacological control is achieved by α-adrenergic blockade to counteract the increased peripheral vascular resistance and reduced circulating volume. Phenoxybenzamine, phentolamine and prazosin have all been used successfully. A β-adrenergic antagonist may be required subsequently to control tachycardia but this may precipitate cardiac failure and acute pulmonary oedema if introduced without α-adrenergic blockade and appropriate fluid replacement. Propranolol, metoprolol and atenolol are useful agents if β-blockade is required. Labetalol is favoured by some physicians. Synthesis of catecholamine may be suppressed actively by administration of methyl-*p*-tyrosine, a tyrosine hydroxylase inhibitor. This drug may be very successful in controlling the disease, but may cause severe side effects including diarrhoea, fatigue and depression.

Preoperative preparation of the patient by α-blockade with phenoxybenzamine may be accomplished by oral administration of increasing dosage of the drug over a period of weeks. In this event, expansion of the capacitance system occurs gradually with normal oral intake of fluid. Alternatively, phenoxybenzamine may be given by i.v. infusion (frequently on a daily basis for the 3 days preceding surgery). In this event, it is necessary to monitor intravascular volume by measurement of CVP and to maintain a normal volume by i.v. infusion of colloids.

Conduct of anaesthesia

Sudden and large fluctuations in arterial pressure occur during surgery for phaeochromocytoma, especially when tumour tissue is handled. Monitoring of ECG, central venous pressure and direct arterial pressure must be instituted *before* induction of anaesthesia.

Premedication should provide sedation and agents used for induction and maintenance should be selected on the basis of cardiovascular stability (Table 36.6).

Table 36.6 Drugs to avoid in patients with phaeochromocytoma

Atropine	Droperidol
Suxamethonium	Morphine
Gallamine	Halothane
d-Tubocurarine	Cyclopropane
Atracurium	Diethyl ether
Pancuronium	

Anaesthesia may be induced by slow administration of thiopentone or etomidate, and maintained with nitrous oxide in oxygen, supplemented by either enflurane or isoflurane. A lipid-soluble opioid, e.g. fentanyl, reduces the risk of excessive hypertension during tracheal intubation and skin incision. Release of catecholamines occurs commonly when the tumour is mobilised, and an arterial vasodilator such as sodium nitroprusside may be required to control arterial pressure. Arterial pressure may decrease after removal of the tumour, although this is uncommon if preoperative preparation has been adequate.

Invasive monitoring should be continued for 12–24 h after surgery and the patient must be nursed in a high-dependency or intensive care unit.

MAJOR VASCULAR SURGERY

Anaesthesia for major vascular surgery is a complex subject. Only the more important features of four vascular operations are described here: elective and emergency repair of abdominal aortic aneurysm, bypass of abdominal aorto-iliac occlusion and carotid artery surgery.

Patients presenting for major vascular surgery have a high incidence of coexisting disease and many exhibit the features of one or more of the following:

1. Hypertension.
2. Ischaemic heart disease.
3. Renal disease.
4. Congestive cardiac failure.
5. Diabetes mellitus.
6. Pulmonary disease.

It is vital that such conditions are treated preoperatively and that the patient presents for surgery only when no further improvement might be expected. The risks of morbidity and death after these operations are increased greatly by the presence of cardiac failure, recent myocardial infarction, hypertension and arrhythmias (see Chs 19 and 41).

Recent general anaesthesia for arteriography should be noted and evidence sought of renal dysfunction following injection of large volumes of radio-opaque dye. Physical examination should include Allen's test on both wrists because radial artery cannulation will be required during anaesthesia for measurement of systemic arterial pressure and sampling of blood for acid–base and blood gas status.

Elective repair of abdominal aortic aneurysm

It is normal practice to prescribe a sedative premedication. Atropine should be avoided if there is evidence of ischaemic heart disease.

On arrival in the anaesthetic room, the patient should be placed on a warming blanket, and arterial pressure measured. In patients with myocardial disease, direct intra-arterial pressure and ECG monitoring should be instituted before induction of anaesthesia. Pre-oxygenation of the lungs is followed by induction of anaesthesia by slow injection of thiopentone. After muscle relaxation, the trachea is intubated (see below) and IPPV continued using humidified gases.

The following procedures are performed before surgery starts:

1. Intravenous access is obtained with at least one 14-gauge cannula for infusion of warmed fluids.
2. Cannulation of a radial artery.
3. Central venous catheterisation for measurement of right atrial pressure.
4. An oesophageal or tympanic membrane temperature probe is inserted for measurement of temperature.
5. Bladder catheterisation for monitoring of urine output.

Three specific stimuli may give rise to cardiovascular instability in patients undergoing aneurysm repair.

1. *Tracheal intubation*. The increase in systemic arterial pressure which accompanies tracheal intubation may be of considerable magnitude and must be minimised to avoid myocardial ischaemia. Attenuation of this response may be produced by the i.v. administration of a β-blocker or a high dose of a lipid-soluble opioid (e.g. alfentanil 500–600 μg) before intubation. Topical anaesthesia to the larynx is not effective.

2. *Cross-clamping of the aorta*. Clamping of the aorta causes a sudden increase in systemic vascular resistance (afterload). This increases cardiac work, and may result in myocardial ischaemia, arrhythmias and left ventricular failure. It may be necessary to administer vasodilators (e.g. sodium nitroprusside or glyceryl trinitrate) during this period to obviate these problems.

3. *Aortic declamping*. Declamping of the aorta causes a sudden decrease in afterload and reperfusion of the lower part of the body. Acid metabolites enter the circulation and may cause vasodilatation and metabolic acidosis. Bleeding is a problem throughout the operation but may be particularly severe at this time as the adequacy of vascular anastomoses is tested. These factors may result in severe hypotension unless circulating volume has been well maintained and transfusion is continued to maintain an adequate CVP. If relative hypervolaemia is produced during the period of clamping by infusion of fluids to produce a CVP of 10–12 cmH_2O (and perhaps administration of SNP), declamping hypotension is not a problem and metabolic acidosis is avoided.

Many patients undergoing this operation are old and have a low metabolic rate. Consequently they are unable to tolerate the large heat loss which occurs through the extensive surgical exposure, which necessitates displacement of the bowel outside the abdominal cavity. All possible measures must be taken to minimise heat loss. These include:

1. Warming of infusion fluids.
2. Warming and humidification of anaesthetic gases.
3. Use of a warming blanket under the patient.
4. Wrapping the bowel in a clear plastic bag.
5. Use of a warm, humid ambient atmosphere in the operating theatre.

In the more compromised patient, e.g. ischaemic heart disease and poor left ventricular function, the use of a pulmonary artery catheter is indicated. This permits measurement of cardiac output and monitoring of left ventricular preload during the more dangerous stages of the operation. Preservation of an optimal left ventricular preload reduces the incidence of precipitous decreases of arterial pressure after declamping of the aorta.

The postoperative period

There is some controversy regarding postoperative artificial ventilation in patients who have undergone elective repair of an aortic aneurysm. This is not employed in most centres unless there is severe impairment of pulmonary or myocardial function, although some anaesthetists use this technique routinely because of the theoretical benefits. Continuous monitoring of the cardiovascular system (especially CVP) is essential during the first 12–24 h, as vasodilatation occurs in response to increasing body temperature. In addition, there may be continued oozing of blood from anastomoses. A satisfactory degree of nursing care is usually available only in a high-dependency or intensive care unit.

Emergency repair of abdominal aortic aneurysm

The principles of management are similar to those discussed above. However, the patient is likely to be grossly hypovolaemic and often arterial pressure is maintained only by the tone of the abdominal muscles acting on the abdominal capacitance vessels. The patient is prepared and anaesthetised on the operating table in theatre. While 100% oxygen is administered by mask, all monitoring lines and two large-bore i.v. cannulae are inserted under local anaesthesia. The surgeon then prepares and towels the patient ready for surgery and it is only at this point that anaesthesia is induced. When muscle relaxation occurs, systemic arterial pressure may decrease precipitously and immediate laparotomy and aortic clamping may be required. Thereafter, the procedure is similar to that for elective repair.

The prognosis is poor for several reasons. There has been no preoperative preparation and the patient may be suffering from concurrent disease. There may have been a period of severe hypotension, resulting in impairment of renal, cerebral or myocardial function. Massive blood transfusion, which in itself carries significant risks (see p. 133) is usually required. In addition, postoperative jaundice is common because of haemolysis of damaged red cells in the circulation and in the large retroperitoneal haematoma which usually develops after aortic rupture.

Bypass of aorto-iliac occlusion

Patients suffering from atherosclerotic arterial disease may present with ischaemic pain in a limb. Many are heavy smokers and suffer from pulmonary disease which results in dyspnoea, productive cough and polycythaemia. Aortic bifurcation grafting is performed to overcome occlusion in the aorta and iliac arteries and to restore flow to the lower limbs. It must be assumed that all patients have widespread arterial disease, even in the presence of a normal ECG. Anaesthetic management is similar to that required for surgery of aortic aneurysm. Where possible, it is normal surgical practice to side-clamp the aorta, maintaining some peripheral flow, and to declamp the arteries supplying the legs in sequence. The metabolic changes and hypotension are thus less severe than those seen during aneurysm surgery.

Peripheral arterial surgery

The commonest peripheral arterial grafts inserted are those between axillary and femoral, or femoral and popliteal, arteries. Because of the prolonged nature of these operations, an IPPV/relaxant anaesthetic technique should be used. Extradural anaesthesia is a useful adjunct, although heparin is often administered i.v. during vascular operations (vide infra) and this may increase the risk of an extradural haematoma if a catheter has been introduced. There may be considerable postoperative blood loss through the walls of open-weave grafts. In patients who have undergone an axillo-femoral graft, it is important to monitor cardiovascular status closely for the first 12 h so that such loss is observed and adequate replacement instituted.

Carotid artery surgery

Patients are selected for carotid artery surgery if symptoms are thought to result from cerebral

Table 36.7 Mortality rates for patients with differing neurological states on presentation for carotid artery surgery

Symptoms	Mortality
Frank stroke with neurological deficit	6%
Transient cerebral ischaemia	↓
Chronic cerebral ischaemia	↓
Asymptomatic carotid bruit	0%

ischaemia secondary to obstruction in the carotid arteries. The underlying pathology is usually atherosclerosis, which presents typically in elderly hypertensive patients. Cerebral autoregulation is deficient and cerebral blood flow tends to be proportional to systemic arterial pressure. The perioperative mortality varies with the severity of the presenting symptoms (Table 36.7).

The main risk of operation is the production of a neurological deficit which was not present before surgery and/or an increase in pre-existing symptoms.

The carotid artery is clamped during surgery. The adequacy of cerebral blood flow during the period of clamping must be assessed at an early stage before proceeding with the endarterectomy. This can be achieved by one of the following methods:

1. Observation of retrograde flow from the opened carotid artery.
2. Determination of the arterial pressure in the occluded distal carotid segment (the 'stump' pressure).
3. Performance of the initial clamping under local anaesthesia and clinical assessment of the patient.
4. Continuous measurement of jugular P_{O_2}.
5. Monitoring of the EEG.

Cerebral perfusion is dependent on collateral circulation, and maintenance of an adequate blood flow is the primary aim of the anaesthetic technique. A moderately high systemic arterial pressure (up to 170 mmHg systolic), a high Pa_{O_2} and normocapnia are desirable. These may be achieved by ventilation of the lungs using an inspired oxygen concentration of 50% in nitrous oxide (100% inspired oxygen produces cerebral vasoconstriction) and the administration of pancuronium to achieve muscle relaxation. An arterial cannula is mandatory for pressure monitoring and sampling for blood gas analysis. Under no circumstances should hypotension be allowed to develop. Cerebral ischaemia may be overcome during the period of clamping by insertion of a temporary shunt which bypasses the site of obstruction. In this way carotid arterial flow is uninterrupted and may even be improved.

After surgery, early assessment of cerebral function is required and residual anaesthetic effects may confuse the diagnosis of intraoperative embolism or ischaemic change. Approximately 30% of patients require control of postoperative hypertension, which may otherwise compromise the graft or cause intracranial haemorrhage. An infusion of trimetaphan, hydralazine or sodium nitroprusside may be required for this purpose.

Heparin

Centres in the UK differ in their use of heparin during vascular surgery. In units where it is used systemically, a dose of 100 units/kg is given i.v. after preclotting the graft (where material such as Dacron is used) and at least one circulation time should elapse before arterial clamping begins. Some vascular surgeons rely solely on the local use of heparinised saline. If i.v. heparin has been employed the anaesthetist may be asked to antagonise the heparin with protamine (0.5 mg/100 units heparin) before the termination of surgery.

CARDIOVERSION

DC cardioversion is an effective treatment for some re-entrant tachyarrhythmias which may produce haemodynamic instability and myocardial ischaemia and which do not respond to other measures. Atrial fibrillation, atrial flutter, supraventricular tachycardia and ventricular tachycardia may be converted to sinus rhythm, although maintenance of sinus rhythm depends usually on the subsequent use of drugs. The technique is not useful in atrial tachycardias (with or without block) or in digitalis-induced tachyarrhythmias.

Cardioversion is a simple and immediate therapy with a low incidence of side effects or complications. It has little effect on contractility, conductivity or excitability of the myocardium.

Patients may present with a chronic arrhythmia for elective cardioversion or as an emergency with an arrhythmia which is life-threatening.

Preanaesthetic assessment

Patients may have serious pre-existing cardiovascular pathology such as rheumatic disease, arteriosclerotic heart disease, myocardial infarction, congestive cardiac failure or cerebrovascular occlusive disease. Digitalis therapy predisposes to post-cardioversion arrhythmias; in some centres, it is withheld for at least 24 h before cardioversion. Accurate knowledge of the medical and drug history, and thorough clinical examination, are essential before selecting the method of anaesthesia. Preanaesthetic sedation reduces circulating endogenous catecholamine concentrations. Atropine should be avoided.

Cardioversion

DC electrical discharge passed through the heart depolarises all excitable myocardial cells and interrupts abnormal pathways and foci. The attendant physician sites the electrodes anterolaterally with the patient supine, or anteroposteriorly with the patient in the lateral position. The paddles should not be sited over the scapula, sternum or vertebrae and the skin must be protected with electrolyte jelly, saline-soaked gauze or any type of conducting pad.

The ECG monitoring lead chosen should demonstrate a clear R wave in order to synchronise the discharge away from the T wave and thus reduce the risk of development of ventricular fibrillation. If the arrhythmia does not convert after the first 50 J discharge, further shocks are given using an increased energy discharge of up to 200 J.

Despite the use of synchronised discharge, ventricular fibrillation may be produced in the presence of hypokalaemia, ischaemia, digitalis intoxication and Q–T prolongation (caused by quinidine, tricyclic antidepressants or hyperalimentation). There is a risk of embolic phenomena in patients with:

1. Mitral stenosis and atrial fibrillation of recent onset.
2. A history of embolic phenomena.
3. A prosthetic mitral valve.
4. Congestive cardiac failure.

Patients with these conditions should receive prophylactic anticoagulants.

Anaesthesia

Treatment should be carried out only in areas specifically designed for the purpose, and with a full range of drugs, resuscitation and monitoring equipment available. These must be checked by the anaesthetist before every list. Patients should be prepared as for a surgical procedure.

Insertion of a cannula into a vein and preoxygenation, together with institution of ECG monitoring and measurement of arterial pressure, should precede induction of anaesthesia with an i.v. agent. The choice of agent is determined by the cardiovascular stability and recovery period required.

As soon as the patient is insensible, the airway is secured and oxygenation maintained with a suitable breathing system. If repeated shocks are required, incremental doses of the anaesthetic may be given (e.g. methohexitone or etomidate).

The patient should be monitored carefully both during anaesthesia and after recovery of consciousness, with particular regard to evidence of hypotension, cardiac dilatation and pulmonary oedema, or systemic or pulmonary embolism.

FURTHER READING

Nimmo W S, Smith G (eds) 1989 Anaesthesia. Blackwell Scientific Publications, Oxford

Vickers M D, Jones R M (eds) 1989 Medicine for Anaesthetists, 3rd edn. Blackwell Scientific Publications, Oxford

37. Hypotensive anaesthesia

Induced hypotension may be defined as the deliberate reduction of systemic arterial pressure in order to reduce bleeding and facilitate surgery. The technique was introduced into anaesthetic practice in the 1940s when the range of agents available was small, spontaneous ventilation was the norm, and uncontrolled hypertension was common amongst surgical patients. As a result of the changes, both evident and theoretical, produced by this technique, the use of induced hypotension has been controversial since its introduction into clinical practice, but despite this, it has retained a place in modern anaesthesia.

A major source of difficulty in practising hypotensive anaesthesia is the inability to measure oxygen supply to vital organs. Arterial pressure is merely one index of perfusion and existing clinical monitors of the balance between oxygen supply and demand (ECG for myocardium, CFM for brain) are insensitive.

The indications for the use of this technique include:

1. Microsurgery, where small quantities of blood may obscure the operative field.
2. Major cancer surgery; a bloodless operative field facilitates clearance of tumour tissue.
3. When it is desirable to reduce the need for blood transfusion either as a result of its concomitant hazards, or because of the patient's objections (e.g. Jehovah's Witness).
4. To improve the safety of vascular surgery by reducing the risk of haemorrhage and anastomotic disruption.
5. To reduce myocardial oxygen demand when oxygen supply is already compromised, e.g. hypertension in patients with ischaemic heart disease undergoing coronary artery bypass procedures.

In order to reduce systemic arterial pressure, the anaesthetist must interfere with the homeostatic control of the circulation. Arterial pressure is determined by intravascular volume, cardiac output and peripheral resistance. Peripheral resistance is controlled principally by the calibre of the resistance vessels; the capacitance vessels play a minor role. The intrinsic tone of these vessels may be altered by local metabolites, circulating catecholamines and the activity of the autonomic nervous system. A negative feedback loop exists which enables changes in arterial pressure to be detected by baroreceptors, which modify the level of sympathetic tone within the circulation. The vasomotor centre acts as the integrator of information.

The techniques for interfering with the physiological control of arterial pressure may be classified under three major headings:

1. Intravascular volume may be reduced by haemorrhage. This technique is dangerous and is only of historical interest.
2. Peripheral resistance may be reduced by blocking part of the negative feedback loop.
3. Cardiac output may be reduced.

If a bloodless field is required, it is generally more appropriate to use a technique which reduces cardiac output. However, blood flow to the surgical field may be reduced by the judicious use of posture, and hypotension induced by drugs which have little *primary* effect on cardiac output. Where hypotension is used for vascular surgery (e.g. intracranial aneurysm), the objective is to reduce the *tension* (and therefore the risk of inadvertent rupture) of the vessel manipulated by the surgeon, and reduction in blood flow is of lesser importance unless there is unexpected haemorrhage.

REDUCTION OF PERIPHERAL RESISTANCE

The sympathetic reflex arc may be blocked at six discrete sites (Fig. 37.1).

1. *Baroreceptors*

A decrease in arterial pressure results normally in an increase in heart rate, mediated by the baroreceptor reflex. The baroreceptors operate over a discrete range of arterial pressure, and their sensitivity to changes in pressure may be reduced by the volatile anaesthetic agents (halothane in particular). Thus, lower levels of arterial pressure may be achieved without reflex tachycardia when halothane is used.

2. *Vasomotor centre*

All general anaesthetics depress the central nervous system resulting in a reduction in sympathetic tone and a decrease in arterial pressure.

3. *Preganglionic sympathetic nerves*

The preganglionic sympathetic nerve fibres (which leave the spinal cord from T1-L2) may be blocked by subarachnoid or extradural anaesthesia. Blockade, of all or part of the sympathetic outflow results in vasodilatation of both resistance and capacitance vessels, the latter promoting venous pooling which enhances the decrease in arterial pressure. The block produced by subarachnoid anaesthesia is more predictable than that achieved with extradural blockade, and total spinal anaesthesia has been used to produce a bloodless field. Lesser degrees of blockade may be employed to produce both analgesia and systemic hypotension. Larger volumes of local anaesthetic drugs are required to achieve neural blockade when the extradural route is used and consequently systemic absorption of the local anaesthetic may contribute to the depression of the circulation. During general anaesthesia, both subarachnoid and extradural analgesia produce more profound hypotension than that seen in the conscious patient.

4. *Sympathetic ganglia*

Transmission through sympathetic ganglia may be blocked by agents which compete with acetylcholine for the postsynaptic receptor sites. A reduction in sympathetic tone results in venous

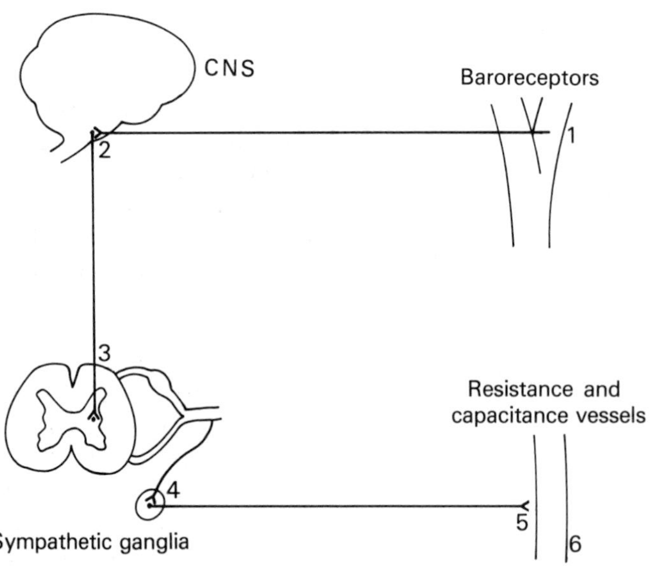

Fig. 37.1 Sites of action of drugs inducing hypotension.

pooling and systemic hypotension. The degree of hypotension produced depends upon the pre-existing sympathetic tone; thus the effects of ganglion blockade are unpredictable. Cerebral and coronary blood vessels are poorly supplied by sympathetic nerves; these vessels do not dilate significantly during sympathetic blockade, and perfusion of the brain and heart is reduced if arterial pressure is reduced in this manner. All autonomic ganglia are blocked, and this may cause unwanted side effects including cycloplegia. As the arterial pressure decreases, compensatory tachycardia may be troublesome and tachyphylaxis occurs rapidly. Tachyphylaxis may be mediated by pathways through the ganglia which are not cholinergic and therefore not blocked by cholinergic antagonists. Release histamine may be an additional problem, causing profound hypotension and bronchospasm.

The ganglion-blocking drugs in current use include hexamethonium, pentolinium and trimetaphan. The last is administered as an i.v. infusion, since it has a short duration of action. The ganglion-blocked man is exquisitely sensitive to postural changes, which result in pooling of blood in the dilated vascular bed.

5. *α-Adrenergic blocking drugs*

The chemical transmitters at the postganglionic sympathetic nerve endings may be antagonised by the α-adrenergic blocking drugs. A common problem with the use of these drugs in the young adult is reflex tachycardia. Phentolamine is a short-acting competitive α-antagonist which may be useful during anaesthesia. Phenoxybenzamine produces a more prolonged blockade, and is reserved usually for the management of phaeochromocytoma. Labetalol (a mixed α-and β-antagonist in the ratio 3:7 respectively) has also been used to produce hypotension during anaesthesia; the β-blockade, which predominates, prevents the development of tachycardia.

6. *Vessel wall*

Several drugs which act as direct vasodilators may be used to induce hypotension. Some have actions which affect predominantly resistance vessels (e.g. sodium nitroprusside), whilst others dilate capacitance vessels (e.g. glyceryl trinitrate). Although many of these drugs could be used during anaesthesia, the most commonly employed for induced hypotension in general surgery is SNP. In patients with severe coronary artery disease, glyceryl trinitrate has been advocated as an alternative, particularly during coronary artery bypass procedures.

(a) Hydralazine dilates predominantly the resistance vessels, producing a reduction in vascular tone which persists for up to 45 min when the drug is administered i.v. This drug is employed commonly for treatment of postoperative hypertension.

(b) Sodium nitroprusside (SNP) is a powerful, rapidly acting, smooth muscle relaxant. This property is attributed to the nitroso radicals which combine with the sulphydryl groupings on the cell membrane of the vessel wall. This interaction stabilises the membrane, and prevents the flux of ionised calcium which is necessary to activate the contractile mechanism in the smooth muscle. SNP acts predominantly upon small resistance vessels, the fourth order arterioles. Its evanescent action entails administration as a continuous infusion. Once prepared, the solution is extremely unstable and it should be protected from light at all times.

General vasodilatation aids tissue perfusion, which may remain adequate even at low levels of arterial pressure. Dilatation of cerebral vessels may cause an increase in intracranial pressure, and SNP should be used with caution in the presence of intracranial hypertension. This problem may be minimised by the slow administration of nitroprusside whilst at the same time reducing intracranial pressure by artificial hyperventilation. Rebound hypertension has been reported, and this has been attributed to the release of renin during the period of hypotension.

Reflex tachycardia is marked, and this tends to maintain cardiac output. The increase in heart rate cannot be prevented completely by β-blockade, and this has led to the suggestion that SNP may have a direct action on the cardiac pacemaker.

Several deaths have been reported in association with the use of SNP, usually after the administration of excessive quantities. Figure 37.2 shows the possible routes of elimination of SNP from the body. If the rate of breakdown of sodium

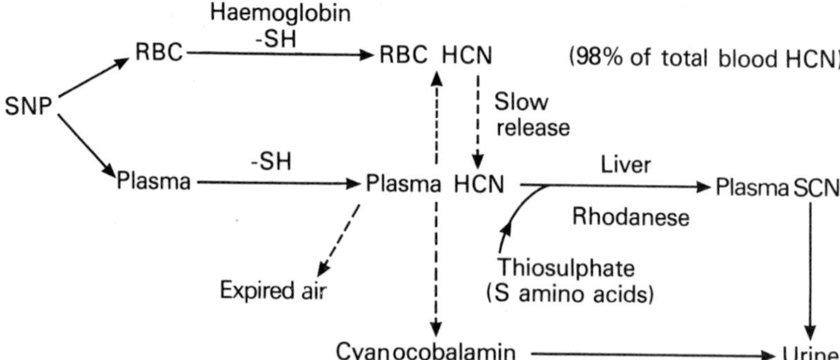

Fig. 37.2 Diagram of nitroprusside metabolism. At the end of the infusion about 98% of the cyanide liberated from the SNP is found in the red cells, from which it is slowly released. The half-life of the plasma cyanide is about 30 min.

nitroprusside to cyanide exceeds the rate of removal of cyanide from the plasma, plasma cyanide concentration increases, cellular respiration is impaired and histotoxic hypoxia results. The total dose of SNP given acutely should be limited to 1.5 mg/kg body weight to avoid this complication. During chronic use the rate of administration should not exceed 4 $\mu g\ kg^{-1}\ min^{-1}$. Various drug combinations have been used in an attempt to limit the dose of SNP. These include captopril, β-blocking agents and a 1:10 mixture of SNP with trimetaphan.

(c) Adenosine and adenosine triphosphate (ATP) are naturally occurring purines. Adenosine is the active purine and causes arteriolar dilatation. However, it is unstable and ATP is used more commonly. ATP produces effects similar to those seen with SNP, except that tachycardia does not occur. There have been only limited clinical trials, and it is not yet certain if ATP is a safe alternative to SNP.

(d) Glyceryl trinitrate (GTN) acts in a manner similar to SNP, stabilising the membrane and reducing vascular tone, but its action is more pronounced on capacitance vessels. The rate of onset of action is slightly slower than that of SNP and rebound hypertension is less marked. It may be given continuously as an infusion but it is absorbed on to plastics and polypropylene and should be administered using a glass syringe and pump. Cerebral blood flow is maintained by direct cerebral vasodilatation, but as with SNP the increase in venous volume leads to an increase in intracranial pressure.

Drugs used to produce a reduction in peripheral resistance are listed in Table 37.1.

Table 37.1 Drugs used for inducing hypotension

Drug	Formulation	Dosage	Duration of action
Trimetaphan	500 mg powder in 500 ml	Slow i.v. infusion of 0.1% solution	1–8 min
Sodium nitroprusside	50 mg in 500 ml of 5% glucose, protected from light	Slow i.v. infusion of 0.01% solution	¼–5 min
Pentolinium		10–20 mg i.v. 5–10 mg in elderly	5–45 min
Hexamethonium		10–40 mg i.v.	3–20 min
Nitroprusside/trimetaphan combination	12.5 mg nitroprusside + 125 mg trimetaphan in 500 ml of 5% glucose	Slow i.v. infusion	2–10 min
Glyceryl trinitrate	10 mg in 100 ml saline	Slow i.v. infusion of 0.01% solution	½–5 min

REDUCTION IN CARDIAC OUTPUT

Cardiac output is reduced either by a reduction in venous return, as occurs with venous pooling, or by a reduction in myocardial contractility. Thus, when hypotension is produced by arteriolar dilatation, cardiac output is maintained well provided that the patient is not postured so as to produce marked pooling of blood in dependent capacitance vessels. Myocardial depressants, including β-blocking drugs and volatile anaesthetic agents, cause both hypotension and a reduction in cardiac output, leading to an *increase* in right atrial filling pressure.

β-Adrenergic blockade

β-adrenergic blockade results in both a decrease in heart rate and a reduction in myocardial contractility. The former action is particularly useful in an induced hypotensive technique as it reduces reflex tachycardia. The majority of β-blockers may be employed, but it is probably wise to use a cardiospecific drug. β-Blocking drugs which have been employed in anaesthesia are shown in Table 37.2.

Halothane

Halothane is a powerful direct myocardial depressant and produces a dose-related decrease in arterial pressure. During spontaneous ventilation, cardiac output and arterial pressure tend to be maintained by the associated increase in Pa_{CO_2}. However, arterial pressure declines normally during spontaneous respiration and hypotension is often marked in the presence of bradycardia. Considerable improvement in arterial pressure is effected by the administration of atropine.

During controlled ventilation with hypocapnia, the use of halothane is associated with a profound reduction in cardiac output; peripheral resistance remains unchanged, with consequent hypotension, and thus halothane should not be used as the sole agent for hypotensive techniques. In low concentrations, it is a useful adjuvant to other hypotensive techniques.

Isoflurane

This is a potent hypotensive agent. It causes some depression of myocardial contractility but its major hypotensive action is caused by reduction in peripheral resistance. Coronary and cerebral vessels dilate, increasing flow, but this may divert blood from areas supplied by diseased narrowed vessels to territory served by normal vessels, resulting in local areas of ischaemia. It is claimed that intracranial pressure does not increase when isoflurane is used during controlled ventilation, even if intracranial compliance has been reduced by the presence of a space-occupying lesion. However, there are isolated reports of intracranial hypertension resulting from the use of isoflurane, and this agent should be avoided if a space-occupying lesion has produced midline shift.

Calcium channel blockers

Calcium channel blockers act on the heart and the resistance vessels. Nifedipine and nicardipine act predominantly on the channels of resistance vessels, lowering arterial pressure. Coronary vasodilatation occurs and subendocardial perfusion is increased.

Table 37.2 β-Blocking drugs employed by i.v. route in anaesthesia as adjuvants to hypotensive anaesthesia, for attenuation of hypertensive response to tracheal intubation or in treatment of appropriate arrhythmias (ISA = Intrinsic sympathomimetic activity)

Drug	Intravenous dose (mg)	Plasma half-life (h)	ISA	Cardioselectivity	Membrane stabilising effect
Labetalol (30% α-blocking)	25–30	4	–	–	+
Metoprolol	1–2	3–4	–	+	±
Oxprenolol	1–2	2	+	–	+
Propranolol	1–2	2–4	–	–	+

ADJUVANTS TO INDUCED HYPOTENSION

Posture

The importance of correct positioning must not be forgotten. There is a decrease in systemic pressure in sites elevated above the level of the heart (2 mmHg for every 2.5 cm). In addition, venous pooling occurs in dependent areas, and this may be enhanced by the use of vasodilating agents.

Intermittent positive pressure ventilation

IPPV reduces venous return by increasing mean intrathoracic pressure. The Pa_{CO_2} usually decreases during controlled ventilation, and this results in low levels of circulating endogenous catecholamines.

Good anaesthesia

Increased bleeding at the surgical site is produced by the patient coughing or straining, by an increased intrathoracic pressure (resulting from increased airway resistance e.g. kinked or inappropriately small tracheal tube), by tachycardia (light anaesthesia) or by hypercapnia resulting from hypoventilation. Thus, induced hypotension must not become a substitute for good anaesthesia which involves meticulous attention to oxygenation, carbon dioxide elimination and analgesia. A scheme for management of induced hypotension is shown in Table 37.3.

Table 37.3 Scheme for inducing hypotension

Assessment	Avoid hypotensive anaesthesia in patients with severe cardiac, respiratory, cardiovascular or renal disease
Premedication	Avoid atropine Objective to produce well-sedated patient Phenothiazine useful
Induction	Thiopentone preferred induction agent Spray larynx with 4% lignocaine Tracheal intubation mandatory
Maintenance	IPPV with at least 50% O_2 in N_2O Pa_{CO_2} 4 kPa (30 mmHg) dTC relaxant of choice Analgesic drugs to maintain good analgesia Halothane (up to 0.5%) or enflurane as required
Posture	Operation site should be elevated Head should *not* be elevated >20%
Hypotensive agents	SNP, GTN, trimetaphan or hexamethonium β-Blocker if tachycardia results
Monitoring	ECG mandatory Peripheral pulse meter or pulse oximeter Arterial pressure — 1 min reading with Dinamap acceptable Direct arterial pressure recording mandatory if hypotension prolonged or gross — permits measurements of Pa_{O_2}, Pa_{CO_2}, pH
Recovery	O_2 mask, FI_{O_2} 0.5 ECG HR and arterial pressure Must not be discharged from recovery room until arterial pressure restored to preinduction level

COMPLICATIONS OF INDUCED HYPOTENSION

A major disadvantage of induced hypotension is that tissue oxygenation may be impaired if arterial pressure is reduced excessively and autoregulation fails. It is therefore important to consider the requirements of the vital organs.

Brain

The brain has high energy requirements and little reserve, so that a reduction in supply of oxygenated blood may have disastrous consequences. Cerebral blood flow remains constant over a wide range of perfusion pressures (mean arterial pressure 60–130 mmHg). The autoregulatory curve is shifted to the right in hypertensive subjects, and to the left when direct vasodilators (including SNP and GTN) are used.

Autoregulation may be lost completely after an insult to the brain; this includes a period of marked hypotension.

Experimental work suggests that when cerebral blood flow is reduced by 50%, ischaemic signs develop, and permanent damage may occur. Patients with pre-existing cerebrovascular disease are less tolerant than normal subjects to this reduction in cerebral blood flow. Some degree of brain protection during hypotensive anaesthesia may be conferred by anaesthetic agents including thiopentone and isoflurane, both of which reduce cerebral metabolism. The level of tolerance varies not only with the patient, but also with the technique chosen. Direct vasodilator agents including SNP and GTN cause potent cerebral vasodilatation, thereby preserving cerebral blood flow to lower levels of arterial pressure.

Monitoring cerebral perfusion during general anaesthesia is difficult and various methods have been employed with limited success. Historically, spontaneous respiration was considered to be a sign of adequate perfusion of vital centres, but this view is no longer held. An approximate index of cerebral perfusion may be obtained by measurement of oxygen extraction by the brain from the oxygen content of jugular venous blood. The cerebral function monitor may be used to demonstrate severe global ischaemia. Despite the limitations of the currently available monitoring techniques, the frequency of reported mishaps remains small, although psychometric testing has shown evidence of temporary cerebral dysfunction after periods of moderate hypotension.

Heart

The myocardium may benefit from a modest reduction in arterial pressure, because myocardial oxygen requirements are also reduced. However, ECG evidence of ischaemia may be detected with increasing frequency when the systolic arterial pressure is below 60 mmHg. The hypertensive subject manifests these changes at higher systolic arterial pressures.

Kidneys

Renal perfusion and glomerular filtration are reduced when the systolic arterial pressure is reduced to levels below 80 mmHg. Oliguria is frequently seen, but is usually only temporary.

Lungs

Physiological deadspace increases as arterial pressure decreases and thus meticulous control of ventilation and oxygenation is required. During induced hypotension, the $F\text{I}_{O_2}$ should not be less than 0.5.

Other

Other problems which may result from hypotensive anaesthesia include:

1. Reactionary haemorrhage.
2. Deep venous thrombosis.
3. Retraction anaemia — ischaemia of the brain produced by surgical retraction. This is magnified by hypotensive anaesthesia.

It is difficult to assess the increase in morbidity and mortality associated with induced hypotension. Lindop, using results pooled from several major surveys, suggested that 2.5% of all patients undergoing hypotensive anaesthesia suffer a non-fatal complication, although their causation is uncertain. Various factors increase morbidity and mortality, including poor patient selection and the hypotensive technique employed. Patients with pre-existing hypertension, cerebrovascular disease, hypovolaemia or anaemia are more likely to suffer complications. Hypotension achieved by myocardial depression results in more complications than other techniques. The complication rate also increases if the mean arterial pressure is reduced below 70 mmHg, the anaesthetist is inexperienced, or there is inadequate monitoring of the patient.

It is mandatory that arterial pressure is measured accurately and frequently, using intra-arterial pressure monitoring when rapid changes in arterial pressure are produced. The ECG must be monitored continuously although it should be remembered that the band width used during anaesthesia is narrower than that of a diagnostic ECG and ischaemic changes may be missed.

Hypoxaemia must be avoided by increasing the FI_{O_2} during the period of hypotension, and ventilation should be controlled to prevent hypercapnia.

The duration of the period of hypotension must be taken into consideration, and also the importance of fine rapid control of the circulation. It may be essential in some surgical procedures to restore arterial pressure quickly to normal levels so that haemostasis may be achieved, but in other types of surgical practice a gradual recovery may be desirable.

Before embarking upon hypotensive anaesthesia, the anaesthetist must be aware of the potential advantages and disadvantages of the technique. In each instance in which this physiological trespass is used, he must be certain that the increased risk to the patient is justified by the improvement in surgical conditions.

FURTHER READING

Cole P 1979 The safe use of sodium nitroprusside. Anaesthesia 33: 473

Enderby G E H (ed) 1985 Hypotensive anaesthesia. Churchill Livingstone, Edinburgh

Ingram G S 1982 Neurosurgical anaesthesia. In: Kaufman L (ed) Anaesthesia review 1. Churchill Livingstone, Edinburgh

Lindop M J 1975 Complications and morbidity of controlled hypotension. British Journal of Anaesthesia 47: 799

38. Neurosurgical anaesthesia

Anaesthesia for intracranial operations requires conditions which maintain perfusion of the brain with blood. This is dependent upon cerebral perfusion pressure (CPP = mean arterial pressure minus intracranial pressure).

Anaesthesia must also facilitate surgical access by reducing brain volume and minimising surgical haemorrhage.

PHYSIOLOGY OF INTRACRANIAL PRESSURE AND CEREBRAL BLOOD FLOW

The intracranial contents comprise the brain (weighing approximately 1400 g), the CSF (approximately 75 ml) and blood (approximately 130 ml). Although these compartments of the intracranial volume are essentially fluid and therefore incompressible, both blood and CSF communicate with extracranial compartments allowing a certain degree of adaptability of intracranial pressure to changes in intracranial volume.

Volume–pressure relationship

In the presence of an expanding intracranial lesion, the intracranial pressure (ICP) changes from its normal value when the adaptive mechanisms of CSF and venous blood displacement have been exhausted.

Figure 38.1 shows that between points 1 and 2 intracranial pressure is normal, although the volume change that can be tolerated is reduced progressively. Beyond point 2, compliance is lost and an increase in volume of any intracranial content results in a very steep increase in intracranial pressure, seen at points 3 and 4.

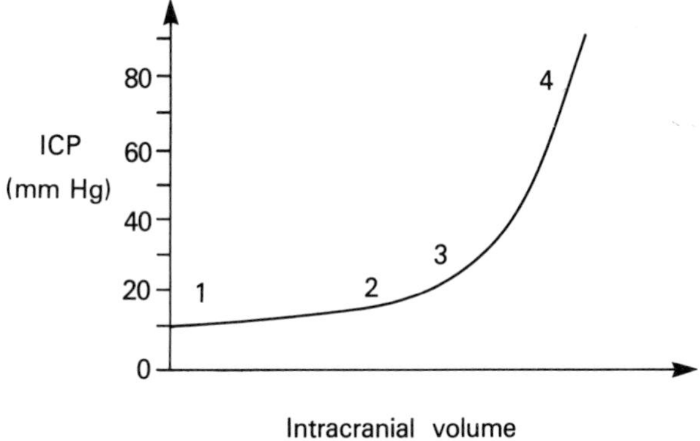

Fig. 38.1 The intracranial pressure/volume relationship.

When the growth of a lesion is slow and its siting allows maximum accommodation, large volumes of tumour may be found in the presence of a relatively normal ICP. Lesions which grow quickly soon exhaust the displacement mechanisms and lead to severe elevations of ICP.

Intracranial volumes

The volume occupied by the brain may be increased by tumour, abscess or haematoma, and augmented by oedema or hyperaemia. CSF is formed at approximately 0.3–0.5 ml/min irrespective of ICP up to pressures of 200 mmH_2O. It is reabsorbed in the arachnoid villi by a purely mechanical process dependent on the pressure gradient between CSF and venous blood in the sinuses.

Intracranial blood volume is increased by cerebral vasodilatation and by obstruction of venous return. The effect on ICP of neck flexion, neck rotation and compression of the jugular veins is shown in Figure 38.2. The normal ICP is 100–150 mmH_2O (or 7–10 mmHg) throughout the CSF in the horizontal position. Jugular bulb pressure is approximately equal to atmospheric pressure. On assuming the erect posture there is an initial decrease in ICP (and increase in lumbar CSF pressure), but ICP is restored rapidly as a result of the decreased rate of absorption of CSF by the arachnoid villi.

CSF pressure is related directly to airway pressure. Large increases in ICP are produced by coughing, straining and the use of positive end-expiratory pressure (PEEP). The effect of positive pressure ventilation seen in Figure 38.3 is caused probably by transmission of intrathoracic pressure through the jugular and vertebral veins.

ICP recordings show fluctuations related to the arterial pulse and respiration. These oscillations reflect changes in the size of the arterioles and to a lesser extent of the choroid plexus. Their amplitude is increased when ICP is elevated and when there is cerebral vasodilatation.

From the relationship between ICP and intracranial volume illustrated in Figure 38.1, it is evident that as the decompensated stage is approached, the brain becomes more vulnerable

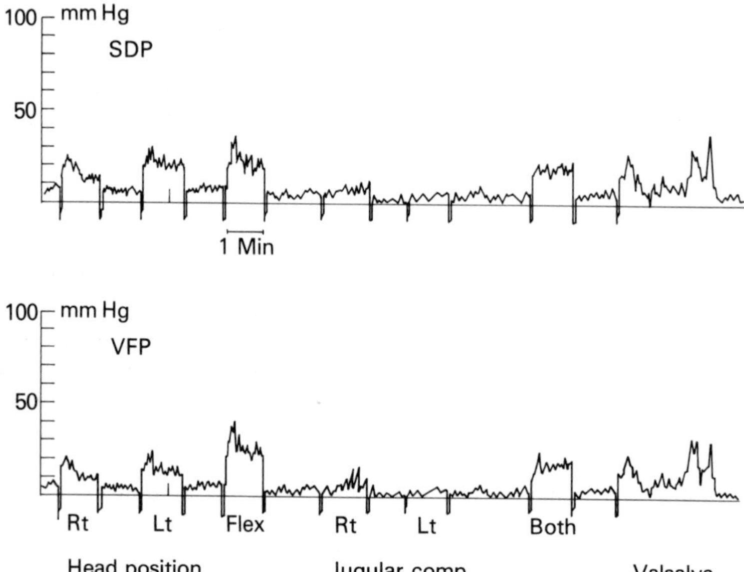

Fig. 38.2 Effect of head movement (right, left lateral movement and flexion), right, left and combined jugular compression and Valsalva manoeuvres on ICP (SDP = subdural pressure, VFP = ventricular fluid pressure).

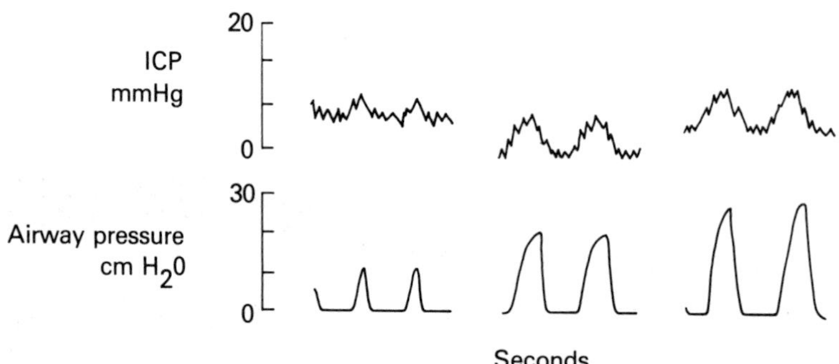

Fig. 38.3 Effects of change in airway pressure on ICP.

to the effects of any cerebral vasodilator, e.g. ketamine, halothane or carbon dioxide, or any other cause of increased intracranial volume, e.g. poor posture. A feature of this phase of the volume–pressure relationship is the appearance of Lundberg A waves on the ICP recording. These are plateaus of large increases in CSF pressure (up to 80 mmHg) often superimposed on a relatively normal baseline pressure. These waves have a duration of 5–20 min. A transient increase in Pa_{CO_2} often precedes the development of A waves, although other factors may be responsible. B waves, with a frequency of approximately 1/min, and C waves of 6/min are seen also in these patients (Fig. 38.4).

Cerebral blood flow (CBF)

Two-thirds of the CBF is transmitted through the carotid arteries and one-third through the vertebral arteries.

Autoregulation

Normally, CBF is approximately 50 ml/100 g of brain tissue per min, and is maintained at this constant rate over a wide range of CPP. The cerebral arteries constrict as the systemic arterial pressure increases and dilate as it diminishes. This phenomenon is termed autoregulation, and in man is effective between mean arterial pressures of 60–130 mmHg; below and above these limits, CBF varies passively with perfusion pressure. Although autoregulation appears to be an intrinsic response of cerebral arteriolar smooth muscle, the sympathetic nervous system influences the range of pressures over which autoregulation is effective.

Autoregulation occurs when CPP is decreased by either hypotension or raised ICP. In states of raised ICP, CBF is preserved until ICP exceeds 30–40 mmHg; at higher pressures, the Cushing response of hypertension maintains perfusion at the cost of further increases in ICP.

The lower limit of autoregulation during hypotension depends on the cause. Hypotension resulting from haemorrhage leads to a loss of autoregulation at higher pressures than during drug-induced hypotension. Halothane hypotension is associated with autoregulation at lower pressures than trimetaphan and much lower than sodium nitroprusside.

In hypertensive patients, there is a rightward shift in autoregulation limits (e.g. 90–160 mmHg); cervical sympathetic stimulation produces a similar elevation. This is illustrated in Figure 38.5.

When the upper limit of autoregulation is exceeded, breakthrough focal haemorrhages and oedema are produced.

Autoregulation is impaired or abolished by hypoxia and this impairment persists for some time in the posthypoxic brain. Hypercapnia, acute intracranial disease and trauma, and drug-induced hypotension to very low levels lead to a persisting loss of autoregulation. Hyperventilation has been shown to restore autoregulation in some patients in whom the disease process had produced a loss of autoregulation at normocapnia.

Metabolic regulation of cerebral blood flow

Increases in specific regional cerebral blood flows are encountered during increased mental activity or voluntary muscle effort. Both global cerebral blood flow and cerebral metabolism are greatly increased by the intense activity of a grand mal convulsion.

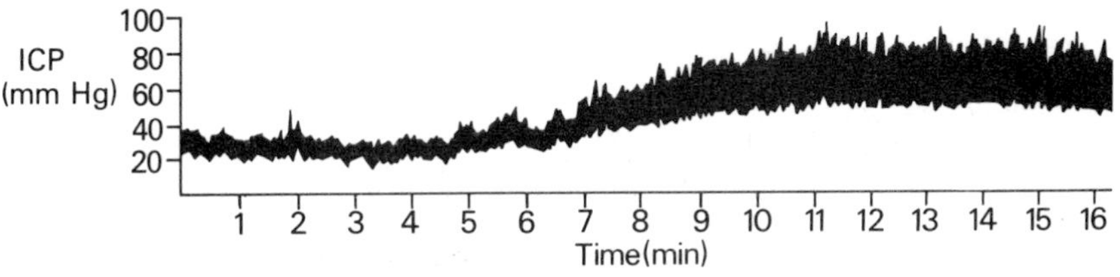

Fig. 38.4 Lundberg A wave in a recording of ICP.

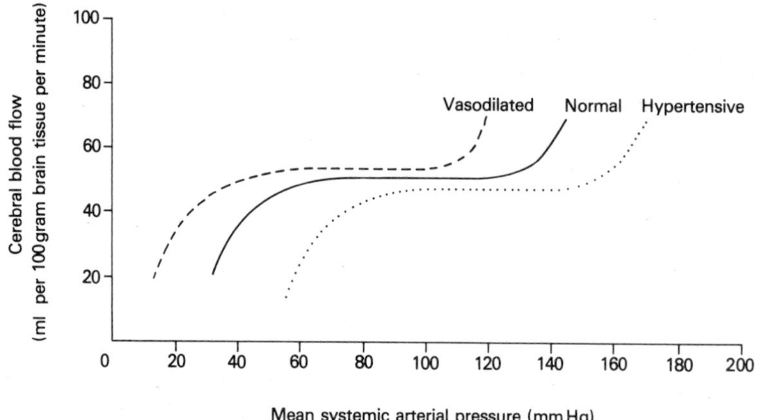

Fig. 38.5 Autoregulation curves in normal, hypertensive and drug-induced hypotensive states.

The regulation of regional CBF to match the metabolic demand of the brain is thought to be mediated by local changes in concentrations of vasodilator metabolites, lactic acid and carbon dioxide, which may act via pH and K^+ in the region of the terminal arterioles. Pain and anxiety also increase CBF and cerebral metabolism; these effects are probably related to the enhanced neuronal function and catecholamine release in the brain associated with arousal.

Metabolic depression leads to a reduction in cerebral blood flow and may be induced by hypothermia, barbiturates, propofol etomidate, diazepam and midazolam.

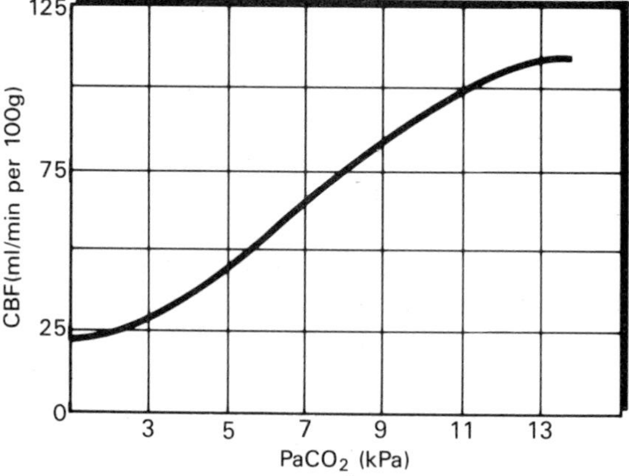

Fig. 38.6 Effect on CBF of change in Pa_{CO_2}.

Carbon dioxide and blood flow changes

The effect of changes of Pa_{CO_2} on cerebral blood flow is shown in Figure 38.6. The greatest response in CBF is at normal Pa_{CO_2}, where a change of 1 kPa results in a 30% change in blood flow. Hyperventilation below 4 kPa has less effect and below 2.6 kPa it is minimal. Less vasodilatation takes place with hypercapnia in excess of 10 kPa.

Hyperventilation below 2.6 kPa is associated with increased desaturation of jugular bulb venous blood, slow waves on the EEG, increasing drowsiness, and evidence of anaerobic glycolysis.

The response of the cerebral circulation to hyperventilation is modified by the arterial pressure. High perfusion pressures are associated with increased responsiveness to hyperventilation whereas hypotension to 50 mmHg abolishes the effect of increased or decreased Pa_{CO_2}.

Oxygen

Hypoxaemia below Pa_{O_2} of 7 kPa is necessary before cerebral vasodilatation occurs. Further hypoxaemia produces marked vasodilatation. The vasoconstrictor effect of hypocapnia is preserved in the presence of arterial hypoxaemia.

CEREBRAL METABOLISM AND $CMRO_2$

Although regional metabolic requirements of the brain vary with the level of cerebral activity, the overall energy consumption of the brain is relatively constant during sleep or active intellectual work. This activity is high; the brain consumes 20% of the oxygen used by a resting subject. To support this metabolism, the brain relies on glucose supplies; there is no store of substrate. There is also active metabolism of amino acids including glutamate, aspartate and γ-aminobutyric acid in addition to the release and inactivation of neurotransmitters.

The energy production of the brain may be equated with its rate of oxygen consumption. The cerebral metabolic rate for oxygen ($CMRO_2$) is the product of the cerebral blood flow and the arteriovenous oxygen content difference.

When there is a failure in oxygen or glucose supply, ATP production falls short of ATP utilisation and $CMRO_2$ does not reveal the nature or extent of this deficit.

Knowledge of regional blood flow and $CMRO_2$ is an inadequate guide to cellular oxygenation because of the considerable tissue heterogeneity in pathological conditions. Tissue P_{O_2} measurements are undergoing rapid development and in the future it may be possible to monitor P_{O_2} at selected cortical sites. Alternative approaches have been developed using fluorimetric techniques to measure $NADH^+$, dual-beam spectrophotometry of cytochrome oxidase redox changes, and optodes (fluorescent oxygen sensitive compounds). Potassium, hydrogen ion, and glucose can also be monitored by tissue electrodes.

EFFECTS OF DRUGS AND TECHNIQUES

The following are under the anaesthetist's control and have profound effects on the neurosurgical patient.

Arterial carbon dioxide tension

Carbon dioxide is the most potent cerebral vasodilator and CBF changes associated with it are linearly related to cerebral blood volume. The decrease in ICP produced by hypocapnia leads to gradual redistribution of the intracranial contents, resulting in an increase in CSF volume which tends to restore ICP; nevertheless, hypocapnia provides good operating conditions at craniotomy. There is no advantage in reducing Pa_{CO_2} below 4 kPa.

Hypercapnia increases ICP as a result of increased CBF and vascular engorgement. Autoregulation is abolished.

Arterial pressure changes

Hypertension

Many neurosurgical patients have focal or global loss of autoregulation and therefore cannot withstand hypertension. Even patients with preserved autoregulation should be protected from hypertensive episodes.

It is recognised that hypertensive incidents occur in response to tracheal intubation, skin incision and other nociceptive stimuli, and also at the end of anaesthesia. Only gradual restoration of normal arterial pressure should be permitted after deliberate hypotension, and control of arterial pressure with maintenance of hypocapnia is desirable in patients with disturbances of autoregulation.

Hypertensive episodes produce the added risk of haemorrhage, especially during aneurysm surgery.

Hypotension

Although reduction in arterial pressure reduces brain bulk at pressures below the limit of autoregulation, it is generally wise to avoid hypotension until satisfactory decompression of the brain has been achieved.

Effect of anaesthetic agents

Inhalational agents including nitrous oxide are cerebral vasodilators and tend to increase CBF and ICP. Hyperventilation almost always prevents the increase in ICP caused by volatile agents and nitrous oxide. Despite increasing CBF, all inhalational anaesthetics, with the possible exception of nitrous oxide, are mild metabolic depressants.

Enflurane increases the likelihood of seizures, especially in combination with extreme hypocapnia. It also induces increased production of CSF and resistance to CSF outflow. Isoflurane seems to be the best of the volatile agents. In common with halothane, it decreases $CMRO_2$, but it produces a smaller increase in CBF and a lesser increase in ICP. It causes less brain swelling than other volatile agents, and the large reduction in $CMRO_2$ greatly offsets the disadvantages of its hypotensive effects. Isoflurane does not increase production of CSF.

Thiopentone, etomidate, diazepam and midazolam produce a reduction in $CMRO_2$ and CBF, and consequently in ICP. Propofol also reduces $CMRO_2$, CBF and ICP; it is likely to prove to be useful both as an anaesthetic induction agent and for maintenance infusions in neurosurgery. Ketamine increases $CMRO_2$, CBF and ICP, although these effects can be prevented by concurrent use of diazepam.

The commonly used opioids have little direct effect on intracranial haemodynamics, although their effect can be devastating if ventilatory depression is permitted to occur.

The muscle relaxants in common use do not affect cerebral metabolism or cerebral blood flow directly; however, their effects on arterial pressure, cardiac output and venous pressure cause indirect effects.

Effect of anaesthetic technique

Increases in central venous pressure are transmitted directly to the intracranial veins and also increase CSF pressure; consequently a slight head-up posture is often indicated. Insufficient expiratory time, high expiratory resistance, coughing, or straining on the tracheal tube increase ICP.

Cerebral venous pressure is reduced only slightly by a subatmospheric expiratory phase and generally if the patient is well relaxed, has a free expiratory pathway and an adequate expiratory time there is little to be gained from a negative phase. PEEP increases ICP, although the effects are usually less than might be expected.

ANAESTHESIA FOR NEUROLOGICAL INVESTIGATIONS

Precise anatomical localisation of intracranial pathology almost always requires sophisticated radiological investigations. The development of computerised axial tomography in 1973 revolutionised neuroradiology and made pneumoencephalography a rarely used technique.

The majority of neuroradiological investigations require the use of contrast medium which carries some intrinsic risks. Nevertheless, as these investigations are essential before surgery, they are justifiable even when performed on very ill patients.

Contrast material occasionally produces anaphylactic or other hypersensitivity reactions and resuscitation facilities should always be available in the X-ray department. Metrizamide is used for intrathecal injection. It is said to be less likely than Myodil to cause anaphylactic reactions but may cause epileptiform convulsions. Known epileptics and patients receiving butyrophenone or phenothiazine derivatives are said to be particularly susceptible to this complication.

Local anaesthetic techniques may be used, with or without sedation, in cooperative adult patients. Small children and nervous, confused or disorientated adult patients usually require general anaesthesia.

Respiratory depressants must be avoided in patients with space-occupying lesions. Many neurosurgical patients require several anaesthetics and therefore agents which are known to produce occasional sensitivity reactions on repeated use should be avoided.

Any patient having a general anaesthetic for neuroradiology requires the same degree of care and the same precautions as when definitive neurosurgery is to be performed.

A detailed description of anaesthesia for neuroradiological procedures is contained in Chapter 30.

ANAESTHESIA FOR NEUROSURGERY

The conduct of anaesthesia should aim to provide good operating conditions with an easily retractable brain and minimal blood loss.

Preoperative assessment

The care of the patient begins some days before major surgery. It is essential to recognise those patients who have an increased ICP, as the adverse effects of anaesthesia are greatly magnified. The presence of papilloedema, depression of consciousness and the degree of neurological deficit must be assessed. If there has been vomiting, there may be dehydration and electrolyte abnormalities, but no attempt should be made to hydrate fully patients with intracranial hypertension before surgery. The general medical condition of the patients and their fitness for anaesthesia must also be assessed.

Many patients are receiving steroid, anticonvulsant or antihypertensive drug therapy. Patients with grossly increased ICP should have ventricular drainage or mannitol therapy before operation. If glioma or other causes of cerebral oedema are present, steroid therapy (e.g. betamethasone 8 mg every 6 h) should be instituted.

Blood should be cross-matched as there is often more than 1 litre of haemorrhage at surgery and replacement with large volumes of crystalloid solutions is contraindicated.

The preoperative visit also allows assessment of the suitability of either the radial or dorsalis pedis artery for cannulation.

Alert patients are naturally apprehensive before a craniotomy and, as opioid and sedative premedication are usually contraindicated, it is important that reassurance and explanation are kind and thoughtful. Atropine 0.6 mg reduces oral secretions, and is frequently prescribed, while diazepam calms the patient and is used widely for premedication of neurosurgical patients. Diazepam has little effect on ICP, is a useful anticonvulsant, and in modest dosage produces little respiratory depression.

Induction of anaesthesia

With suitable preoperative care, few patients arrive in the anaesthetic room with grossly increased ICP. The induction technique should prevent hypoxaemia and hypercapnia and employ agents which reduce ICP, e.g. thiopentone, propofol or etomidate. The depth of anaesthesia achieved at induction should limit the responses of arterial pressure and ICP to laryngoscopy and intubation. A β-adrenergic receptor blocker or lignocaine 1–2 mg/kg administered i.v. at this stage may also be used to attenuate further the pressor responses. Preoxygenation, hyperventilation and full muscular relaxation should be achieved before attempting intubation in order to avoid coughing and straining.

Rapid gentle intubation of the trachea should be performed after spraying the larynx and upper trachea with local anaesthetic solution (e.g. lignocaine 4%). A non-kinkable tracheal tube is recommended and should be fixed to the face with meticulous care, after checking that it is positioned correctly. A nasogastric tube is a useful precaution in long operations which may be associated with gastric dilatation. A pharyngeal pack is necessary in patients in whom a leak of blood or CSF into the nasopharynx is anticipated.

Monitoring

1. Arterial pressure and heart rate. Direct cannulation of the radial artery at the wrist or the dorsalis pedis artery is usually indicated. This permits arterial pressure and heart rate to be displayed and provides access for arterial blood gas analysis. Newer non-invasive techniques are improving in reliability and may lessen the need for invasive monitoring in some patients.
2. Electrocardiogram.
3. Temperature — oesophageal or rectal.
4. Central venous pressure. A central venous line is indicated in operations where severe bleeding is expected. If the sitting position is used it is considered essential in certain centres that the catheter is placed in the right atrium or ventricle.
5. A precordial or oesophageal stethoscope is useful and is indicated especially in operations performed in the sitting position, and in craniotomies in infants.
6. Expired carbon dioxide concentration.
7. Other monitoring may include ICP, EEG or a processed derivative, blood gas measurements and measurements of CBF.

Transfusion and heat loss

An i.v. infusion of compound sodium lactate should be started and should incorporate a blood warming device. It is useful to prepare a second separate infusion for use with mannitol or hypotensive agents.

Heat loss is reduced by the use of a 'space rescue' blanket — a polyester sheet surrounded by laminates of aluminium foil. The impermeable material prevents heat loss from convection and evaporation and the aluminium prevents radiant heat loss. Alternatively, the patient may be placed on, and covered by, water circulation blankets.

Neurosurgical patients are at great risk of developing postoperative deep vein thrombosis. As there is some anxiety regarding the use of prophylactic heparin or dextran 70 because of the risks of bleeding, mechanical methods should be used for minimising stagnation of blood in the legs.

Iatrogenic injury

Care must be taken to protect the eyes by covering the closed lids with waterproof non-irritant adhesive plaster. There must be no stretching of peripheral nerves, and vulnerable skin pressure areas including the forehead, ears and nose must be protected.

Position for surgery

The surgical position is chosen to provide operative access and should allow good venous drainage from the site of operation by elevation of the head above the heart. Care should be taken to avoid excessive flexion or rotation of the neck, which might obstruct the neck veins.

Most craniotomies are performed in the supine brow-up position; temporal and posterior fossa craniotomies are satisfactory in the lateral or lateral/prone position with some rotation of the neck depending on the site of the lesion. The full prone position gives adequate exposure for many posterior fossa and cervical spine operations, but meticulous care must be taken to support the body on the iliac crests and the chest in order to leave a free, uncompressed abdomen and vena cava.

In many centres, the sitting position is still preferred to provide optimal access for posterior fossa surgery, despite a 5% reported incidence of marked postural hypotension, necessitating vasopressor therapy in 40% of patients. Air embolism occurs in 2 to 40% of patients (depending on the sensitivity of the method of detection). Many authorities believe that the use of the sitting position for posterior fossa surgery should be discouraged strongly and that it should not be used for cervical spine surgery.

It is kinder to shave the head under anaesthesia with the patient in the surgical position rather than before operation. Finally the patient should be inspected to check the position of the tracheal tube, its fixation and that of the anaesthetic tubing and other equipment.

Maintenance of anaesthesia

The basic technique for most craniotomies is hyperventilation with 70% nitrous oxide in oxygen to an arterial P_{CO_2} of 3.3 to 4 kPa. Muscle relaxation is maintained with incremental doses of a non-depolarising neuromuscular blocking agent given regularly to prevent any possibility of coughing or straining. An adequate depth of anaesthesia may be maintained if nitrous oxide is supplemented with fentanyl. It is safer to supplement anaesthesia with isoflurane or an alternative volatile agent during hypocapnia than to allow a lightly anaesthetised patient to suffer awareness or hypertensive episodes during surgical stimulation.

Currently there is great interest in the replacement of inhalational anaesthetic agents by a total i.v. technique. Barbiturates and propofol lower intracranial pressure, and in expert hands problems of hypotension and delayed recovery do not seem to be unacceptable.

Active reduction of intracranial pressure

When the ICP is high or when the dura is tight and the brain swollen, the ICP must be lowered by pharmacological and occasionally mechanical means.

Mannitol in a 20% solution may be given in a dosage of 0.25–0.5 g/kg body weight. In this dosage, serum osmolality increases of over 10 mmol/kg may be expected and the acute effects on ICP are comparable to those achieved by higher doses. Effective reduction of ICP occurs within 5 min of starting the infusion, and the improvement in the volume–pressure relationship lasts for up to 2 h. Mannitol is also helpful in making the brain softer and more easily retractable.

A disadvantage of mannitol is the associated transient hypervolaemia which may increase surgical bleeding.

Loop diuretics (e.g. frusemide in a dose of 1 mg/kg) produce a brisk diuresis and a reduction in brain bulk. In less urgent situations 30% glycerol may be given by mouth. Unfortunately, high concentrations of glycerol produce haemolysis and haemoglobinuria when administered i.v.

When osmotic therapy is anticipated, a catheter should be placed in the bladder.

ICP reduction may also be achieved by ventriculostomy. In patients in whom only a small increase of ICP is present and there is communicating hydrocephalus, e.g. aneurysm surgery, drainage may be achieved via an indwelling lumbar spinal needle. However, drainage should be limited in volume and to a rate of less than 5 ml/min, otherwise arterial hypertension and cardiac arrhythmias are common and a rebound increase in ICP may occur.

Recovery from anaesthesia

Patients who are expected to have a high risk of developing convulsions should be given phenytoin 250 mg by slow i.v. injection during anaesthesia. When cerebral oedema is anticipated after surgery, betamethasone or dexamethasone therapy should be started.

At the end of the operation, problems may arise as a result of depression of consciousness, damage to cranial nerves (limiting the patient's ability to maintain a safe airway), and central respiratory depression.

After major procedures in which oedema is expected, or where autoregulation is likely to be grossly impaired, it is wise to continue hyperventilation into the postoperative period.

In patients in whom spontaneous ventilation is to be preferred, residual neuromuscular blockade should be antagonised with neostigmine and atropine. The increased sensitivity of neurosurgical patients to opioids makes it advisable to administer naloxone routinely to reverse residual effects.

The ability of the patient to breathe and maintain an airway spontaneously must be assessed and no carbon dioxide retention, hypoxia or asphyxia permitted otherwise serious brain swelling will occur.

SPECIFIC OPERATIONS

Intracranial vascular surgery

Before operation, hypertension should be treated and after subarachnoid haemorrhage epsilon aminocaproic acid therapy instituted to reduce the risk of further haemorrhage.

Induction of anaesthesia as described above should prevent surges of arterial pressure. After dural exposure, CSF may be withdrawn via a needle in the lumbar subarachnoid space.

Ventilation should be adjusted to maintain normocapnia, as extremely low grey matter blood flows are encountered when hypocapnia is superimposed on the vasoconstriction associated with intracranial aneurysms.

The use of the operating microscope and hypotensive anaesthesia provide excellent operating conditions for surgical dissection of the aneurysmal sac and have led to the gradual abandonment of hypothermia in most neurosurgical units in the United Kingdom.

Halothane or isoflurane may be used as the primary hypotensive agent, or used in addition to infusion of sodium nitroprusside or trimetaphan.

Hypophysectomy

Removal of the pituitary gland is performed for tumours of the gland and for treatment of metastatic hormone-sensitive tumours. Hormone replacement with cortisone should be started before operation; other hormone problems, e.g. diabetes insipidus or mellitus, may require therapy postoperatively.

Tracheal intubation in patients with acromegaly can be difficult and introducers and an extra long laryngoscope blade should be available. Patients with carcinomatosis are often anaemic and cachectic and may have multiple bone metastases, pleural effusions and ascites. They should quickly be rendered as healthy as possible and the anaesthetic risk accepted, as there is often a gratifying response to surgery.

After hypophysectomy, a few patients develop severe hypothalamic disturbances of temperature and circulatory regulation.

AIR EMBOLISM

Air embolism occurs in 2 to 40% of patients in the sitting position, the reported incidence being related to the sensitivity of the method of detection. The severity of the embolism is determined by the rate and volume of air entrained and the ability of the circulation to withstand the insult. Air bubbles expand in the presence of nitrous oxide, whilst 100% oxygen reduces the hazard.

Detection

Monitoring with a stethoscope reveals a drum-like resonance to the heart sounds and this becomes 'millwheel' with larger volumes of air. The Doppler ultrasonic flowmeter is the most sensitive detection device but many instruments are still unshielded from diathermy interference.

Expired carbon dioxide concentration decreases and arterial pressure and ECG changes are common. Pulmonary artery pressure increases during embolism before circulatory collapse; this haemodynamic variable is measured commonly in the USA.

Treatment of air embolism comprises surgical sealing of the open veins, accompanied by jugular vein compression and an increase in intrathoracic pressure. A G-suit may be used to increase venous pressure, and aspiration of the right heart via the central venous catheter enables air to be removed directly. Oxygen, vasopressors and external or internal cardiac massage may also be required.

HEAD INJURIES

Anaesthetists are involved in the care of patients with head injury because they are asked to provide anaesthesia for extracranial surgery in patients who have suffered minor head injuries, anaesthesia for intracranial surgery in more severe head injuries, and also to assist or supervise the resuscitation and medical care of comatose patients.

Anaesthesia for patients with head injury

All patients with head injury have some oedema of the brain with damage to its blood vessels and some degree of loss of autoregulation. An anaesthetic with a volatile agent using spontaneous ventilation is likely to produce a severe increase in ICP and neurological deterioration in the patient. Patients having minor procedures performed require the same anaesthetic standards as those undergoing neurosurgery.

First aid

Unconscious patients should be nursed in the semiprone position; the airway should be cleared of blood, vomit, false teeth, etc. It is essential to take great care when moving the head or neck as cervical spine injuries are commonly associated with head injuries. If cough and swallowing reflexes are impaired, tracheal intubation is mandatory. It is wise to pass a large nasogastric tube, and, as far as possible, empty the stomach. Hypotension is rare in closed head injuries and suggests associated injuries.

Clinical assessment using the Glasgow coma scale (Table 38.1) should include an initial baseline assessment, and additional investigations may be required including X-ray, CAT scan and arterial blood gas analysis.

Mannitol should not be used routinely but may help to prevent deterioration during patient transfer or postpone 'coning' when a patient appears to be deteriorating rapidly.

Immediate surgery is required in those patients in whom there is a rapid decline in conscious level or sudden development of unilateral neurological signs. Most operations are performed for suspected or proven haematoma, depressed fractures or CSF rhinorrhoea not associated with simple malar fractures.

Intensive care

Special care is necessary in all patients with head injury where airway care is required, if a lapar-

Table 38.1 The Glasgow coma scale is based upon eye opening, verbal and motor response. Each response on the scale is given a number (high for normal and low for impaired responses). The responsiveness of the patient is expressed by summation of the numbers. The lowest score is 3; the highest is 15.

Eyes open		Spontaneously	4
		To verbal command	3
		To pain	2
		No response	1
Best motor response	To verbal command	Obeys	6
	To painful stimulus*	Localises pain	5
		Flexion — withdrawal	4
		Flexion — abnormal (decorticate rigidity)	3
		Extension (decerebrate rigidity)	2
		No response	1
Best verbal response**		Orientated and converses	5
		Disorientated and converses	4
		Inappropriate words	3
		Incomprehensible sounds	2
		No response	1
TOTAL			3–15

* Apply knuckle to sternum, observe arms
** Arouse patient with painful stimulus if necessary

otomy has been performed and in those with combinations of head and chest, spinal or jaw injury.

Control of raised ICP

Many patients with severe head injury develop an elevation of ICP. This may result from the development of a subdural or extradural haematoma, but occurs also in patients with no mass lesion, or in patients whose haematoma has been drained. In the first 24 h following head injury, the cerebral vasculature in damaged areas of brain dilates (vasoparesis), resulting in an increased cerebral blood volume. Later, both extracellular and intracellular oedema develop, increasing the volume of fluid inside the skull. Measures to control raised ICP are designed either to reduce cerebral blood volume, or to decrease the volume of intracerebral water.

Position. In order to encourage venous drainage, the patient should be nursed with the head and shoulders elevated at about 15° to the horizontal. The head should be straight, as kinking of neck veins occurs if cervical rotation is permitted.

Oxygenation. An arterial oxygen tension of at least 13 kPa should be maintained. Secondary cerebral damage may occur if areas of damaged brain with impaired capillary blood flow are subjected to hypoxaemia, and further cerebral vasodilatation occurs if Pa_{O_2} decreases below 7 kPa.

Controlled ventilation. Elective controlled hyperventilation is used widely in patients whose head injury results in persistent intracranial hypertension. It is also indicated in hyper- or hypoventilating or hypoxaemic patients, e.g. where $Pa_{CO_2} < 3$ kPa, or $Pa_{O_2} < 10$ kPa with an FI_{O_2} of 0.4. Neurological indications include status epilepticus or decerebrate spasms which have not responded to conventional therapy, and combined head and chest injuries.

When controlled ventilation is instituted, it is essential to prevent coughing and straining, and achieve good oxygenation and moderate hypocapnia (Pa_{CO_2} 3.5–4 kPa). Arterial oxygenation and carbon dioxide clearance must be maintained with the minimal airway pressure and the least value of PEEP, whenever the latter is necessary in the presence of severe lung dysfunction.

When elective ventilation is required, continuous ICP monitoring must be instituted.

Sedation. In the patient receiving IPPV, sedation is usually necessary, despite the resulting difficulty in clinical assessment of the nervous system. A continuous infusion of an opioid agent (e.g. papaveretum 10–20 mg/h) is often sufficient to prevent arterial hypertension, coughing and straining. Neuromuscular blocking agents may be useful if moderate doses of opioids are inadequate to prevent transient elevation of ICP, and are most effective if administered as a continuous infusion. Bolus doses of i.v. anaesthetic agents may be required in addition immediately before turning or physiotherapy.

Steroids. The use of steroids in patients with head injury does not influence control of ICP, or the eventual outcome of the patient.

Diuretics. Mannitol 0.25–0.5 g/kg, administered over 15–30 min, may be used to reduce the volume of intracranial water if the general trend of ICP is rising. Mannitol extracts water from normal brain, and does not reduce cerebral oedema per se. Serum osmolality must be monitored if frequent doses of mannitol are administered, and if the value exceeds 320 mosmol/kg, further mannitol should be withheld. Frusemide or bumetanide may be used, and these agents reduce CSF formation in addition to reducing intracerebral water. Serum electrolyte concentrations should be monitored closely.

Fluid balance. Normal fluid requirements and appropriate electrolytes should be administered. Dehydration does not assist in control of ICP.

The development of diabetes insipidus should be suspected if urine output increases in the absence of diuretic administration. Confirmation may be obtained by biochemical analysis of urine, and measurements of serum electrolyte concentrations and osmolality. Vasopressin should be administered as necessary.

Metabolic depression. When the management described fails to control ICP, but there are grounds for hope that the patient's condition may be reversible, metabolic depression may be undertaken using an infusion of an i.v. anaesthetic agent.

It is necessary to monitor directly arterial and central venous pressure to ensure that volume replacement is adequate. Access to a central vein is essential as dopamine may be required occasionally to counteract drug-induced circulatory depression.

Pentobarbitone, thiopentone and gamma hydroxybutyric acid have been used. In all instances the cerebral perfusion pressure should be maintained at 60–70 mmHg using circulatory support if necessary.

Phenytoin has protective effects on the brain as a result of its anticonvulsant properties and perhaps its ability to reduce CSF K^+ accumulation during hypoxia.

Although the use of these agents is often valuable in helping to control ICP, there is little evidence at present that this form of therapy has produced any great improvement in the outcome of these very ill patients.

Anticonvulsants

Anticonvulsants are required prophylactically in patients with depressed skull fractures with dural penetration, in those with early convulsions, and following acute subdural haematoma. Usually, phenytoin suffices, but if fits persist diazepam, phenobarbitone or other agents may be required. The metabolism of the brain is increased greatly during convulsions and therefore all fits must be treated vigorously. Monitoring the EEG is helpful.

FURTHER READING

Campkin T V, Turner J M 1980 Neurosurgical anaesthesia and intensive care. Butterworths, London

Greenbaum R 1976 General anaesthesia for neurosurgery. British Journal of Anaesthesia 48: 773

Greenbaum R 1987. A practical approach to head injuries, including intracranial pressure monitoring and protection of damaged tissue. Anaesthesia for neurosurgery (International practice and research). Jewkes D (ed) Baillières Clinical Anaesthesiology. Vol. 1, No. 2

Jennett B, Teasdale G 1981 Management of head injuries. F A Davis, Philadelphia

Jones P W 1981 Hyperventilation in the management of cerebral oedema. Intensive Care Medicine 7: 205

Levy W J, Shapiro H M, Maruchak G, Meathe E 1980 Automated EEG processing for intraoperative monitoring: a comparison of techniques. Anesthesiology 53: 223

McDowall D G 1975 The influence of anaesthetic drugs and techniques on intracranial pressure. In: Gordon E (ed) A basis and practice of neuroanaesthesia. Excerpta Medica, Amsterdam

Marshall L F, Smith R W, Shapiro H M 1979 The outcome with aggressive treatment in severe head injuries. Journal of Neurosurgery 50: 20

Silver I A 1979 The significance of clinical assessment of brain tissue oxygenation in different pathological conditions: an overview. Federation Proceedings 38: 2495

39. Anaesthesia for thoracic surgery

In the early twentieth century, thoracic surgery was confined predominantly to the treatment of tuberculosis and empyema. Advances in anaesthetic practice permitted thoracoplasty, and subsequently lung resection and pneumonectomy, to be performed with increasing safety. With the introduction of antibiotics and antituberculous agents, surgical intervention has become progressively less common for pulmonary tuberculosis and bronchiectasis. The most common conditions presenting currently for thoracic surgery are carcinoma of bronchus, carcinoma of oesophagus, metastatic disease, and a variety of benign processes.

PREOPERATIVE ASSESSMENT

General assessment of the preoperative patient is considered in Chapter 19. In this section, only factors specific to thoracic surgery are discussed.

History

Dyspnoea

This common symptom may indicate disease of lungs or airways, cardiac disease or anaemia. Attempts should be made to relate dyspnoea to a specified degree of activity, e.g. climbing a flight of stairs, walking on the level, etc. The degree of dyspnoea in an individual may vary considerably, particularly if it is associated with disease of small airways, e.g. asthma or chronic bronchitis, when it may be accompanied by wheezing. Dyspnoea may result also from mucosal oedema, secretions, premature small airways closure, or alveolar fibrosis and infiltration.

Cough

A dry cough usually indicates irritation of the large airways, but if persistent may be caused by serious pathology, e.g. compression of the trachea or main bronchi by glands. A productive cough is of greater importance, as material in the bronchial tree may spread infection, or cause obstruction and collapse of areas of lung. Sputum should be obtained for bacteriological examination.

Haemoptysis

Large haemoptyses are uncommon, but have important anaesthetic implications, as the area responsible may require isolation using a technique of bronchial intubation in order to prevent contamination of the entire respiratory tree. Bronchiectasis and cavitating tuberculosis may cause severe haemoptysis, as may some tumours, particularly after biopsy. Minor degrees of haemoptysis are common in inflammatory and neoplastic disease of the lung.

Dysphagia

Severe dysphagia has two important sequelae; the patient rapidly becomes malnourished and cachectic, and the oesophagus above the lesion dilates and may contain large volumes of previously ingested food which may be regurgitated when the patient becomes unconscious.

Examination

Careful examination of the respiratory system is essential in patients presenting for thoracic surgery.

Cyanosis may be present, either centrally because of severe pulmonary disease, or peripherally in the distribution of superior vena caval drainage if that vessel is obstructed. Asymmetry of chest wall movement should be noted, together with any deviation of the trachea. If an intercostal drain is in place, the presence of an air leak should be noted, and its magnitude assessed. Stridor may be present if there is major obstruction of the trachea.

Percussion may demonstrate the presence of a pleural effusion or a major area of lung collapse.

Auscultation may reveal mild tracheal stridor, or partial obstruction of a main or lobar bronchus. More generalised airways obstruction is indicated by widespread rhonchi, often heard only during expiration. Fine crepitations suggest disease of peripheral airways or alveoli; coarse crepitations are associated more usually with secretions in large airways, and may disappear after coughing.

The mouth and neck should be examined carefully. Features which suggest difficulty in tracheal intubation are likely to result in severe hindrance to the introduction of a bronchial or double lumen tube. Loose, prominent or capped teeth may interfere with, or be damaged during, rigid bronchoscopy or oesophagoscopy.

Preoperative investigations

Routine

Full blood count, serum urea and electrolyte concentrations, and blood glucose estimations are requested normally. A coagulation screen and liver function tests may be indicated. An ECG is essential.

Radiological

Good quality posteroanterior and lateral X-rays of chest are helpful in demonstrating localised disease of the lungs, and distortion of the tracheobronchial tree. Tomography provides more detailed information on a lesion or malformation of the bronchial anatomy. Computerised axial tomography (body scan), nuclear magnetic resonance imaging and radionuclide scanning are used increasingly. Bronchography, using radio-opaque contrast medium to display the tracheobronchial tree, is employed particularly in patients with bronchiectasis. A barium swallow is required to define lesions of the oesophagus.

Pulmonary function tests

Objective assessment of pulmonary function is essential to assess the extent of impairment of lung function and as an aid in predicting the ability of a patient to survive pneumonectomy.

Reduction in forced vital capacity (FVC) indicates a restrictive defect. A low forced expiratory volume in one second ($FEV_{1.0}$), reduced $FEV_{1.0}$/FVC ratio, and decreased peak expiratory flow rate (PEFR) suggest the presence of obstructive disease of the airways. Additional information may be obtained by displaying flow–volume loops (see Ch. 2, Fig. 2.9). Reversibility of airways obstruction should be ascertained by repeating these tests after administration of a bronchodilator, e.g. salbutamol. Measurement of gas transfer using carbon monoxide, and in particular, calculation of the gas transfer coefficient (gas transfer per unit of ventilated lung volume) provides information on gas exchange which may be useful in predicting the extent of postoperative hypoxaemia. Arterial blood gas analysis is necessary in all patients with moderate or severe lung disease in order to select an appropriate inspired oxygen concentration during and after surgery, and to detect patients with hypercapnia, in whom excessive inspired oxygen concentrations may reduce respiratory drive.

Regional lung function is assessed using radioisotope techniques, and aids decisions concerning pulmonary resection; overall lung function is unlikely to be impaired significantly if the resectable area has poor function.

Interpretation of lung function tests is not always easy, particularly with regard to prediction of postoperative problems. It is important to consider measurements in comparison with those predicted for a patient on the basis of height and weight (see Appendix XI(b), pp. 751–2). In general, if the FVC, $FEV_{1.0}$/FVC, and gas transfer are less than 50% of predicted values, prognosis after pneumonectomy is poor. If PEFR is less than 70% of predicted, or $FEV_{1.0}$/FEV less than

60%, complications may be anticipated after any form of pulmonary surgery. However, many factors not amenable to measurement are likely to influence the outcome, including motivation of the patient, coexisting non-pulmonary disease, and the occurrence of surgical complications.

PREPARATION FOR SURGERY

If possible, patients should stop cigarette smoking in order to reduce bronchial secretions. Antibiotics may be required if infected sputum is present. Bronchodilator drugs, preferably inhaled, may reduce airway obstruction considerably. Occasionally, corticosteroids may be required to reduce bronchospasm.

Preoperative physiotherapy is used to help clear bronchial secretions, and to encourage all patients to practise breathing exercises which are required in the postoperative period.

Rehydration, electrolyte correction and i.v. nutrition are often necessary in patients with oesophageal obstruction. Oesophageal lavage may be advisable in patients with a grossly dilated oesophagus.

Perioperative digitalisation is used in a number of centres for older patients undergoing thoracotomy. Low-dose heparin therapy has become popular to reduce the incidence of deep venous thrombosis and its sequelae.

An explanation should be given to the patient of the procedure which is to be undertaken, and of the postoperative environment. In particular, it is wise to warn the patient of the presence of chest drains and postoperative pain.

Premedication

The choice of premedication, if any, is one of personal preference, although an anticholinergic agent is advisable prior to bronchial instrumentation.

DIAGNOSTIC PROCEDURES

Fibreoptic bronchoscopy

The fibreoptic bronchoscope (Fig. 39.1) may be introduced through the nose, injecting local anaesthetic solution through the injection port under direct vision as the instrument is advanced. In the anaesthetised patient, the bronchoscope may be introduced through a tracheal tube by insertion through a diaphragm (Fig. 39.2) which minimises leakage of gas during ventilation. Artificial ventilation should be maintained throughout bronchoscopy. Ventilation is impaired significantly unless the internal diameter of the tube is more than 2 mm larger than the diameter of the bronchoscope. Techniques of ventilation using jet devices may be dangerous if expiration through

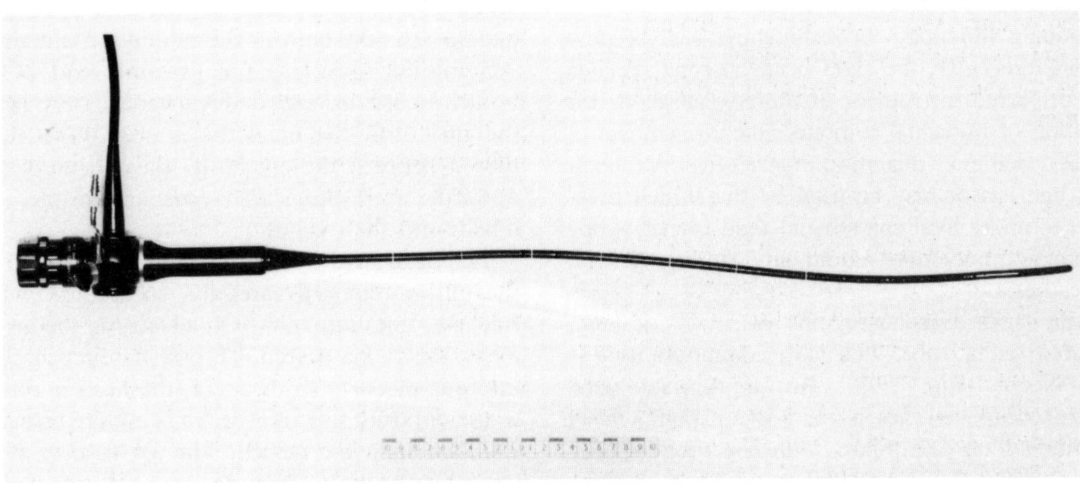

Fig. 39.1 The fibreoptic bronchoscope.

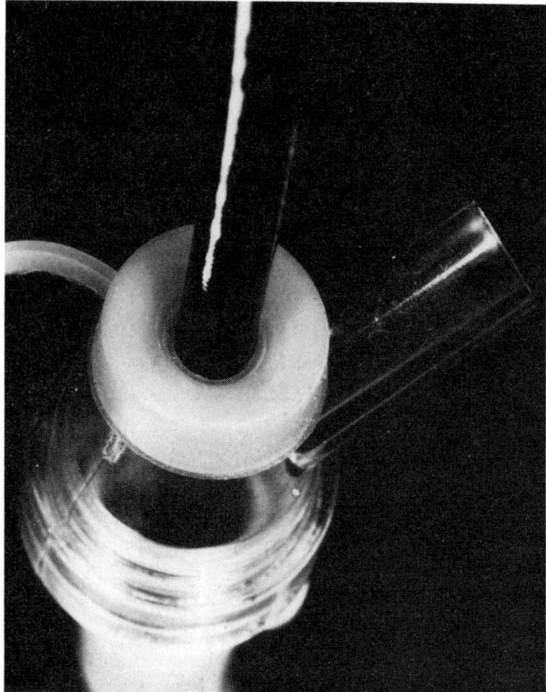

Fig. 39.2 Diaphragm used to ensure an airtight seal during fibreoptic bronchoscopy in patients receiving IPPV.

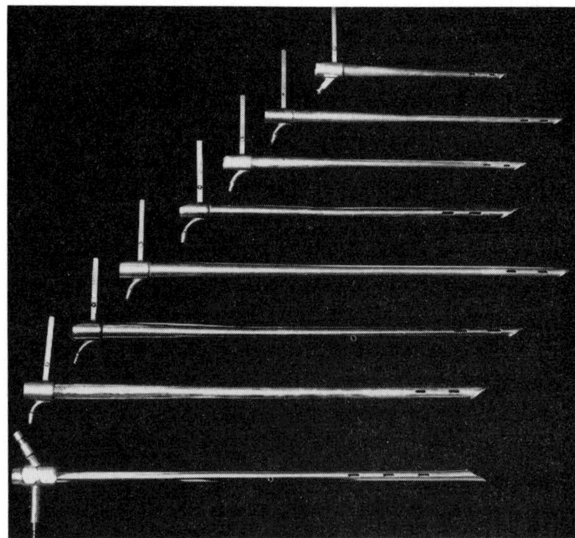

Fig. 39.3 Negus bronchoscopes.

the tracheal tube is impeded by the presence of the bronchoscope, resulting in very high pressures in the lower trachea and bronchi.

Rigid bronchoscopy

Although fibreoptic bronchoscopy has become popular recently, the rigid bronchoscope remains the preferred instrument of thoracic surgeons for location of bronchial tumours and for removal of foreign bodies or dilatation of strictures. Although this instrument may be used by the skilled practitioner under local anaesthesia, rigid bronchoscopy is carried out more commonly during general anaesthesia.

The rigid bronchoscope is essentially a long, tapered, metal tube. The most commonly used is the Negus (Fig. 39.3). An appropriate sized bronchoscope is chosen, and the patient's head positioned on one pillow with the neck slightly flexed. The head is extended on the neck. A gauze swab is placed on the patient's upper teeth or gums, and the middle finger of the bronchoscopist's left hand positioned on the patient's upper left second incisor (or the corresponding position in the edentulous patient). The bronchoscope is held in the right hand and introduced into the mouth alongside the operator's left middle finger, ensuring that the instrument is in the midline at the alveolar margin. The index finger and thumb of the left hand support the bronchoscope as it is advanced, keeping it clear of the teeth. The bronchoscope is passed backwards in the mouth until the uvula is visualised. The tip of the bronchoscope and the portion at the alveolar margin are now both in the midline. Maintaining this midline position, the proximal end of the bronchoscope is angled downwards, thus lifting the tip, until the epiglottis is seen. The tip is passed beneath the epiglottis, then forwards and upwards until the vocal cords are visible, and finally into the trachea.

The head of the table may now be lowered, or the pillow removed carefully, so that the whole trachea comes into view. On advancing the instrument, the carina is seen. To pass the bronchoscope into one of the main bronchi, the head is rotated to the opposite side in order to bring the bronchus into line with the mouth. The appearance of the carina and main bronchi as seen through a bronchoscope are shown in Figure 1.15.

Rigid bronchoscopy may induce bronchospasm or cardiac arrhythmias, and interfere with ventilation. Thus, the anaesthetic technique should provide adequate analgesia and muscle relaxation to permit introduction of the instrument and abolish reflexes from stimulation of the respiratory tract. Adequate gas exchange must be maintained. Rapid recovery of consciousness is desirable to enable the patient to cough up secretions or blood.

Topical analgesia is used occasionally, the technique being similar to that described for tracheal intubation in Chapter 32.

Inhalational anaesthesia using halothane or ether is used by some anaesthetists for rigid bronchoscopy in children. The child is anaesthetised deeply using the volatile agent, and bronchoscopy performed with the patient breathing air spontaneously through the instrument. The depth of anaesthesia lightens progressively, fairly rapidly with halothane but more slowly if ether is used, and the bronchoscope may have to be removed intermittently to allow the level of anaesthesia to be deepened.

More commonly, i.v. anaesthesia is used. Following preoxygenation, light narcosis is induced using an i.v. anaesthetic agent, e.g. methohexitone. Suxamethonium is used to provide muscle relaxation. The lungs are inflated with oxygen by facemask, and bronchoscopy undertaken. Incremental doses of i.v. anaesthetic agent and suxamethonium are given as indicated. Artificial ventilation is achieved usually using an injector, which produces a high-pressure jet of gas down the bronchoscope. Either oxygen or Entonox may be used as the driving gas. The jet of gas entrains air and produces inflation of the lungs. Expiration occurs through and round the bronchoscope. An appropriate size of jet must be selected (Table 39.1). High-frequency positive pressure ventilation (HFPPV), at rates of 100–300 breaths/min, may be used during bronchoscopy. This technique eliminates air entrainment and allows ventilation with an undiluted anaesthetic gas mixture.

Table 39.1 Appropriate sizes, and typical maximum inflation pressures, with Venturi bronchoscope injectors

Patient	Size (s.w.g.)	Pressure (cmH_2O)
Adult (poor compliance)	14	50
Adult	16	25
Child (over 12 years)	17	20
Child (under 12 years)	19	15

Oesophagoscopy

Fibreoptic oesophagoscopy is undertaken normally in the sedated patient. The rigid oesophagoscope is inserted under general anaesthesia. Features of importance to the anaesthetist are the potential for regurgitation on induction of anaesthesia, and the risk of damage to teeth or the cervical spine as the instrument is introduced. A rapid-sequence induction technique should be used, and ventilation controlled after tracheal intubation. The cuff of the tracheal tube may require deflation temporarily to enable the oesophagoscope to pass through the cricopharyngeal sphincter.

The most serious complication of oesophagoscopy is perforation of the oesophagus, and a chest X-ray is required after the procedure before any fluids are allowed by mouth.

Mediastinoscopy

This procedure permits direct inspection and biopsy of mediastinal lesions, in particular lymph nodes. The mediastinoscope is introduced through a small suprasternal incision. Complications include haemorrhage, pneumothorax, haemothorax, air embolism and recurrent laryngeal nerve damage. The most commonly used anaesthetic technique employs tracheal intubation and controlled ventilation.

Bronchography

The commonest indication for bronchography is investigation of the extent of bronchiectasis. The patient may already have compromised respiratory function and copious infected sputum.

Bronchography is performed usually using the oil-based radio-opaque contrast medium propyliodine (Dionosil) to outline the tracheobronchial tree. The procedure may be undertaken in the conscious patient under local anaesthesia, either by injecting contrast medium through a catheter placed in the trachea, or by allowing it to trickle over the back of the tongue. General anaesthesia is required for children and uncooperative adults. The anaesthetic management of patients undergoing bronchography is described in Chapter 30.

CHEST WALL INTEGRITY

If chest wall integrity is lost, either as a result of trauma or surgical intervention, abnormal chest wall movement and gas distribution occur. In the patient with a damaged chest wall, e.g. crush injury, paradoxical movement of the chest wall is seen, with inward movement of the rib cage during inspiration and the reverse during expiration. During inspiration, the lung on the unaffected side expands, but fills with gas partly from the trachea, and partly from the lung on the abnormal side, which deflates. During expiration, the normal lung deflates, but part of the expired gas passes into the lung on the affected side, which expands. This pattern of ventilation, termed 'pendulum breathing' or Pendelluft, results in progressive hypoxaemia and hypercapnia. A similar pattern occurs if the chest wall is opened surgically. Thus spontaneous ventilation is inappropriate if integrity of the chest wall is to be lost, and positive pressure ventilation should be employed.

ONE-LUNG ANAESTHESIA

Distribution of ventilation and perfusion

In the awake, spontaneously breathing subject in the lateral position, the dependent lung is better perfused than the upper lung because of the effects of gravity. The dependent diaphragm is pushed higher than the upper during expiration by the weight of the abdominal contents. As a result, it contracts more efficiently, so that ventilation of the dependent lung is also better than that of the upper lung. Thus, ventilation and perfusion are reasonably well matched in both lungs. However, in the anaesthetised patient, functional residual capacity (FRC) is reduced and the upper lung receives greater ventilation, whereas perfusion remains better in the lower lung. Similarly, during controlled ventilation, the upper lung is ventilated preferentially as the compliance of the dependent lung is reduced by the weight of the abdominal contents and mediastinum. Perfusion of the upper lung may be greater than during spontaneous ventilation in the lateral position because the higher intra-alveolar pressure in the dependent lung diverts blood to the upper lung. Nevertheless, there is increased ventilation/perfusion mismatch whether ventilation is controlled or not.

In order to improve surgical access, the upper lung may be allowed to collapse, whereupon it acts as a source of true shunt because it still receives a proportion of the right ventricular output, but no ventilation. The dependent lung receives the major portion of pulmonary blood flow, and the entire minute ventilation. Ventilation and perfusion are unlikely to be matched perfectly throughout the dependent lung, and the total calculated intrapulmonary shunt therefore varies from 25 to 40% when the upper lung is collapsed. Paradoxically, higher values tend to be found in patients with normal lungs, because a diseased lung, even if it contains a focal lesion, tends to have a reduced blood supply. During pulmonary surgery, the more diseased lung is uppermost, and the dependent lung receives an increased proportion of total pulmonary blood flow. In contrast, a patient undergoing oesophageal surgery may have two healthy lungs, and intrapulmonary shunt during one-lung anaesthesia may be very high.

Increased intrapulmonary shunting causes a decrease in arterial oxygen tension. Although there is no degree of hypoxaemia which may be regarded as safe, it is generally felt that an arterial P_{O_2} of approximately 9 kPa is acceptable; this results in an oxygen saturation of approximately 90%. In order to achieve this or a higher Pa_{O_2} during one-lung ventilation, a number of techniques may be employed. It is recommended generally that an inspired oxygen concentration of 40% be provided initially on switching to one-lung anaesthesia. Higher concentrations may be necessary if there is clinical or blood gas evidence of hypoxaemia. However, concentrations of oxygen in excess of 60% are unlikely to produce a substantial increase in Pa_{O_2}, and may, unexpectedly, increase intrapulmonary shunt by decreasing the normal hypoxic vasoconstriction in poorly ventilated areas of the dependent lung. Although blood flow to the unventilated lung decreases because of an increase in vascular resistance, this does not occur to a significant extent in the first few hours after lung collapse, and a large intrapulmonary shunt persists throughout the course of one-lung anaesthesia.

Blood flow through the collapsed lung may be reduced by restricting intra-alveolar pressure, thereby encouraging blood flow through the dependent lung. Thus, positive end-expiratory pressure (PEEP), which might be expected to improve arterial oxygenation by increasing FRC in the dependent lung, may increase shunt by diverting blood to the unventilated lung. In some patients, it may be necessary to supply oxygen under a small positive pressure (0.3–0.5 kPa; 3–5 cmH_2O) to the unventilated lung. This permits diffusion oxygenation of the blood perfusing that lung, and reduces arterial hypoxaemia.

Because of the increased inspired oxygen concentration required to prevent arterial hypoxaemia, only 40–60% nitrous oxide should be administered. In order to ensure adequate anaesthesia, this should be supplemented with a volatile agent (halothane, isoflurane, or enflurane), i.v. opioid drugs, or a combination of the two. Opioids may be administered through an extradural catheter to provide intraoperative analgesia, although a volatile agent should be used in conjunction with nitrous oxide in order to prevent awareness.

Although deadspace:tidal volume ratio may diminish when one-lung ventilation starts, the increase in intrapulmonary shunt results in impaired carbon dioxide excretion. The net result is that carbon dioxide elimination remains essentially unchanged if minute ventilation is kept constant on changing to one-lung ventilation.

Apparatus for one-lung anaesthesia

Bronchial blockers

A bronchial blocker is simply a suction catheter with an inflatable balloon at its distal end. It is used to isolate, and to permit aspiration of secretions from, one lung or lobe. After introduction through a bronchoscope, the balloon is inflated, and a tracheal tube inserted to permit ventilation of the unblocked areas of lung. Bronchial blockers are seldom used now, having been superseded by double-lumen tubes, but they have occasional indications, e.g. for control of haemorrhage.

Single-lumen bronchial tubes

Some single-lumen bronchial tubes may be introduced blindly into position, while others are designed to be inserted under direct vision over a bronchoscope. These latter types are useful if bronchial anatomy is distorted. A single-lumen tube is passed into the main bronchus of the non-operated lung. This lung may be isolated by inflation of the balloon at the distal end of the tube, or both lungs may be ventilated, although unequally, by deflation of this balloon, and inflation of the tracheal cuff.

In infants, bronchial intubation may be required occasionally, and can be achieved by the use of a tracheal tube cut 1 cm longer than normal, and of the same diameter or 1 mm smaller than would be used normally for tracheal intubation.

Double-lumen tubes

Double-lumen tubes (Fig. 39.4) are the commonest type of endobronchial apparatus in current use. Their purpose is to provide separate channels for ventilation and suction of both lungs. The lumen on one side is shaped at its distal end to enter and occupy one or other main bronchus, while the second lumen ends in the trachea. In order to permit clamping and transection of the main bronchus during pneumonectomy, a right-sided tube is used for operations on the left lung, although it may occlude the upper lobe bronchus despite the slit in the bronchial cuff (Fig. 39.5), because the location of the right upper lobe bronchus is variable. A left-sided tube is used when surgery of the right lung is planned, or when non-pulmonary surgery is undertaken. Double-lumen tubes may be awkward to introduce through the larynx, and may not enter the desired bronchus if the anatomy is distorted. However, when

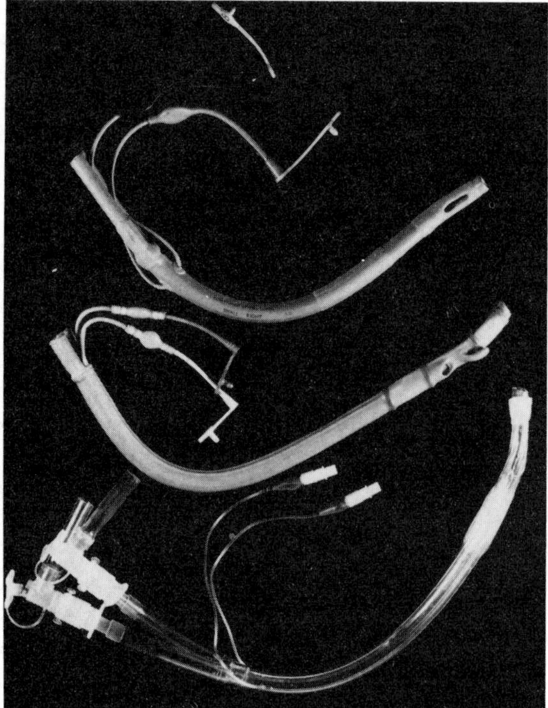

Fig. 39.4 Double-lumen tubes. Top to bottom: right-sided Robertshaw, Carlen (left-sided, with carinal hook), left-sided Bronchocath (disposable, PVC).

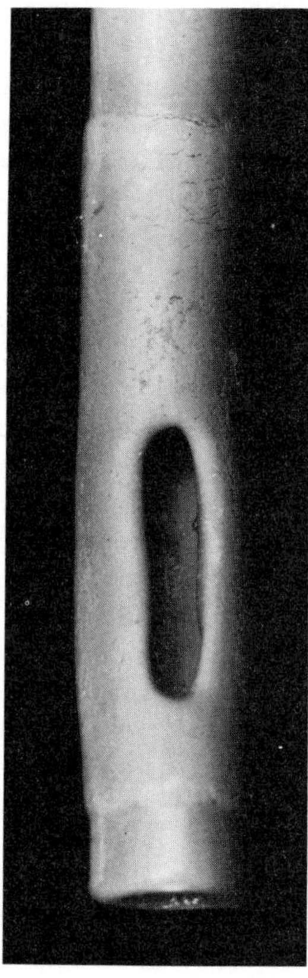

Fig. 39.5 Orifice in bronchial lumen of right-sided Robertshaw double-lumen tube to permit ventilation of right upper lobe.

correctly positioned, they permit access to both lungs, provide even ventilation, and are less likely to be dislodged than a single-lumen tube.

THORACOTOMY

Anaesthetic technique

(Modifications to the technique described here are required in the presence of a bronchopleural fistula, empyema, lung cyst or pneumothorax. These modifications are detailed in the appropriate sections of this chapter.)

Induction of anaesthesia may be achieved using an appropriate i.v. agent. Although some anaesthetists prefer to use suxamethonium if a double-lumen tube is to be introduced, others use a large dose of non-depolarising relaxant (e.g. vecuronium 0.1 mg/kg, alcuronium 0.3 mg/kg), as comparable relaxation ensues in 2–3 min, and thoracotomy is seldom of shorter duration than that of the relaxant.

A large-gauge i.v. cannula is essential for infusion of fluids and blood (which is usually required).

Maintenance of anaesthesia is achieved normally using a combination of nitrous oxide/oxygen, i.v. opioid and volatile anaesthetic. The choice may be influenced by the need for one-lung anaesthesia. The depth of anaesthesia required is comparable to that for abdominal surgery.

Monitoring

Monitoring of ECG, heart rate and arterial pressure is mandatory. Arterial pressure may be measured indirectly with a sphygmomanometer or oscillotonometer, although in the lateral position pressure recordings from the dependent arm may be unreliable because of compression by the thorax. Direct arterial pressure measurement using an intra-arterial cannula is indicated in the poor-risk patient, or if severe haemorrhage or mediastinal retraction are anticipated. This technique also allows sampling for blood gas analysis, and is useful if severe hypoxaemia is expected. Pulse oximetry is valuable, especially during one-lung anaesthesia. Central venous pressure monitoring may be necessary when major surgery, associated with heavy bleeding, is planned. Monitoring of temperature is important in children, or if prolonged surgery is anticipated in adults. In these situations, a warming blanket and blood warmer should be used, and inspired gases require warming and humidification.

Position

Pulmonary surgery is undertaken normally with the patient in the lateral position (Fig. 39.6), with the diseased side uppermost. Care must be taken to avoid nerve damage in the upper arm by avoiding excess traction, and a pillow should be placed between the legs to prevent pressure damage.

Some surgeons prefer the patient to be positioned prone, in the Parry Brown position (Fig. 39.7). The shoulders and pelvis are supported to prevent pressure on the abdomen, which increases intra-abdominal pressure, impairs expansion of the lung bases, and reduces venous return to the heart. The arm on the operated side hangs over the edge of the operating table so that the scapula is pulled away from the site of surgery. This position allows drainage of secretions from the diseased lung towards the trachea without soiling the other lung.

Oesophageal surgery is undertaken usually with the patient in the lateral or semilateral position.

At the end of thoracotomy, the pleural cavity is drained (although not always after pneumonectomy) to ensure that air or fluid does not accumulate in the postoperative period. If the lung has been collapsed, it is reinflated before the

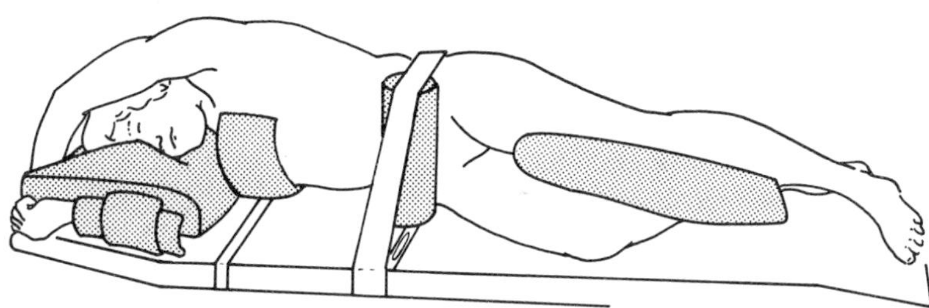

Fig. 39.6 Patient in lateral position for thoracic surgery.

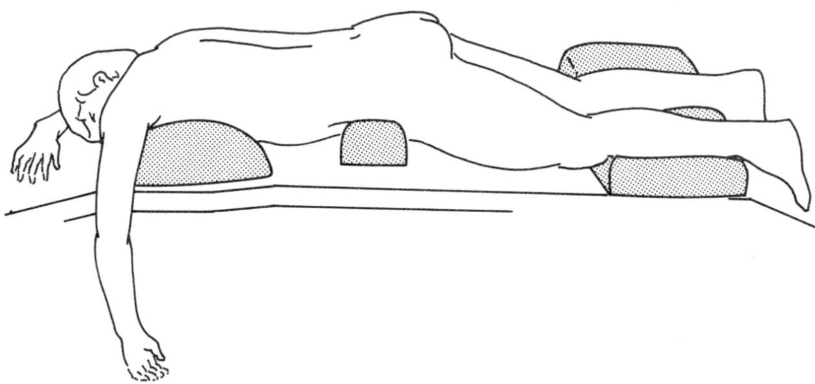

Fig. 39.7 Patient in Parry Brown position for thoracic surgery.

thorax is closed so that re-expansion may be confirmed under direct vision. After closure of the thorax, the drains are connected to an underwater seal, which permits drainage of air or fluid with minimal resistance, and allows measurement of volumes of drained fluid or blood. As IPPV is continued, air is expelled from the pleural space, and the lung expands to fill the cavity.

It is usual to allow patients to breathe spontaneously after thoracotomy, and residual effects of neuromuscular blocking drugs are therefore antagonised. Secretions are aspirated via a suction catheter passed through the tracheal tube. When adequate spontaneous ventilation has returned, and the patient has regained control of reflexes, pharyngeal secretions are aspirated and the tracheal (or double-lumen) tube removed.

Postoperative care

Pulmonary function may be reduced considerably after thoracotomy. The lungs may be affected by chronic disease, a lobe or lung may have been excised, and the remaining lung tissue has been manipulated and retracted, resulting in patchy oedema and contusion, and an increase in pulmonary secretions. Blood or infected material from a resected area may contaminate the remaining lung. Pain from the incision and chest drain sites inhibits chest wall movement, and, together with any accumulation of fluid or air in the pleural cavity, may reduce expansion and encourage atelectasis and collapse.

Although mechanical ventilation in the postoperative period permits expansion of the lungs, aspiration of secretions and adequate analgesia and sedation (without fear of ventilatory depression), there are disadvantages, particularly after pulmonary surgery. Air leaks from the surface of the lung or from the resected bronchial stump may be augmented by IPPV. Continued tracheal intubation may result in increased risk of chest infection. However, elective mechanical ventilation is necessary occasionally in debilitated patients after oesophageal resection, and in patients with severely impaired lung function following pulmonary surgery.

In all patients, adequate oxygenation and ventilation should be ensured. An increased inspired oxygen concentration of 40% (unless the patient is chronically hypercapnic) is advisable to prevent arterial hypoxaemia, together with humidification of the inspired gases to prevent inspissation of secretions, and physiotherapy to aid lung expansion and coughing. Effective analgesia is essential. An opioid analgesic administered intermittently by the i.m. route is easy to prescribe, but provides sporadic analgesia, and may cause depression of ventilation. Patient-controlled i.v. infusions of opioid analgesic drugs provide more continuity of analgesia. Blockade of the intercostal nerves during thoracotomy either with a local anaesthetic agent or using cryoanalgesia reduces the requirements for systemic analgesic drugs. Paravertebral or extradural nerve block with a local anaesthetic agent is extremely effective, while extradural or intrathecal opioids may provide profound analgesia with virtually no cardiovascular complications, although there is a risk of late respiratory depression. Extradural catheter techniques permit administration of repeated doses of drug, but require careful monitoring, and should be contemplated only if the patient is nursed in a high dependency or intensive care area.

SURGERY RELATED TO THE LUNG

Removal of inhaled foreign body

Inhalation of foreign bodies is not uncommon in children. Obstruction of the larynx results in acute obstruction, but smaller objects wedge more distally and may result either in valvular obstruction with emphysema of the affected lobe or segment, or more commonly in total obstruction leading to distal consolidation and collapse. Eighty per cent of foreign bodies lodge in the right lung. There may be considerable reaction and oedema at the site of obstruction, particularly when an irritant object, e.g. a peanut, has been inhaled.

The patient may have a degree of respiratory obstruction, pulmonary infection and hypoxaemia. An inhalational induction is preferable in children, particularly if respiratory obstruction is present, and a selection of tracheal tubes should be available. Removal of the foreign body is performed through a rigid bronchoscope, and may be extremely difficult, particularly if bronchial oedema is present. Laryngeal stridor is not uncommon during recovery, and the patient must be observed closely for at least 12 h.

Lobectomy

The usual indications for lobectomy are:

1. *Bronchial neoplasm.*
2. *Bronchiectasis.* Lobectomy is indicated if haemoptyses occur repeatedly or infection cannot be controlled.
3. *Infection.* Although it is now relatively rare, tuberculosis is the most common infective condition under this heading.

Lobectomy may be a straightforward procedure with few surgical problems, but it may be difficult and result in severe haemorrhage in the presence of invading tumour, chronic infection or pleural adhesions. In many centres, isolation of the affected lung is achieved using a single or double-lumen bronchial tube in the healthy lung. This permits aspiration of secretions, deflation of the affected lung when required, and reflation of the remaining lobes before closure of the chest. When the lobe has been removed, the bronchus is clamped and divided, and the remnant either sutured or stapled. The pleural cavity may be filled with saline, and inflation of the affected lung to a pressure of 3–4 kPa (30–40 cmH_2O) is undertaken to ensure that no significant air leak exists. Depending on the experience and requirements of the surgeon, bronchial division and closure may not require cessation of ventilation of the affected lung for any significant period of time, and a standard tracheal tube may be satisfactory unless there is a need to protect the healthy lung from secretions, or sleeve resection of the main bronchus is anticipated because of tumour close to the origin of the lobar bronchus.

Pneumonectomy

Bronchial carcinoma not confined to a single lobe is the normal indication for this operation. Pneumonectomy may be performed either in the prone or lateral position. Bronchial intubation is usually selected if the lateral position is used. Mediastinal manipulation may result in arrhythmias, and haemorrhage may be considerable. The main bronchus is divided and sutured, and tested for air leaks as described above.

After pneumonectomy, the pleural space fills with serosanguinous fluid, and this is allowed to accumulate. Thus, the pleural cavity is not always drained. If a drain is inserted at operation, it is connected to an underwater seal, and left open to drain air and fluid while the patient is returned to the supine position. After a chest X-ray has confirmed that the mediastinum is central, the drain is clamped, but the clamps are removed for a short period every hour during the 24 h following surgery to ensure that neither air nor excess fluid is accumulating.

If the pleural space is not drained, the following procedure is undertaken when the patient has been returned to the supine position at the end of surgery; a needle is inserted through the chest wall, connected to a three-way stopcock and manometer, and air removed or injected until the intrapleural pressure is normal, indicating that the mediastinum is central. The risks of leaving the cavity undrained are that air may accumulate under pressure if the bronchial stump leaks, and that massive haemorrhage may go unrecognised. Drainage may, however, increase the risk of infection.

Normally, the empty pleural space fills gradually with serosanguinous fluid, and fibrosis occurs subsequently, pulling the diaphragm into the thorax and the mediastinum across to the operated side. If fluid accumulates too rapidly, mediastinal distortion and compression of the remaining lung result in a combination of hypotension, right ventricular failure and hypoxaemia. Central venous pressure is often high because of mediastinal distortion, although the patient is usually hypovolaemic because of fluid loss. Mediastinal displacement causing cardiorespiratory distress may occur also if the space fills too slowly with fluid as air is absorbed.

Sputum retention and respiratory failure are not uncommon after pneumonectomy; mortality is increased significantly if mechanical ventilation is required. Arrhythmias and pericarditis are also frequent complications, probably because of mediastinal manipulation. The incidence of supraventricular arrhythmias is reduced if the patient is digitalised during the perioperative period.

Other complications of major surgery, e.g. myocardial infarction and renal failure, may occur. The mortality after left pneumonectomy is 7–10%, and may be as high as 20% after excision of the larger right lung.

Bronchopleural fistula

A connection between the tracheobronchial tree and the pleural cavity may result from trauma, neoplasm, rupture of an intrapulmonary cavity (e.g. abscess), or from breakdown of a bronchial stump or anastomosis after surgery. Bronchopleural fistulae are almost always complicated by the collection of infected fluid in the pleural cavity. This results in a number of problems of importance to the anaesthetist. The patient may be cachectic and dehydrated, and pulmonary function may be impaired considerably. Careful preoperative assessment is essential, although surgical intervention may be urgent. In addition to factors related to the general condition of the patient, two specific dangers exist:

1. The remaining healthy lung is at risk of contamination by the infected contents of the pleural space.
2. Positive pressure applied to the affected bronchial tree may result either in passage of the inspired gas out through the chest drain resulting in little or no effective alveolar ventilation, or, if the drain is only partially patent, in an increase in intrapleural pressure with the danger that infected material may be squeezed into the tracheobronchial tree with consequent pulmonary contamination.

Only anticholinergic premedication is prescribed. The patient is placed in a semisitting, semilateral position with the affected side dependent. Bronchial intubation is essential if possible. The optimum method of induction of anaesthesia is controversial. Some anaesthetists feel that an inhalational induction is the safest technique, as spontaneous ventilation is maintained until the bronchial or double-lumen tube is in position and the damaged lung isolated. However, deep anaesthesia is required, and this may have cardiovascular complications in the semirecumbent position. In addition, prolonged attempts at intubation may result in coughing, which increases intrapleural pressure and may spread infected material through the lungs. Consequently, many anaesthetists who are practised at bronchial intubation prefer to preoxygenate the lungs, induce anaesthesia with an i.v. agent, and produce muscle paralysis with suxamethonium. Intubation is carried out when spontaneous ventilation has ceased.

When the tube is in position, the healthy lung is ventilated, and infected material from the affected bronchial tree aspirated. A non-depolarising muscle relaxant is administered, and one-lung anaesthesia maintained as described above. After surgery, attempts are made to restore spontaneous ventilation, although this may be precluded by the patient's condition.

Drainage of empyema

An empyema is a collection of purulent material in the pleural cavity. It is associated usually with an infective process in the lung, although it may occur also after oesophageal perforation or as a complication of thoracotomy. Initial treatment is with appropriate antibiotics and drainage through an intercostal drain. This is inserted under local anaesthesia. Drainage may be incomplete, however, and a chronic empyema may develop with fibrosis of the surrounding pleura. Resection of one or more ribs may be required in order to obtain satisfactory drainage. An empyema is often accompanied by a bronchopleural fistula, and this determines anaesthetic management (vide supra).

Lung cysts and bullae

These are thin-walled, air-filled cavities within the lung which may be congenital, the consequence of previous infection, or the result of emphysema. Their connection with the bronchial tree may be valvular. Large cysts may present problems during unrelated surgery. IPPV may result in rupture of a thin-walled cyst. Enlargement of the cyst may occur if a valvular connection is present. Nitrous oxide may also enlarge a cyst because nitrogen is less soluble in blood.

Rupture of a cyst results very rapidly in respiratory distress. Gross enlargement of a cyst may produce a similar effect. The two may be indistinguishable clinically, and a chest drain should be inserted if respiratory distress occurs. A persistent air leak is likely to develop if an enlarged cyst is drained, and may also follow rupture of a cyst.

During anaesthesia for resection of a lung cyst, attention must be given to prevention of rupture of the cyst, in addition to the problems associated with thoracotomy. Bronchial blocking or intubation permit selective ventilation of the normal lung, although tracheal intubation and gentle positive pressure ventilation is regarded by some anaesthetists as a satisfactory technique.

Lung abscess

The majority of lung abscesses are amenable to treatment with antibiotics, and usually rupture into a bronchus from which the contents are expectorated, or into the pleura resulting in an empyema and bronchopleural fistula. Surgery for an abscess may result in its rupture during anaesthesia. A double-lumen tube should be used to ensure that contamination of the unaffected lung does not take place, and so that infected material can be aspirated.

Pleurectomy and pleurodesis

Pleurectomy is performed through an anterolateral thoracotomy. Pleurodesis is achieved by the introduction of iodised talc through a thoracoscope, or by abrasion of the pleura with a gauze swab through a small thoracotomy incision. The usual indication for these procedures is repeated spontaneous pneumothorax.

The patient presenting for pleurectomy may have a pneumothorax, and may have underlying pulmonary disease. If the pleural cavity is not drained, the pneumothorax may be increased in size by nitrous oxide, or by IPPV if an air leak is present or a lung cyst ruptured. However, the time period between induction of anaesthesia and exposure of the pleural cavity is short. It is seldom necessary to avoid the use of nitrous oxide, and gentle IPPV may be used until the chest wall is open. A double-lumen tube is not necessary unless a large air leak is present. Haemorrhage may be considerable, and postoperative pain is severe.

NON-PULMONARY SURGERY

Diaphragmatic hernia

Anaesthesia for repair of a congenital diaphragmatic hernia in the neonate is discussed in Chapter 34. A congenital hernia may present in adults, but the condition is associated more commonly in adult life with trauma. It may be possible to repair the hernia from the abdomen, but thoracotomy is often necessary. The lung may be compressed by distended bowel, and pulmonary function impaired as a result. Electrolyte abnormalities may be present because of intestinal obstruction. If the stomach has herniated into the thorax, the risk of reflux of gastric contents is increased.

Repair of hiatus hernia

A hiatus hernia may require repair using a thoracic approach through a left thoracotomy. The patient may be obese. It should be assumed that regurgitation of gastric contents may occur because of incompetence of the lower oesophageal sphincter. Antacids should be continued preoperatively, and H_2-antagonists may be given with premedication to increase pH of the gastric contents. Preoxygenation of the lungs should be carried out before induction of anaesthesia, and cricoid pressure applied until the airway is secure. A tracheal tube is usually adequate, and is easier and faster to position than a double-lumen tube. However, in some centres, a left-sided double-lumen tube is used and the left lung deflated to permit better surgical access. One-lung anaesthesia in the patient with normal lungs may result in severe hypoxaemia (vide supra).

Oesophageal myotomy

Oesophageal myotomy (Heller's operation) is indicated in the presence of achalasia. This disorder of oesophageal motility results in gross dilatation of the oesophagus and the collection in it of large volumes of undigested food. The patient may have pulmonary disease as a result of repeated aspiration of oesophageal contents. The principal risk during anaesthesia is that of aspiration, and the anaesthetic management is similar to that described for repair of hiatus hernia.

Surgery for carcinoma of oesophagus

Inoperable carcinoma of oesophagus causes progressive obstruction, resulting eventually in complete dysphagia. Insertion of an oesophageal tube (e.g. Celestin) may provide some palliation. Bypass of the tumour may be accomplished by mobilisation of the stomach through a laparotomy and, after passing the stomach behind the sternum, anastomosis to the upper oesophagus in the neck.

Tumours of the middle and lower thirds of the oesophagus may be resectable. This is a major procedure, undertaken in a patient who may be cachectic, hypoproteinaemic and anaemic. In addition, pulmonary function may be impaired by repeated aspiration of oesophageal contents. Preoperative nutrition, either enteral or parenteral, may be advisable in the cachectic patient. Premedication should be appropriate for the nutritional state of the patient.

Carcinoma of the lower third of the oesophagus is resected through a left thoracoabdominal incision. If the lesion is in the middle third, the operation may be performed in two stages; initially, abdominal organs are mobilised through a laparotomy, and the patient is turned into the left lateral position in order that the resection can be completed, and the anastomosis performed, through a right thoracotomy. Irrespective of the surgical approach, a left-sided double-lumen tube is used and the lung on the side of the thoracotomy collapsed intermittently to allow surgical access to the oesophagus. Haemorrhage may be considerable, and cardiovascular problems may result from retraction of the vena cava or heart. An indwelling arterial cannula and central venous catheter are required. The procedure is often of prolonged duration, and precautions should be taken to prevent hypothermia.

FURTHER READING

Gothard J W W (ed) 1987 Thoracic anaesthesia. Clinical anaesthesiology: international practice and research. Baillière-Tindall, London

Gothard J W W, Branthwaite M A 1982 Anaesthesia for thoracic surgery. Blackwell Scientific Publications, Oxford

Kaplan J A (ed) 1983 Thoracic anesthesia. Churchill Livingstone, New York

Marshall B E, Longnecker D E, Fairley H B (eds) 1988 Anesthesia for thoracic procedures. Blackwell Scientific Publications, Boston

40. Anaesthesia for cardiac surgery

The cardiac surgical theatre, with its profusion of personnel, monitors and support equipment, is often intimidating to the trainee anaesthetist. However, the principles of anaesthetic care are similar to those pertaining elsewhere, the differences lying in the specific operations undertaken and the fact that essential organ perfusion is achieved artificially when the heart itself is the object of surgery. Operations are termed 'open heart' when the function of the heart and the lungs are assumed by an extracorporeal pump and gas exchange unit (cardiopulmonary bypass, or CPB). During 'closed' operations, cardiac and pulmonary functions remain intact, and anaesthetic management is similar to that for thoracic surgery (Ch. 39).

Excluding the insertion of pacemakers, more than 20 000 cardiac operations are undertaken each year in the UK in NHS hospitals. These include approximately 3000 for congenital abnormalities, 5000 for acquired valvular disease, 12 000 for ischaemic heart disease plus a miscellany of aortic and pericardial surgery, and a number of heart or heart and lung transplants.

Congenital cardiac abnormalities

These occur at a rate of 6–8 per 1000 live births. Correction of almost a third of these lesions, including patent ductus arteriosus or coarctation, may be undertaken by 'closed' operation but the remainder, including atrial and ventricular septal defects, valve abnormalities and cyanotic lesions such as Fallot's tetralogy, require CPB.

Acquired valvular disease

This type of cardiac lesion has become less common as a result of the reduced incidence of rheumatic fever. Stenosis or incompetence still occur and most commonly involve the mitral and aortic valves. Although closed valvotomy is possible, surgery usually comprises replacement with an artificial valve. This may be a mechanical prosthesis with a ball or tilting disc, or a tissue valve (usually a pig valve) specially mounted and prepared (heterograft). Less commonly, a human valve (homograft) is used. Prosthetic valves are reliable but necessitate the patient receiving anticoagulants for life. This is not usually necessary when porcine heterografts are used and, although there are some doubts about their durability, these valves are becoming more popular.

Ischaemic heart disease

The concept of revascularising ischaemic myocardium was introduced approximately 20 years ago with the insertion of a portion of saphenous vein from aorta to coronary artery distal to a stenosis (Fig. 40.1). Since then, coronary artery bypass grafting has become the most commonly performed cardiac operation. However, there is some controversy regarding the indications for this operation. Although angina is relieved in 80–90% of patients, life expectancy may not be increased in all groups when compared with medical treatment. Only in left main and triple vessel disease has life expectancy been shown clearly to have been prolonged as a result of surgery.

EXTRACORPOREAL CIRCULATION (ECC)

The essential components of ECC comprise:

1. Pumps.
2. An oxygenator.
3. Connecting tubes and filters.
4. Fluid prime of these components.

These are arranged normally as shown in Figure 40.2. Blood from the venous side of the circulation, usually from the venae cavae, is drained by gravity to a venous reservoir and thence to a gas exchange unit (oxygenator), where oxygen is delivered to, and carbon dioxide removed from, the blood. This 'arterialised' blood is pumped into

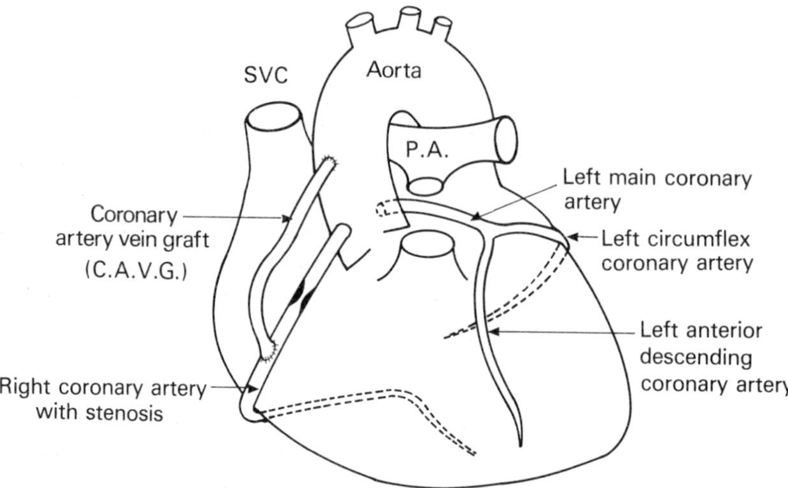

Fig. 40.1 Diagrammatic representation of coronary arteries and CAVG. 'Triple' vessel disease includes right, left circumflex and left anterior descending arteries.

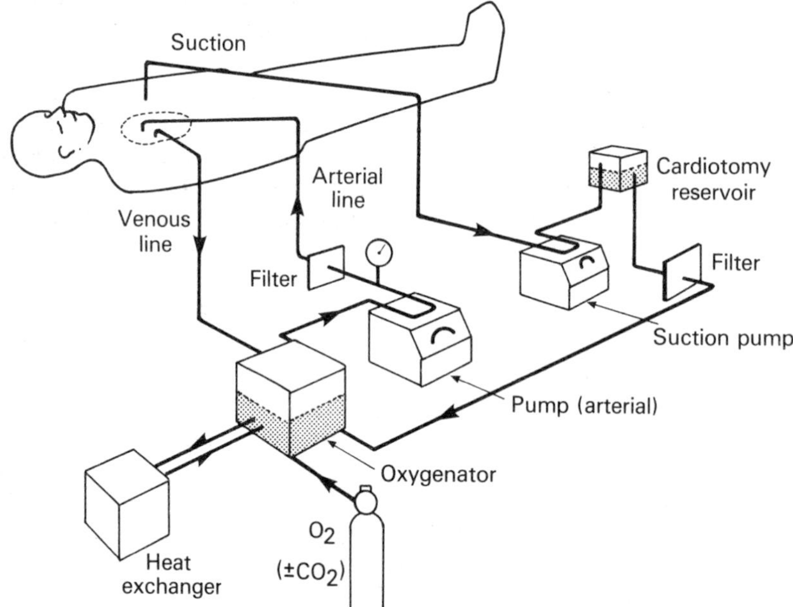

Fig. 40.2 Components of extracorporeal circuit.

the arterial side of the circulation, usually into the ascending aorta. The heart and lungs are thus 'bypassed' or isolated and their function maintained temporarily by mechanical equipment remote from the body. Most systems include a heat exchanger in the oxygenator to vary the temperature of blood rapidly, and suction to drain redundant or spilled blood in or around the bypassed heart and return it to the venous reservoir for oxygenation and thence to the circulation.

Pumps (Fig. 40.3)

The majority of pumps are of the roller variety, which displace blood around the circuit by intermittent compression of the circuit tubing during each sweep.

Traditionally, these pumps have produced a 'continuous' or steady arterial wave form, but by intermittent acceleration of the roller head, a 'pulsatile' wave form may be achieved which mimics normal physiological blood flow and is claimed to reduce postoperative organ dysfunction.

Oxygenator

There are two types of oxygenator:

1. *Direct contact oxygenators*

Disc oxygenators consist of rotating discs which dip into blood; the film of blood on the disc is rotated through a flow of oxygen. These have been superseded by the 'bubble' oxygenator in which oxygen is bubbled through venous blood (Fig. 40.3). Bubble oxygenators are the most commonly used devices at present. They are produced relatively cheaply, are disposable and are of small internal volume. They usually include a venous reservoir and an integral heat exchanger. However, 'bubbling' results in damage to red cells and platelets, and consumption of coagulation factors. Their use is limited to a few hours as the extent of damage is time-dependent.

2. *Membrane oxygenators*

These comprise a semipermeable membrane which separates gas and blood phases, and through which gas exchange occurs. In comparison with bubble oxygenators, damage to blood components is reduced. Membrane oxygenators have been used in certain circumstances to support the circulation for several days.

Connecting tubes, filters, manometer, suction

These must be sterile and non-toxic, and should damage blood as little as possible during passage through the circuit.

A defoaming unit is included in bubble oxygenators but, in addition, a unit should be incorporated in the arterial line to remove gas emboli which would pass directly to the aorta. Suction pumps are supplied to vent blood collecting in the pulmonary circulation or left ventricle during bypass, and also to remove spilled blood from the pericardial sac. The blood is collected in the 'cardiotomy' reservoir, filtered and returned to the main circuit. This suction also causes damage to blood components.

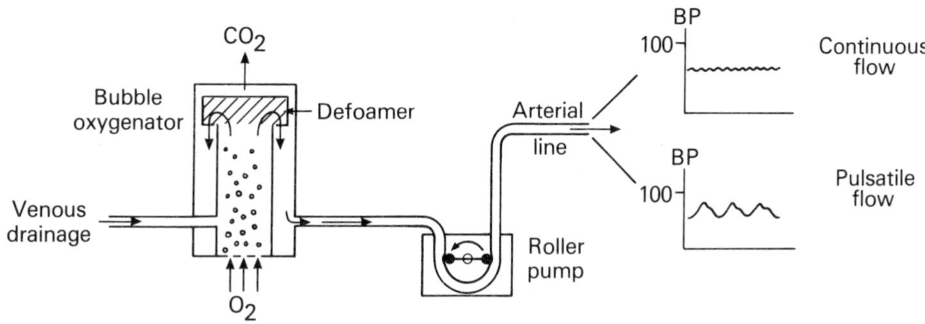

Fig. 40.3 Diagrammatic representation of oxygenator and arterial pump.

Fluid prime

Originally it was anticipated that connection of the circulation to an external circuit would necessitate the extracorporeal circuit being filled with anticoagulated whole blood. However, this is expensive and may lead to incompatibility reactions. In addition, it became clear that the use of whole blood to fill the external circuit was unnecessary, as the body tolerates a relatively low haematocrit. When CPB is commenced and the patient's blood mixes with an ECC comprising clear fluid (fluid prime), the haematocrit decreases to approximately 20–25%. Although oxygen content is reduced, availability may be increased by improved organ blood flow resulting from reduced blood viscosity. In certain patients (low body weight, children, or those with a low preoperative haemoglobin in whom dilution would reduce the haematocrit to below 20%), blood may be added to the prime. In the normal adult, 'clear' primes are used almost exclusively and comprise crystalloid solutions, e.g. glucose or Ringer lactate. Most cardiac surgical units have individual recipes for addition to the prime, e.g. plasma, dextran, mannitol, sodium bicarbonate and potassium, to achieve an isosmolar solution of physiological pH.

PREOPERATIVE ASSESSMENT

The majority of patients presenting for cardiac surgery have undergone comprehensive cardiological investigation and are usually receiving medications. In addition to the routine investigations undertaken before any operation, certain specialised techniques are employed to assess the cardiac lesion and degree of resultant dysfunction. The results of these investigations permit the anaesthetist to identify patients at particular risk in whom extra care and monitoring are required.

Exercise electrocardiography

Various stress protocols are employed whereby a standard exercise test is used to provoke ischaemic changes and symptoms. Changes in rhythm, rate, arterial pressure and conduction are recorded. The anaesthetist may identify the most useful ECG leads to monitor during surgery and notes the rate–pressure product (heart rate × systolic arterial pressure) at which evidence of ischaemia occurs.

Cardiac catheterisation

Considerable information may be obtained from catheterisation:

1. Evidence of failing function or of gradients across stenosed valves may be identified by pressure monitoring.
2. Oximetry of blood at different sites indicates if shunts are present (Fig. 40.4).
3. Cardiac output may be measured.
4. The injection of radio-opaque dye into aorta or ventricles assesses incompetence of valves and the efficiency of ventricular contraction (ejection fraction) and wall motion.

The ejection fraction (EF) =

$$\frac{\text{end-diastolic volume} - \text{end-systolic volume}}{\text{end-diastolic volume}}$$

5. Injection of dye into coronary arteries defines the anatomy of the coronary circulation and the degree of patency or sites of stenosis.

Echocardiography

Ultrasound is used to identify myocardial motion and valvular function. Although ventricular function may be assessed and EF estimated, this

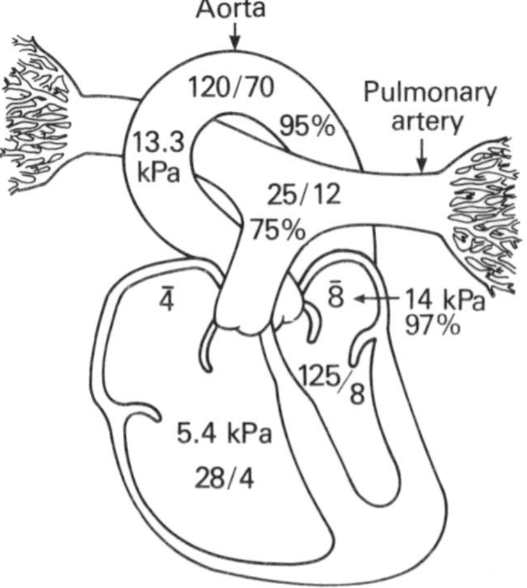

Fig. 40.4 Diagram of catheterisation values in normal adult: pressures (mmHg), oxygen saturations (%) and tensions (kPa).

technique is most useful in identifying the degree of valvular abnormality.

Radionuclide imaging

By imaging the activity of an appropriate radioisotope as it passes through the heart or into the myocardium, ventricular function and myocardial perfusion may be assessed. Technetium images blood volume and may be used to demonstrate abnormal wall motion and EF. Thallium, which is taken up by the myocardium, may be used to assess regional blood flow. These techniques may be employed before and after exercise and/or therapy.

Preoperative drug therapy

Digitalis. Most centres discontinue digoxin-24–48 h before surgery to diminish digoxin-associated arrhythmias after surgery.

β-Blocking agents. Continued administration of these drugs up to the time of surgery is desirable unless evidence of overdosage is present. Discontinuation may increase the risk of perioperative infarction.

Calcium antagonists. These drugs have a negative inotropic effect but, as with the β-blockers, it is preferable to continue therapy throughout the preoperative period.

Nitrates should be continued, and may be included in the premedication if indicated.

Diuretics should be continued until the day before surgery.

Anticoagulants are usually stopped several days before surgery to permit coagulation to return towards normal. If a high risk of embolism is present, anticoagulants should be continued and coagulation defects treated postoperatively.

Other investigations before surgery

Haemoglobin. Should be adequate (>11 g/dl) to prevent excessive haemodilution on bypass.

Coagulation. Prothrombin time should be measured before surgery. Specific defects require correction before surgery or alternatively the appropriate blood products should be made available.

Electrolytes. In particular, serum K^+ should be within normal limits.

Urea and creatinine. Raised concentrations indicate an increased risk of renal failure postoperatively. Adequate urine output should be ensured during and after operation.

Liver function tests. Abnormal values may indicate evidence of congestive cardiac failure.

Pulmonary function tests. In patients complaining of dyspnoea, spirometry should be undertaken to measure vital capacity and forced expiratory volume. If $FEV_{1.0}/FVC$ is less than 60%, more extensive tests are indicated including assessment of the effect of bronchodilators and arterial blood gas analysis.

ASSESSMENT OF RISK

The mortality rate associated with cardiac surgery is diminishing but is still significant. Many units have reduced the mortality rate to 1–2% for uncomplicated coronary vein grafts but valve surgery is usually associated with a mortality of 4–5%. When more extensive surgery is undertaken, e.g. multiple valve replacement or coronary artery vein graft (CAVG) plus valve replacement, mortality rate increases.

Patients with an increased risk of perioperative complications may be identified during preoperative assessment. Patients who are classified as the New York Heart Association's functional class III or IV, in which symptoms occur with minimal activity or at rest, may be expected to experience problems. Increased risk is associated with the following factors:

1. Age > 65 years.
2. Unstable angina or infarction within 6 months prior to surgery.
3. Emergency surgery or reoperation.
4. Poor left ventricular function as shown by:

(a) LVEDP > 18 mmHg
(b) ejection fraction < 30%
(c) cardiac index < 2 litre min^{-1} m^{-2}
(d) dyskinetic wall motion.

5. Raised pulmonary artery pressures (mean PAP > 25 mmHg especially after exercise).
6. Evidence of right ventricular failure.
7. Other system disease, e.g. diabetes.

MONITORING

Extensive and accurate monitoring is essential throughout the perioperative period for the safe practice of cardiac surgery.

ECG

ECG should be monitored throughout the perioperative period. The ideal system is one which allows simultaneous multiple lead monitoring or at least switching between lead II and V_5 for accurate identification of ischaemia. Rate and rhythm should also be observed.

Systemic arterial pressure

Arterial cannulation is mandatory, and permits not only direct measurement but also sampling of arterial blood for biochemical analysis. The preferred site is a radial artery.

Central venous and left atrial pressures

Right-sided filling pressure should be monitored by a cannula placed into the superior vena cava.

Controversy exists regarding the necessity to monitor left heart filling pressure in all patients. If time permits, a direct left atrial line can be inserted at surgery as an aid to terminating bypass and improving postoperative care but it is often desirable to insert a flow-directed pulmonary artery catheter at or before induction to measure pulmonary capillary wedge pressure (PCWP). In the USA there is enthusiasm for commencing full invasive monitoring before anaesthesia but most anaesthetists in the UK undertake this only in poor-risk patients.

Cardiac output (CO)

CO may be measured by thermal or dye dilution, most conveniently in association with measurement of PCWP and PAP using a pulmonary artery catheter. Calculation of cardiac output and cardiac index together with the derivatives of stroke work, pulmonary and systemic vascular resistances and tissue oxygen flux, permits the most accurate assessment of cardiological therapy.

EEG

A simple guide to cerebral activity and perfusion may be obtained from the cerebral function monitor although interpretation is difficult in the hypothermic patient.

Temperature

Core temperature should be monitored from the nasopharynx. It is helpful also to monitor the peripheral temperature from the first toe to assess core–peripheral temperature gradients and peripheral perfusion.

Biochemical analysis

Facilities should be available for immediate analysis of blood gases, acid-base balance, serum potassium and blood glucose concentrations.

Haematological analysis

Measurement of packed cell volume and coagulation status should be available. Activated clotting time (ACT) can be measured quickly in the operating theatre using the Haemochron apparatus (normal = 100–120 s) but access to the haematology laboratory should be rapid for assessment of a full clotting screen. It is also salutary to measure free haemoglobin on occasion as an indicator of erythrocyte damage during extracorporeal circulation.

Display

ECG, pressure waveforms, and a digital output of heart rate and pressures should be displayed clearly on a screen visible to both surgeon and anaesthetist. The facility to produce a hard copy of ECG and pressures is necessary for records and accurate diagnosis.

PATHOPHYSIOLOGICAL CONSIDERATIONS

The anaesthetist should have a clear understanding of the fundamental principles of cardiac physiology. Accurate monitoring reveals alterations in cardiac function and permits the anaesthetist to manipulate those factors which ensure adequate pump output (Fig. 40.5) and myocardial blood supply.

Preload and contractility determine the amount of work that the heart can perform. In the failing heart the afterload determines how much work is expended in overcoming pressure compared with that used to provide forward flow. Thus, cardiac output may be increased either by increasing preload or contractility, or by reducing afterload. However, oxygen consumption is raised by increasing heart rate, contractility, preload and afterload.

Augmentation of cardiac output by increasing preload or contractility may thus have a detrimental effect on oxygen balance. Reduction of afterload, however, may increase cardiac output while simultaneously reducing oxygen demand.

Adequate coronary perfusion demands maintenance of diastolic aortic pressure at an adequate level. Oxygen supply to the myocardium occurs predominantly in diastole and is dependent on the gradient between diastolic aortic pressure and intraventricular pressure, and on diastolic time. The portion of myocardium most at risk of developing ischaemia is the left ventricular endocardium. The endocardial viability ratio (EVR) (Fig. 40.6)

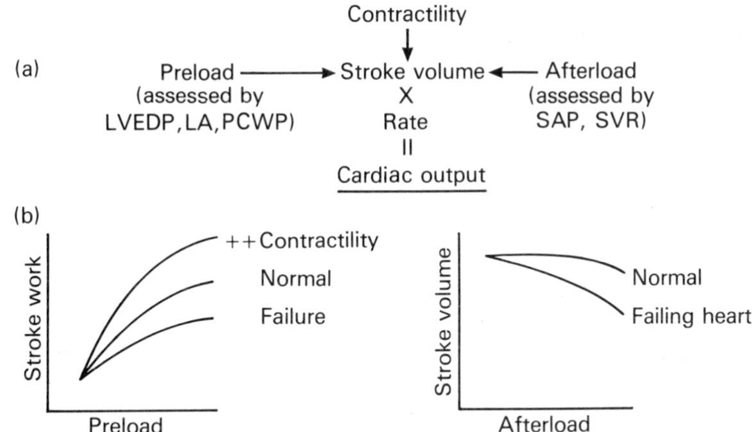

Fig. 40.5 Important aspects of mechanical function.

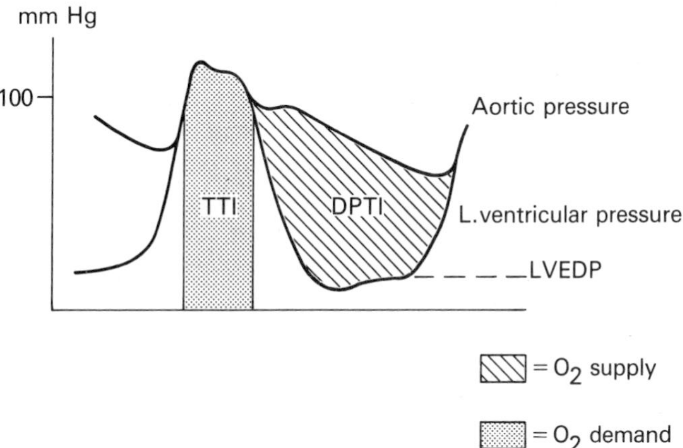

Fig. 40.6 Endocardial viability ratio (EVR) $= \frac{\text{diastolic pressure time index (DPTI)}}{\text{tension time index (TTI)}}$

is a useful index of oxygen balance. Normally, the EVR exceeds 1, but if the ratio decreases below 0.7, ischaemia is likely to develop.

The rate–pressure product (RPP) (heart rate × systolic arterial pressure) is a useful clinical measurement of oxygen demand. This simple index may predict the point at which ischaemia occurs in the conscious exercising patient. During anaesthesia, RPP should be maintained below the conscious ischaemic value.

Care of the patient suffering from ischaemic heart disease therefore necessitates attempts to reduce oxygen demand and maintain oxygen supply. In general, patients with valvular stenosis require adequate preload and do not tolerate rapid reduction in peripheral resistance. Aortic stenosis presents a high afterload to the left ventricle and also renders coronary perfusion particularly sensitive to systemic hypotension. Incompetent valves tend to perform better if afterload is maintained at a low level. Abnormal heart rates are not tolerated well by a heart with any valvular lesion.

ANAESTHETIC TECHNIQUE

There is no single preferred anaesthetic technique for cardiac surgery. The choice of particular agents is less important than the care with which the drug is administered and its effects monitored.

Premedication

As far as the patient is concerned, the most important preoperative preparation is a full explanation of what is about to occur and the development of rapport with, and confidence in, the nursing and medical staff.

Most patients (particularly those with poor cardiovascular reserve) may be sedated preoperatively with an oral benzodiazepine (lorazepam 2–4 mg, temazepam 20–30 mg). Opioid premedication may diminish cardiovascular and respiratory reserves.

In the particularly anxious patient, heavy sedation may be required to prevent increases in heart rate and arterial pressure before operation. Tranquillisers, e.g. diazepam, may be prescribed on a regular basis several days before operation and premedication undertaken with papaveretum (10–20 mg) and hyoscine (0.2–0.4 mg) i.m. 1–2 h before transfer to theatre.

Atropine should be avoided in cardiac patients because of its potent chronotropic effect. Patients receiving glyceryl trinitrate (GTN) may benefit from its administration as a skin paste or patch at the time of premedication.

Induction

All drugs and equipment should be prepared and ready and the theatre and bypass circuit available for immediate use before the arrival of the patient in the anaesthetic room. Two anaesthetists should be available at induction.

Before induction, ECG electrodes should be applied and the ECG displayed, arterial pressure recorded and large-gauge venous cannulae inserted under local anaesthesia. The lungs should be preoxygenated.

Induction may be undertaken with any standard agent in a small dose (e.g. thiopentone 1–3 mg/kg), or with large doses of opioids (e.g. morphine 1–4 mg/kg, fentanyl 10–50 μg/kg) in combination with benzodiazepines to obtain unconsciousness. Exponents of the latter technique claim greater cardiovascular stability especially if nitrous oxide is avoided, and this may be valuable in the poor-risk patient. A combination of these techniques may be used; consciousness is obtunded by an opioid in moderate dose and hypnosis produced by a small dose of an induction agent.

As consciousness is lost, a muscle relaxant is administered and ventilation supported when necessary. Atracurium or vecuronium may be associated with bradycardia, especially in the β-blocked patient. Pancuronium is preferred. The objective is to undertake tracheal intubation without cardiovascular stimulation and thus adequate analgesia/anaesthesia is required. It is customary to spray the cords and trachea with local anaesthetic solution. A low-pressure high-volume cuffed tracheal tube should be used. Positive pressure ventilation is continued usually with 50% nitrous oxide in oxygen.

Percutaneous cannulation of the radial artery and internal jugular veins is performed. A multi-lumen catheter or two central lines should be used for monitoring and infusion. Nasopharyngeal and peripheral temperature probes are applied and a urinary catheter inserted. Mechanical ventilation is continued with a breathing system which contains a humidifier.

Previously identified 'poor-risk' patients may require more extensive monitoring of pressures and cardiac output before induction, and these are established under local anaesthesia. Induction should be undertaken in theatre with the full team ready for immediate surgery. Adequate sedation must be provided during insertion of invasive monitoring lines.

Maintenance — prebypass

During this period, surgical procedure involves preparation of the patient, skin incision, sternotomy, and insertion of arterial and venous bypass cannulae. Anaesthetic management is designed to maintain stability of heart rate and arterial pressure, particularly at moments of profound stimulation, notably skin incision and sternotomy. Additional i.v. analgesic drug or inhalational anaesthetic should be given before stimulation. Large doses of morphine, alfentanil or fentanyl are required to obtund the effects of surgical stimulation. The use of volatile anaesthetic agents, (halothane, isoflurane or enflurane) is effective, although their negative inotropic actions may be undesirable and arrhythmias precipitated, particularly in those with poor ventricular function. In addition, isoflurane is suspected of causing diversion or 'steal' of blood from ischaemic areas of myocardium and its avoidance has been recommended in patients undergoing revascularisation. However, this is a controversial area.

The alternative to deepening anaesthesia/analgesia is to counteract hypertension with vasodilators (phentolamine 1–2 mg, or infusion of sodium nitroprusside 1–5 $\mu g\ kg^{-1}\ min^{-1}$ or glyceryl trinitrate 0.5–5 $\mu g\ kg^{-1}\ min^{-1}$ and to treat tachycardia with β-blockers (e.g. oxprenolol 0.25–1 mg).

Whatever method is employed the rate–pressure product should not be allowed to exceed approximately 12 000 or the critical ischaemic level determined previously during preoperative assessment.

Arterial blood gases, serum K^+ concentration and haematocrit should be measured when surgery is under way and conditions are stable. If possible, the activated clotting time (ACT) should be estimated. Before cannulation for bypass lines, heparin (3–4 mg/kg) should be injected into a secure central line of proven patency. In some units, the surgeon injects heparin directly into the left atrium before cannulation. ACT measurement should be repeated shortly after injection of heparin; the value should exceed 4 times normal. Cardioplegia should be prepared, and stored at 4°C.

When preparations are complete, the bypass pump is started and circulation is assumed by the extracorporeal circuit.

Maintenance — on bypass

Two factors complicate the provision of anaesthesia during cardiopulmonary bypass. Firstly, the dilutional effect of the crystalloid prime reduces the concentration of drugs administered previously, and secondly, by short-circuiting the lungs, bypass prevents the continuation of inhalational anaesthesia. Therefore, anaesthesia is maintained usually by the administration of bolus doses of an opioid. Additional adjuvants include benzodiazepines, a continuous i.v. infusion of a short-acting anaesthetic agent or more rarely the administration of a volatile agent into the gas flow of the oxygenator. Additional doses of muscle relaxant are required also. When full pump oxygenator flow is reached and ventricular ejection ceases, ventilation is suspended and the lungs maintained in inflation with a slight positive pressure (5 cmH_2O). If possible, air should be employed for this manoeuvre as nitrogen helps to prevent atelectasis.

Surgery is preceded usually by cross-clamping the aorta to isolate the heart and prevent backflow. In the case of valvular surgery, the appropriate valve is exposed, excised and a new valve sutured in place. During coronary artery vein grafting, the distal anastomoses are usually completed first and, following release of the cross-clamp to permit restoration of myocardial perfusion, the proximal anastomoses are constructed using a portion of the aorta isolated by a side-clamp (Fig. 40.7).

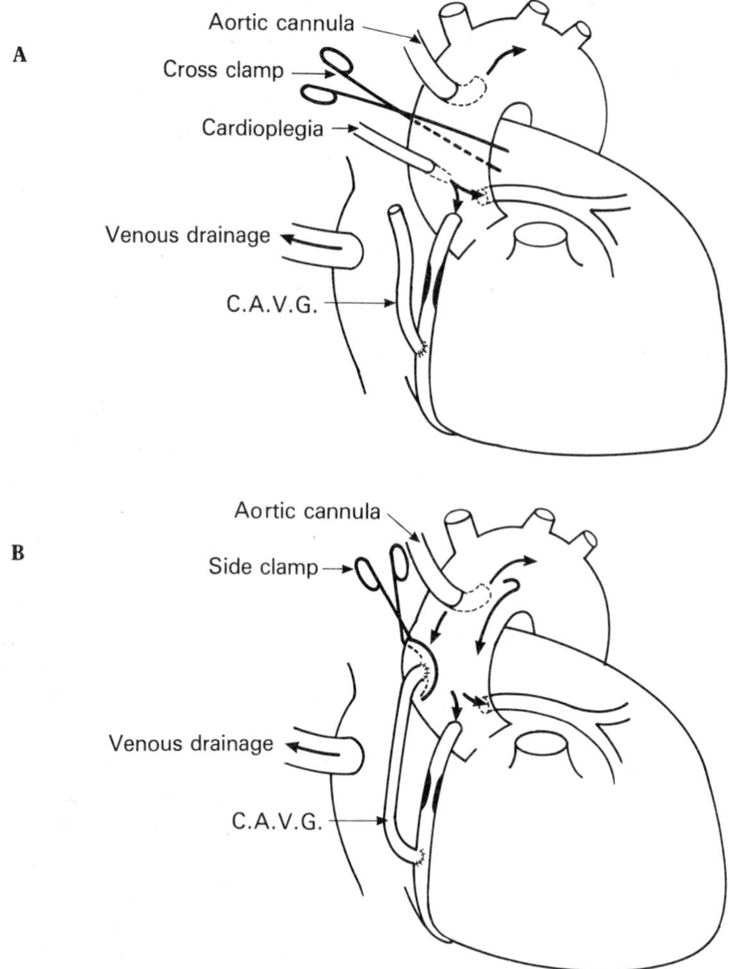

Fig. 40.7 Arrangement of cross-clamp, cardioplegia and anastomoses.

Myocardial preservation

Most surgical techniques on the heart require an immobile heart with empty chambers. On bypass, the aorta is cross-clamped between the aortic cannula and the aortic valve, thus isolating the heart from the flow of oxygenated blood. During aortic cross-clamping, the myocardium is at risk of ischaemic damage unless measures are taken to reduce myocardial oxygen consumption. Currently, techniques of myocardial preservation include hypothermia to reduce basal metabolic rate and cardiac arrest to reduce oxygen requirements to a minimum. Arrest is achieved by injecting 500–1000 ml of cardioplegic solution around the coronary arteries and arresting the heart in diastole. Many cardioplegic solutions are available, but the majority contain potassium and a membrane stabilising agent, e.g. procaine. Cooling is achieved by the use of chilled cardioplegia and by pouring cold fluid (4°C) into the pericardial sac and into the heart chambers if they have been opened.

If the heart is cooled to 15°C it withstands total ischaemia for approximately 1 h. The technique used most commonly at present involves moderate hypothermia of the body to 25–30°C and local cooling of the myocardium to a temperature of 15–18°C. This technique is very successful but depends on meticulous attention to detail. If prolonged cross-clamp times are required, cardioplegic cooling must be repeated if evidence of spontaneous cardiac contraction is seen or the temperature of the heart increases above 18°C.

Perfusion on bypass

At normothermia, a pump flow of 2.4 litre min^{-1} m^{-2} of body surface area is required to prevent inadequate perfusion of the body. The pressure achieved within the vascular system is dependent on pump output and systemic vascular resistance. Controversy exists regarding optimum perfusion pressure. However, it has been suggested that essential organs, in particular brain, are damaged if perfusion is maintained below 50 mmHg mean arterial pressure.

Following the institution of bypass, there are usually marked decreases in peripheral resistance and arterial pressure, which in most instances resolve spontaneously in 5–10 min. If this does not occur, arterial pressure may be increased by raising systemic resistance with a sympathomimetic agent, e.g. methoxamine 1–5 mg. Frequently, systemic resistance increases during and after bypass as a result of increasing plasma concentrations of catecholamines, renin–angiotensin and thromboxane. If the mean arterial pressure exceeds 100 mmHg, the use of vasodilators may be required.

Perfusion is difficult to assess clinically, especially in the hypothermic patient, and often the most useful monitor of adequate organ perfusion is urine output. The cerebral function monitor may be useful in assessing the adequacy of pressure and perfusion.

Coagulation control. Adequate anticoagulation must be maintained during CPB. If the Haemochron is available, ACT should be measured every 30 min and extra heparin administered if ACT decreases below 400 s. If this facility is not available, half the initial dose of heparin should be given every hour.

Oxygen delivery. Arterial blood samples should be obtained regularly, and blood gases and haematocrit measured.

Oxygen carriage is dependent on haemoglobin concentration in addition to adequate oxygen tension. Haematocrit may be permitted to decrease to 20% but further reduction should be prevented by the addition of packed cells or blood to the bypass circuit.

Acid–base balance. The development of metabolic acidosis suggests that perfusion is inadequate and if necessary (base deficit > 6–8 mmol/litre), sodium bicarbonate should be administered.

Serum potassium. Serum K^+ concentration should be maintained above 4.5 mmol/litre by the administration of KCl (10–20 mmol).

Restoration of spontaneous heart beat

When the cross-clamp has been removed, oxygenated blood flows again into the coronary arteries, washing out cardioplegia and repaying the oxygen debt. In most instances, the heart regains activity spontaneously; in a minority of patients it starts to beat in sinus rhythm, but reverts usually to ventricular fibrillation. Internal defibrillation is required to convert fibrillation to sinus rhythm and is successful only if pH, oxygenation and temperature are approaching normal values. The heat exchanger in the oxygenator is used to raise the temperature of blood but peripheral temperature is often depressed for some time. If a spontaneous heart beat cannot be maintained, pacing wires should be attached to the epicardium to initiate activity artificially.

At this stage, full bypass flow is maintained and although the heart is beating there is little ejection from the ventricles. It is wise at this time to pause, ensure that all air has been vented from the heart chambers, wait until core temperature exceeds 36°C and rest the heart before it is required to pump again.

Termination of bypass

When body temperature exceeds 36°C, metabolic indices are normal and a regular heart beat present, the establishment of spontaneous cardiac output is attempted. This is undertaken by diverting an increasing volume of venous blood into the right atrium past the extracorporeal cannulae by constricting the venous return line to the pump. Blood is now passing again through the pulmonary circulation and mechanical ventilation should be restarted. One hundred per cent oxygen should be employed, as the gas-exchanging efficiency of the lung is unknown at this stage and in addition any air bubbles which have not been vented enlarge in volume if nitrous oxide is introduced.

If pump flow has been pulsatile, it is advisable to revert to a continuous output at this time; any output or ejection from the left ventricle is seen as a 'blip' on the arterial pressure trace after a QRS complex. If the myocardium is contracting satisfactorily, pump flow is reduced cautiously and the heart, now receiving all the venous return, achieves normal output. At this time, 5 mmol $CaCl_2$ (repeated if necessary) may provide a useful if temporary inotropic stimulus.

Although arterial pressure is the most easily measured index of successful termination of bypass, it should be remembered that this is a derivative of cardiac output and peripheral resistance. The former is measured fairly easily and where there is doubt regarding pump efficiency, cardiac output (and thus cardiac index) should be assessed.

Peripheral resistance may be derived when cardiac output is measured but is assessed clinically by observing peripheral perfusion, core–peripheral temperature gradient and urine output. Peripheral resistance is increased consistently during bypass and much of the care of patients henceforth is directed towards producing increased peripheral dilatation and perfusion.

If ECC is discontinued successfully, preload should be optimised (left atrial pressure 12–15 mmHg) by infusion of as much as possible of the residual fluid contained in the pump circuit. This is facilitated by the administration of vasodilators, e.g. SNP and GTN. If cardiac output is inadequate, the circulation is reassumed by the extracorporeal pump and the heart allowed more time to recover.

Low output

If the heart is unable to generate sufficient output to maintain body perfusion after the preload has been optimised, further action is required. An increase in contractility is produced by inotropes. The simplest is a bolus of $CaCl_2$ but the most commonly employed are dobutamine or dopamine (2–20 $\mu g\ kg^{-1}\ min^{-1}$) by infusion. Adrenaline (0.05–0.2 $\mu g\ kg^{-1}\ min^{-1}$) or, if heart rate is slow, isoprenaline (0.02–0.2 $\mu g\ kg^{-1}\ min^{-1}$), may be indicated in some patients.

Although all these drugs augment cardiac output they tend to precipitate tachyarrhythmias. Adrenaline and dopamine also cause vasoconstriction in high doses. In addition, all these agents increase myocardial oxygen demand. They may precipitate infarction in patients with ischaemic heart disease.

An alternative approach is to assist output by reducing the afterload with vasodilators. As described previously, reduced afterload not only reduces oxygen demand, but also, in the failing ventricle, augments forward flow into the aorta. Diastolic pressure must not be reduced excessively (<55 mmHg) as oxygen supply to the ventricle is jeopardised. Infusion of fluid may be required during dilatation to maintain preload at adequate levels. In acute low-output syndromes, vasodilators are usually prescribed in addition to inotropes and the drugs may have a cumulative effect in raising cardiac index, permitting a reduction in the dosage of inotropes. Sodium nitroprusside, which reduces both preload and afterload, may cause a 'steal' from areas of ischaemic myocardium. Glyceryl trinitrate, which reduces predominantly preload, does not appear to have this effect and is the dilator of choice in patients with myocardial ischaemia, although some patients appear to be resistant to its hypotensive action.

The success of these manoeuvres should not be measured by the level of arterial pressure attained but by evidence of increased flow to tissues, particularly increased cardiac output and peripheral temperatures, and increasing urine output. It should be remembered, however, that both drugs may affect ventilation/perfusion ratios adversely and may aggravate hypoxaemia.

If these pharmacological methods fail to produce an adequate cardiac output, the intra-aortic balloon pump (IABP) may be used.

Intra-aortic balloon pump. The principle of the IABP is illustrated in Figure 40.8. If the balloon in the aorta is inflated immediately after systole,

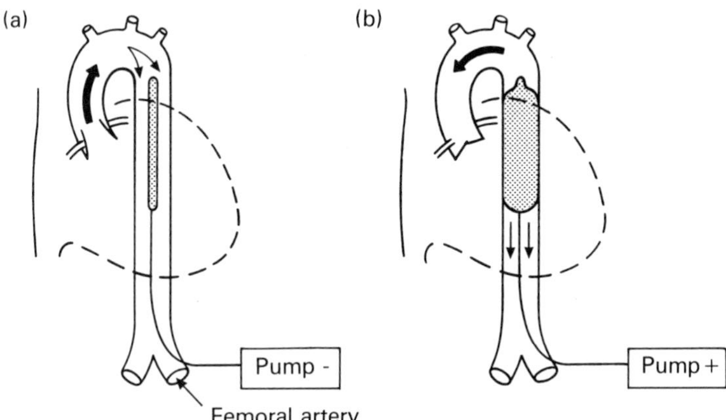

Fig. 40.8 Intra-aortic balloon pump (IABP). (a) systole (b) diastole.

diastolic filling pressure is augmented and myocardial oxygen balance improved. Inflation also displaces blood from the aorta and increases peripheral flow. The balloon is deflated immediately before systole and this creates a low pressure in the aorta as ventricular output starts, reducing afterload (and thus oxygen consumption) and at the same time augmenting output. The use of the IABP has decreased recently as surgery, anaesthesia, and in particular myocardial preservation techniques have improved. However, it is remarkably successful in some patients with a persistent low-output syndrome.

Coagulation control

When the bypass cannulae have been removed, residual effects of heparin are antagonised with protamine. Traditionally 1.5 mg protamine has been administered per 1 mg heparin, but this does not take into account the short half-life of heparin (1.5–2 h) and much smaller doses of protamine may be adequate to regain normal coagulability after a bypass lasting 1–2 h. The dosage may be titrated using the ACT. The drug should be given slowly, especially if there is residual hypovolaemia or raised pulmonary vascular resistance. Protamine may produce systemic hypotension rapidly, as a result of peripheral vasodilatation, but may cause pulmonary vasoconstriction also. In excessive dosage, it has anticoagulant effects.

Heparin is not the only factor which may cause bleeding during and after bypass. Contact of blood with bubbles in the oxygenator and with foreign surfaces in the bypass circuit and suction tubing causes consumption of clotting factors and of platelets. Thus if heparin appears to have been antagonised satisfactorily and unexplained bleeding persists, a full clotting screen should be performed, including estimation of platelet numbers. Clotting factors may be replaced by the infusion of fresh frozen plasma and/or cryoprecipitate, and platelet concentrate should be infused if the platelet count is less than 60×10^9/litre.

From the surgical standpoint, the period following termination of bypass is concerned with prevention of haemorrhage and closure of the chest with drains in situ. In addition to the maintenance of patient comfort, the anaesthetist must ensure the efficiency of myocardial pumping, oxygen balance and peripheral perfusion together with correction of metabolic, biochemical, haematological or temperature abnormalities.

CONTROL OF THE CIRCULATION AFTER BYPASS

Despite the use of measures to protect the myocardium during bypass, the heart suffers some deterioration in function and has reduced contractility for several hours. Thus it operates on a lower Frank Starling curve (Fig. 40.5) and requires a higher preload to produce the same output. Usually, a left atrial pressure of approximately 15 mmHg is optimal. The contractility of the myocardium improves in the first 3–4 h after bypass and this increased efficiency permits reduction in preload.

In addition, the peripheral circulation remains vasoconstricted for several hours postoperatively. In patients with reasonable ventricular function, hypertension often occurs after bypass, especially in operations involving the aortic valve or revascularisation. The increased afterload results in additional myocardial oxygen consumption and tends to reduce cardiac output.

Reduction of peripheral resistance and systemic arterial pressure by a vasodilator (e.g. SNP or GTN) protects suture lines from damage, decreases oxygen demand, increases cardiac output if preload is not reduced excessively, improves peripheral perfusion and accelerates warming. The use of vasodilators in the early postoperative period is increasing and is now regarded as beneficial in the majority of patients.

Other aspects of maintenance after bypass

In addition to maintaining cardiac function and oxygen supply to the tissues during this period, the anaesthetist should ensure that normality is regained as soon as possible, and maintained, in respect of the following:

1. *Temperature*

Core temperature is raised easily on bypass via the oxygenator. However the efficiency of rewarming the peripheral tissues depends on the patient's weight, total flow rate and peripheral perfusion. After bypass there is often a decrease in core temperature (afterdrop). More efficient rewarming and reduction in afterdrop may be achieved by the use of a warming mattress.

2. *Biochemical monitoring*

Essential monitoring includes measurement of blood gas tensions, acid–base balance, serum K^+ concentration and haematocrit.

3. *Cardiac rhythm*

Heart block. Epicardial pacing lines should be inserted if AV dissociation occurs. Infusion of isoprenaline may improve ventricular rate and output as a temporary measure.

Supraventricular arrhythmias. Direct current cardioversion is the most convenient treatment when the chest is open. After chest closure, digoxin or verapamil are of value.

Ventricular arrhythmias. The threshold for arrhythmias is reduced by hypokalaemia, and serum K^+ concentration should be maintained above 4.5 mmol/litre. If ventricular arrhythmias persist, lignocaine is the drug of choice although β-blockers may be useful, but should be administered cautiously.

Transfer to postoperative ITU

It is normal to prolong the same level of support and monitoring undertaken during surgery into the postoperative period. The duration of this care depends on the individual patient's response to surgery and speed of recovery.

Transfer of the patient from theatre to the ITU may involve journeys along corridors and into lifts. It is essential that controlled ventilation is continued and ECG and arterial pressure monitored during transfer. Hypertension often occurs as a result of stimulation during movement, as anaesthesia for the latter part of surgery is maintained at a light level. In addition infusion of vasodilators may be interrupted during transfer. A bolus dose of opioid is often advisable before transfer.

POSTOPERATIVE INTENSIVE THERAPY

The surgical team should have a well-practised routine for the care of patients after surgery. Ventilation of the lungs with a volume-preset ventilator (preferably with the facility for intermittent mandatory ventilation) and full cardiovascular monitoring should be instituted immediately.

The principles of care in this phase are similar to those described for the period of anaesthesia after termination of bypass.

Haemodynamic care

On return to ITU, most patients are cold, vasoconstricted and exhibit a tendency to hypertension. Attention is directed towards achieving vasodilatation, reduction of afterload and maintenance of preload. Blood is required if the haematocrit is less than 35%. Urine output should be maintained with diuretics or low-dose dopamine (1–4 $\mu g\ kg^{-1}\ min^{-1}$) if necessary but usually a spontaneous diuresis occurs in response to the crystalloid load received in theatre. Potassium concentrations should be monitored carefully, and abnormalities corrected.

The majority of patients stabilise and regain adequate peripheral perfusion over the succeeding 3–4 h, permitting the level of cardiovascular support to be reduced.

In a minority of patients, low cardiac output requires the continued use of inotropes, vasodilators and, if necessary, IABP for some time.

Blood loss

This should be measured accurately. If excessive (300–400 ml/h), it may be necessary to re-operate on the patient. Attention to the coagulation system is required and further protamine or coagulation factors prescribed as necessary. The most sinister complication of excessive bleeding is cardiac tamponade which requires rapid thoracotomy and evacuation of blood from the chest. If deterioration is rapid, this must be undertaken in the ITU.

Ventilation

Respiratory dysfunction is manifest as an increase in venous admixture. This is common after cardiac surgery and persists for several days. Usually ventilation is assisted for 6–12 h after operation in order to obviate the work of breathing and maximise oxygenation. Adequate analgesia is prescribed more safely, and return to theatre, if required, is more convenient and rapid. However, recent experience suggests that the time of mechanical ventilation may be reduced safely and continued only for the period of postoperative haemodynamic instability, which in most patients lasts 3–6 h. Thus when the patient's arterial pressure and peripheral perfusion are satisfactory, the temperature exceeds 36°C core and 30°C peripheral, urine output is more than 30 ml/h, blood loss less than 100 ml/h, and the patient is conscious and can maintain satisfactory blood gases with an inspired oxygen concentration of less than 40%, a trial of spontaneous ventilation is indicated. If respiratory volumes are adequate and the patient is not distressed, the trachea may be extubated.

There are some patients in whom these criteria are not achieved, and ventilation is continued. High inspired oxygen concentrations should be avoided if possible by the use of PEEP to maintain an arterial oxygen tension of approximately 10 kPa (75 mmHg) if cardiovascular function permits.

Analgesia

The anaesthetic technique employed determines the timing of administration of postoperative analgesia. Even after high-dose opioid techniques, patients usually show some sign of response in the first 2–3 h after surgery. It is useful to assess cerebral function at this stage in case damage has occurred, but it is inadvisable to distress the patient, as reflex hypertension may occur. The most commonly used method of pain relief is the use of i.v. opioids either by bolus or continuous infusion. Often the addition of a tranquilliser (diazepam 5 mg or midazolam 2–5 mg) is advantageous in maintaining the patient comfortable but rousable. The uses of inhalational sedation with isoflurane and infusion of a short-acting i.v. anaesthetic agent, e.g. propofol, are being investigated, and may offer valuable options for patients who are difficult to sedate. Regional analgesic techniques are not popular since coagulation defects are common but the use of pre-bypass intrathecal opioids or postoperative extradural analgesia has been reported.

As important as pharmacological support is the human rapport which should be achieved between attending staff and patient.

FURTHER READING

Gothard J W W 1987 Anaesthesia for cardiac surgery. Blackwell Scientific Publications, Oxford

Kaplan J A 1987 Cardiac anaesthesia. Grune and Stratton, New York

Nimmo W S, Smith G (eds) 1989 Anaesthesia. Blackwell Scientific Publications, Oxford

Ream A K, Fogdall R P 1982 Acute cardiovascular management: anesthesia and intensive care. J B Lippincott, Philadelphia

Streisand J B, Wong H C 1988 Anaesthesia for coronary artery bypass graft. British Journal of Anaesthesia 61: 97–104

Tarhan S 1988 Cardiovascular anaesthesia and postoperative care. Year Book Medical Publishers, Chicago

41. Intercurrent disease and anaesthesia

Many patients presenting for surgery suffer from unrelated disease, for which they may be receiving drug treatment. The course of this disease may be modified by anaesthesia and surgery, while the disease process itself may influence the effects of anaesthesia.

The aims of anaesthetic management in such patients are:

1. To assess the extent of the medical problem.
2. To ensure that the patient's condition is optimised in the time available before surgery (this may vary widely between emergency and elective surgery).
3. To conduct anaesthesia and postoperative care using drugs and techniques which interact least with the medical condition.

To achieve these aims, all patients who present for surgery require a full clinical history and examination. A past medical history, including previous anaesthesia, drug and allergy history and examination of previous anaesthetic records (if available) may be particularly important. In addition, special investigations may be necessary depending on the age and fitness of the patient and the nature of the surgery (see Ch. 19).

CARDIOVASCULAR DISEASE

General principles

Anaesthesia for patients with cardiovascular disease involves the application of a number of basic principles:

1. Adequate oxygenation must be maintained throughout.
2. Cardiac output must be maintained at a level commensurate with adequate tissue perfusion.
3. Systemic arterial pressure must be adequate to maintain cerebral and coronary circulation and preserve renal and hepatic function.
4. The balance of myocardial oxygen supply and demand must be preserved, thus minimising the risk of perioperative ischaemia and infarction (Table 41.1).

Table 41.1 Factors affecting myocardial oxygen supply and consumption

Supply	*Consumption*	
Coronary perfusion pressure (diastolic pressure — LVEDP)	H.R.	
Arterial oxygen tension	Contractility	
Haemoglobin concentration	Wall tension	1. LVEDP 2. Arterial pressure 3. Contractility
Coronary vascular resistance – intraluminal obstruction – external compression 1. H.R. 2. LVEDP – autoregulation — dependent on myocardial O_2 consumption	External Work	1. Cardiac output 2. Arterial Pressure

This demands a knowledge of the physiological mechanisms governing cardiac output, myocardial oxygen availability and consumption, and the adjustments that occur in disease states. An understanding of the effects of i.v. and volatile anaesthetic agents, and muscle relaxants allows a choice to be made of appropriate drugs and techniques. Reversible risk factors (e.g. cardiac failure or hypertension) must be detected and treated preoperatively.

Preoperative assessment

History

Symptoms which suggest cardiovascular disease include dyspnoea, chest pain, palpitations, ankle swelling and intermittent claudication. Severity of symptoms assessed by a history of exercise tolerance is the most useful estimate of severity of cardiovascular disease.

Past medical history and previous medical records usually reveal the nature and severity of disease. A number of factors relating to history, clinical examination and proposed surgery are associated with an increased risk of perioperative cardiac complications, such as myocardial infarction (Table 19.4). For example, the date of a previous myocardial infarction must be noted and elective surgery should not be performed within 6 months of that date. Unstable angina may be associated also with an increased risk of perioperative infarction, and should be treated before elective surgery. Previous thromboembolic disease necessitates prophylactic measures, e.g. low-dose heparin, Dextran 70, or intermittent calf compression.

Concurrent drug treatment

Digoxin. The dose should be assessed on the basis of age, weight and renal function, and reduced in the elderly, in patients with impaired renal function or if the plasma digoxin concentration exceeds the therapeutic range. Serum potassium concentration should be measured, especially when there is concurrent diuretic therapy, and symptoms of digoxin toxicity, e.g. nausea and vomiting, should be sought. Heart rate and rhythm require assessment. In excessive dosage, especially with concurrent hypokalaemia, ventricular arrhythmias or heart block may occur.

Diuretics. Serum potassium concentration should be checked, and hypokalaemia corrected.

Anticoagulants. Where long-term therapy is indicated, perioperative control must be monitored closely. Warfarin should be stopped 48 h preoperatively, and the prothrombin time monitored daily; it should not be greater than 1.5 times control at the time of surgery. For emergency surgery, or if undue bleeding occurs, fresh frozen plasma is indicated. Postoperatively, for minor surgery, warfarin may be restarted the following day, while for major surgery a heparin infusion may be used to maintain anticoagulation (with control by thrombin time estimations) until warfarin therapy is restarted. This allows reversal of anticoagulation with protamine 1 mg for every 100 units of heparin if bleeding occurs. Protamine should be administered slowly to avoid hypotension.

β-Adrenergic blockers. In most instances, β-blockade should be maintained throughout the perioperative period. Sudden preoperative cessation may be associated with rebound angina, myocardial infarction, arrhythmia or hypertension postoperatively. Intravenous atropine may be given prior to induction or, if undue bradycardia occurs, intraoperatively. β-Blockers may contribute to and mask the signs of hypoglycaemia.

Calcium channel blockers. These drugs block the slow influx of calcium ions which contribute to depolarisation. *Verapamil*, which acts predominantly on the AV node, is used in the management of supraventricular tachyarrhythmias, angina and hypertrophic obstructive cardiomyopathy. As it increases AV block, concurrent use with digoxin or β-blockers should be avoided, as should halothane anaesthesia. *Nifedipine*, which acts predominantly on vascular smooth muscle, is used in the management of angina, hypertension and as a preload reducer in left ventricular failure. It should be used cautiously in patients on β-blocker therapy. There is some evidence that the risk of myocardial ischaemia is increased as a result of coronary steal when isoflurane is used in patients receiving nifedipine.

Examination

Preoperative cardiovascular examination should include measurement of heart rate and rhythm, arterial pressure, assessment of peripheral perfusion and detection of signs of cardiac failure. Hypertension and cardiac murmurs are not infrequently a chance finding, and require further assessment before surgery.

Investigations

In addition to routine haematological and biochemical investigations, an ECG is important as a baseline before surgery for the diagnosis of arrhythmias, to provide confirmatory evidence of ischaemic heart disease and to assess the severity of cardiac disease, e.g. hypertension, cor pulmonale and valvular heart disease.

Chest X-ray provides information on heart and chamber sizes, the state of the pulmonary vasculature and evidence of pulmonary oedema and infection.

Ultrasound examination (echocardiography) is useful in diagnosing valve lesions, and detection of pericardial effusions.

Cardiac catheterisation and coronary angiography are rarely indicated before routine surgery.

Preoperative treatment

Cardiac failure, arrhythmias, hypertension and angina should be controlled before surgery. Anaemia should be treated, if necessary with blood transfusion, at least 48 h before surgery. Haemoglobin concentration should be greater than 10 g/dl.

Premedication

In ischaemic heart disease and hypertension, premedication should be adequate to allay anxiety. The combination of papaveretum and hyoscine is often satisfactory. In patients with low or fixed cardiac output states (e.g. mitral or aortic stenosis, constrictive pericarditis), and congestive cardiac failure, premedication should be light, e.g. oral temazepam. In poor-risk patients, it may be preferable to avoid preanaesthetic medication.

Anaesthesia

In practical terms, this involves maintenance of a normal heart rate, and an arterial pressure adequate to maintain coronary perfusion and oxygenation without increasing cardiac work and thus myocardial oxygen requirements. Excessive myocardial depression should be avoided.

The high-risk periods during anaesthesia are:

1. *Induction.* Most induction agents are cardiovascular depressants, and in patients with low or fixed cardiac output, hypertension or hypovolaemia, hypotension may occur. Etomidate has least cardiovascular effects. Of the numerous neuromuscular-blocking drugs, atracurium and vecuronium produce least (and negligible) cardiovascular effects.
2. *Intubation.* Tracheal intubation is associated commonly with hypertension.
3. *Postoperative period.* Rebound hypertension occurs commonly in association with pain and peripheral vasoconstriction. Good analgesia is necessary with careful attention to intravascular volume.

Careful monitoring is essential and must always include heart rate, arterial pressure and ECG. The common ECG configuration used for anaesthetic monitoring is standard limb lead II. Whilst this is useful for differentiating arrhythmias, myocardial ischaemia occurs most commonly in the left ventricle and is detected more sensitively with a CM_5 configuration (Fig. 21.2). In high-risk patients undergoing major surgery, intra-arterial cannulation and CVP measurements are indicated. Pulmonary capillary wedge pressure measurement is useful in patients with severe left ventricular failure, shock, or for surgery where major blood loss is anticipated. Monitoring should be instituted before induction, and maintained throughout the immediate postoperative period (if necessary in the ITU).

Hypertension

Untreated hypertension is associated with increased perioperative morbidity and mortality, and increased risks of cerebrovascular accident and myocardial infarction. As arterial pressure increases with age, an acceptable maximum pressure is difficult to define, but elective surgery should rarely be undertaken when the resting diastolic pressure exceeds 110 mmHg. Control of hypertension is achieved using a thiazide diuretic, with the possible addition of a β-blocker and an ACE inhibitor, e.g. captopril. A calcium channel blocker, e.g. nifedipine may be used also in more severe cases.

Where hypertension is a chance preoperative finding, surgery should be delayed until investigation and treatment have been instituted.

Endocrine and renal causes should be excluded. Complications of hypertension, e.g. myocardial ischaemia, cardiac failure and renal impairment, should be sought, and unstable angina and cardiac failure controlled before surgery. Antihypertensive therapy should be continued throughout the perioperative period.

Anaesthesia

Premedication should be generous with, for example, papaveretum and hyoscine. Anaesthetic management should be directed towards avoidance of hypotension and, more particularly, hypertension. Thus close monitoring of arterial pressure and ECG is required from before induction through anaesthesia and the postoperative period. Blood loss should also be monitored carefully, and deficits replaced promptly.

Hypertensive patients are particularly vulnerable to the development of hypotension following induction of anaesthesia or following establishment of subarachnoid or extradural blockade. Etomidate has least cardiovascular effects, but thiopentone is acceptable if administered carefully. Propofol may produce excessive hypotension. Ketamine is contraindicated in anaesthetic dosages. Pancuronium should be avoided in severe hypertension; atracurium and vecuronium are suitable but *d*-tubocurarine or alcuronium may cause severe but transient hypotension.

Tracheal intubation commonly causes hypertension, tachycardia and arrhythmias. Pre-induction administration of a β-blocker or rapidly acting opioid (fentanyl 5 μg/kg or alfentanil 20 μg/kg) may attenuate this response.

For maintenance of anaesthesia, a nitrous oxide/oxygen/opioid/relaxant technique is appropriate in most instances. Halothane and enflurane possess marked cardiovascular depressant effects, and require careful administration. However, they are suitable for minor procedures with a spontaneous breathing technique.

Intraoperatively, nodal arrhythmias occur commonly, and may produce a decrease in cardiac output. Depending on heart rate, i.v. atropine, β-blocker or decrease of the inspired halothane concentration may be effective in treating arrhythmias. β-Blockers prevent the physiological heart rate response to intraoperative blood loss, while vasodilators prevent vasoconstriction. Thus careful monitoring of blood and fluid loss and CVP is important, and prompt replacement of fluid deficits is necessary to avoid undue hypotension. Local anaesthetic preparations containing catecholamine vasoconstrictors should be avoided.

Postoperative hypertension occurs frequently, partly as a result of inadequate analgesia, and partly because of peripheral vasoconstriction which occurs during prolonged surgery with associated heat loss and bleeding. Plasma adrenaline concentrations may be increased markedly. Hypertension increases myocardial work and oxygen demand, and may cause subendocardial ischaemia or infarction in patients with left ventricular hypertrophy or enlargement. Good analgesia is essential, and continuous extradural analgesia is safe in treated hypertensive patients if closely monitored.

Hypertension should be treated promptly; labetalol titrated in 10–20 mg i.v. bolus doses is usually effective. In the presence of peripheral vasoconstriction, a vasodilator, e.g. titrated i.v. boluses of chlorpromazine 2.5–5 mg, phentolamine 2.5 mg or hydralazine 5–10 mg, are usually effective. All hypotensive therapy requires careful arterial pressure monitoring. β-Blocker therapy is indicated in the presence of tachycardia.

If the patient has been managed preoperatively with oral β-blockers, a long-acting agent, e.g. atenolol or nadolol, should be given before surgery, and oral treatment recommenced on the day after surgery. In some instances, nasogastric administration or i.v. infusion may be necessary.

With propranolol, the i.v. daily dose is approximately one-tenth of the oral dose.

Ischaemic heart disease

Five per cent of patients over 35 years of age have symptomless ischaemic heart disease. In patients who have had a previous myocardial infarction, anaesthesia and surgery within 3 months of infarction carry a 40% risk of perioperative reinfarction. This rate decreases to 15% at 3–6 months and 5% thereafter. Mortality from postoperative infarction is 40–60%. Elective surgery should be postponed until at least 6 months after infarction unless it is urgent.

Unstable angina is associated also with increased risk of perioperative myocardial infarction and should be controlled with β-blockade, nitrates or a calcium channel blocker before surgery. There is no evidence that the incidence of postoperative infarction is reduced by using local or regional anaesthetic techniques.

Factors which precipitate further infarction are those which increase myocardial work and thus oxygen requirement, or which decrease coronary blood flow (Table 41.1).

Anaesthesia

Preoperatively, congestive cardiac failure should be treated with diuretics and, if necessary, digoxin. The increase in oxygen consumption resulting from increased contractility is balanced by the beneficial effects on myocardial oxygen supply and demand achieved by decreased left ventricular end-diastolic pressure. Anaemia should be corrected. Premedication should be adequate to allay anxiety. Anaesthetic management demands the same close monitoring, avoidance of tachycardia and bradycardia, maintenance of normotension or slight hypotension and careful choice of anaesthetic agent which is necessary in the hypertensive patient. β-Blockade should be maintained and this necessitates care in fluid replacement and concurrent drug administration.

Halothane depresses contractility and myocardial oxygen consumption, but coronary blood flow is depressed to a proportionately lesser extent. Thus halothane is tolerated well in small concentrations. However, high concentrations of halothane may produce excessive myocardial depression with a profound decrease in cardiac output, increased LVEDP and myocardial ischaemia. These effects may be potentiated by β-blockade. Normocapnia should be maintained, since hypercapnia may provoke arrhythmias, while hypocapnia causes peripheral and coronary vasoconstriction, and shifts the oxygen dissociation curve to the left.

Enflurane dilates the peripheral circulation in addition to depressing myocardial contractility. Overall, it causes a decrease in arterial pressure comparable with that resulting from administration of halothane.

Isoflurane causes less reduction in cardiac output than enflurane or halothane. It is a potent vasodilator and has been implicated as a cause of coronary 'steal' in patients with myocardial ischaemia. Although there is some dispute about the importance of this effect at high doses, it is likely that small concentrations of isoflurane (<0.5%) do not cause coronary steal.

Interactions between calcium channel blockers and volatile anaesthetic agents may cause serious hypotension (Table 41.2).

Postoperative monitoring, management of analgesia, and arterial pressure control must be meticulous.

Congestive cardiac failure

Anaesthesia and surgery in patients with cardiac failure carry an increased risk of morbidity and mortality. The cause of the failure should be elucidated, and treatment instituted before surgery.

Table 41.2 Cardiovascular effects of calcium channel blockers and volatile anaesthetic agents. Use of a volatile agent with similar actions to a concurrently administered calcium channel blocker may result in hypotension

Drugs	Predominant effect
Nifedipine Isoflurane	Reduced systemic vascular resistance (SVR)
Verapamil Halothone	Reduced cardiac contractility and impaired AV conduction
Diltiazem Enflurane	Intermediate effect on SVR, contractility and

Left heart failure causes pulmonary congestion and oedema, decreases pulmonary compliance, increasing respiratory work and resulting in hypoxaemia and hypocapnia. Causes include hypertension, aortic valve disease, mitral valve disease, ischaemic heart disease and cardiomyopathy (hypertrophic obstructive cardiomyopathy, HOCM and congestive cardiomyopathy). It is often precipitated by arrhythmias, e.g. atrial fibrillation in mitral stenosis.

Treatment involves diuretic therapy and, in some instances, digitalisation. In addition, specific therapy is required for the cause of failure, e.g. arrhythmias. The outflow obstruction seen in HOCM responds to β-blockade. If failure is refractory to digoxin and diuretic therapy, venodilatation with glyceryl trinitrate or isosorbide dinitrate decreases preload and may decrease pulmonary congestion.

Right heart failure may be secondary to left heart failure, chronic lung disease (cor pulmonale), idiopathic pulmonary hypertension or pulmonary stenosis. ECG evidence of right atrial and ventricular hypertrophy raises the suspicion of pulmonary hypertension. Hypoxia in such patients causes a marked increase in pulmonary vascular resistance provoking right ventricular failure. Acute right heart failure occurs commonly when patients with chronic obstructive airways disease suffer an acute infective exacerbation with hypoxaemia. Preoperative treatment of infection is important, and intra- and postoperative maintenance of the airway and avoidance of hypoxia are imperative.

Biventricular failure is also associated with fluid overload and hypoalbuminaemia, e.g. in renal or hepatic disease.

Low subarachnoid and extradural blockade may be useful in some patients with cardiac failure, as the sympathetic block produces venodilatation and reduction in preload.

Shock

Surgery should not be undertaken until adequate resuscitation of the patient has been undertaken. In cases of severe haemorrhage, only initial resuscitation may be possible before surgery, and resuscitation continued during operation until bleeding is controlled. Such patients require adequate oxygenation and ventilation, with blood gas measurements. Monitoring required during resuscitation and anaesthesia includes arterial pressure, heart rate, CVP and urine output, while the core–peripheral temperature gradient provides a useful indication of peripheral perfusion. Pulmonary artery catheterisation for measurement of PCWP and cardiac output is usually necessary to monitor the effects of fluid and inotrope therapy in the shocked patient.

Anaesthesia in shock

Adequate venous access with large-bore cannulae should be ensured before induction of anaesthesiae. Minimal doses of induction agent should be employed. Etomidate is associated with least cardiovascular disturbance, but other agents, e.g. thiopentone, may be used with care in very low dosage. Ketamine increases myocardial work and may increase oxygen demand excessively in an ischaemic myocardium, but is useful in patients with hypovolaemic shock resulting from trauma. A nitrous oxide/oxygen/opioid/relaxant technique, using vecuronium (or pancuronium), is usually well tolerated. The management of shock is discussed in Chapters 32 and 42.

Arrhythmias (see also Ch. 23, p. 412)

Arrhythmias occurring preoperatively should be treated before surgery (which should be postponed if necessary). The most commonly occurring arrhythmia is probably atrial fibrillation, which is caused usually by ischaemic heart disease, mitral valve disease or thyrotoxicosis. The ventricular rate should be controlled with digoxin. If the ventricular rate is normal, digoxin should usually be started preoperatively to prevent an increase in ventricular rate during operation.

Intraoperative arrhythmias

Approximately 12% of patients undergoing anaesthesia develop arrhythmias but this frequency increases to 30% in patients with cardiovascular disease. Treatment may not be required, depending on the nature of the arrhythmia and its effect on cardiac output. Single supraventricular or ventricular ectopic beats, and slow supraventricular rhythms do not require treatment unless cardiac output is compromised.

Factors affecting intraoperative arrhythmias include:

1. Spontaneous ventilation. Raised Pa_{CO_2} may cause ventricular extrasystoles.
2. Hypoxaemia. Initially this caused tachycardia, then bradycardia.
3. Anaesthetic agents. Cyclopropane and halogenated hydrocarbons, e.g. trichloroethylene and halothane, are associated with an increased incidence of ventricular arrhythmias, especially if Pa_{CO_2} is raised.
4. Catecholamines. Local anaesthetic preparations containing adrenaline may provoke ventricular arrhythmias especially in patients anaesthetised with halothane in the presence of a raised Pa_{CO_2}. A maximum of 100 μg of adrenaline (10 ml of 1:100 000 solution) may be injected over any 10-min period. Enflurane is less likely to be associated with adrenaline-induced arrhythmias, and isoflurane even less so.
5. Hypokalaemia may be associated with ventricular arrhythmias especially in the presence of digoxin. Hyperkalaemia delays ventricular conduction, with eventual cardiac arrest.
6. Reflex arrhythmias tend to occur during light anaesthesia as a result of sympathetic or parasympathetic stimulation. They include tachyarrhythmias in response to laryngoscopy and intubation (diminished by β-blockers), ventricular arrhythmias following dental extraction (blocked partially by local anaesthetic infiltration), and the oculocardiac reflex (blocked partially by atropine). Reflex arrhythmias in general are prevented by deepening anaesthesia.

Treatment of intraoperative arrhythmias depends on the nature of the arrhythmia. Supraventricular tachycardia may be treated with i.v. verapamil or β-blockers, but concurrent administration of these two drugs should be avoided. Cardioversion may be performed if these drugs are ineffective or if cardiac failure is present, as this may be aggravated by verapamil or β-blockers. If digoxin has been used in an attempt to control atrial flutter or fibrillation, it is advisable to administer lignocaine before cardioversion to prevent ventricular arrhythmias. Ventricular tachycardia responds to i.v. lignocaine 50–100 mg followed by an infusion, but if unsuccessful mexiletine, procainamide, phenytoin or β-blockers may be tried. Other measures include correction of hypercapnia, hypoxaemia or hypokalaemia, and reduction of the inspired halothane concentration.

Heart block

The extent of the conduction deficit should be determined preoperatively by ECG monitoring. If the patient has syncopal attacks, or is in cardiac failure, long-term pacing is indicated.

If the patient with heart block presents for surgery without a pacemaker in situ, preoperative insertion of a temporary pacing line is indicated usually in:

1. Complete heart block.
2. Second-degree heart block, of Mobitz Type 2 variety.
3. First-degree heart block with bifascicular block (right bundle branch block with left anterior or posterior hemiblock).

A decision on whether long-term pacing is indicated or not may be made by a cardiologist after the immediate postoperative period. During anaesthesia, ECG should be monitored continuously, a standby pacemaker should be available and care should be taken to avoid undue blood loss or vasodilatation as heart rate is unable to increase.

Diathermy should be avoided if possible since it may interfere with pacemaker function. Where unavoidable, the diathermy plate should be sited as far away as possible from the pacemaker generator. Temporary generators and demand permanent generators are most often affected. Demand pacemakers should be converted to fixed-rate before surgery if the use of diathermy is essential. During transurethral prostatectomy, the 'cutting' current may affect the pacemaker while the 'coagulation' current has no effect. With some pacemakers, the reverse may occur. Diathermy should be used in short bursts only. If first-degree heart block only is present, not necessitating external pacing, drugs which slow AV conduction should be avoided, e.g. β-blockers, digoxin, verapamil.

Sick sinus syndrome

This term covers a number of conduction defects which affect the sino-atrial node, ranging from sinus bradycardia to sinus arrest. Sino-atrial block may be associated with runs of supraventricular tachycardia (so called tachycardia–bradycardia syndrome). Long-term pacing is indicated if the patient has syncopal episodes. Sinus bradycardia responds usually to atropine while in complete sino-atrial block, atropine accelerates nodal escape rhythm. In the tachycardia–bradycardia group, temporary pacing is indicated to cover anaesthesia and surgery, since treatment of tachycardia with, for example, a β-blocker, calcium channel blocker or digoxin, may provoke severe bradycardia.

Valvular heart disease

Aortic stenosis

Isolated aortic stenosis is associated most commonly with calcification, often on a congenital bicuspid valve. In rheumatic heart disease, aortic stenosis occurs rarely in the absence of mitral disease, and is combined usually with incompetence. The diagnosis is suggested by the findings of an ejection systolic murmur, low pulse pressure, and clinical and ECG evidence of left ventricular hypertrophy. Aortic systolic murmurs in elderly patients are ascribed frequently to aortic sclerosis, and an assessment of the degree of stenosis rests on examination of pulse waveform, pulse pressure and ECG evidence of left ventricular hypertrophy. On chest X-ray, heart size is normal until late in the disease, while symptoms of angina, effort syncope and left ventricular failure indicate advanced disease.

Perioperative mortality is increased in patients with aortic stenosis; arrhythmias are common and are associated with precipitous decreases in cardiac output. The myocardial oxygen balance is upset by the decreases in coronary perfusion pressure and subendocardial blood flow, and the increase in ventricular afterload. Successful management demands precise maintenance of heart rate, arterial pressure and myocardial contractility. Bradycardia causes a decrease in cardiac output because stroke volume is fixed; tachycardia decreases the time available for coronary filling and therefore both should be avoided. Vasodilatation causes severe hypotension since cardiac output cannot be increased significantly and thus coronary perfusion pressure is reduced.

Most anaesthetic induction agents, and 'first-generation' muscle relaxants (*d*-tubocurarine, pancuronium, alcuronium) must be used with extreme caution. The relaxant of choice would be atracurium or vecuronium. Volatile agents which depress ventricular contractility (halothane, enflurane) may also seriously decrease cardiac output; in addition, halothane predisposes to arrhythmias. Replacement of blood must be prompt. Intensive monitoring is important and should include measurement of intra-arterial pressure and, in severe instances, PCWP measurement.

Mitral stenosis

This is usually a manifestation of rheumatic heart disease. Characteristic features include atrial fibrillation, arterial embolism, pulmonary oedema, pulmonary hypertension and right heart failure. Acute pulmonary oedema may follow the onset of atrial fibrillation.

Patients with mitral stenosis who present for surgery are frequently receiving digoxin, diuretics and anticoagulants. Preoperative control of atrial fibrillation, treatment of pulmonary oedema and management of anticoagulant therapy (see Ch. 7, p. 131) is necessary. During anaesthesia, control of heart rate is important. Tachycardia reduces diastolic ventricular filling and thus cardiac output, while bradycardia also results in a decreased cardiac output because stroke output is limited. As with aortic stenosis, drugs which produce vasodilatation may cause severe hypotension.

As a result of pre-existing pulmonary hypertension, patients are particularly vulnerable to hypoxaemia, including transient episodes. Both hypoxaemia and acidosis are potent pulmonary vasoconstrictors and may produce immediate right ventricular failure. Thus opioid analgesics should be prescribed cautiously, and airway obstruction avoided.

Aortic incompetence

Acute aortic incompetence resulting, for example, from subacute bacterial endocarditis or Marfan's syndrome, causes rapid left ventricular failure and requires emergency valve replacement.

Chronic aortic incompetence is asymptomatic for many years. Left ventricular dilatation occurs, with eventual left ventricular failure.

Patients with mild to moderate aortic incompetence without left ventricular failure or massive ventricular dilatation tolerate anaesthesia well. A slightly increased heart rate of approximately 100 beats/min is desirable since this reduces left ventricular dilatation. Bradycardia causes ventricular distension and should be avoided. Vasodilator therapy increases net forward flow by decreasing afterload, and is useful in severe aortic incompetence; however, careful monitoring is required, preferably with PCWP measurement, if severe hypotension is to be avoided.

Mitral incompetence

Acute mitral incompetence commonly results from subacute bacterial endocarditis, or myocardial infarction with papillary muscle dysfunction or ruptured chordae tendineae. Acute pulmonary oedema results, and urgent valve replacement is required.

Chronic mitral incompetence is associated commonly with mitral stenosis. In pure mitral incompetence, left atrial dilatation occurs with a minimal increase in pressure. The degree of regurgitation may be reduced by reducing the size of the left ventricle and the impedance to left ventricular ejection. Thus inotropic agents and vasodilators may be useful. A slight increase in heart rate is desirable except if there is concomitant stenosis.

Subacute bacterial endocarditis

This is caused predominantly by the *viridans* group of streptococci, occasionally by Gram-negative organisms or enterococci and also by staphylococci, especially after cardiac surgery or in drug addicts. *Coxiella burnetti* also accounts for a few cases. Patients with rheumatic or congenital heart disease, including asymptomatic lesions, e.g. bicuspid aortic valve, are at risk. Infection is caused by transient bacteraemia, most frequently after dental extraction or genitourinary investigation or surgery.

Antibiotic cover should be given for all surgical procedures in vulnerable patients. Appropriate regimens are detailed in Appendix IV(d) (p. 733). Cloxacillin or an alternative antistaphylococcal agent should be included in regimens for cardiac surgery.

Role of local and regional anaesthesia in cardiovascular disease

In appropriate patients with cardiovascular disease, local infiltration, or peripheral nerve or plexus blocks provide satisfactory anaesthesia with little risk of side effects. However, local anaesthetic preparations containing adrenaline produce tachycardia and should be avoided in patients with severe cardiovascular disease.

Patients undergoing lower abdominal, pelvic or lower limb surgery may be managed satisfactorily with low subarachnoid or extradural anaesthesia. With higher blocks, sympathetic block produces vasodilatation, reducing preload and afterload on the heart. While controlled vasodilatation may have beneficial effects in ischaemic heart disease, hypertension and cardiac failure, patients anaesthetised with subarachnoid or extradural blockade must be managed very carefully in respect of posture, fluid preloading and replacement to avoid undue hypotension. The sympathetic blockade may produce severe hypotension in patients with untreated hypertension, low cardiac output states, constrictive pericarditis, severe valvular disease or a fixed heart rate resulting from heart block or β-blocker therapy. However, patients with congestive cardiac failure may benefit from the preload reduction caused by sympathetic block, and patients with peripheral vascular disease may benefit from peripheral vasodilatation.

High subarachnoid or extradural blockade is contraindicated in patients with cardiovascular disease.

By and large, for anaesthetists with little experience in regional anaesthesia, SAB and extradural blocks should be avoided in patients with severe cardiac disease.

RESPIRATORY DISEASE

Successful anaesthetic management of the patient with respiratory disease is dependent on accurate assessment of the nature and extent of functional impairment, and an appreciation of the effects surgery may have on pulmonary function.

Assessment

History

Of the six cardinal symptoms of respiratory disease (cough, sputum, haemoptysis, dyspnoea, wheeze and chest pain) dyspnoea provides the best indication of functional impairment. Specific questioning is required to elicit the extent to which activity is limited by dyspnoea. Dyspnoea at rest or on minor exertion clearly indicates severe disease. A cough productive of purulent sputum indicates active infection. Chronic copious sputum production may indicate bronchiectasis. A history of heavy smoking or occupational exposure to dust may suggest pulmonary pathology.

A detailed drug history is important. Long-term steroid therapy within three months of the date of surgery necessitates high-dose cover for the perioperative period and may cause hypokalaemia. Bronchodilators should be continued during the perioperative period. Patients with cor pulmonale may be receiving digoxin and diuretics.

Examination

A full physical examination is required with emphasis on detecting signs of airways obstruction, increased work of breathing, active infection which can be treated preoperatively, and evidence of right heart failure. Presence of obesity, cyanosis or dyspnoea is noted. In addition, a simple forced expiratory manoeuvre may reveal prolonged expiration.

Investigations

Chest X-ray. The preoperative chest X-ray is a poor indicator of functional impairment but is important for several reasons:

1. As a baseline for assessing postoperative radiographs.
2. To discover any localised disease of lungs and pleura not detected on clinical examination, e.g. neoplasm, collapse, consolidation, effusion.
3. To reveal underlying generalised lung disease in patients presenting with acute pulmonary symptoms, e.g. pulmonary fibrosis, emphysema.

ECG. This may indicate right atrial or ventricular hypertrophy (P pulmonale in II; dominant R wave in III, V_{1-3}) while associated ischaemic heart disease is common.

Haematology. Polycythaemia occurs secondary to chronic hypoxaemia, while anaemia aggravates tissue hypoxia. Leucocytosis may indicate active infection.

Sputum culture is essential in patients with chronic lung disease or suspected acute infection.

Pulmonary function tests (see Appendix XI, p. 75). Peak expiratory flow rate, forced expiratory volume in 1 s ($FEV_{1.0}$), and forced vital capacity (FVC) may be measured easily at the bedside. The $FEV_{1.0}$:FVC ratio is decreased in obstructive lung disease and normal in restrictive disease. In the presence of obstructive disease, the test should be repeated 5–10 min after administration of a bronchodilator aerosol to provide an indication of reversibility.

Fuller investigation involves measurement of FRC, RV and TLC.

Blood gas measurement is indicated where the pulmonary function tests are markedly abnormal, for example, in obstructive disease where the $FEV_{1.0}$ is less than 1.5 litres. A raised Pa_{CO_2} is a prognostic indication that pulmonary complications are likely to develop postoperatively. With a Pa_{CO_2} of 6.7 kPa (50 mmHg) or greater, elective postoperative ventilation may be required after all but minor surgery. The combination of a low preoperative Pa_{O_2} and dyspnoea at rest is associated with a high risk of the need for elective ventilation after abdominal surgery.

Effects of anaesthesia and surgery

Fitness for anaesthesia and surgery in patients with respiratory disease depends on the type and magnitude of surgery. The effects of anaesthesia alone on respiratory function are generally minor and short-lived, but may tip the balance towards respiratory failure in patients with severe disease. These effects include mucosal irritation by anaesthetic agents, ciliary paralysis, introduction of infection by aspiration or tracheal intubation and respiratory depression by relaxants, opioid analgesics or volatile anaesthetic agents. In addition, anaesthesia is associated with a decrease in FRC, especially in the elderly and in obese patients, which leads to basal airways closure and shunting of blood through underventilated areas of lung. This effect resolves within a few hours after anaesthesia.

Following thoracic and upper abdominal surgery the decrease in FRC is more profound and persists for 5–10 days after surgery with a parallel increase in $(A-a)P_{O_2}$ (see Fig. 24.3). Complications including atelectasis and pneumonia occur in approximately 20% of these patients. Clearly patients with pre-existing respiratory disease are at much greater risk undergoing upper abdominal rather than limb, head and neck or lower abdominal surgery.

Chronic obstructive airways disease

Chronic bronchitis is characterised by the presence of productive cough for three months in two successive years. Airways obstruction is caused by bronchial oedema and hypersecretion of mucus. In the postoperative period, pulmonary atelectasis and pneumonia result if sputum is not cleared. Chronic airways disease may be classified into two groups: the bronchitic group (blue bloaters) and the emphysematous group (pink puffers), although in practice most patients have mixed pathologies. The former group is characterised by hypoxaemia, hypercapnia and right ventricular failure while patients in the latter group are usually markedly dyspnoeic.

Preoperative management

This should include:

1. Detection and treatment of active infection. Ampicillin, amoxycillin, trimethoprim or co-trimoxazole are usually appropriate, the common infecting organisms being *Str. pneumoniae* and *H. influenzae*. Sputum for culture and sensitivities should be obtained to allow appropriate choice of antibiotic. Chest physiotherapy and humidification of inspired gases aid expectoration.

2. Treatment of airway obstruction. Some patients respond to bronchodilator therapy, either β_2-agonist (e.g. salbutamol), anticholinergic agent (e.g. ipratropium bromide), or phosphodiesterase inhibitor (e.g. aminophylline). Existing bronchodilator therapy should be continued perioperatively, while in patients not receiving bronchodilators a trial of oral aminophylline (Phyllocontin) 225 mg b.d. and salbutamol 200 μg or ipratropium 40 μg (2 puffs) by inhalation may decrease airways obstruction. Steroids may occasionally improve airways obstruction.

3. Chest X-ray examination to exclude spontaneous pneumothorax or emphysematous bullae.

4. Treatment of congestive cardiac failure. Biventricular failure resulting from concurrent ischaemic heart disease and cor pulmonale frequently complicates chronic pulmonary disease. Digoxin and diuretics are indicated.

5. Obese patients. Weight reduction should be encouraged before elective surgery.

6. Ideally, smoking should be stopped for 6 weeks before elective surgery.

Premedication. Opioids should be avoided if severe disease exists. Atropine is useful if copious secretions are present. Diazepam is satisfactory to allay anxiety.

Regional anaesthesia

Regional anaesthesia for operations on head, neck or limbs offers freedom from respiratory side effects, while avoiding the complications of general anaesthesia. Low subarachnoid or extradural anaesthesia for lower abdominal and pelvic surgery have a similar advantage. However, if the block is sufficiently high to affect the intercostal muscles, peak expiratory flow rate is reduced and the ability to expectorate is impaired. Overall, the morbidity resulting from general anaesthesia for such operations is low, and it is only, perhaps, in the respiratory cripple that any significant advantage accrues from the use of a regional technique. In these patients, sedation should be kept to a minimum.

In upper abdominal and thoracic surgery, where

changes in respiratory function are more profound and prolonged, there is no evidence that extradural anaesthesia is associated with a lower morbidity than general anaesthesia. The advantages accruing from avoidance of volatile anaesthetics, muscle relaxants and opioids are balanced by the effect of extradural blockade on expiratory muscles, decreasing vital capacity. However, the use of extradural analgesia postoperatively may reduce postoperative hypoxaemia by diminishing the decrease in FRC, and result in fewer pulmonary complications.

General anaesthesia

Two approaches may be taken in the presence of severe chronic obstructive disease:

1. *Elective spontaneous ventilation*. This involves using minimal sedation, avoiding opioid analgesics and maintaining spontaneous ventilation, usually with a face mask. Tolerance to tracheal intubation is improved by spraying the larynx with local anaesthetic solution. Analgesia is provided best by a local or regional technique.
2. *Elective artificial ventilation*. A deliberate decision is made to undertake IPPV during anaesthesia and for a variable period after operation, and at least until elimination of muscle relaxants and anaesthetic agents has occurred. This also permits optimal provision of analgesia without fear of opioid-induced depression of ventilation. This technique is usually preferred if the preoperative Pa is greater than 6.7 kPa (50 mmHg) or if major thoracic or abdominal surgery is planned.

Intravenous fluid should be administered with care during the perioperative period. After surgery, salt and water retention occurs, and in combination with overenthusiastic fluid administration, and perhaps a decrease in cardiac output, may result in an increase in lung water which in turn may cause small airway closure, and hypoxaemia.

There is an increased risk of pneumothorax, especially if high inflation pressures are used.

Postoperative care

Elective postoperative controlled ventilation allows adequate oxygenation, analgesia without respiratory depression, clearance of secretions by physiotherapy, tracheal suction and, if necessary, fibreoptic bronchoscopy. Cardiac output and peripheral perfusion may be optimised and fluid overload corrected before restoration of spontaneous ventilation. Unless there is pre-existing pulmonary infection, a period of 24 h elective controlled ventilation is usually adequate. Institution of analgesia by regional (e.g. intercostal, paravertebral, or extradural) blockade often allows earlier return to spontaneous ventilation when the respiratory depressant effects of anaesthetics and relaxants have terminated.

Oxygen. With spontaneous ventilation, controlled oxygen is required using a 24% or 28% Ventimask with frequent checks on arterial blood gases to ensure an adequate Pa_{O_2}(> 8 kPa) without excessive CO_2 retention (Pa_{CO_2} < 7.5–8 kPa). Hypoxaemia may seriously aggravate existing pulmonary hypertension, and precipitate right ventricular failure.

Analgesia. Simple, non-opioid analgesics, and/or local and regional techniques should be used if possible. Fifty per cent nitrous oxide in oxygen (Entonox) is useful for physiotherapy and painful procedures. Opioid analgesics are best administered, where necessary, in small i.v. doses, e.g. morphine 2 mg, under direct supervision.

Physiotherapy, bronchodilators and antibiotics should be continued postoperatively. Doxapram by infusion (2 mg/kg over a period of 30 min to 4 h) may decrease marginally the extent of postoperative alveolar collapse and infection, although the evidence for this is controversial.

A technique of percutaneous cricothyroid puncture and insertion of a small-diameter tube into the trachea (minitracheotomy) permits aspiration of secretions while preserving the ability of the patient to cough and speak. However, a number of potentially serious complications, including severe haemorrhage, have been reported.

The application of continuous positive airway pressure (CPAP) via a close-fitting facemask in the spontaneously breathing patient increases FRC and reduces the incidence of atelectasis in postoperative patients with pulmonary disease. It may reduce the need for mechanical ventilation, although it is not tolerated well by all patients.

Restrictive lung disease

This category includes a wide range of conditions which affect the lung and chest wall. Lung diseases include sarcoidosis and fibrosing alveolitis, while lesions of chest wall include kyphoscoliosis and ankylosing spondylitis. Pulmonary function tests reveal a decrease in both $FEV_{1.0}$ and FVC with a normal $FEV_{1.0}$/FVC ratio and a decreased FRC and TLC. Small airways closure occurs during tidal ventilation, with resultant shunting and hypoxaemia. Lung or chest wall compliance is decreased; thus work of breathing is increased and the ability to cough and clear secretions impaired. There is an increased risk of postoperative pulmonary infection.

Anaesthesia causes little additional decrease in lung volumes, and is tolerated well provided hypoxaemia is avoided. Postoperatively, however, inadequate basal ventilation and retention of secretions may occur, partly as a result of pain, opioid analgesics and the residual effects of anaesthetic agents. High concentrations of oxygen may be used without risk of respiratory depression. A short period of mechanical ventilation may be necessary in patients with severe disease to allow adequate analgesia and clearing of secretions. High extradural anaesthesia should be avoided in these patients since it causes a further reduction in VC.

Bronchiectasis

The patient should be admitted several days before surgery and regular postural drainage carried out. Appropriate antibiotics, based on sputum culture, should be prescribed. Disease localised in one lung should be isolated using a double-lumen tube.

Bronchial carcinoma

Patients with bronchial carcinoma frequently suffer from coexisting chronic bronchitis. In addition, there is frequently infection and collapse of the lung distal to the tumour. Patients with bronchial carcinoma may have a myasthenic syndrome (see p. 674), while oat cell tumours may secrete a number of hormones, among the commonest being ACTH, producing Cushing's syndrome, and ADH, producing dilutional hyponatraemia.

Tuberculosis

Tuberculosis should be considered in patients with persistent pulmonary infection, especially if associated with haemoptysis or weight loss. If active disease is present, all anaesthetic equipment should be sterilised after use to avoid cross-infection of other patients.

Bronchial asthma

This common disease, which affects all age groups, is characterised by recurrent generalised airways obstruction, caused by bronchial smooth muscle spasm, mucous plugs and bronchial oedema. Asthma may be classified into two types: *extrinsic*, where an external allergen is demonstrable, and *intrinsic*. Intrinsic asthma tends to occur in adults, is more chronic and continuous and often requires long-term steroid therapy.

Preoperative management

The current state of the patient's disease is assessed by:

1. History: frequency and severity of attacks, factors provoking attacks, drug history.
2. Examination: presence or absence of rhonchi, prolonged expiratory phase, overdistension, evidence of infection.
3. Pulmonary function testing: $FEV_{1.0}$/FVC before and after inhalation of bronchodilator. Blood gas analysis may be required in severe disease.

Elective surgery should not be undertaken until asthma is well controlled. This involves the use of one or more of a number of drugs: sodium cromoglycate, to control the allergic component;

bronchodilators (phosphodiesterase inhibitors, e.g. aminophylline, and β_2-adrenoceptor agonists, e.g. salbutamol) and steroids, systemic or inhaled. Pulmonary infection requires treatment where appropriate. An appropriate bronchodilator regimen in the preoperative period comprises salbutamol 200 μg (2 puffs) 4 times daily by inhaler, possibly in combination with oral aminophylline (Phyllocontin) 225 mg b.d. Patients with intrinsic asthma sometimes respond well to ipratropium bromide, an anticholinergic agent, 40 μg (2 puffs) by inhaler. A dose of bronchodilator should be given with the premedication 1 h before induction of anaesthesia.

Patients with severe asthma, who are receiving topical or systemic steroid therapy, or not responding to conventional bronchodilator therapy, require systemic steroid therapy to cover the anaesthetic and postoperative periods. Prednisolone 40–100 mg daily may be given preoperatively, hydrocortisone 100 mg i.m. with premedication, and 100 mg 4 times daily for the first postoperative day. An equivalent dose of oral prednisolone (Table 41.3) should be substituted when oral intake is resumed, and the dose reduced gradually as the severity of asthma permits.

Premedication should consist of a sedative agent, e.g. diazepam, with atropine to block vagal reflex-induced bronchospasm. Pethidine and promethazine are also satisfactory.

Anaesthesia

The volatile agents halothane and ether are bronchodilators, and therefore well tolerated. Bronchoconstriction may be triggered by tracheal intubation or by surgical stimuli during light anaesthesia. The larynx and trachea should be sprayed with local anaesthetic and adequate depth of anaesthesia maintained. Drugs which are associated with histamine release (*d*-tubocurarine and morphine) are best avoided; vecuronium and pethidine or fentanyl are preferable. β-Blocking drugs should also be avoided.

With controlled ventilation, a prolonged expiratory phase is required if there is evidence of severe airways obstruction; the inspiratory time should be adequate to avoid unduly high inflation pressures. Pneumothorax is a possible complication and requires early detection and prompt drainage. Humidification is necessary if ventilation is prolonged.

If bronchospasm occurs, aminophylline 250–500 mg or salbutamol 125–250 μg should be administered by slow i.v. injection under ECG monitoring. Thereafter an infusion of aminophylline, up to 5 mg/kg 6-hourly, or salbutamol, possibly in combination with nebulised salbutamol by positive pressure ventilation (solution of 50–100 μg per ml of water) should be maintained until improvement occurs. Intravenous hydrocortisone 100–200 mg should be given simultaneously, although it has no immediate effect. Intravenous ketamine has also been used with success when other agents have failed to relieve acute bronchospasm.

Postoperative management consists of close respiratory monitoring, continued treatment of bronchospasm and provision of adequate analgesia, humidified oxygen and physiotherapy. Salbutamol is administered best by nebulisation (2.5 mg in 2.5 ml saline 4–6-hourly) and aminophylline by i.v. infusion (0.5–0.8 mg kg^{-1} h^{-1}. There is no loss of carbon dioxide responsiveness in asthmatic patients and high inspired oxygen concentrations are tolerated well.

GASTROINTESTINAL DISEASE

Dysphagia

Patients with dysphagia resulting from oesophageal stricture or achalasia may be severely malnourished and fluid-depleted. Fluid and electrolyte depletion should be corrected preoperatively, and anaesthetic drug dosage should be reduced appropriately to avoid hypotension at induction of anaesthesia.

There may be a considerable quantity of food debris in the oesophagus, and the usual precautions should be taken to avoid regurgitation and aspiration at induction.

Hiatus hernia

There is a risk of regurgitation and inhalation of gastric contents, especially in obese patients. In addition to the usual measures to avoid aspiration, administration of a histamine H_2-receptor antagonist, e.g. ranitidine, together with 0.3 M sodium citrate 30 ml 5 min before induction may decrease the risk of pneumonitis if aspiration occurs.

Intestinal obstruction

The principal anaesthetic problems in these patients are extreme fluid and electrolyte depletion with consequent risk of cardiovascular collapse on induction of anaesthesia, and the increased risk of vomiting and inhalation of gastric contents. A large nasogastric tube should be used to empty the stomach as effectively as possible before induction. The tube itself should be removed to allow effective cricoid pressure to be applied.

Patients who have severe vomiting and diarrhoea also pose problems in relation to fluid and electrolyte depletion. All such patients undergoing surgery require appropriate fluid and electrolyte replacement preoperatively; the volume and composition depend on blood urea and electrolyte measurements and CVP monitoring.

Subarachnoid and extradural anaesthesia should be avoided if significant fluid depletion is suspected.

LIVER DISEASE

Anaesthesia and surgery may affect liver function adversely even in previously normal patients. In addition, liver dysfunction may have effects on the conduct of anaesthesia, for example on the metabolism of anaesthetic drugs.

Preoperative assessment should be directed towards detection of jaundice, ascites, oedema and signs of hepatic failure (encephalopathy with flapping tremor). Routine preoperative investigations should include a coagulation screen, measurement of haemoglobin concentration, white cell and platelet counts, and concentrations of serum bilirubin, alkaline phosphatase, transaminase, urea, electrolytes, proteins (including albumin) and blood sugar. Blood should also be taken for detection of hepatitis B antigen. If positive, appropriate measures must be taken to protect theatre staff from possible contamination.

Particular problems relevant to the anaesthetist include:

1. ***Acid–base and fluid balance.*** Many patients are overloaded with fluid. Hypoalbuminaemia results in oedema and ascites, and predisposes to pulmonary oedema. Secondary hyperaldosteronism produces sodium retention and hypokalaemia. Diuretic therapy, often including spironolactone, may also affect serum potassium concentration. In hepatic failure, a combined respiratory and metabolic alkalosis may occur, which shifts the oxygen dissociation curve to the left, impairing tissue oxygenation.
2. ***Hepatorenal syndrome.*** Jaundiced patients are at risk of developing postoperative renal failure. This may be precipitated by hypovolaemia. Prevention involves adequate preoperative hydration, with i.v. infusion for at least 12 h before surgery, and close monitoring of urine output, intra- and postoperatively. Intravenous 20% mannitol 100 ml is recommended immediately preoperatively, and is indicated postoperatively if the hourly urine output decreases below 50 ml. Close cardiovascular monitoring is essential.
3. ***Bleeding problems.*** Production of clotting factors II, VII, IX and X is reduced as a result of decreased vitamin K absorption. Production of factor V and fibrinogen is also reduced. Thrombocytopenia occurs if portal hypertension is present. Vitamin K should be administered and fresh frozen plasma given to cover surgery, with regular checks made on coagulation. Infusion of platelet concentrate is indicated to cover surgery in cases of severe thrombocytopenia or if there is overt bleeding in a thrombocytopenic patient.
4. ***Drug metabolism.*** Impairment of liver function slows elimination of drugs including anaesthetic induction agents, opioid analgesics, benzodiazepines, suxamethonium, local anaesthetic agents and many others. Since the duration of action of many of these is determined initially by redistribution, prolongation of action may not become apparent until a subsequent dose has been given. Altered plasma protein concentrations affect drug binding, and may account for resistance to *d*-tubocurarine and pancuronium in liver failure.

In addition, a large number of drugs have toxic effects on the liver. Rarely, halothane is associated with postoperative hepatitis, usually when administered more than once within a period of a few weeks. The mechanism appears to be induction of reductive enzymes in the liver, which, in the presence of hypoxia, causes an increase in hepatotoxic reductive metabolites. A single halothane anaesthetic is safe in patients with liver disease provided cardiac output and hepatic blood flow are not depressed unduly. Halothane should not be employed within 3 months of a previous halothane anaesthetic, or if there is a history of unexplained jaundice after any previous halothane anaesthetic. If postoperative jaundice occurs, other causes should be sought before accepting a diagnosis of halothane hepatitis.

5. ***Hepatic failure.*** In such patients, all sedative drugs should be administered with extreme care, as they aggravate encephalopathy. All opioids and benzodiazepines are eliminated by the liver. Benzodiazepines are probably the best sedatives to use in small doses, the short-acting midazolam being first choice. Patients with hepatic failure require intensive management, including close metabolic, fluid and electrolyte monitoring. Hypoglycaemia, which occurs as a result of depleted liver glycogen stores, should be avoided by the administration of glucose infusion, and sodium intake should be restricted. Amino acids, fat emulsions and fructose should be avoided. Mechanical ventilation is often required, and this diminishes the risks of sedative administration.

Conduct of anaesthesia

If liver function is severely impaired, no premedication should be given. Otherwise, a light benzodiazepine premedication is suitable.

The liver is particularly vulnerable to hypotension and hypoxia. During anaesthesia, cardiac output should be maintained as stable as possible. Blood loss should be replaced promptly, and overall fluid balance maintained with CVP monitoring. Drugs which depress cardiac output, including halothane, enflurane, isoflurane and β-blockers, should be used with caution to avoid decreasing hepatic blood flow unduly.

Vecuronium and atracurium are the muscle relaxants of choice because of their cardiovascular stability and short duration of action; atracurium may prove to be preferable because its elimination is independent of liver and renal function. Opioid analgesic drugs should be administered with caution unless ventilatory support is planned postoperatively. Pethidine may be preferable to morphine, and is best titrated initially against pain in small i.v. doses, e.g. 20 mg, in the immediate postoperative period.

Controlled ventilation to a normal Pa_{CO_2} is important, as hypocapnia is associated with decreased hepatic blood flow. Hypoxaemia should be avoided throughout, with blood gas monitoring if necessary into the postoperative period.

RENAL DISEASE

Renal dysfunction has a number of important implications for anaesthesia, and therefore full assessment is required before even minor surgical procedures are contemplated.

Measurement of blood urea and electrolyte concentrations should be undertaken before all major surgery and in all elderly or potentially unhealthy patients; a raised blood urea demonstrated preoperatively may be the first indication of renal disease. Severity of renal dysfunction may be assessed further by measurement of serum creatinine and creatinine clearance, urinary:plasma osmolality ratio and urinary urea and electrolyte excretion.

Preanaesthetic assessment of the patient should be directed to a number of specific problems which require correction before embarking on anaesthesia:

1. *Fluid balance.* In both acute and chronic renal failure, fluid overload may occur. In acute failure, the overload develops suddenly and is uncompensated. In chronic failure, overload may be controlled with diuretic therapy or dialysis. Congestive cardiac failure and hypertension may result from overload, and must be treated before induction of anaesthesia. This may require dialysis or haemofiltration.

In patients with nephrotic syndrome, hypoalbuminaemia results in oedema and ascites. Circulating blood volume in these patients is often decreased, and care should be taken at induction of anaesthesia to avoid hypotension.

2. *Electrolyte disturbances.* Sodium retention occurs in renal failure, and through increased

secretion of ADH is associated with water retention, oedema and hypertension. Hyponatraemia is common also in renal disease. It is caused usually by reduced renal tubular ability to conserve sodium, e.g. in pyelonephritis or analgesic nephropathy. Hyponatraemia occurs also in patients with renal failure as a result of vomiting and diarrhoea or diuretic therapy.

Hyperkalaemia occurs typically in renal failure, frequently in association with metabolic acidosis. A raised serum potassium may be controlled in the short term by infusion of glucose and insulin: 80 ml of 50% glucose, with 20 units of soluble insulin may be given for acute control, followed by an infusion of 50% glucose with insulin as required using a modified sliding scale governed by BM-test blood sugar estimation. In the longer term, correction of the metabolic acidosis with sodium bicarbonate, and administration of an ion-exchange resin, e.g. calcium polystyrene sulphonate in a dose of 15 g t.i.d. orally or as a 30 g retention enema, are useful in controlling hyperkalaemia. Administration of calcium chloride antagonises the cardiac effects of potassium. Dialysis is required if these measures are ineffective. Suxamethonium should be avoided in hyperkalaemic patients in view of its effect of releasing potassium from muscle cells. An increase of up to 0.6 mmol/litre may be expected in normal dosage. Hyperkalaemia is associated with delayed myocardial conduction and ultimately cardiac arrest.

Hypokalaemia commonly occurs in patients receiving diuretic therapy. These patients require preoperative measurement of serum potassium, and replacement if necessary. Hypokalaemia is associated with ventricular irritability, notably in patients taking digoxin.

3. *Cardiovascular effects.* Hypertension may occur for a number of reasons. A raised plasma renin concentration occurring as a result of decreased perfusion of the juxtaglomerular apparatus results in hypertension through increased secretion of angiotensin and aldosterone.

Fluid retention also causes hypertension by increasing the circulating blood volume. Conversely, hypertension from other causes results in renal impairment. The precise cause of hypertension in these patients should be sought and the hypertension treated. Anaesthesia for hypertensive patients is discussed on page 647.

Both pulmonary and peripheral oedema may occur from a combination of fluid overload, hypertensive cardiac disease and hypoproteinaemia. Cardiac failure should be treated preoperatively.

Uraemia may cause pericarditis and a haemorrhagic pericardial effusion, which may embarrass cardiac output and require aspiration.

4. *Neurological effects.* Uraemia causes drowsiness and eventually coma. Electrolyte disturbances and rapid fluid shifts, e.g. during dialysis, may also affect conscious level. Sedative drugs including morphine should be used with care in these patients. In addition, a combined motor and sensory peripheral neuropathy may occur in uraemic patients.

5. *Haematology.* Patients with chronic renal failure suffer from normochromic anaemia, which results from marrow depression, partly as a result of erythropoietin deficiency. They also have an increased incidence of gastrointestinal bleeding and so an iron deficiency component may be present. These patients are well compensated, with an increased cardiac output; excessive preoperative blood transfusion should be avoided.

6. *Other factors.* Patients with chronic renal failure are frequently undernourished. They tend to be vulnerable to infection. Patients who have received a renal transplant and are immunosuppressed are particularly vulnerable to low-grade pathogens, e.g. *Pneumocystis carinii.* Patients undergoing chronic haemodialysis are not infrequently carriers of hepatitis-B antigen, and if so appropriate precautions should be taken by theatre staff.

7. *Drug treatment.* Many patients with renal disease are receiving diuretics, antihypertensive therapy, including β-blockers, and digoxin. The doses of drugs excreted renally, e.g. digoxin and aminoglycoside antibiotics, should be reduced; monitoring of plasma concentrations is useful in determining appropriate dosage.

Anaesthesia

A light premedication with benzodiazepine or opioid analgesic is satisfactory. Minor procedures, e.g. to establish vascular access for dialysis, are carried out most satisfactorily under regional anaesthesia; brachial plexus block for upper limb and combined femoral and sciatic block for lower limb.

Patients who suffer from acute renal failure, and those on long-term dialysis for chronic renal failure, may require dialysis before surgery to correct fluid overload, acid-base disturbances and hyperkalaemia. Ideally, there should be some delay before surgery to allow correction of anticoagulation.

The i.v. cannula for induction and fluid infusion should be sited in the contralateral limb from the arteriovenous shunt or fistula (in those patients undergoing dialysis) and care should be taken to protect the shunt during the operation. Careful monitoring of arterial pressure and ECG is required, and CVP measurement is indicated in patients who are clinically fluid-overloaded. Intravenous fluid administration should be cautious, and in some instances titrated against CVP measurements. Excessive sodium administration should be avoided, and potassium-containing solutions avoided completely in renal failure. If the patient is anaemic preoperatively, intraoperative blood loss should be replaced promptly.

Drugs excreted primarily via the kidneys should be used with caution in renal failure. In anaesthetic practice, the principal drugs involved are the muscle relaxants. Atracurium (elimination of which is independent of kidney and liver function, and which has minimal cardiovascular effects) would appear to be the relaxant of choice. All other relaxants depend to some extent on renal elimination and should be avoided. In addition other drugs including morphine are conjugated in the liver before excretion in the urine. Depending on the activity of the conjugated metabolite, these drugs may have adverse effects following repeated doses. Morphine-6-glucuronide, and active metabolite of morphine, accumulates in renal failure and may result in prolongation of clinical effects after administration of morphine.

Methoxyflurane should be avoided in renal impairment, as the concentrating ability of the kidney is reduced by the effect of fluoride ion on the distal tubule. Enflurane is also metabolised to fluoride ion, although to a much lesser extent and should be used with caution in patients with severe renal impairment.

Postoperative renal failure

This is not infrequently a problem in patients undergoing major surgery which involves large blood loss, in surgery following trauma and in septic patients. Avoidance of renal failure in these patients involves close monitoring of the cardiovascular state including CVP and urinary output, avoidance of hypotension, adequate fluid and blood replacement and the use of low-dose dopamine infusion. Inotropic support may be required to maintain adequate cardiac output. Jaundiced patients are also at risk of developing acute renal failure — the hepatorenal syndrome.

Stimulation of urinary output by an osmotic diuretic (mannitol 100 ml of 20% solution over 15 min and repeated once if no response occurs), followed by dopamine 2–5 μg kg^{-1} min^{-1} by infusion should be undertaken if no diuresis occurs after correction of fluid depletion and attainment of cardiovascular stability. If severe fluid overload exists, high-dose i.v. frusemide should also be given.

Postoperative oliguria may also be the result of postrenal causes. Patients with prostatic enlargement are particularly liable to develop acute retention. Examination to exclude a full bladder, and catheterisation, should always be carried out in the anuric postoperative patient.

CONNECTIVE TISSUE DISORDERS

Rheumatoid arthritis

Rheumatoid arthritis is a multisystem disease, with a number of implications for anaesthesia which must be considered on preoperative assessment:

1. *Airway problems.* The arthritic process may involve the temporomandibular joints, rendering laryngoscopy and intubation difficult. The cervical spine may be fixed, or subluxed, and thus unstable, especially when the patient is anaesthetised and paralysed. Crico-arytenoid involvement should be suspected if hoarseness or stridor is present.

2. *Respiratory function.* Costochondral involvement causes a restrictive defect with reduced vital capacity. Pulmonary involvement with interstitial

fibrosis produces $\dot{V}/\dot{Q}$ abnormalities, a diffusion defect and thus hypoxaemia.

3. *Cardiovascular system.* Endocardial and myocardial involvement may occur. Coronary arteritis, conduction defects and peripheral arteritis are other features. Immobility caused by arthritis may mask symptoms of cardiorespiratory disease.

4. *Anaemia.* A chronic anaemia, hypo- or normochromic, but refractory iron, occurs. Preoperative transfusion to approximately 10 g/dl is advisable before major surgery. Treatment with salicylates or other non-steroidal anti-inflammatory drugs may cause gastrointestinal blood loss.

5. *Renal failure,* or nephrotic syndrome, may occur as a result of amyloidosis.

6. *Steroid therapy.* Many patients are receiving long-term steroid therapy and require augmented steroid cover for the perioperative period (see p. 667). They are more vulnerable to postoperative infection. Thus, routine preoperative investigation should include full blood count, urea and electrolytes, chest X-ray and ECG. Other investigations, e.g. pulmonary function tests and cervical spine X-rays, may be required in certain instances.

Conduct of anaesthesia

Particular care should be taken with venepuncture and placing of i.v. infusions because of atrophy of skin and subcutaneous tissues and fragility of veins. Careful positioning of the patient on the operating table is required since these patients may have multiple joint involvement. Padding may be required to prevent pressure sores.

The anaesthetist should be prepared for difficult intubation, and spinal, extradural or regional techniques are useful for many limb or lower abdominal operations because they obviate the need for tracheal intubation.

Other collagen diseases

Scleroderma

Scleroderma (systemic sclerosis) is characterised by many of the above features including restricted mouth opening, lower oesophageal involvement with increased risk of regurgitation, pulmonary involvement, renal failure, steroid therapy and peripheral vascular disease.

Systemic lupus erythematosus

Anaemia, renal and respiratory involvement may be severe. Steroid therapy is usual.

Polyarteritis

There is diffuse vasculitis, with possible coronary involvement, and neuropathy. Pulmonary involvement and steroid therapy are additional problems.

Ankylosing spondylitis

The rigid spine makes intubation difficult, and spinal and extradural anaesthesia may be technically impossible. Costovertebral joint involvement restricts chest expansion.

Marfan's syndrome

This is a disorder of connective tissue of autosomal dominant inheritance, which is characterised by long, thin extremities, high arched palate, lens subluxation and aortic and mitral regurgitation. Regurgitation may be severe, and the valve lesions may be complicated by subacute bacterial endocarditis. Antibiotic cover is necessary therefore for dental and other surgical procedures.

NUTRITIONAL PROBLEMS

Obesity

Obesity poses a number of problems to the anaesthetist and surgeon:

1. *Cardiovascular function.* Obesity is associated with increased blood volume, cardiac work, hypertension and cardiomegaly. Atherosclerosis and coronary artery disease are common. Diabetes may coexist.

2. *Respiratory function.* Vital capacity and functional residual capacity are decreased. Closing volume is increased. As a result, increased shunting occurs through underventilated dependent lung regions with consequent hypoxaemia. These changes, brought about by abdominal splinting of the diaphragm, are accentuated in the supine,

Trendelenburg and lithotomy positions. Lung/chest wall compliance is decreased, the work of breathing increased, and increased oxygen consumption and CO_2 production cause hyperventilation.

3. *Other factors*. Surgery is technically more difficult, with heavy blood loss, and increased incidences of wound infection and wound dehiscence. Hiatus hernia with risk of regurgitation is more common, and maintenance of the airway and tracheal intubation may be more difficult.

Obese patients require careful preoperative respiratory and cardiovascular assessment (see p. 340). The inspired oxygen concentration should be increased to 40%. Fluid balance should be monitored carefully. Elective postoperative ventilation should be considered, especially after abdominal surgery. Pulmonary, thromboembolic and wound complications are more common, and appropriate prophylactic measures and/or early recognition and treatment are important.

Pickwickian syndrome

Pickwickian syndrome is characterised by a combination of obesity, episodic somnolence and hypoventilation with cyanosis, polycythaemia, pulmonary hypertension and right ventricular failure. Avoidance of hypoxia is important, and elective postoperative ventilation may be necessary, especially after abdominal surgery.

Malnutrition

As a result of persistent anorexia, dysphagia or vomiting, malnourished patients may be severely fluid and electrolyte depleted. Anaemia and hypoproteinaemia are common.

Preoperative correction of fluid and electrolyte deficits is required with CVP monitoring in severe cases. Infusion of albumin may be advisable in some instances to raise the colloid osmotic pressure. Doses of induction agents should be administered carefully to avoid hypotension, while smaller doses of relaxants are required, vecuronium or atracurium being the agent of choice.

ENDOCRINE DISEASE

Pituitary disease

The clinical features of pituitary disease depend on the local effects of the lesion and its effect on the secretion of pituitary hormones. Local effects include headache and visual field disturbances. The effects on hormone secretion depend on the cells involved in the pathological process.

Acromegaly

Acromegaly is caused by increased secretion of growth hormone from eosinophil cell tumours of the anterior pituitary. If this occurs before fusion of the epiphyses, gigantism results. Problems for the anaesthetist include:

1. Upper airway obstruction resulting from an enlarged mandible, tongue and epiglottis, thickened pharyngeal mucosa and laryngeal narrowing. Maintenance of a clear airway and intubation may be difficult, and postoperative care of the airway must be meticulous.
2. Cardiac enlargement, hypertension and congestive cardiac failure occur commonly and require preoperative treatment.
3. Growth hormone increases blood sugar. Hyperglycaemia should be controlled perioperatively.
4. Thyroid and adrenal function may be impaired because of decreased release of TSH and ACTH. Thyroxine and steroid replacement may be required.

Treatment involves hypophysectomy which requires steroid cover preoperatively, and steroid, thyroxine and possibly ADH replacement thereafter.

Cushing's disease

Cushing's disease results from basophil adenomas, which secrete ACTH (vide infra).

Hypopituitarism (Simmonds disease)

Causes include infarction following postpartum haemorrhage, chromophobe adenoma, tumours of surrounding tissues (e.g. craniopharyngioma), skull fractures and infection. Clinical features include loss of axillary and pubic hair, amenorrhoea, features of hypothyroidism and adrenal insufficiency, including hypotension, but with a striking pallor in contrast with the pigmentation of Addison's disease (see p. 666).

The fluid and electrolyte disturbances are not as marked as in primary adrenal failure as a result of intact aldosterone production, but may be unmasked by surgery, trauma or infection.

Anaesthesia in these patients requires steroid cover (p. 667), cautious administration of induction agent and volatile anaesthetic agents, and careful cardiovascular monitoring. Vecuronium or atracurium is probably the relaxant of choice.

Diabetes insipidus

This is caused by disease or damage affecting the hypothalamic–posterior pituitary axis. Commonest causes are pituitary tumours, craniopharyngiomas, basal skull fracture, infection, or as a sequel to pituitary surgery.

Dehydration follows excretion of large volumes of dilute urine. Patients require fluid replacement and treatment with vasopressin (DDAVP — desmopressin 2–4 μg i.m. daily).

Thyroid disease

Goitre

Thyroid swelling may result from iodine deficiency (simple goitre), autoimmune (Hashimoto's) thyroiditis, adenoma, carcinoma or thyrotoxicosis. Nodules of the thyroid gland may be 'hot' (secreting thyroxine) or 'cold'.

The goitre may occasionally cause respiratory obstruction. Retrosternal goitre may in addition cause superior vena caval obstruction. The presence of a goitre should alert the anaesthetist to the possibility of tracheal compression or displacement. A preoperative X-ray of neck and thoracic inlet may be useful, and a selection of small-diameter tracheal tubes should be available. Preoperative assessment of thyroid function is essential.

Thyrotoxicosis

This is characterised by excitability, tremor, tachycardia and arrhythmias (commonly atrial fibrillation), weight loss, heat intolerance and exophthalmos. Diagnosis is confirmed by measurement of total serum thyroxine and T_3 resin uptake.

Elective surgery should not be carried out in hyperthyroid patients; they should first be rendered euthyroid with carbimazole or radioactive iodine. However, urgent surgery and elective subtotal thyroidectomy may be carried out safely in hyperthyroid patients using β-adrenergic blockade alone or in combination with potassium iodide to control thyrotoxic symptoms and signs. Emergency surgery carries a significant risk of thyrotoxic crisis. Control is best achieved in these circumstances by i.v. potassium iodide and β-blockers. If patients are unable to absorb oral medication, i.v. infusion is indicated (for propranolol, the daily i.v. dose is approximately one-tenth of the oral dose).

The dosages of sedative drugs for premedication, and of anaesthetic agents, should be increased to compensate for faster distribution and elimination. Spinal nerve block reduces the effects of hyperthyroidism, provided solutions containing adrenaline are not used. Larger than normal doses of sedative drugs are required to avoid anxiety when procedures are carried out under regional anaesthesia.

Preparation for thyroidectomy. Previous conventional management involved at least 6–8 weeks' administration of carbimazole to render the patient euthyroid, followed by potassium iodide 60 mg t.i.d. for 10 days to decrease the vascularity of the gland.

Many anaesthetists now use β-blockers to prepare the hyperthyroid patient for thyroidectomy. Propranolol 160–480 mg daily for 2 weeks preoperatively and a further 7–10 days postoperatively provides adequate control in most patients. However, control with β-blockers depends on maintaining an adequate plasma concentration of the drug. Since β-blockers, in common with other drugs, are cleared faster in thyrotoxic patients, propranolol should be prescribed more frequently (e.g. 4 times daily). Alternatively, a long-acting β-blocker, e.g. nadolol 160 mg once daily (including the morning of surgery), provides satisfactory control, and avoids the problem of impaired drug absorption immediately after operation. A combination of β-blocker and potassium iodide 60 mg t.i.d provides reliable control in even the most severely thyrotoxic patient.

Hypothyroidism

This may result from primary thyroid failure, Hashimoto's thyroiditis, as a consequence of thyroid surgery, or secondary to pituitary failure. The diagnosis is suggested by tiredness, cold intolerance, loss of appetite, dry skin and hair loss. It may be confirmed by the finding of a low serum thyroxine concentration, associated, in primary thyroid failure, with a raised serum TSH.

Basal metabolic rate is decreased. Cardiac output is decreased, with little myocardial reserve and hypothermia is usually present. Treatment is with thyroxine, which should be started in a small dose of 0.05–0.1 mg daily. Rapid correction of hypothyroidism may be achieved using i.v. triiodothyronine, but this is inadvisable in elderly patients and those with ischaemic heart disease, as the sudden increase in myocardial oxygen demand may provoke infarction. ECG monitoring is advisable.

Elective surgery should be avoided in myxoedematous patients, but if emergency surgery is necessary close cardiovascular, ECG and blood gas monitoring is essential. Drug distribution and metabolism are slowed and thus all anaesthetic agents must be administered in reduced dosage.

Disease of the adrenal cortex

Clinical syndromes are associated with increased and decreased secretion of cortisol or aldosterone.

Hypersecretion of cortisol (Cushing's syndrome)

Most instances are caused by pituitary adenomas which secrete ACTH and thus cause bilateral adrenocortical hyperplasia (Cushing's disease). In 20–30% of patients, an adrenocortical adenoma or carcinoma is present. Rarely, an oat-cell carcinoma of bronchus secreting ACTH is the cause. ACTH or corticosteroid therapy present a similar picture. Clinical features include obesity, hypertension, myopathy, diabetes mellitus and hypokalaemia. Depending on the cause, treatment may involve hypophysectomy or adrenalectomy.

Anaesthetic management of these patients involves preoperative treatment of hypertension and congestive cardiac failure, and correction of hypokalaemia. Intraoperative management is directed towards careful monitoring of arterial pressure, and maintenance of cardiovascular stability, with careful choice and administration of anaesthetic agents and muscle relaxants. Etomidate and atracurium or vecuronium would be an appropriate choice of induction agent and relaxant. Postoperative steroid cover is required for hypophysectomy adrenalectomy (vide infra). Fludrocortisone 0.1–0.3 mg daily is required after bilateral adrenalectomy.

Hypersecretion of aldosterone (Conn's syndrome)

Conn's syndrome is caused by an adenoma of the zona glomerulosa of the adrenal cortex and presents with hypertension, hypernatraemia, hypokalaemia and polyuria. Anaesthetic management involves preoperative treatment of hypertension, the administration of spironolactone and potassium replacement, while intra- and postoperative monitoring of arterial pressure is essential.

Adrenocortical hypofunction

Primary adrenocortical insufficiency (Addison's disease) may be caused by an autoimmune process, tuberculosis, amyloid, metastatic carcinoma, following bilateral adrenalectomy or, acutely, from haemorrhage into the glands in association with meningococcal septicaemia. Secondary failure results from hypopituitarism or prolonged corticosteroid therapy. In secondary failure resulting from pituitary insufficiency, aldosterone secretion is maintained and fluid and electrolyte disturbances less marked.

Clinical features include weakness, weight loss, pigmentation, hypotension, vomiting, diarrhoea and dehydration. Hypoglycaemia, hyponatraemia and hyperkalaemia are characteristic biochemical findings. The stress of infection, trauma or surgery provokes profound hypotension. Diagnosis is made by measurement of plasma cortisol concentrations, the response to ACTH stimulation and to insulin-induced hypoglycaemia.

All surgical procedures in these patients must be covered by increased steroid administration (vide infra). Patients with acute adrenal insufficiency require urgent fluid and sodium replacement with arterial pressure and CVP monitoring, glucose infusion to combat hypoglycaemia and hydrocortisone 100 mg 6-hourly i.v. Antibiotics are advisable to cover the possibility that infection has provoked the crisis. In cases of primary adrenal failure, mineralocorticoid replacement with fludrocortisone is required. If emergency surgery is required in acute adrenal failure, all precautions necessary for anaesthetising the shocked patient should be taken (p. 536).

Congenital adrenal hyperplasia (adrenogenital syndrome)

This is associated with overproduction of androgens as a result of deficiency of hydroxylase enzyme required for production of cortisol. Hydrocortisone treatment overcomes adrenal insufficiency and, by suppressing ACTH production, decreases androgen accumulation. Augmented steroid cover is required for surgery in these patients.

Steroid therapy

Replacement therapy in cases of primary adrenocortical failure and hypopituitarism is given as oral hydrocortisone 20 mg in the morning and 10 mg in the evening. Fludrocortisone 0.05–0.1 mg daily is given additionally to replace aldosterone in primary adrenocortical failure. Equivalent doses of other steroid preparations are shown in Table 41.3. Prednisolone and prednisone have less mineralocorticoid effect, while betamethasone and dexamethasone have none. Requirements increase vastly following infection, trauma or surgery.

Corticosteroids are prescribed also for a wide range of medical conditions including asthma and collagen diseases. Prolonged therapy suppresses adrenocortical function.

Table 41.3 Equivalent doses of glucocorticoids

Betamethasone	3 mg
Cortisone acetate	100 mg
Dexamethasone	3 mg
Hydrocortisone	80 mg
Methylprednisolone	16 mg
Prednisolone	20 mg
Prednisone	20 mg
Triamcinolone	16 mg

Steroid cover for anaesthesia and surgery

Indications for augmented perioperative steroid cover include:

1. Patients with pituitary–adrenal insufficiency, on steroid replacement therapy.
2. Patients undergoing pituitary or adrenal surgery.
3. Patients on steroid therapy for more than 2 weeks before surgery.
4. Patients on steroid therapy for more than 1 month in the year before surgery.

Topical fluorinated steroid preparations applied widely to the skin may be absorbed sufficiently to produce adrenal suppression.

Preoperative assessment should involve appropriate fluid and electrolyte correction. Evidence of infection should be sought in patients on long-term steroid therapy.

Corticosteroid cover for operation should be given as follows:

1. Minor diagnostic procedures: single dose of hydrocortisone 100 mg i.m. 1 h preoperatively.
2. Intermediate operations (e.g. inguinal herniorrhaphy): hydrocortisone 100 mg i.m. with premedication; 100 mg 6-hourly for 24 h.
3. Major surgery: hydrocortisone 100 mg 6-hourly for 72 h starting with premedication.

The requirements may need to be increased if infection is present, or be continued beyond 3 days if infection or the effects of major trauma persist. Oral administration may be resumed after 24 h.

If steroids are prescribed for asthma or other medical conditions, the perioperative dosage may require modification according to the activity of the disease.

Disease of the adrenal medulla

Phaeochromocytoma

See page 588.

DIABETES MELLITUS

Fifty per cent of all diabetic patients present for surgery during their lifetime, usually for ophthalmic or vascular disease or for drainage of an abscess. Perioperative morbidity and mortality are greater in diabetic than in non-diabetic patients. This may result partly from controllable factors such as regulation of perioperative blood glucose, but unavoidable complications of diabetes, such as ischaemic heart disease and infection, may affect anaesthetic management.

The problems of managing diabetics who undergo surgery are associated with its attendant period of starvation and the metabolic effects of surgery. The aim is to minimise the metabolic disturbance by ensuring an adequate glucose, calorie and insulin intake, thus controlling hyperglycaemia and reducing proteolysis, lipolysis and production of lactate and ketones.

Adequate control of blood glucose concentration must be established preoperatively and maintained until oral feeding is resumed after operation. Hypoglycaemia, which may not be detectable readily in the anaesthetised patient, must be avoided. Modern techniques for frequent monitoring of blood glucose (Dextrostix, Ames; BM-Test-Glycemie, Boehringer-Mannheim, preferably used in conjunction with a reflectance colorimeter) have simplified management considerably.

Precise management depends upon the nature of the diabetes and its treatment (insulin-dependent or maturity-onset), on the magnitude of the surgery contemplated (including the estimated time to resumption of oral intake) and on the time available for control of the diabetes.

Preoperative assessment

Preoperative assessment is aimed at evaluating (a) blood glucose control, (b) the treatment regimen used and (c) the presence of complications.

Control of blood glucose

This is assessed by inspection of the patient's urine-testing records, by random blood glucose measurements and by a 24-h blood glucose profile in patients receiving insulin. Whenever possible, blood glucose should be maintained between 6 and 10 mmol/litre; insulin dosage should be adjusted to achieve this, with the introduction of twice-daily short and intermediate-acting insulins if necessary. Blood urea and electrolyte concentrations should be checked.

Treatment regimens

Oral hypoglycaemic agents are of two types. The sulphonylureas stimulate release of insulin from the pancreatic islets. Chlorpropamide has a very prolonged duration of action and may cause hypoglycaemia unless it is withdrawn 48 h before surgery. A change to a shorter-acting agent such as glipizide, gliclazide or glibenclamide is preferable.

Biguanides, which increase peripheral uptake of glucose and decrease gluconeogenesis, are used in obese maturity-onset diabetics either alone or in combination with sulphonylureas. These agents may cause lactic acidosis, usually, but not exclusively, in patients with renal or hepatic impairment. This complication carries a high mortality; consequently, metformin, the only biguanide now available, should be discontinued at least 24 h before surgery.

The last dose of oral hypoglycaemic agent should be administered 24 h before surgery and no further treatment is required until the morning of surgery if blood glucose control is satisfactory.

Insulin. Some of the newer insulin preparations in common use are listed in Table 41.4. The best control is achieved by twice-daily injections of short-acting and intermediate-acting insulin. The type of preparation must be noted, and if a change is made in the type of insulin (bovine, porcine, human) the dose must be adjusted, because increased sensitivity to the latter two may lead to hypoglycaemia. Insulin with the human sequence of amino acids is produced either biosynthetically (chain recombinant DNA technology using

Table 41.4 Newer insulin preparations

Proprietary name	Type and Source	Onset (h)	Peak action (h)	Duration of action (h)	Dosage
Humulin S	Short-acting, soluble, CRB	0.5	1–3	5–7	t.i.d. alone or b.d. + intermediate preparation
Human Velosulin	Short-acting, soluble, EMP	0.5	1–3	8	
Actrapid MC	Short-acting, soluble, porcine	0.5	2–5	8	
Humulin ***I***	Intermediate, isophane, CRB	1.0	2–8	18–20	b.d. + short-acting preparation
Insulatard	Intermediate, isophane, porcine	1.5	4–12	24	b.d. + short-acting preparation
Semitard	Insulin zinc suspension amorphous semilente, porcine	1.5	5–10	16	b.d. + short-acting preparation
Humulin M2	Mixed 20% soluble, 80% isophane, CRB	0.5	1–8	14–16	b.d.
Mixtard 30/70	Mixed 30% soluble, 70% isophane, porcine	0.5	4–8	24	b.d.
Monotard MC	Long-acting, insulin zinc suspension, 30% amorphous, 70% crystalline, lente, porcine	2.5	7–15	22	daily or b.d.
Humulin Zn	Long-acting, insulin zinc suspension, crystalline CRB	3	6–14	20–24	daily or b.d.

bacteria — CRB) or semi-synthetically (by enzyme modification of porcine material — EMP) from purified porcine insulin. The biosynthetic preparations are less expensive than purified porcine, and may become the principal commercial preparations. Insulin with the human sequence is associated with a less severe degree of antigenicity and is thus the preparation of choice for newly diagnosed diabetics and for patients requiring short-term therapy (e.g. in the perioperative period).

In well-controlled diabetics, it is not necessary to change to a short-acting insulin regimen on the day before surgery, provided that the dose of the intermediate or long-acting insulin is not excessive (40 units of long-acting or 24-unit evening dose of intermediate insulin); all too often a change of regimen results in poorer control.

The poorly controlled diabetic. Whether the patient is normally insulin-dependent or not, elective surgery should be delayed until improved control is achieved by administration of short-acting insulin three times daily. If surgery is urgent, a glucose, insulin and potassium regimen (Table 41.5) should be instituted to achieve rapid blood glucose control.

Complications

1. *Cardiovascular disorders* (coronary artery, cerebrovascular and peripheral vascular) are common in diabetics, and there is an increased risk of perioperative myocardial infarction. Careful preoperative assessment of cardiovascular function, appropriate choice of anaesthetic technique and precise perioperative monitoring are essential (page 645).

2. *Renal disease.* Microvascular damage produces glomerulosclerosis with proteinuria, oedema and eventually chronic renal failure. Anaesthetic implications of renal disease are discussed on page 660.

3. *Ocular problems.* Cataracts, exudative or proliferative retinopathy, vitreous haemorrhage and retinal detachment may occur. In the long term, good blood glucose control has been shown to reduce the frequency of such complications.

4. *Infection.* Diabetics are prone to infection

and an increased risk of septicaemia and abscess formation. Infection is associated with increased insulin requirements, which return to normal on its eradication, e.g. after surgical drainage of an abscess.

5. *Neuropathy*. Chronic, sensory peripheral neuropathies are common; mononeuropathies and acute motor neuropathies (amyotrophy) are associated with poor control of blood glucose. Loss of sensation together with peripheral vascular disease can lead to ulceration after trivial trauma; consequently, care in positioning patients in the operating theatre is important. Local anaesthetic nerve or plexus blocks should be avoided in patients with an acute neuropathy as neurological deficits may be attributed to the local anaesthetic solution.

6. *Autonomic neuropathy* may cause postoperative urinary retention or vasomotor instability, e.g. postural hypotension or hypotension during anaesthesia. IPPV or subarachnoid or extradural blockade may be associated with severe hypotension; adequate preoperative hydration, precise cardiovascular monitoring and careful anaesthetic management are essential.

Concurrent drug therapy

Thiazide diuretics, frusemide, diazoxide, adrenergic agents (e.g. salbutamol) and corticosteroids tend to increase the blood glucose concentration. Hypotensive drugs, e.g. ganglion blockers and β-adrenergic blockers, tend to potentiate hypoglycaemia and mask its clinical signs. Blood glucose should be monitored if any of these drugs is administered, and insulin dosage altered accordingly.

Some drugs, including phenylbutazone, displace sulphonylureas from protein-binding sites and potentiate their hypoglycaemic effect.

Perioperative diabetic management

A combination of glucose and insulin is the most satisfactory method of overcoming the deleterious metabolic consequences of starvation and surgical stress in the diabetic patient.

Although satisfactory control of blood glucose may be achieved using a no-glucose/no-insulin regimen, the raised blood urea concentration which occurs often in the postoperative period is indicative of increased protein breakdown, accompanying lipolysis and ketosis. Minor procedures may be carried out at the start of an operating list by delaying the morning dose of insulin until a late breakfast is taken after recovery from anaesthesia. A low-dose insulin infusion on its own (0.5 units/h by syringe pump) is effective for minor surgery, but is not adequate for major surgery.

Subarachnoid and extradural anaesthesia have some advantages in the diabetic patient; avoidance of general anaesthesia allows hypoglycaemia to be recognised, while early resumption of oral diet eases postoperative management.

Tables 41.5 and 41.6 (both of which are based on Alberti's recommendations) describe schemes for the precise management of patients receiving oral hypoglycaemic agents or insulin therapy who require minor or major surgery. Minor surgery includes endoscopic procedures and body surface surgery.

The combination of intravenous glucose solution

Table 41.5 Perioperative management of the maturity-onset diabetic

Preoperative	
Check random glucose, urea and electrolyte concentrations	
Poor control:	Start insulin (t.i.d. soluble) and delay surgery Urgent surgery: glucose/insulin infusion (Table 41.6)
Good control:	Chlorpropamide — change to a shorter-acting agent All agents terminated 24 h preoperatively
Day of surgery	
Check fasting blood glucose (BM stix, Dextrostix)	
No oral hypoglycaemic agent	
Minor surgery:	If blood glucose <10 mmol/litre, no specific therapy
Major surgery:	Treat as insulin-dependent diabetic (Table 41.6)
Postoperative	
Check blood glucose (BM stix, Dextrostix)	
Minor surgery:	Restart oral hypoglycaemic agent with first meal.
Major surgery:	Treat as insulin-dependent diabetic (Table 41.6) When oral diet resumed, t.i.d. soluble insulin 8–12 units before each meal; restart oral therapy when daily requirement less than 20 units

Table 41.6 Perioperative management of the insulin-dependent diabetic

Preoperative
- Blood glucose profile; urea and electrolytes; urine ketones
- Adjust insulin therapy; most patients b.d. soluble + isophane
- Poor control: change to t.i.d soluble insulin and delay surgery
- Urgent surgery: glucose/insulin infusion (vide infra)

Day of surgery
- Check fasting blood glucose; repeat 2-hourly
- No subcutaneous insulin
- Start infusion of 10% glucose (500 ml) with soluble (Humulin S) insulin 10 units and KCl 10 mmol at 0800 h to run 4–6-hourly
- Adjust insulin in bag as follows depending on blood glucose:
  - <4 mmol/litre: no insulin
  - 4–6 mmol/litre: insulin 5 units/500 ml glucose 10%
  - 6–10 mmol/litre: infusion as above
  - 10–20 mmol/litre: insulin 15 units/500 ml glucose 10%
  - >20 mmol/litre: insulin 20 units/500 ml glucose 10%
- Adjust potassium dosage depending on plasma K^+ concentration
  - <3 mmol/litre: add KCl 20 mmol
  - >5 mmol/litre: omit KCl

Postoperative
- Check blood glucose 2–6-hourly; check urea and electrolytes daily
- Continue 4–6-hourly infusions until oral diet re-established
- If delayed, change to decreased volume of 20–50% glucose with independent insulin infusion by syringe pump
- When oral diet resumed, t.i.d. soluble insulin s.c.; daily dosage as preoperative
- When requirements stable, restart normal regimen

with insulin added to the bag is a safety precaution; one cannot be infused inadvertently without the other and thus hyperglycaemia, and more particularly hypoglycaemia, are avoided. Glucose 10% is used to provide adequate carbohydrate and energy without excessive volume. The glucose/insulin solution should be administered through an intravenous cannula separate from that used for other intravenous fluids; it is preferable to use an infusion pump to regulate the rate of infusion.

This scheme provides 250 g of glucose (1000 kcal) and an average of 50 units of insulin over 24 h. If the patient has high insulin demands normally or is obese, additional insulin may be required (e.g. 5 units/bag more than the amount stated in Table 41.6). Patients who normally receive oral hypoglycaemic agents may be more sensitive, and require less insulin.

Blood transfusion may increase insulin requirements as the elevated citrate concentration stimulates gluconeogenesis. Ringer's lactate (Hartmann's) solution elevates blood glucose concentration for the same reason and should be avoided.

If control is difficult to achieve with this regimen because of postoperative complications such as sepsis or a result of steroid therapy, blood glucose may be controlled by a separate insulin infusion delivered by a syringe pump, with regulation of the insulin infusion rate determined on 2-hourly blood glucose measurements.

Emergency surgery; diabetic ketoacidosis

Diabetic ketoacidosis results from inadequate insulin dosage or increased insulin requirements, precipitated often by infection, trauma or surgical stress. Diabetics who require emergency surgery often have a grossly elevated blood glucose concentration and occasionally overt ketoacidosis. Such patients require rehydration, correction of sodium depletion, correction of subsequent potassium depletion and i.v. soluble (humulin S) insulin by infusion at an initial rate of 4–8 units/h.

Initial fluid replacement should consist of isotonic (0.9%) saline: 1 litre in the first 30 min, 1 litre in the next hour and a further litre over the next 2 h. If the plasma sodium concentration is greater than 150 mmol/litre, 0.45% saline should be used.

Progress is monitored by regular measurements of blood glucose, sodium and potassium concentrations, and arterial pH and blood gases. Correction of acidosis is required only if the arterial pH is less than 7.10, in which case 50 mmol of sodium bicarbonate should be given. Cellular potassium depletion is present from the outset, but hyperkalaemia or normokalaemia may be found initially because potassium shifts out of cells in the presence of acidosis. Potassium replacement should not be started until the plasma concentration begins to decrease with the correction of the acidosis. An infusion of glucose 5% should be given when the blood glucose concentration decreases to approximately 15 mmol/litre. When rehydration is under way, and some reversal of acidosis and hyperglycaemia has been achieved, surgery may be carried out while management of the diabetes is continued intra- and postoperatively.

NEUROLOGICAL DISEASE

There are several points of significance:

1. *Medicolegal.* Perioperative alteration in neurological deficit may be attributed to anaesthesia. This may render subarachnoid or extradural anaesthesia inadvisable in some patients.

2. *Respiratory impairment.* Motor neuropathy from various causes, e.g. motor neurone disease, acute polyneuritis (Guillain-Barré syndrome), disorders of the neuromuscular junction and high spinal cord lesions may produce respiratory inadequacy. These patients are sensitive to anaesthetic agents, opioids and relaxants, and if intraoperative IPPV is undertaken a period of elective postoperative ventilation may be necessary until full recovery from the effects of anaesthesia has occurred. If possible, procedures should be carried out under local or regional block. If bulbar muscles are involved, protection of the airway from regurgitation and aspiration may require prolonged tracheal intubation or tracheostomy. Surgery should be postponed if a chest infection is present preoperatively.

3. *Altered innervation of muscle, and potassium shifts.* An altered ratio of intracellular to extracellular potassium tends to produce a sensitivity to non-depolarising, and resistance to depolarising relaxants. If there is widespread denervation of muscle in lower motor neurone disease, e.g. in Guillain-Barré syndrome, disorganisation of the motor end-plate occurs, resulting in hypersensitivity to acetylcholine and suxamethonium, with increased permeability of muscle cells to potassium. A similar potassium efflux occurs in the presence of direct muscle damage, widespread burns involving muscle, upper motor neurone lesions, spinal cord lesions with paraplegia, and tetanus. In upper motor neurone and spinal cord lesions, the reason for this shift is less clear.

The resulting increase in serum potassium after suxamethonium may be 3 mmol/litre (in comparison with 0.5 mmol/litre in the normal patient) and may occur from 24 h after acute muscle denervation or damage until 6–12 months later. In such patients, suxamethonium is clearly contraindicated.

4. *Autonomic disturbances* may occur as part of a polyneuropathy, e.g. diabetes, Guillian-Barré syndrome and porphyria. Sympathetic stimulation, for example during light anaesthesia, tracheal intubation or following administration of pancuronium or catecholamines, may produce severe hypertension and arrhythmias. More commonly, blood loss, head-up posture or IPPV may be associated with severe hypotension.

5. *Increased intracranial pressure.* Elective surgery should be postponed if raised intracranial pressure (ICP) is suspected, until investigation and treatment have been undertaken. Anaesthetic agents which cause an increase in cerebral blood flow must be avoided. Hypercapnia must also be avoided and controlled ventilation to a Pa_{CO_2} of approximately 4 kPa (30 mmHg) is indicated. This is discussed fully in Chapter 38.

6. *Cerebrovascular disease.* In patients with suspected widespread cerebrovascular disease, the principal aim of anaesthetic management should be to maintain normotension and normocapnia. Although hypercapnia increases cerebral blood flow, it may produce 'steal' from ischaemic to well-perfused areas of brain. Hypocapnia decreases cerebral blood flow and is also contraindicated.

Epilepsy

In most patients with epilepsy, no identifiable cause can be found. Epilepsy may also be associated with birth injury, hypoglycaemia, hypocalcaemia, drug withdrawal, fever, head injury, cerebrovascular disease and cerebral tumour, the most likely cause depending on the age of onset. Epilepsy developing after the age of 20 years usually indicates organic brain disease.

Anaesthesia

Patients should be maintained on anticonvulsant therapy throughout the perioperative period. Some anaesthetic agents, e.g. enflurane and methohexitone, have cerebral excitatory effects and should be avoided. Thiopentone is a potent anticonvulsant and is the i.v. induction agent of choice. Local anaesthetic agents may cause convulsions at lower than normal concentrations and the safe maximum dose should be reduced.

The anticonvulsants phenobarbitone and phenytoin induce hepatic enzymes and accelerate elimination of drugs metabolised by the liver.

In cases of late-onset epilepsy, where increased ICP may be present as a result of tumour, controlled ventilation is advisable to avoid any increase in ICP.

Multiple sclerosis

Deterioration of symptoms tends to occur after surgery, but no particular anaesthetic technique is implicated. It is usually advisable to avoid extradural and subarachnoid anaesthesia, if only for medicolegal reasons, but there is no evidence that these techniques affect the disease adversely and they may be used if indicated strongly, provided that a full explanation has been given to the patient.

If a larger motor deficit of recent onset is present, there may be increased potassium release from muscle following suxamethonium, which should thus be avoided.

Peripheral neuropathies

These may exhibit axonal 'dying back' degeneration or segmental demyelination. They are classified by anatomical distribution, the commonest being a symmetrical peripheral polyneuropathy. Motor, sensory and autonomic fibres are involved. Causes include:

1. Metabolic (diabetes, porphyria).
2. Nutritional deficiency.
3. Toxic (heavy metals, drugs).
4. Collagen disease.
5. Carcinoma.
6. Infective.

Problems for the anaesthetist include the effects of autonomic neuropathy, and respiratory and bulbar involvement.

Acute inflammatory polyneuropathy (Guillain-Barré syndrome)

This polyneuropathy appears some days after a pyrexial illness. Progression is very variable, ranging from near total paralysis in 24 h to progression over several weeks. Respiratory and bulbar muscles may be affected, and if so tracheal intubation followed by tracheostomy and IPPV are required. Autonomic neuropathy may result in hypotension following institution of IPPV. This may be minimised by adequate fluid preloading and gradual increases in minute volume. Suxamethonium should be avoided.

Motor neurone disease (Progressive muscular atrophy, amyotrophic lateral sclerosis, progressive bulbar palsy)

Motor neurone disease is characterised by slow onset and progressive deterioration in motor function. Several patterns of motor loss occur with both upper and lower motor neurone loss. Problems for the anaesthetist include sensitivity to all anaesthetic agents and muscle relaxants, respiratory inadequacy and laryngeal incompetence. Local anaesthetic techniques may be useful. Mechanical ventilation should be avoided if possible, as the motor deficit is irreversible.

Hereditary ataxias

Friedreich's ataxia is the most common. Spinocerebellar, corticospinal and posterior columns are involved, and the course of the disease is slowly progressive. Problems for the anaesthetist include scoliosis, respiratory failure and cardiomyopathy with cardiac failure and arrhythmias.

Spinal cord lesions with paraplegia

Release of potassium from muscle cells by suxamethonium precludes its use within 6–12 months of cord injury.

Huntington's chorea

It has been reported that thiopentone may cause prolonged apnoea, while abnormal serum cholinesterase may prolong the action of suxamethonium.

Myasthenia gravis

This disease occurs usually in young adults and is characterised by episodes of increased muscle fatiguability, caused by decreased numbers of acetylcholine receptors at the neuromuscular junction. Treatment involves anticholinesterase (pyridostigmine 60 mg q.i.d. or neostigmine 15 mg q.i.d.) and a vagolytic agent (atropine or propantheline) to block the muscarinic effects. Steroid therapy is useful in some cases and thymectomy may benefit many patients considerably, especially young women with myasthenia of recent onset.

The chief problems concern adequacy of ventilation, ability to cough and clear secretions, and the increased secretions resulting from anticholinesterase therapy. If there is evidence of respiratory infection, surgery should be postponed. Serum potassium concentration should be normal, as hypokalaemia potentiates myasthenia. Local and regional anaesthesia, including low subarachnoid or extradural block, may be suitable alternatives to general anaesthesia, although the maximum dose of local anaesthetic agents should be reduced because of their neuromuscular blocking action. The minimum possible dose of induction agent should be used and relaxants should be avoided if possible. For major procedures requiring relaxation, the anticholinesterase may be omitted for 4 h preoperatively, and a small dose of relaxant may be given if necessary. Vecuronium and atracurium are the relaxants of choice because of their short durations of action, and should be administered in a reduced dose (10–20% of normal). Suxamethonium has a variable effect in myasthenia and is best avoided.

Postoperatively, the patient's lungs should be ventilated electively for 24–48 h after major surgery. Good chest physiotherapy and tracheal suction are required. Steroid cover is required if appropriate. If extreme muscle weakness occurs, i.v. atropine 0.6–1.2 mg and neostigmine 1–2 mg may be given. Care must be taken to titrate the doses of anticholinesterase carefully, or a cholinergic crisis, characterised by a depolarising neuromuscular block, with sweating, salivation, and pupillary constriction may occur. Edrophonium may be used to test the end-plate response to acetylcholine.

A myasthenic state may also be associated with carcinoma, thyrotoxicosis, Cushing's syndrome, hypokalaemia and hypocalcaemia. In these patients, non-depolarising relaxants should be avoided, or used in reduced dosage.

Familial periodic paralysis

This is also associated with prolonged paralysis after non-depolarising muscle relaxants.

Progressive muscular dystrophy

Several types of muscular dystrophy exist, of varying patterns of heredity and described according to their anatomical distribution. Muscular weakness occurs, and must be distinguished from myasthenia and lower motor neurone disease. The anaesthetic complications comprise sensitivity to relaxants, opioids and other sedative and anaesthetic drugs, and liability to respiratory infection. Myocardial involvement may occur.

Dystrophia myotonica

This is a disease of autosomal dominant inheritance characterised by muscle weakness and muscle contraction persisting after the termination of voluntary effort. Other features may include frontal baldness, cataract, sternomastoid wasting, gonadal atrophy and thyroid adenoma. Problems which affect anaesthetic management include:

1. ***Respiratory muscle weakness.*** Respiratory function should be fully assessed preoperatively. Respiratory depressant drugs, e.g. thiopentone or opioids, should be used with care; there is sensitivity also to non-depolarising relaxants. Elective postoperative IPPV may be required. Postoperative care of the airway must be meticulous because of muscle weakness. Chest infections are common.
2. ***Cardiovascular effects.*** Arrhythmias are common, particularly during anaesthesia, and may result in cardiac failure. Careful monitoring is essential.
3. ***Muscle spasm.*** This may be provoked by administration of depolarising muscle relaxants or anticholinesterases. Suxamethonium and neostigmine should thus be avoided. The spasm is not abolished by non-depolarising relaxants.

MISCELLANEOUS DISORDERS

Carcinoid syndrome

See Chapter 36, page 586.

Myeloma

This neoplastic condition affects plasma cells and has a number of points of significance to the anaesthetist:

1. Widespread skeletal destruction occurs and careful handling of the patient on the operating table is essential. Pathological fractures are common.
2. Bone pain may be severe and often requires large doses of analgesics. Thus, tolerance to opioids may occur.
3. Hypercalcaemia occurs as a result of bony destruction, and may precipitate renal failure.
4. Anaemia is almost invariable, and preoperative blood transfusion is often necessary.
5. Infection. Patients are liable to infection, including chest infection, especially during cytotoxic therapy.
6. Bleeding disorders. During cytotoxic therapy, thrombocytopenia is common.
7. Increased plasma immunoglobulin concentrations may raise blood viscosity, predisposing to arterial and venous thrombosis. Drug binding may be affected, e.g. resistance to D-tubocurarine may occur.
8. Neurological manifestations include spinal cord and nerve root compression.

Porphyria

The porphyrias are an inherited group of disorders of porphyrin metabolism characterised by increased acivity of δ-aminolaevulinic acid synthetase with excessive production of porphyrins or their precursor. In the UK, *acute intermittent porphyria* is the most common type. It is characterised by acute attacks which may arise spontaneously or be precipitated by infection, starvation, pregnancy or administration of some drugs. Inheritance is Mendelian dominant and thus a family history of porphyria requires further investigation. Clinical features include:

1. *Gastrointestinal:* abdominal pain and tenderness, vomiting, constipation, and occasionally diarrhoea.
2. *Neurological:* a motor and sensory peripheral neuropathy is common. It may involve bulbar and respiratory muscles. Epileptic fits and psychological disturbance may occur.
3. *Cardiovascular:* hypertension and tachycardia often occur during the attacks. Hypotension has been reported also.
4. *Fever and leucocytosis* occur in 25–30% of patients.

Drugs which provoke the attack include alcohol, barbiturates, chlordiazepoxide, steroid hormones, chlorpropamide, pentazocine, phenytoin and sulphonamides.

Anaesthesia in such patients is directed to avoiding drugs which may provoke attacks. Induction with ketamine or possibly propofol, followed by muscle relaxation with suxamethonium, *d*-tubocurarine or gallamine, ventilation with nitrous oxide, halothane and oxygen and analgesic supplementation with morphine or pethidine is satisfactory. If fits occur, diazepam is a suitable anticonvulsant, while chlorpromazine, promethazine or promazine are suitable sedatives.

FURTHER READING

Aitkenhead A R, Grant I S 1983 Intercurrent disease and medication. In: Henderson J J, Nimmo W S (eds) Practical regional anaesthesia. Blackwell Scientific Publications, Oxford

Alberti K G M M, Thomas B J B 1979 The management of diabetes during surgery. British Journal of Anaesthesia 51: 693

Bevan D R 1979 Renal function in anaesthesia and surgery. Academic Press, London

Bevan D R 1979 Shy-Drager syndrome. A review and a description of anaesthetic management. Anaesthesia 34: 866

Bevan D R 1978 Symposium on clinical assessment. British Journal of Anaesthesia 50: 1

Brown B R 1981 Anesthesia and the patient with liver disease. Davis, Philadelphia

Fisher A, Waterhouse T D, Adams A P 1975 Obesity: its relation to anaesthesia. Anaesthesia 30: 633

Foëx P 1982 Anaesthesia and cardiovascular disease: the importance of preoperative assessment. In: Atkinson R S, Langton Hewer C (eds) Recent advances in anaesthesia and analgesia 14. Churchill Livingstone, Edinburgh

Goldman L 1988 Assessment of the patient with known or suspected ischaemic heart disease for non-cardiac surgery. British Journal of Anaesthesia 61: 38

Hamilton W F D, Forest A L, Gunn A, Peden W R, Feely J 1984 Beta-adrenoceptor blockade and anaesthesia for thyroidectomy. Anaesthesia 39: 335

Jones R M, Healy T E J 1980 Anaesthesia and demyelinating disease. Anaesthesia 35: 879
Jones R M, Rosen M, Seymour L 1987 Smoking and anaesthesia. Anaesthesia 42: 1
Katz J, Benumof J, Kadis L B 1981 Anesthesia and uncommon diseases. W B Saunders, Philadelphia
Lamberty J M, Rubin B K 1985 The management of anaesthesia for patients with cystic fibrosis. Anaesthesia 40: 448
Mason R A, Steane P A 1976 Carcinoid syndrome: its relevance to the anaesthetist. Anaesthesia 31: 228
Nimmo W S 1986 Should a fasting patient receive his medication? Survey of Anesthesiology 30: 382
Philbin D M 1979 Anesthetic management of the patient with cardiovascular disease. International Anesthesiology Clinics 17, 1. Little, Brown, Boston
Prys-Roberts C 1980 Hypertension, ischaemic heart disease and anesthesia. International Anesthesiology Clinics 18, 4. Little, Brown, Boston
Prys-Roberts C 1984 Anaesthesia and hypertension. British Journal of Anaesthesia 56: 711
Smith G B, Shribman A J 1984 Anaesthesia and severe skin disease. Anaesthesia 39: 443
Strunin L 1977 The liver and anaesthesia. W B Saunders, London
Stoelting R K, Dierdorf S R 1983 Anesthesia and coexisting disease. Churchill Livingstone, New York
Vickers M D, Jones R M 1989 Medicine for anaesthetists, 3rd edn. Blackwell Scientific Publications, Oxford
Weatherill D, Spence A A 1984 Anaesthesia and disorders of the adrenal cortex. British Journal of Anaesthesia 56: 741
Welbourn R B, Joffe S N 1977 The apudomas. Recent advances in surgery, 9. Churchill Livingstone, Edinburgh

42. The intensive therapy unit

The intensive therapy unit (ITU) is the hospital facility within which the highest level of continuous patient care and treatment is provided. Approximately 1–2% of acute beds are used for this purpose and are organised usually into units of four to eight beds, as this is considered to be the optimal size.

The nature of the patient care carried out in the ITU has led to the development of designs which differ considerably from hospital to hospital. A much greater area needs to be allocated to each bed than in ordinary wards because several nurses must treat patients simultaneously and bulky items of equipment often need to be accommodated. Each bed area is supplied with oxygen and piped suction (two outlets of each per bed), medical compressed air and sometimes nitrous oxide (or Entonox). At least 12 electric power sockets are required and these should be connected to the emergency standby generator. Sufficient local storage space is required to make the nurse self-sufficient for common procedures such as administration of drugs and tracheal aspiration. Each bed area should be equipped with a self-inflating resuscitation bag to enable the staff to maintain artificial ventilation in case the mechanical ventilator fails.

WHO SHOULD BE ADMITTED?

Patients admitted to the unit should be those whose lives are in imminent danger but in whom, it is believed, the immediate risk may be averted by active and often invasive therapeutic efforts. A wide range of pathological conditions may lead to such a state but all involve failure, or the threat of failure, of the respiratory and/or circulatory systems. In addition, dysfunction of one or more of the renal, gastrointestinal, hepatic, haematological and neurological systems may be present, but involvement of one of these systems alone is rarely a reason for admission to the ITU.

Patients admitted to the ITU require active and aggressive therapy for either (a) appropriate management of a diagnosed condition, or (b) resuscitation while a definitive diagnosis is made. Critically ill patients benefit usually from prompt rather than delayed admission to the unit, and early notification of such patients elsewhere in the hospital is to be encouraged.

Admission should not be sought for patients whose basic condition is essentially untreatable, e.g. the patient whose lungs are destroyed almost completely by chronic bronchitis and emphysema and who cannot be cured by artificial ventilation. It should be appreciated that it is easier to institute heroic therapeutic efforts than to withdraw them if it becomes clear that restoration of a patient's ability to lead an independent existence is impossible. It should be noted that it is unethical and almost certainly unlawful to treat a patient against his or her volition.

STAFFING CONSIDERATIONS

The ITU consultant

Difficult therapeutic and ethical policy decisions may be required at any time in the ITU. It is essential that they are taken by one whose previous experience is such as to allow a reasonable assessment of the likely outcome, and whose therapeutic expertise is likely to give the patient the optimal chance of recovery. The ITU consultant, if not physically present in the unit, must always be available by telephone and should not be involved in any activity which precludes his or her attendance there within 30 min. Because of the critical nature of the ITU patients' illnesses, the ITU consultant will expect to be informed immediately of any significant change in their condition. The consultant's basic specialty is relatively unimportant.

The roles of the ITU resident

Communications

Although medical involvement with therapy in the ITU is greater than anywhere else in the hospital except the operating theatre, it should be appreciated that the majority of patient care activities are undertaken by nursing staff. The route by which complex instructions and information are transmitted between medical and nursing staff is of vital importance. A system in which a relatively junior clinician serves as a 'final common pathway' for all instructions works well in practice provided that the doctor involved is present within the unit at all times so that the nurses may obtain clarification of instructions, report changes in status and receive immediate help in emergencies. Nurses shoulder a greater degree of clinical responsibility if their confidence is sustained by a continuous medical presence, and this has important consequences for maintaining therapeutic momentum. In addition, a great deal of frustration is engendered by a system in which the nurses are required to contact one or more doctors outside the unit on each occasion that an unexpected alteration occurs in a patient's condition.

Confusion is minimised if the nursing staff take orders only from the unit staff and not directly from visiting clinicians, however eminent, and even if they are nominally in charge of the patient. This is to ensure that the nurses who execute orders are able to confer with the person who wrote them in case of difficulties. In addition, many patients may be under the care of several clinical teams (e.g. multiply injured patients may be treated by a selection from the orthopaedic, general, neuro-, dental, plastic or urological surgeons), so that it is essential that one individual is available to draw attention to, and when necessary harmonise, often conflicting therapeutic regimens. The ITU resident, because of his continuous presence in the unit, should be better informed about the patient's recent diagnostic results, physiological status and therapeutic responses than any visiting clinician and should attempt to use his current knowledge to guide treatment along rational lines.

The department which provides the unit staff differs from hospital to hospital; units serving primarily a single specialty (e.g. cardiac surgery or neurosurgery units) are staffed usually by the specialty involved, whereas most general ITUs are staffed by the anaesthetic department, which is well used to providing round-the-clock emergency services.

Therapeutic functions

As the person on the spot, the resident is the first doctor called in by the nursing staff. It is necessary for him to decide rapidly whether the problem is one with which he can cope, or if more experienced help should be obtained. The number of occasions when immediate emergency action is required should be relatively small for patients already under the care of experienced ITU nurses (e.g. unforeseen circulatory collapse, accidental tracheal extubation) but resuscitative measures are often required for patients being admitted to the unit. In these latter circumstances, the ITU must be forewarned about likely admissions (e.g. by the ambulance service or accident department, operating theatre or wards); the resident should then have time for discussion with the ITU consultant before the patient's arrival.

It follows that most calls to the unit are the result of alterations in measurements rather than a major catastrophe. Tracheal intubation and obtunded consciousness make direct communication with many patients extremely difficult, so that assessment of their problems is based primarily on clinical observation and interpretation of patterns of change in physiological status. The resident should remember that the majority of intensive therapy nurses (and especially the sisters and charge nurses) have an enormous amount of bedside experience with critically ill patients, and considerable reliance should be placed on their observations.

ASSESSMENT OF PATIENTS

When called to a patient, the resident should begin to assess the situation by observing the patient and asking himself questions such as:

1. What changes have occurred since I last saw the patient?
2. Is the patient alert or inert?
3. Is the patient cooperative or confused?
4. Is the patient comfortable or distressed?
5. Is the patient pale or flushed?
6. Is the patient pink or cyanosed?

Simple observations such as these may offer the resident some insight into the severity of the patient's problem, and should always be undertaken before seeking additional information from the ITU chart.

As considerable information is gathered on the patient undergoing intensive care, comprehensive charts are required for its display. The charts should be accessible easily to the nursing staff who complete them and to the medical staff who refer to them. They should provide a record of changes in physiological variables (so that significant alterations are recognised easily), of drugs administered to the patient and of intake and output of fluid. It is desirable that a complete record of what has happened to the patient is collected on a single, although necessarily somewhat complex, chart. Medical orders, which inevitably include discretionary elements, should be charted separately. Many units record the results of laboratory tests on a separate chart because of the different time-base for these investigations.

In attempting to evaluate unit performance, information may be collected on the physiological status of patients on admission and their subsequent progress (e.g. APACHE II score) and on therapeutic activities within the unit (e.g. TISS scores). However, the lack of statistical precision of these scores makes them unsuitable for use in reaching therapeutic decisions on individual patients.

Clinical guidelines

The following sections present a set of systematic guidelines designed to help the resident in his assessment of the patient's condition. As unusual problems occur commonly during intensive therapy, the flow charts and the suggested actions are obviously not comprehensive. However, the proposed order of evaluation of the different physiological variables may prove useful as a check-list in most circumstances.

RESPIRATORY PROBLEMS

Who should receive artificial ventilation?

Patients who are unable to maintain adequate levels of oxygenation or who develop hypercapnia may be candidates for artificial ventilation, provided that their pulmonary pathology is potentially reversible. Ventilatory failure may have developed already (in which case arterial blood gas values are abnormal), or may be judged as likely to occur (when blood gas values may be normal but the patient is exhausted).

Hypoxaemia

The commonest indication for ventilating a patient's lungs artificially in the ITU is inability to maintain a satisfactory Pa_{O_2}. There are many pathological conditions which produce hypoxaemia but all have the same basic problem — that of an area or areas of lung which have a greater pulmonary blood flow than alveolar ventilation. Blood flow through areas of lung from which ventilation is absent completely is said to be 'shunted', and hypoxaemia caused by this mechanism shows little improvement when the inspired oxygen concentration is increased. Some clinical conditions which are associated frequently with hypoxaemia, and their common responses to therapy, are listed in Table 42.1. Central cyanosis (seen best in the lips) always shows that significant hypoxaemia is present, but if moderate anaemia (Hb $>$ 10 g/dl) is present, as it is in many ITU patients, severe hypoxaemia ($Pa_{O_2} < 6$ kPa) may occur without obvious cyanosis.

Table 42.1 Some causes of hypoxaemia and usual responses to therapy.

Clinical condition	Response to therapy O_2 by mask	IPPV	Need for PEEP
1. Pulmonary oedema			
(a) cardiac	Fair	Good	Uncommon
(b) permeability	Poor	Fair	Often needed
2. Asthma (bronchodilators may make worse)	Good	Good but technically very difficult	Uncommon
3. Chronic bronchitis	Fair (Ventimask)	Good	Uncommon
4. Emphysema	Good (Ventimask)	Good	Rare, beware pneumothorax
5. Pneumonia			
(a) lobar	Poor	Poor	Try, often dissappointing
(b) broncho-	Fair	Good	Useful
6. Pulmonary contusion	Fair	Fair	Often needed, beware pneumothorax
7. Right to left intracardiac shunts	Poor	Disastrous	Never
8. Retained secretions	Poor	Good, access for suction important	Helpful
9. 'Exhaustion'	Not accepted	Good	Uncommon

The initial treatment of hypoxaemia is the administration of oxygen by face mask. At least 40% oxygen should be given, either by means of a fixed-performance mask (e.g. 40, 50 or 60% Ventimask), or by supplying at least 6 litres/min of oxygen to a variable-performance mask (e.g. Hudson). Low-concentration fixed-performance masks and other devices which deliver 24–35% oxygen should be reserved for use in patients with chronic lung conditions and in whom hypoxic drive may be maintaining ventilation. The effect of oxygen therapy should be assessed by arterial blood gas analysis after no more than 30 min. If Pa_{O_2} remains below 7 kPa in patients with previously healthy lungs, the oxygen concentration should be increased and blood gases resampled after a further 20 min. In addition, measures to combat infection, pulmonary oedema or bronchospasm should be introduced as appropriate, analgesia given if indicated and chest physiotherapy started. Artificial ventilation is required if Pa_{O_2} does not remain above 7–8 kPa.

Patients who are unable to maintain adequate oxygenation often have a pulmonary problem which is associated with other pathology. Persisting inability to cough effectively because of pain and/or weakness leads to retention of secretions and progressive alveolar collapse. The prophylactic use of tracheal intubation and IPPV has become common in patients who normally produce significant quantities of bronchial secretions and whose ability to cough has been impaired by injury or operation to the chest and/or upper abdomen. Patients in whom pain rather than weakness is the major defect may often be managed more conservatively if first-class pain relief is provided (e.g. by regional analgesia, injections of opioid into the extradural space or i.v. infusion of opioid), together with skilful physiotherapy. Cannulation of the trachea via the cricothyroid membrane with a small-bore tube (minitracheotomy) may help also by allowing access to the tracheobronchial tree for aspiration of retained secretions.

Because of the lower intensity of nursing care provided currently on most general wards, it is appropriate to admit such a patient to the ITU solely to obtain the medical and nursing supervision necessary to manage the analgesic technique safely. Many surgeons regularly 'book' patients into the ITU after major operations which are associated with ventilatory problems, e.g. thoraco-abdominal gastrectomy or oesophagectomy, major vascular surgery.

Hypercapnia

Carbon dioxide clearance is related directly to alveolar ventilation. Causes of inadequate ventilation together with the likely duration of the disability are listed in Table 42.2; it may be inappropriate to start IPPV in clinical situations where ventilatory insufficiency cannot be reversed by therapy. Patients whose dysfunction is described in the lower part of Table 42.2 are likely to make vigorous efforts to maintain normocapnia, while those in whom the dysfunction can be described broadly as 'neurological' are usually unable to help themselves significantly. Artificial ventilation is required usually if Pa_{CO_2} exceeds 7 kPa in patients who habitually maintain a Pa_{CO_2} in the normal range (4.7–5.3 kPa), or if Pa_{CO_2} increases by more than 2 kPa above the patient's usual level.

Exhaustion is indicated by a laboured pattern of rapid, shallow breathing which is accompanied often by deterioration in the level of consciousness. This situation may occur in a wide range of clinical conditions, including cardiac failure and severe septicaemia, when the institution of artificial ventilation may be followed by an improvement in oxygenation, a reduction in pulse rate and reversal of a trend towards metabolic acidosis. When it occurs in conjunction with myocardial failure, a disproportionate amount of the limited cardiac output is used to maintain ventilation, and institution of artificial ventilation may allow adequate perfusion of vital organs to be resumed. Artificial ventilation is probably required if the respiratory rate remains at or above 45 breaths/min for more than 1 h.

Table 42.2 Some causes of inadequate spontaneous ventilation

Site of dysfunction	Common causes	Probable duration of inadequacy
A. Patients usually unable to increase ventilation (appear passive)		
1. Respiratory centre	Brain injury (coning)	Permanent
	Pharmacological depression (e.g. opioids, barbiturates)	Hours (depends on drug)
2. Upper motor neurones	High spinal damage (above C4)	Permanent
3. Lower motor neurones	Poliomyelitis	Weeks but may be permanent
	Polyneuritis	Months
	Tetanus	Weeks
4. Neuromuscular junction	Myasthenia gravis	Weeks or months
	Neuromuscular blockers	Minutes or hours
5. Respiratory muscles	Myopathies, dystrophies	Permanent
B. Patients who attempt to increase ventilation (appear dyspnoeic)		
6. Chest wall		
(a) deformity	Kyphoscoliosis	Permanent
	Burn eschars	Until incised
(b) damage	Rib fractures	Days or weeks
7. Lungs — reduced compliance	Pulmonary fibrosis	Permanent
	ARDS	Days or weeks
8. Airways — increased resistance	Upper airway obstruction: croup, epiglottitis	Until relieved
	Lower airway obstruction: asthma, bronchitis and emphysema	Days Permanent

Institution of mechanical ventilation

Tracheal intubation

To enable IPPV to be carried out effectively, a cuffed tube must be placed in the trachea either via the mouth or nose or directly through a tracheostomy. In the emergency situation, an oral tracheal tube is usually inserted. If the patient is conscious, anaesthesia should be induced carefully with an i.v. induction agent, and muscular relaxation produced, usually with suxamethonium. If the patient is unconscious, a muscle relaxant alone may be necessary (but not obligatory) to facilitate the passage of the tube; an i.v. induction agent and muscle relaxant should always be used in patients with a severe head injury to prevent an increase in intracranial pressure during laryngoscopy and intubation. As many patients may be hypoxaemic, it is essential that 100% oxygen is administered before intubation. The tube should be inserted by the route which is associated with the least delay once muscle relaxation has been induced.

Cricoid pressure should be applied to minimise the risk of aspirating gastric contents. A sterile, disposable plastic tube with a low-pressure cuff should be used. The tube should be cut so that the top of the cuff lies not more than 3 cm below the vocal cords. The incompressible plastic connector should lie between the incisor teeth if an oral tube is used, or in the external nares if nasal intubation is selected. The head should be placed in a neutral or slightly flexed position (on one pillow) after tracheal intubation, and a chest X-ray taken to ensure that the tip of the tube lies at least 5 cm above the carina.

Bronchial intubation is the commonest dangerous complication during artificial ventilation as the tracheal tube may migrate down the trachea when the patient is moved for normal nursing procedures. Intubation of the right main bronchus cannot be detected reliably by observation of chest movements or by auscultation of the chest because of the exaggerated transmission of breath sounds during IPPV, although absent or asynchronous chest movement may occur when pulmonary collapse has taken place. Bronchial intubation is one of the causes of a sudden decrease in compliance, and restlessness and coughing occur if the end of the tube irritates the carina. If this is suspected, the tube should be withdrawn gradually by up to 5 cm while lung compliance and chest expansion are observed carefully. The position of the tube should always be confirmed with a chest radiograph.

Tracheostomy is mandatory only when the upper airway or larynx is obstructed and intubation is not possible (e.g. occasional cases of epiglottitis or laryngeal trauma). The operation is employed more commonly as a planned procedure to make management easier and more comfortable in patients who require ventilation for prolonged periods, e.g. tetanus, poliomyelitis and some chest injuries. In such cases it is performed as a formal operation under general anaesthesia after the airway has been secured using a tracheal tube.

Adjusting the ventilator

There are two main types of ventilator in common use; those which deliver a preset tidal volume and those which develop a set pressure during each inspiration. In most units, volume-preset machines predominate, and subsequent comments and instructions refer to this general type of ventilator. The ITU resident should familiarise himself with the controls and facilities of ventilators available in the unit — preferably with an experienced colleague when the machine is not attached to a patient!

The ventilator should be adjusted initially to deliver a tidal volume of 12–15 ml/kg body weight (approximately 1000 ml for a 70-kg patient) and a minute volume of 8–10 litres/min. An initial inspired oxygen concentration of 40% is appropriate for most patients, but an initial concentration of 50% or more should be selected in patients who are already hypoxaemic despite oxygen therapy. If controllable, the inspiratory time should be approximately half the expiratory time. After approximately 10 min, arterial blood gases should be measured, and the inspired oxygen concentration adjusted if necessary.

Management of the ventilated patient

The aims of IPPV are to maintain adequate oxygenation of the tissues with an inspired oxygen concentration of less than 50% and to maintain the Pa_{CO_2} at a satisfactory level. Most patients find the process of receiving artificial ventilation uncomfortable, principally because of irritation from the oral or nasal tracheal tube. This discomfort is accentuated by movement, particularly of the head. If hypoxaemia or hypercapnia is present, the respiratory centre stimulates ventilatory efforts which are not synchronised with those of the ventilator. In conditions with decreased lung compliance, e.g. ARDS, patients tend to breathe rapidly even when blood gases are normal and the respiratory centre is depressed with large doses of opioids.

Arterial oxygenation during IPPV

Arterial oxygenation is controlled by manipulating the inspired oxygen concentration and by varying the end-expiratory pressure. Figure 42.1 describes measures that may be employed to maintain the arterial oxygen within the desired limits (Pa_{O_2} 10–15 kPa and $Sa_{O_2} > 95\%$). Concentrations of oxygen exceeding 50–60% should be avoided for more than a few hours because of the risk of oxygen-induced pulmonary damage.

The application of positive end-expiratory pressure (PEEP), or the use of a respiratory pattern in which the inspiratory time exceeds the expiratory time (reversed I/E ratio), are methods of increasing the FRC and improving arterial oxygenation. Both methods have inherent dangers:

1. They raise the mean intrathoracic pressure, thereby tending to impair transpulmonary blood flow and reduce cardiac output. Consequently, oxygen delivery to vital organs may be reduced.
2. They increase peak inspiratory pressure and make rupture of alveoli more likely (vide infra).

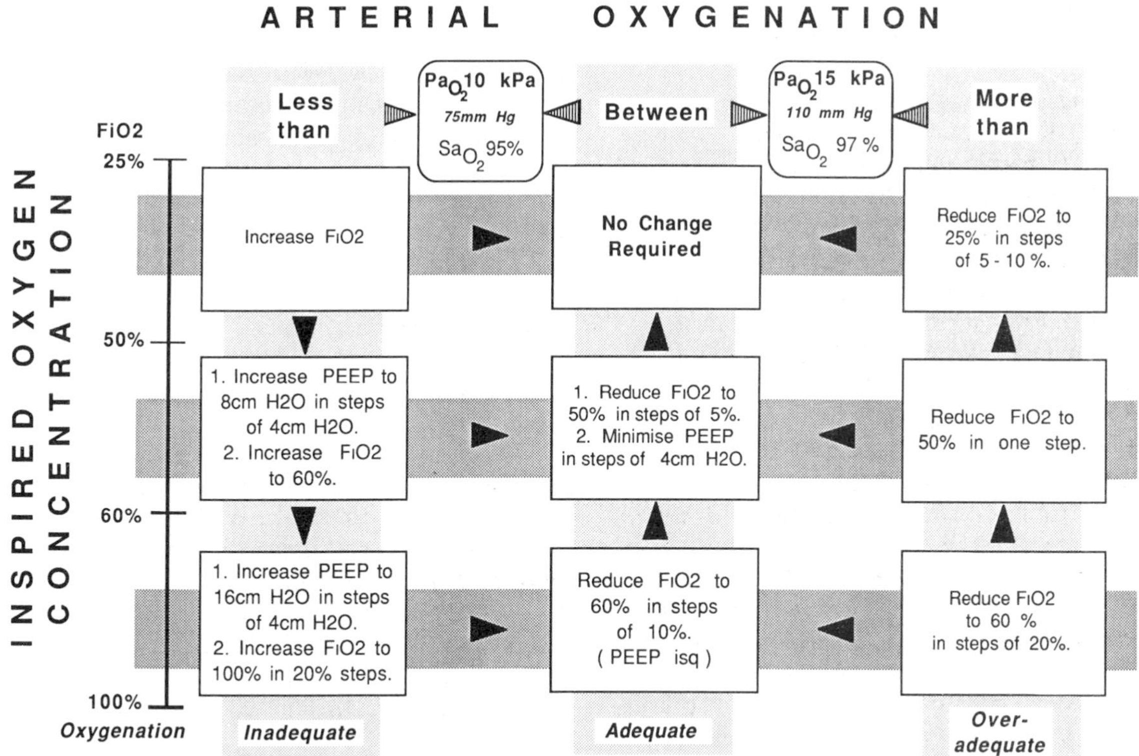

Fig. 42.1 Control of arterial oxygenation. To use this diagram:
1. Measure the inspired oxygen concentration ($F\text{I}_{O_2}$) and arterial blood gases and find appropriate box on diagram.
2. Adjust $F\text{I}_{O_2}$ and/or positive end-expiratory pressure (PEEP) as suggested. Where more than one action is proposed, proceed in the order described. In general, the greater the deviation from adequacy, the larger the steps required.
3. Repeat measurements after 20–30 min and re-adjust if necessary. NB: If P_{O_2} is measured on samples of mixed (or central venous) blood before and after adding or increasing PEEP, effect of PEEP on cardiac output and oxygen flux may be assessed (see text).

The effects of PEEP on the circulation should be monitored by observing trends in arterial pressure and by measuring changes in the oxygen concentration in mixed (or central) venous blood. The supply of oxygen available to the body (the oxygen flux) is the product of the cardiac output and the arterial oxygen content. PEEP often increases the arterial oxygen content but may depress cardiac output so that oxygen flux is reduced. If this happens, and total body oxygen consumption remains unchanged, less oxygen is returned to the heart and the concentration in the mixed (or central) venous blood decreases. If venous oxygen saturation does decrease after the application of (or increase in the level of) PEEP, then:

1. PEEP should be reduced by 4 cmH_2O.
2. Inspired oxygen concentration should be increased by 10%.
3. Measurements of arterial and venous Po_2 should be repeated after 20 min.

Carbon dioxide tension

It is desirable to minimise the changes in the Pa_{CO_2} (especially if initially elevated), as a rapid reduction leads to a marked decrease in cardiac output and arterial pressure. In patients with a normal or low Pa_{CO_2} before IPPV, minute volume should be adjusted to produce a Pa_{CO_2} of 4–4.5 kPa, a level at which spontaneous ventilatory efforts should be minimal. If the pre-IPPV Pa_{CO_2} is high, Pa_{CO_2} should not be reduced by more than 1 kPa/h, and, if raised chronically (e.g. in chronic bronchitis), to not less than 5.5–6 kPa.

If the Pa_{CO_2} is below 4 kPa, minute volume should be reduced by lowering respiratory rate. Because Pa_{CO_2} increases relatively slowly, at least 1 h should elapse before contemplating further changes in minute volume.

A scheme for the assessment of the patient undergoing ventilation is shown in Figure 42.2.

'Fighting the ventilator'

When a patient attempts to breathe out of phase with the ventilator, the first priority is to exclude and if necessary correct, any hypoxaemia or hypercapnia (Figs 42.1 and 42.2). When these have been excluded, two possible approaches to the problem should be considered.

Many modern ventilators allow a considerable range of adjustments so that the characteristics of the ventilatory cycle may be altered to suit the patient and reduce the need for heavy sedation. Intermittent mandatory ventilation (IMV), or its variants (see Ch. 2), are modes of ventilation which are often useful in allowing the patient to continue with some spontaneous ventilatory effort whilst ensuring that a background of mechanical ventilation is continued. It may be 'dialled in' on more sophisticated ventilators, but may be applied also with simpler machines by using a lightly loaded bypass valve. As the total minute volume (and hence Pa_{CO_2}) is effectively under the patient's control during IMV, it is important that muscle relaxants should have been discontinued for some hours and that only moderate doses of respiratory depressants (e.g. opioid analgesics) are being administered.

Alternatively, and especially if oxygenation is precarious, it may be necessary to inhibit spontaneous ventilatory efforts by administering central respiratory depressants (e.g. morphine in a dose of up to 20 mg/h by continuous infusion). Neuromuscular blocking drugs should be used only as a last resort to control the hypoxaemic patient who does not settle after sedation. If it is necessary to use these drugs, sedative agents *must* be given at the same time.

If patients who are improving start to 'fight the ventilator', it may be appropriate to wean them from IPPV.

Reassurance, analgesia and sedation

All but a few patients require some sedation or analgesia while receiving IPPV through a tracheal tube. Ideally, patients should require only light sedation, except when unpleasant or painful procedures are performed, so that they can understand and cooperate with therapy. The experienced ITU nurse explains exactly what is happening, reassures and develops methods of communication that do not distress the voiceless patient. Such explanations should be brief, as attention span is short in the sick, and should be repeated frequently, because memory is impaired. A sympathetic approach by all ITU staff can often

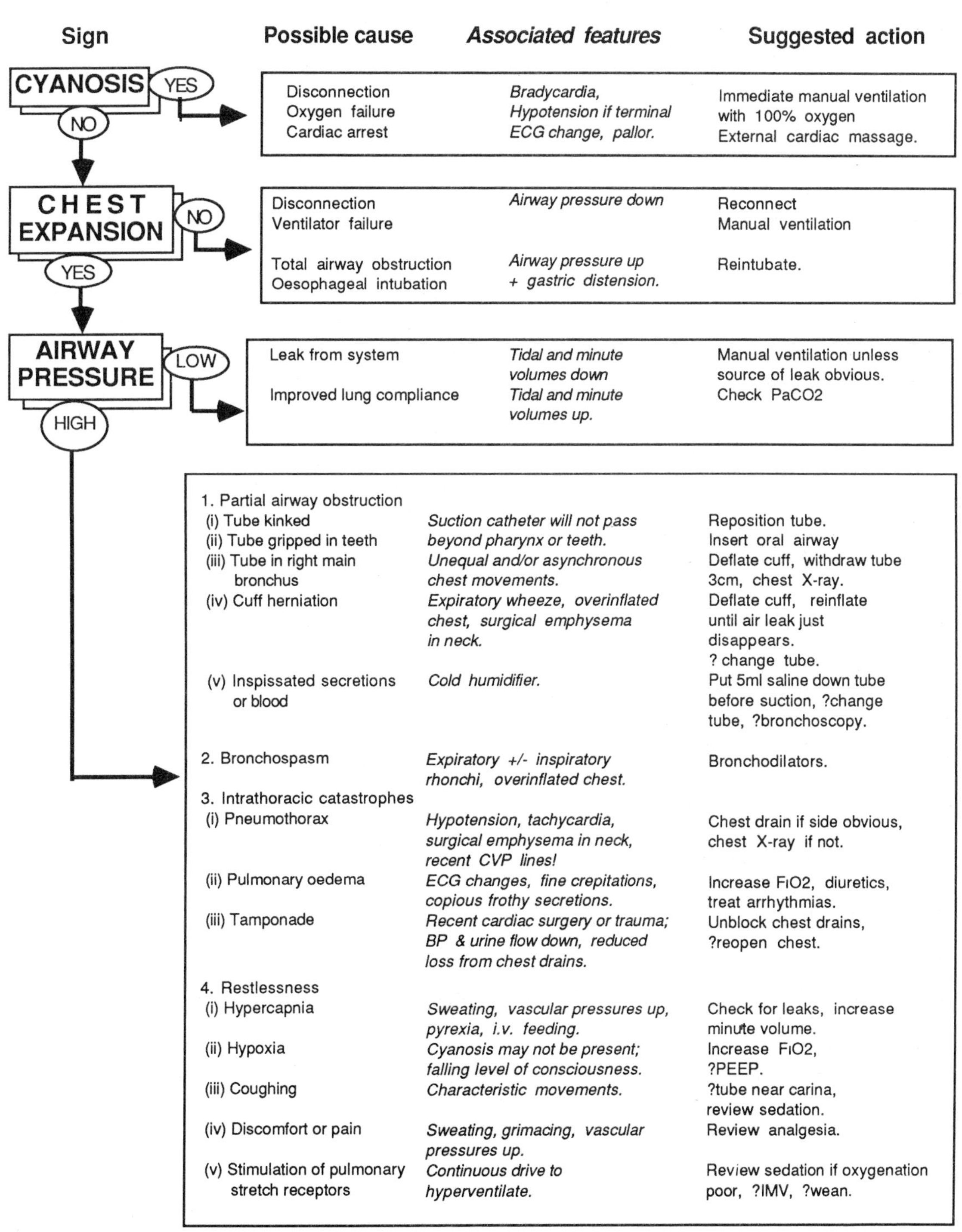

Fig. 42.2 Check-list for the artificially ventilated patient.

reduce sedation requirements considerably.

Analgesics. These should be given if the patient has injuries or wounds which normally merit such drugs, or complains of the tracheal tube (vide supra). They should be given by continuous infusion with additional boluses if painful procedures are undertaken.

Sedatives. Benzodiazepines are often used to provide additional sedation in combination with analgesics. Midazolam is often used by continuous infusion (2–10 mg/h), as it has a shorter action than other drugs in this group. However, it may accumulate in some patients and cause very prolonged sedation and respiratory depression. Disorientation and cardiovascular depression may also occur with these drugs.

Intravenous anaesthetic agents. Continuous infusions of anaesthetic induction agents have been used to provide sedation for long periods, but further research is required into the effects of long-term administration of these drugs before they can be recommended. At present, propofol has been shown to be effective and safe when infused for up to 24 h, with rapid recovery when it is discontinued. Chlormethiazole by continuous infusion may be a useful hypnotic agent in confused patients with hepatic problems in whom opioids are relatively contraindicated. Haloperidol may calm the otherwise almost uncontrollable hyperactivity and confusion observed sometimes (usually at night) in patients with chronic obstructive airways disease.

Other drugs. Nitrous oxide may be used to provide short-term sedation and analgesia but should not be used for more than a few hours because of depressant effects on bone marrow. Isoflurane is effective in concentrations of 0.1–0.6% but the effects of long-term (>24 h) administration are not known.

Complications of artificial ventilation

While IPPV may often be a life-saving procedure, the technique is not without risk to the patient and should be employed only if appropriate, and then for the minimum time required.

Pulmonary barotrauma

Rupture of alveoli may occur in any patient who receives artificial ventilation but is most likely when high mean airway pressures are required because of poor lung compliance or because PEEP has been applied (both commonly occur together). Air is forced into the substance of the lung and then either into the pleural cavity, when a pneumothorax occurs, and/or up through the hilum and into the mediastinum. Pneumothoraces are likely particularly if there has been previous trauma to the lung, as in chest injuries, and tension develops almost inevitably if IPPV is continued. Drainage of the pleural cavity is mandatory in any patient who develops a pneumothorax while receiving IPPV.

Mediastinal emphysema is diagnosed usually on X-ray, but may appear as surgical emphysema in the neck. As there is no specific treatment for mediastinal emphysema, its significance is chiefly as a warning that a leak has occurred and that a pneumothorax may develop, although a chest drain is not yet required. Airway pressures should be reduced either by reducing PEEP (and raising $F\text{I}_{O_2}$), by lowering tidal volume to 10 ml/kg body weight or perhaps by switching to a high-frequency ventilator if one is available.

It should be noted that surgical emphysema appears first at a site close to the leak. Consequently, in a traumatised patient who presents initially with emphysema in the neck, particular attention should be paid to the cervical structures (larynx, pharynx, oesophagus) before assuming that the air has tracked up from the thorax.

Weaning from IPPV

Artificial ventilation should be prolonged only for specific reasons. It should be routine to consider weaning the patient each day.

Patients who are otherwise stable should be weaned as soon as:

1. Pulmonary function seems likely to be adequate during spontaneous ventilation.
2. Neuromuscular strength and coordination seem to be sufficient to maintain an adequate minute volume and to permit coughing.

As pulmonary efficiency is usually slightly worse, at least initially, after discontinuing IPPV and because it is difficult to give an inspired oxygen concentration of more than approximately 60% through a facemask, patients whose lung function is usually normal should be able to achieve a Pa_{O_2} of more than 10 kPa with an inspired oxygen concentration of 40% or less. If the lungs are damaged permanently (e.g. in chronic lung disease), less effective oxygenation may have to be accepted both during, and particularly after, IPPV.

The indications for weaning, tracheal extubation and reinstituting IPPV are shown in Table 42.3. It is probably safer to wean patients from IPPV and to extubate the trachea early in the day rather than in the late afternoon or evening, as less medical and nursing supervision tends to be available at night.

In general, the shorter the period of ventilation, the simpler the weaning procedures; weaning over a period of several days may be necessary after prolonged IPPV, particularly for neuromuscular disorders.

Table 42.3 Guidelines for weaning, extubation and restarting IPPV

1. *When can weaning be started?*

If, when on IPPV (or IMV) and general condition stable (e.g. temperature < 38°C, Hb > 10 g/dl)

(a) HR < 100 beats/min in adults (can safely be more in children)

AND (b) Pa_{O_2} > 10 kPa, FI_{O_2} < 0.45 and PEEP < 5 cmH_2O

AND (c) Pa_{CO_2} < 6 kPa with minute volume < 10 litres/min (or V_D/V_T < 50%)

AND (d) Spontaneous tidal volume > 7 ml/kg

If answers to a + b + c are YES but d is NO, start or continue IMV.

2. *When may the trachea be extubated?*

If patient cooperative and able to cough:

If unconscious and tolerating tube, leave trachea intubated

If uncooperative or intolerant of tube, extubate if IPPV not required (see below)

3. *When does IPPV need to be restarted?*

(Assess patient after 5–10 min of spontaneous ventilation, then at 30 min intervals)

Restart IPPV if:

(a) RESPIRATORY RATE climbs steadily for 3 sucessive 30 min periods

OR (b) it exceeds 45/min

OR (c) HEART RATE climbs steadily for 3 successive 30 min periods

OR (d) it exceeds 130 beats/min

OR (e) HYPOXAEMIA develops (Pa_{O_2} < 8 kPa) (except some chronic chest failure patients)

OR (f) HYPERCAPNIA develops (Pa_{CO_2} > 1.5 kPa above pre-IPPV level)

OR (g) LEVEL OF CONSCIOUSNESS deteriorates.

If one of these conditions does apply, consider WHY spontaneous ventilation cannot be maintained. Bronchospasm and/or pulmonary oedema are important factors which may be overlooked

Adult respiratory distress syndrome (ARDS)

ARDS is the final common pathway of many severe pulmonary insults (e.g. shock, septicaemia, contusion, fat embolism or aspiration of gastric contents). The syndrome is characterised by tachypnoea, cyanosis and diffuse pulmonary infiltrates visible on the X-ray. The most significant pathological feature of ARDS is increased capillary permeability which permits fluid to leak into the interstitial tissues of the lung and results in severe (non-cardiac) pulmonary oedema. In severe cases, the pulmonary leak of proteinaceous fluid progresses rapidly to fibrosis over a few days and irreversible pulmonary failure ensues.

ARDS is difficult to reverse, and treatment is therefore supportive and aimed at preventing further damage. Occasionally, definitive treatment may be available for the primary cause (e.g. laparotomy and drainage of intraperitoneal abscess for septicaemia), but the condition usually develops more insidiously so that curative treatment is impossible.

Mechanical ventilation is nearly always required, although oxygen via a face mask or continuous positive airways pressure (CPAP) may be sufficient to ensure adequate oxygenation in mild cases. If IPPV is used, PEEP is usually added and may improve oxygenation dramatically by reducing interstitial oedema. High inspired oxygen concentrations and minute volumes may be required to achieve barely adequate gas exchange; however, if an inspired oxygen concentration greater than 60% is needed with more than 10 cmH_2O of PEEP to maintain arterial oxygenation, prognosis is poor. Fluid overload must be avoided, haemodynamic status controlled and plasma oncotic pressure maintained. Corticosteroid (methylprednisolone 2 g 6-hourly for 24 h), if given early, may reduce capillary leakage and prevent ARDS developing in susceptible patients but is contraindicated when major sepsis is present.

Despite aggressive therapy, the mortality from ARDS remains high (approximately 50%). Patients with ARDS rarely die from respiratory failure as modern techniques of ventilatory support can usually maintain (just) adequate gas exchange. The pathophysiology of this condition is not confined to the lung and multisystem organ failure may develop during the days after the onset of pulmonary failure. The combination of respiratory, cardiac and renal failure carries a particularly poor prognosis.

As in many illnesses, prevention is better than cure and early diagnosis and treatment of possible precipitating causes of ARDS are likely to have a much greater effect in improving outcome than prolonged aggressive treatment of the established condition.

CARDIOVASCULAR FAILURE

Although actual or expected ventilatory failure is the commonest reason for admission to the general ITU, cardiovascular failure is a frequent finding in the critically ill patient. When associated with pulmonary problems, the effects of cardiovascular insufficiency may be exacerbated because of reduced oxygenation of blood.

Cardiovascular failure may be acute or chronic. When it develops rapidly (e.g. heart failure after myocardial infarction or peripheral circulatory failure after haemorrhage), it is known as 'shock' and, unless the condition is corrected rapidly, admission to the ITU is necessary. Chronic cardiovascular failure is one of the main *raisons d'être* of many departments of medicine (especially cardiology) and surgery (especially cardiac and vascular surgery), but patients who are receiving treatment for one of the varieties of chronic cardiovascular failure should be placed on a 'short list' for ITU admission if they present with unrelated complaints or complications.

Cardiovascular monitoring

Patients are often admitted to the ITU because their cardiovascular status is unpredictable and potentially unstable, making continuous availability of information essential. All patients in the ITU should be monitored with an ECG which displays both the electrical signal and heart rate. The ECG monitoring system in the coronary care unit is often more complex and may include circuits to recognise, count and display frequency histograms of various arrhythmias.

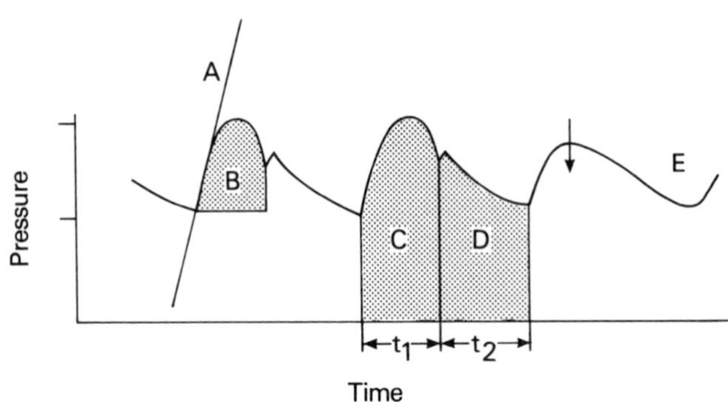

Fig. 42.3 Information to be gained from the arterial pressure signal.

Visible sign	*Physiological effect*
A — Rate of pressure increase	myocardial contractility
B — Area under pulse pressure	stroke volume
C — Systolic pressure × time (t_1)	myocardial oxygen consumption
D — Diastolic pressure × time (t_2)	myocardial oxygen supply
E — Loss of waveform detail	catheter occlusion (flush it!)

Arterial pressure may be measured intermittently by a conventional or automated sphygmomanometer, or continuously by direct intra-arterial recording from the radial, brachial, dorsalis pedis or femoral arteries. Percutaneous arterial cannulation is used widely to monitor arterial pressure (Figs 42.3 and 42.4) and to give ready access to arterial blood samples. Enormous technical efforts are being made to design non-invasive systems which will make invasive procedures less necessary, but, at present, their accuracy and dependability are inadequate in critical situations.

Central venous pressure (CVP) may be measured from a catheter introduced into the superior vena cava or right atrium and connected to either a water or electronic manometer. If the latter is used, care must be taken to calibrate it in the more appropriate 'cmH_2O' rather than 'mmHg'.

Pulmonary artery pressure may be measured using a flow-directed catheter (see Ch. 21). The information gained from measurement of pulmonary capillary wedge pressure permits distinction between pulmonary oedema from high left atrial pressure and that caused by increased permeability of pulmonary capillaries. This may be helpful particularly in patients with multiple injuries and pulmonary problems, severe septicaemia or actual or incipient left ventricular failure.

Cardiovascular assessment

A scheme to aid the ITU resident in assessment of the cardiovascular status is shown in Tables 42.4 and 42.5. Further information which may be obtained from the arterial pressure waveform is indicated in Figures 42.3 and 42.4. A wide range of therapeutic agents is available to modify the behaviour of the cardiovascular system. Some of those used commonly in the ITU are listed and classified under their major effects in Table 42.6.

Shock (acute cardiovascular failure)

In shock, there is an acute failure of the circulatory system to supply adequate nutrients to the tissues and to remove metabolites. Under these circumstances, cell death occurs eventually as a result of impairment of vital membrane functions and abnormal cell metabolism. This sequence of events may follow severe haemorrhage (from a traumatic or surgical cause) and may occur also after loss of fluid from the gastrointestinal tract.

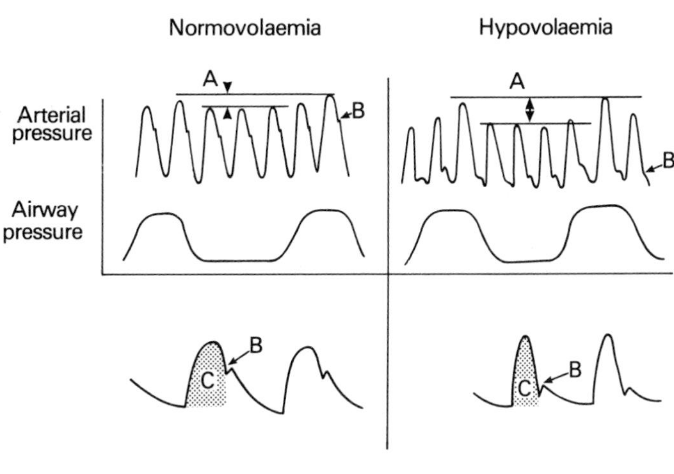

Fig. 42.4 Effect of hypovolaemia on arterial pressure signal.

Table 42.4 Cardiovascular check-list.
Check the primary variables, (systemic arterial pressure (SAP), heart rate (HR), ECG and urine flow) first. Look at (1) absolute values, (2) trends (up, down, variable), (3) relationships with one another — particularly SAR and HR.
Use secondary variables (CVP/neck veins, core–peripheral temperature differences, pulmonary artery pressure (PAP) and pulmonary capillary wedge pressure (PCWP) to distinguish between various possibilities

SAP and HR relationship	Common causes	Confirmatory findings	Suggested action
HR up, SAP up	Sympathetic activation with pain, arousal, etc.	Restlessness, CVP up, PAP up	Review sedation and analgesia
HR down, SAP down	1. Heart block	ECG change	Isoprenaline, pacemaker
	2. Severe hypoxaemia	Cyanosis	Reconnect ventilator or oxygen. Manual IPPV
	3. Response to sedative or analgesic drugs	Recent drug administration	Reduce subsequent doses of drug
HR down, SAP up	Rising intracranial pressure	Deteriorating level of consciousness, enlarging pupils	Hyperventilate, diuretics, mannitol
HR up, SAP down	1. Shock (a) Hypovolaemic	CVP and urine flow down, limbs poorly perfused	Infuse colloid
	(b) septic (early)	CVP and urine flow down, limbs well perfused	Infuse colloid, release pus, give antibiotics
	2. Tamponade after heart surgery	CVP up, urine flow and lung compliance down	Unblock drains, reopen chest
	3. Pneumothorax	Restlessness, lung compliance down	Chest drain
	4. Tachyarrhythmias	ECG change, CVP up	Antiarrhythmics
	5. Pulmonary embolus	Chest pain, cyanosis, CVP up, ?ECG changes	O_2 ?Pulmonary angiography
	6. Allergic reaction	?Rash, recent drug or blood administration	Antihistamines, infuse colloid, ?steroids

In cardiogenic shock, the heart is unable to maintain a sufficiently high output; this occurs most commonly after severe myocardial infarction. Septic shock may complicate overwhelming infections of many types but results most frequently from Gram-negative infections.

Pathophysiology

In the early stages of circulatory insufficiency, the sympathetic nervous system is activated, and constriction of veins and arteries maintains arterial pressure and perfusion of vital organs (brain, heart and kidneys). These compensatory mechanisms provide a short period during which aggressive treatment may prevent further development of the more severe and irreversible features of shock. If effective treatment is not started, poor perfusion leads to tissue hypoxia and anaerobic metabolism. The resultant acidosis causes relaxation of precapillary sphincters despite maximal sympathetic activity. However, the postcapillary sphincters remain constricted and fluid becomes sequestrated in tissues. The progressive loss of intravascular volume eventually causes hypoperfusion of the previously protected vital organs; respiratory and renal failure develop, followed later by hepatic, cardiac and eventually neurological failure.

Table 42.5 Cardiovascular indicators.
It is often not possible to measure some cardiovascular variables directly, so that it is necessary to use other variables to indicate indirectly what changes are occurring. Changes which are normally undesirable are indicated in the table below. Welcome changes are normally accompanied by alterations in the 'indicator observations' in the opposite direction

Undesirable change	Indicator observations
1. Cardiac output DOWN	Urine flow DOWN. Core–peripheral temperature difference UP
2. Blood volume DOWN	CVP and PCWP DOWN. Inspiratory to expiratory difference in systolic SAP ('paradox') UP (see Fig. 42.4). Dicrotic notch LOWER on arterial pressure waveform (see Fig. 42.4). LARGE SAP fall in response to IPPV, sedatives or analgesics
3. Right ventricular function DETERIORATING	CVP UP. PAP DOWN. Peripheral oedema INCREASING
4. Left ventricular function DETERIORATING	PCWP or left atrial pressure UP. Arterial SAP DOWN. Pulmonary oedema INCREASING. Oxygenation DETERIORATING
5. Peripherial vascular resistance INCREASING	Core–peripheral temperature difference UP. STEEPER pressure decay during diastole
6. Myocardial oxygen demand UP	HR UP. SAP UP. Product of HR × SAP UP
7. Myocardial oxygen supply DOWN	HR UP. Diastolic arterial pressure DOWN

Septic shock

Septic, Gram-negative, bacteraemic or endotoxic shock are names which have been given to a clinical state which may appear following localised or systemic bacterial, fungal or viral infections. The commonest sources of infection are the gastrointestinal tract, particularly after laparotomy, and the urogenital tract, especially after instrumentation. Infections of the respiratory and biliary tracts may also be implicated.

Table 42.6 A summary of cardiovascular drugs and their starting doses

A. INOTROPES	
These stimulate the myocardium and increase cardiac output. Often used to raise SAP and increase urine flow	
(a) Sympathomimetics	
1. Dopamine	i.v. inf. (2–5 μg kg^{-1} min^{-1} for renal effect, 10–20 μg kg^{-1} min^{-1} for max. pressor effect)
2. Dobutamine	i.v. inf. (up to 15 μg kg^{-1} min^{-1}
3. Noradrenaline	i.v. inf. (5–10 μg/min)
(NB: much larger doses of these drugs are required if the patient has received β-blocking drugs)	
(b) Non-sympathomimetics	
1. Digoxin	Slow i.v. (0.5–1.0 mg in 5 min) (beware hypokalaemia)
2. Calcium	i.v. bolus (10 ml of 10% Ca gluconate)
B. CHRONOTROPES	
These increase the heart rate but a pacemaker is required in heart block.	
1. Atropine	i.v. bolus (0.2–0.6 mg)
2. Isoprenaline	i.v. inf. (0.5–10 μg/min)
C. ANTIARRHYTHMICS	
(a) For VENTRICULAR arrhythmias.	
Before treatment, check that the CVP catheter is not stimulating the heart. All these drugs depress cardiac contractility and tend to reduce SAP	
1. Lignocaine	i.v. bolus (100 mg) + inf. (1–4 mg/min)
2. Disopyramide	Slow i.v. (up to 2 mg/kg) + inf. (400 μg kg^{-1} h^{-1})
3. Practolol	Slow i.v. (up to 5 mg)
4. Mexiletine	Slow i.v. (200 mg in 10 min) + inf. (250 mg in 1 h)
(b) For SUPRAVENTRICULAR tachyarrhythmias	
1. Digoxin	i.v. bolus (0.5–1 mg)
2. Amiodarone	Slow i.v. (via CVP) (150 mg in 30 min and repeat)
3. Verapamil	Slow i.v. (5 mg) + inf. (5–10 mg/h)
D. ANTIHYPERTENSIVES	
(a) Vasodilators.	
These lower peripheral vascular resistance and reduce afterload	
1. Hydralazine	Slow i.v. (20–40 mg and repeat)
2. Nitroprusside	i.v. inf. (0.5–5 μg kg^{-1} min^{-1})
3. Glyceryl trinitrate	i.v. inf. (10–150 μg/min)
4. Isosorbide dinitrate	i.v. inf. (30–120 μg/min)
5. Phenoxybenzamine	i.v. bolus (20–100 mg)
6. Phentolamine	i.v. inf. (0.2–2 mg/min)
(b) β-Adrenergic blockers.	
These reduce myocardial contractility and may increase afterload	
1. Labetalol	i.v. bolus (10–50 mg) + inf. (2 mg/min) (also has α-blocking effects)
2. Atenolol	Slow i.v. (150 μg/kg over 20 min)
3. Metoprolol	slow i.v. (5 mg in 5 min)
4. Oxprenolol	slow i.v. (5 mg in 10 min)

Microorganisms isolated from patients with this condition are usually Gram-negative gut bacteria, e.g. *Escherichia coli*, *Klebsiella* or *Proteus* spp. In a small but significant minority, Gram-positive organisms such as *Staphylococcus aureus* or *Pneumococcus* may be found. Patients who are immunocompromised or receiving chemotherapy are particularly liable to develop septic shock from infection with *Candida* or other fungi.

Septic shock is extremely rare outside hospital and occurs usually as a complication of existing clinical problems. Its occurrence and mortality are related to the severity of the underlying condition. It is commonest at the extremes of life, in patients in whom resistance to infection is low and after splenectomy (when pneumococcal infection is common).

Characteristically, the patient appears warm and well perfused in early septic shock, with a normal or often elevated cardiac output but a low arterial pressure because of reduced peripheral resistance ('warm phase'). If shock persists, a hypodynamic cardiovascular state develops in which cardiac output and blood volume decrease, systemic and pulmonary resistances increase ('cold phase'), and the chances of recovery decrease sharply. In the 'warm' phase, the increased temperature and cardiovascular activity are accompanied by a marked increase in metabolic requirements although, paradoxically, oxygen extraction by the tissues is reduced so that the arteriovenous oxygen content difference is low. Among the factors postulated to contribute to the impaired oxygen utilisation are the opening of arteriovenous capillary 'shunts' in tissues and uncoupling of the normal processes that link energy production and oxygenation. In the 'cold' phase, the pathophysiological picture resembles more closely that seen in hypovolaemic shock.

Treatment

In shock of all types, the primary aim of treatment is to restore and maintain an adequate flow of well-oxygenated blood. Thus, the initial step in management of the shocked patient is to ensure that arterial blood is well saturated (>95%). Fluid should be given rapidly through a large i.v. cannula to restore the circulating volume. At least two-thirds of the fluid should be administered as colloid solutions; whole blood is preferred if blood has been lost, although substitutes (e.g. Haemaccel) may be used in septic shock or while awaiting the definitive replacement fluid. Inotropic support and vasodilators (see Table 41.6) may assist in restoring the circulation, and renal function should be encouraged with diuretics (e.g. frusemide) or low-dose dopamine.

In septic shock, blood should be obtained for culture before antibiotics are administered. In this serious condition, large doses of broad-spectrum antibiotics are appropriate (e.g. cefuroxime + gentamicin + metronidazole). It is essential that every appropriate diagnostic technique, including laparotomy, be employed in the search for the source of infection. Collections of pus must be evacuated despite the patient's critical condition, otherwise bacteraemia recurs and progressive multiorgan failure ensues.

OTHER SYSTEMS

Many ITU patients are at risk of multiple organ failure and the expert knowledge of many different specialists should be available when required. Bacteriologists, nephrologists and cardiologists, amongst others, are frequent visitors to an ITU to provide advice on patient management. In some hospitals, however, specialist opinions may not be available and it falls to the ITU team to provide care for the more common problems.

Renal failure

The development of renal failure can be prevented in most ITU patients at risk by judicious use of fluids, low-dose dopamine infusion (see Table 42.6) and diuretic therapy. Peritoneal dialysis can be carried out in all units if haemodialysis is unavailable or inappropriate. Continuous arteriovenous haemofiltration (CAVH) is a new technique which may be undertaken in most units and is valuable in reducing fluid overload in patients with inadequate renal function. CAVH may be used also in some patients in oliguric renal failure to control electrolyte abnormalities while recovery is awaited.

Nutrition

It is often difficult to maintain an adequate nutritional intake in ITU patients. In acute illness, resuscitation is more important usually than nutrition for the first 24–48 h, but after this time efforts should be made to provide enough food for recovery to occur. Enteral nutrition by nasogastric tube should be used whenever possible but paralytic ileus, other gastrointestinal disturbances or the effects of analgesic and sedative drugs often prevent this in ITU patients. Parenteral nutrition should be undertaken as a planned procedure with the intention of providing a balanced intake of amino acids, carbohydrates, fats, vitamins and trace elements. Parenteral 'diet' in these patients usually requires day-to-day adjustment, and daily monitoring of blood and urinary biochemistry is essential. Hospital pharmacists often keep information on preparations available for parenteral nutrition.

DEATH IN THE ITU

The mortality rate amongst patients admitted to the ITU is higher than that elsewhere in hospital. This is inevitable in view of the pathological processes which make it necessary to provide artificial assistance for one or more of the vital systems, but it is to be hoped that fewer patients die than if the facilities of the ITU were not available. In order to maintain the morale and sense of purpose of the unit staff, it is essential that the need for therapy be the main criterion for admission to the unit rather than the imminence of death.

In a significant proportion of cases, the patient is unable to overcome the pathological processes in spite of maximal therapeutic support, and this becomes apparent when the patient fails to improve sufficiently to become independent of the measures employed to support ventilation and/or perfusion. The prognosis deteriorates markedly the longer IPPV is required and the more systems require support. The maintenance of a physiologically satisfactory status quo by means of artificial support does not augur well and the appropriate message must be transmitted to the relatives. It must be stressed repeatedly to them that improvement is required to give significant hope of survival, because the patient must be able not only to throw off the effects of the initial insult, but also to resist the infective episodes which often complicate the recovery period. Failure to improve is followed usually by slow deterioration in the efficiency of previously unaffected organs, and by a poor response to supportive measures introduced to counteract the effects of this deterioration.

In terms of predicting which patients are unlikely to survive, those who are comatose and unresponsive after severe brain damage are amongst the easier to distinguish. The signs of 'brain death' are well described (Pallis 1983), and a scheme of assessment is included in Table 42.7. Formal assessment must be carried out twice by two senior clinicians, at least one of whom must be a consultant.

Table 42.7 Recognition of brain stem death. Brain stem death may be assumed if (a) the answer to each of the ten questions is 'NO', and (b) if the assessment is repeated, with the same results, after at least 4 h. If the answer to any of the questions is 'YES' or 'DON'T KNOW', active treatment must be continued

1. Is there any doubt as to the cause of the coma and brain damage (e.g. trauma, cerebrovascular accident, drowning)?
2. Has the patient received (or taken) any drugs which could have either depressed the central nervous system (e.g. alcohol, sedatives, hypnotics, analgesics), or impaired his or her muscular capabilities (e.g. muscle relaxants)?
3. Are there any metabolic or endocrine disturbances which could affect neural function (e.g. blood glucose changes, uraemia, hepatic dysfunction)?
4. Is the patient's temperature less than 35°C? (Midbrain failure is often followed by a rapid fall in temperature, but hypothermia itself may induce coma. If the temperature is below 35°C, active warming must be started and further cooling minimised with 'space blankets')
5. Do the pupils react to light?
6. Are there corneal reflexes?
7. Do the eyes move during or after caloric testing?
8. Are there motor responses in the cranial nerve distribution in response to painful stimulation of the face, trunk or limbs?
9. Does the patient gag, cough or otherwise move following the passage of a suction catheter into the nose, mouth or bronchial tree?
10. Does the patient show any respiratory activity at all when the arterial carbon dioxide tension exceeds 7 kPa (checked on an arterial sample)?

FURTHER READING

Hinds C J 1987 Intensive care — a concise textbook. Baillière Tindall, London

Oh T E 1985 Intensive care manual. Butterworths, Sydney

Pallis C 1983 The ABC of brain stem death. British Medical Association, London

Tinker J, Rapin M (eds) 1983 Care of the critically ill patient. Springer Verlag, Berlin

43. Relief of chronic pain

Most pain is mild, transitory and of little consequence. Sometimes it may warn of a curable condition, but on occasions it may not be possible to discover the cause, or the cause may be untreatable, and the pain may persist. It is this type of pain that becomes chronic or intractable, and is the stock-in-trade of pain relief clinics.

Patients with chronic pain may be allocated broadly to two groups: (a) those with a normal expectation of life and who are often difficult to treat and (b) those with a short expectation of life (usually resulting from neoplastic disease) and who are normally easier to treat.

Patients seen in a pain relief clinic present usually with one of the following categories of pain.

Neurological

1. Postherpetic neuralgia.
2. Trigeminal neuralgia.
3. Nerve entrapment syndromes, including back pain and scar pain.
4. Disseminated sclerosis.
5. Central pain syndromes: 'stroke' pain, thalamic pain syndrome, and phantom limb pain.
6. Pain from neuroma formation: stump pain.

Vascular

1. Migraine.
2. Claudication.
3. Raynaud's disease.

Orthopaedic

1. Back pain and sciatica.
2. Arthritis.
3. A variety of vague pains associated usually with the cervical or lumbar spine and often defying conventional diagnosis.

Neoplastic

1. Arising from primary tumour.
2. Induced by metastases.
3. Resulting from treatment, e.g. necrosis after radiotherapy.

Unknown or undiagnosable cause

Atypical facial pain

Psychogenic pain

This is defined usually as pain occurring without the presence of an obvious physical cause. However, central pain may also have no obvious cause, which leads to confusion. The distinction is even more intangible as psychogenic pain may result from the existence of some minor disorder, undetectable by normal means, or may be produced by some past injury. It is thought that when pain has been experienced, it leaves within the nervous system a memory which is suppressed by inhibitory mechanisms. It is only when these inhibitory mechanisms are removed, usually by psychological factors, that pain becomes apparent.

Szasz wrote: 'the notions of physical and mental pain are meaningless. The "common-sense" view that regards this matter as if there were two types of pain — one organic and another psychogenic — is misleading and responsible for numerous pseudoproblems in the borderland between medicine and psychology'.

However, it is important to delineate the relative importance of psychological and physical mechanisms in a patient's pain experience as this influences treatment. Sometimes, distinctive qualities are noted in the pain of patients with psychiatric illness (e.g. in the form of hallucinations) but such cases are not common clinically.

ASSESSMENT OF PATIENTS WITH CHRONIC PAIN

A full history should be obtained and a full clinical examination undertaken (not just of the painful area). Radiological or other investigations may be indicated.

The patient's description of the pain is important. Some pains are described so similarly by different individuals as to be diagnostic, e.g. the pain of trigeminal neuralgia. The patient's choice of words and the vividness of his description provides a pointer to diagnosis (e.g. the burning pain of causalgia) and reflects also the patient's emotional state and his ethnic and cultural background.

Many pain analysis questionnaires exist, but that suggested by Bond is easy to remember and covers all the essential points.

Before treatment of a patient with chronic pain is attempted, it is important that a firm diagnosis is reached and to establish that the patient's pain cannot be relieved by treatment of the cause. This may involve consultation with many other disciplines. In some patients, however, no diagnosis can be made in spite of extensive and lengthy investigations, and these patients have to be accepted and treated symptomatically in the way that seems most appropriate to their pain.

Some attempt should be made to assess the patient's personality and psychological status. Two formal measurements of personality are available: the Minnesota Multiphasic Personality Inventory (MMPI) and the Eysenck Personality Inventory (EPI). Those personality traits which are important in evaluating the patient with chronic pain include susceptibility to anxiety and/or depression, and the existence of hysterical, hypochondriacal or obsessional traits. Most patients suffering from chronic pain exhibit some degree of anxiety or, more usually, depression. These may present as an obvious neurosis, in which case the patient should be referred for full psychiatric assessment.

METHODS OF MANAGEMENT OF CHRONIC PAIN

Simple measures

For centuries, rest has been used to relieve pain and suffering and this is still an important measure. This may involve resting the whole patient or just the painful part. Splinting and immobilisation often relieve pain arising from joints or pathological fractures, without the need for potent analgesic drugs.

The relief of anxiety occasioned by pain may produce considerable diminution in intensity of pain. Anxiety may be relieved more effectively by simple and careful explanation than by anxiolytic drugs.

The injection of tender areas in myofascial syndromes with mixtures of local anaesthetic and steroids is often effective, as may be the use of cold pain-relieving sprays, heat or percussion.

Drugs

For reasons of finance and availability of facilities, the majority of patients with chronic pain are treated with drugs prescribed usually by the general practitioner.

Analgesic drugs

Many analgesic drugs may be used (Table 43.1). Prescription of an analgesic regimen for a patient with chronic pain requires the following considerations:

What potency of drug does the patient require? Not all patients need potent opioid analgesics and although the risk of dependence is usually overstated, these drugs should be avoided if possible in patients with a normal expectation of life. However, in general, pain severity (mild, moderate and severe) matches analgesic requirements: low (aspirin); medium (codeine); high (morphine).

Table 43.1 Analgesic drugs in common use

1. *Low potency: antipyretic analgesics*	
Salicylates	Aspirin
Aniline derivatives	Paracetamol
Anthranillic acid derivatives	Mefenamic acid
Indole derivatives	Indomethacin
Pyrazolone derivatives	Phenylbutazone
2. *Medium potency*	
Medium duration	
Morphine derivatives	Codeine
	Dihydrocodeine
Methadone derivatives	Dextropropoxyphene
Benzmorphinan derivatives	Pentazocine
3. *High potency: opioid analgesics*	
Long acting	
Slow-release morphine	
Buprenorphine	
Oxycodone	
Medium duration	
Morphine	
Diamorphine	
Phenazocine	
Levorphanol	
Methadone	
Short acting	
Dextromoramide	

Dose of drug and frequency of administration. The object of treating chronic pain is to provide complete pain relief. The correct dose of an analgesic drug is that dose which relieves the pain for an acceptable period of time without unacceptable side effects. The drug should be administered frequently enough to ensure that the patient remains pain-free.

Route of administration. Ideally, drugs are given orally and injections should be avoided if at all possible. Some drugs (e.g. buprenorphine, phenazocine) may be given sublingually and others (e.g. morphine, diamorphine, oxycodone) by suppository.

Potential duration of treatment. This is evident usually from the aetiology of the pain and influences the choice of drug.

Specific types of pain. Some types of pain or disease are treated most appropriately by a specific group of drugs. Analgesic drugs either interfere with the production of peripheral pain-producing substances including prostaglandins and kinins (e.g. aspirin and non-opioid analgesics) or act on central mechanisms at endorphin receptors, often including perceptual mechanisms and emotional response to pain (e.g opioid analgesics). Studies of osseous metastases have demonstrated that prostaglandin E_2 (PGE_2) is implicated in the mediation of pain, and prostaglandin inhibitors alone or combined with opioid analgesics provide better pain relief than opioid analgesics alone.

Having established adequate pain relief, the patient should be reassessed at intervals, as it is often possible to reduce analgesic drug dosage slowly without pain reappearing. Reappearance of pain on a previously satisfactory drug regimen requires reassessment of the patient before therapy is modified.

Other drugs used in the management of patients with chronic pain

Psychotropic drugs. Analgesic activity appears to be present in most of the tricyclic antidepressant drugs, but is most noticeable in agents which enhance 5-hydroxytryptamine (5-HT) activity by preventing reuptake into presynaptic stores (e.g. amitriptyline, clomipramine). Pain relief may take up to two weeks to appear. The antidepressant effect is useful in many patients.

Some of the phenothiazines possess analgesic activity, particularly when used in combination with a tricyclic antidepressant. Currently there is interest in enhancement of these effects with transmitter precursors including L-tryptophan.

Anticonvulsants. These drugs have membrane stabilising properties and the principal use is for the treatment of epilepsy. Carbamazepine was the first drug to be used for trigeminal neuralgia and has proved particularly successful. However, anticonvulsants are useful also in other conditions with a 'shooting' component to the pain, e.g. postherpetic neuralgia.

Steroids. Steroids may be useful in several ways:

1. They interfere with the synthesis of prostaglandins.
2. They may reduce oedema in neoplastic tissue (either primary tumour or metastasis), so relieving pain by reducing pressure on adjacent pain-sensitive structures.
3. They are very effective by the extradural or intrathecal route in treatment of low back pain

and sciatica. The mechanism of action is not clear, but may be a result of reduction of oedema in nerve roots and adjacent structures.

Cytotoxic drugs. Cytotoxic drugs may reduce the size of tumour tissue and relieve pressure on adjacent structures.

Nerve blocks

Blockade of a peripheral pain pathway reduces or obviates the need for potent analgesic drugs and unwanted effects of these agents. Nerve blocks are appropriate for pain confined to an area with a discrete nerve supply.

Blockade of nerves may be carried out at various sites (Fig. 43.1) either temporarily with local anaesthetic for diagnostic or prognostic purposes or permanently or semipermanently for therapeutic purposes (with neurolytic solutions, radiofrequency or cryotherapeutic lesions).

The practice of nerve blocking techniques has been improved greatly by the use of the image intensifier and nerve stimulator.

Before undertaking a permanent nerve block the consequent effects should be assessed by an initial local anaesthetic block. This confirms the presumptive effect of the block (which does not always conform to anticipated effects) and permits the patient to experience effects including anaesthesia, which may result.

Not infrequently the duration of pain relief afforded by local anaesthetic blocks outlasts the duration of action of the local anaesthetic. The reasons for this are not clear.

The following are some of the more common useful blocks.

Somatic nerve blocks

Spinal nerves may be blocked paravertebrally from the cervical to the sacral region, although the precise technique varies with the region. In all instances, the use of an image intensifier is advisable to ensure accurate placement of needles.

It is unusual to require a block of more than a limited number of nerves in order to ascertain which are responsible for transmitting the patient's pain. It is important that the block is discrete, i.e. not involving adjacent nerves, and so provides an unequivocal response, especially when a subsequent permanent block is contemplated.

If permanent block of a single nerve is contemplated, this is carried out most conveniently with

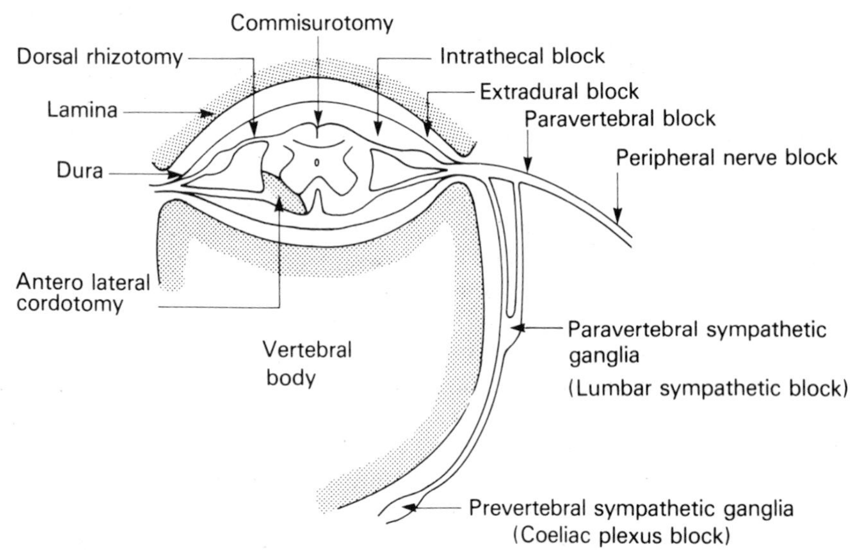

Fig. 43.1 Potential sites for interrupting pain pathways.

a radiofrequency lesion (if necessary in the dorsal root ganglion).

Trigeminal nerve and its branches

Blockade of the peripheral branches of the trigeminal nerve is often helpful in the management of facial pain.

Diagnostic blocks are performed with local anaesthetic followed by a neurolytic drug (alcohol, phenol) or, increasingly, the production of a radiofrequency lesion. The standard approaches are described in textbooks of local anaesthesia. Additional help is obtained from an image intensifier.

These blocks may be helpful for the pain of trigeminal neuralgia and that of head and neck malignancy, although blockade of the peripheral branches of the trigeminal nerve is often insufficient and trigeminal rhizotomy may be required (vide infra).

Extradural blocks

Extradural blocks may be performed at any level of the spinal cord from cervical to caudal. Blocks may be either therapeutic or diagnostic for distinguishing between low back pain of organic or psychogenic origin.

In patients with a limited life expectancy, the block may be repeated with a neurolytic solution (usually phenol), but comparatively large doses are required and the block is less precise than that obtained by intrathecal injection, which is usually preferred.

Mention has been made earlier of the use of extradural steroids, usually methylprednisolone, for the treatment of low back pain and sciatica. This indication probably accounts for the largest number of extradural blocks carried out in pain clinics. Useful pain relief is achieved in at least 60% of patients although the block may need to be repeated.

The pain of spinal nerve compression from spinal metastases may also respond dramatically to extradural steroids, presumably as a result of reduction of oedema and consequent reduction in compression of nerve roots.

Intrathecal blocks

One of the most important historical developments in the management of pain of malignant origin was the introduction in 1931 of intrathecal neurolysis with alcohol. This was refined subsequently by Maher, who used a hyperbaric solution of phenol in glycerine (in place of hypobaric alcohol).

The technique is ideally suited to those patients with pain confined to a few dermatomes, and although simple, requires meticulous attention to detail. After full explanation of the technique and description of possible side effects, lumbar puncture is performed under local anaesthesia with the patient lying on the painful side on an adjustable table.

A 22 G spinal needle (the finest through which it is possible to inject the viscous phenol in glycerine solution) is inserted with the bevel pointing downwards to just penetrate the dura. The patient is then rotated approximately 45° backwards so that the dorsal roots are most dependent (Fig. 43.2) and phenol in glycerine injected in small increments. Between each increment, the patient is questioned for the presence of altered sensations.

Usually the patient experiences a sensation of warmth or paraesthesiae in the area supplied by the roots bathed in phenol. If this coincides with the area in which the patient experiences pain, then the positioning is correct; if not, the table is tipped in order to move the solution in either a cephalad or caudad direction by gravity.

Further increments (maximum 1.0 ml) are injected until analgesia exists in the painful area. Occasionally patients do not experience paraesthesia and the only indication of the effect of the phenol is the development of anaesthesia, which must be sought in case it does not conform to the correct area.

Side effects are confined usually to loss of sensation, which is frequently inevitable, but this may be accompanied by paraesthesia, lasting usually for only a few days. Motor block is rare, but if it occurs is probably the result of incorrect positioning.

A more common complication with blocks of sacral roots is disturbance of sphincter action.

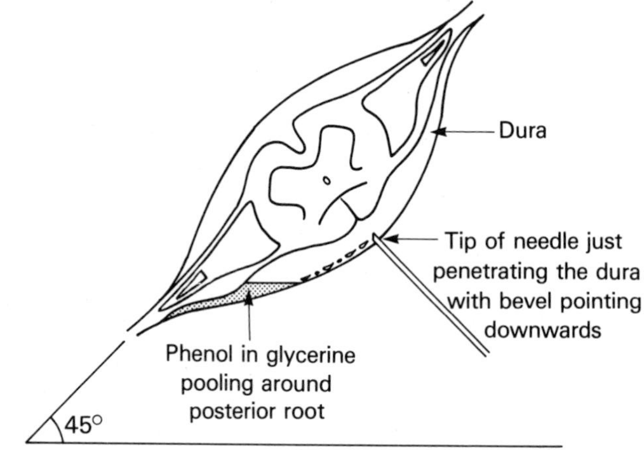

Fig. 43.2 Intrathecal phenol block.

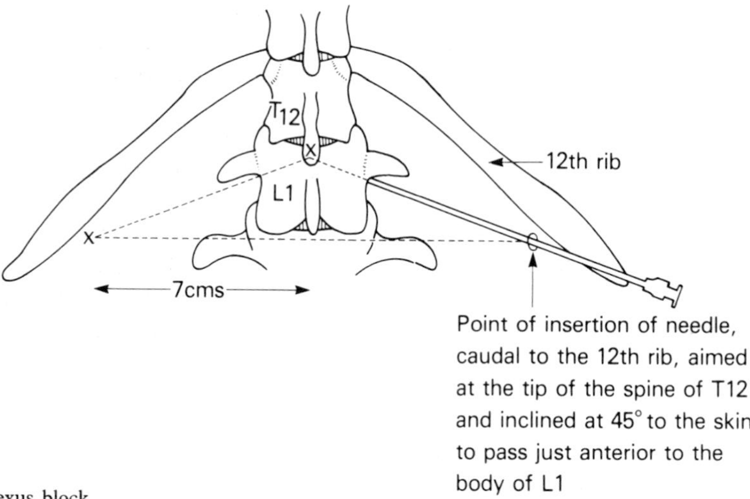

Fig. 43.3 Coeliac plexus block.

Provided that the block is unilateral this is uncommon unless there are pre-existing sphincter problems. The resulting urinary retention requires catheterisation, but bladder function usually returns to normal within 2-3 weeks. Spinal headache is surprisingly rare.

The mean duration of analgesia is 3-4 months, but there is considerable variation. However, the technique is repeated easily if necessary.

Autonomic blocks

1. *Stellate ganglion block.* Stellate ganglion block is helpful in managing pain of vascular origin in the upper limb. Repeated blocks with local anaesthetic may be effective, but neurolytic blockade should be undertaken only by the expert because of the adjacent structures and the risks of intravascular or intrathecal injection.

2. *Coeliac plexus block.* Pain resulting from intra-abdominal malignancy (especially neoplasms of pancreas or stomach) is ablated readily by blocking the coeliac plexus with alcohol. The use of an image intensifier makes the positioning of needles more precise. The surface landmarks are shown in Figure 43.3. A 12.5 cm needle is inserted below the 12th rib at a point level with the spinous process of L1. Depending on whether or not the

angle of the 12th rib is wide or narrow, the point of insertion of the needle varies in distance (5–10 cm) from the midline, but the further from the midline the easier it is to direct the point of the needle medially in front of the vertebral body of L1.

The needle is inserted at an angle of approximately 45° to the skin and directed medially and slightly cephalad towards the spine of T12 so as to pass just in front of the upper part of the body of L1. Needles are inserted bilaterally for a complete block and require insertion usually to a depth of approximately 10 cm. Twenty-five ml of 50% alcohol are injected through each needle. This injection is painful and should be preceded by local anaesthetic; alternatively the patient should be sedated.

The only significant complication of this technique is hypotension. This is occasionally profound and may be prolonged. It may be ameliorated by the use of elastic stockings and if necessary an abdominal binder.

3. *Lumbar sympathetic block*. Lumbar sympathetic block with phenol solution (chemical sympathectomy) may be useful for the relief of pain resulting from vascular insufficiency of the lower limbs. However, improvement in blood flow tends to be in the superficial tissues. Claudication may not be improved, and may even be worsened as a result of shunting of blood away from muscles.

The pain of claudication may be relieved by lumbar plexus block using a strength of neurolytic solution which blocks mainly small C fibres.

Radiofrequency lesions

Radiofrequency current may be used to produce lesions within the nervous system. This is a relatively recent technique which has proved very useful.

The radiofrequency electrode comprises an insulated needle with a small exposed tip. A high-frequency alternating current flows from the electrode tip to the tissues, producing ionic agitation and a frictional heating effect in tissue adjacent to the tip of the probe. The magnitude of this heating effect is monitored by a thermistor in the tip of the electrode.

Damage to nerve fibres sufficient to block conduction occurs at temperatures above 45°C although in practice most lesions are made with a probe tip temperature of 60°–80°C. The size of the lesion is determined by the size of the exposed electrode tip and the duration and magnitude of heating. The lesion produced comprises all areas heated to 45°C or higher.

Because the lesion is small (average size 10 mm × 7 mm) most radiofrequency lesion generators are equipped with a nerve stimulator to aid accurate placement of the probe. Radiofrequency lesions may be made in almost any peripheral nerve or within the central nervous system (percutaneous cervical cordotomy, midbrain tractotomy, thalamotomy, etc.).

An example of the use of radiofrequency lesions is the treatment of trigeminal neuralgia.

Trigeminal neuralgia is managed normally with one of the anticonvulsant drugs, e.g. carbamazepine. However, in a proportion of patients the pain is not controlled or the patient finds the side effects of the drugs intolerable. These patients are treated by radiofrequency trigeminal rhizotomy. Under local or general anaesthesia an electrode is passed through the foramen ovale under image intensifier control so that the tip is amongst the trigeminal rootlets behind the ganglion (Fig. 43.4).

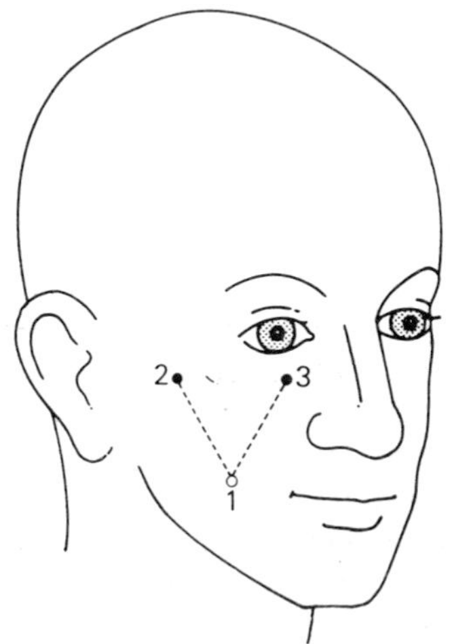

Fig. 43.4 Landmarks for trigeminal rhizotomy.
1 — Point of electrode insertion 2.5–3 cm lateral to labial commisure.
2 — A point 3 cm anterior to the external auditory meatus.
3 — A point below the medial border of the pupil with the patient looking straight ahead.

If anaesthetised, the patient is allowed to awaken and gentle electrical stimulation of the rootlets produces paraesthesia in the division in which the electrode lies. If this does not coincide with the distribution of the patient's pain, the patient is reanaesthetised if necessary, and the electrode manipulated until stimulation coincides with the area of pain.

Incremental radiofrequency lesions are made, monitoring the degree of sensory loss after each lesion. Results of this technique are excellent, affording patients good pain relief with minimal sensory loss.

Cryotherapy

Lesions may also be produced in the nervous system by cold. The cryoprobe consists of an insulated needle, but of larger gauge than the radiofrequency electrode. Cooling is produced by the Joule–Thompson effect using nitrous oxide as the refrigerant. The probe also carries a nerve stimulator for accurate localisation of the nerve.

Nerve destruction is produced by the disruptive effect of the formation of ice crystals within the cells and is enhanced by the application of more than one freeze–thaw cycle. The probe tip may reach a temperature as low as −80°C.

Blocking of peripheral nerves by cryotherapy appears to be completely reversible and this may offer advantages in some situations. The technique has been used not only in chronic pain patients, but also for postoperative pain relief, e.g. at thoracotomy by cryotherapy of intercostal nerves.

Electrical nerve stimulation

It has been known for centuries that an electrical current (from electric catfish, rays, eels, etc.) can relieve pain. More recently, the use of electrical stimulation techniques has been based on the gate control theory of pain which is still accepted as valid, although it has undergone several revisions and has been criticised (see Ch. 5).

The simplest method of applying electrical stimulation to the nervous system is transcutaneous nerve stimulation (TNS). A small battery-powered stimulator is used to apply an electrical stimulus to the skin via flexible carbon electrodes.

The stimulator supplies a square wave or spike pulse with variable voltage, pulse width and frequency. Stimulation is applied at an intensity which the patient finds comfortable, with the electrodes positioned over the painful area, on either side of it, or over nerves supplying the area. The initial response is often good, but judgement of the efficacy of the technique should be delayed for a month or two as the placebo response rate is high. Adverse effects are minimal and are confined usually to allergic responses to the electrodes, gels or tapes, although electrical burns occur occasionally.

Electrical stimulation applied to the dorsal columns is also effective in relieving pain. Electrodes may be implanted either surgically over the dorsal columns or positioned in the extradural space via a Tuohy needle. Many patients obtain worthwhile pain relief. However, long-term results have been disappointing, possibly as a result of poor patient selection.

Stimulation by implanted electrodes of the periaqueductal and paraventricular grey matter of the brain, and also of various regions of the thalamus, have been successful in abolishing pain, but these techniques are still experimental.

Acupuncture

For four thousand years the Chinese have known that the insertion of needles at specific points of the body may produce analgesia. Understandably this has been treated with some scepticism by Western physicians. However, there now seems little doubt that acupunture or 'needle effect' has a useful part to play in the management of pain.

The precise mechanism of action of acupuncture analgesia is uncertain. However, naloxone reverses the effects of acupuncture and injection of naloxone into the periaqueductal grey matter of animals also reduces the effect. Increases in CSF endorphin concentrations have also been demonstrated. Furthermore, lesions of the anterolateral tracts prevent the occurrence of acupuncture analgesia. It appears, therefore, that acupuncture analgesia is mediated via Aβ, Aδ and C fibres which, via the anterolateral tracts, relay to the periaqueductal grey matter and nucleus raphe magnus. It is possible that descending inhibitory pathways are then activated. There is also a correlation between acupuncture points and trigger points in myofascial syndromes.

Acupuncture points are described usually by the Chinese nomenclature, which provides a useful shorthand. They appear to be areas of low skin electrical resistance (in comparison with surrounding skin) and may be detected by a variety of 'point detectors' which assess electrical resistance.

Modern acupuncture needles are of stainless steel and approximately 30 G. The points for treatment are selected and the needles (which should be sterile) inserted to depths varying from a few millimetres to several centimetres, according to the point.

For acupuncture analgesia to be effective, patients should experience a sensation known as Te-Ch'i. It is described variously as a numbing, tingling or heavy sensation spreading from the acupuncture site. The needle should be manipulated until this sensation is elicited.

Stimulation of the points may be achieved simply by insertion of the needles, or by manual stimulation by rotation between thumb and finger, electrical stimulation which may last 20 min or more, or a combination of these manoeuvres. Patients usually appreciate some change in level of pain, either during or shortly after treatment. This may last for a variable length of time, but it is customary to give a course of treatments. Acupunture is now accepted generally as having a useful place in the pain relief clinic.

Pituitary alcohol injection

It has been known for many years that hormonal manipulations influence the course of malignant disease and associated pain.

Oophorectomy, adrenalectomy and hypophysectomy are all used in attempts to induce regression of hormone-dependent tumours, but have the disadvantage of being major operative procedures in patients whose general condition may be poor.

Chemical hypophysectomy is a technique designed to ablate the pituitary with minimal upset to the patient, and is achieved by injecting absolute alcohol into the gland. This is a remarkably simple and safe method of treating the pain of malignant disease and also, unlike other methods of pain control, carries the potential for regression of the tumour.

Cordotomy and other neurosurgical procedures

Interruption of pathways in the central nervous system appears superficially to be an attractive way of relieving pain, as the lesion produced should not recover normal function and pain relief should be permanent.

In practice this is not so; pain returns eventually, although it is not clear if this is induced by regeneration or by development of alternative pathways. Nevertheless, neurosurgical procedures are useful for some patients with a limited expectation of life.

In general, the closer to the periphery the surgical section of the pain pathway, the more certain is the subsequent pain relief; the more central the section, the more uncertain is pain relief because of the existence of multiple pain pathways. Section of peripheral nerve is followed rapidly by axonal regeneration, and dorsal root section also has a failure rate for reasons which are not understood fully.

Anterolateral cordotomy is probably the most widely used surgical procedure for the relief of pain. The anterolateral tracts of the cord are sectioned midway between root levels, and anaesthesia for pain and temperature are obtained on the contralateral side of the body, from three to four dermatomes below the level of section.

This technique has been refined in the form of a percutaneous technique at C1-2 level. A spinal needle is introduced under local anaesthesia into the neck approximately 1 cm below and posterior to the mastoid process. It is aimed under radiographic control at the space between the first and second cervical vertebrae so that its tip pierces the dura just anterior to the dentate ligament. This is identified by injecting Myodil emulsion, and if the position is correct, a fine electrode, insulated except at the tip, is introduced through the needle into the spinal cord. The position of the electrode is checked by stimulation, when the patient should experience paraesthesia in the painful region on the opposite side of the body. If this occurs, incremental lesions are produced using radiofrequency current.

The patient develops anaesthesia to pain and temperature on the contralateral side in a zone dependent on the size and placement of the lesion.

Percutaneous cervical cordotomy with radiofrequency current may be undertaken in patients who are a relatively poor risk, because unlike surgical cordotomy, it does not entail a major surgical procedure.

Radiotherapy

Pain is often a feature of malignant disease, and if radiotherapy is given in the expectation of curing the patient's disease, relief of pain is incidental. However, even when there is no prospect of curing the patient, palliative radiotherapy may be valuable for controlling pain.

Reduction in tumour bulk often relieves pain by relief of pressure on adjacent nerves and other structures. This applies also to metastases, particularly those in bone. A similar effect may be achieved by the use of cytotoxic drugs and hormones.

Psychiatric aspects of pain relief

It is important that a pain relief clinic should have the help and advice of a skilled psychiatrist who is interested in the problems of patients with pain. The need for a psychiatrist illustrates the many facets of chronic pain and emphasises that the division between organic and psychogenic pain is largely false. His functions are threefold:

1. To diagnose and treat patients presenting with frank psychiatric syndromes.
2. To offer advice and guidance on the use of psychotropic drugs, psychotherapy, hypnosis and other specialised techniques.
3. To recognise personality disorders and patterns of behaviour which are maladaptive, and advise on treatment.

The psychiatrist is of great help also in the support of patients in whom treatment appears impossible, but for whom the pain clinic may at least play a useful supportive role, preventing their endless search for further consultation and treatments.

FURTHER READING

Bond M R 1978 Psychological and psychiatric aspects of pain. Anaesthesia 33: 355
Bond M R 1979 Pain. Its nature and treatment. Churchill Livingstone, Edinburgh
Budd K 1978 Psychotropic drugs in the treatment of chronic pain. Anaesthesia 33: 531
Budd K 1982 Pain. Update postgraduate series. Update Publications, London.
Lipton S 1979 Relief of pain in clinical practice. Blackwell Scientific Publications, Oxford
Swerdlow M 1978 Relief of intractable pain. Excerpta Medica, Amsterdam
Szasz T S 1957 Pain and pleasure. Basic Books, New York
Trimble M R 1981 Neuropsychiatry. John Wiley & Sons, New York
Wood K M 1978 The use of phenol as a neurolytic agent. A review. Pain 5: 205

44. Cardiopulmonary resuscitation

Cardiopulmonary resuscitation (CPR) is required when the supply of oxygen to the brain is insufficient to maintain function. Oxygen delivery is dependent upon cardiac output, haemoglobin concentration and saturation of haemoglobin with oxygen, which depends predominantly on respiratory function. CPR is required most commonly after cardiac arrest, respiratory arrest or a combination of the two.

Cerebral hypoxia

The brain is more sensitive to hypoxia than any other organ, including the heart. It has a limited facility for anaerobic metabolism and cannot store oxygen. Hypoxaemia is tolerated remarkably well in the normal individual, as cerebral blood flow (CBF) increases substantially to compensate for reduced oxygen carriage in blood. In contrast, ischaemia (e.g. circulatory arrest), or hypoxaemia in a patient unable to increase CBF (e.g. cerebrovascular atherosclerosis or a low cardiac output state) result in the rapid onset of anaerobic metabolism. The cerebral cortex is damaged permanently by ischaemia of more than 3–4 min duration. Thus, although a patient may survive an episode of circulatory arrest, permanent impairment of cerebral function may result if cerebral oxygen delivery is not restored within 3–4 min of the initial cessation of blood flow. The commonest cause of brain damage after cardiac arrest is delay in starting resuscitation. Therefore, when circulatory arrest has occurred, it is essential to start CPR as rapidly as possible.

Signs of cardiac arrest

These are shown in Figure 44.1. During surgery it may be difficult to distinguish between profound hypotension and circulatory arrest. If neither surgeon nor anaesthetist can find a pulse, external cardiac massage must be instituted.

MANAGEMENT OF CARDIAC ARREST

The aim of resuscitation is to restore oxygen delivery to the body tissues, in particular the

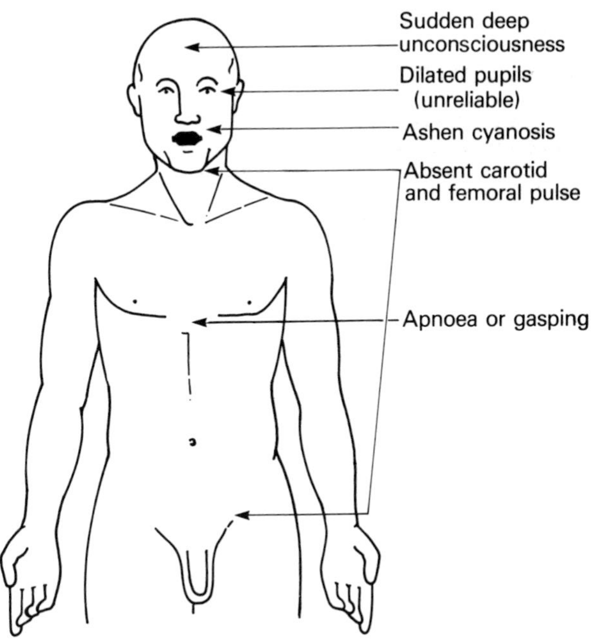

Fig. 44.1 The signs of cardiac arrest. Sudden loss of consciousness and absence of major pulses are sufficient to justify diagnosis.

brain, as soon as possible. Until a spontaneous circulation is restored, circulation must be maintained by external cardiac massage and oxygenation by artificial ventilation (Basic Life Support, BLS).

External cardiac massage (ECM)

ECM is the only manoeuvre that perfuses the body with blood if circulatory arrest has occurred, and it must be started immediately. The only exception is cardiac arrest resulting from hypoxaemia or asphyxia, when ventilation takes priority. That is because:

1. The lungs normally contain sufficient oxygen to prevent serious desaturation of blood for at least 30 s, or longer if the patient's lungs were preoxygenated.
2. The brain is more tolerant to hypoxaemia than ischaemia.
3. External cardiac massage is normally easier to institute than artificial ventilation.
4. If instituted immediately before the heart becomes deoxygenated, cardiac massage may itself restart the heart.

Mechanism of blood flow

'Old' CPR. This assumes that the heart behaves as a simple pump during external cardiac massage. During the compression phase, the heart is squeezed between the sternum and the vertebral column, the valves act normally and blood is ejected into the aorta and the pulmonary artery. The heart refills with blood between compressions and oxygenation occurs in the lungs. With 'old' CPR, the lungs are ventilated once after every five cardiac compressions.

'New' CPR. When external cardiac compression and ventilation are timed to coincide, cyclical increases occur in intrathoracic pressure. This results in improved forward flow in comparison with 'old' CPR, i.e. raised intrathoracic pressure acts as a pump in series with the heart. However, venous pressure is increased also by 'new' CPR. Although forward flow in the aorta and carotid arteries increases, CBF does not, and may be impaired. Improved survival has not been demonstrated using 'new' CPR, and the technique is no longer recommended.

Recommended technique for external cardiac massage

This is shown in Figure 44.2. Ideally, the patient should lie on a hard surface, but cardiac massage must not be delayed until such a surface is found.

With two operators, the sternum should be compressed 60 times per minute and one ventilation given after every five cardiac compressions. For a single operator, it is less tiring to inflate the lungs twice after every 15 compressions. The time

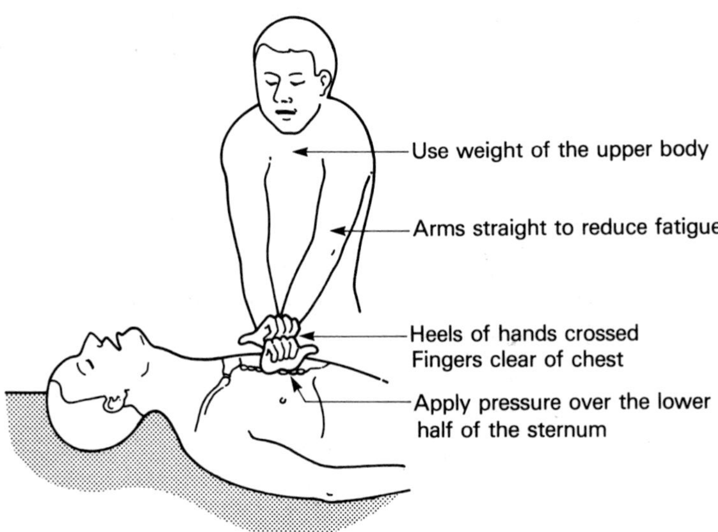

Fig. 44.2 External cardiac massage.

at which resuscitation is started should be noted; this is important for medicolegal and prognostic purposes.

If cardiopulmonary arrest occurs in the operating theatre, the surgeon should be informed, the table tilted head-down, all anaesthetic agents discontinued and the patient's lungs ventilated with 100% oxygen. Internal cardiac massage is more effective than ECM; if the abdomen is open, the surgeon should be asked to make an incision in the diaphragm and massage the heart directly.

The airway and artificial ventilation

The simplest technique of artificial ventilation is expired-air resuscitation using either the mouth-to-mouth or mouth-to-nose method. This option is always available, requires no special equipment and can be started immediately. Expired air contains 16–18% oxygen and results in a Pa_{O_2} of approximately 10 kPa and oxygen saturation of approximately 89% in a patient with normal lungs.

Oxygen 100% should be given as soon as possible, but operator expired-air resuscitation should never be delayed whilst equipment is found for administration of oxygen.

Technique of operator expired-air resuscitation

The operator clears the airway by extending the patient's neck. If necessary, the angles of the jaw are pulled forward. These manoeuvres prevent the tongue from falling back against the posterior pharyngeal wall.

The patient's nose is pinched closed, the operator takes a deep breath, and applying his lips closely over the patient's lips so as to obtain an airtight seal, exhales slowly but forcefully, feeling his expired air enter the patient's chest and watching it expand (Fig. 44.3). The operator then removes his lips and allows the patient to exhale passively. The aesthetics of this technique may be improved if the operator places a handkerchief over the patient's face.

If mouth-to-mouth ventilation proves difficult, mouth-to-nose ventilation should be performed. The operator closes the patient's mouth whilst inflating the lungs via the nose and then the patient's mouth is opened to permit passive expiration to occur.

Other problems which may arise include failure to maintain a patent airway, failure to keep an airtight seal, gastric distension and regurgitation. Suction apparatus should be at hand to remove vomitus.

Transmission of infection is a theoretical hazard during operator expired-air resuscitation. Ventilation masks such as the Laerdal pocket mask with one-way valve may offer some protection, but resuscitation should not be delayed if such a device is not available.

Bag and mask ventilation

In an emergency, a self-inflating bag may be used. These units save operator fatigue and deliver either room air, which has a higher $F_{I_{O_2}}$ than expired air, or room air with added oxygen. A

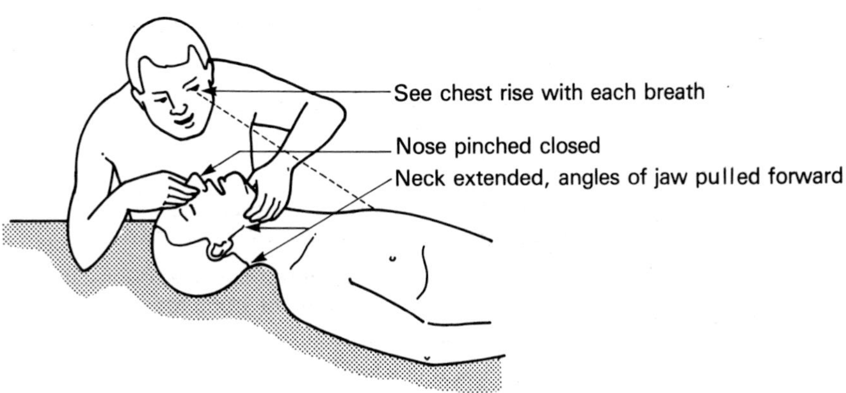

Fig. 44.3 Operator expired-air resuscitation.

Guedel or nasopharyngeal airway is a useful aid to inflation of the lungs and may help also to maintain patency of the airway in the spontaneously breathing patient. A transparent facemask allows early detection of vomit. In the operating theatre, a facemask is used in combination with a standard anaesthetic breathing system.

Tracheal intubation

This renders resuscitation easier and more efficient and is always desirable. A cuffed tube positioned correctly protects the lungs, guarantees an airway and permits the administration of 100% oxygen more easily. However, it is not essential as a first step unless the airway cannot be maintained by other means, e.g. in the presence of facial trauma or if regurgitation has occurred.

Acute upper airway obstruction

If upper respiratory tract obstruction cannot be obviated by tracheal intubation and the situation is desperate, the options are:

1. *Cricothyrotomy.* The cricothyroid membrane is incised transversely (Fig. 44.4) and the resulting airway maintained with any available piece of tubing, e.g. a 6.0-mm plain tracheal tube. A minitracheotomy using a guarded blade, introducing stilette and precut tracheal tube is a suitable alternative, although the technique may be difficult to perform in the obese patient.

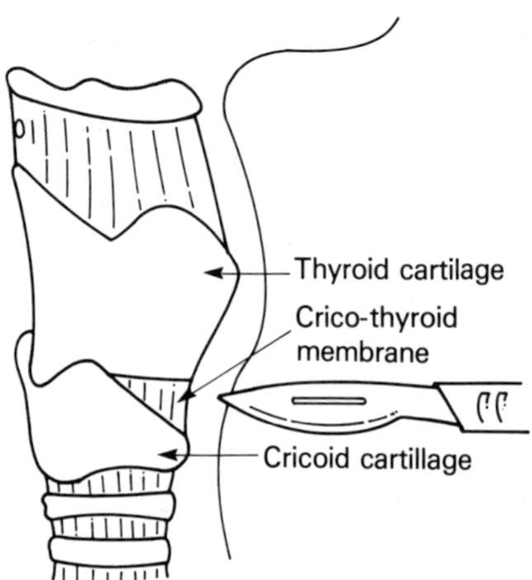

Fig. 44.4 The site for laryngotomy. The soft area between the thyroid and cricoid cartilages is palpated easily and is relatively avascular.

2. *Cricothyroid puncture.* Two large-bore i.v. cannulae, e.g. 12- or 14-gauge, are inserted via the cricothyroid membrane. A standard 15-mm paediatric tracheal tube connector, e.g. size 3.0 or 3.5, is connected to the end of one cannula and the patient's lungs are inflated gently by means of a self-inflating bag. The second cannula vents expired gas to the atmosphere.

3. *Tracheostomy.* This may be very difficult as an emergency in the patient without a tracheal tube in situ.

Re-establishment of a spontaneous circulation of oxygenated blood (advanced life support, ALS)

With the brain protected by an artificial circulation, measures to restart adequate spontaneous cardiac contractions must be instituted at once without interrupting external cardiac compression or artificial ventilation.

Intravenous infusion

Intravenous access is necessary not only to administer drugs but also to correct the relative hypovolaemia which may occur in acute circulatory failure. In cardiac arrest resulting from haemorrhage, massive transfusion is necessary. If blood is not available, infusion of crystalloid or colloid solutions may be life-saving. Adrenaline 1 mg should be administered i.v. (1 ml of 1:1000 or 10 ml of 1:10 000). This dose is repeated every 2–5 min until spontaneous cardiac action is restored. Adrenaline may help to restart the heart regardless of the cause of the arrest. In addition, its α-effect increases perfusion pressure and thus myocardial and cerebral blood flow during ECM. The β-effect is less important during cardiac massage but helps to maintain cardiac output after spontaneous heart action has been restored. Adrenaline also facilitates defibrillation and is beneficial in both asystole and electromechanical dissociation. There is no evidence that the intratracheal route of administration results in a significant increase in plasma adrenaline concentrations after cardiac arrest in man, unless very large doses are used.

Correction of metabolic acidosis

Only the minimum necessary dose of sodium bicarbonate should be given. During CPR, lactic acid may accumulate in areas of poor perfusion. However, the worst effects of metabolic acidosis are not seen until after the circulation has been restored. Excessive bicarbonate administration during CPR may lead to hypokalaemia, hyperosmolality, hypercapnia and intracellular acidosis. Victims of abrupt cardiac arrest who are resuscitated promptly do not need sodium bicarbonate. Generally, no more than 50 mmol of sodium bicarbonate should be given without prior blood gas analysis. In the short term, efficient ventilation controls acidosis better than sodium bicarbonate.

ECG monitoring

This should be instituted as soon as possible. If a major pulse is still absent, the likely patterns are:

1. Ventricular fibrillation (VF) (or ventricular tachycardia (VT) with no cardiac output).
2. Asystole.
3. Electromechanical dissociation (EMD).

Management of ventricular fibrillation/ventricular tachycardia

An immediate DC countershock of 200 J produces simultaneous depolarisation of all myocardial fibres. The SA node should then assume the initiation of contractions if the myocardium is well oxygenated and not acidotic. One paddle should be applied to the right of the upper half of the sternum and the other just below the left nipple, and good electrical contact ensured by the use of electrode jelly or conducting gel pads. All attendants must stand clear of the patient and the bed before discharge.

Failure to defibrillate. If the first shock is unsuccessful, defibrillation should be attempted again with 200 then 360 J. If VF persists, adrenaline 1 mg should be given i.v. before the fourth shock (360 J). If a fifth shock (360 J) is necessary, lignocaine 100 mg should be given first. In refractory cases where VF persists despite efficient BLS and correction of blood gas and electrolyte abnormalities, bretylium 500 mg i.v. should be considered. Bretylium increases the fibrillation threshold and facilitates defibrillation. However, the maximum effect is delayed for 15 min. In addition, bretylium may cause hypotension.

The witnessed arrest. Immediate DC countershock is indicated in sudden witnessed monitored VF, e.g. in the operating theatre or ITU. It should be considered within the first 30 s of a witnessed but unmonitored arrest unless the cause is obviously hypoxaemia, asphyxia or haemorrhage. It is futile and time-wasting to attempt to defibrillate an anoxic heart.

Management of asystole

Asystole commonly follows hypoxaemia, exsanguination or excessive cholinergic activity. It is associated with a poorer prognosis than VF. Adrenaline 1 mg i.v. should be given, followed by atropine 2 mg. Isoprenaline 100 μg i.v. may be effective because of its β-effect. In asystole secondary to exsanguination, α-adrenergic agents, e.g. methoxamine or phenylephrine, which increase coronary and cerebral perfusion pressures may be useful adjuncts to volume replacement. Calcium is not useful for the management of asystolic cardiac arrest.

Pacing. If asystole persists despite repeated doses of myocardial stimulants, internal pacing should be attempted. A bipolar electrode is passed transvenously into the right ventricle via the antecubital, internal jugular or subclavian veins. Transthoracic pacing is often disappointing. Oesophageal pacing is almost always unsuccessful.

Management of electromechanical dissociation

In EMD, there is no cardiac output despite a normal or near-normal ECG. In common with asystole, it has a worse prognosis than VF. Primary EMD is a failure of excitation–contraction coupling and may follow inferior myocardial infarction. Secondary EMD has a physical cause, e.g. pneumothorax, cardiac tamponade, pulmonary embolus or exsanguination. After physical causes have been eliminated, adrenaline 1 mg i.v. and isoprenaline 100 μg i.v. should be tried. Calcium may be of value if the QRS complex is of more than 0.12 s duration. BLS must be continued with the minimum of interruption until heart action is restored.

The return of spontaneous heart action

Restoration of spontaneous cardiac action is signalled by the return of peripheral pulses and circulation. Spontaneous respiration and the return of consciousness usually follow. It is useful to mark the position of the femoral pulse during resuscitation. If it disappears at any time, cardiac massage and artificial ventilation must be resumed at once.

Doses of drugs used in CPR are shown in Table 44.1.

Table 44.1 Doses of some drugs used by the i.v. route in CPR (70-kg adult)

Drug	Dose
Adrenaline	1 mg (1 ml 1:1000 or 10 ml 1:10 000) every 2–5 min
Atropine	1 mg
Bretylium	500 mg
Calcium chloride	5–10 mmol
Digoxin	0.5 mg stat. then 0.25 mg 6-hourly until digitalised
Dopamine	Infusion of 2–10 μg kg^{-1} min^{-1} (200 mg in 500 ml at 5–25 standard drops/min)
Isoprenaline	100 μg stat. then infusion of 0.02–0.04 μg/kg^{-1} min^{-1} (2 mg in 500 ml at 5–100 standard drops/min.
Lignocaine	100 mg stat. then infusion of 1–4 mg/min
Phenylephrine	2–5 mg
Sodium bicarbonate	50 mmol (8.4% solution contains 1 mmol/ml)
Verapamil	5–10 mg

NOTE: suggested dilutions of dopamine and isoprenaline are for emergency use by standard infusion set (15 drops/ml). For longer term use, more concentrated solutions should be used either by microdrop infusion set (60 dros/ml) or by syringe pump.

Aftercare

After a spontaneous circulation has been restored, the time should be noted and recorded in the case sheet, together with notes on the cause of the arrest and the presence of any complications, e.g. inhalation of vomit. Sometimes, recovery is rapid and complete, particularly if resuscitation is prompt and the period of arrest brief. However, some degree of organ failure often persists and requires treatment.

Cardiovascular system

Cardiac output may remain unsatisfactory as a result of cardiogenic shock and may be so poor that unconsciousness persists (vide infra). A low cardiac output may result from:

1. *Poor myocardial contractility*, e.g. after myocardial infarction or pulmonary embolus. Dopamine 2–10 μg kg^{-1} min^{-1} by infusion is the treatment of choice. In this dose range, it has little vasoconstrictor effect and causes a preferential increase in renal blood flow. The optimal preload for the failing heart should be ensured by the cautious administration of colloid (Haemaccel, Gelofusine or human albumin solution) as guided by the CVP. A normal CVP does not exclude the possible development of pulmonary oedema.
2. *Hypovolaemia*. This requires further transfusion guided by CVP measurement.
3. *Arrhythmias*. These require treatment if:

(a) cardiac output is compromised; or
(b) they are electrically unstable and therefore predispose to a further episode of circulatory arrest.

Emergency management is summarised in Table 44.2. All arrhythmias are potentiated by disturbances in blood gas or potassium homeostasis.

Respiratory system

Lung dysfunction is produced during resuscitation for reasons which may include inhalation of vomit, lung contusion, fractured ribs and pneumothorax. Pulmonary oedema may occur in the presence of heart failure and after head injury, drowning or smoke inhalation. Oxygen therapy for 24 h should follow any episode of circulatory arrest. If overt respiratory failure supervenes, more intensive treatment is required, including possibly a period of artificial ventilation. All patients should have a chest X-ray and blood gas analysis after resuscitation.

Central nervous system

Efficient cardiac massage and ventilation provide sufficient oxygen delivery to protect the brain from damage, although not to prevent depression of function. If efficient resuscitation was started immediately after circulatory arrest occurred and was continued until restoration of an adequate spontaneous cardiac output, the patient should regain consciousness fairly quickly. Recovery tends to be delayed after prolonged arrest or when general anaesthesia is involved.

Patients may fail to recover consciousness for the following reasons:

1. Low cardiac output (vide supra).
2. Brain damage, which may be present if resuscitation was delayed or if the circulatory arrest was precipitated by hypoxaemia.

Management of brain damage

The aim of treatment is to provide optimal conditions for recovery of cerebral cells and prevention of secondary neuronal damage.

General measures

Airway obstruction occurs readily in the unconscious patient and leads to hypoxaemia and hypercapnia, which aggravate cerebral damage. In addition, cough and swallowing reflexes are

Table 44.2 Management of important arrhythmias during CPR

Arrhythmia	Significance	Treatment
Ventricular fibrillation	No cardiac output	DC shock 200 J (see text)
Ventricular tachycardia	Cardiac output ↓ or absent, may precipitate VF	If cardiac output reasonable, lignocaine. If pulseless, DC shock 200 J
Ventricular ectopics	May herald VF/VT if frequent, multifocal or R-on-T	Suppress with lignocaine
Complete heart block	May cause profound hypotension or herald asystole	Isoprenaline infusion until transvenous pacemaker in situ
2° Heart block, Mobitz type II	May progress to complete block	Transvenous pacemaker
Atrial fibrillation Atrial flutter	Cardiac output ↓ from: loss of atrial contraction, fast ventricular rate	1. Synchronised DC shock 50 J if patient deteriorating 2. Digitalisation 3. Verapamil
Supraventricular tachycardia	As atrial fibrillation	1. Carotid sinus massage 2. Verapamil 3. Synchronised DC shock 50 J if patient deteriorating 4. Digitalisation
Asystole Electromechanical dissociation	No cardiac output	Adrenaline (see text)
Bradycardia	Cardiac output ↓	Atropine

depressed. Continued tracheal intubation protects the lungs, secures the airway and renders it easy to institute mechanical ventilation if respiration becomes inadequate. With the airway secure, epileptiform fits which increase $CMRO_2$ may be treated safely with anticonvulsants. In general, if the patient can tolerate the tracheal tube, it should be left in situ. The unconscious patient whose trachea is not intubated should be nursed in the lateral position to assist drainage of oral secretions. Arterial pressure should be maintained in the normal range to ensure adequate cerebral perfusion pressure, and haematocrit in the low normal range to optimise oxygen delivery. Tissue hydration and blood biochemistry should be maintained as normal; there is no evidence that dehydration is beneficial. An increase in body temperature increases $CMRO_2$ and should be avoided. Depth of coma should be assessed regularly.

Specialised treatment

1. *Hyperventilation.* Mild passive hyperventilation to a Pa_{CO_2} of 4 kPa helps to minimise increases in intracranial pressure secondary to cerebral oedema, although there is no evidence that cerebral damage after cardiac arrest is reduced by hyperventilation if the patient is able to achieve adequate gas exchange when breathing spontaneously. Control of ventilation may be achieved with the aid of muscle relaxants or cerebral depressants. A head-up tilt assists cerebral venous drainage.

2. *Osmotherapy.* Increasing the plasma osmolality decreases intracranial water content and thus ICP. Mannitol (0.25 g/kg initially) is often used. Mannitol increases the circulating blood volume and may be dangerous in the presence of pulmonary oedema or a high CVP. In this situation, frusemide or bumetanide may be more appropriate.

3. *Steroids.* There is no evidence that steroids are beneficial after cardiac arrest.

4. *Barbiturates and CNS depressants.* Thiopentone and diazepam are often used in conventional doses to provide sedation, facilitate control of ventilation and suppress seizures. Both these drugs must be used with care after circulatory arrest. In particular, large loading doses of barbiturates are contraindicated, as they produce profound cardiovascular depression. There is no evidence that they protect the brain after cardiac arrest.

5. *Calcium antagonists.* The role of these drugs after cardiac arrest awaits clarification. At the present time, there is no evidence that they are of value in man.

Prevention of cardiac arrest

The commonest causes of cardiac arrest during surgery are hypoxaemia and haemorrhage. Hypoxaemia may occur with alarming rapidity during periods of apnoea or respiratory obstruction, particularly in obstetric patients and young children; in the latter, bradycardia is an important premonitory sign. Steady haemorrhage may pass unnoticed until the patient deteriorates suddenly. Other causes include overdosage with hypotensive or local anaesthetic agents, exogenously administered adrenaline and the use of i.v. induction agents in the presence of hypovolaemia. Vagal reflexes may be involved in surgery on the eye, rectum, carotid sheath or upper respiratory tract.

Generally, the outcome after abrupt cardiac arrest is good provided that treatment is prompt and effective.

Initiating and terminating CPR

In the first instance, all patients should be resuscitated unless the medical or nursing notes indicate that a contrary decision has been reached. If it becomes apparent when resuscitation has started that CPR would be inappropriate (e.g. because the patient is in the terminal stages of an incurable disease), it should cease.

Future cerebral function cannot be predicted accurately during CPR and suspicion of brain damage is no justification for terminating resuscitation. When in doubt, CPR should be continued until there is no doubt that the patient will fail to recover. Good recovery has taken place after 1–2 h of continuous CPR.

FURTHER READING

Evans T R 1986 ABC of resuscitation. British Medical Association, London

Greenbaum R 1985 Resuscitation. In: Kaufman L (ed) Anaesthesia review 3. Churchill Livingstone, Edinburgh

Grenvik A, Safar P (eds) 1981 Brain failure and resuscitation. Clinics in critical care medicine 2. Churchill Livingstone, New York

Safar P, Bircher N 1988 Cardiopulmonary cerebral resuscitation. Laerdal Medical, Stavanger

Standards for cardiopulmonary resuscitation (CPR) and emergency cardiac care (ECC) 1986 Journal of the American Medical Association 255: 2905

Appendices

David R. Derbyshire

Appendix	*Subject*
I	Abbreviations
	(a) Abbreviations used in text and appendices
	(b) SI units
II	Anaesthetic agents — physical properties
III	Chemical pathology — biochemical values
IV	Cardiovascular system
	(a) Normal variables — ECG times — haemodynamic variables
	(b) Drugs for infusion
	(c) Drugs for use at cardiac arrest
	(d) Antibacterial prophylaxis
V	Sizes of tracheal and tracheostomy tubes
VI	Fluid balance
	(a) Fluid composition of body compartments
	(b) Fluid and electrolyte requirements
	(c) Intraoperative fluid requirements
	(d) Composition of common i.v. fluids
VII	Gas flows for spontaneous ventilation and intermittent positive pressure ventilation in anaesthetic breathing systems
VIII	Haematology
	(a) Normal values
	(b) Coagulation tests
	(c) Abnormal coagulation
	(d) Coagulation screen
IX	Paediatrics
	(a) Dosage of drugs in common anaesthetic use
	(b) Fluid and electrolyte balance
X	Renal function tests
XI	Respiratory function tests
	(a) Spirogram
	(b) Tables of $FEV_{1.0}$, FVC, $FEV_{1.0}$/FVC and PEFR
	(c) Adult and neonatal values

APPENDIX I(a)
Abbreviations

α	adrenoceptor type (after Ahlquist)
ABO	nomenclature for blood groups (after Landsteiner)
ACD	acid citrate dextrose
ACE	angiotensin converting enzyme
ACh	acetylcholine
ACT	activated clotting time
ACTH	adrenocorticotrophic hormone
ADH	antidiuretic hormone
ADP	adenosine diphosphate
AHF	antihaemophilic factor (factor VIII)
AIDS	acquired immune deficiency syndrome
AMP	adenosine monophosphate
ANS	autonomic nervous system
ARDS	adult respiratory distress syndrome
ASA	American Society of Anesthesiologists
ATP	adenosine triphosphate
AV	atrioventricular
β	adrenoceptor type (after Ahlquist)
B	bone marrow dependent (as in B cells)
BCR	British corrected ratio (for oral anticoagulants)
BM	Boehringer Mannheim (makers of BM Stix blood glucose testing strips)
BP	boiling point
BP	*British Pharmacopoeia*
BSA	body surface area
BZ	benzodiazepine
C	cervical or coccygeal vertebra
°C	degrees Celsius
C_x	clearance of x
C	compliance
$CaCO_3$	calcium carbonate
cAMP	cyclic adenosine monophosphate
CaO	calcium oxide
CAT	computerised axial tomography
CAVG	coronary artery vein graft
CBF	cerebral blood flow
CC	closing capacity
CCT	central conduction time
CCU	coronary care unit
CDH	Christiansen Douglas Haldane (effect)
CFAM	cerebral function analysing monitor
CFM	cerebral function monitor
CHO	carbohydrate
CI	cardiac index (cardiac output/body surface) area
CK	creatine kinase
Cl	clearance (of drug)
cm	centimetre (10^{-2} m; not a unit in the SI system)
cmH_2O	centimetres of water
$CMRO_2$	cerebral metabolic rate for oxygen
CMV	cytomegalovirus
CNS	central nervous system
C_0	concentration at time = 0
CO	cardiac output
CO_2	carbon dioxide
cp	centipoise
CPAP	continuous positive airways pressure
CPB	cardiopulmonary bypass
CPD	citrate phosphate dextrose
CPD–A	citrate phosphate dextrose with adenine
CPK	creatine phosphokinase
CPP	cerebral perfusion pressure

CPPV	continuous positive pressure ventilation
CPR	cardiopulmonary resuscitation
^{51}Cr	chromium atom — isotope weight 51 daltons ('radiolabelled')
CSF	cerebrospinal fluid
C_{ss}	concentration at steady state
C_t	concentration at time t
CV	closing volume
CVP	central venous pressure
Δ	delta — minimal increment (of)
D	dose (of drug)
d	density
D & C	dilatation and curettage (of uterus)
DAP	diastolic arterial pressure
DC	direct current
DCR	dacrocystorhinostomy
DDAVP®	desmopressin
DHSS	Department of Health and Social Security
DIC	disseminated intravascular coagulation
DNA	deoxyribonucleic acid
Dopa	deoxyphenylalanine
2,3-DPG	2,3-diphosphoglycerate
dTC	dextrotubocurarine
DVT	deep vein thrombosis
ECC	extracorporeal circulation ('heart bypass')
ECF	extracellular fluid
ECG	electrocardiogram
ECM	external cardiac massage
ECT	electroconvulsive therapy
EEC	European Economic Community
EEG	electroencephalogram
EDTA	ethylene diamine tetra-acetic acid
EF	ejection fraction
EMD	electromechanical dissociation
EMG	electromyogram
EMMV	extended mandatory minute ventilation
EMO	Epstein and Macintosh (of Oxford)
ENT	ear, nose and throat
EP	evoked potential
EPI	Eysenck personality inventory
EPP	end-plate potential
EUA	examination under anaesthesia
EVR	endocardial viability ratio
F	Faraday's constant

FDP	fibrin degradation products
$Fe^{2+(3+)}$	iron ionised — ferrous (ferric) ion
$FEV_{1.0}$	forced expiratory volume (in 1 s)
FF	filtration fraction
FFP	fresh frozen plasma
$F_{I_{O_2}}$	fractional inspired oxygen concentration
FRC	functional residual capacity
FSH	follicle stimulating hormone
FVC	forced vital capacity
G-6-PD	glucose-6-phosphate dehydrogenase
GABA	γ-aminobutyric acid
GFR	glomerular filtration rate
GH	growth hormone
GI	gastrointestinal
GTN	glyceryl trinitrate
h	hour
H^+	hydrogen ion
H_1	histamine — type 1 receptor
H_2	histamine — type 2 receptor
HAFOE	high air flow oxygen enrichment
Hb	haemoglobin
HbA	adult haemoglobin
Hb_{Barts}	Saint Bartholomew's haemoglobin (γ-thalassaemia)
HbF	fetal haemoglobin
HbNH	carbamino haemoglobin
HBsAg	hepatitis B surface antigen
hCG	human chorionic gonadotrophin
HCO_3^-	bicarbonate ion
H_2CO_3	carbonic acid
Hct	haematocrit
He	helium
HFDV	high-frequency forced diffusion ventilation
HFJV	high-frequency jet ventilation
HFOV	high-frequency oscillatory ventilation
HFPPV	high-frequency positive pressure ventilation
HFV	high-frequency ventilation
5-HIAA	5-hydroxyindole acetic acid
HIV	human immunodeficiency virus
HLA	human lymphocyte associated
HOCM	hypertrophic obstructive cardiomyopathy
HPA	hypothalamo-pituitary axis
hPL	human placental lactogen

HR	heart rate
5-HT	5-hydroxytryptamine (serotonin)
Hz	hertz (cycles per second)
I	infusion rate
IABP	intra-aortic balloon pump
ICP	isometric contraction period; intracranial pressure
I/E	inspiratory/expiratory
IgA	immunoglobulin type A (γ-globulin A)
IgE	immunoglobulin type E (γ-globulin E, reagin)
IgG	immunoglobulin type G (γ-globulin G)
i.m.	intramuscular
IMV	intermittent mandatory ventilation
IOP	intraocular pressure
IPPV	intermittent positive pressure ventilation
IRP	isometric relaxation period
ISA	intrinsic sympathomimetic activity
ITU	intensive therapy unit
i.v.	intravenous
IVC	inferior vena cava
IVRA	intravenous regional anaesthesia
J	joule
K	kelvin
K^+	potassium ion
KCCT	kaolin cephalin clotting time
kg	kilogram
K_i^+	potassium ion (inside cell)
K_o^+	potassium ion (outside cell)
kPa	kilopascal
l	length
L(*n*)	lumbar vertebra (number *n*)
LAP	left atrial pressure
LATS	long-acting thyroid stimulator
lb/in^2	pounds per square inch
LDH	lactate dehydrogenase
LH	luteinising hormone
LMN	lower motor neurone
log	logarithm(ic)
LOS	lower oesophageal sphincter
LSCS	lower segment Caesarean section
LVEDP	left ventricular end-diastolic pressure
μ	micro (10^{-6})
μV	microvolts
M	molar (strength of solution)
mA	milliampere
MAC	minimum alveolar concentration (for anaesthesia)
MAO	monoamine oxidase
MAOI	monoamine oxidase inhibitor
MAP	mean arterial pressure
M.C.	'Mary Caterill' (name of proprietary mask)
MC	monocomponent — 'free of impurities' (as in insulin)
MCV	mean corpuscular volume
MEPP	miniature end-plate potential
mg	milligram
Mg^{2+}	magnesium ion
MI	myocardial infarction
min	minute
ml	millilitre
mm	millimetre
mmHg	millimetres of mercury
MMPI	Minnesota Multiphasic Personality Inventory
MMV	mandatory minute ventilation
mN	millinewton
mol	mole
mosm	milliosmole
MRI	magnetic resonance imaging
ms	millisecond
mV	millivolt
MVP	mean venous pressure
MW	molecular weight
η	viscosity
N	newton (unit of force)
N/A	not available; not applicable
N_2O	nitrous oxide
Na	sodium
Na^+	sodium ion
Na-K-ATPase	sodium and potassium dependent adenosine triphosphatase
NEEP	negative end-expiratory pressure
NH_3	ammonia
NH_4^+	ammonium ion
NHS	National Health Service (United Kingdom)
NMR	Nuclear magnetic resonance
NSAID	non-steroidal anti-inflammatory drug
NTD	neural tube defects
O_2	oxygen
ODC	oxyhaemoglobin dissociation curve
osmol	osmole
π	pi (= 3.14159)

π_{BC} oncotic pressure in Bowman's capsule
π_{CAP} oncotic pressure in capillary
P electrocardiographic nomenclature
P_{50} needed for 50% saturation (of haemoglobin)
Pa pascal (unit of pressure)
P_A alveolar partial pressure (of gas)
P_a arterial partial pressure (of gas)
PAH *para*-aminohippuric acid
PAP pulmonary artery pressure
P_{BC} hydrostatic pressure in Bowman's capsule
P_{CAP} hydrostatic pressure in capillary
PCWP pulmonary capillary 'wedge' pressure
PE pulmonary embolus
$P_{\bar{E}}$ mean expired partial pressure
$P_{E'}$ end-expired partial pressure
PEEP positive end-expiratory pressure
PEFR peak expiratory flow rate
PF pathological fibrinolysis
PG(X) prostaglandin type (X)
pH hydrogen ion activity (−logarithm to base 10 of the measured hydrogen ion concentration)
P_I inspired partial pressure
PIFR peak inspiratory flow rate
pK_a expression of dissociation constant in an equilibrium — (−logarithm to base 10 of the dissociation constant)
PMGV piped medical gases and vacuum systems
ppm parts per million
PRN pro re nata ('as needed')
PRP platelet-rich plasma
PTA plasma thromboplastin antecedent (factor IX)
PTTK partial thromboplastin time, kaolin
PVC polyvinyl chloride
PVR pulmonary vascular resistance
$\dot{Q}_t$ total liquid flow in unit time
ρ rho (= density)
r radius (of circle)
R universal gas constant
RA_x renal artery concentration of x
RAP right atrial pressure
RBF renal blood flow
RDS respiratory distress syndrome
Re Reynolds' number (dimensionless)
REM Rapid eye movement
Rh(x) Rhesus blood group (major phenotype x)
RLF retrolental fibroplasia
RPF renal plasma flow
RPP rate–pressure product
RV residual volume
RV_x renal vein concentration of x
s second
SA sinoatrial
SAB subarachnoid block
SAP systolic arterial pressure
s.c. subcutaneous
SDP subdural pressure
SG specific gravity
SI Système International d'Unités
SIMV synchronised intermittent mandatory ventilation
SNP sodium nitroprusside
SRS–A slow-reacting substance of anaphylaxis
SVC superior vena cava
SVP saturated vapour pressure
T thymus-dependent (T cells)
T temperature
$T_{\frac{1}{2}\alpha}$ α half-life (distribution half-time)
$T_{\frac{1}{2}\beta}$ β half-life (elimination half-time)
T_3 tri-iodothyronine
T_4 thyroxine
TA titratable acid
TBG thyroxine binding globulin
TcP_{O_2} transcutaneous oxygen partial pressure
TLC total lung capacity
Tm tubular maximal reabsorption
TMJ temporomandibular joint
TNS transcutaneous nerve stimulation
TO4 train of four
TPR total systemic peripheral resistance
TWC total water content
URT upper respiratory tract
V volt
V volume
$\dot{V}$ volume per unit time (gas flow)
v velocity
V4R mobile chest lead in electrocardiography (position 4 reversed)

VC	vital capacity
V_D	deadspace (ventilation)
$V_{D(ANAT)}$	anatomical deadspace
$V_{D(PHYS)}$	physiological deadspace
VF	ventricular fibrillation
VFP	ventricular fluid pressure
VIC	vaporiser in circuit
VIE	vacuum insulated evaporator
VOC	vaporiser out of circuit
VT	ventricular tachycardia
V_T	tidal volume
W	watt

APPENDIX I(b)
SI System

The Système International d'Unités (SI system) has been developed to reduce the large number of units in everyday physical use to a much smaller number, with standard symbols.

The seven base units are derivatives of the MKS system of physical measurement.

Length	metre	m
Mass	kilogram	kg
Time	second	s
Electric current	amp	A
Thermodynamic temperature	kelvin	K
Amount of substance	mole	mol
Luminous intensity	candela	cd

Any other units are derived units and may be expressed by multiplicaton or division of base units.

Volume	cubic metre	—	m^3	
Force	newton	N	$kg\ m\ s^{-2}$ =	$J\ m^{-1}$ (J/m)
Work	joule	J	$kg\ m^2\ s^{-2}$ =	N m (Nm)
Power (rate of work)	watt	W	$kg\ m^2\ s^{-3}$ =	$J\ s^{-1}$ (J/s)
Pressure (force/area)	pascal	Pa	$kg\ m^{-1}s^{-2}$ =	$N\ m^{-2}$ (N/m^2)

The solidus (/) has been used in preference to X^{-1}, either of which is specified in the standard.

Non-standard units such as the litre, day, hour and minute may be used with SI but are not part of the standard.

Volume

The SI unit of volume is the cubic metre, but for medical purposes the litre (1 dm^3) is retained.

Temperature

A temperature difference of 1 kelvin is numerically equivalent to 1 degree Celsius. In everyday use the degree Celsius is retained. The Fahrenheit scale is no longer used medically and is being phased out of use with the general public.

The magnitude of a unit is expressed by the additions of standard prefixes and symbolic prefixes. The magnitude of SI units usually changes by 10^3 per step.

Fraction	SI prefix	Symbol	*Multiple*	SI prefix	Symbol
10^{-1}	deci	d	10	deca	da
10^{-2}	centi	c	10^2	hecto	h
10^{-3}	milli	m	10^3	kilo	k
10^{-6}	micro	μ	10^6	mega	M
10^{-9}	nano	n	10^9	giga	G
10^{-12}	pico	p	10^{12}	tera	T
10^{-15}	femto	f			
10^{-18}	atto	a			

It can be seen that the SI handling of 'kilogram' is non-standard; the name of the base unit already contains a preficacial multiple. Names of decimal multiples and submultiples of the unit of mass are formed by attaching prefixes to the word 'gram'.

Moles

$$\text{moles} = \frac{\text{weight in g}}{\text{molecular weight}}$$

thus, 1 mole $H_2O = \frac{18\ g}{18}$

18 g H_2O = 1 mole

For univalent ions, moles and equivalents are numerically equal, but for multivalent ions the number of equivalents must be divided by the valency to obtain the molar value. Thus 10 mEq Ca^{2+} = 5 mmol Ca^{2+}.

Moles/osmoles

Strictly the SI unit of osmolality should be the mole, this representing the calculated number of particles/molecules in solution. However, the osmole is used also; this is the measured osmolality (the number of osmotically active particles per kilogram of solution). Thus, the molar value for osmolality is theoretical, while the osmolar value is empirical.

APPENDIX II
Anaesthetic agents — physical properties

Name	Formula	MW	BP (°C)	SVP KPa	SVP (at 20°C) mmHg	MAC (%)	Flam. in O_2(%)	Ostwald coefficients of solubilities at 37°C H_2O/Gas	Oil/Gas	Blood/Gas	Oil/H_2O
Chloroform	$CHCl_3$	119	61	21.3	160	0.5	0	40	260	10	100
Cyclopropane	$CH_2CH_2CH_2$	42	−33	638	4800	9.2	2–60	0.20	11.5	0.45	34.4
Enflurane	$CHFCl.CF_2$ O CF_2H	184.5	56	23.3	175	1.68	6	0.78	98	1.9	120.1
Ether (diethyl)	C_2H_5 O C_2H_5	74	35	56.5	425	1.9	2–82	13	65	12	3.2
Ethyl chloride	C_2H_5Cl	64.5	13	131	988	2.0	4–67	1.2	—	3.0	—
Fluroxene	CF_3CH_2 O $CH.CH_2$	126	43	38	286	3.5	4	0.85	48	1.4	90
Halothane	$CF_3CHClBr$	197	50	32.3	243	0.8	0	0.8	220	2.5	220
Isoflurane	CF_3CHCl O CF_2H	184.5	49	33.2	250	1.15	6	0.62	97	1.4	174
Methoxyflurane	$CHCl_2.CF_2$ O CH_3	165	105	3	23	0.2	5–28	4.5	950	13	400
Nitrous oxide	N_2O	44	−88	(5300)	(39 800)	105	0	0.44	1.4	0.47	3.2
Trichloroethylene	$CHCl.CCl_2$	131	87	8	60	0.17	9–65	1.7	960	9.0	400

APPENDIX III
Chemical pathology — biochemical values

These values are given for example only — each reporting laboratory provides 'normal values' for its own population and method. This is especially true of enzyme assays. Values given are those obtained from Chemical Pathology in Leicester, where these are available. No inference should be made about the molecular weight of a substance by reference to US and SI values

Name	*US units*	*SI units*
Adrenaline	100 pg/ml	0.55 nmol/litre
Amino acid nitrogen	4–8 mg%	3–6 mmol/litre
Ammonia	80–110 μg%	47–65 μmol/litre
Amylase	80–180 Somogyi units%	70–300 i.u./litre
Base excess	± 2 mEq/litre	± 2 mmol/litre
Bicarbonate — actual	22–30 mEq/litre	22–30 mmol/litre
standard	21–25 mEq/litre	21–25 mmol/litre
Bilirubin — total	0.3–1.1 mg%	3–18 μmol/litre
Buffer base (pH 7.4, Pa_{CO_2} 5.3 Hb 15 g/dl)	48 mEq/litre	48 mmol/litre
Calcium — total	8.5–10.5 mg%	
	(4.5–5.7 mEq/litre)	2.25–2.6 mmol/litre
— ionised	4–5 mg%	1.0–1.25 mmol/litre
Chloride	95–105 mEq/litre	95–105 mmol/litre
Cholesterol	140–300 mg%	3.6–7.8 mmol/litre
Cholinesterase, plasma (pseudo-cholinesterase)	Dibucaine number >80% usually normal Dibucaine number <20% usually homozygote for atypical cholinesterase	
Copper	80–150 μg%	13–24 nmol/litre
Urinary copper	15–50 μg/24 h	0.2–0.8 μmol/24 h
Cortisol —		
0900 } RIA tech	9–23 μg/litre	
2400 } RIA tech	<7.2 μg%	
neonatal	30 μg/litre	200–650 nmol/litre
(competitive protein-binding tech.)		<200 nmol/litre 330–1700 nmol/litre
Creatine (phospho)kinase (CK)	100 i.u./litre — male	25–200 i.u./litre
	60 i.u./litre — female	25–200 i.u./litre
Creatinine	0.5–1.4 mg%	45–120 μmol/litre

Name	*US units*	*SI units*
Fibrinogen	150–400 mg%	1.5–4.0 g/litre
Folate	3–20 ng/ml	3–20 μg/litre 2.1–27 nmol/litre
Glucose —		
fasting	55–85 mg%	3.0–4.6 mmol/litre
post prandial	<180 mg%	<10 mmol/litre
γ-glutamyl transpeptidase	7–25 i.u./litre	10–55 i.u./litre
Hydroxybutyrate dehydrogenase (HBD)		100–240 i.u./litre
Iodine — total	3.5–8.0 μg/litre	273–624 nmol/litre
^{131}I uptake	20–50% of administered dose in 24 h	
Iron	80–160 μg%	14–30 μmol/litre
Iron binding capacity	250–400 μg%	45–69 μmol/litre
Lactate	0.6–1.8 mEq/litre	0.6–1.8 mmol/litre
Lactate dehydrogenase	30–90 i.u./litre	100–300 i.u./litre
Lead		<1.8 μmol/litre
Magnesium	1–2 mg% 1.5–2.0 mEq/litre	0.7–1.0 mmol/litre
Methaemoglobin	<3% of total haemoglobin	
Nitrogen (non-protein) (urea + urate + creatinine + creatine)	18–30 mg%	12.8–21.4 mmol/litre
Noradrenaline	200 pg/ml	1.25 nmol/litre
Osmolality	280–300 mosmol/kg	280–300 mmol/kg
Phosphate	2.0–4.5 mg% 3.0–6.0 mg% (children) <8.1 mg% (neonatal)	0.8–1.4 mmol/litre 1.0–1.8 mmol/litre (children) <2.6 mmol/litre (neonatal)
Phosphatase —		
acid (total)	1–5 KA units%	1–9 i.u./litre
acid (prostatic)		0–3 i.u./litre
alkaline	3–13 KA units%	17–100 i.u./litre
Potassium	3.4–5.3 mEq/litre	3.4–5.3 mmol/litre
Protein — total	6.0–8.0 g%	60–80 g/litre
albumin	3.5–5.0 g	35–50 g/litre
globulin	1.5–3.0 g%	15–30 g/litre
Pyruvate	0.4–0.7 mg%	34–80 μmol/litre
Sodium	133–148 mEq/litre	133–148 mmol/litre
Thyroxine (T_4)	4.7–11 μg%	52–140 nmol/litre
Transaminase:		
Aspartate transaminase — AST	5–40 units/ml	5–30 i.u./litre
Alanine transaminase — ALT		2–53 i.u./litre
Transferrin	220–400 mg%	2.2–4.0 g/litre
Triglycerides (fasting)	71–160 mg%	0.8–1.8 mmol/litre
Triiodothyronine (T_3)	90–170 ng%	0.8–2.5 nmol/litre

Name	*US units*	*SI units*
T_3 uptake	95–117%	95–117%
Urea	15–48 mg%	2.7–7.0 mmol/litre
Urea nitrogen (BUN)	10–20 mg%	1.6–3.3 mmol/litre
Urate — men	4–9.5 mg%	240–590 μmol/litre
women	3–7.5 mg%	170–460 μmol/litre

APPENDIX IV(a)
Cardiovascular system

NORMAL VALUES FOR VARIABLES

Blood flows	*% of cardiac output*	*Flow (ml/min) (70-kg man)*
Heart	4	200
Brain	14	700
Liver	25	1250
Kidneys	24	1200
Lung	3	150
Muscle	19	950
Skin	5	250
Fat	5	250
Remainder	1	50
Total	100	5000

ECG TIMES

P wave	<0.10 s
PR interval	0.12–0.20 s
QRS time	0.05–0.08 s
QT time	0.35–0.40 s
T wave	<0.22 s

PRESSURES (mmHg)

	Range	*Mean*
Central venous (CVP)	0–8	4
Right atrial (RA)	0–8	4
Right ventricular (RV)		
systolic	14–30	25
end-diastolic (RVEDP)	0–8	4
Pulmonary arterial (PA)		
systolic	15–30	23
diastolic	5–15	3
mean ($\overline{PAP}$)	10–20	15
Pulmonary artery wedge (PAWP)		
mean	5–15	10
Left artrial (LA)	4–12	7
Left ventricular (LV)		
systolic	90–140	120
end-diastolic (LVEDP)	4–12	7

DERIVED HAEMODYNAMIC VARIABLES

Variable		*Typical value* (70 kg)
Cardiac output (CO)	SV × HR	5 litres/min
Cardiac index (CI)	$\frac{CO}{BSA}$	3.2 litres min^{-1} m^{-2}
Stroke volume (SV)	$\frac{CO}{HR} \times 1000$	80 ml

Variable		*Typical value* (70 kg)
Stroke index (SI)	$\frac{SV}{BSA}$	50 ml/m^2
Systemic vascular resistance (SVR)	$\frac{MAP - CVP}{CO} \times 80$	1000–1200 dyne s cm^{-5} (not SI unit)
Pulmonary vascular resistance (PVR)	$\frac{\overline{PAP} - LAP}{CO}$	60–120 dyne s cm^{-5} (not SI unit)
Left ventricular stroke work index (LVSWI)	$\frac{1.36\,(MAP - LAP)}{100} \times SI$	50–60 g m m^{-2}
Rate–pressure product (RPP)	$SAP \times HR$	9600
Ejection fraction (EF)	$\frac{ESV - EDV}{EDV}$	>0.6

APPENDIX IV(b)

VASOACTIVE INFUSIONS

Sympathomimetic drugs

Drug	*Dilution into 500 ml glucose 5%*	*Typical dosage range*
Adrenaline (low — α, β_{1+2}) (higher — α)	5 mg = 10 μg/ml	Start 0.02–0.05 μg kg^{-1} min^{-1} Most respond to less than 0.2 μg kg^{-1} min^{-1} Greater than 0.5 μg kg^{-1} min^{-1} leads to excess vasoconstriction
Dobutamine (β_1)	250 mg = 500 μg/ml	0.5–20 μg kg^{-1} min^{-1}
Dopamine (low — δ) (moderate — $\delta + \beta_2 + \beta_1$) (high — α, β_1)	200 mg = 400 μg/ml OR 800 mg = 1600 μg/ml	 0.5–5 μg kg^{-1} min^{-1} (low) 5–10 μg kg^{-1} min^{-1} (moderate) $>$15 μg kg^{-1} min^{-1} (high)
Isoprenaline ($\beta_1 + \beta_2$)	4 mg = 8 μg/ml	0.02–0.4 μg kg^{-1} min^{-1}
Metaraminol (α)	50 mg = 100 μg/ml	0.1–1 μg kg^{-1} min^{-1} infrequent use as infusion
Noradrenaline (α, β_1)	4 mg = 8 μg/ml	0.05–0.2 μg kg^{-1} min^{-1}
Phenylephrine (α)	25 mg = 50 μg/ml	0.1–0.5 μg kg^{-1} min^{-1}
Salbutamol (β_2)	5 mg = 10 μg/ml	0.1–0.5 μg kg^{-1} min^{-1}

Miscellaneous

Drug	*Dilution into 500 ml glucose 5%*	*Typical dosage range*
Disopyramide (membrane stabilisation)	500 mg into 450 ml glucose 5% or saline 0.9% = 1000 μg/ml	5–7 μg kg^{-1} min^{-1} after loading dose — see data sheet or BNF
Flecainide (membrane stabilisation)	150 mg into 500 ml glucose 5% or saline 0.9% = 300 μg/ml	4 μg kg^{-1} min^{-1} after loading dose — see data sheet or BNF

Drug	*Dilution into 500 ml glucose 5%*	*Typical dosage range*
Glyceryl trinitrate (VENOUS and arteriolar dilator) NB: Do not use with PVC giving set	50–100 mg into 500 ml glucose 5% or saline 0.9% = 100–200 μg/ml	10–200 μg/min ($0.2–3\ \mu g\ kg^{-1}\ min^{-1}$)
Isosorbide dinitrate (VENOUS and arteriolar dilator) NB: Do not use with PVC giving set	50 mg into 450 ml glucose 5% or saline 0.9% = 100 μg/ml	30–120 μg/min ($0.6–2\ \mu g\ kg^{-1}\ min^{-1}$)
Lignocaine (membrane stabilisation)	1 g into 500 ml glucose 5% or saline 0.9% = 2 mg/ml = 2000 μg/ml	$25–50\ \mu g\ kg^{-1}\ min^{-1}$ after loading dose — see data sheet or BNF
Mexiletine (membrane stabilisation)	250 mg into 500 ml glucose 5% or saline 0.9% = 500 μg/ml	500 μg/min after loading dose — see data sheet
Sodium nitroprusside (arteriolar and venous dilator) NB: Protect from light	50 mg into 500 ml glucose 5% = 100 μg/ml	$0.5–8\ \mu g\ kg^{-1}\ min^{-1}$ (for hypertensive crisis) $0.1–1.5\ \mu g\ kg^{-1}\ min^{-1}$ (during hypotensive anaesthesia)

APPENDIX IV(c)

DRUGS USED AT CARDIAC ARREST

Drug	*Dose*	*Action*
Adrenaline 1:1000 (1 mg/ml) 1:10000 (1 mg/10 ml)	100 μg–1 mg i.v. or intracardiac	α- and β-receptor stimulator. May cause ventricular tachycardia or fibrillation
Atropine 0.5–1.2 mg/ml	0.6–1.8 mg	Mainly via vagal nucleus, 'blocks vagus'. Decreases vagal tone and increases heart rate especially when due to sinus bradycardia
Bretylium 50 mg/ml	5–10 mg/kg	Prolongs action potential. 'Pharmacological defibrillator'. Used in refractory ventricular fibrillation
Calcium chloride 10% (0.68 mmol Ca^{2+}/ml) Calcium gluconate 10% (0.225 mmol Ca^{2+}/ml) (Physical incompatibility with bicarbonate)	10 ml	Inotropic. May cause ventricular asystole in tonic contraction
Disopyramide 10 mg/ml	50–150 mg	Membrane stabilisation. ↓ tendency for tachyarrhythmias (inc. digitalis-induced)
Lignocaine 2% 20 mg/ml	100 mg	Membrane stabilisation. ↓ tendency for tachyarrhythmias
Mexiletine 25 mg/ml	100 mg	Membrane stabilisation. ↓ tendency for tachyarrhythmias (inc. digitalis-induced)
Phenytoin 50 mg/ml	50–100 mg	Membrane stabilisation. Especially in digitalis-induced arrhythmia. Disopyramide or mexiletine may be preferred
Metoprolol 1 mg/ml	5 mg	β-blocker — for SVT. Do not give VERAPAMIL subsequently

Drug	*Dose*	*Action*
Sodium bicarbonate 8.4% 1 mmol/ml (incompatible with Ca^{2+})	50 mmol	Corrects acidosis. Allows easier recovery of spontaneous activity
Verapamil 2.5 mg/ml NOT with β-blockers	5–10 mg	Calcium antagonist. Supraventricular tachyarrhythmias such as Wolff–Parkinson–White syndrome

APPENDIX IV(d)

ANTIBACTERIAL PROPHYLAXIS

Prevention of endocarditis in patients with heart valve lesions, septal defect, patent ductus arteriosus or prosthetic valve.

Dental procedures under local anaesthesia including patients with a prosthetic heart valve but not those who have had endocarditis — amoxycillin 3 g orally 1 h preoperatively and amoxycillin 500 mg orally 6 h later:
— if penicillin-allergic, erythromycin stearate 1.5 g 1 h preoperatively then erythromycin stearate 500 mg 6 h later.
Patients who have had endocarditis — amoxycillin + gentamicin i.m. as below under general anaesthesia.

Dental procedures under general anaesthesia — NO SPECIAL RISK
Either amoxycillin 1 g i.m. before induction, then amoxycillin 500 mg orally 6 h later.
or amoxycillin 3 g orally 4 h before induction then amoxycillin 3 g orally as soon as possible after procedure
or amoxycillin 3 g orally + probenecid 1 g orally 4 h before induction.
SPECIAL RISK (those with a prosthetic heart valve or who have had endocarditis) — amoxycillin 1 g i.m. plus gentamicin 1.5 mg/kg i.m. immediately before induction, then amoxycillin 500 mg orally 6 h later.
Patients who are penicillin-allergic or already taking a penicillin, vancomycin 1 g infused i.v. over 60 min before induction and gentamicin 1.5 mg/kg i.v. before induction.
NOTE: These high-dose (3 g) amoxycillin regimens are considered suitable for patients who have recently received penicillins.

Genito-urinary and colonic procedures
Amoxycillin 1 g i.m. plus gentamicin 1.5 mg/kg i.m. immediately before induction then amoxycillin 500 mg orally or i.m. 6 h later.
Patients who are penicillin-allergic, vancomycin 1 g infused i.v. over 60 min before induction and gentamicin 1.5 mg/kg i.v. immediately before induction.
Metronidazole as a suppository or by i.v. infusion may also be added.

APPENDIX V
Tracheal and tracheostomy tube size

Age (years)	TT and tracheostomy tube size int. diam. (mm)	TT length (cm) Oral	TT length (cm) Nasal
0–3 month	3.0	10	
3–6 month	3.5	12	15
6–12 month	3.5	12	15
2	4.0	13	16
3	4.0	13	16
4	4.5	14	17
5	5.0	14	17
6	5.5	15	18
7	5.5	15	18
8	6.0	16	19
9	6.0	16	19
10	6.5	17	20
11	6.5	17	20
12	7.0	18	21
13	7.0	18	21
14	7.5	21	24
15	7.5	21	24
16	8.0	21	24
17	9.0	22	25
18	9.5	22	25
20	9.5	23	26

Below 8–10 years, non-cuffed tubes should be used.
It is always advisable to have available a tube one size smaller than calculated.

APPENDIX VI(a)
Fluid balance

FLUID COMPOSITION OF BODY COMPARTMENTS

Typical blood volumes		*Total water content (TWC)*
Infant	90 ml/kg body weight	60% ♂ (55% ♀) of body weight (18–40 years)
Child	80 ml/kg body weight	55% ♂ (46% ♀) of body weight (>60 years)
Adult male	70 ml/kg body weight	*Volume of ECF* 35% TWC
Adult female	60 ml/kg body weight	*Volume of ICF* 65% TWC

APPENDIX VI(b)

FLUID, ELECTROLYTE AND NUTRITIONAL REQUIREMENTS

Minimum daily requirements per kg for adults and children and infants.

	Adults (per kg)	*Children and infants (per kg)*
Water	30–45 ml	100–150 ml
Energy	30–50 kcal (0.15–0.21 MJ)	90–125 kcal (0.38–0.5 MJ)
Protein	0.7–1.0 g	2.2–2.5 g
Na^+	1–1.4 mmol	1–2.5 mmol
K^+	0.7–0.9 mmol	2 mmol
Ca^{2+}	0.11 mmol	0.5–1 mmol
Mg^{2+}	0.04 mmol	0.15 mmol
Fe^{2+}	1 μmol	2 μmol
Mn^{2+}	0.1 μmol	0.3 μmol
Zn^{2+}	0.7 μmol	1.0 μmol
Cu^+	0.07 μmol	0.3 μmol
Cl^-	1.3–1.9 mmol	1.8–4.3 mmol

Neonates

See Appendix IX (b)

APPENDIX VI(c)

INTRAOPERATIVE FLUID REQUIREMENTS — ADULT

	(1) Initial volume	1.5 ml kg^{-1} h^{-1} for duration of preoperative starvation
+	(2) Maintenance	1.5 ml kg^{-1} h^{-1}
+	(3) Operative insensible loss	e.g. 1–2 litres for abdominal surgery
+	(4) Blood loss	replace with blood when loss exceeds 20% of estimated blood volume

APPENDIX VI(d)

COMPOSITION OF COMMON I.V. FLUIDS

Crystalloids

Name	*pH*	*Calculated* osmolality*	*Ions mmol/litre* Na^+	K^+	Cl^-	HCO_3^-	*Misc.*	*CHO g/litre*	*Protein g/litre*	*MJ/ litre*
Sodium chloride 0.9%	5.0	308	154	0	154	0	0	0	0	0
Glucose 5%	4.0	280	0	0	0	0	0	50	0	0.84
Glucose 4% + Saline 0.18%	4.5	286	31	0	31	0	0	40	0	0.67
Glucose 5% + Saline 0.45%	4.5	430	77	0	77	0	0	50	0	0.84
Lactated Ringer's (Hartmanns solution)	6.5	280	131	5	112	29 (as lact.)	Mg^{2+} 1 Ca^{2+} 1	0	0	0.038
Sodium bicarbonate 8.4%	8.0	2000	1000	0	0	1000	0	0	0	0

* = Calculated value. Assumes total dissociation of ions.

Colloids

Name	pH	Oncotic pressure (mmH_2O)	Ionic content/litre Na^+	K^+	Cl^-	Misc.	CHO g/litre	Protein g/litre	MJ/ litre	Typical half-life in plasma
Gelatin (succinylated, Haemaccel, Hoechst)	7.4	370	145	5.1	145	Ca^{2+} 6.25 PO_4^{2-} Trace SO_4^{2-} Trace	0	35	0	5 h
Gelatin (polygeline, Gelofusin, Consol. Chemicals)	7.4	465	154	0.4	125	Ca^{2+} 0.4 Mg^{2+} 0.4	0	40	0	4 h
Dextran 70 in NaCl 0.9%	4–7	268	154	0	154	0	0	0	0	12 h
Dextran 70 in glucose 5%	3.5–7	268	0	0	0	0	50	0	0.84	12 h
Hetastarch (Hespan, Du Pont)	5.5	310	154	0	154	0	0	0	0	17 days
Human albumin solution (HAS) (PPF) — 4%	7.4 (100 ml 20% salt poor also available — ionic content varies with manufacturer)	275	150	2	120	—	—	—	40	

Whole blood	usually >6.5	Depends upon donor values. K^+ increases with storage time
Plasma reduced blood	usually >6.5	Depends on donor values. K^+ is higher than whole blood — but *quantity* of K^+ is similar
Packed cells	usually >6.5	Usually low Na^+ and K^+ load cf. whole blood, due to late separation of plasma from red cells

Accepted safe storage times at 4°C for whole blood depend upon type of preservative and (in the case of packed cells) time of separation.

Heparinised blood — only available for special applications
Acid citrate dextrose (ACD) — 21 days
Citrate phosphate dextrose (CPD) — 28 days
Citrate phosphate dextrose adenine (CPD–A_1) — 35 days

APPENDIX VII
Gas flows in anaesthetic breathing systems

	Spontaneous ventilation	*IPPV*
Magill (Mapleson A) (not suitable for children <6 years)	MV (theoretically V_A) 70 ml kg^{-1} min^{-1}	MV × 2.5
Bain (Mapleson D) (suitable for children)	150–200 ml kg^{-1} min^{-1}	70 ml kg^{-1} min^{-1} for Pa_{CO_2} of 5.3 kPa 100 ml kg^{-1} min^{-1} for Pa_{CO_2} of 4.3 kPa
Ayre's T piece (Mapleson E)	2 × MV	As for Bain circuit Minimum 3 litres/min

NORMAL VENTILATION VALUES FOR RESTING AWAKE SUBJECTS

Weight	*Minute volume — MV (ml)*	*Tidal volume (ml)*	*Frequency (breaths/min)*
Neonate 2 kg	480	14–16	30–45
3 kg	600	17–24	25–40
10 kg	1680	80	21
20 kg	3040	160	19
30 kg	4080	240	17
40 kg	4800	320	15
50 kg	5200	400	13
60 kg	5280	480	11
70 kg	5600	560	10

APPENDIX VIII(a)
Haematology

NORMAL VALUES

Haemoglobin	men	13.5–18.0	g/dl
	women	11.5–16.5	
	10–12 years	11.5–14.8	
	12/12	11.0–13.0	
	3/12	9.5–12.5	
	full term	13.6–19.6	
Red blood cell count (RBC)	men	$4.5–6.0 \times 10^{12}$/litre	
	women	$3.5–5.0 \times 10^{12}$/litre	
White blood cell count (WBC)		$4.0–11.0 \times 10^{9}$/litre	
Neutrophils		40–70%	
Lymphocytes		20–45%	
Monocytes		2–10%	
Eosinophils		1–6%	
Basophils		0–1%	
Platelet count		$150–400 \times 10^{9}$/litre	
Reticulocyte count		0–2% of RBC	
Sedimentation rate	men	0–15 mm in 1 h	
	women	0–20 mm in 1 h	
Plasma viscosity		1.50–1.72 cp	
Packed cell volume (PCV) / Haematocrit (Hct)	men	0.4–0.55	
	women	0.36–0.47	
Mean corpuscular volume (MCV)		76–96 fl	
Mean corpuscular haemoglobin concentration (MCHC)		31–35 g/dl	
Mean corpuscular haemoglobin (MCH)		27–32 pg	

APPENDIX VIII(b)

NORMAL VALUES FOR COAGULATION TESTS

Activated clotting time — ACT (Haemochron type)	80–135 s
Antithrombin III	>80% normal
Bleeding time (platelet function)	2–9 min
Clotting time (largely replaced by ACT)	3–11 min
Fibrinogen — plasma	1.5–4 g/litre
Fibrin degradation products — FDP	<10 mg/litre (μg/ml)
APTT/PTTK — heparin therapy value	2 times normal
Partial thromboplastin time — PTT	35–45 s
Platelet count	150–400 × 10^9/litre
Prothrombin time	12–14 s
(International normalized ratio — INR) therapeutic range	2–4
Reptilase clotting time. Heparin independent	<thrombin time + 4 s
Thrombin time	c. 15 s
Thrombotest — normal	70–130%
— therapeutic	5–15%

APPENDIX VIII(c)

ABNORMAL COAGULATION TESTS

Consumption coagulopathy — disseminated intravascular coagulation (DIC)

Early — decreased platelets
— increased fibrin degradation products
— Presence of { thrombin/antithrombin complexes
fibrinopeptide A }

Late — abnormal PTT
— abnormal prothrombin time

Dilutional coagulopathy or massive blood transfusion

Increased prothrombin time — >20 s
Decreased Thrombotest — <30%

Abnormal liver

Early — decreased activity of vit. K-dependent tests — PT — (PTT — later)
Late — massive derangement of some or all coagulation tests

APPENDIX VIII(d)

Coagulation screen

What? When? What to do?

What to check?

Prothrombin time — PT
Partial thromboplastin time — PTT
Thrombin time — TT
Platelet count
— IF all normal consider checking bleeding time and, in neonates, factor XIII concentration

When to check?

Elective patient
with suspicious history (bleeding after cuts, previous surgery or dental extractions; easy bruising)
with family history of bleeding problems
receiving anticoagulants — warfarin, heparin or ASPIRIN, for example
with intercurrent illness such as obstructive jaundice, liver disease, uraemia or leukaemia

Emergency patient or intraoperative patient
with excessive bleeding despite apparent vascular integrity

What to do?

PT & PTT prolonged

?Drug effect (warfarin/coumarin)	→	FFP ?? Vitamin K
?Obstructive jaundice	→	Vitamin K
?Liver disease	→	FFP ?Vitamin K
?Haemorrhagic disease of the newborn	→	Vitamin K
?Factor II, V, X deficiency	→	Cryoprecipitate FFP
IF TT is also prolonged: ?Fibrinogen deficiency	→	Cryoprecipitate FFP
?Are FDP's increased? DIC	→	Treat cause FFP Platelets ?Cryoprecipitate

PTT prolonged		
?heparin therapy	→	Stop therapy ?Reverse effect with protamine
?Factor VIII deficiency Haemophilia	→	Factor VIII concentrate
?Von Willebrand's disease	→	Vasopressin Cryoprecipitate
?Factor IX deficiency	→	Factor IX concentrate
?Factor XI or XII deficiency	→	FFP
PT prolonged (with normal PTT)		
?Factor VII deficiency	→	FFP
Platelet count decreased ($<100 \times 10^9$*/litre*)		
?Peripheral destruction		
immune	→	Steroids
DIC	→	Treat cause Platelets FFP ?Cryoprecipitate
?Inadequate production		
marrow failure	→	Platelets
Bleeding time prolonged		
?Von Willebrand's disease	→	Cryoprecipitate Vasopressin
?Functional platelet disorder		
inherited	→	Platelets
acquired	→	Platelets
?Uraemia	→	Dialysis Cryoprecipitate
?Drugs		

If still confused/uncertain then ASK your haematologist or pathologist!

APPENDIX IX(a)
Paediatrics

DOSES OF DRUGS IN PAEDIATRIC ANAESTHESIA

Premedication	
Atropine	20μg/kg
Hyoscine	20 μg/kg
Glycopyrrolate	5 μg/kg
Diazepam	200–400 μg/kg
Droperidol	100 μg/kg
Trimeprazine	2–4 mg/kg
Intravenous induction	
Thiopentone	5–6 mg/kg
Methohexitone	1 mg/kg
Etomidate	300 μg/kg
Ketamine	2 mg/kg
Propofol	2–2.5 mg/kg
Other induction routes	
Thiopentone rectal	30 mg/kg
Methohexitone rectal	25 mg/kg
Ketamine intramuscular	10 mg/kg
Neuromuscular blocking drugs	
Suxamethonium	1–2 mg/kg
Tubocurarine	500–600 μg/kg
Pancuronium	80–100 μg/kg
Alcuronium	250–300 μg/kg
Atracurium	300–500 μg/kg
Vecuronium	100 μg/kg
Reversal	
Neostigmine	50–80 μg/kg
Atropine	20–40 μg/kg
Analgesics	
Morphine	200 μg/kg
Papaveretum	300 μg/kg

Fentanyl	0.5–1.5 μg/kg
Alfentanil	2.5–5 μg/kg

Local analgesics (maximum safe dose)

Lignocaine	5 mg/kg (≡ 1 ml 0.5% solution/kg)
Bupivacaine	2 mg/kg (≡ 0.8 ml 0.25% solution/kg)
Prilocaine	6 mg/kg (≡ 1.2 ml 0.5% solution/kg)

APPENDIX IX(b)

POSTOPERATIVE FLUID AND ELECTROLYTE REQUIREMENTS IN INFANCY AND CHILDHOOD

Weight	*Rate*
Up to 10 kg	100 ml kg^{-1} day^{-1}
10 to 20 kg	1000 ml + 50 × [wt (kg) − 10] ml kg^{-1} day^{-1}
20 to 30 kg	1500 ml + 25 [wt (kg) − 20] ml kg^{-1} day^{-1}

Fluid requirements in the first week of life

Day	*Rate*
1	0
2, 3	50 ml kg^{-1} day^{-1}
4, 5	75 ml kg^{-1} day^{-1}
6	100 ml kg^{-1} day^{-1}
7	120 ml kg^{-1} day^{-1}

FLUID AND ELECTROLYTE REQUIREMENTS IN INFANCY AND CHILDHOOD

	Age	*(years)*									
	1 week	1	2	3	4	5	6	7	8	9	10
Weight (kg)	3.5	10	13	15	17	19	21	23	25	28	32
Insensible water loss (ml kg^{-1} day^{-1})	30	27.5	27	26.5	26	25	24	23	22	21	20
Water requirement (ml kg^{-1} day^{-1})	150	100	100	90	90	90	70	70	70	70	70
Na^+ requirement (mmol kg^{-1} day^{-1})	4	3	2.5	2	2	1.9	1.9	1.9	1.8	1.75	1.7
K^+ requirements (mmol kg^{-1} day^{-1})	2.5	2	2	2	2	1.75	1.75	1.5	1.5	1.5	1.5

These are basal requirements. Additional fluid (10–20%) is required during major surgery, in addition to replacement of overt losses. During the postoperative period, fluid requirements are increased in the presence of pyrexia. Fluid and electrolyte balance should be adjusted after measurement of serum electrolyte concentrations and serum osmolality.

APPENDIX X
Renal function tests

Clearance tests

Inulin clearance ≏ glomerular filtration	100–150 ml/min
PAH clearance ≏ renal plasma flow	560–830 ml/min
Creatinine clearance ≏ glomerular filtration rate (overestimates low GFR)	104–125 ml/min

Blood tests

Serum/plasma

Osmolality	280–300 mosmol/kg
Creatinine	45–120 μmol/litre
Urea	2.7–7.0 mmol/litre
Urea nitrogen	1.6–3.3 mmol/litre

Urine tests

Osmolality	300–1200 mosmol/kg
Creatinine	8.85–17.7 mmol/24 h
Sodium	50–200 mmol/24 h

Comparative urinary values

	SG	*Osmolality*	*U/P urea ratio*	*U/P osmolality*
Normal	1000–1040	300–1200	>20:1	>2.0:1
Prerenal failure	>1022	>400	>20:1	>2.0:1
Renal failure:				
Early	1010	<350	<14:1	<1.7:1
Late			<5:1	<1.1:1

APPENDIX XI(a)
Respiratory function tests

ABBREVIATIONS COMMONLY USED

Primary symbols

C = concentration of gas — blood phase
D = diffusing capacity
F = fractional concentration in the dry gas phase
P = partial pressure — gas
Q = volume of blood
R = respiratory exchange ratio
S = saturation of haemoglobin with oxygen or carbon dioxide
V = volume of gas
$\dot{X}$ = dot above symbol indicates 'per unit time'
$\bar{X}$ = bar above symbol indicates 'mean value'

Examples: Pa_{O_2} = partial pressure — arterial — oxygen.

Secondary symbols

Usually typed as subscripts, capital letters indicate gaseous phase; lower case letters indicate liquid phase.

A = alveolar
B = barometric
D = dead space
E = expired
I = inspired
T = tidal
a = arterial
c = capillary (pulmonary capillary)
v = venous

LUNG SPIROMETRY

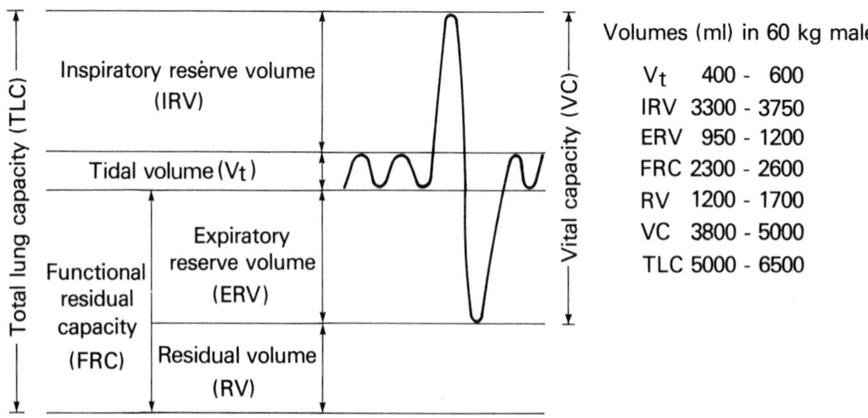

Fig. XI(a) Lung volumes in an average healthy male adult.

APPENDIX XI(b)

PULMONARY FUNCTION TESTS — FEMALES

Age (years)	*Height (cm)*	*$FEV_{1.0}$ (litres)*	*FVC (litres)*	*$FEV_{1.0}/FVC$ (%)*	*PEFR (litres/min)*
20	145	2.60	3.13	81.0	377
	152	2.83	3.45	81.0	403
	160	3.09	3.83	81.0	433
	168	3.36	4.20	81.0	459
	175	3.59	4.53	81.0	489
30	145	2.45	2.98	79.9	366
	152	2.68	3.30	79.9	392
	160	2.94	3.68	79.9	422
	168	3.21	4.05	79.9	448
	175	3.44	4.38	79.9	478
40	145	2.15	2.68	77.7	345
	152	2.38	3.00	77.7	371
	160	2.64	3.38	77.7	401
	168	2.91	3.75	77.7	427
	175	3.14	4.08	77.7	457
50	145	1.85	2.38	75.5	324
	152	2.08	2.70	75.5	350
	160	2.34	3.08	75.5	380
	168	2.61	3.45	75.5	406
	175	2.84	3.78	75.5	436
60	145	1.55	2.08	73.2	303
	152	1.78	2.40	73.2	329
	160	2.04	2.78	73.2	359
	168	2.31	3.15	73.2	385
	175	2.54	3.48	73.2	415
70	145	1.25	1.78	71.0	282
	152	1.48	2.10	71.0	308
	160	1.74	2.48	71.0	338
	168	2.01	2.85	71.0	364
	175	2.24	3.18	71.0	394

PULMONARY FUNCTION TESTS — MALES

Age (years)	*Height (cm)*	$FEV_{1.0}$ *(litres)*	*FVC (litres)*	$FEV_{1.0}/FVC$ *(%)*	*PEFR (litres/min)*
20	160	3.61	4.17	82.5	572
	168	3.86	4.53	82.5	597
	175	4.15	4.95	82.5	625
	183	4.44	5.37	82.5	654
	191	4.69	5.73	82.5	679
30	160	3.45	4.06	80.6	560
	168	3.71	4.42	80.6	584
	175	4.00	4.84	80.6	612
	183	4.28	5.26	80.6	640
	191	4.54	5.62	80.6	665
40	160	3.14	3.84	76.9	536
	168	3.40	4.20	76.9	559
	175	3.69	4.62	76.9	586
	183	3.97	5.04	76.9	613
	191	4.23	5.40	76.9	636
50	160	2.83	3.62	73.1	512
	168	3.09	3.98	73.1	534
	175	3.38	4.40	73.1	560
	183	3.66	4.82	73.1	585
	191	3.92	5.18	73.1	608
60	160	2.52	3.40	69.4	488
	168	2.78	3.76	69.4	509
	175	3.06	4.18	69.4	533
	183	3.35	4.60	69.4	558
	191	3.61	4.96	69.4	579
70	160	2.21	3.18	65.7	464
	168	2.47	3.54	65.7	484
	175	2.75	3.96	65.7	507
	183	3.04	4.38	65.7	530
	191	3.30	4.74	65.7	551

APPENDIX XI(c)

LUNG FUNCTION: ADULT AND NEONATAL VALUES

Examples

	Adult (65 kg)	*Neonate (3 kg)*
V_D	2.2 ml/kg	2–3 ml/kg
V_T	7–10 ml/kg	5–7 ml/kg
$\dot{V}_E$	85–100 ml kg^{-1} min^{-1}	100–200 ml kg^{-1} min^{-1}
Vital capacity	50–55 ml/kg	33 ml/kg
Respiratory rate	12–18 breath/min	25–40 breaths/min
Pa_{O_2}	12.6 kPa (95 mmHg)	9 kPa (68 mmHg)
Pa_{CO_2}	5.3 kPa (40 mmHg)	4.5 kPa (33 mmHg)

Index

Abbreviations, 716–20
Abdominal surgery, respiratory system changes, 430–2
ABO antigens, 120
ABO blood groups, 133–4
Abortion *see* Termination of pregnancy, Miscarriage
Absorption, of drugs, 142
Absorption atelectasis due to oxygen, 171
Accident and emergency departments, 494
Accidents, anaesthetic, 330–1
Acetazolamide, 506
Acetylcholine
  antagonists, 214, 215–18
  central nervous system, 84
  neuromuscular transmission, 212–13
Acetylsalicylic acid, 127, 202
Acid-base balance, 398–403
  liver disease, 659
  monitoring, 384
  renal regulation, 74–5
Acidosis, 400–2
  vs acidaemia, 399
Acquired immunodeficiency syndrome, 327
Acromegaly, 664
  tracheal intubation, 611
Action potentials
  cardiac, 251–2
  neurones, 79
Activated clotting time, 634
Active scavenging systems, 315
Acupuncture, 702–3
Acute epiglottitis, 570
Acute infective polyneuropathy, 673
Acute upper airway obstruction, 708
Adams valve, 274, 295
Adaptation of sensory nerves, 87
Addison's disease, 666–7
Adenoidectomy, 496
Adenoids, 10
Adenosine triphosphate, 598
Adhesive arachnoiditis, 461
Adjustable pressure-limiting valves, 301
Admission
  day-case surgery, 522
  intensive care units, indications, 677, 680
Adrenal gland
  cortex
    disease, 666–7
    etomidate affecting, 185
    neonatal, 122
  medulla
    response limitation, 344
Adrenaline, 83–4, 226, 230
  arrhythmias caused by halothane, 162
  cardiopulmonary resuscitation, 708
  control of systemic circulation, 47
  with local anaesthetic drugs, 265–6, 266
  ophthalmic surgery, 506
Adrenergic agonist drugs, 232–3
Adrenergic fibres, sympathetic, control of systemic circulation, 45–6
Adrenergic receptors, 83–4
β-Adrenoceptor agonists, 244–5
Adrenoceptor antagonists
  α-, 237–8, 250, 597
  β-, 233–7, 597
    for arrhythmias, 253
    concurrent therapy, 645
    for hypotensive anaesthesia, 599
    for thyroidectomy, 665–6
Adrenogenital syndrome, 667
Adult respiratory distress syndrome, 687–8
  steroids, 254
Advanced life support, 708–10
Adverse effects
  diazepam, 205
  drugs in pregnancy, 123, 124
  etomidate, 186
  ketamine, 187–8
  local anaesthetic drugs, 259, 261–2
  methohexitone, 183
  oxygen, 171
  pethidine, 198
  propofol, 184–5
  spinal opioids, 201
  suxamethonium, 219
  thiopentone, 180–2
Adverse reactions to β-adrenoceptor antagonists, 237
Aerosols for β-adrenoceptor agonists, 244–5
Affective disorders, 85–6
Afferent spinal cord pathways, sensory, 88–90
Age and preoperative risk assessment, 340
Agent-specific connectors for vaporisers, 299
Agitation in recovery period, 424
Agonists, 141
Air, bulk storage, 292
Air embolism, 414–15
  in neurosurgery, 612
  and nitrous oxide, 170
Air encephalography, 511
Airway, 7
  burns, 584, 585
  cardiopulmonary resuscitation, 707
  dentistry, 577
  compliance, 25
  ENT surgery, 495
  epithelial receptors, 24
  mask anaesthesia, 355
  obstruction, 405–6
    acute upper, 708
    contraindication to thiopentone, 181
    postoperative, 425–6
    use of helium, 278
  paediatrics, 563–5
  pressure, measurement, 376
  resistance, 28
  stretch receptors, 24
Airways (instruments), 321
Alarms
  oxygen failure, 300–1
  ventilator disconnection, 376
Alcohol
  clinical history, 334
  injection, pituitary, 703
  withdrawal, 517

Alcuronium, 217
Aldosterone, 74
  hypersecretion, 666
Alfentanil, 199
Alimentary system, *see* Gastrointestinal system
Alkalosis, 401–2
  vs alkalaemia, 400
Allen's test, 444
Allergy *see* Hypersensitivity
Althesin, 189
Altitude, effect on chemoreceptor response, 24
Alveolar air equations, 34
Alveolar–capillary diffusion, 35
Alveolar deadspace, 31–2
Alveoli, 'fast' and 'slow', 27
Alzheimer's disease, 86
Amethocaine, 263
γ-Amino butyric acid, 82
Aminoglycosides, effect on neuromuscular transmission, 81
para-Aminohippuric acid, 65
Aminophylline, 243–4
Amiodarone, 253
Amnesia, benzodiazepines, 203
Amnesic drugs, 343
Anaemia, 125–7
  blood flow, 44
  neonatal physiological, 119–20
  renal disease, 661
Anaesthetic agents
  cardiac function, effect on, 60
  inhalational *see* Inhalational anaesthetic agents
  intravenous *see* Intravenous anaesthetic agents
  mode of action, 101–3
  neurosurgery, 607–8
Anaesthetic apparatus, 291–321
Anaesthetic machines, 294–309
  dentistry, 573–5
  safety features, 299–301
Anaesthetic nurses, 329
Anaesthetic rooms, 324–5
Analeptic drugs, 208
Analgesia
  after cardiac surgery, 643
  chronic obstructive airways disease, 656
  on controlled mechanical ventilation, 684–6
  ketamine, 188
  labour, 542–8
  sequential, 100
  spinal with opioids, 200–1
Analgesic action of morphine, 195
Analgesics, 193–203
  for chronic pain, 696–7
  for local anaesthetic techniques, 464
  postoperative for day-case surgery, 524
  variability of effects, 450–1
Anaphylactic reactions to blood transfusion, 136
Anatomical deadspace, 30, 31, 32
Anatomical shunt, 30
Ancillary staff, 329
Aneroid pressure gauges, 275
Angina, β-adrenoceptor antagonists for, 235–6
Angiography
  cerebral, 510–11
  pulmonary, 442
Angiotensin, effect in pregnancy, 112
Angiotensin converting enzyme inhibitors, 250
Angiotensin II, 74
  role in control of systemic circulation, 47
Ankylosing spondylitis, 490
Anoxia *see* Hypoxia, Hypoxaemia
Antacids, 241, 549
Antagonists, 141
  acetylcholine, 214, 215–18
  α-adrenoceptor, 237–8, 250
  β-adrenoceptor *see* β-adrenoceptor antagonists
  benzodiazepines, 206
  histamine H_2-receptor, 241–2, 549
  opioid, 201–2
  parasympathetic, 239–40
Antepartum haemorrhage, 553
Anterior spinal artery syndrome, 461
Anterolateral cordotomy for chronic pain, 703–4
Antiarrhythmic drugs, 250–3
Antibacterial prophylaxis, 733
Antibiotics
  neuromuscular transmission, effects on, 81
  preoperative for subacute bacterial endocarditis, 341
Anticholinergic drugs
  deadspace, effect on, 32
  premedication, 343, 346
Anticholinesterase drugs, 220
  and local anaesthetic drugs, 262
  parasympathomimetic effects, 239
Anticoagulants, 131–2
  concurrent therapy, 645
  monitoring, 385
  oral
    for DVT, 440, 442
    and spinal anaesthesia, 476
Anticonvulsant effect of benzodiazepines, 203
Anticonvulsants
  head injuries, 614
  and local anaesthetic drugs, 262
  for neuralgia, 697
Antidepressants, 85–6, 514
Antidiuretic hormone, 75
  inappropriate secretion syndrome, 397
Antiemetics, 242, 343
  for intraocular surgery, 505
Antigens, red cell, 120
Antihistamines, 242, 255
Anxiety, relief of, 342–3
Anxiolysis due to benzodiazepines, 203
Aortic aneurysm, abdominal, 590
Aortic incompetence, 653
Aortic stenosis, 652
Aorto-iliac occlusion, bypass, 591
Aortography, translumbar, 511–12
Apneusis, 23
Apparatus
  anaesthetic, 291–321
    see also Anaesthetic machines
  for scavenging, 314
Apudomas, 586–9
Aqueous theory of general anaesthesia, 101
Aqueous volume, 503
Arachnoid mater, 18
Arachnoiditis, adhesive, 461
Armoured latex tracheal tube, 318
Arrhythmias, 250–1, 650–2
  β-adrenoceptor antagonists affecting, 235
  anaesthesia, 413–14
  cardiac glycosides, 247
  dentistry, 577–8
  halothane, 161–2
  postoperative, 438
    cardiac surgery, 642
  suxamethonium, 219
Arterial cannulation, 369–71
  complications, 444
Arterial embolism, 414
Arterial grafting, 591
Arterial injection of thiopentone, 180, 351
Arterial oxygenation during IPPV, 683
Arterial pressure, systemic *see* Systemic arterial pressure
Arterial supply, upper respiratory airway, 9, 11
Arterial thrombosis, 444
Arteries
  ascending pharyngeal, 10
  brachial, 3
  cerebral, 108
  coronary, 54
  maxillary, 9–10
  radial, 1
  renal, 65
  subclavian, 4
  ulnar, 1, 3
Arteriosonde, 369
Arteriovenous shunt for dialysis, 662
Arthritic diseases, 490
Artificial noses, 285, 416
ASA Physical Status Scale, 338–9
Ascending pharyngeal artery, 10
Asepsis for local anaesthetic techniques, 464
L-Aspartate as neurotransmitter, 82
Asphyxia, neonatal, 119
Aspirin, 127, 202

Asthma, 406, 657–8
  airway resistance, 30
  pethidine premedication, 198
Asystole, management, 709
Ataxias, hereditary, 673
Atelectasis, 432
  due to oxygen, 171
Atracurium, 218
Atrial natriuretic peptide, 74
Atrial receptors, 49
Atropine, 239–40
Audit, 332
Autonomic nerve blockade for chronic pain, 700–1
Autonomic nervous system, 91–3
  control of systemic circulation, 45–7
  drugs affecting, 225–40
  pregnancy, 112
Autonomic neuropathy, 670, 672
Autoregulation
  cerebral blood flow, 605
  renal circulation, 66
Avogadro's hypothesis, 271
Awake intubation, 532–4
  local anaesthesia for, 477
Awareness, 331–2, 359, 381–2, 551
Axillary block, 479
Axons
  see also Nerve fibres
Axons
  action of anaesthetic agents, 101–2
Ayre's T-piece, 305–6, 563

Back pressure
  in flowmeters, 296
  in vaporisers, 284
Bag and mask ventilation in cardiopulmonary resuscitation, 707–8
Bain system, 304–5
Barbiturates, 177–83
  for cerebral oedema, 712
Baricity of local anaesthetic solutions, 471
Barium enema for intussusception, 512
Baroreceptors, arterial, 49
Barotrauma, pulmonary, 686
Basal nuclei, 92, 95–6
Base excess, 400
Basilic vein, 2
Benzocaine, 263
Benzodiazepines, 203–6
  antagonists, 206
  central nervous system, effect on, 85
  premedication, 344–5
Berg analyser, 106
Bethanechol, 239
Bicarbonate, 39
  administration, 401
  standard, 400
  tubular transport, 71–2
Biliary colic due to morphine, 196
Biliary excretion of drugs, 147–8
Birth canal, nerve supply, 541–2
Blind nasal intubation, 532
Blood, viscosity, 44
Blood–brain barrier, 98, 145
Blood coagulation *see* Coagulation
Blood cross-matching, 135
Blood flow, 43–4
  cardiopulmonary resuscitation, 706
  cerebral, 605–6
    ECT affecting, 515
  coronary, 54–5
  renal, 65–6
Blood gases, 38, 616
  monitoring, 384
  ophthalmic surgery, 502
  preoperative analysis, 338, 654
Blood glucose
  monitoring, 384
  preoperative estimation, 338
Blood grouping, 135
Blood groups, 133–4
Blood loss, 415
  burns surgery, 585
  emergency anaesthesia, 528
  measurement, 375
Blood patch, extradural, 547
Blood pressure *see* Systemic arterial pressure
Blood storage, 134–5
Blood transfusion, 133–6
  emergency, 536
  massive, 538
    coagulation, effect on, 384
  neonate, 556–7
  neurosurgery, 609
  platelets, 128
  reactions, 136, 419
  requests, 342–3
Blood volume in neonate, 556
Bobbin flowmeters, 279
Body plethysmography, 40
Bohr effect, 39
Bohr–Enghoff equation, 31
Bone
  cement, 491
  Paget's disease, 490
Bougies, gum elastic, 320
Boyle's law, 271
Brachial artery, 3
Brachial plexus block, 476–8
Bradycardia
  causes, 344
  neonate, 556, 566
  squint surgery, 505
Brain damage, management, 711–12
Brain stem, 94–6
  death, 693
Breathing systems, 301
  gas flows, 740
Bretylium, 253
Bronchi, 15–17
Bronchial asthma *see* Asthma
Bronchial blockers, 621
Bronchial carcinoma, 657
Bronchial intubation, inadvertent, 406, 682
Bronchial tubes, 621–2
Bronchiectasis, 657
Bronchiolitis, 570
Bronchodilators, 243–5
Bronchography, 512
Bronchopleural fistula, 626
Bronchopulmonary segments, 16–17
Bronchoscopy, 617–19, 619–20
  anatomy, 17
  Bronchospasm, 355, 406, 658
  postoperative, 426–7
Brown fat in neonate, 559
Buffers, 399
Bulk supply of gases, 291–2
Bullae, 626–7
Bunsen solubility coefficient, 285
Bupivacaine, 265
  extradural anaesthesia, 474
  postoperative local anaesthesia, 455
  solutions for subarachnoid anaesthesia, 471
Buprenorphine, 198
  postoperative pain, 452
Burns, 584–5
Burst suppression, 104
Butyrophenones, 206–7
  premedication, 345
Bypass, for aorto-iliac occlusion, 591
Bypass valves, oxygen, 300

Caesarian section, 548–52
  antacids, 241
  choice of anaesthetic technique, 551
Calcitonin, neonatal, 124
Calcium, role in neuromuscular transmission, 212
Calcium channel blocking drugs, 249–50
  concurrent therapy, 645, 649
  for hypotensive anaesthesia, 599
Cannulation, arterial, 369–71
  complications, 444
Capacitance vessels, 48
Capillary bed, blood flow control, 44–5
Capnography, 379–81
Captopril, 250
Carbamino compounds of haemoglobin, 40
Carbon dioxide, 172
  excretion, monitoring, 379–81
  with local anaesthetic drugs, 266
  narcosis, 171
  pneumoperitoneum, 487–8
  tension
    and cerebral blood flow, 606, 607
    chemoreceptors, effect on, 24
    controlled mechanical ventilation, 684
  transport, 39–40

Carcinoid tumours, 586–8
Carcinoma
  bronchus, 657
  oesophagus, 628
Cardiac action potentials, 251–2
Cardiac arrest, 705–13
  drugs, 731–2
  paediatrics, 570
  prevention, 712
Cardiac catheterisation, 632
  normal values, 54
Cardiac conducting system, 51–2
Cardiac conduction defects, 651
  postoperative, 438
Cardiac cycle, 51–4
Cardiac failure
  see also Cardiovascular failure
Cardiac failure, 59–60, 649–50
  adrenergic agonist drugs, 232–3
Cardiac function
  assessment, 57
  cardiac surgery, 634–6, 641–2
Cardiac glycosides, 246–8
Cardiac imaging with radioisotopes, 633
Cardiac muscle, 50, 56
Cardiac output, 55–6
  cardiac surgery, 634
  heart rate affecting, 57
  IPPV affecting, 36
  low after cardiopulmonary bypass, 640
  measurement, 58, 280
  monitoring, 374–5
  neonate, 556
  reduction for hypotensive anaesthesia, 599
Cardiac surgery, 629–44
Cardiac tamponade, 643
Cardiac valves, 50
Cardiff inhaler, 157, 453–4
Cardioplegia, 638
Cardiopulmonary bypass, 637–42
  see also Extracorporeal circulation
Cardiopulmonary resuscitation, 705–13
Cardioselectivity of beta-adrenoceptor antagonists, 234
Cardiovascular check-lists, 690–1
Cardiovascular disease, concurrent, 645–54
Cardiovascular failure, 688–92
  see also Cardiac failure
Cardiovascular physiology, 43–61
  pregnancy, 111–12
Cardiovascular system
  aftercare after cardiac arrest, 710
  carbon dioxide affecting, 172
  drugs affecting
    benzodiazepines, 203
    beta-adrenoceptor antagonists, 235
    diethyl ether, 159
    dobutamine, 232
    droperidol, 207
    enflurane, 163, 166–7
    halothane, 161–2, 166–7
    isoflurane, 164, 166–7
    ketamine, 187
    methohexitone, 182
    morphine, 195–6
    nitrous oxide, 170
    pethidine, 198
    propofol, 184
    sympathomimetic, 229
    thiopentone, 179, 181
  ECT affecting, 515
  extradural anaesthesia affecting, 467
    in pregnancy, 112
  monitoring, 363–75
    on intensive care units, 688
  neonatal, 117–18, 556
  normal values, 727–8
  oxygen affecting, 171
  parasympathetic stimulation, 238
  in recovery period, 421, 436
  renal disease, 661
  subarachnoid anaesthesia affecting, 466
Cardioversion, 592–3
  benzodiazepines, 204
Carotid artery surgery, 591–2
Casualty departments, 494
Catecholamines, 226, 230–2
Catheterisation
  arterial, 370
  cardiac, 54, 632
  pulmonary artery, 373–4
  venous, 371
Cauda equina, 19
Caudal anaesthesia, 475–6
  labour, 544
  postoperative pain, 455
Cell membranes, 64, 77–8
Cement, bone, 491
Central chemoreceptors, 24
Central conduction time, 107
Central nervous system
  acetylcholine, 84
  aftercare after cardiac arrest, 711
  complications of induced hypotension, 600–1
  drugs affecting
    benzodiazepines, 85
    diethyl ether, 158
    droperidol, 207
    enflurane, 163
    ketamine, 186
    methohexitone, 182
    propofol, 183–4
    thiopentone, 178–9
  electrical stimulation, 702
  hyperbaric oxygen affecting, 172
  monitoring, 381–2
  neonate, 560
  in recovery period, 421, 423–4
  renal disease, 661
Central venous pressure, 57
  cardiac surgery, 634
  monitoring, 371
Cephalic vein, 2
Cerebellar pathways, 91
Cerebral angiography, 510–11
Cerebral arteries, 108
Cerebral blood flow, 605–6
  ECT affecting, 515
Cerebral cortex, evoked potentials, 106–7
Cerebral function monitors, 104–5, 106, 382
Cerebral hypoxia, 705
Cerebral metabolic rate for oxygen, 606–7
Cerebral oedema
  management, 712
  steroids, 255
Cerebral pathology in recovery period, 424
Cerebrospinal fluid, 97–8
  pressure, 603–5
Cerebrovascular disease, 672
Cervical cordotomy, percutaneous for chronic pain, 704
Cervical spine X-rays, preoperative, 338
Charles' law, 271
Check-lists, cardiovascular, 690–1
Chemical hypophysectomy, 703
Chemical pathology, normal values, 724–6
Chemical properties of local anaesthetic drugs, 262
Chemoreceptors, 23–4, 49
Chest wall
  compliance, 26
  integrity, 620
Chest X-rays, preoperative, 337, 654
'Chloride' shift, 40
Chloroform, 156–7
  vapour pressure/temperature curve, 283
Chloroprocaine, 263
Chlorpromazine, 208
Cholinergic fibres, sympathetic, control of systemic circulation, 47
Cholinergic receptors, 84
Cholinesterase, plasma, 218–19
Chorda tympani nerve, 10–11
Choroidal volume, 502
Christiansen–Douglas–Haldane effect, 40
Chronic obstructive airways disease, 406, 655–6
  airway resistance, 30
  chemoreceptor response, effect on, 24
  controlled oxygen therapy, 435
  lung function tests, 40
Chronic pain, relief, 695–704
Cimetidine, 241–2
  in premedication, 345
Cinchocaine, 265
Circle of Willis, 108
Circle systems, 307–9

Circuits *see* Breathing systems
Circulation
  coronary, 54–5
  peripheral, 43–9
  renal, 65–6
  systemic, blood flow control, 45–7
Clark electrodes, 379
Classification
  antiarrhythmic drugs, 252
  breathing systems, 301
  electrical insulation, 287–8
  nerve fibres (Gasser), 87
  neuromuscular blockade, 214
  ventilators, 313
Clausen harness, 355
Cleanliness, zones in operating theatre suites, 323–4
Cleft palate, 568
Clinical history, 333–6
Clinics, outpatient anaesthetic assessment, 333
Closed circuits, 306
Closed gas spaces, effect of nitrous oxide, 170
Closing capacity, 28
Coagulation, 128–32
  control, cardiopulmonary bypass, 639, 641
  disorders
    in liver disease, 659
    postoperative, 436–7
  massive blood transfusion affecting, 384
  monitoring, 384
  pregnancy, 113
  tests, 742–5
    preoperative, 338
Coagulopathies, 130
Coanda effect, 280
Cocaine, 257, 263
Coeliac plexus block, 700–1
Collagen diseases, 662–3
Collapse, alveolar, *see* Atelectasis
Colonic procedures, antibacterial prophylaxis, 733
Colour coding of gas cylinders, 294
Coma after head injuries, 612–13
Combustion, support, 289
Committee on Safety of Medicines, on halothane, 162
Communication, 332
  in intensive therapy units, 678, 684
Compartment models for pharmacokinetics, 148–50
Compartmental distribution of total body water, 390
Compartments, fluid, 63–4
Compliance of respiratory system, 25–8
Complications
  anaesthesia, 405–19
  arterial cannulation, 444
  controlled mechanical ventilation, 686
  after day-case surgery, 524
  diabetes mellitus, 669
  extradural anaesthesia, 474–5
    labour, 547
  induced hypotension, 600–2
  subarachnoid anaesthesia, 472
  tracheal intubation, 358–9
Compressed air, bulk storage, 292
Computerised tomography, 507–8
  investigation of venous admixture, 35
Concentration effect of nitrous oxide, 169
Concentrators, oxygen, 171, 292
Conchae, nasal, 8
Concurrent diseases
  cardiovascular, 645–54
  hepatic, 659
  renal, 660–2
  respiratory, 654–8
Condenser humidifiers, 285, 416
Conducting system, cardiac, 51–2
Conduction defects in recovery period, cardiac, 438
Conduction of nerve impulses, 78–80, 257–9
Conductivity of floors of operating rooms, 289
Confidential Enquiries into Maternal Deaths, 548–9
Confidential Enquiry into Perioperative Deaths, 329–30
Conflagrations, 288
Confusion, postoperative, 424
Congenital adrenal hyperplasia, 667
Congenital cardiac abnormalities, operations, 629
Connections for extracorporeal circulation, 631
Connectors
  tracheal tubes, 318–19, 357
  vaporisers, 299
Conn's syndrome, 666
Consent, informed, 341
Constant-pressure and -flow generators, 311
Constant-pressure flowmeters, 278–9
Consultants for intensive therapy units, 677–8
Continuous infusions of opioids for postoperative pain, 453
Continuous positive airway pressure, 36
  in restrictive lung disease, 657
Contraceptives, oral, 486
  withdrawal, 334
Contractility of cardiac muscle, 56
Contraction coupling, muscle excitation, 213
Contraindications
  diethyl ether, 160
  ECT, 516
  enflurane, epilepsy, 163
  etomidate, 186
  extradural anaesthesia, 468
    labour, 545
  ketamine, 188
  local anaesthetic techniques, 461
  subarachnoid anaesthesia, 468
  thiopentone, 181
Contrast media, 510–11
Controlled mechanical ventilation
  see also Ventilation
Controlled mechanical ventilation, 36–8, 309–13, 682–7
  burns, 585–6
  cardiac function, effect on, 61
  for increased intracranial pressure, 613
  indications in intensive therapy units, 679–81
  after repair of aortic aneurysm, 590
  after thoracotomy, 624
Controlled oxygen therapy, 435–6
Controlled ventilation in paediatrics, 568–70
Conus medullaris, 19
Coplan's tube, 496
Cordotomy for chronic pain, 703–4
Coronary artery bypass grafting, 629
Coronary artery disease and isoflurane, 164
Coronary circulation, 54–5
Cortex, cerebral, 96–7
Cortical nephrons, 65
Corticosteroids *see* Steroids
Cortisol, hypersecretion, 666
Cough, 615
Counter-current mechanism, 72
Coupling, negative and positive, 228
Cranial nerves, 93–4, 96
  see also Olfactory nerve, Trigeminal nerve
Creatine kinase, 417
Creatinine, plasma, 67
Cricoid pressure, 532, 549
Cricothyroid puncture, 657
Cricothyrotomy, 708
Cricotracheal ligament, 15
Critical incidents, 330–1
Critical temperature, 271
Critical volume hypothesis, 101
Cross-matching, blood, 135
Cryoprecipitate, 135
Cryotherapy, 702
  for postoperative pain, 457
Cuffs on tracheal tubes, 317–18, 356
Curare, 217, 503
Curtiss method, anaesthesia of nose, 498
Cushing's syndrome, 666
Cutaneous sensation, modalities, 88
Cyanide formation, 597
Cyclic adenosine monophosphate, 227–8
Cycling of controlled mechanical ventilation, 312–13
Cyclizine, 242

Cyclopropane, 158
  flammability, 289
Cylinders, gas 293–4
  carbon dioxide, 172
  nitrous oxide, 168
  oxygen, 170
  pressures, 271–2
Cystoscopy, 489
Cysts of lung, 626–7

Dacryocystorhinostomy, 505–6
Daily fluid requirements, 392
Dalton's law, 271, 286
Day-case anaesthesia, 519–25
  for gynaecological surgery, 486
DC countershock defibrillation, 709
Deadspace
  physiological in neonate, 555
  respiratory, 30, 31
Death in intensive care units, 693
Decamethonium, 219–20
Deep venous thrombosis, 440–1
  prevention in neurosurgery, 610
Defibrillation, DC countershock, 709
Deficits, fluid, 392, 393, 415–16
Defoaming units for extracorporeal circulation, 631
Deglutition, 12
  neonates, 121
Dehydration, 393, 395
  neonates, 558
Delayed ventilatory depression
  due to fentanyl, 199
  due to spinal opioids, 201
Delirium tremens, 517
Delivery, monitoring
  gases, 378
  inhalational anaesthetic agents, 381
Demand regulators, pressure, 275
Demyelinating diseases, evoked potentials, 107
Dental anaesthesia, 573–81
Dentistry
  antibacterial prophylaxis, 733
  benzodiazepines, 204
Depolarising neuromuscular blocking drugs, 215, 218–19
Depression, endogenous, 85
Desensitisation to drugs, 142
Deslanoside, 247
Detonations, 288
Deviation of nasal septum, 10
Dew point, 285
Dextrans
  with local anaesthetic drugs, 266
  plasma volume expanders, 137
  reactions, 419
Diabetes insipidus, 614, 665
Diabetes mellitus, 668–72
Dialysis, 662
Diamorphine, 197
Diaphragmatic hernia, 567, 627
Diathermy, 289
Diazepam, 204–5
  for cerebral oedema, 712
Diazoxide, 249
Diclofenac, 202
Diethyl ether, 153, 158–60
  flammability, 288–9
  vapour pressure/temperature curve, 283
Differential nerve blockade, 466
Diffusion, through membranes, 285–6
Diffusion hypoxia due to nitrous oxide, 170, 429
Digitoxin, 248
Digoxin, 246–7
  concurrent therapy, 645
Dilatation and curettage, 487
2,3-Diphosphoglycerate, 39
Discharge after day-case surgery, 524
Disconnection alarm, ventilator, 376
Disopyramide, 252
Disseminated intravascular coagulation, 129–30
  platelet therapy, 133
Dissociation curve, oxyhaemoglobin, 39
Diuretics, 245–6
  loop, 611, 614
  osmotic, 395
    ophthalmic surgery, 503
Divinyl ether, 154–6
Dobutamine, 231–2
Domperidone, 243
Dopamine, 231
  in postoperative renal failure, 662
  receptors, 84
Dopaminergic fibres, control of systemic circulation, 47
Doppler ultrasound, 369, 375
Dorsal column-medial lemniscus system, 89–90
Dorsal columns, electrical stimulation, 702
Dorsal metatarsal veins, 5
Dorsal motor nucleus of vagus nerve, 17
Dorsal venous arch of hand, 2
Dosage
  see also Administration
Dosage
  of opioids, 194–5
  vs response, to drugs, 140–1
Double-lumen bronchial tubes, 621–2
Down's syndrome, 516
Doxapram, 208, 407
Drainage, thoracic, 625, 626
Drawover systems, 306
Drawover vaporisers, 297
Drill for failed tracheal intubation, 410
Droperidol, 207, 345
Drugs
  adverse effects in pregnancy, 123, 124
  for cardiac arrest, 710, 731–2
  cardiovascular system, 691
  diabetes mellitus, 670
  doses in paediatrics, 746–7
  interactions, 150, 334–6
    ophthalmic surgery, 506
    psychiatry, 513
  metabolism in liver disease, 659–60
Dura mater, 18
Dural tap, inadvertent, 475, 547
Dye dilution methods for cardiac output, 58
Dynamic compliance, 26–7, 40
Dyskinesia due to methohexitone, 183
Dysphagia, 615, 658
Dyspnoea, 615
Dystrophia myotonica, 674

Ears, surgery, 499–500
East–Radcliffe ventilator, 311
Echocardiography, 632–3
  two-dimensional, 375
Eclampsia, 552–3
Ecothiopate, 219, 506
Ectopic pregnancy, 488–9
Edrophonium, 220
Efferent spinal cord pathways, motor, 90
Elastic recoil, pulmonary, 26
Elderly patients, glycopyrronium, 424
Elective Caesarian section, extradural anaesthesia, 549–50
Electrical safety, 287–8, 326
Electrical stimulation, 702
  for postoperative pain, 457
Electrocardiography, 52
  cardiac surgery, 634
  exercise, 632
  hyperkalaemia, 398
  monitoring, 363–5
    in cardiopulmonary resuscitation, 709
  neonatal, 118
  preoperative, 338
  pulmonary embolism, 441
Electrochemical gradients, 78
Electroconvulsive therapy, 507, 514–16
Electrodes, Clark, 379
Electroencephalogram, 103–7
  with ketamine, 187
Electrolytes, 63
  balance, 389–98
  estimation, preoperative, 337
  monitoring, 384
  normal values, 736
  renal disease, 660
  requirements in paediatrics, 748
Electromagnetic flowmeters, 280
Electromechanical dissociation, management, 709–10
Electromyography
  evoked, 224
  scalp, 382
Electrophysiology of heart, 51–3
Embolism, 414
  air, *see* Air embolism
  after cardioversion, 593
  pulmonary, 441–2

Emergence from anaesthesia, 361
  delirium, 186, 187
  after emergency surgery, 535
Emergency anaesthesia, 527–39
Emergency blood transfusion, 536
Emergency surgery
  aortic aneurysm, 591
  Caesarian section, extradural anaesthesia, 550
  diabetes mellitus, 671
  trauma, 493–4
EMLA, *see* entectic mixture of local anaesthetics
EMMA multigas analyser, 381
EMO vaporiser, 297–8
Emphysema, mediastinal, 686
Empyema, drainage, 626
Enalapril, 250
Encephalography, 511
End-diastolic pressure, 57
End-organs, 87–8
End-tidal CO_2 tension, 379–81
Endocrine disease, concurrent, 664
Endocrine glands, effect of morphine, 196
Endogenous depression, 85
Endogenous opioids, 100–1
Endoscopy, benzodiazepines, 204
Endotracheal tubes *see* Tracheal tubes
Enema, barium, for intussusception, 512
Enflurane, 163–4, 165–7
  in renal failure, 662
  vapour pressure/temperature curve, 283
Enkephalins, 100
ENT surgery, 495–500
Entonox
  labour, 544
  postoperative pain, 456–7
  storage, 272
Entonox valve, 275
Enzyme induction, 146–7
Enzyme inhibition, 140, 147
Epidural space *see* Extradural space
Epiglottitis, acute, 570
Epilepsy, 86, 672–3
  contraindication to enflurane, 163
  electroencephalogram, 104
Epistaxis, 499
Epithelial receptors in airways, 24
Equipment
  see also Apparatus
Equipment
  for recovery wards, 422
  Essential monitoring, 385–6
Ether *see* Diethyl ether, Divinyl ether
Ethyl chloride, 154
Ethylene, 154
Etidocaine, 265
Etomidate, 176, 185–6
  in emergency anaesthesia for major trauma, 537
Eustachian tube, 8
Eutectic mixture of local anaesthetics, 266, 484
Evacuation of retained products of conception, 487
Evaporation, fluid loss, 415–16
Evoked electromyography, 224
Evoked potentials in cerebral cortex, 106–7
Examination, physical, 333, 336–7
Examination under anaesthesia, eye, 505
Excretion
  carbon dioxide, monitoring, 379–81
  drugs, 147
Exercise electrocardiogram, 632
Exhaustion, 681
Exomphalos, 567–8
Expiratory valves, 301
Expired volume, measurement, 377
Expirography, marker gas, 28
Explosions, 288, 326
Extended mandatory minute volume, 37
External cardiac massage, 706–7
External jugular vein, 4
Extracellular fluid, 63–4
  composition, 390
Extracorporeal circulation, 630–2
  see also Cardiopulmonary bypass
Extradural anaesthesia, 472–5
  Caesarian section, 549–50
  chronic pain, 699
  cardiovascular system, effects on, 61, 467
    in pregnancy, 112
  contraindications, 468
  labour, 545–8
  postoperative pain, 455
Extradural blood patch, 547
Extradural opioids
  labour, 543–4
  postoperative pain, 456
Extradural space, 20
Extraocular surgery, 505
Extrapyramidal system, 90–1
Extubation, 360
  doxapram for laryngeal spasm, 407
  after tonsillectomy, 495
Eye
  drugs affecting
    ketamine, 187
    morphine, 196
    suxamethonium, 219
    thiopentone, 179
  parasympathetic stimulation, 239
  surgery, 501–6
  trauma, 446

F receptors, 24
Facemasks *see* Masks
Faciomaxillary trauma, 536
Failed tracheal intubation, drill, 410, 551–2
Failure of pregnancy, 552
Familial periodic paralysis, 674
'Fast' alveoli, 27
Felypressin, 266
Femoral nerve block, 481–2
  for postoperative pain, 455
Femur, fracture of neck, 493
Fentanyl, 199
  transdermal for postoperative pain, 454
Fetal haemoglobin, 120
Fibreoptic bronchoscopy, 617–18
Fibrinogen uptake, radioactive, 440
Fibrinolysis, 129
  in pregnancy, 113
Fick principle, 279–80
  for cardiac output, 58
  measurement of renal plasma flow, 65
Field block for inguinal hernia repair, 481
'Fighting the ventilator', 684
Filley's equation, 34
Filling ratios for cylinders of nitrous oxide, 272
Filtration fraction, 67–8
Filum terminale, 18
Fires, 288–9
First-pass metabolism, 143
Fitness for anaesthesia, 333
Fixed-orifice flowmeters, 278
Fixed-performance oxygen therapy devices, 433–4
Flammability of inhalational anaesthetic agents, 288–9
Flecainide, 253
Fleisch pneumotachograph, 279
Flexible metal tracheal tubes, 318
Floors of operating rooms, conductivity, 289
Flow, 276–80
  blood, 43–4
  gas, 29
  generators, 310–11
  meters, 278–80, 296–7
  restrictors, 295
Fluid balance, 63–4, 389–94
  burns, 584–5
  liver disease, 659
  monitoring, 384
  neonate, 557–8
  normal values, 735
  renal disease, 660
Fluid deficits, 392, 415–16
  emergency anaesthesia, 528–9
Fluid management
  in emergency surgery, 535
  in neonate, 557–8
  perioperative, 393–4
Fluid overload, 416
Fluid priming for extracorporeal circulation, 632
Fluid requirements
  daily, 392
  intraoperative in adults, 737
  in paediatrics, 748
Fluids, Physics, 270–81
Flumazenil, 206

Folate requirements in pregnancy, 113
Foramina, intervertebral, 18
Forced expired volume, 40
Forced vital capacity, 40
Forceps, intubating, Magill, 319
Foreign body, inhaled, removal, 624–5
Formulae, inhalational anaesthetic agents, 155–6
Fractures, 493–4
Fresh frozen plasma, 131
Friedreich's ataxia, 673
Fuel cell oxygen analysers, 378
Fuels, 288–9
Functional residual capacity, 40
  vs closing capacity, 28
  general anaesthesia affecting, 30
  neonate, 555
  postoperative, 430, 655

GABA, 82
Gag reflex, pathways, 11
Gags, mouth, 320
Gallamine, 217
Galvanic oxygen analysers, 378
Ganglion blockade, sympathetic, 596–7
Gas exchange
  respiratory, inefficiency, 30–6
  tests, 40–1
Gas spaces, closed, nitrous oxide affecting, 170
Gases
  see also Blood gases
Gases
  blood, 38
  flow, 29
    in breathing systems, 740
  humidification, 285
  measurement of volumes, 278
  monitoring delivery, 378
  physics, 270–5, 278–9
  solution, 285
  supplies
    bulk, 291–2
    safety checks, 293
    to anaesthetic machines, 294
    to ventilators, 313
Gasser, H. S., classification of nerve fibres, 87
Gastric contents, inhalation, 351, 361, 529–31, 548–9
Gastric emptying, 530–1
Gastrointestinal disease, concurrent, 658–9
Gastrointestinal system
  drugs affecting
    diethyl ether, 159
    morphine, 196
    pethidine, 198
  neonatal, 121
  parasympathetic stimulation, 238
  pregnancy, 113–14
  subarachnoid anaesthesia affecting, 467
Gastroschisis, 567–8
Gate control theory of pain, 99–100
Gauge pressure, 272
Gauges, pressure, aneroid, 275
Gelatins as plasma volume expanders, 136
Gelofusine, 136, 137
General anaesthesia
  mechanisms, 101–3
  pulmonary function, effect on, 28, 30
  venous admixture, effect on, 35
Generator potentials, 87
Genitourinary surgery
  anaesthesia, 485–9
  antibacterial prophylaxis, 733
Glial cells, 77
Glomerular filtration, 66–8
Glomerulotubular balance, 70
Glomus cells, 24
Glucocorticoids, 667
Glucose
  blood
    monitoring, 384
    preoperative estimation, 338
  5% infusion, effect, 391
  reabsorption, 70–1
  transfer across placenta, 117
L-Glutamate as neurotransmitter, 82
Glycerol for reduction of intracranial pressure, 611
Glyceryl trinitrate, 598
Glycine as neurotransmitter, 82
Glycopyrronium, 240, 424
Glycosides, cardiac, 246–8
Glycosuria, renal, 71
Goitres, 665
Goldman Cardiac Risk Index, 340
Grafting, arterial, 591
Graham's law, 286
Granulomata, laryngeal, 446
Grouping, blood, 135
Guedel, A. E.
  airway, 321
  signs of anaesthesia, 353–4
Guillain-Barré syndrome, 673
Gum elastic bougies, 321
Gynaecological surgery, anaesthesia, 485–9

Haemaccel *see* Polygeline
Haematocrit for extracorporeal circulation, 632
Haematology, 125–37
  neonatal, 119–20
  nitrous oxide affecting, 170
  normal values, 741–2
  oxygen affecting, 172
  pregnancy, 112–13
Haematomata, postoperative, 444
Haemoglobin, 39
  carbamino compounds, 40
  fetal, 120
  neonate, 556–7
  preoperative estimation, 337
Haemoglobinopathies, 126–7
Haemophilias, 130–1, 490
Haemoptysis, 615
Haemorrhage, 415
  antepartum, postpartum, 553
  after tonsillectomy, 496
Haemostasis, 127–33
Hagen-Poiseuille law, 29, 44, 277
Haldane effect, 40
Haloperidol, 207
Halothane, 160–3, 165–7
  cardiac arrhythmias, 413
  hypotensive anaesthesia, 599
  in liver disease, 659–60
  liver toxicity, 162, 443–4
  thymol in, 299
  vapour pressure/temperature curve, 283
Hamburger shift, 40
Hand, dorsal venous arch, 2
Harness systems, 319, 355
Head, plastic surgery, 583–4
Head injuries, 612–14
  evoked potentials, 107
Headache
  postoperative, 445
  after spinal anaesthesia, 472, 547
Heart, 49–61
  block, 651
  complications of induced hypotension, 601
  drugs affecting
    beta-adrenoceptor antagonists, 235
    chloroform, 156
    inhalational anaesthetic agents, 649
  electrophysiology, 51–3
  neonatal, 118
  in pregnancy, 111
  rate, 57
  restoration of beat, 639
  see also Cardiac
Heat, physics, 281
Heat capacity, 281–2
Heat loss, 383–4
  burns, 586
  neonate, 559
  neurosurgery, 609–10
  repair of aortic aneurysm, 590–1
Heidbrink valve, 272
Helium, use in airway obstruction, 278
Heller's operation, 627–8
Henderson–Hasselbalch equation, 399
Henry's law, 285
Heparin, 132
  DVT and pulmonary embolism, 442
  patients on anticoagulants, 131
  spinal anaesthesia, 476
  vascular surgery, 592
Hepatic disease
  administration of thiopentone, 181
  coagulopathy, 132
  concurrent, 659
Hepatic dysfunction
  halothane-associated, 162
  postoperative, 443–4

Hepatic encephalopathy, 86
Hepatic failure, 660
Hepatic function
  neonate, 560
  pregnancy, 114
  preoperative tests, 337
Hepatic toxicity of inhalational anaesthetic agents, 443–4
Hepatitis B, 327
Hepatitis due to halothane, 443–4
Hepatorenal syndrome, 659
Hering–Breuer reflex, 24
Hernia, diaphragmatic, 567
Hetastarch (Hespan), 137
Hexobarbitone, 189
Hiatus hernia, 627, 658–9
Hiccups, 407
High air flow oxygen enrichment devices, 433–4
High altitude, effect on chemoreceptor response, 24
High-frequency positive pressure ventilation for bronchoscopy, 619
High-frequency ventilation, 37–8, 313
High-risk patient, ketamine, 188
Histamine H_2-receptor antagonists, 241–2, 549
Histamine receptors, 84
Histamine release due to morphine, 196
History, clinical, 333–6
History of anaesthesia in obstetrics, 541
Hoarseness, postoperative, 446
Hofmann degradation, 218
Homeostasis, 63
Hormonal status, monitoring, 384
Hormones, placental, 117
Hüfner's constant, 39
Human albumin solution, 137
Human immunodeficiency virus, 131, 327
  antibody, 135
Humidification of gases, 282, 285
Humidifiers, condenser, 416
Humidity, 284–5
  in operating theatre suites, 325
Huntington's chorea, 673
Hyaline membrane disease *see* Respiratory distress syndrome
Hyaluronidase, 266
Hydralazine, 249, 597
Hydrocephalus, 568
Hydrogen ions
  concentrations, 398–9
  excretion, 74–5
Hydrostatic pressure, 64
α-Hydroxybutyric acid, 189
Hydroxyethyl starch, 137
5-Hydroxytryptamine, 84
Hygrometers, 284–5
Hyoscine, 239–40
Hyperbaric oxygen, effect on central nervous system, 172
Hypercapnia, 681
Hyperglycaemia in recovery period, 424
Hyperkalaemia, 398
  cardiac arrhythmias, 413–14
  suxamethonium, 84, 219
Hypernatraemia, 394–5
Hyperpyrexia, malignant, 355, 384, 417, 490
Hypersensitivity, effects of sympathomimetic drugs, 230
Hypersensitivity reactions, 418
  intravenous anaesthetic agents, 189–90
  local anaesthetic drugs, 262
  steroids for, 254–5
  thiopentone, 181
Hypertension
  beta-adrenoceptor antagonists for, 236
  during anaesthesia, 411–12
  concurrent, 647–9
  labour, 552–3
  neurosurgery, 607
  postoperative, 437–8
  preoperative risk assessment, 339–40
  preoperative therapy, 341
Hyperthyroidism, neonatal, 123
Hyperventilation
  cerebral blood flow, effect on, 603, 606
  for cerebral oedema, 712
Hypervolaemia, 416
Hypo-osmolar syndrome, 424
Hypocapnia, effect on systemic circulation, 47
Hypoglycaemia in recovery period, 423
Hypoglycaemic agents, oral, 668
Hypokalaemia, 397–8
  and cardiac arrhythmias, 413
Hyponatraemia, 395–7
Hypophysectomy, 611–12
  chemical, 703
Hypopituitarism, 664–5
Hypotension, 410–11
  emergency anaesthesia in major trauma, 537
  extradural anaesthesia, 547, 550
  induced, complications, 600–2
  local anaesthetic techniques, 460
  neurosurgery, 607
  postoperative, 436–7
  subarachnoid anaesthesia, 466–7, 472
  thiopentone, 180
Hypotensive anaesthesia, 595–602
Hypothermia, 416
  for cardiac surgery, 638
Hypothyroidism, 666
Hypoventilation, 31
  postoperative, 424–8, 429
Hypovolaemia, 59, 415–16
  aortic aneurysm, 591
  burns, 584–5
  emergency anaesthesia, 527–8
  major trauma, 536, 537
  postoperative, 436–7
Hypoxaemia, 679–81
  neonatal, 119
  postoperative, 428–30
Hypoxia
  cerebral, 705
  diffusion, due to nitrous oxide, 170
  systemic circulation, effect on, 47
Hysterectomy, abdominal, 488
Hysteresis, pulmonary, 26

Idiopathic respiratory distress syndrome, 119
Ignition, sources, 289
Immunity, neonatal, 120
Impedance, 287
Impedance cardiography, thoracic, 375
Impulses, nerve, conduction, 78–80, 257–9
Inappropriate antidiuretic hormone secretion, syndrome, 397
Inappropriate intravenous therapy, syndrome, 396
Incidents, critical, 330–1
Indomethacin, 202
Induced hypotension, complications, 600–2
Induction, enzyme, 146–7
Induction of anaesthesia, 349–51
  cardiac surgery, 636
  concurrent cardiovascular disease, 647
  day-case surgery, 522–3
  dentistry, 575–6, 578
  emergency anaesthesia, 531–4, 537
  neurosurgery, 609
  ophthalmic surgery, 503
  paediatrics, 563–5
Infection in operating theatre suites, 327
Information processing by nervous system, 81
Informed consent, 341
Infrared analysers, 381
Infusion fluids, 391–2, 738–9
Infusions
  cardiopulmonary resuscitation, 708
  labour, 543
  neonate, 558, 566
  opioids for postoperative pain, 453
  vasoactive, 729–30
Inguinal hernia repair, field block, 480
Inguinal perivascular technique for lumbar plexus block, 483
Inhalation of gastric contents, 351, 361, 529–31, 548–9
Inhalational anaesthesia
  absorption of drugs, 143–5
  bronchoscopy, 619
  for intubation, 357
  spontaneous ventilation, 353–5

Inhalational anaesthetic agents, 153–70
flammability, 288–9
heart, effects on, 649
intraocular pressure, 503
liver toxicity, 443–4
monitoring delivery, 381
paediatrics, 560–1
physical properties, 723
pollution, 313, 326–7
postoperative pain, 456–7
in shock, 537–8
Inhalational analgesia in labour, 544
Inhalational induction of anaesthesia, 349–50, 532
Inhaled foreign body, removal, 624–5
Inhibition, enzyme, 147
Initiating and terminating cardiopulmonary resuscitation, 712
Injection technique, local anaesthetic drugs, 261
Injectors
for ventilation for bronchoscopy, 619
monitoring, 382–4
Venturi, 280–1
Inotropism, negative, 235
Inspiration/expiration ratio, reversed, 683
Inspiratory assist, 37
Inspired volume, measurement, 377
Instructions to patients for day-case surgery, 520–1
Insulation, electrical, classification, 287–8
Insulin, 668–9
Insurance risk of anaesthetic practice, 329
Intensive care
benzodiazepines, 204
after cardiac surgery, 642–3
paediatrics, 568–70
propofol, 185
units, 677–94
Interactions, drug, 150
Intercostal nerve block for postoperative pain, 455
Intercurrent see Concurrent
Intermittent mandatory ventilation, 37
Intermittent positive pressure ventilation, 36, 682
after emergency surgery, 536
intraocular surgery, 504
weaning, 686
Internal jugular vein, 4
cannulation, 371
Internal vertebral venous plexus, 20
International System of units, 269–70, 721–22
Interscalene block, 480
Interspinous ligaments, 17–18
Interstitial fluid, 63
Interstitial pressure, 64
Intervertebral foramina, 18
Intestinal obstruction, 659
neonate, 568
Intra-aortic balloon pump, 640–1
Intracellular fluid, 63, 391
Intracranial pressure, 603–5
increased, 355, 608–9, 613
reduction, 610–11, 613–4
Intracranial tumours, evoked potentials, 107
Intracranial vascular surgery, 611
Intracranial volumes, 603
Intramuscular absorption of drugs, 143
Intramuscular opioids for postoperative pain, 451–3
Intraocular pressure, 501, 503
Intraocular surgery, anaesthetic techniques, 504–5
Intraoperative fluid requirements in adults, 737
Intrapleural pressure, 26
Intrathecal neurolysis, 699–700
Intravenous anaesthesia, total, 185, 188–9
Intravenous anaesthetic agents, 146, 175–91
hypersensitivity reactions, 189–90
paediatrics, 561
Intravenous induction of anaesthesia, 350–1
Intravenous infusions *see* Infusions
Intravenous opioids, bolus for postoperative pain, 453
Intravenous regional anaesthesia, 259, 464–5
Intravenous sedation for dentistry, 579–80
Intravenous therapy, inappropriate, syndrome, 396
Intrinsic activity of drugs, 141
Intrinsic sympathomimetic activity of β-adrenoceptor antagonists, 234
Intubating forceps, Magill, 319–20
Intubation
awake, 477, 532–4
bronchial, 621–2
inadvertent, 406, 682
oesophageal, 410
tracheal *see* Tracheal intubation
Intussusception (paediatric), barium enema, 512
Inulin, 67
Investigations
for emergency anaesthesia, 529
preoperative, 337
Ion exchange resins, 661
Ion pumps, 78
Ipratropium, 240, 245
Iron requirements in pregnancy, 112–13
Irreversible shock, 59
ISA see Intrinsic sympathomimetic activity
Ischaemic heart disease
concurrent, 649
postoperative, 439
surgery for, 629
Isoflurane, 164–5, 165–7
for hypotensive anaesthesia, 599
Isolation circuits, 288
Isoprenaline, 230–1

Jaundice
neonatal, 121–2
obstructive, preoperative therapy, 341–2
Joint Subcommittee on Dental Anaesthesia, 580
Joints, prosthetic, 491
Juxtamedullary nephrons, 65

Kell antibody, 120, 134
Kelvin unit of temperature, 281
Ketamine, 176, 186–8
for burns, 586
emergency anaesthesia in major trauma, 537
paediatrics, 561–2
Ketoacidosis, 671
Krause end bulbs, 88
Kyphoscoliosis, 490

Labetalol, 238, 597
Laboratories in operating theatre suites, 328
Labour
analgesia, 542–8
hypertension, 552–3
infusions, 543
physiology, 115
Lack system, 303–4
Laminae, Rexed, 98
Laminar flow, 29, 276–7
Laparoscopy, 486, 487–8
Laplace equation, 26
Laryngectomy, 497
Laryngopharynx, 11, 12
Laryngoscopes, 316–17, 356
Laryngoscopy, 357–8
Laryngotracheobronchitis, 570
Larynx, 12–15
granulomata, 446
obstruction, 405
oedema, postoperative, 426
spasm, 354–5, 361, 407
postoperative, 426, 568–9
thiopentone, 179
sprays, 319
Laser surgery, 498
Lateral position, 351, 489
Lateral recovery position, 360
Leakage currents, 288
Leakage in flowmeters, 296
Left atrial filling pressure in cardiac surgery, 634
Letters, explanatory for day-case surgery, 520–1
Leucocyte counts in neonates, 120

Leukaemia, platelet therapy, 132
Levallorphan, 202
Level of consciousness
  head injuries, 612
  postoperative, 423
Levorphanol, 200
Ligamenta flava, 17
Ligamentum denticulatum, 19
Ligands, 82
Lighting of operating theatre suites, 325–6
Lignocaine, 263
  for arrhythmias, 252–3
  for extradural anaesthesia, 474
  for subarachnoid anaesthesia, 471
Limb plethysmography, 279
Limiting valves, 301
Lingual nerve, 10
Lipid solubility theory of general anaesthesia, 101
Lithium, 514
Lithotomy position, 351, 486–7
Litigation, 329
Liver
  enflurane affecting, 163
  halothane affecting, 162
  see also Hepatic
Lobectomy, 625
Local anaesthesia, 534
  awake intubation, 477, 533
  choice of agent, 266–7
  chronic obstructive airways disease, 655–6
  concurrent cardiovascular disease, 653–4
  day-case surgery, 523
  equipment, 462
  labour, 544–5
  orthopaedic surgery, 492
  paediatrics, 483–4, 568
  postoperative, 454–6
    paediatrics, 568
  techniques, 459–84
Local anaesthetic drugs, 257–67
  test doses, 460
  toxicity, 459–60
Local anaesthetic solutions, baricity, 471
Long saphenous vein, 5–6
Loop diuretics for reduction of intracranial pressure, 611, 614
Loops of Henle, 72–3
Lorazepam, 206
Lorrain–Smith effect, 171
Lower limb
  peripheral nerve blockade, 481–2
  plastic surgery, 584
  superficial veins, 5
  venepuncture, 6
Lower oesophageal contractility, 382
Lower oesophageal sphincter, 530
Lower respiratory airway, 15–17
Lumbar plexus blockade, 701
  inguinal perivascular technique, 483
Lumbar puncture, 20, 468–71
Lundberg waves, 605
Lymphatic drainage
  larynx, 14
  upper respiratory airway, 10

MAC, *see* minimum alveolar concentration
Macintosh curved blade laryngoscope, 316
Magill attachment, 301–3
Magill intubating forceps, 319
Magnesium, effect in neuromuscular transmission, 81, 212
Magnetic resonance imaging, 107–8, 508–10
Mains electricity, 287
Maintenance
  extradural anaesthesia in labour, 548
  general anaesthesia, 353
    cardiac surgery, 637
    day-case surgery, 523
    emergency surgery, 534
    neurosurgery, 610–11
Major trauma, 536–9
Malignant hyperpyrexia, 355, 384, 417, 490
Malnutrition, 664
Mandatory minute ventilation, 37
Mannitol
  postoperative renal failure, 662
  reduction of intracranial pressure, 611, 613–14
Manometers, 275
  for CVP, 372
Mapleson classification of breathing systems, 301–6
Marfan's syndrome, 663
Marker gas expirography, 28
Mask anaesthesia, maintenance of airway, 355
Mask ventilation in cardiopulmonary resuscitation, 707–8
Masks, 319
  laryngeal, 319
  oxygen, 280–1, 433–5
  Rendell–Baker–Soucek, 563
Mass spectrometers, 381
Massive blood transfusion, 538
  coagulation, effect on, 384
Maternal physiology, 111–16
Maxillary artery, 9–10
Maxillectomy, 499
Mean arterial pressure, 49
Mechanical transduction in end-organs, 87
Mechanical ventilation *see* Controlled mechanical ventilation
Mechanisms
  general anaesthesia, 101
  local anaesthetic drugs, 259
Meconium, 121
Medial cutaneous nerve of forearm, 3
Median basilic vein, 3
Median cephalic vein, 3
Median nerve, 3
Mediastinal emphysema, 686
Mediastinoscopy, 619
Medicolegal environment, 329
Medishield S60M regulator, 274
Medulla, 94–5
Membrane potential, 79
Membrane receptors, 82–5
Membrane stabilising activity of β-adrenoceptor antagonists, 234
Membranes, diffusion, 285–6
Meningeal spaces, 20
Mental subnormality, 516
Mepivacaine, 263
Meptazinol, 200
Metabolic acidosis, 400–1
Metabolic alkalosis, 401–2
Metabolic control of cerebral blood flow, 605–6
Metabolic depression for reduction of intracranial pressure, 614
Metabolic effects of diethyl ether, 159
Metabolic effects of sympathomimetic drugs, 229
Metabolic rate for oxygen, cerebral, 606–7
Metabolism
  drugs, 146
    enflurane, 163, 165
    halothane, 165
    isoflurane, 164
    in liver disease, 659–60
    local anaesthetic drugs, 260
    thiopentone, 180
  monitoring, 382–4
Metacarpal veins, 1–2
Methadone, 200
Methaemoglobinaemia and prilocaine, 265
Methohexitone, 176, 182–3
Methoxyflurane, 157
  nephrotoxicity, 442–3
  in renal failure, 662
  vapour pressure/temperature curve, 283
Metoclopramide, 243
  in premedication, 344
Metrizamide, 608
Mexiletine, 253
Microlaryngoscopy, 496–7
Microshock, 28.,
Microsurgery, 584
Mid-tarsal block, 482
Midazolam, 205
Midbrain, 95–6
Middle ear surgery, 499–500
Miniature end-plate potentials, 212
Minimum alveolar concentration, 153–4, 353
  nitrous oxide, 168
  paediatrics, 560
Minimum effective analgesic concentration, 451
Minimum infusion rate in total intravenous anaesthesia, 189
Minitracheotomy, 708
Minoxidil, 249
Miosis due to morphine, 196

Miscarriage, 552
Mitral incompetence, 653
Mitral stenosis, 652
Mixer flowmeter, Quantiflex, 296–7
Moffatt's method, topical anaesthesia of nose, 498
Monitoring, 363–86
  cardiac surgery, 634, 636–7
  cardiopulmonary resuscitation, 709
  cardiovascular system on intensive care units, 688
  controlled mechanical ventilation, 309
  delivery of inhalational anaesthetic agents, 381
  dentistry, 577
  emergency anaesthesia in major trauma, 537
  extradural anaesthesia in labour, 546–7
  neonate, 556, 559–60
  neurosurgery, 609
  paediatrics, 565
  recovery wards, 422–3
  thoracotomy, 622–3
Monitors, cerebral function, 104–5, 106
Monoamine oxidase inhibitors, 334, 514
Monoamines as neurotransmitters, 82
Morbidity
  anaesthesia, 330–2
  ECT, 516
Morphine, 195–7
Mortality, anaesthesia, 329–31
  obstetrics, 548
Motor efferent spinal cord pathways, 90
Motor neurone disease, 673
Motor neuropathies, respiratory impairment, 672
Mounting of vaporisers, 300
Mouth, 10–11
  gags, 320
Mucous membrane of laryngopharynx, 12, 14
Multiple sclerosis, 673
Multisite expansion hypothesis, 102
Muscarinic cholinergic receptors, 84
Muscle, cardiac, 50
  contractility, 56
Muscle disease, administration of thiopentone, 181
Muscle excitation contraction coupling, 213
Muscle relaxants *see* Relaxants
Muscle tone
  benzodiazepines affecting, 203
  ketamine affecting, 187
  signs of return, 359–60
Muscles
  drugs affecting
    diethyl ether, 159
    enflurane, 167
    halothane, 162, 167
    isoflurane, 167
    of laryngopharynx, 12
    pharyngeal constrictor, 11
    respiratory, 25
Muscular dystrophy, 674
Myasthenia gravis, 673–4
Myelin sheaths, 80
Myeloma, 675
Myelomeningocoele, 568
Myeloneuropathy due to nitrous oxide, 170
Myocardial infarction
  postoperative, 439–40
  preoperative risk assessment, 339
  secondary prevention, 236–7
Myocardial preservation, 638–9
Myocardium, oxygen supply, 645
Myotomy of oesophagus, 627–8
Myotonia and suxamethonium, 219
Myringotomy, 499
Myxoedema, administration of thiopentone, 182

Nalbuphine, 200
Nalorphine, 202
Naloxone, 201–2
  in recovery period, 427
Narcosis, carbon dioxide, 171
Narcotics *see* Opioids
Nasal intubation, 358
  blind, 532
Nasal polyps, 10
Nasal septum, deviation, 10
Nasal surgery, 498–9
Nasolacrimal duct, 8
Nasopharynx, 8
  airways, 321
Natriuretic factor, 70
Nausea
  morphine, 196
  postoperative, 445
NBPM *see* Nucleus parabrachialis medialis
Near-infra-red spectrophotometry, 108
Nebulisers, 285
  β-adrenoceptor agonists, 244–5
Neck
  plastic surgery, 583–4
  venepuncture, 4
Necrosis due to thiopentone, 180
Negative coupling, 228
Negative end-expiratory pressure, 36
Negative inotropism, 235
Negus bronchoscope, 618
Neonate
  anaesthesia, 566
  jaundice, 121–2
  physiology, 117–24, 555
Neostigmine, 220
  parasympathomimetic effects, 239
Nephrons, 65
Nephrotoxicity of methoxyflurane, 157, 442–3
Nerve blockade
  autonomic, 700–1
  peripheral, 477–84
    for chronic pain, 698
Nerve fibres
  classification (Gasser), 87
  conduction velocities, 80
Nerve impulses, conduction, 78–80, 257–9
Nerve stimulation, 702
Nerve stimulators, 221–4, 463
Nerves
  autonomic to upper respiratory airway, 9
  birth canal and uterus, 541–2
  chorda tympani, 10–11
  laryngeal, 14
  lingual, 10
  medial cutaneous of forearm, 3
  median, 3
  olfactory, 8
  pharyngeal plexus, 11
  phrenic, 4
  pulmonary plexus, 17
  recurrent laryngeal, 14
  trigeminal, 8
  vagus, 14
Nervous system
  monitoring, 381–2
  neonatal, 122
  physiology, 77–109
  sensory, 87–90
  see also Central nervous system, Autonomic nervous system
Neuralgia, anticonvulsants for, 697
Neuritis, due to local anaesthetic techniques, 461
Neuroglial cells, 77
Neuroleptanalgesia and neuroleptanaesthesia, 206
Neurological diseases, 672–4
Neuromuscular blockade
  assessment, 220–4
  residual, 427–8
  reversal, 220, 360
Neuromuscular blocking drugs, 211–24
  see also Relaxants
Neurones, 77–80
Neuropathies
  diabetic, 670
  motor, respiratory impairment, 672
  peripheral, 673
Neuropeptides, 82
Neurophysiology, 77–109
Neuroradiology, 608
Neurosurgery, 603–14
  for chronic pain, 703–4
Neurotransmitters, 81–7
Newtonian fluids, 276
Nicotinic cholinergic receptors, 84
Nifedipine, 249–50
  concurrent therapy, 645
Nikethamide, 208
Nitrates, organic, 249
Nitroprusside, sodium, 248–9, 597
Nitrous oxide, 168–71
  bulk storage, 292

Nitrous oxide (*contd*)
  diffusion hypoxia, 429
  and air encephalography, 511
  filling ratios for cylinders, 272
  and middle ear surgery, 500
  pressures in cylinders, 271
  support of combustion, 289
Nociception, 99
Nodes of Ranvier, 80
Non-return valves, 300
Non-steroidal anti-inflammatory drugs, 202–3
  platelets, effects on, 127
Noradrenaline, 83–4, 226, 230
  control of systemic circulation, 47
Normal values
  cardiac catheterisation, 54
  cardiovascular system, 727–8
  chemical pathology, 724–6
  electrolytes, 736
  fluid balance, 735
  haematology, 741–2
  nutrition, 736
Nose, 7–10
  artificial, 285, 416
Nuclear magnetic resonance, 107–8, 508–10
Nuclei
  basal, 92, 95–6
  respiratory, 23
Nucleus, dorsal motor of vagus nerve, 17
Nucleus ambiguus, 23
Nucleus parabrachialis medialis, 23
Nurse anaesthetists, 329
Nutrients, transfer across placenta, 117
Nutrition
  in intensive care units, 693
  normal values, 736
  in pregnancy, 114

Obesity, 663–4
Obstetrics, 541–53
Obstruction
  airway *see* Airway obstruction
  intestinal, 659
    neonate, 568
Obstructive jaundice, preoperative therapy, 341–2
Octreotide, 587
Oculocephalic reflex, 96
Oedema, laryngeal, postoperative, 426
Oesophagoscopy, 619
Oesophagus
  atresia, 567
  carcinoma, 628
  intubation, 410
  lower, contractility, 382
  myotomy, 627–8
  stethoscopes, 376
Ohm's law, 287
Olfactory nerve, 8
Olfactory region, 7
Oncotic pressure, 287
One-lung anaesthesia, 620–2
Open heart surgery, 629–44
Operating department assistants, 329
Operating rooms, 325–7
  conductivity of floors, 289
Operating theatre suites, 323–8
Operator expired-air resuscitation, 707
Ophthalmic surgery, 501–6
Opioid antagonists, 201–2
Opioid receptors, 193–4
Opioids, 193–202
  endogenous, 100–1
  intraocular pressure, 503
  postoperative pain, 450–4
  premedication, 345
  spinal, 200–1
    labour, 543–4
    postoperative pain, 456
    reduced respiratory drive, 427
Oral absorption of drugs, 142, 150
Oral anticoagulant therapy, 440, 442
  and spinal anaesthesia, 476
Oral cavity, 10
Oral contraceptives, 486
  withdrawal, 334
Oral hypoglycaemic agents, 668
Oral opioids for postoperative pain, 454
Orifices, flow, 278
Oropharynx, 11
  airways (instruments), 321
Orthopaedic surgery, 490–4
Oscillometry, 369
Oscillotonometer of Von Recklinghausen, 368–9
Osmolality, 389
Osmolar clearance, 75–6
Osmolar regulation, renal, 75–6
Osmolarity, 389
  vs osmolality, 287
Osmosis, 286–7, 389
Osmotherapy for cerebral oedema, 712
Osmotic diuretics, 395
  ophthalmic surgery, 503
Osmotic pressure, 64
Ostwald solubility coefficient, 285
Outlets, PMGV systems, 293
Outpatients
  administration of thiopentone, 182
  anaesthetic assessment clinics, 333
  dental anaesthesia, 574–8
  methohexitone, 183
Overload, fluid, 416
Oxford tracheal tube, 318
Oximetry, pulse, 365–7
Oxygen, 171–2
  bulk storage, 292
  bypass valves, 300
  cerebral metabolic rate, 606–7
  concentrators, 292
  delivery, monitoring, 378
  failure warning devices, 300–1
  for high subarachnoid anaesthesia, 466
  pressures in cylinders, 271
  supply to myocardium, 645
  tension
    cerebral blood flow, 606
    chemoreceptors, effect on, 24
  therapy, 433–6, 680
    chronic obstructive airways disease, 656
    Venturi masks, 280–1
  transport, 38–9
Oxygenation, arterial during IPPV, 683
Oxygenators for extracorporeal circulation, 631
Oxyhaemoglobin dissociation curve, 39
Oxytocin, 116

Pacing in cardiopulmonary resuscitation, 709
Pacinian corpuscles, 88
Packed cells, 135–6
Paediatrics, 555–71
  doses of drugs, 746–7
  eutectic mixture of local anaesthetics, 266
  fluid requirements, 748
  induction of anaesthesia, 563–5
    day-case surgery, 522–3
  ketamine, 188
  local anaesthesia, 482–3
  microlaryngoscopy, 497
  radiotherapy, 512–13
Paget's disease of bone, 490
Pain, 98–101
  chronic, 695–704
  cutaneous, 88
  postoperative, 449–57
  suxamethonium, 219, 446–7
Palatine tonsils, 11
Pancreas, neonatal endocrine, 123–4
Pancuronium, 217
Papaveretum, 198
para-Aminohippuric acid, 65
Paracervical block, 545
Paracetamol, 203
Paradoxical sleep, 104
Paralysis of recurrent laryngeal nerve, 14
Paranasal sinuses, 8, 499
Paraplegia, suxamethonium, 492
Parasympathetic antagonists, 239–40
Parasympathetic nerve supply
  larynx, 14
  salivary glands, 11
  upper respiratory airway, 9
Parasympathetic nervous system, 92, 225
  drugs, 238–40
Parathyroid glands, neonatal, 124
Paravertebral block for postoperative pain, 455
Parry Brown position, 623
Partial agonists, 141
Partial pressures, Dalton's law, 271
Partial thromboplastin time with kaolin, 132

Passive scavenging systems, 315–16
Patient-controlled analgesia, 453–4
Patients
selection for day-case surgery, 519–20
selection for local anaesthetic techniques, 461
transfer to operating theatre suite, 323–4
Peak expiratory flow rate, 40
Pendelluft, 620
Penetrating eye injury, 505
Penile block, 480
Pentolinium, 598
Peptic ulcers, histamine H_2-receptor antagonists, 241–2
Peptides as neurotransmitters, 82
Percutaneous arterial catheterisation, 370
Percutaneous cervical cordotomy, 704
Percutaneous venous catheterisation, 371
Perforating veins, 5
Perfusion
on cardiopulmonary bypass, 639
monitoring, 367
Peridural space *see* Extradural space
Perioperative fluid therapy, 393–4
Perioperative myocardial infarction, 339
Peripheral blood flow, measurement, 47–8
Peripheral chemoreceptors, 23–4
Peripheral circulation, 43–9
Peripheral nerve blockade, 476–83, 698
Peripheral neuropathies, 673
Peripheral pulse, monitoring, 365
Peripheral resistance
in pregnancy, 111
total systemic, 49
Perphenazine, 242
Personality
assessment, 696
pain, effect on, 450
Pethidine, 198
labour, 543
Phaeochromocytoma, 588–9
alpha-adrenoceptor antagonists, 237–8
Pharmacodynamics, 139–48
opioids, 194
Pharmacokinetics, 139, 148–50
β-adrenoceptor antagonists, 234–5
etomidate, 175–7, 186
ketamine, 175–7, 187
local anaesthetic drugs, 259–61
methohexitone, 175–7, 182
morphine, 194, 197
nitrous oxide, 168
non-depolarising acetylcholine antagonists, 215–16
opioids, 194
propofol, 175–7, 184
thiopentone, 175–7, 179–80
Pharmacology in neonate, 560
Pharyngeal tonsils, 10
Pharyngolaryngectomy, 497–8
Pharyngotympanic tube, 8
Pharynx, anatomy, 11
Phenoperidine, 200
Phenothiazines, 207–8, 242–3, 514
for premedication, 345–6
Phenoxybenzamine, 589
Phentolamine, 597
Phenytoin for cardiac arrhythmias, 253
Phosphate transport, tubular, 71
Photoplethysmography, 365
Phrenic nerve, 4
Physical assessment of patients in intensive therapy units, 679
Physical examination, 333, 336–7
Physical properties
inhalational anaesthetic agents, 723
local anaesthetic drugs, 262
Physics, 269–90
Physiological anaemia, neonatal, 119–20
Physiological jaundice, 121
Physiology
cardiac function in cardiac surgery, 634–6
cardiovascular, 43–61
labour, 115
maternal, 111–16
neonatal, 117–24, 555
nervous system, 77–109
neuromuscular transmission, 211–14
renal, 63–76
respiratory, 23–41
Physiotherapy, preoperative, 341
Pia mater, 18–19
Pickwickian syndrome, 664
Pierre Robin syndrome, 568
Pin index system, 294
Pipecuronium, 218
Piped medical gases and vacuum systems, 291–3
Pirenzepine, 240
Piriform fossae, 12
Pituitary gland
alcohol injection, 703
neonatal, 122
in pregnancy, 115
Placenta, 116–17
transfer of local anaesthetic drugs, 261
Placenta praevia and abruption, 553
Plasma, 64
fresh frozen, 131
Plasma cholinesterase, 218–19
Plasma skimming, 44
Plasma volume expanders, 136
Plasma-reduced cells, 135–6
Plasmapheresis and plasma cholinesterase deficiency, 219
Plastic surgery, 583–6
Platelet count and spinal anaesthesia, 476
Platelets, 127–8
therapy, 132–3
Plenum vaporisers, 297
Plethysmography
body, 40
limb, 279
pulse, 365
Pleural surgery, 627
Pneumomediastinum, 408
Pneumonectomy, 625–6
Pneumonia, 432
Pneumoperitoneum, 487–8
Pneumotachographs, 279, 378
Pneumotactic centre, 23
Pneumothorax, 407–8, 627
due to local anaesthetic techniques, 460
postoperative, 428
tension, 537
Pollard's tube, 497
Pollution by inhalational anaesthetic agents, 313, 326–7
Polygeline, 136, 137
reactions, 419
Polyps, nasal, 10
Polyradiculoneuritis, 673
Pons, 23, 95
Pop-off valves, 301
Porphyria for surgery, 181, 186, 675
Positioning, 351–2
dentistry, 577
hypotensive anaesthesia, 600
neurosurgery, 610
thoracotomy, 623
Positive coupling, 228
Positive end-expiratory pressure, 36, 683–4
effect in one-lung anaesthesia, 621
Posterior longitudinal ligament of spine, 17
Postoperative analgesics for day-case surgery, 524
Postoperative care, 421–47
cardiac surgery, 641–3
chronic obstructive airways disease, 656
diabetes mellitus, 670–1
emergency surgery, 535–6
local anaesthetic techniques, 464
paediatrics, 568
thoracotomy, 624
Postoperative fluid and electrolyte requirements in paediatrics, 748
Postoperative haemorrhage after tonsillectomy, 496
Postoperative hepatic dysfunction, 443–4
Postoperative pain, 449–57
Postoperative renal dysfunction, 442–3
Postoperative renal failure, 662
Postpartum haemorrhage, 553
Postponement of surgery, causes, 340
Posture *see* Positioning
Potassium, 63
balance, 397–8
Power spectrum analysis of electroencephalogram, 104–6

Prazosin, 250
Precipitation of vecuronium by thiopentone, 180
Preganglionic sympathetic blockade by spinal anaesthesia, 596
Pregnancy, 111–16
  adverse effects of drugs, 123, 124
  anaesthesia, 334, 485–6
  diethyl ether affecting, 159
  ectopic, 488–9
  failure, 552
  halothane affecting, 162
  termination, 486, 487, 552
Premedication, 342–7
  airway resistance, effect on, 30
  benzodiazepines, 204
  cardiac surgery, 636
  compliance, effect on, 28
  day-case surgery, 522
  gynaecological surgery, 486
  local anaesthetic techniques, 462
  neurosurgery, 609
  ophthalmic surgery, 503
  paediatrics, 563
  regimens, 344
Preoperative assessment, 333–41
  cardiac surgery, 632–3
  concurrent cardiovascular disease, 645–7
  diabetes mellitus, 668–9
  ECT, 515
  emergency anaesthesia, 527
  local anaesthetic techniques, 461
  neurosurgery, 608
  paediatrics, 562–3
  thoracic surgery, 615
Preoperative investigations, 654
Preoperative management
  asthma, 657–8
  chronic obstructive airways disease, 655
  diabetes mellitus, 670–1
Preoperative therapy for respiratory system, 432
Pressure
  changes in extradural space, 20
  in cylinders, 271–2
  demand regulators, 275
  gauges, aneroid, 275
  generators, 310–11
  reducing valves, 273–4, 295
  relief valves, 272–3, 295–6, 300
  reversal of general anaesthesia, 101
  systemic arterial *see* Systemic arterial pressure
  units, 269, 272
Prilocaine, 265
  for intravenous regional anaesthesia, 465
Priming, for extracorporeal circulation, 632
Procainamide, 252
Procaine, 257, 263
Prochlorperazine, 243
Progressive muscular dystrophy, 674
Prolactin in pregnancy, 115
Promethazine, 208
Prone position, 351
Propanidid, 189
Propofol, 176, 183–5
Prostate, resection, 489
Prosthetic joints, 491
Protein binding of drugs, 145
  local anaesthetics, 261
Protein C, 129
Proteins, effect of anaesthetic agents, 102
Proton pump leak theory of general anaesthesia, 103
Pseudohyponatraemia, 64, 395
Psychiatry, 507, 513–17
  pain relief, 704
Psychogenic pain, 695–6
Psychotropic drugs for chronic pain, 697
Pterygopalatine ganglion, 9
Pudendal block, 544
Pulmonary angiography, 442
Pulmonary artery pressure
  see also Pulmonary capilliary wedge pressure
Pulmonary artery pressure monitoring, 372
  pregnancy, 111
Pulmonary barotrauma, 686
Pulmonary capilliary wedge pressure, 58
Pulmonary compliance, 25–8
Pulmonary disease
  preoperative risk assessment, 340
  restrictive, 490
Pulmonary elastic recoil, 26
Pulmonary embolism, 441–2
Pulmonary function tests, 40, 616, 749–53
  preoperative, 338, 654
Pulmonary hysteresis, 26
Pulmonary oxygen toxicity, 171
Pulmonary plexus of nerves, 17
Pulmonary vascular resistance, neonatal, 118
Pulse, peripheral, monitoring, 365
Pulse oximetry, 365–7
Pump failure, 537
Pumping effect in vaporisers, 284
Pumps for extracorporeal circulation, 631
Puncture, spinal, 17–22, 20
Pyloric stenosis, 567
Pyramidal tract, 90
Pyridostigmine, 220
  parasympathomimetic effects, 239

Quantiflex mixer flowmeter, 296–7
Quartz crystal oscillators, 381
Quinidine, 252

Radial artery, 1
Radioactive fibrinogen uptake, 440
Radiofrequency lesions, 701–2
Radioisotopes
  cardiac imaging, 633
  for glomerular filtration rate, 67
  for renal plasma flow, 65
Radiology, 507–12
  preoperative, 337–8
  thorax, 337, 616, 654
Radiotherapy, 507, 512–13
  for chronic pain, 704
Ranitidine, 241–2
Rapid eye movement sleep, 104
Rapid-sequence induction of emergency anaesthesia, 531–2
Rapport, establishment, 333
Rate-limited tubular transport, 70–2
Reabsorption, renal
  glucose, 70–1
  sodium, 68
Rebreathing systems, 306
Reception areas of operating theatre suites, 324
Receptors
  acetylcholine, 213
  adrenaline, 226–7
  drugs, 140
  epithelial in airways, 24
  F, 24
  membrane, 82–5
  opioid, 193–4
  stretch, airway, 24
Records
  anaesthetic, 332, 363
  intensive therapy unit, 679
Recovery, 361
  day-case surgery, 523–4
  enflurane, halothane, isoflurane, 165
  neurosurgery, 611
  propofol, 185
Recovery period, 421–47
Recovery position, lateral, 360
Recovery rooms, 328
Recovery wards, 422
Rectal opioids for postoperative pain, 454
Recurrent laryngeal nerve, 14
Red cell antigens, 120
Red cell concentrates, 135–6
Reducing valves, pressure, 273–4, 295
Rees' modification of Ayre's T-piece, 306
Referred pain, 88
Reflexes
  brain stem, 96
  gag, pathways, 11
  Hering-Breuer, 24
  vagal, reduction, 344
Refractory periods, 79
Regional anaesthesia *see* Local anaesthesia, Intravenous regional anaesthesia
Regnault's hygrometer, 285
Regulators
  pressure demand, 275
    see also pressure reducing valves

Regurgitation *see* Inhalation of gastric contents
Reimplantation, 584
Relative analgesia, 579
Relative humidity, 284–5
Relaxant anaesthesia, 359–61
  for intubation, 357
  for orthopaedic surgery, 493
Relaxants
  see also Neuromuscular blocking drugs
  Relaxants
  ECT, 515–16
  neonate, 566
  paediatrics, 562
Relief of chronic pain, 695–704
Relief valves, 272–3, 295–6, 300
Removal of inhaled foreign body, 624–5
Renal blood flow, 65–6
Renal disease
  administration of thiopentone in, 181
  concurrent, 660–2
Renal dysfunction, postoperative, 442–3
Renal excretion of drugs, 147
Renal failure
  anaesthesia, 486
  in intensive care unit, 692
Renal function
  in neonate, 557
  tests, 749
Renal glycosuria, 71
Renal physiology, 63–76
  in pregnancy, 114–15
Renal surgery, 489
Renal system, neonatal, 122
Renal toxicity of methoxyflurane, 157, 442–3
Rendell–Baker–Soucek masks, 563
Renin, 47
Renin-angiotensin system, 74
Resident doctors for intensive therapy units, 678
Residual neuromuscular blockade in recovery period, 427–8
Residual volume, 28, 40
Resistance, airway, 28
Respiratory acidosis and alkalosis, 402
Respiratory depression, 427
Respiratory disease, concurrent, 654–8
Respiratory distress syndrome
  adult, 254, 687–8
  idiopathic, 119
  neonatal, 570
Respiratory impairment due to motor neuropathies, 672
Respiratory obstruction, 405–7
Respiratory physiology, 23–41
  neonatal, 118–19
  in pregnancy, 112
Respiratory system
  aftercare after cardiac arrest, 710–11
  anaesthesia affecting, 654–5
  changes after abdominal surgery, 430–2
  complications of induced hypotension, 601
  drugs affecting
    benzodiazepines, 203
    buprenorphine, 198
    diethyl ether, 159
    enflurane, halothane, isoflurane, 165–6
    fentanyl, 199
    halothane, 161, 165–6
    ketamine, 187
    methohexitone, 182
    morphine, 195
    thiopentone, 179
  examination for thoracic surgery, 616
  oxygen affecting, 171
  subarachnoid anaesthesia affecting, 466
  monitoring, 375–81
  neonate, 555
  parasympathetic stimulation, 238
  preoperative therapy, 432
  recovery period, 422, 424–32
Respirometer, Wright, 377–8
Response *vs* dose of drugs, 140–1
Rest, 696
Resting potential, 79
Restoration of heart beat, 639
Restrictive lung disease, 490, 657
Resuscitation
  cardiopulmonary, 705–13
  equipment for local anaesthetic techniques, 462
  major trauma, 536
  paediatrics, 570
Retention of secretions in recovery period, 430
Reticular formation, 96
Retrolental fibroplasia, 172
Return of muscle tone, signs, 359–60
Reversal of neuromuscular blockade, 220, 360
  after emergency surgery, 535
Reversed inspiration/expiration ratio, 683
Rewarming after cardiac surgery, 642
Rexed laminae, 98
Reynolds' number, 29, 277
Rhesus antigens, 120
Rhesus blood groups, 134
Rheumatoid arthritis, 490, 662–3
Rigid bronchoscopy, 618–19
Riley's equation, 34
Risk assessment
  cardiac surgery, 633
  preoperative, 338–40
Ropivacaine, 265
Rotameter, 279

Safety
  checks for gas supplies, 293
  electrical, 287–8
  features in anaesthetic machines, 300–301
  in operating theatre suites, 326–7
Salbutamol, 658
Salivary glands, parasympathetic nerve supply, 11
Saturated vapour pressures, 282
Scalp electromyograms, 382
Scavenging, 313–16
  terminal outlets, 293
Schizophrenia, 86
Schwann cells, 80
Sciatic nerve block, 481
Scoliosis, correction, 492
Second gas effect of nitrous oxide, 169
Second messengers, 140, 227–8
Secretions
  reduction, 343
  retention in recovery period, 430
Sedation
  benzodiazepines, 203
  controlled mechanical ventilation, 684–6
  dentistry, 578–80
  for increased intracranial pressure, 613
  ketamine, 188
  local anaesthetic techniques, 464
  propofol, 185
Seebeck effect, 281
Selectatec block, 300
Sellick's manoeuvre, 532
Semi-active scavenging systems, 315
Sensation, cutaneous, modalities, 88
Sensory-motor modulation systems, effect of anaesthetic agents, 103
Sensory nervous system, 87–90
Septic shock, 691–2
  postoperative, 437
  steroids, 254
Septum, nasal, 7
  deviation, 10
Sequential analgesia, 100
Sequestration of fluid, 393
Serotonin, 84
Shivering, postoperative, 446
Shock, 528, 650, 688, 689
  inhalational anaesthetic agents, 537–8
  irreversible, 59
  septic, 691–2
    postoperative, 437
    steroids, 254
Short saphenous vein, 5
Shunt
  anatomical, 30
  controlled oxygen therapy, 435–6
  due to low ventilation/perfusion ratio, 34
  one-lung anaesthesia, 621
  postoperative, 429
Shunt, arteriovenous, for dialysis, 662
Sick sinus syndrome, 652
Sickledex tests, preoperative, 338

Signs
anaesthesia (Guedel), 353–4
inadequate ventilation, 360
return of muscle tone, 359–60
Single-lumen bronchial tubes, 621
Sinus tachycardia in recovery period, 438
Sinuses, paranasal, 8, 499
Sitting position for surgery, 352
Sizes of tracheal tubes, 734
Sleep, 104
'Slow' alveoli, 27
Smoking, 334
Smooth muscle, effects of sympathomimetic drugs, 229
Soda lime, 306–7
reaction of trichloroethylene, 157
Sodium, 63–4
in antacids, 241
balance, 394–7
infusion, distribution, 391
pump, 78
reabsorption, 68
Sodium bicarbonate
administration, 401
cardiopulmonary resuscitation, 709
Sodium citrate in premedication, 344
Sodium nitroprusside, 597
Sodium-potassium exchange, renal, 73–4
Solution of gases, 285
Somatostatin, 587
Sore throat, postoperative, 445–6
'Space rescue' blankets, 610
Special investigations
for emergency anaesthesia, 529
preoperative, 337
Specific heat capacity, 282
Spectrophotometry, near-infra-red, 108
Sphygmomanometry, 276
Spill valves, 301
Spinal anaesthesia
in concurrent cardiovascular disease, 653–4
hypotension, 411
preganglionic sympathetic blockade, 596
Spinal cord pathways, 88–93
Spinal opioids, 200–1
postoperative pain, 456
reduced respiratory drive, 427
Spinal puncture, 17–22
Spine
fracture, 493
posterior longitudinal ligament, 17
surgery, 491–2
Spinocerebellar degeneration, 673
Spinothalamic tract, 89–90
Spirometers, 40
Splenectomy and platelet therapy, 132–3
Spontaneous ventilation, inhalational anaesthesia, 353–5
for orthopaedic surgery, 492
Sprays, laryngeal, 320
Squint surgery, 505
Staff
accommodation in operating theatre suites, 328
intensive therapy units, 677–9
recovery wards, 422
Stages of anaesthesia, 353–4
Standard bicarbonate, 400
Starling resistor, 32
Starling's forces, 64
Starling's law, 56
Static compliance *vs* dynamic compliance, 26–7
Static electricity, 289, 326
in flowmeters, 296
Static lung compliance, 25
Stellate ganglion block, 700
Steroid therapy
for chronic pain, 697–8
concurrent, 663, 667
Steroids, 253–5
Stethoscopes
oesophageal, 376
paediatrics, 565
Stilettes, 321
Stimulants, ventilatory, 208
Stimulators, nerve, 221–4
Stoichiometric mixtures, 289
Storage
blood, 134–5
bulk gases, 292
Entonox, 272
nitrous oxide, 168
oxygen, 170
Strabismus, surgery, 505
Straight blade laryngoscopes, 316
Stress ulcers, antacids, 241
Stretch receptors, airway, 24
Structural formulae of inhalational anaesthetic agents, 155–6
Subacute bacterial endocarditis, 653
preoperative antibiotics, 341
Subarachnoid anaesthesia
see also Intrathecal neurolysis
Subarachnoid anaesthesia, 465–72
Caesarian section, 550–1
cardiac function, effect on, 61
conduct, 468–72
Subarachnoid opioids
labour, 543–4
postoperative pain, 456
Subarachnoid space, 22
Subclavian arteries, 4
Subclavian perivascular approach for supraclavicular block, 480
Subclavian veins, 3–4
cannulation, 371
Subcutaneous absorption of drugs, 143
Subdural space, 21–2
Sublingual opioids for postoperative pain, 454
Subnormality, mental, 516
Substance P, 100
Succinylated gelatin, 136, 137
Suction pumps for extracorporeal circulation, 631
Sufentanil, 200
Superficial veins
lower limb, 5
upper limb, 1–3
Supine position for surgery, 352
Supraclavicular block, 479
Supraglottic structures, airway obstruction, 405
Supraventricular arrhythmias in recovery period, 438
Surfactant, 26, 118–19
Surgery, positioning, 351–2
Surgical stimulation, effect on cardiac function, 61
Suxamethonium, 218–19
avoidance in burns, 586
hyperkalaemia, 84
intraocular pressure, 503
neurological disease, 672
pain, 219, 446–7
and paraplegia, 492
Swallowing *see* Deglutition
Sympathetic control of renal blood flow, 65
Sympathetic fibres, control of systemic circulation, 45–6, 47
Sympathetic ganglion blockade, 596–7
Sympathetic nerve supply to upper respiratory airway, 9
Sympathetic nervous system, 225–8
Sympathetic response, limitation, 344
Sympathetic stimulation, effect on cardiac contractility, 57
Sympathetic system, 91–2
Sympathomimetic drugs, 228–33
see also β-Adrenoceptor agonists
Synapses, 80–1
action of anaesthetic agents, 102–2
Synchronised intermittent mandatory ventilation, 37
Syndrome of inappropriate antidiuretic hormone secretion, 397
Syndrome of inappropriate intravenous therapy, 396
Systemic analgesics in labour, 543
Systemic arterial pressure
control, 48
measurement, 276
monitoring, 368–71
neonate, 556
ophthalmic surgery, 503
pregnancy, 111
reduction, 595–600
Systemic circulation
blood flow control, 45–7
on cardiopulmonary bypass, 639
Systemic peripheral resistance, total, 49

Tachycardia, postoperative, 438
Tachyphylaxis, 142

Tachyphylaxis (*contd*)
suxamethonium, 218
Taste, 11
Te-Ch'i, 703
Tec vaporisers, 297, 299
Tecota inhaler, 158
Teeth
see also Dental
Teeth
examination, 337
trauma, 446
Temazepam, 205
Temperature
after cardiac surgery, 642
compensation in vaporisers, 284
Kelvin unit, 281
monitoring, 383–4
neonate, 558–60
operating theatre suites, 325
sensation, 88
Tension pneumothorax, 537
Teratogenesis and nitrous oxide, 170
Terminal outlets of PMGV systems, 293
Terminating cardiopulmonary resuscitation, 712
Termination of pregnancy, 486, 487, 552
Test doses of local anaesthetic drugs, 460
Tetanic contraction, 213–14
use in assessment of neuromuscular blockade, 223–4
Thalassaemias, 120, 126–7
Theophylline, 243–4
Thermal dilution methods for cardiac output, 58
Thermistor measurement of cardiac output, 374–5
Thermistor probes, 383–4
Thermometry, 281
Thiamylal sodium, 183
Thiopentone, 146, 176, 178–82
arterial injection, 351
Third space loss, 393
Thoracic impedance cardiography, 375
Thoracic inlet X-rays, preoperative, 338
Thoracic surgery, 615–28
Thoracotomy, 622–4, 625–6
Thorax
compliance, 25–8
radiology, 616
3-in-l block *see* Lumbar plexus blockade
Threshold stimuli, 79
Throat packs in dentistry, 576
Thrombocytopenia, autoimmune, 132–3
Thrombophlebitis, postoperative, 444
Thrombosis
arterial, 444
deep venous, 440–1
Thymol in halothane, 299
Thyroid gland
goitres, 665
myxoedema, 182
neonatal, 122–3
pregnancy, 116
Thyroidectomy, 665
Thyrotoxicosis, 665
Timolol maleate, 506
Tissue hypoxia in recovery period, 430
'To-and-fro' system, 307
Tocainide, 253
Tolerance to drugs, 142
Tongue, 10
Tonicity, 389
Tonsillectomy, 495–6
Tonsils
palatine, 11
pharyngeal, 10
tubal, 10
Top-up injections in extradural anaesthesia, 550
Topical anaesthesia of nose, 498
Total body water, compartmental distribution, 390
Total intravenous anaesthesia, 185, 188–9
bronchoscopy, 619
neurosurgery, 610
Total lung capacity, 40
Total spinal anaesthesia, 475, 547
Total systemic peripheral resistance, 49
Total thoracic compliance, 26
Touch, 88
Tourniquets, 491
and local anaesthetic techniques, 464, 465
Toxicity of local anaesthetic drugs, 261–2, 459–60
Trachea, 15
Tracheal extubation after tonsillectomy, 495
Tracheal intubation, 355–9
acromegaly, 611
cardiopulmonary resuscitation, 708–8
for controlled mechanical ventilation, 682
day-case surgery, 523
dentistry, 578
difficult, 408–10
equipment, 349
failed, drill, 410
in Caesarian section, 551–2
neonate, 566
neurosurgery, 609
paediatrics, 564–5, 568
plastic surgery to head and neck, 583–4
Tracheal tubes, 317, 356–7
airway obstruction, 405–6
damage by lasers, 498
for nasal surgery, 498–9
sizes, 734
Tracheo-oesophageal fistula, 567
Tracheostomy, 682
Training in dental anaesthesia, 580
Transcutaneous CO_2 tension measurement, 380–1
Transcutaneous electrical stimulation
for chronic pain, 702
for postoperative pain, 457
Transcutaneous oxygen tension measurement, 379
Transdermal drugs
absorption, 144
fentanyl for postoperative pain, 454
local anaesthetic, 266
Transduction, mechanical in end-organs, 87
Transfer factor, alveolar-capillary, 35, 40
Transfer of patient to operating theatre suite, 323–4
Transfusion *see* Blood transfusion Platelets; therapy
Translumbar aortography, 511–12
Transmural pressure *vs* lung compliance, 25
Transport
carbon dioxide, 39–40
oxygen, 38–9
Transport, tubular, rate-limited, 70–2
Transurethral resection of prostate, 489
Trauma
see also Head injuries
Trauma
emergency surgery, 493–4
eyes, 446
major, 536–9
teeth, 446
Trendelenburg position, 351–2, 487
Trichloroethylene, 157–8
vapour pressure/temperature curve, 283
Tricyclic antidepressants, 85–6, 514
Trigeminal nerve, 8
blockade for chronic pain, 699
Trigeminal rhizotomy, radiofrequency, 701–2
Triggering, ventilation, 36
Trimetaphan, 598
Triservice apparatus, 306
Trolleys, 324
Tubal tonsil, 10
Tuberculosis, 657
Tubes
bronchial, 621–2
Coplan's, 496
Pollard's, 497
tracheal *see* Tracheal tubes
Tubocurarine, 217
and intraocular pressure, 503
Tubular function, renal, 68
Tubular transport, rate-limited, 70–2
Tumours
intracranial, evoked potentials, 107
see also Carcinoma
Tuohy needle, 473
Turbulent flow, 277, 278
TURP syndrome, 424
Two-dimensional echocardiography, 375

Ulcers, stress, antacids, 241
Ulnar artery, 1, 3
Ultrasound, Doppler, 369, 375
Unblocked segment, 547–8
Unilateral block, 547—8
Units, International System, 269–70
'Universal blood donors and recipients', 133
Upper airway obstruction, acute, 708
Upper limb
  peripheral nerve blocks, 476–80
  plastic surgery, 584
  superficial veins, 1–3
Upper respiratory airway, anatomy, 7–10
Uraemia, 661
  platelets, effects on, 128
Urea
  preoperative estimation, 337
  tubular transport, 72
Uric acid, tubular transport, 72
Urinary retention due to local anaesthetic techniques, 460
Urinary tract, parasympathetic stimulation, 238
Urine output
  after cardiac surgery, 643
  monitoring, 367
Urological procedures, 489
Uterus
  nerve supply, 541
  pregnancy, 115

Vacuum, piped medical, 292
Vaginal procedures, major, 488
Vagus, 14
  dorsal motor nucleus, 17
  reflexes, reduction, 344
  role in ventilation, 23
Valsalva manoeuvre, 49
Valves
  adjustable pressure-limiting, 301
  cardiac, 50
  Entonox, 275
  non-return, 300
  oxygen bypass, 300
  pressure reducing, 273–4, 295
  pressure relief, 272–3
Valvular disease
  acquired, operations, 629
  concurrent, 652–3
Vaporisers, 282–4, 297–9
  in circle systems, 308–9
  mounting, 300
Variable-orifice flowmeters, 278–9
Variable-performance oxygen therapy devices, 434
Variable-pressure flowmeters, 278
Vascular surgery, 589–92
  intracranial, 611
Vascular volume, 502
Vascular waterfall, 32
Vasoactive infusions, 729–30
Vasoconstrictors with local anaesthetic drugs, 265–6
Vasodilatation, peripheral, in pregnancy, 112
Vasodilators, 237–8, 248–50, 597
Vasomotor centre, 46, 49
Vasopressin, 75
Vasovagal attacks, 460
Vecuronium, 180, 217–18
Veins
  coronary, 54
  jugular, 4
  laryngopharynx, 11
  larynx, 14
  lower limb, 5
  oropharynx, 11
  pharyngeal plexus, 11
  renal, 65
  subclavian, 3–4
  upper limb, 1–3
  upper respiratory airway, 10
Venepuncture
  lower limb, 6
  neck, 4
  upper limb, 1–4
Venous admixture, 34
Venous arch, dorsal, of hand, 2
Venous catheterisation, percutaneous, 371
Venous embolism, 414
Venous plexus, internal vertebral, 20
Venous pressure
  eye, 502
  pregnancy, 111
Ventilation
  after cardiac surgery, 643
  cardiopulmonary resuscitation, 707
  control, 23
  controlled, paediatrics, 568–70
  controlled mechanical *see* Controlled mechanical ventilation
  inadequate, signs, 360
  intraocular surgery, 504–5
  monitoring, 375–8
  neonate, 566
  of operating theatre suites, 325
  using injectors for bronchoscopy, 619
  work, 25
Ventilation/perfusion mismatch, 31, 32, 33–5, 620
  postoperative, 429
Ventilators, 309–13
  adjustment, 682
  disconnection alarm, 376
Ventilatory depression
  delayed
    due to fentanyl, 199
    due to spinal opioids, 201
  due to buprenorphine, 198
Ventilatory drive, postoperative reduction, 427
Ventilatory failure, 681
  postoperative, 430–2
Ventilatory stimulants, 208
Ventricular arrhythmias, postoperative, 438
Ventricular failure, postoperative, 437
Ventricular fibrillation, caused by electricity, 287
Ventricular fibrillation/tachycardia, management, 709
Ventriculography, 511
Ventriculostomy, 611
Venturi injectors, 280–1
Venturi masks, 433–4
Venturi scavenging systems, 315
Verapamil, 249–50, 252, 253
  concurrent therapy, 645
Vertebral canal, 17
Vertebral venous plexus, internal, 20
Vestibule, nasal, 7
Vestibulo-ocular reflex, 96
Vinesthene, 154–6
Viruses
  AIDS, 131, 327
    antibody, 135
  hepatitis B, 327
  transfer across placenta, 117
Viscosity, 276
  blood, 44
Vitalograph, 40
Vitamin B_{12}
  requirements in pregnancy, 113
  synthesis, nitrous oxide affecting, 170
Vitreous volume, 503
Vocal folds, 14
Volumes
  gases, measurement, 278
  intracranial, 603
Vomiting, 12
  due to morphine, 196
  in emergency anaesthesia, 529–31
  postoperative, 445
Von Recklinghausen oscillotonometer, 368–9

Warfarin, 131
Warning devices, oxygen failure, 300–1
Water
  balance, 391
  body, 63–4
  transfer across placenta, 116
Waterfall, vascular, 32
Waters' system, 307
Weaning from controlled mechanical ventilation, 36–7, 686
Work of ventilation, 25
Wright peak flow meter, 40, 279
Wright respirometer, 377–8
Wylie Report, 580

Xanthine bronchodilators, 243–4

Zones of cleanliness in operating theatre suites, 323–4